Recommended Dietary Allowances (RDA) and Adequate Intakes (AI) for Vitamins

Age (yr)	Thiamin RDA (mg/day)	Riboflavin RDA (mg/day)	Niacin RDA (mg/day)[a]	Biotin AI (µg/day)	Pantothenic acid AI (mg/day)	Vitamin B_6 RDA (mg/day)	Folate RDA (µg/day)[b]	Vitamin B_{12} RDA (µg/day)	Choline AI (mg/day)	Vitamin C RDA (mg/day)	[illegible]n A [illegible]µg/day)[c]	[illegible]min D [illegible](µg/day)[d]	[illegible]amin E [illegible]A (mg/[illegible]y)[e]	[illegible]itamin K AI (µg/day)
Infants														
0–0.5	0.2	0.3	2	5	1.7	0.1	65	0.4	125	40	[illegible]	[illegible]	[illegible]	[illegible]
0.5–1	0.3	0.4	4	6	1.8	0.3	80	0.5	150	50	[illegible]	[illegible]	[illegible]	2.5
Children														
1–3	0.5	0.5	6	8	2	0.5	150	0.9	200	15	[illegible]	[illegible]	[illegible]	30
4–8	0.6	0.6	8	12	3	0.6	200	1.2	250	25	400	[illegible]	[illegible]	55
Males														
9–13	0.9	0.9	12	20	4	1.0	300	1.8	375	45	600	15	11	60
14–18	1.2	1.3	16	25	5	1.3	400	2.4	550	75	900	15	15	75
19–30	1.2	1.3	16	30	5	1.3	400	2.4	550	90	900	15	15	120
31–50	1.2	1.3	16	30	5	1.3	400	2.4	550	90	900	15	15	120
51–70	1.2	1.3	16	30	5	1.7	400	2.4	550	90	900	15	15	120
>70	1.2	1.3	16	30	5	1.7	400	2.4	550	90	900	20	15	120
Females														
9–13	0.9	0.9	12	20	4	1.0	300	1.8	375	45	600	15	11	60
14–18	1.0	1.0	14	25	5	1.2	400	2.4	400	65	700	15	15	75
19–30	1.1	1.1	14	30	5	1.3	400	2.4	425	75	700	15	15	90
31–50	1.1	1.1	14	30	5	1.3	400	2.4	425	75	700	15	15	90
51–70	1.1	1.1	14	30	5	1.5	400	2.4	425	75	700	15	15	90
>70	1.1	1.1	14	30	5	1.5	400	2.4	425	75	700	20	15	90
Pregnancy														
≤18	1.4	1.4	18	30	6	1.9	600	2.6	450	80	750	15	15	75
19–30	1.4	1.4	18	30	6	1.9	600	2.6	450	85	770	15	15	90
31–50	1.4	1.4	18	30	6	1.9	600	2.6	450	85	770	15	15	90
Lactation														
≤18	1.4	1.6	17	35	7	2.0	500	2.8	550	115	1200	15	19	75
19–30	1.4	1.6	17	35	7	2.0	500	2.8	550	120	1300	15	19	90
31–50	1.4	1.6	17	35	7	2.0	500	2.8	550	120	1300	15	19	90

NOTE: For all nutrients, values for infants are AI. The glossary on the inside back cover defines units of nutrient measure.

[a]Niacin recommendations are expressed as niacin equivalents (NE), except for recommendations for infants younger than 6 months, which are expressed as preformed niacin.

[b]Folate recommendations are expressed as dietary folate equivalents (DFE).

[c]Vitamin A recommendations are expressed as retinol activity equivalents (RAE).

[d]Vitamin D recommendations are expressed as cholecalciferol and assume an absence of adequate exposure to sunlight.

[e]Vitamin E recommendations are expressed as α-tocopherol.

Recommended Dietary Allowances (RDA) and Adequate Intakes (AI) for Minerals

Age (yr)	Sodium AI (mg/day)	Chloride AI (mg/day)	Potassium AI (mg/day)	Calcium RDA (mg/day)	Phosphorus RDA (mg/day)	Magnesium RDA (mg/day)	Iron RDA (mg/day)	Zinc RDA (mg/day)	Iodine RDA (µg/day)	Selenium RDA (µg/day)	Copper RDA (µg/day)	Manganese AI (mg/day)	Fluoride AI (mg/day)	Chromium AI (µg/day)	Molybdenum RDA (µg/day)
Infants															
0–0.5	120	180	400	200	100	30	0.27	2	110	15	200	0.003	0.01	0.2	2
0.5–1	370	570	700	260	275	75	11	3	130	20	220	0.6	0.5	5.5	3
Children															
1–3	1000	1500	3000	700	460	80	7	3	90	20	340	1.2	0.7	11	17
4–8	1200	1900	3800	1000	500	130	10	5	90	30	440	1.5	1.0	15	22
Males															
9–13	1500	2300	4500	1300	1250	240	8	8	120	40	700	1.9	2	25	34
14–18	1500	2300	4700	1300	1250	410	11	11	150	55	890	2.2	3	35	43
19–30	1500	2300	4700	1000	700	400	8	11	150	55	900	2.3	4	35	45
31–50	1500	2300	4700	1000	700	420	8	11	150	55	900	2.3	4	35	45
51–70	1300	2000	4700	1000	700	420	8	11	150	55	900	2.3	4	30	45
>70	1200	1800	4700	1200	700	420	8	11	150	55	900	2.3	4	30	45
Females															
9–13	1500	2300	4500	1300	1250	240	8	8	120	40	700	1.6	2	21	34
14–18	1500	2300	4700	1300	1250	360	15	9	150	55	890	1.6	3	24	43
19–30	1500	2300	4700	1000	700	310	18	8	150	55	900	1.8	3	25	45
31–50	1500	2300	4700	1000	700	320	18	8	150	55	900	1.8	3	25	45
51–70	1300	2000	4700	1200	700	320	8	8	150	55	900	1.8	3	20	45
>70	1200	1800	4700	1200	700	320	8	8	150	55	900	1.8	3	20	45
Pregnancy															
≤18	1500	2300	4700	1300	1250	400	27	12	220	60	1000	2.0	3	29	50
19–30	1500	2300	4700	1000	700	350	27	11	220	60	1000	2.0	3	30	50
31–50	1500	2300	4700	1000	700	360	27	11	220	60	1000	2.0	3	30	50
Lactation															
≤18	1500	2300	5100	1300	1250	360	10	13	290	70	1300	2.6	3	44	50
19–30	1500	2300	5100	1000	700	310	9	12	290	70	1300	2.6	3	45	50
31–50	1500	2300	5100	1000	700	320	9	12	290	70	1300	2.6	3	45	50

NOTE: For all nutrients, values for infants are AI. The glossary on the inside back cover defines units of nutrient measure.

Tolerable Upper Intake Levels (UL) for Vitamins

Age (yr)	Niacin (mg/day)[a]	Vitamin B_6 (mg/day)	Folate (µg/day)[a]	Choline (mg/day)	Vitamin C (mg/day)	Vitamin A (IU/day)[b]	Vitamin D (µg/day)	Vitamin E (mg/day)[c]
Infants								
0–0.5	—	—	—	—	—	600	25	—
0.5–1	—	—	—	—	—	600	38	—
Children								
1–3	10	30	300	1000	400	600	63	200
4–8	15	40	400	1000	650	900	75	300
9–13	20	60	600	2000	1200	1700	100	600
Adolescents								
14–18	30	80	800	3000	1800	2800	100	800
Adults								
19–70	35	100	1000	3500	2000	3000	100	1000
>70	35	100	1000	3500	2000	3000	100	1000
Pregnancy								
≤18	30	80	800	3000	1800	2800	100	800
19–50	35	100	1000	3500	2000	3000	100	1000
Lactation								
≤18	30	80	800	3000	1800	2800	100	800
19–50	35	100	1000	3500	2000	3000	100	1000

[a]The UL for niacin and folate apply to synthetic forms obtained from supplements, fortified foods, or a combination of the two.
[b]The UL for vitamin A applies to the preformed vitamin only.
[c]The UL for vitamin E applies to any form of supplemental α-tocopherol, fortified foods, or a combination of the two.

Tolerable Upper Intake Levels (UL) for Minerals

Age (yr)	Sodium (mg/day)	Chloride (mg/day)	Calcium (mg/day)	Phosphorus (mg/day)	Magnesium (mg/day)[d]	Iron (mg/day)	Zinc (mg/day)	Iodine (µg/day)	Selenium (µg/day)	Copper (µg/day)	Manganese (mg/day)	Fluoride (mg/day)	Molybdenum (µg/day)	Boron (mg/day)	Nickel (mg/day)	Vanadium (mg/day)
Infants																
0–0.5	—	—	1000	—	—	40	4	—	45	—	—	0.7	—	—	—	—
0.5–1	—	—	1500	—	—	40	5	—	60	—	—	0.9	—	—	—	—
Children																
1–3	1500	2300	2500	3000	65	40	7	200	90	1000	2	1.3	300	3	0.2	—
4–8	1900	2900	2500	3000	110	40	12	300	150	3000	3	2.2	600	6	0.3	—
9–13	2200	3400	3000	4000	350	40	23	600	280	5000	6	10	1100	11	0.6	—
Adolescents																
14–18	2300	3600	3000	4000	350	45	34	900	400	8000	9	10	1700	17	1.0	—
Adults																
19–50	2300	3600	2500	4000	350	45	40	1100	400	10,000	11	10	2000	20	1.0	1.8
51–70	2300	3600	2000	4000	350	45	40	1100	400	10,000	11	10	2000	20	1.0	1.8
>70	2300	3600	2000	3000	350	45	40	1100	400	10,000	11	10	2000	20	1.0	1.8
Pregnancy																
≤18	2300	3600	3000	3500	350	45	34	900	400	8000	9	10	1700	17	1.0	—
19–50	2300	3600	2500	3500	350	45	40	1100	400	10,000	11	10	2000	20	1.0	—
Lactation																
≤18	2300	3600	3000	4000	350	45	34	900	400	8000	9	10	1700	17	1.0	—
19–50	2300	3600	2500	4000	350	45	40	1100	400	10,000	11	10	2000	20	1.0	—

[d]The UL for magnesium applies to synthetic forms obtained from supplements or drugs only.
NOTE: An Upper Limit was not established for vitamins and minerals not listed and for those age groups listed with a dash (—) because of a lack of data, not because these nutrients are safe to consume at any level of intake. All nutrients can have adverse effects when intakes are excessive.

SOURCE: Adapted from the *Dietary Reference Intakes series*, National Academies Press. National Academies of Sciences.

Understanding Nutrition

Custom Edition

Ellie Whitney | Sharon Rady Rolfes

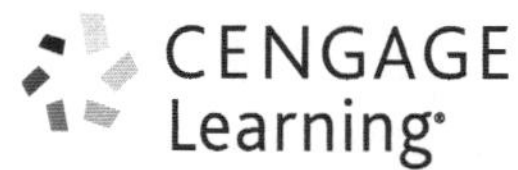

Australia • Brazil • Japan • Korea • Mexico • Singapore • Spain • United Kingdom • United States

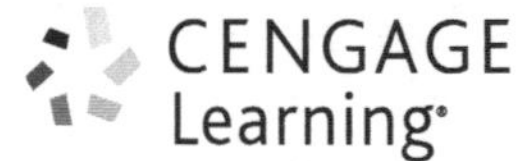

Understanding Nutrition: Custom Edition

Understanding Nutrition, 14 Edition
Whitney | Rolfes

For product information and technology assistance, contact us at
Cengage Learning Customer & Sales Support, 1-800-354-9706

For permission to use material from this text or product,
submit all requests online at **cengage.com/permissions**
Further permissions questions can be emailed to
permissionrequest@cengage.com

This book contains select works from existing Cengage Learning resources and was produced by Cengage Learning Custom Solutions for collegiate use. As such, those adopting and/or contributing to this work are responsible for editorial content accuracy, continuity and completeness.

ISBN: 978-1-377-04958-0

WCN: 01-100-101

Cengage Learning
20 Channel Center Street
Boston, MA 02210
USA

Cengage Learning is a leading provider of customized learning solutions with office locations around the globe, including Singapore, the United Kingdom, Australia, Mexico, Brazil, and Japan. Locate your local office at: **www.international.cengage.com/region.**

Cengage Learning products are represented in Canada by Nelson Education, Ltd.

For your lifelong learning solutions, visit **www.cengage.com/custom.**

Visit our corporate website at **www.cengage.com.**

Brief Contents

Preface

Nutrition is a science. The details of a nutrient's chemistry or a cell's biology can be overwhelming and confusing to some, but it needn't be. When the science is explained step by step and the facts are connected one by one, the details become clear and understandable. By telling stories about fat mice, using analogies of lamps, and applying guidelines to groceries, we make the science of nutrition meaningful and memorable. That has been our mission since the first edition—to reveal the fascination of science and share the excitement of nutrition with readers. We have learned from the thousands of professors and more than a million students who have used this book through the years that readers want an *understanding* of nutrition so they can make healthy choices in their daily lives. We hope that this book serves you well.

A Book Tour of This Edition

Understanding Nutrition presents the core information of an introductory nutrition course. The early chapters introduce the nutrients and their work in the body, and the later chapters apply that information to people's lives—describing the role of foods and nutrients in energy balance and weight control, in physical activity, in the life cycle, in disease prevention, in food safety, and in hunger.

The Chapters Chapter 1 begins by exploring why we eat the foods we do and continues with a brief overview of the nutrients, the science of nutrition, recommended nutrient intakes, assessment, and important relationships between diet and health. Chapter 2 describes the diet-planning principles and food guides used to create diets that support good health and includes instructions on how to read a food label. In Chapter 3 readers follow the journey of digestion and absorption as the body breaks down foods into nutrients. Chapters 4, 5, and 6 describe carbohydrates, fats, and proteins—their chemistry, roles in the body, and places in the diet. Then Chapter 7 shows how the body derives energy from these three nutrients. Chapters 8 and 9 continue the story with a look at energy balance, the factors associated with overweight and underweight, and the benefits and dangers of weight loss and weight gain. Chapters 10, 11, 12, and 13 complete the introductory lessons by describing the vitamins, the minerals, and water—their roles in the body, deficiency and toxicity symptoms, and sources.

The next seven chapters weave that basic information into practical applications, showing how nutrition influences people's lives. Chapter 14 describes how physical activity and nutrition work together to support fitness. Chapters 15, 16, and 17 present the special nutrient needs of people through the life cycle—pregnancy and lactation; infancy, childhood, and adolescence; and adulthood and the later years. Chapter 18 focuses on the dietary risk factors and recommendations associated with chronic diseases, and Chapter 19 addresses consumer concerns about the safety of the food and water supply. Chapter 20 closes the book by examining hunger and the global environment.

The Highlights Every chapter is followed by a highlight that provides readers with an in-depth look at a current, and often controversial, topic that relates to its companion chapter. For example, Highlight 4 examines the scientific evidence behind some of the current controversies surrounding carbohydrates and their role in weight gain and weight loss. New to this edition are Critical Thinking Questions designed to encourage readers to develop clear, rational, open-minded, and informed thoughts based on the evidence presented in the highlight.

Special Features The art and layout in this edition have been carefully designed to be inviting while enhancing student learning. For example, numbered steps have been added to several figures to clarify sequences and processes. In addition, special features help readers identify key concepts and apply nutrition knowledge. For example, when a new term is introduced, it is printed in bold type, and a **definition** is provided. These definitions often include pronunciations and derivations to facilitate understanding. The glossary at the end of the book includes all defined terms.

definition (DEF-eh-NISH-en): the meaning of a word.
- **de** = from
- **finis** = boundary

LEARNING GPS

The opening page of each chapter provides a Learning GPS that serves as an outline and directs readers to the main heads (and subheads) within the chapter. Each main head is followed by a Learn It—a learning objective for the content covered in that section. The Learn It also appears within the text at the start of each main section as well as at the start of each Review It. After reading the chapter, students will be able to demonstrate competency in the Learn It objectives.

Nutrition in Your Life

The opening paragraph of each chapter—called Nutrition in Your Life—introduces the chapter's content in a friendly and familiar way. This short paragraph closes with a preview of how readers might apply that content to their daily lives by inviting them to use the Nutrition Portfolio section at the end of the chapter.

Nutrition Portfolio

The Nutrition Portfolio section at the end of each chapter prompts readers to consider whether their personal choices are meeting the goals presented in the chapter. Most of these assignments include instructions that use the Diet & Wellness Plus program. Such tools help students assess their current choices and make informed decisions about healthy options.

› REVIEW IT Each major section within a chapter concludes with a Review It paragraph that summarizes key concepts. Similarly, Review It tables cue readers to important summaries.

Also featured in this edition are the 2010 *Dietary Guidelines for Americans*, which are introduced in Chapter 2 and presented throughout the text whenever their subjects are discussed. Look for the following design.

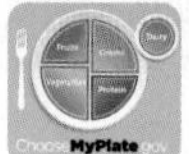

> DIETARY GUIDELINES FOR AMERICANS
These guidelines provide science-based advice to promote health and to reduce the risk of chronic disease through diet and physical activity.

>How To

Many of the chapters include "How To" features that guide readers through problem-solving tasks. For example, a "How To" in Chapter 1 presents the steps in calculating energy intake from the grams of carbohydrate, fat, and protein in a food.

› TRY IT Each "How To" feature ends with a "Try It" activity that gives readers an opportunity to practice these new lessons.

STUDY CARD 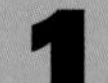 1

› STUDY IT To review the key points of this chapter and take a practice quiz, go to the Study Cards at the end of the book.

Study cards appear at the back of the text—one for each chapter. The Study It side of each card presents a review of the chapter's core concepts, and perhaps a table or figure to remind readers of key points. The Test It side of the study card provides essay and multiple-choice questions to help prepare students for exams.

The Appendixes

The appendixes are valuable references for a number of purposes. Appendix A summarizes background information on the hormonal and nervous systems, complementing Appendixes B and C on basic chemistry, the chemical structures of nutrients, and major metabolic pathways. Appendix D describes measures of protein quality. Appendix E provides detailed coverage of nutrition assessment, and Appendix F presents the estimated energy requirements for men and women at various levels of physical activity. Appendix G presents the 2008 *Choose Your Foods: Exchange List for Diabetes.* Appendix H is a 4000-item food composition table. Appendix I lists nutrition recommendations from the World Health Organization (WHO), and Appendix J presents the 2020 Healthy People nutrition-related objectives. Appendix K features aids to calculations, a short tutorial on converting metric measures and handling basic math problems commonly found in the world of nutrition.

The Inside Covers

The inside covers put commonly used information at your fingertips. The inside front covers (pp. A–C) present the current nutrient recommendations; the inside back covers feature the Daily Values used on food labels and a glossary of nutrient measures (p. Y on the left) as well as suggested weight ranges for various heights (p. Z on the right).

Notable Changes in This Edition

Because nutrition is an active science, staying current is paramount. Just as nutrition research continuously adds to and revises the accepted body of knowledge, this edition builds on the science of previous editions with the latest in nutrition research. Much has changed in the world of nutrition and in our daily lives since the first edition. The number of foods has increased dramatically—even as we spend less time than ever in the kitchen preparing meals. The connections between diet and disease have become more apparent—and consumer interest in making smart health choices has followed. More people are living longer and healthier lives. The science of nutrition has grown rapidly, with new "facts" emerging daily. In this edition, as with all previous editions, every chapter has been revised to enhance learning by presenting current information accurately and attractively. For all chapters and highlights we have:

- Reviewed and updated content
- Created several new figures and tables and revised others to enhance learning
- Added Critical Thinking Questions to the highlights
- Revised figures to reflect new food and supplement labels and tables to include nutrients of concern (vitamin D, calcium, potassium, and iron)

Chapter 1

- Created table to summarize ways to describe six classes of nutrients
- Introduced *registered dietitian nutritionist (RDN)*, another term to describe an RD

Chapter 2

- Revised figure comparing nutrient density of two breakfasts to include potassium and vitamin D
- Introduced new food labels and revised figure to illustrate differences
- Introduced front-of-package labeling and added figure to illustrate

Chapter 3

- Introduced *microbiome* and revised section on gastrointestinal bacteria

Chapter 4

- Revised table showing nutrients in sugars and other foods to include potassium and vitamin D
- Created tables to define glucose for normal and diabetes; to show the glycemic index of a few common foods; to list the functions of sugars in foods; to present ways to prevent dental caries
- Included fructose metabolism in the highlight

Chapter 5

- Created tables to define blood lipids for heart health; to list fat choices among protein foods and among milk products; to show omega-3 fatty acid quantities in a variety of fish and seafood
- Created new figure on how to read fish oil supplement labels
- Added definitions for resistin and adiponectin

Chapter 6

- Expanded discussion on the association between dietary protein and body weight

Chapter 7

- Created new figure illustrating labels on beer, wine, and liquor

Chapter 8

- Discussed "3500 kcalorie rule" and its limitations
- Created new tables for estimating energy expended on basal metabolism and on thermic effect of foods and for percent body fat at various BMI
- Revised section on female athlete triad to include new expanded term—Relative Energy Deficiency in Sports (RED-S)—and created new table of its adverse consequences
- Added discussion of food addiction to section on binge eating disorder

Chapter 9

- Added discussion of brite adipocytes to section on brown adipocyte tissue and uncoupling proteins
- Updated table on FDA-approved weight loss drugs
- Revised figure on gastric surgery used to treat obesity
- Deleted discussion and figure on unrealistic expectations
- Created new table of national strategies to prevent obesity
- Updated table on popular weight loss diets

Chapter 11

- Added a paragraph on "golden rice," a genetically modified rice used in the worldwide fight against vitamin A deficiency
- Added details on vitamin D's non-bone-related roles
- Rewrote the introduction to vitamin E
- Rewrote the food sources of vitamin K paragraph to include the terms phylloquinone (vitamin K_1) and menaquinone (vitamin K_2)

Chapter 12

- Revised calcium balance figure

Chapter 13

- Created table of factors influencing iron absorption

Chapter 14

- Reorganized, shortened, and rewrote section on Developing Fitness

- Reorganized, clarified, and rewrote section entitled Energy Systems and Fuels to Support Activity
- Enhanced and reorganized table of primary fuels used for activities of different intensities and durations
- Created new table comparing symptoms of heat stroke and hypothermia
- Added discussion and definition of beta-alanine to highlight on ergogenic aids

Chapter 15

- Created several new tables: benefits of WIC, risk factors for gestational diabetes, signs and symptoms of pre-eclampsia, complications from smoking during pregnancy, tips to prevent listeriosis
- Reorganized sections on fetal programming and fetal development of chronic diseases

Chapter 16

- Created several new tables: protective factors in breast milk, tips for picky eaters, examples of foods and non-food items children can choke on, iron recommendations for adolescents
- Added information about fluoride and formula preparation
- Added brief discussion about new AAP guidelines for reduced, low-fat, and fat-free milk for toddlers
- Added discussion of new school meal initiatives

Chapter 17

- Created new figure comparing healthy lens with cataract lens

Chapter 18

- Created new tables for selected nutrient roles in immune function and criteria for diagnosis of diabetes
- Revised, reworked, and updated tables for recommendations and strategies to reduce the risk of CVD and recommendations and strategies to reduce the risk of cancer
- Emphasized role of obesity throughout the chapter as major risk for other chronic diseases
- Included information related to 2013 American College of Cardiology/American Heart Association guidelines for assessment of CVD risk and lifestyle modifications for reducing risk of heart disease
- Added discussion and definitions of fasting plasma glucose test and A1C test for diabetes

Chapter 19

- Added brief discussion in Nutritional Adequacy of Foods section on ultraprocessed foods
- Added a paragraph in the Environmental Contaminants section on arsenic
- Added more information throughout Pesticide section on children's health and consumers' perceptions
- Added brief discussion in Food Additives section comparing natural and artificial additives
- Added a paragraph in Food Additives section on edible packaging

Chapter 20

- Added discussion on controversy surrounding whether SNAP participants should be allowed to purchase soft drinks and other non-nutritious foods and beverages
- Added tips to reduce food waste to the How To feature on p. 667
- Added discussion on eco-friendly products and packaging to the highlight

Student and Instructor Resources

MindTap: A new approach to highly personalized online learning. Beyond an eBook, homework solution, digital supplement, or premium website, MindTap is a digital learning platform that works alongside your campus LMS to deliver course curriculum across the range of electronic devices in your life. MindTap is built on an "app" model allowing enhanced digital collaboration and delivery of engaging content accross a spectrum of Cengage and non-Cengage resources.

Instructor Companion Site: Everything you need for your course in one place! This collection of book-specific lecture and class tools is available online via www.cengage.com/login. Access and download PowerPoint presentations, images, instructor's manual, videos, and more.

Test Bank with Cognero: Cengage Learning Testing Powered by Cognero is a flexible, online system that allows you to:

- author, edit, and manage test bank content from multiple Cengage Learning solutions
- create multiple test versions in an instant
- deliver tests from your LMS, your classroom, or wherever you want

Diet & Wellness Plus: Diet & Wellness Plus helps you understand how nutrition relates to your personal health goals. Track your diet and activity, generate reports, and analyze the nutritional value of the food you eat. Diet & Wellness Plus includes over 55,000 foods as well as custom food and recipe features. The new Behavior Change Planner helps you identify risks in your life and guides you through the key steps to make positive changes.

Global Nutrition Watch: Bring currency to the classroom with Global Nutrition Watch from Cengage Learning. This user-friendly website provides convenient access to thousands of trusted sources, including academic journals, newspapers, videos, and podcasts, for you to use for research projects or classroom discussion. Global Nutrition Watch is updated daily to offer the most current news about topics related to nutrition.

Closing Comments

We have taken great care to provide accurate information and have included many references at the end of each chapter and highlight. To keep the number of references manageable over the decades, however, many statements that appeared in previous editions with references now appear without them. All statements reflect current nutrition knowledge, and the authors will supply references upon request. In addition to supporting text statements, the end-of-chapter references provide readers with resources for finding a good overview or more details on the subject. Nutrition is a fascinating subject, and we hope our enthusiasm for it comes through on every page.

Ellie Whitney
Sharon Rady Rolfes
January 2015

Acknowledgments

To produce a book requires the coordinated effort of a team of people—and, no doubt, each team member has another team of support people as well. We salute, with a big round of applause, everyone who has worked so diligently to ensure the quality of this book.

We thank our partners and friends, Linda DeBruyne and Fran Webb, for their valuable consultations and contributions; working together over the past 30 years has been a most wonderful experience. We especially appreciate Linda's research assistance on several chapters. Special thanks to our colleagues Kathy Pinna for her insightful comments and Sylvia Crews for her careful review of the math explanations in Appendix K. Thank you to Taylor Newman for clarifying content and providing a student's perspective, Chelsea Mackenzie for assisting in numerous office tasks, and Marni Jay Rolfes for offering behind-the-scenes editorial suggestions.

We also thank those who prepared content for instructor and student resources: Samantha Yunko, instructor resources, internet exercises, and case studies; Pat Colsher, case studies; and Jennifer Peterson, PowerPoint slides. Thanks also to Miriam Myers, and the folks at Axxya Systems for their assistance in creating the food composition appendix and developing the computerized Diet & Wellness Plus program that accompanies this book.

Our heartfelt thanks to our editorial team for their efforts in creating an outstanding nutrition textbook—Peggy Williams for gently pushing through resistance for changes that enhance this edition in amazing ways; Nedah Rose for her calming presence, delightful humor, and thoughtful suggestions; Carol Samet for her management of this project; Tom Ziolkowski for his energetic efforts in marketing; Miriam Myers for her dedication in developing online resources and study tools; John Sarantakis and Christine Myaskovsky for their assistance in obtaining permissions; and Casey Lozier and Kellie Petruzzelli for their competent editing of ancillaries.

We also thank Gary Hespenheide and John Walker for creatively designing these pages; Jill Traut for her diligent attention to the innumerable details involved in production; Priya Subbrayal for selecting photographs that deliver nutrition messages attractively; Debbie Stone for copyediting close to 1000 manuscript pages; Heather Mann for proofreading close to 1000 final text pages; and Cheryl Duksta for composing a thorough and useful index. To the hundreds of others involved in production and sales, we tip our hats in appreciation.

We are especially grateful to our friends and families for their continued encouragement and support. We also thank our many reviewers for their comments and contributions.

Reviewers of *Understanding Nutrition*

Becky Alejandre
American River College

Janet B. Anderson
Utah State University

Sandra D. Baker
University of Delaware

Angelina Boyce
Hillsborough Community College

Lynn S. Brann
Syracuse University

Shalon Bull
Palm Beach Community College

Dorothy A. Byrne
University of Texas, San Antonio

John R. Capeheart
University of Houston, Downtown

Leah Carter
Bakersfield College

James F. Collins
University of Florida

Diane Curis
Los Rios Community College District

Lisa K. Diewald
Montgomery County Community College

Kelly K. Eichmann
Fresno City College

Shannon Fenster
Bellevue College

Shawn Flanagan
University of Iowa

Mary Flynn
Brown University

Betty J. Forbes
West Virginia University

Sue Fredstrom
Minnesota State University, Mankato

Trish Froehlich
Palm Beach Community College

Stephen P. Gagnon
Hillsborough Community College

Leonard Gerber
University of Rhode Island

Jill Golden
Orange Coast College

Barbara J. Goldman
Palm Beach State College

Kathleen Gould
Towson University

Margaret Gunther
Palomar College

Charlene Hamilton
University of Delaware

D. J. Hennager
Kirkwood Community College

Catherine Hagen Howard
Texarkana College

Ernest B. Izevbigie
Jackson State University

Craig Kasper
Hillsborough Community College

Shawnee Kelly
Pennsylvania State University

Younghee Kim
Bowling Green State University

Rebecca A. Kleinschmidt
University of Alaska Southeast

Vicki Kloosterhouse
Oakland Community College

Donna M. Kopas
Pennsylvania State University

Susan M. Krueger
University of Wisconsin, Eau Claire

Barbara Lange
College of Central Florida

Melissa Langone
Pasco-Hernando Community College

Grace Lasker
Lake Washington Institute of Technology

Darlene M. Levinson
Oakland Community College, Orchard Ridge

Kimberly Lower
Collin County Community College

Melissa B. McGuire
Maple Woods Community College

Diane L. McKay
Tufts University

Anne Miller
De Anza College

Anahita M. Mistry
Eastern Michigan University

Lisa Morse
Arizona State University

Mithia Mukutmoni
Sierra College

Steven Nizielski
Grand Valley State University

Yvonne Ortega
Santa Monica College

Jane M. Osowski
University of Southern Mississippi

Sarah Panarello
Yakima Valley Community College

Ryan Paruch
Tulsa Community College

Jill Patterson
Pennsylvania State University

Gina Pazzaglia
West Chester University

Julie Priday
Centralia College

Kelsey Rami
South Dakota State University

Jennifer Rogers
University of Iowa

Kathy L. Sedlet
Collin County Community College

Vidya Sharma
San Antonio College

Melissa Shock
University of Central Arkansas

Krista M. Simonetti
Maricopa County College

LuAnn Soliah
Baylor University

Kenneth Strothkamp
Lewis & Clark College

Andrea Villarreal
Phoenix College

Terry Weideman
Oakland Community College, Highland Lake

H. Garrison Wilkes
University of Massachusetts, Boston

Lynne C. Zeman
Kirkwood Community College

Maureen Zimmerman
Mesa Community College

Understanding Nutrition

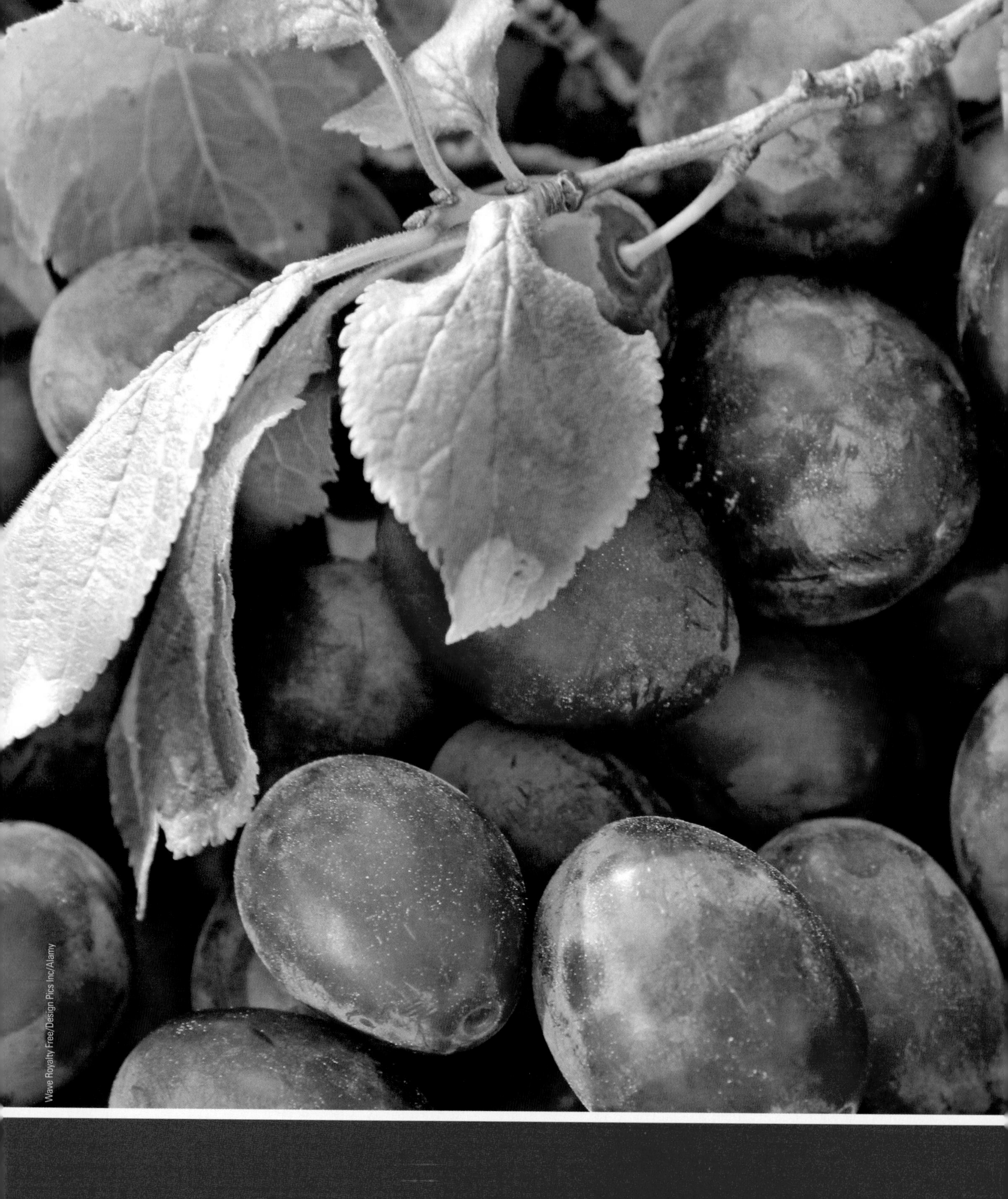
Wave Royalty Free/Design Pics Inc/Alamy

1

An Overview of Nutrition

LEARNING GPS

Nutrition in Your Life

Believe it or not, you have probably eaten at least 20,000 meals in your life. Without any conscious effort on your part, your body uses the nutrients from those foods to make all its components, fuel all its activities, and defend itself against diseases. How successfully your body handles these tasks depends, in part, on your food choices. Nutritious food choices support healthy bodies. In the Nutrition Portfolio at the end of this chapter, you can see how your current food choices are influencing your health and risk of chronic diseases.

Nutrition has always played a significant role in your life. Every day, several times a day, you select **foods** that influence your body's health. Each day's food choices may benefit or harm health only a little, but over time, the consequences of these choices become major. That being the case, paying close attention to good eating habits now supports health benefits later. Conversely, carelessness about food choices can contribute to **chronic diseases.** Of course, some people will become ill or die young no matter what choices they make, and others will live long lives despite making poor choices. For most of us, however, the food choices we make will benefit or impair our health in proportion to the wisdom of those choices.

Although most people realize food habits affect health, they often choose foods for other reasons. After all, foods bring pleasures, traditions, and associations as well as nourishment. The challenge, then, is to combine favorite foods and fun times with a nutritionally balanced **diet.** Take a moment to review the definition and note that *diet* does *not* mean a restrictive food plan designed for weight loss. It simply refers to the foods and beverages a person consumes. Whether it's a vegetarian diet, a weight-loss diet, or any other kind of diet depends on the types of foods and beverages a person chooses.

nutrition: the science of the nutrients in foods and their actions within the body. A broader definition includes the study of human behaviors related to food and eating.

foods: products derived from plants or animals that can be taken into the body to yield energy and nutrients for the maintenance of life and the growth and repair of tissues.

chronic diseases: diseases characterized by slow progression and long duration. Examples include heart disease, diabetes, and some cancers.

- **chronos** = time

diet: the foods and beverages a person eats and drinks.

1.1 Food Choices

> LEARN IT Describe how various factors influence personal food choices.

People decide what to eat, when to eat, how much to eat, and even whether to eat in highly personal ways based on a complex interaction of genetic, behavioral, or social factors rather than on an awareness of nutrition's importance to health.[1] A variety of food choices can support good health, and an understanding of human nutrition helps you make sensible selections more often.

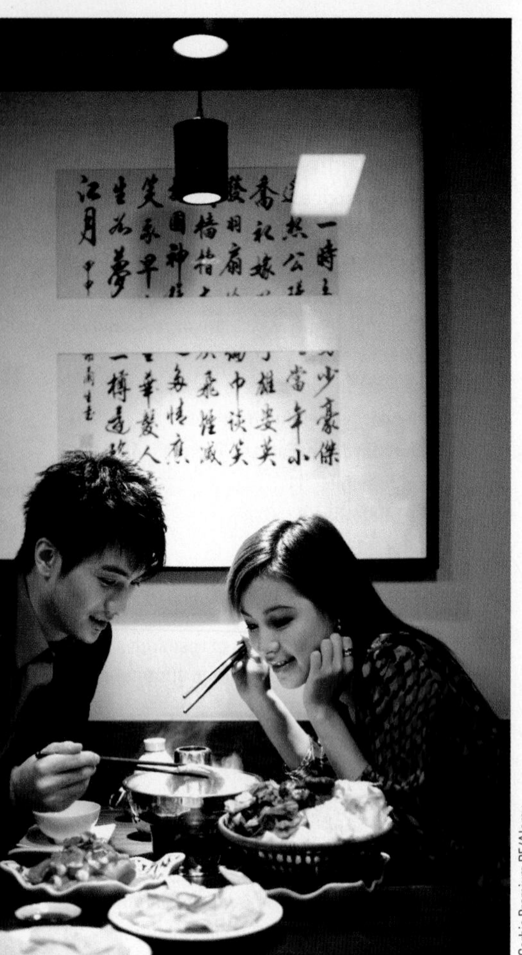

An enjoyable way to learn about a culture is to taste the ethnic foods.

Preferences As you might expect, the number one reason most people choose certain foods is taste—they like the flavor. Two widely shared preferences are for the sweetness of sugar and the savoriness of salt.[2] High-fat foods also appear to be a universally common preference. Other preferences might be for the hot peppers common in Mexican cooking or the curry spices of Indian cuisine. Research suggests that genetics may influence taste perceptions and therefore food likes and dislikes.[3] Similarly, the hormones of pregnancy seem to influence food cravings and aversions (see Chapter 15).

Habit People sometimes select foods out of habit. They eat cereal every morning, for example, simply because they have always eaten cereal for breakfast. Eating a familiar food and not having to make any decisions can be comforting.

Ethnic Heritage and Regional Cuisines Among the strongest influences on food choices are ethnic heritage and regional cuisines. People tend to prefer the foods they grew up eating. Every country, and in fact every region of a country, has its own typical foods and ways of combining them into meals. These cuisines reflect a unique combination of local ingredients and cooking styles. Chowder in New England is made with clams, but in the Florida Keys conch is the featured ingredient. The Pacific Northwest is as famous for its marionberry pie as Georgia is for its peach cobbler. Philly has its cheesesteaks and New Orleans has its oyster po'boys. The "American diet" includes many ethnic foods and regional styles, all adding variety to the diet.

Enjoying traditional **ethnic foods** provides an opportunity to celebrate a person's heritage. People offering ethnic foods share a part of their culture with others, and those accepting the foods learn about another's way of life. Developing **cultural competence** honors individual preferences and is particularly important for professionals who help others plan healthy diets.

Social Interactions Most people enjoy companionship while eating. It's fun to go out with friends for a meal or share a snack when watching a movie together. Meals are often social events, and sharing food is part of hospitality. Social customs invite people to accept food or drink offered by a host or shared by a group—regardless of hunger signals. Chapter 9 describes how people tend to eat more food when socializing with others.

Availability, Convenience, and Economy People often eat foods that are accessible, quick and easy to prepare, and within their financial means. Consumers who value convenience frequently eat out, bring home ready-to-eat meals, or have food delivered. Even when they venture into the kitchen, they want to prepare a meal in 15 to 20 minutes, using less than a half dozen ingredients—and those "ingredients" are often semiprepared foods, such as canned soups and frozen foods.

Consumer emphasis on convenience limits food choices to the selections offered on menus and products designed for quick preparation. Whether decisions based on convenience meet a person's nutrition needs depends on the choices made. Eating a banana or a candy bar may be equally convenient, but the fruit provides more vitamins and minerals and less sugar and fat.

Rising food costs have shifted some consumers' priorities and changed their shopping habits.[4] They are less likely to buy higher-priced convenience foods and

ethnic foods: foods associated with particular cultural groups.

cultural competence: having an awareness and acceptance of cultures and the ability to interact effectively with people of diverse cultures.

more likely to buy less-expensive store brand items and prepare home-cooked meals. In fact, more than 70 percent of meals are prepared in the home.[5] Those who frequently prepare their own meals report more positive emotions and healthier food choices.[6] They tend to eat fast food less often and are more likely to meet dietary guidelines for fat, calcium, fruits, vegetables, and whole grains. Not surprisingly, when eating out, consumers choose low-cost fast-food outlets over more expensive fine-dining restaurants. Foods eaten away from home, especially fast-food meals, tend to be high in kcalories, total fat, saturated fat, and *trans* fat—which can contribute to a variety of health problems.[7]

Unfortunately, healthful diets that include plenty of fruits and vegetables tend to be more costly than less healthful diets featuring foods containing solid fats and added sugars.[8] These low-cost foods are often high in kcalories and low in nutrients.[9] Consumers can improve the quality of their diets without increasing their spending by choosing more plant-based foods, such as nuts, legumes, and whole grains, and fewer refined grains, red and processed meats, and high-fat milk products.[10]

Positive and Negative Associations People tend to like particular foods associated with happy occasions—such as hot dogs at ball games or cake and ice cream at birthday parties. By the same token, people can develop aversions and dislike foods that they ate when they felt sick or that they were forced to eat in negative situations. Similarly, children learn to like and dislike certain foods when their parents use foods as rewards or punishments. Negative experiences can have long-lasting influences on food preferences. More than 50 years after World War II, veterans who had experienced intense combat in the Pacific dislike Chinese and Japanese food significantly more than their peers who were not engaged in battle or those who fought elsewhere.

Emotions Emotions guide food choices and eating behaviors.[11] Some people cannot eat when they are emotionally upset. Others may eat in response to a variety of emotional stimuli—for example, to relieve boredom or depression or to calm anxiety. A depressed person may choose to eat rather than to call a friend. A person who has returned home from an exciting evening out may unwind with a late-night snack. These people may find emotional comfort, in part, because foods can influence the brain's chemistry and the mind's response. Carbohydrates and alcohol, for example, tend to calm, whereas proteins and caffeine are more likely to stimulate. Eating in response to emotions and stress can easily lead to overeating and obesity, but it may be helpful at times. For example, sharing food at times of bereavement serves both the giver's need to provide comfort and the receiver's need to be cared for and to interact with others as well as to take nourishment.

Values Food choices may reflect people's religious beliefs, political views, or environmental concerns. For example, some Christians forgo meat on Fridays during Lent (the period prior to Easter), Jewish law includes an extensive set of dietary rules that govern the use of foods derived from animals, and Muslims fast between sunrise and sunset during Ramadan (the ninth month of the Islamic calendar). Some vegetarians select foods based on their concern for animal rights. A concerned consumer may boycott fruit picked by migrant workers who have been exploited. People may buy vegetables from local farmers to save the fuel and environmental costs of foods shipped from far away. They may also select foods packaged in containers that can be reused or recycled. Some consumers accept or reject foods that have been irradiated, grown organically, or genetically modified, depending on their approval of these processes (see Chapter and Highlight 19 for a complete discussion).

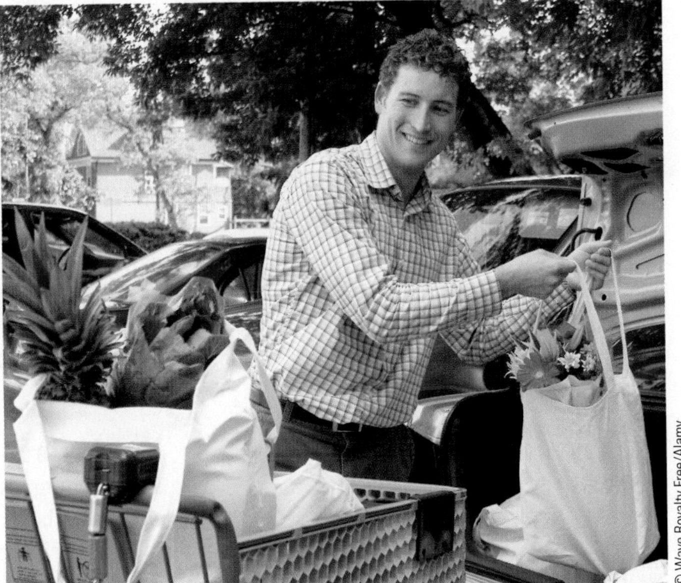

To enhance your health, keep nutrition in mind when selecting foods. To protect the environment, shop at local markets and reuse cloth shopping bags.

Body Weight and Image Sometimes people select certain foods and supplements that they believe will improve their physical appearance and avoid those they believe might be detrimental. Such decisions can be beneficial when based on sound nutrition and fitness knowledge, but decisions based on fads or carried to extremes undermine good health, as pointed out in later discussions of eating disorders (Highlight 8) and dietary supplements commonly used by athletes (Highlight 14).

Nutrition and Health Benefits Finally, of course, many consumers make food choices they believe will improve their health.[12] Food manufacturers and restaurant chefs have responded to scientific findings linking health with nutrition by offering an abundant selection of health-promoting foods and beverages.[13] Foods that provide health benefits beyond their nutrient contributions are called **functional foods.** Functional foods include whole foods as well as fortified, enriched, or enhanced foods.[14] Whole foods—as natural and familiar as oatmeal or tomatoes—are the simplest functional foods. In some cases, foods have been modified to provide health benefits, perhaps by lowering the *trans* fat contents. In other cases, manufacturers have fortified foods by adding nutrients or **phytochemicals** that provide health benefits (see Highlight 13). Examples of these functional foods include orange juice fortified with calcium to help build strong bones and margarine made with a plant sterol that lowers blood cholesterol.

Consumers typically welcome new foods into their diets, provided that these foods are reasonably priced, clearly labeled, easy to find in the grocery store, and convenient to prepare. These foods must also taste good—as good as the traditional choices. Of course, a person need not eat any "special" foods to enjoy a healthy diet; many "regular" foods provide numerous health benefits as well. In fact, "regular" foods such as whole grains; vegetables and legumes; fruits; seafood, meats, poultry, eggs, nuts, and seeds; and milk products are among the healthiest choices a person can make.

› REVIEW IT Describe how various factors influence personal food choices.
A person selects foods for a variety of reasons. Whatever those reasons may be, food choices influence health. Individual food selections neither make nor break a diet's healthfulness, but the balance of foods selected over time can make an important difference to health.[15] For this reason, people are wise to think "nutrition" when making their food choices.

Foods bring pleasure—and nutrients.

functional foods: foods that have a potentially beneficial effect on health when consumed as part of a varied diet on a regular basis at effective levels.

phytochemicals (FIE-toe-KEM-ih-cals): nonnutrient compounds found in plants. Some phytochemicals have biological activity in the body.

- **phyto** = plant

energy: the capacity to do work. The energy in food is chemical energy. The body can convert this chemical energy to mechanical, electrical, or heat energy.

nutrients: chemical substances obtained from food and used in the body to provide energy, structural materials, and regulating agents to support growth, maintenance, and repair of the body's tissues. Nutrients may also reduce the risks of some diseases.

1.2 The Nutrients

› LEARN IT Name the six major classes of nutrients and identify which are organic and which yield energy.

Biologically speaking, people eat to receive nourishment. Do you ever think of yourself as a biological being made of carefully arranged atoms, molecules, cells, tissues, and organs? Are you aware of the activity going on within your body even as you sit still? The atoms, molecules, and cells of your body continuously move and change, even though the structures of your tissues and organs and your external appearance remain relatively constant. The ongoing growth, maintenance, and repair of the body's tissues depend on the **energy** and the **nutrients** received from foods.

Nutrients in Foods and in the Body

Amazingly, our bodies can derive all the energy, structural materials, and regulating agents we need from the foods we eat. This section introduces the nutrients that foods deliver and shows how they participate in the dynamic processes that keep people alive and well.

Nutrient Composition of Foods Chemical analysis of a food such as a tomato shows that it is composed primarily of water (95 percent). Most of the solid materials are carbohydrates, lipids (fats), and proteins. If you could remove these materials, you would find a tiny residue of vitamins, minerals, and other

> FIGURE 1-1 **Body Composition of Healthy-Weight Men and Women**

The human body is made of compounds similar to those found in foods—mostly water (60 percent) and some fat (18 to 21 percent for young men, 23 to 26 percent for young women), with carbohydrate, protein, vitamins, minerals, and other minor constituents making up the remainder. (Chapter 8 describes the health hazards of too little or too much body fat.)

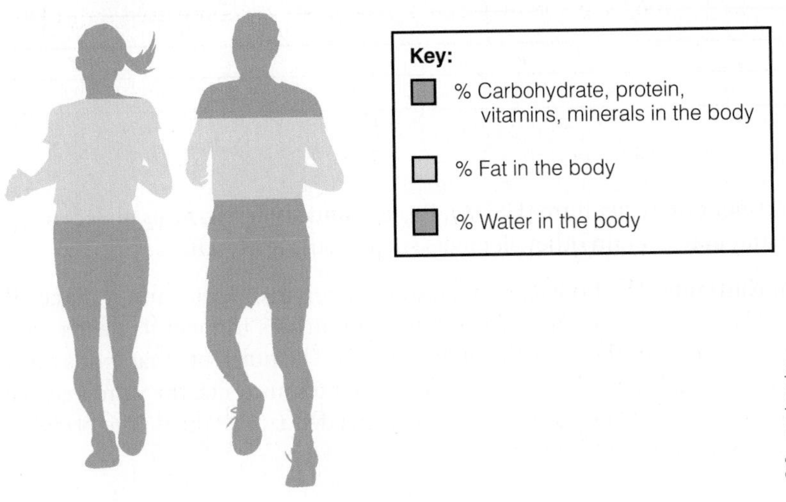

compounds. Water, carbohydrates, lipids, proteins, vitamins, and some of the minerals found in foods represent the six classes of nutrients—substances the body uses for the growth, maintenance, and repair of its tissues.

This book focuses mostly on the nutrients, but foods contain other compounds as well—fibers, phytochemicals, pigments, additives, alcohols, and others. Some are beneficial, some are neutral, and a few are harmful. Later sections of the book touch on these compounds and their significance.

Nutrient Composition of the Body A chemical analysis of your body would show that it is made of materials similar to those found in foods (see Figure 1-1). A healthy 150-pound body contains about 90 pounds of water and about 20 to 45 pounds of fat. The remaining pounds are mostly protein, carbohydrate, and the major minerals of the bones. Vitamins, other minerals, and incidental extras constitute a fraction of a pound.

Chemical Composition of Nutrients The simplest of the nutrients are the minerals. Each mineral is a chemical element; its atoms are all alike. As a result, its identity never changes. For example, iron may have different electrical charges, but the individual iron atoms remain the same when they are in a food, when a person eats the food, when the iron becomes part of a red blood cell, when the cell is broken down, and when the iron is lost from the body by excretion. The next simplest nutrient is water, a compound made of two elements—hydrogen and oxygen. Minerals and water are **inorganic** nutrients—which means they do not contain carbon.

The other four classes of nutrients (carbohydrates, lipids, proteins, and vitamins) are more complex. In addition to hydrogen and oxygen, they all contain carbon, an element found in all living things; they are therefore called **organic** compounds (meaning, literally, "alive").* This chemical definition of *organic* differs from the agricultural definition. As Chapter 19 explains, organic farming refers to growing crops and raising livestock according to standards set by the

* Note that this definition of *organic* excludes coal, diamonds, and a few carbon-containing compounds that contain only a single carbon and no hydrogen, such as carbon dioxide (CO_2), calcium carbonate ($CaCO_3$), magnesium carbonate ($MgCO_3$), and sodium cyanide (NaCN).

inorganic: not containing carbon or pertaining to living organisms. The two classes of nutrients that are inorganic are minerals and water.

- **in** = not

organic: in chemistry, substances or molecules containing carbon-carbon bonds or carbon-hydrogen bonds that are characteristic of living organisms. The four classes of nutrients that are organic are carbohydrates, lipids (fats), proteins, and vitamins.

TABLE 1-1 The Six Classes of Nutrients

Nutrient	Organic	Inorganic	Energy-yielding	Macronutrient	Micronutrient
Carbohydrates	✓		✓	✓	
Lipids (fats)	✓		✓	✓	
Proteins	✓		✓	✓	
Vitamins	✓				✓
Minerals		✓			✓
Water		✓			

US Department of Agriculture (USDA). Protein and some vitamins also contain nitrogen and may contain other elements such as sulfur as well.

Essential Nutrients The body can make some nutrients, but it cannot make all of them. Also, it makes some in insufficient quantities to meet its needs and, therefore, must obtain these nutrients from foods. The nutrients that foods must supply are **essential nutrients.** When used to refer to nutrients, the word *essential* means more than just "necessary"; it means "needed from outside the body"—normally, from foods.

The Energy-Yielding Nutrients: Carbohydrate, Fat, and Protein

In the body, three of the organic nutrients can be used to provide energy: carbohydrate, fat, and protein. In contrast to these **energy-yielding nutrients**, vitamins, minerals, and water do not yield energy in the human body.

Carbohydrate, fat, and protein are sometimes called *macronutrients* because the body requires them in relatively large amounts (many grams daily). In contrast, vitamins and minerals are *micronutrients*, required only in small amounts (milligrams or micrograms daily). Table 1-1 summarizes some of the ways the six classes of nutrients can be described.

TABLE 1-2 kCalorie Values of Energy Nutrients

Nutrients	Energy
Carbohydrate	4 kcal/g
Fat	9 kcal/g
Protein	4 kcal/g

NOTE: Alcohol contributes 7 kcal/g that can be used for energy, but it is not considered a nutrient because it interferes with the body's growth, maintenance, and repair.

Energy Measured in kCalories The energy released from carbohydrates, fats, and proteins can be measured in **calories**—tiny units of energy so small that a single apple provides tens of thousands of them. To ease calculations, energy is expressed in 1000-calorie metric units known as kilocalories (shortened to kcalories, but commonly called "calories"). When you read in popular books or magazines that an apple provides "100 calories," it actually means 100 kcalories. This book uses the term *kcalorie* and its abbreviation *kcal* throughout, as do other scientific books and journals. The "How To" on p. 9 provides a few tips on "thinking metric."

Energy from Foods The amount of energy a food provides depends on how much carbohydrate, fat, and protein it contains. When completely broken down in the body, a gram of carbohydrate yields about 4 kcalories of energy; a gram of protein also yields 4 kcalories; and a gram of fat yields 9 kcalories (see Table 1-2).* The "How To" on p. 10 explains how to calculate the energy available from foods.

Because fat provides more energy per gram, it has a greater **energy density** than either carbohydrate or protein. Figure 1-2 on p. 10 compares the energy density of two breakfast options, and later chapters describe how foods with a high energy density help with weight *gain*, whereas those with a low energy density help with weight *loss*.

One other substance contributes energy—alcohol. Alcohol, however, is not considered a nutrient. Unlike the nutrients, alcohol does not sustain life. In fact, it interferes with the growth, maintenance, and repair of the body. Its only common characteristic with nutrients is that it yields energy (7 kcalories per gram) when metabolized in the body.

essential nutrients: nutrients a person must obtain from food because the body cannot make them for itself in sufficient quantity to meet physiological needs; also called *indispensable nutrients.* About 40 nutrients are currently known to be essential for human beings.

energy-yielding nutrients: the nutrients that break down to yield energy the body can use:

- Carbohydrate
- Fat
- Protein

calories: a measure of *heat* energy. Energy provided by foods and beverages is measured in *kilocalories* (1000 calories equal 1 kilocalorie), abbreviated *kcalories* or *kcal.* One kcalorie is the amount of heat necessary to raise the temperature of 1 kilogram (kg) of water 1°C. The scientific use of the term *kcalorie* is the same as the popular use of the term *calorie.*

energy density: a measure of the energy a food provides relative to the weight of the food (kcalories per gram).

*For those using kilojoules: 1 g carbohydrate = 17 kJ; 1 g protein = 17 kJ; 1 g fat = 37 kJ; and 1 g alcohol = 29 kJ.

>How To

Think Metric

Like other scientists, nutrition scientists use metric units of measure. They measure food energy in kilocalories, people's height in centimeters, people's weight in kilograms, and the weights of foods and nutrients in grams, milligrams, or micrograms. For ease in using these measures, it helps to remember that the prefixes imply 1000. For example, a *kilo*gram is 1000 grams, a *milli*gram is 1/1000 of a gram, and a *micro*gram is 1/1000 of a milligram.

Most food labels and many recipes provide "dual measures," listing both household measures, such as cups, quarts, and teaspoons, and metric measures, such as milliliters, liters, and grams. This practice gives people an opportunity to gradually learn to "think metric."

A person might begin to "think metric" by simply observing the measure—by noticing the amount of soda in a 2-liter bottle, for example. Through such experiences, a person can become familiar with a measure without having to do any conversions.

The international unit for measuring food energy is the joule—the amount of energy expended when 1 kilogram is moved 1 meter by a force of 1 newton. The joule is thus a measure of work energy, whereas the kcalorie is a measure of heat energy. While many scientists and journals report their findings in kilojoules (kJ), many others, particularly those in the United States, use kcalories (kcal). To convert energy measures from kcalories to kilojoules, multiply by 4.2; to convert kilojoules to kcalories, multiply by 0.24. For example, a 50-kcalorie cookie provides 210 kilojoules:

$$50 \text{ kcal} \times 4.2 = 210 \text{ kJ}$$

Appendix K provides assistance and conversion factors for these and other units of measure.

Volume: Liters (L)

1 L = 1000 milliliters (mL)
0.95 L = 1 quart
1 mL = 0.03 fluid ounces
240 mL = 1 cup

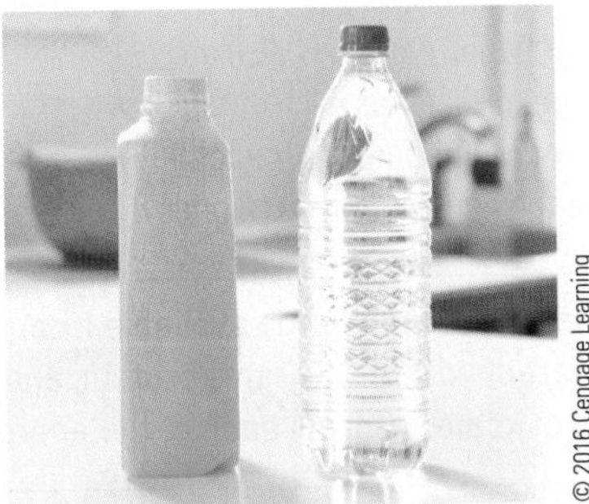

A liter of liquid is approximately one US quart. (Four liters are only about 5 percent more than a gallon.)

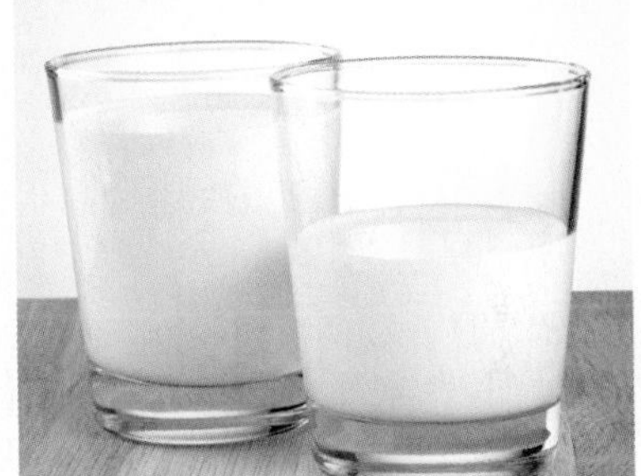

One cup of liquid is about 240 milliliters; a half-cup of liquid is about 120 milliliters.

Weight: Grams (g)

1 g = 1000 milligrams (mg)
1 g = 0.04 ounce (oz)
1 oz = 28.35 g (or 30 g)
100 g = 3½ oz
1 kilogram (kg) = 1000 g
1 kg = 2.2 pounds (lb)
454 g = 1 lb

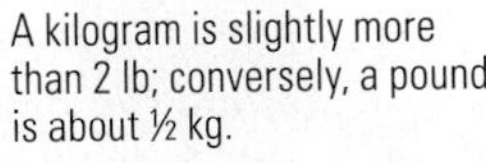

A kilogram is slightly more than 2 lb; conversely, a pound is about ½ kg.

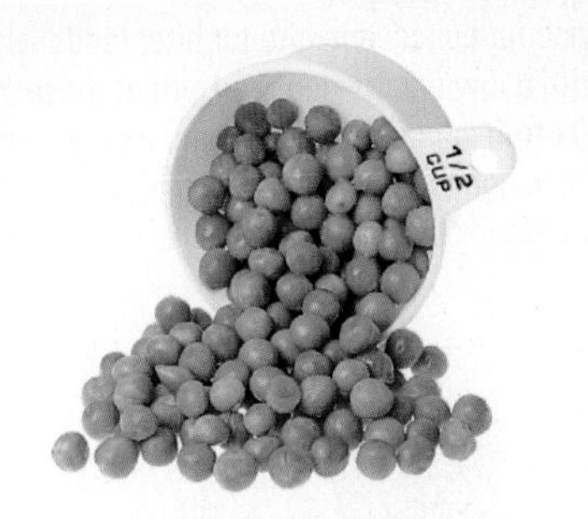

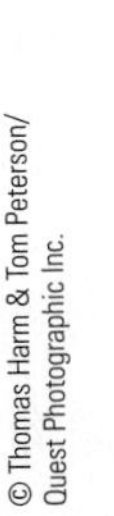

A half-cup of vegetables weighs about 100 grams; one pea weighs about ½ gram.

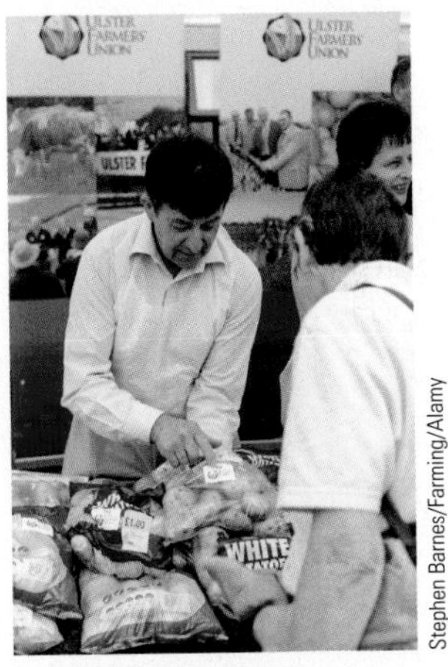

A 5-pound bag of potatoes weighs about 2 kilograms, and a 176-pound person weighs 80 kilograms.

> TRY IT Convert your body weight from pounds to kilograms and your height from inches to centimeters.

Most foods contain the energy-yielding nutrients, as well as vitamins, minerals, water, and other substances. For example, meat contains water, fat, vitamins, and minerals as well as protein. Bread contains water, a trace of fat, a little protein, and some vitamins and minerals in addition to its carbohydrate. Only a few foods are exceptions to this rule, the common ones being sugar (pure carbohydrate) and oil (essentially pure fat).

>How To

Calculate the Energy Available from Foods

To calculate the energy available from a food, multiply the number of grams of carbohydrate, protein, and fat by 4, 4, and 9, respectively. Then add the results together. For example, 1 slice of bread with 1 tablespoon of peanut butter on it contains 16 grams carbohydrate, 7 grams protein, and 9 grams fat:

$$\begin{aligned} 16 \text{ g carbohydrate} \times 4 \text{ kcal/g} &= 64 \text{ kcal} \\ 7 \text{ g protein} \times 4 \text{ kcal/g} &= 28 \text{ kcal} \\ 9 \text{ g fat} \times 9 \text{ kcal/g} &= 81 \text{ kcal} \\ \text{Total} &= 173 \text{ kcal} \end{aligned}$$

From this information, you can calculate the percentage of kcalories each of the energy nutrients contributes to the total. To determine the percentage of kcalories from fat, for example, divide the 81 fat kcalories by the total 173 kcalories:

$$81 \text{ fat kcal} \div 173 \text{ total kcal} = 0.468 \text{ (rounded to 0.47)}$$

Then multiply by 100 to get the percentage:

$$0.47 \times 100 = 47\%$$

Dietary recommendations that urge people to limit fat intake to 20 to 35 percent of kcalories refer to the day's total energy intake, not to individual foods. Still, if the proportion of fat in each food choice throughout a day exceeds 35 percent of kcalories, then the day's total surely will, too. Knowing that this snack provides 47 percent of its kcalories from fat alerts a person to the need to make lower-fat selections at other times that day.

> TRY IT Calculate the energy available from a bean burrito with cheese (55 grams carbohydrate, 15 grams protein, and 12 grams fat). Determine the percentage of kcalories from each of the energy nutrients.

> FIGURE 1-2 **Energy Density of Two Breakfast Options Compared**

Gram for gram, ounce for ounce, and bite for bite, foods with a high energy density deliver more kcalories than foods with a low energy density. Both of these breakfast options provide 500 kcalories, but the cereal with milk, fruit salad, scrambled egg, turkey sausage, and toast with jam offers three times as much food as the doughnuts (based on weight); it has a lower energy density than the doughnuts. Selecting a variety of foods also helps to ensure nutrient adequacy.

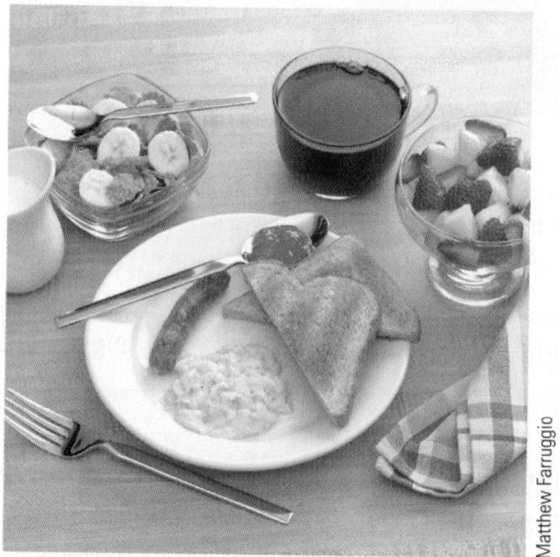

Matthew Farruggio

LOWER ENERGY DENSITY
This 450-gram breakfast delivers 500 kcalories, for an energy density of 1.1 (500 kcal ÷ 450 g = 1.1 kcal/g).

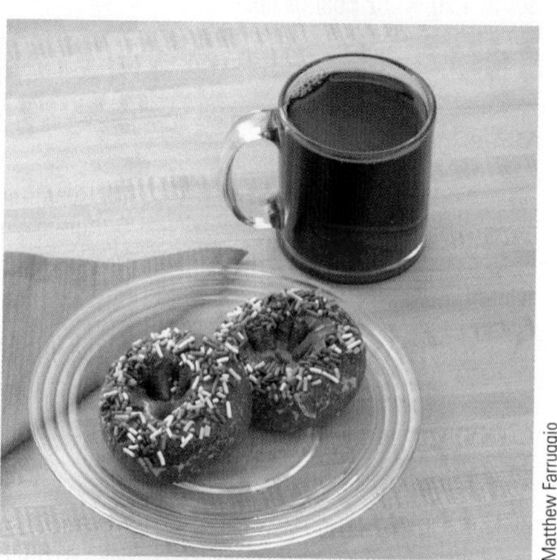

Matthew Farruggio

HIGHER ENERGY DENSITY
This 144-gram breakfast delivers 500 kcalories, for an energy density of 3.5 (500 kcal ÷ 144 g = 3.5 kcal/g).

Energy in the Body When the body uses carbohydrate, fat, or protein to fuel its activities, the bonds between the nutrient's atoms break. As the bonds break, they release energy. Some of this energy is released as heat, but some is used to send electrical impulses through the brain and nerves, to synthesize body compounds, and to move muscles. Thus the energy from food supports every activity from quiet thought to vigorous sports.

If the body does not use these nutrients to fuel its current activities, it converts them into storage compounds (such as body fat), to be used between meals and overnight when fresh energy supplies run low. If more energy is consumed than expended, the result is an increase in energy stores and weight gain. Similarly, if less energy is consumed than expended, the result is a decrease in energy stores and weight loss.

When consumed in excess of energy needs, alcohol, too, can be converted to body fat and stored. When alcohol contributes a substantial portion of the energy in a person's diet, the harm it does far exceeds the problems of excess body fat. (Highlight 7 describes the effects of alcohol on health and nutrition.)

Other Roles of Energy-Yielding Nutrients In addition to providing energy, carbohydrates, fats, and proteins provide the raw materials for building the body's tissues and regulating its many activities. In fact, protein's role as a fuel source is relatively minor compared with both the other two energy-yielding nutrients and its other roles. Proteins are found in structures such as the muscles and skin and help to regulate activities such as digestion and energy metabolism. (Chapter 6 presents a full discussion on proteins.)

The Vitamins

The **vitamins** are also organic, but they do not provide energy. Instead, they facilitate the release of energy from carbohydrate, fat, and protein and participate in numerous other activities throughout the body.

Each of the 13 vitamins has its own special roles to play.* One vitamin enables the eyes to see in dim light, another helps protect the lungs from air pollution, and still another helps make the sex hormones—among other things. When you cut yourself, one vitamin helps stop the bleeding and another helps repair the skin. Vitamins busily help replace old red blood cells and the lining of the digestive tract. Almost every action in the body requires the assistance of vitamins.

Vitamins can function only if they are intact, but because they are complex organic molecules, they are vulnerable to destruction by heat, light, and chemical agents. This is why the body handles them carefully, and why nutrition-wise cooks do, too. The strategies of cooking vegetables at moderate temperatures for short times and using small amounts of water help to preserve the vitamins.

The Minerals

In the body, some **minerals** are put together in orderly arrays in such structures as bones and teeth. Minerals are also found in the fluids of the body, which influences fluid balance and distribution. Whatever their roles, minerals do not yield energy.

Only 16 minerals are known to be essential in human nutrition.** Others are being studied to determine whether they play significant roles in the human body. Still other minerals, such as lead, are environmental contaminants that displace the nutrient minerals from their workplaces in the body, disrupting body functions. The problems caused by contaminant minerals are described in Chapter 13.

---

*The water-soluble vitamins are vitamin C and the eight B vitamins: thiamin, riboflavin, niacin, vitamins B_6 and B_{12}, folate, biotin, and pantothenic acid. The fat-soluble vitamins are vitamins A, D, E, and K. The water-soluble vitamins are the subject of Chapter 10 and the fat-soluble vitamins, of Chapter 11.

**The major minerals are calcium, phosphorus, potassium, sodium, chloride, magnesium, and sulfate. The trace minerals are iron, iodine, zinc, chromium, selenium, fluoride, molybdenum, copper, and manganese. Chapters 12 and 13 are devoted to the major and trace minerals, respectively.

vitamins: organic, essential nutrients required in small amounts by the body for health.

minerals: inorganic elements. Some minerals are essential nutrients required in small amounts by the body for health.

Because minerals are inorganic, they are indestructible and need not be handled with the special care that vitamins require. Minerals can, however, be bound by substances that interfere with the body's ability to absorb them. They can also be lost during food-refining processes or during cooking when they leach into water that is discarded.

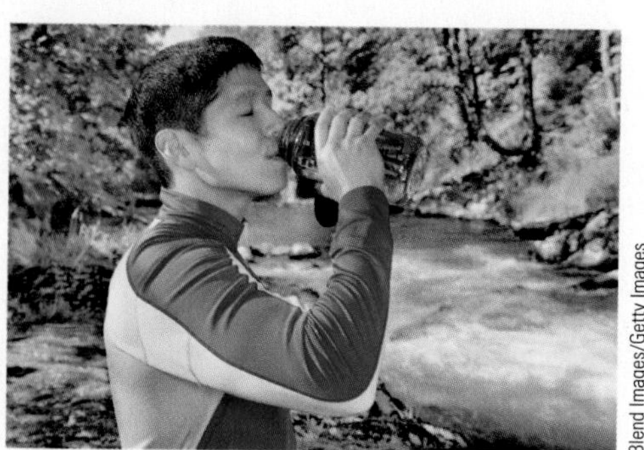

Blend Images/Getty Images

Water is an essential nutrient and naturally carries varying amounts of several minerals.

Water Water provides the environment in which nearly all the body's activities are conducted. It participates in many metabolic reactions and supplies the medium for transporting vital materials to cells and carrying waste products away from them. Water is discussed fully in Chapter 12, but it is mentioned in every chapter. If you watch for it, you cannot help but be impressed by water's participation in all life processes.

› REVIEW IT Name the six major classes of nutrients and identify which are organic and which yield energy.

Foods provide nutrients—substances that support the growth, maintenance, and repair of the body's tissues. The six classes of nutrients include:

- Carbohydrates
- Lipids (fats)
- Proteins
- Vitamins
- Minerals
- Water

Foods rich in the energy-yielding nutrients (carbohydrate, fat, and protein) provide the major materials for building the body's tissues and yield energy for the body's use or storage. Energy is measured in kcalories—a measure of heat energy. Vitamins, minerals, and water do not yield energy; instead they facilitate a variety of activities in the body.

Without exaggeration, nutrients provide the physical and metabolic basis for nearly all that we are and all that we do. The next section introduces the science of nutrition with emphasis on the research methods scientists have used in uncovering the wonders of nutrition.

1.3 The Science of Nutrition

› LEARN IT Explain the scientific method and how scientists use various types of research studies and methods to acquire nutrition information.

The science of nutrition is the study of the nutrients and other substances in foods and the body's handling of them. Its foundation depends on several other sciences, including biology, biochemistry, and physiology. As sciences go, nutrition is young, but as you can see from the size of this book, much has happened in nutrition's short life. And it is currently experiencing a tremendous growth spurt as scientists apply knowledge gained from sequencing the human **genome**. The integration of nutrition, genomics, and molecular biology has opened a whole new world of study called **nutritional genomics**—the science of how nutrients affect the activities of genes and how genes affect the interactions between diet and disease. Highlight 6 describes how nutritional genomics is shaping the science of nutrition, and examples of nutrient–gene interactions appear throughout later chapters of the book.

Conducting Research Consumers sometimes depend on personal experience or reports from friends to gather information on nutrition. Such a personal account of an experience or event is known as an **anecdote** and is not accepted as reliable scientific information (see the glossary on p. 13 for definitions of research terms). In contrast, researchers use the scientific method to guide their work (see Figure 1-3). As the figure shows, research always begins with a problem or a question. For example, "What foods or nutrients might protect against the common cold?" In search of an answer, scientists make an educated guess **(hypothesis)**, such as "foods rich in vitamin C reduce the number of common colds." Then they systematically conduct research studies to collect data that will

genome (GEE-nome): the complete set of genetic material (DNA) in an organism or a cell. The study of genomes is called *genomics*.

nutritional genomics: the science of how nutrients affect the activities of genes (*nutrigenomics*) and how genes affect the interactions between diet and disease (*nutrigenetics*).

> **FIGURE 1-3 The Scientific Method**

Research scientists follow the scientific method. Note that most research generates new questions, not final answers. Thus the sequence begins anew, and research continues in a somewhat cyclical way.

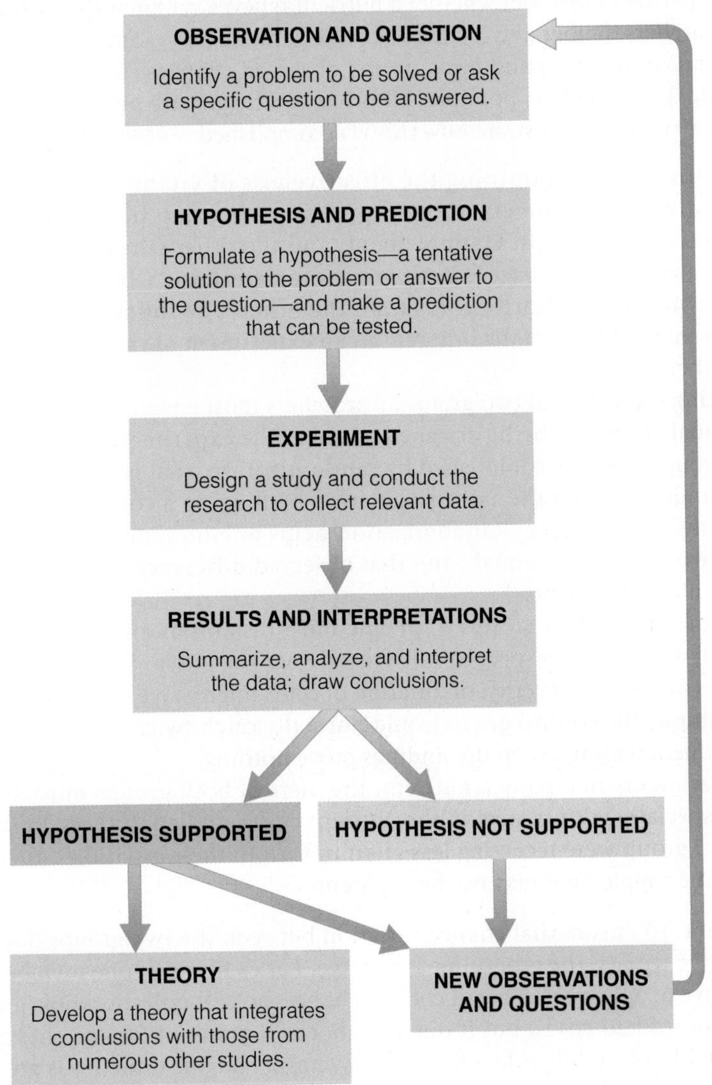

GLOSSARY OF RESEARCH TERMS

anecdote: a personal account of an experience or event; not reliable scientific information.

blind experiment: an experiment in which the subjects do not know whether they are members of the experimental group or the control group.

control group: a group of individuals similar in all possible respects to the experimental group except for the treatment. Ideally, the control group receives a placebo while the experimental group receives a real treatment.

correlation (CORE-ee-LAY-shun): the simultaneous increase, decrease, or change in two variables. If A increases as B increases, or if A decreases as B decreases, the correlation is *positive.* (This does not mean that A causes B or vice versa.) If A increases as B decreases, or if A decreases as B increases, the correlation is *negative.* (This does not mean that A prevents B or vice versa.) Some third factor may account for both A and B.

double-blind experiment: an experiment in which neither the subjects nor the researchers know which subjects are members of the experimental group and which are serving as control subjects, until after the experiment is over.

experimental group: a group of individuals similar in all possible respects to the control group except for the treatment. The experimental group receives the real treatment.

hypothesis (hi-POTH-eh-sis): an unproven statement that tentatively explains the relationships between two or more variables.

peer review: a process in which a panel of scientists rigorously evaluates a research study to ensure that the scientific method was followed.

placebo (pla-SEE-bo): an inert, harmless medication given to provide comfort and hope; a sham treatment used in controlled research studies.

placebo effect: a change that occurs in response to expectations about the effectiveness of a treatment that actually has no pharmaceutical effects.

randomization (RAN-dom-ih-ZAY-shun): a process of choosing the members of the experimental and control groups without bias.

replication (REP-lih-KAY-shun): repeating an experiment and getting the same results.

subjects: the people or animals participating in a research project.

theory: a tentative explanation that integrates many and diverse findings to further the understanding of a defined topic.

validity (va-LID-ih-tee): having the quality of being founded on fact or evidence.

variables: factors that change. A variable may depend on another variable (for example, a child's height depends on his age), or it may be independent (for example, a child's height does not depend on the color of her eyes). Sometimes both variables correlate with a third variable (a child's height and eye color both depend on genetics).

test the hypothesis. Some examples of various types of research designs are presented in Figure 1-4. Because each type of study has strengths and weaknesses, some provide stronger evidence than others, as Figure 1-4 explains.

In attempting to discover whether a nutrient relieves symptoms or cures a disease, researchers deliberately manipulate one variable (for example, the amount of vitamin C in the diet) and measure any observed changes (perhaps the number of colds). As much as possible, all other conditions are held constant. The following paragraphs illustrate how this is accomplished.

Controls In studies examining the effectiveness of vitamin C, researchers typically divide the **subjects** into two groups. One group (the **experimental group**) receives a vitamin C supplement, and the other (the **control group**) does not. Researchers observe both groups to determine whether one group has fewer, milder, or shorter colds than the other. The following discussion describes some of the pitfalls inherent in an experiment of this kind and ways to avoid them.

In sorting subjects into two groups, researchers must ensure that each person has an equal chance of being assigned to either the experimental group or the control group. This is accomplished by **randomization**; that is, the subjects are chosen randomly from the same population by flipping a coin or some other method involving chance. Randomization helps to eliminate bias and ensure that the two groups are "equal" and that observed differences reflect the treatment and not other factors.[16]

Importantly, the two groups of people must be similar and must have the same track record with respect to colds to rule out the possibility that observed differences in the rate, severity, or duration of colds might have occurred anyway. If, for example, the control group would normally catch twice as many colds as the experimental group, then the findings prove nothing.

In experiments involving a nutrient, the diets of both groups must also be similar, especially with respect to the nutrient being studied. If those in the experimental group were receiving less vitamin C from their usual diet, then any effects of the supplement may not be apparent.

Sample Size To ensure that chance variation between the two groups does not influence the results, the groups must be large. For example, if one member of a group of five people catches a bad cold by chance, he will pull the whole group's average toward bad colds; but if one member of a group of 500 catches a bad cold, she will not unduly affect the group average. Statistical methods are used to determine whether differences between groups of various sizes support a hypothesis.

Placebos If people who take vitamin C for colds *believe* it will cure them, their chances of recovery may improve. Taking pills believed to be beneficial may shorten the duration and lessen the severity of illness regardless of whether the pills contain active ingredients.[17] This phenomenon, the result of expectations, is known as the **placebo effect.** In experiments designed to determine vitamin C's effect on colds, this mind-body effect must be rigorously controlled. Severity of symptoms is often a subjective measure, and people who believe they are receiving treatment may report less severe symptoms.

One way experimenters control for the placebo effect is to give pills to all participants. Those in the experimental group, for example, receive pills containing vitamin C, and those in the control group receive a **placebo**—pills of similar appearance and taste containing an inactive ingredient. This way, the expectations of both groups will be equal. It is not necessary to convince all subjects that they are receiving vitamin C, but the extent of belief or unbelief must be the same in both groups. A study conducted under these conditions is called a **blind experiment**—that is, the subjects do not know (are blind to) whether they are members of the experimental group (receiving treatment) or the control group (receiving the placebo).

> FIGURE 1-4 Examples of Research Designs

EPIDEMIOLOGICAL STUDIES research the incidence, distribution, and control of disease in a population. Epidemiological studies include cross-sectional, case-control, and cohort studies.

Strengths:
- Can narrow down the list of possible causes
- Can raise questions to pursue through other research

Weaknesses:
- Cannot control variables that may influence the development or the prevention of a disease
- Cannot prove cause and effect

CROSS-SECTIONAL STUDIES

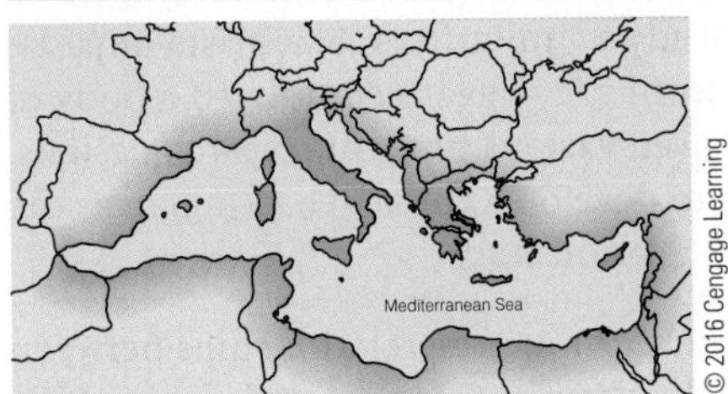

Researchers observe how much and what kinds of foods a group of people eat and how healthy those people are. Their findings identify factors that might influence the incidence of a disease in various populations.

Example. Many people in the Mediterranean region drink more wine, eat more fat from olive oil, and yet have a lower incidence of heart disease than northern Europeans and North Americans.

CASE-CONTROL STUDIES

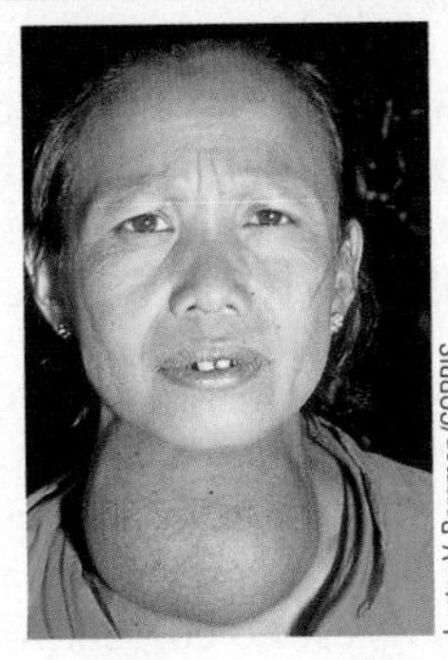

Researchers compare people who do and do not have a given condition such as a disease, closely matching them in age, gender, and other key variables so that differences in other factors will stand out. These differences may account for the condition in the group that has it.

Example. People with goiter lack iodine in their diets.

COHORT STUDIES

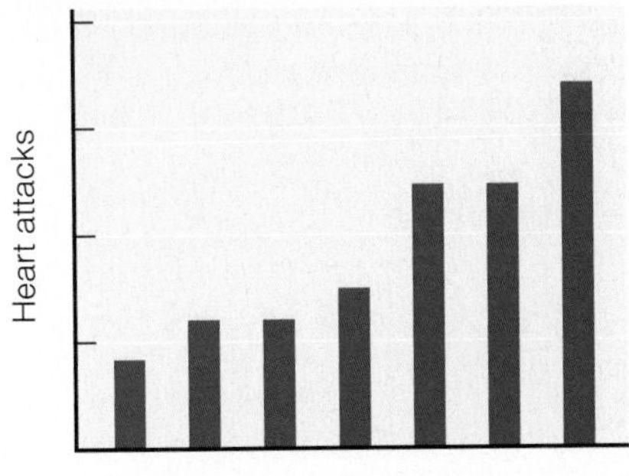

Researchers analyze data collected from a selected group of people (a cohort) at intervals over a certain period of time.

Example. Data collected periodically over the past several decades from more than 5000 people randomly selected from the town of Framingham, Massachusetts, in 1948 have revealed that the risk of heart attack increases as blood cholesterol increases.

EXPERIMENTAL STUDIES test cause-and-effect relationships between variables. Experimental studies include laboratory-based studies—on animals or in test tubes (in vitro)—and human intervention (or clinical) trials.

Strengths:
- Can control conditions (for the most part)
- Can determine effects of a variable
- Can apply some findings on human beings to some groups of human beings

Weaknesses:
- Cannot apply results from test tubes or animals to human beings
- Cannot generalize findings on human beings to all human beings
- Cannot use certain treatments for clinical or ethical reasons

LABORATORY-BASED ANIMAL STUDIES

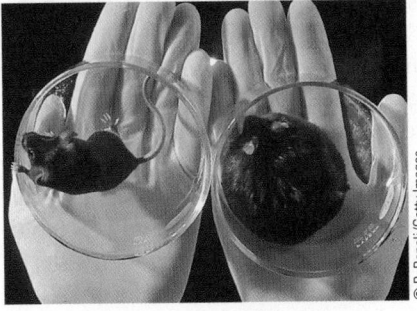

Researchers feed animals special diets that provide or omit specific nutrients and then observe any changes in health. Such studies test possible disease causes and treatments in a laboratory where all conditions can be controlled.

Example. Mice fed a high-fat diet eat less food than mice given a lower-fat diet, so they receive the same number of kcalories—but the mice eating the fat-rich diet become severely obese.

LABORATORY-BASED IN VITRO STUDIES

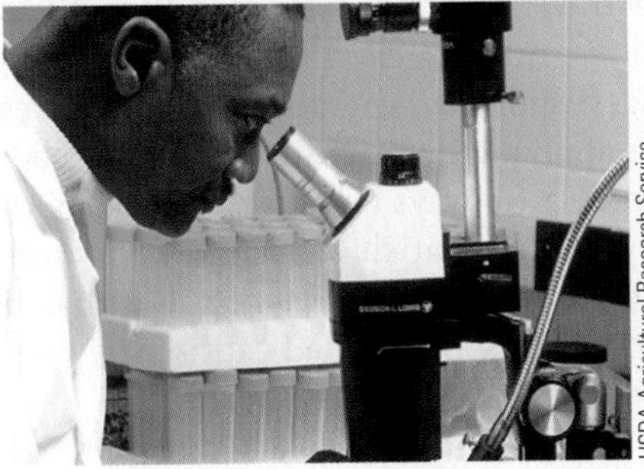

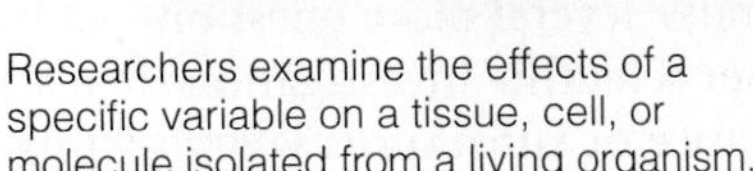

Researchers examine the effects of a specific variable on a tissue, cell, or molecule isolated from a living organism.

Example. Laboratory studies find that fish oils inhibit the growth and activity of the bacteria implicated in ulcer formation.

HUMAN INTERVENTION (OR CLINICAL) TRIALS

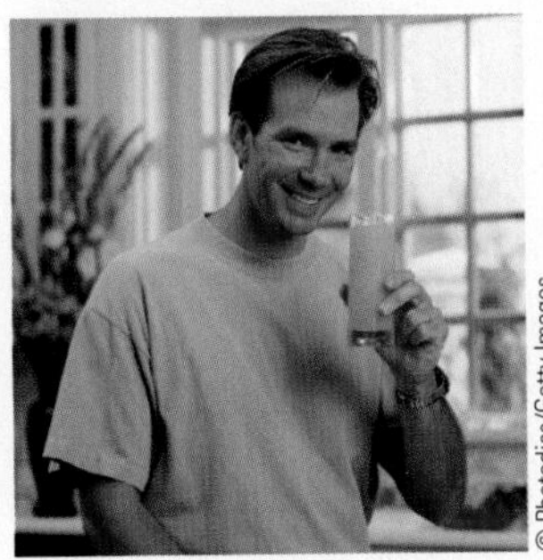

Researchers ask people to adopt a new behavior (for example, eat a citrus fruit, take a vitamin C supplement, or exercise daily). These trials help determine the effectiveness of such interventions on the development or prevention of disease.

Example. Heart disease risk factors improve when men drink fresh-squeezed orange juice daily for 2 months compared with those on a diet low in vitamin C—even when both groups follow a diet high in saturated fat.

Double Blind When both the subjects and the researchers do not know which subjects are in which group, the study is called a **double-blind experiment.** Being fallible human beings and having an emotional and sometimes financial investment in a successful outcome, researchers might record and interpret results with a bias in the expected direction. To prevent such bias, the pills are coded by a third party, who does not reveal to the experimenters which subjects are in which group until all results have been recorded.

Analyzing Research Findings

Research findings must be analyzed and interpreted with an awareness of each study's limitations. Scientists must be cautious about drawing any conclusions until they have accumulated a body of evidence from multiple studies that have used various types of research designs. As evidence accumulates, scientists begin to develop a **theory** that integrates the various findings and explains the complex relationships.

Correlations and Causes Researchers often examine the relationships between two or more **variables**—for example, daily vitamin C intake and the number of colds or the duration and severity of cold symptoms. Importantly, researchers must be able to observe, measure, or verify the variables selected. Findings sometimes suggest no **correlation** between variables (regardless of the amount of vitamin C consumed, the number of colds remains the same). Other times, studies find either a **positive correlation** (the more vitamin C, the more colds) or a **negative correlation** (the more vitamin C, the fewer colds). Notice that in a positive correlation, both variables change in the same direction, regardless of whether the direction is "more" or "less"—"the more vitamin C, the more colds" is a positive correlation, just as is "the less vitamin C, the fewer colds." In a negative correlation, the two variables change in opposite directions: "the less vitamin C, the more colds" or "the more vitamin C, the fewer colds." Also notice that a positive correlation does not necessarily reflect a desired outcome, nor does a negative correlation always reflect an unwanted outcome.

Correlational evidence proves only that variables are associated, not that one is the cause of the other. To actually prove that A causes B, scientists have to find evidence of the *mechanism*—that is, an explanation of how A might cause B.

Cautious Conclusions When researchers record and analyze the results of their experiments, they must exercise caution in their interpretation of the findings. For example, in an epidemiological study, scientists may use a specific segment of the population—say, men 18 to 30 years old. When the scientists draw conclusions, they are careful not to generalize the findings to men and women of all ages. Similarly, scientists performing research studies using animals are cautious in applying their findings to human beings. Conclusions from any one research study are always tentative and take into account findings from studies conducted by other scientists as well. As evidence accumulates, scientists gain confidence about making recommendations that affect people's health and lives. Still, their statements are worded cautiously, such as "A diet high in fruits and vegetables *may* protect against *some* cancers."

Quite often, as scientists approach an answer to one research question, they raise several more questions, so future research projects are never lacking. Further scientific investigation then seeks to answer questions, such as "What substance or substances within fruits and vegetables provide protection?" If those substances turn out to be the vitamins found so abundantly in fresh produce, then "How much is needed to offer protection?" "How do these vitamins protect against cancer?" "Is it their action as antioxidant nutrients?" "If not, might it be another action or even another substance that accounts for the protection fruits and vegetables provide against cancer?" (Highlight 11 explores the answers to these questions and reviews recent research on antioxidant nutrients and disease.)

TABLE 1-3 Parts of a Research Article

- *Abstract:* The abstract provides a brief overview of the article.
- *Introduction:* The introduction clearly states the purpose of the current study and provides a comprehensive review of the relevant literature.
- *Methodology:* The methodology section defines key terms and describes the study design, subjects, and procedures used in conducting the study.
- *Results:* The results report the findings and may include tables and figures that summarize the information.
- *Discussion*: The discussion draws tentative conclusions that are supported by the data and reflect the original purpose as stated in the introduction. Usually, it answers a few questions and raises several more.
- *References*: The references reflect the investigator's knowledge of the subject and should include an extensive list of relevant studies (including key studies several years old as well as current ones).

Publishing Research The findings from a research study are submitted to a board of reviewers composed of other scientists who rigorously evaluate the study to ensure that the scientific method was followed—a process known as **peer review.** The reviewers critique the study's hypothesis, methodology, statistical significance, and conclusions. They also note the funding source, recognizing that financial support may bias scientific conclusions. If the reviewers consider the conclusions to be well supported by the evidence—that is, if the research has **validity**—they endorse the work for publication in a scientific journal where others can read it. This raises an important point regarding information found on the Internet: much gets published without the rigorous scrutiny of peer review. Consequently, readers must assume greater responsibility for examining the data and conclusions presented—often without the benefit of journal citations. Highlight 1 offers guidance in determining whether website information is reliable. Table 1-3 describes the parts of a typical research article.

Even when a new finding is published or released to the media, it is still only preliminary and not very meaningful by itself. Other scientists will need to confirm or disprove the findings through **replication.** To be accepted into the body of nutrition knowledge, a finding must stand up to rigorous, repeated testing in experiments performed by several different researchers. What we "know" in nutrition results from years of replicating study findings. Communicating the latest finding in its proper context without distorting or oversimplifying the message is a challenge for scientists and journalists alike. For a helpful scientific overview of current topics in nutrition, look for review articles in scholarly journals such as *Nutrition Reviews.* Similar to a review article, a meta-analysis study uses the power of a computer to combine and reanalyze the results of many previously published studies on a single topic. Keep in mind that a meta-analysis study is useful in providing an overview of the averages, but its results may not apply to all individuals or cases.[18]

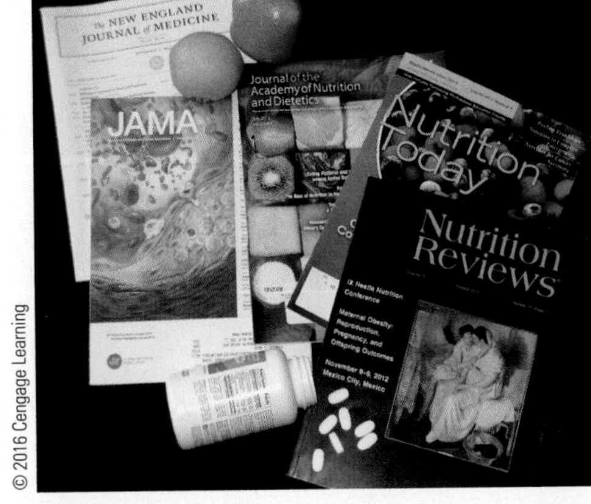

Knowledge about the nutrients and their effects on health comes from scientific studies.

With each report from scientists, the field of nutrition changes a little—each finding contributes another piece to the whole body of knowledge. People who know how science works understand that single findings, like single frames in a movie, are just small parts of a larger story. Over years, the picture of what is "true" in nutrition gradually changes, and dietary recommendations change to reflect the current understanding of scientific research. Highlight 5 provides a detailed look at how dietary fat recommendations have evolved over the past several decades as researchers have uncovered the relationships between the various kinds of fat and their roles in supporting or harming health.

› REVIEW IT Explain the scientific method and how scientists use various types of research studies and methods to acquire nutrition information.

Scientists learn about nutrition by conducting experiments that follow the protocol of scientific research. In designing their studies, researchers randomly assign control and experimental groups, seek large sample sizes, provide placebos, and remain blind to treatments. Their findings must be reviewed and replicated by other scientists before being accepted as valid.

The characteristics of well-designed research have enabled scientists to study the actions of nutrients in the body. Such research has laid the foundation for quantifying how much of each nutrient the body needs.

1.4 Dietary Reference Intakes

› LEARN IT Define the four categories of the DRI and explain their purposes.

Using the results of thousands of research studies, nutrition experts have produced a set of standards that define the amounts of energy, nutrients, other dietary components, and physical activity that best support health. These recommendations are called **Dietary Reference Intakes (DRI),** and they reflect the collaborative efforts of researchers in both the United States and Canada.*[19] The inside front cover of this book provides a handy reference for DRI values.

Establishing Nutrient Recommendations The DRI Committee consists of highly qualified scientists who base their estimates of nutrient needs on careful examination and interpretation of scientific evidence. These recommendations apply to healthy people and may not be appropriate for people with diseases that increase or decrease nutrient needs. The next several paragraphs introduce the four categories of the DRI, explain their purposes, and discuss specific aspects of how the committee goes about establishing these values:

- Estimated Average Requirements (EAR)
- Recommended Dietary Allowances (RDA)
- Adequate Intakes (AI)
- Tolerable Upper Intake Levels (UL)

Estimated Average Requirements (EAR) The committee reviews hundreds of research studies to determine the **requirement** for a nutrient—how much is needed in the diet. The committee selects a different criterion for each nutrient based on its roles in supporting various activities in the body and in reducing disease risks.

An examination of all the available data reveals that each person's body is unique and has its own set of requirements. Men differ from women, and needs change as people grow from infancy through old age. For this reason, the committee clusters its recommendations for people into groups based on gender and age. Even so, the exact requirements for people of the same gender and age are likely to be different. Person A might need 40 units of a particular nutrient each day; person B might need 35; and person C might need 57. Looking at enough people might reveal that their individual requirements fall into a symmetrical distribution, with most near the midpoint and only a few at the extremes (see the left side of Figure 1-5). Using this information, the committee determines an **Estimated Average Requirement (EAR)** for each nutrient—the average amount that appears sufficient for half of the population. In Figure 1-5, the EAR is shown as 45 units.

Recommended Dietary Allowances (RDA) Once a nutrient *requirement* is established, the committee must decide what intake to *recommend* for everybody—the **Recommended Dietary Allowance (RDA).** As you can see by the distribution in Figure 1-5, the EAR (shown in the figure as 45 units) is probably closest to everyone's need. If people consumed exactly the average requirement of a given nutrient each day, however, approximately half of the population would develop deficiencies of that nutrient—in Figure 1-5, for example, person C would be among them. Recommendations are therefore set greater than the EAR to meet the needs of most healthy people.

Small amounts greater than the daily requirement do no harm, whereas amounts less than the requirement may lead to health problems. When people's

*The DRI reports are produced by the Food and Nutrition Board, Institute of Medicine of the National Academies, with active involvement of scientists from the United States and Canada.

Dietary Reference Intakes (DRI): a set of nutrient intake values for healthy people in the United States and Canada. These values are used for planning and assessing diets and include:

- Estimated Average Requirements (EAR)
- Recommended Dietary Allowances (RDA)
- Adequate Intakes (AI)
- Tolerable Upper Intake Levels (UL)

requirement: the lowest continuing intake of a nutrient that will maintain a specified criterion of adequacy.

Estimated Average Requirement (EAR): the average daily amount of a nutrient that will maintain a specific biochemical or physiological function in half the healthy people of a given age and gender group.

Recommended Dietary Allowance (RDA): the average daily amount of a nutrient considered adequate to meet the known nutrient needs of practically all healthy people; a goal for dietary intake by individuals.

> **FIGURE 1-5 Estimated Average Requirements (EAR) and Recommended Dietary Allowances (RDA) Compared**

Each square in the graphs below represents a person with unique nutritional requirements. (The text discusses three of these people—A, B, and C.) Some people require only a small amount of nutrient X and some require a lot. Most people, however, fall somewhere in the middle.

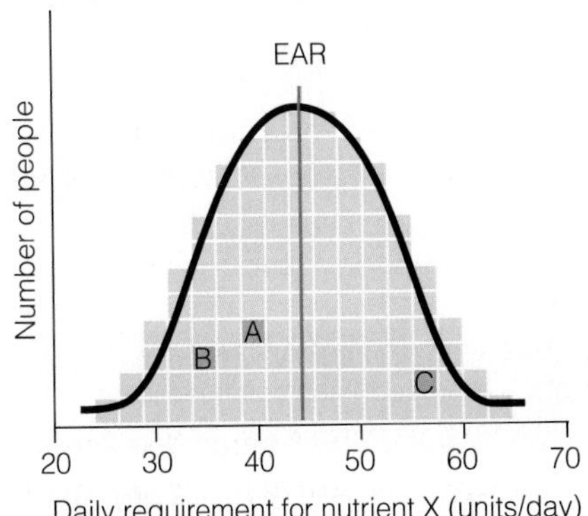

The Estimated Average Requirement (EAR) for a nutrient is the amount that meets the needs of about half of the population (shown here by the red line).

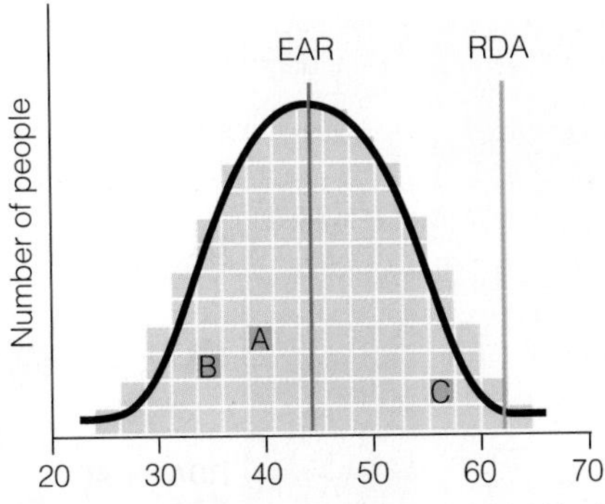

The Recommended Dietary Allowance (RDA) for a nutrient (shown here in green) is set well above the EAR, meeting the needs of about 98% of the population.

nutrient intakes are consistently **deficient** (less than the requirement), their nutrient stores decline, and over time this decline leads to poor health and deficiency symptoms. Therefore, to ensure that the nutrient RDA meet the needs of as many people as possible, the RDA are set near the top end of the range of the population's estimated requirements.

In this example, a reasonable RDA might be 63 units a day (see the right side of Figure 1-5). Such a point can be calculated mathematically so that the needs of about 98 percent of a population are included. Almost everybody—including person C whose needs were more substantial than the average—would consume enough of the nutrient if they met this dietary goal. Relatively few people's requirements would exceed this recommendation, and even then, they wouldn't exceed by much.

Adequate Intakes (AI) For some nutrients, such as vitamin K, there is insufficient scientific evidence to determine an EAR (which is needed to set an RDA). In these cases, the committee establishes an **Adequate Intake (AI)** instead of an RDA. An AI reflects the average amount of a nutrient that a group of healthy people consumes. Like the RDA, the AI may be used as nutrient goals for individuals.

Although both the RDA and the AI serve as nutrient intake goals for individuals, their differences are noteworthy. An RDA for a given nutrient is based on enough scientific evidence to expect that the needs of almost all healthy people will be met. An AI, on the other hand, must rely more heavily on scientific judgments because sufficient evidence is lacking. For this reason, AI values are more tentative than RDA values. The table on the inside front cover identifies which nutrients have an RDA and which have an AI. Later chapters present the RDA and AI values for vitamins and minerals.

Tolerable Upper Intake Levels (UL) As mentioned earlier, the recommended intakes for nutrients are generous, yet they may not be sufficient for every individual for every nutrient. Nevertheless, it is probably best not to exceed these recommendations by very much or very often. Individual tolerances for high doses of nutrients vary, and somewhere beyond the recommended intake is a point beyond which a nutrient is likely to become toxic. This point is known as the **Tolerable Upper Intake Level (UL).** It is naïve—and inaccurate—to think of recommendations as minimum amounts. A more accurate view is to see a person's nutrient

deficient: inadequate; a nutrient amount that fails to meet the body's needs and eventually results in deficiency symptoms.

Adequate Intake (AI): the average daily amount of a nutrient that appears sufficient to maintain a specified criterion; a value used as a guide for nutrient intake when an RDA cannot be determined.

Tolerable Upper Intake Level (UL): the maximum daily amount of a nutrient that appears safe for most healthy people and beyond which there is an increased risk of adverse health effects.

> **FIGURE 1-6 Inaccurate versus Accurate View of Nutrient Intakes**

The RDA (or AI) for a given nutrient represents a point that lies within a range of appropriate and reasonable intakes between toxicity and deficiency. Both of these recommendations are high enough to provide reserves in times of short-term dietary inadequacies, but not so high as to approach toxicity. Nutrient intakes above or below this range may be equally harmful.

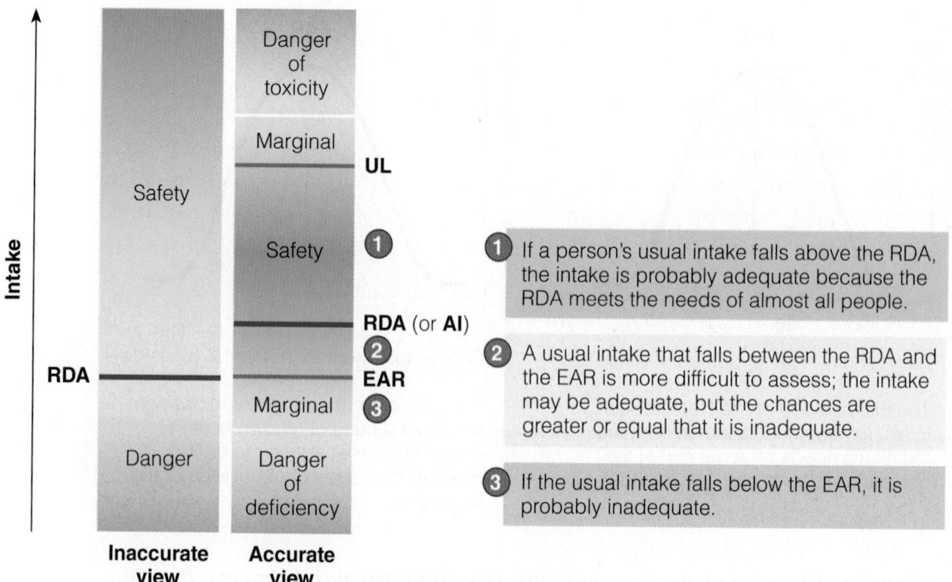

needs as falling within a range, with marginal and danger zones at each end for intakes that are either inadequate or excessive (see Figure 1-6).

Paying attention to upper levels is particularly useful in guarding against the overconsumption of nutrients, which may occur when people use large-dose dietary supplements and fortified foods regularly. Later chapters discuss the dangers associated with excessively high intakes of vitamins and minerals, and the inside front cover (p. C) presents tables of upper levels for selected nutrients.

Establishing Energy Recommendations

In contrast to the RDA and AI values for nutrients, the recommendation for energy is not generous. Excess energy cannot be readily excreted and is eventually stored as body fat. These reserves may be beneficial when food is scarce, but they can also lead to obesity and its associated health consequences.

Estimated Energy Requirement (EER) The energy recommendation—called the **Estimated Energy Requirement (EER)**—represents the average dietary energy intake (kcalories per day) that will maintain energy balance in a person who has a healthy body weight and level of physical activity. Balance is key to the energy recommendation. Enough food energy is needed to sustain a healthy and active life, but too much can lead to weight gain and obesity. Because *any* amount in excess of energy needs will result in weight gain, no upper level for energy has been determined.

Acceptable Macronutrient Distribution Ranges (AMDR) People don't eat energy directly; they derive energy from foods containing carbohydrates, fats, and proteins. Each of these three energy-yielding nutrients contributes to the total energy intake, and those contributions vary in relation to one another. The DRI committee has determined that the composition of a diet that provides adequate energy and nutrients and reduces the risk of chronic diseases is:

- 45 to 65 percent kcalories from carbohydrate
- 20 to 35 percent kcalories from fat
- 10 to 35 percent kcalories from protein

Estimated Energy Requirement (EER): the average dietary energy intake that maintains energy balance and good health in a person of a given age, gender, weight, height, and level of physical activity.

These values are known as **Acceptable Macronutrient Distribution Ranges (AMDR).**

Using Nutrient Recommendations Although the intent of nutrient recommendations seems simple, they are the subject of much misunderstanding and controversy. Perhaps the following facts will help put them in perspective:

1. Estimates of adequate energy and nutrient intakes apply to *healthy* people. They need to be adjusted for malnourished people or those with medical problems who may require supplemented or restricted dietary intakes.
2. *Recommendations* are not minimum requirements, nor are they necessarily optimal intakes for all individuals. Recommendations can target only "most" of the people and cannot account for individual variations in nutrient needs—yet. Given the recent explosion of knowledge about genetics, the day may be fast approaching when nutrition scientists will be able to determine an individual's optimal nutrient needs. Until then, qualified health-care professionals can help determine if recommendations should be adjusted to meet individual needs. (Highlight 1 introduces the college-educated food and nutrition specialists who are qualified to evaluate people's nutritional health and needs.)
3. Most nutrient goals are intended to be met through diets composed of a variety of *foods* whenever possible. Because foods contain mixtures of nutrients and nonnutrients, they deliver more than just those nutrients covered by the recommendations. Excess intakes of vitamins and minerals are unlikely when they come from foods. Using dietary supplements to meet nutrient goals raises the risks of toxicity.
4. Recommendations apply to *average* daily intakes. Trying to meet the recommendations for every nutrient every day is difficult and unnecessary. The length of time over which a person's intake can deviate from the average without risk of deficiency or overdose varies for each nutrient, depending on how the body uses and stores the nutrient. For most nutrients (such as thiamin and vitamin C), deprivation would lead to rapid development of deficiency symptoms (within days or weeks); for others (such as vitamin A and vitamin B_{12}), deficiencies would develop more slowly (over months or years).
5. Each of the DRI categories serves a unique purpose. For example, the EAR are most appropriately used to develop and evaluate nutrition programs for *groups* such as schoolchildren or military personnel. The RDA (or AI if an RDA is not available) can be used to set goals for *individuals*. The UL serve as a reminder to keep nutrient intakes less than amounts that increase the risk of toxicity—not a common problem when nutrients derive from foods, but a real possibility for some nutrients if supplements are used regularly. With these understandings, professionals can use the DRI for a variety of purposes.[20]

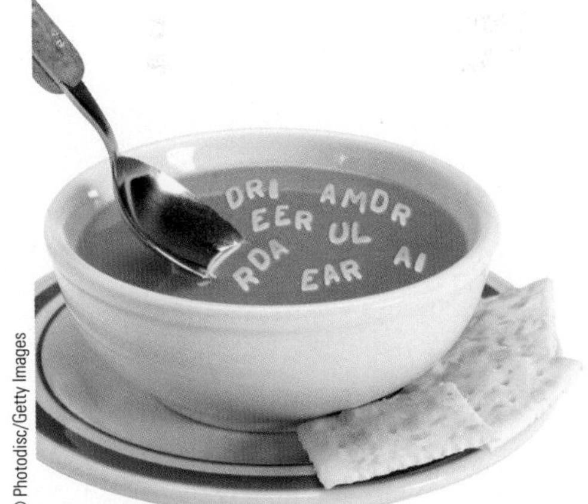

The DRI "alphabet soup" of nutrient intake standards makes sense when you learn their purposes.

Comparing Nutrient Recommendations At least 40 different nations and international organizations have published nutrient standards similar to those used in the United States. Slight differences may be apparent, reflecting differences both in the interpretation of the data from which the standards were derived and in the food habits and physical activities of the populations they serve.

Many countries use the recommendations developed by two international groups: FAO (Food and Agriculture Organization) and WHO (World Health Organization). The FAO/WHO nutrient recommendations are considered sufficient to maintain health in nearly all healthy people worldwide and are provided in Appendix I.

Acceptable Macronutrient Distribution Ranges (AMDR): ranges of intakes for the energy nutrients that provide adequate energy and nutrients and reduce the risk of chronic diseases.

› REVIEW IT Define the four categories of the DRI and explain their purposes.
The Dietary Reference Intakes (DRI) are a set of nutrient intake values that can be used to plan and evaluate diets for healthy people. The Estimated Average Requirement (EAR) defines the amount of a nutrient that supports a specific function in the body for half of the population. The Recommended Dietary Allowance (RDA) is based on the Estimated Average Requirement and establishes a goal for dietary intake that will meet the needs of almost all healthy people. An Adequate Intake (AI) serves a similar purpose when an RDA cannot be determined. The Estimated Energy Requirement (EER) defines the average amount of energy intake needed to maintain energy balance, and the Acceptable Macronutrient Distribution Ranges (AMDR) define the proportions contributed by carbohydrate, fat, and protein to a healthy diet. The Tolerable Upper Intake Level (UL) establishes the highest amount that appears safe for regular consumption.

1.5 Nutrition Assessment

› LEARN IT Explain how the four assessment methods are used to detect energy and nutrient deficiencies and excesses.

What happens when a person doesn't consume enough or consumes too much of a specific nutrient or energy? If the deficiency or excess is significant over time, the person experiences symptoms of **malnutrition.** With a deficiency of energy, the person may display the symptoms of **undernutrition** by becoming extremely thin, losing muscle tissue, and becoming prone to infection and disease. With a deficiency of a nutrient, the person may experience skin rashes, depression, hair loss, bleeding gums, muscle spasms, night blindness, or other symptoms. Similarly, over time, regular intakes in excess of needs may also have adverse effects. With an excess of energy, the person may become obese and vulnerable to diseases associated with **overnutrition,** such as heart disease and diabetes. With a sudden nutrient overdose, the person may experience hot flashes, yellowing skin, a rapid heart rate, low blood pressure, or other symptoms.

Malnutrition symptoms—such as diarrhea, skin rashes, and fatigue—are easy to miss because they resemble the symptoms of other diseases. But a person who has learned how to use assessment techniques to detect malnutrition can identify when these conditions are caused by poor nutrition and can recommend steps to correct it. This discussion presents the basics of nutrition assessment; many more details are offered in later chapters and in Appendix E.

Nutrition Assessment of Individuals

To prepare a **nutrition assessment,** a trained health-care professional uses:

- Historical information
- Anthropometric measurements
- Physical examinations
- Laboratory tests

Each of these methods involves collecting data in various ways and interpreting each finding in relation to the others to create a total picture.

Historical Information One step in evaluating nutrition status is to obtain information about a person's history with respect to health status, socioeconomic status, drug use, and diet. The health history reflects a person's medical record and may reveal a disease that interferes with the person's ability to eat or the body's use of nutrients. The person's family history of major diseases is also noteworthy, especially for conditions such as heart disease that have a genetic tendency to run in families. Economic circumstances may show a financial inability to buy foods or inadequate kitchen facilities in which to prepare them. Social factors such as marital status, ethnic background, and educational level also influence food choices and nutrition status. A drug history, including all prescribed and

malnutrition: any condition caused by excess or deficient food energy or nutrient intake or by an imbalance of nutrients.
- **mal** = bad

undernutrition: deficient energy or nutrients.

overnutrition: excess energy or nutrients.

nutrition assessment: a comprehensive analysis of a person's nutrition status that uses health, socioeconomic, drug, and diet histories; anthropometric measurements; physical examinations; and laboratory tests.

over-the-counter medications, may highlight possible interactions that lead to nutrient deficiencies (as described in Highlight 17). A diet history that examines a person's intake of foods, beverages, and dietary supplements may reveal either a surplus or inadequacy of nutrients or energy.

To take a diet history, the assessor collects data about the foods a person eats. The data may be collected by recording the foods the person has eaten over a period of 24 hours, 3 days, or a week or more or by asking what foods the person typically eats and how much of each. The days in the record must be fairly typical of the person's diet, and portion sizes must be recorded accurately. To determine the amounts of nutrients consumed, the assessor usually enters the foods and their portion sizes into a computer using a diet analysis program. This step can also be done manually by looking up each food in a table of food composition such as Appendix H in this book. The assessor then compares the calculated nutrient intakes with the DRI to determine the probability of adequacy. Alternatively, the diet history might be compared against standards such as the USDA Food Patterns or *Dietary Guidelines* (described in Chapter 2).

An estimate of energy and nutrient intakes from a diet history, when combined with other sources of information, can help confirm or rule out the *possibility* of suspected nutrition problems. A sufficient intake of a nutrient does not guarantee adequacy, and an insufficient intake does not always indicate a deficiency. Such findings, however, warn of possible problems.

Anthropometric Measurements A second technique that may help to reveal nutrition problems is taking **anthropometric** measures such as height and weight. The assessor compares a person's measurements with standards specific for gender and age or with previous measures on the same individual. (Chapter 8 presents information on body weight and its standards, and Appendix E includes growth charts for children.)

Measurements taken periodically and compared with previous measurements reveal patterns and indicate trends in a person's overall nutrition status, but they provide little information about specific nutrients. Instead, measurements out of line with expectations may reveal such problems as growth failure in children, wasting or swelling of body tissues in adults, and obesity—conditions that may reflect energy or nutrient deficiencies or excesses.

Physical Examinations A third nutrition assessment technique is a physical examination looking for clues to poor nutrition status. Visual inspection of the hair, eyes, skin, posture, tongue, and fingernails can provide such clues. In addition, information gathered from an interview can help identify symptoms. The examination requires skill because many physical signs and symptoms reflect more than one nutrient deficiency or toxicity—or even nonnutrition conditions. Like the other assessment techniques, a physical examination alone does not yield firm conclusions. Instead, physical examinations reveal possible imbalances that must be confirmed by other assessment techniques, or they confirm results from other assessment measures.

Laboratory Tests A fourth way to detect a developing deficiency, imbalance, or toxicity is to take samples of blood or urine, analyze them in the laboratory, and compare the results with normal values for a similar population. Laboratory tests are most useful in uncovering early signs of malnutrition before symptoms appear. In addition, they can confirm suspicions raised by other assessment methods.

Iron, for Example The mineral iron can be used to illustrate the stages in the development of a nutrient deficiency and the assessment techniques useful in detecting them. The **overt,** or outward, signs of an iron deficiency appear at the end of a long sequence of events. Figure 1-7 on p. 24 describes what happens in the body as a nutrient deficiency progresses and shows which assessment methods can reveal those changes.

anthropometric (AN-throw-poe-MET-rick): relating to measurement of the physical characteristics of the body, such as height and weight.

- **anthropos** = human
- **metric** = measuring

overt (oh-VERT): out in the open and easy to observe.

- **ouvrir** = to open

> FIGURE 1-7 **Stages in the Development of a Nutrient Deficiency**

Internal changes precede outward signs of deficiencies. Outward signs of sickness, however, need not appear before a person takes corrective measures. Laboratory tests can help determine nutrient status in the early stages.

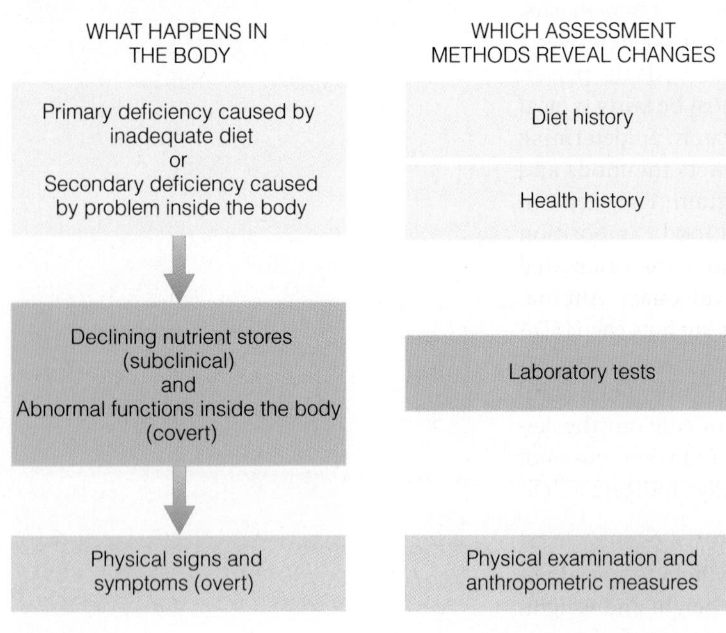

First, the body has too little iron—either because iron is lacking in the person's diet (a **primary deficiency**) or because the person's body doesn't absorb enough, excretes too much, or uses iron inefficiently (a **secondary deficiency**). A diet history provides clues to primary deficiencies; a health history provides clues to secondary deficiencies.

Next, the body begins to use up its stores of iron. At this stage, the deficiency might be described as a **subclinical deficiency.** It exists as a **covert** condition, and although it might be detected by laboratory tests, outward signs are not yet apparent.

Finally, the body's iron stores are exhausted. Now, it cannot make enough iron-containing red blood cells to replace those that are aging and dying. Iron is needed in red blood cells to carry oxygen to all the body's tissues. When iron is lacking, fewer red blood cells are made, the new ones are pale and small, and every part of the body feels the effects of oxygen shortage. At this point in time, the overt symptoms of deficiency appear—weakness, fatigue, pallor, and headaches, reflecting the iron-deficient state of the blood. A physical examination and interview will reveal these symptoms.

Nutrition Assessment of Populations To assess a population's nutrition status, researchers conduct surveys using techniques similar to those used on individuals. The data collected are then used by various agencies for numerous purposes, including the development of national health goals.

National Nutrition Surveys National nutrition surveys gather information about the population's dietary, nutritional, and related health status. One

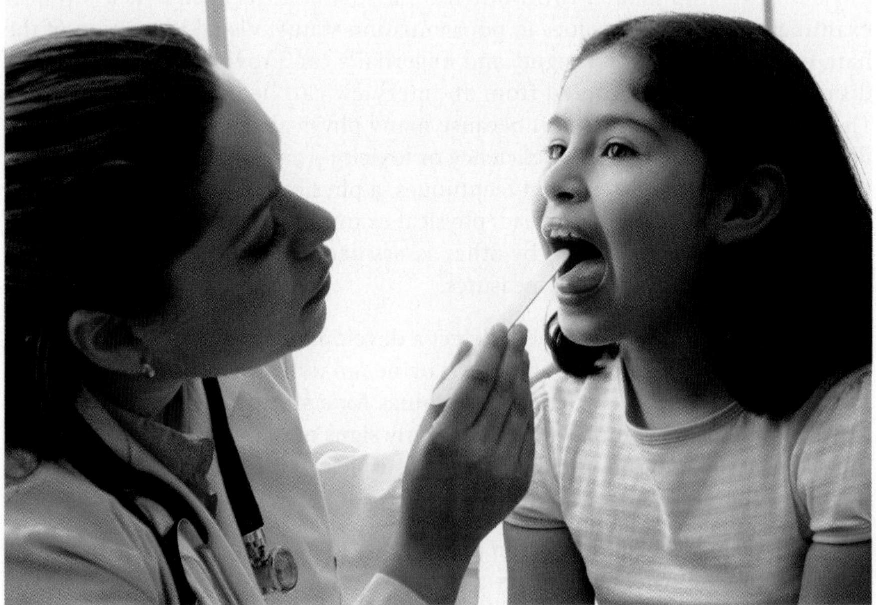

A peek inside the mouth provides clues to a person's nutrition status. An inflamed tongue may indicate a deficiency of one of the B vitamins, and mottled teeth may reveal fluoride toxicity, for example.

primary deficiency: a nutrient deficiency caused by inadequate dietary intake of a nutrient.

secondary deficiency: a nutrient deficiency caused by something other than an inadequate intake such as a disease condition or drug interaction that reduces absorption, accelerates use, hastens excretion, or destroys the nutrient.

subclinical deficiency: a deficiency in the early stages, before the outward signs have appeared.

covert (KOH-vert): hidden, as if under covers.

- **couvrir** = to cover

survey collects data on the kinds and amounts of foods people eat.* Another survey examines the people themselves, using anthropometric measurements, physical examinations, and laboratory tests.** The data provide valuable information on several nutrition-related conditions, such as growth retardation, heart disease, and nutrient deficiencies. National nutrition surveys often oversample high-risk groups (low-income families, pregnant women, adolescents, the elderly, African Americans, and Mexican Americans) to glean an accurate estimate of their health and nutrition status.

The resulting wealth of information from the national nutrition surveys is used for a variety of purposes. For example, Congress uses this information to establish public policy on nutrition education, food assistance programs, and the regulation of the food supply. Scientists use the information to establish research priorities. The food industry uses these data to guide decisions in public relations and product development. The Dietary Reference Intakes and other major reports that examine the relationships between diet and health depend on information collected from these nutrition surveys. These data also provide the basis for developing and monitoring national health goals.

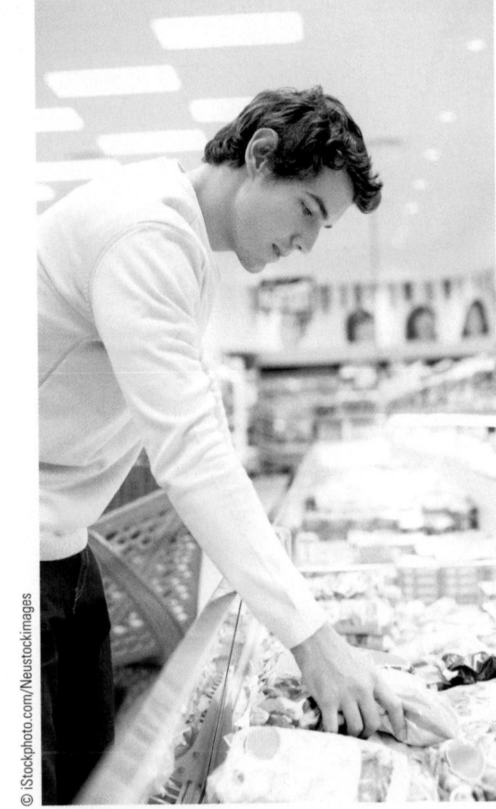

National surveys provide valuable information about the kinds of foods people eat.

National Health Goals The **Healthy People** program sets priorities and guides policies that "increase the quality and years of healthy life" and "eliminate health disparities." At the start of each decade, the program sets goals for improving the nation's health during the next ten years. Nutrition is one of many topic areas, each with numerous objectives. Table 1-4 lists the nutrition and weight status

TABLE 1-4 Healthy People 2020 Nutrition and Weight Status Objectives

- Increase the proportion of adults who are at a healthy weight
- Reduce the proportion of adults who are obese
- Reduce iron deficiency among young children and females of childbearing age
- Reduce iron deficiency among pregnant females
- Reduce the proportion of children and adolescents who are overweight or obese
- Increase the contribution of fruits to the diets of the population aged 2 years and older
- Increase the variety and contribution of vegetables to the diets of the population aged 2 years and older
- Increase the contribution of whole grains to the diets of the population aged 2 years and older
- Reduce consumption of saturated fat in the population aged 2 years and older
- Reduce consumption of sodium in the population aged 2 years and older
- Increase consumption of calcium in the population aged 2 years and older
- Increase the proportion of worksites that offer nutrition or weight management classes or counseling
- Increase the proportion of physician office visits that include counseling or education related to nutrition or weight
- Eliminate very low food security among children in US households
- Prevent inappropriate weight gain in youth and adults
- Increase the proportion of primary care physicians who regularly measure the body mass index (BMI) of their patients
- Reduce consumption of kcalories from solid fats and added sugars in the population aged 2 years and older
- Increase the number of states that have state-level policies that incentivize food retail outlets to provide foods that are encouraged by the *Dietary Guidelines*
- Increase the number of states with nutrition standards for foods and beverages provided to preschool-aged children in childcare
- Increase the percentage of schools that offer nutritious foods and beverages outside of school meals

NOTE: Nutrition and Weight Status is one of 38 topic areas, each with numerous objectives. Several of the other topic areas have nutrition-related objectives, and these are presented in Appendix J.

SOURCE: www.healthypeople.gov

Healthy People: a national public health initiative under the jurisdiction of the US Department of Health and Human Services (DHHS) that identifies the most significant preventable threats to health and focuses efforts toward eliminating them.

*This survey is called *What We Eat in America*.

**This survey is known as the National Health and Nutrition Examination Survey (NHANES).

objectives for 2020, and Appendix J lists nutrition-related objectives from other topic areas.

Progress in meeting the 2010 goals was mixed. A few objectives were met, about half made some progress, and several showed no progress—or even moved in the wrong direction.[21] The objective to reduce average blood cholesterol levels was achieved, but objectives to eat more fruits, vegetables, and whole grains and to increase physical activity showed little or no improvement. Trends in overweight and obesity actually worsened. Clearly, "what we eat in America" must change if we hope to meet the Healthy People goals.

National Trends What do we eat in America and how has it changed over the past 45 years? The short answer to both questions is "a lot." We eat more meals away from home, particularly at fast-food restaurants. We eat larger portions. We drink more sweetened beverages and eat more energy-dense, nutrient-poor foods such as candy and chips. We snack frequently. As a result of these dietary habits, our energy intake has risen and, consequently, so has the incidence of overweight and obesity. Overweight and obesity, in turn, profoundly influence our health—as the next section explains.

> **› REVIEW IT** Explain how the four assessment methods are used to detect energy and nutrient deficiencies and excesses.
> People become malnourished when they get too little or too much energy or nutrients. Deficiencies, excesses, and imbalances of nutrients lead to malnutrition diseases. To detect malnutrition in individuals, health-care professionals use a combination of four nutrition assessment methods.Reviewing historical information on diet and health may suggest a possible nutrition problem. Laboratory tests may detect a possible nutrition problem in its earliest stages, whereas anthropometric measurements and physical examinations pick up on the problem only after it causes symptoms. National surveys use similar assessment methods to measure people's food consumption and to evaluate the nutrition status of populations.

1.6 Diet and Health

› LEARN IT Identify several risk factors and explain their relationships to chronic diseases.

Foods play a vital role in supporting health. Early nutrition research focused on identifying the nutrients in foods that would prevent such common diseases as rickets and scurvy, the vitamin D– and vitamin C–deficiency diseases. With this knowledge, developed countries have successfully defended against nutrient deficiency diseases. World hunger and nutrient deficiency diseases still pose a major health threat in developing countries, however, but not because of a lack of nutrition knowledge (as Chapter 20 explains). More recently, nutrition research has focused on chronic diseases associated with energy and nutrient excesses. Chronic diseases are responsible for 7 out of 10 deaths among US adults. Once thought to be "rich countries' problems," chronic diseases have now become epidemic in developing countries as well—contributing to three out of five deaths worldwide.[22]

TABLE 1-5 Leading Causes of Death in the United States

	Percentage of Total Deaths
1. **Heart disease**	23.7
2. **Cancers**	22.9
3. Chronic lung diseases	5.7
4. **Strokes**	5.1
5. Accidents	4.9
6. Alzheimer's disease	3.4
7. **Diabetes mellitus**	2.9
8. Pneumonia and influenza	2.1
9. Kidney disease	1.8
10. Suicide	1.5

NOTE: The diseases highlighted in bold have relationships with diet.

SOURCE: Deaths: Preliminary data for 2011, *National Vital Statistics Reports*, October 10, 2012, Centers for Disease Control and Prevention, www.cdc.gov/nchs.

Chronic Diseases Table 1-5 lists the ten leading causes of death in the United States. These "causes" are stated as if a single condition such as heart disease caused death, but most chronic diseases arise from multiple factors over many years. A person who died of heart disease may have been overweight, had high blood pressure, been a cigarette smoker, and spent years eating a diet high in saturated fat and getting too little exercise.

Of course, not all people who die of heart disease fit this description, nor do all people with these characteristics die of heart disease. People who are overweight might die from the complications of diabetes instead, or those who smoke might die of cancer. They might even die from something totally unrelated to any of these factors, such as an automobile accident. Still, statistical studies have shown that certain conditions and behaviors are linked to certain diseases.

Table 1-5 highlights four of the top seven causes of death as having a link with diet. Notice that these four diseases—heart disease, cancers, strokes, and diabetes—account for more than half of the deaths each year.

Risk Factors for Chronic Diseases Factors that increase or reduce the *risk* of developing chronic diseases can be identified by analyzing statistical data. A strong association between a **risk factor** and a disease means that when the factor is present, the *likelihood* of developing the disease increases. It does not mean that all people with the risk factor will develop the disease. Similarly, a lack of risk factors does not guarantee freedom from a given disease. On the average, though, the more risk factors in a person's life, the greater that person's chances of developing the disease. Conversely, the fewer risk factors in a person's life, the better the chances for good health.

Risk Factors Persist Risk factors tend to persist over time. Without intervention, a young adult with high blood pressure will most likely continue to have high blood pressure as an older adult, for example. Thus, to minimize the damage, early intervention is most effective.

Risk Factors Cluster Risk factors tend to cluster. For example, a person who is obese may be physically inactive, have high blood pressure, and have high blood cholesterol—all risk factors associated with heart disease. Multiple risk factors act synergistically to increase the risk of disease dramatically. Intervention that focuses on one risk factor often benefits the others as well. For example, physical activity can help reduce weight. Physical activity and weight loss will, in turn, help to lower blood pressure and blood cholesterol.

Risk Factors in Perspective The most prominent factor—contributing to one of every five deaths each year in the United States—is tobacco use, followed closely by diet and activity patterns, and then alcohol use (see Table 1-6). Risk factors such as smoking, poor dietary habits, physical inactivity, and alcohol consumption are personal behaviors that can be changed. Decisions to not smoke, to eat a well-balanced diet, to engage in regular physical activity, and to drink alcohol in moderation (if at all) improve the likelihood that a person will enjoy good health. Other risk factors, such as genetics, gender, and age, also play important roles in the development of chronic diseases, but they cannot be changed. Health recommendations acknowledge the influence of such factors on the development of disease, but they must focus on the factors that are changeable.

Health Behaviors in the United States Despite evidence linking certain behaviors with chronic diseases, many Americans continue to engage in unhealthy behaviors.[23] An estimated 20 percent of US adults consume five or more drinks in a single day at least once a year; 20 percent are cigarette smokers; 40 percent are physically inactive; 60 percent are either overweight or obese; and 30 percent average 6 hours or less of sleep per day.[24] For the two out of three Americans who do not smoke or drink alcohol excessively, the one choice that can influence long-term health prospects more than any other is diet.

TABLE 1-6 Factors Contributing to Deaths in the United States

Factors	Percentage of Deaths
Tobacco	18
Poor diet/inactivity	15
Alcohol	4
Microbial agents	3
Toxic agents	2
Motor vehicles	2
Firearms	1
Sexual behavior	<1
Illicit drugs	<1

SOURCE: A. H. Mokdad and coauthors, Actual causes of death in the United States, 2000, *Journal of the American Medical Association* 291 (2004): 1238–1245, with corrections from *Journal of the American Medical Association* 293 (2005): 298.

› REVIEW IT Identify several risk factors and explain their relationships to chronic diseases.

Within the range set by genetics, a person's choice of diet influences long-term health. Diet has no influence on some diseases but is linked closely to others. Personal life choices, such as engaging in physical activity and using tobacco or alcohol, also affect health for the better or worse.

risk factor: a condition or behavior associated with an elevated frequency of a disease but not proved to be causal. Leading risk factors for chronic diseases include obesity, cigarette smoking, high blood pressure, high blood cholesterol, physical inactivity, and a diet high in saturated fats and low in vegetables, fruits, and whole grains.

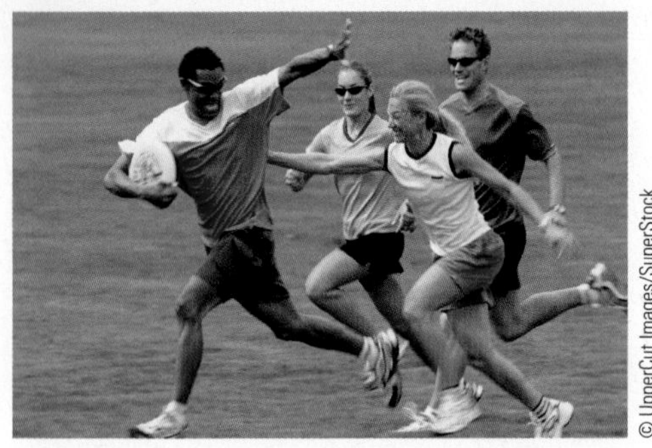
© UpperCut Images/SuperStock

Physical activity can be both fun and beneficial.

The next several chapters provide many more details about nutrients and how they support health. Whenever appropriate, the discussion shows how diet influences each of today's major diseases. Dietary recommendations appear again and again, as each nutrient's relationships with health are explored. Most people who follow the recommendations will benefit and can enjoy good health into their later years.

Nutrition Portfolio

Each chapter in this book ends with simple Nutrition Portfolio activities that invite you to review key messages and consider whether your personal choices are meeting the dietary goals introduced in the text. By using the information you are recording in Diet & Wellness Plus (the dietary tracking software that accompanies this text) and keeping a journal of these Nutrition Portfolio assignments, you can examine how your knowledge and behaviors change as you progress in your study of nutrition.

Your food choices play a key role in keeping you healthy and reducing your risk of chronic diseases. After you have recorded at least one day's foods in Diet & Wellness Plus, look at that day's choices and record your answers to the following in your journal:

- Identify the factors that most influence your food choices for meals and snacks.
- List the chronic disease risk factors and conditions (listed in the definition of *risk factor*, p. 27) that you have.
- Describe lifestyle changes you can make to improve your chances of enjoying good health.

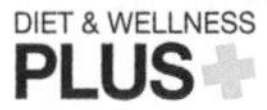

To complete this exercise, go to your Diet and Wellness Plus at **www.cengagebrain.com.**

› STUDY IT To review the key points of this chapter and take a practice quiz, go to the study cards at the end of the book.

REFERENCES

1. E. R. Grimm and N. I. Steinle, Genetics of eating behavior: Established and emerging concepts, *Nutrition Reviews* 69 (2011): 52–60.
2. A. Drewnowski and coauthors, Sweetness and food preference, *Journal of Nutrition* 142 (2012): 1142S–1148S; J. E. Hayes, B. S. Sullivan, and V. B. Duffy, Explaining variability in sodium intake through oral sensory phenotype, salt sensation and liking, *Physiology and Behavior* 100 (2010): 369–380.
3. J. E. Hayes and R. S. Keast, Two decades of supertasting: Where do we stand? *Physiology and Behavior* 104 (2011): 1072–1074.
4. Food Marketing Institute, US grocery shopper trends 2012: Executive summary, www.fmi.org/research, 2012.
5. A. E. Sloan, Not too basic, *Food Technology* 65 (2011): 21.
6. J. Lu, C. Huet, and L. Dube, Emotional reinforcement ass a protective factor for healthy eating in home settings, *American Journal of Clinical Nutrition* 94 (2011): 254–261.
7. A. Jaworowska and coauthors, Nutritional challenges and health implications of takeaway and fast food, *Nutrition Reviews* 71 (2013): 310–318; J. E. Todd, L. Mancino, and B. Lin, The impact of food away from home on adult diet quality, *Economic Research Report* ERR-90, February 2010.
8. C. D. Rehm, P. Monsivais, and A. Drewnowski, The quality and monetary value of diets consumed by adults in the United States, *American Journal of Clinical Nutrition* 94 (2011):1333–1339; C. N. Mhurchu, Food costs and healthful diets: The need for solution-oriented research and policies, *American Journal of Clinical Nutrition* 92 (2010): 1007–1008.
9. A. Drewnowski, The cost of US foods as related to their nutritive value, *American Journal of Clinical Nutrition* 92 (2010): 1181–1188.
10. A. M. Bernstein and coauthors, Relation of food cost to healthfulness of diet among US women, *American Journal of Clinical Nutrition* 92 (2010): 1197–1203.
11. C. Jacquier and coauthors, Improving the effectiveness of nutritional information policies: Assessment of unconscious pleasure mechanisms involved in food-choice decisions, *Nutrition Reviews* 70 (2012): 118–131.
12. International Food Information Council Foundation, *2013 Food & Health Survey*, www.foodinsight.org.
13. J. P. Koplan and K. D. Brownell, Response of the food and beverage industry to the obesity threat, *Journal of the American Medical Association* 304 (2010): 1487–1488.
14. Position of the Academy of Nutrition and Dietetics: Functional foods, *Journal of the Academy of Nutrition and Dietetics* 113 (2013): 1096–1103.
15. Position of the Academy of Nutrition and Dietetics: Total diet approach to healthy eating, *Journal of the Academy of Nutrition and Dietetics* 113 (2013): 307–317.
16. Laura Mauri, Why we still need randomized trials to compare effectiveness, *New England Journal of Medicine* 366 (2012): 1538–1540.
17. B. Barrett and coauthors, Placebo effects and the common cold: A randomized controlled trial, *Annals of Family Medicine* 9 (2011): 312–322.
18. S. M. Chang, Should meta-analyses trump observational studies? *American Journal of Clinical Nutrition* 97 (2013): 237–238.

19. P. R. Trumbo and coauthors, Dietary Reference Intakes: Cases of appropriate and inappropriate uses, *Nutrition Reviews* 71 (2013): 657–664; S. A. Atkinson, Defining the process of Dietary Reference Intakes: Framework for the United States and Canada, *American Journal of Clinical Nutrition* 94 (2011): 655S–657S.
20. Practice paper of the American Dietetic Association: Using the Dietary Reference Intakes, *Journal of the American Dietetic Association* 111 (2011): 762–770.
21. E. J. Sondik and coauthors, Progress toward the Healthy People 2010 goals and objectives, *Annual Review of Public Health* 31 (2010): 271–281.
22. B. M. Popkin, L. S. Adair, and S. W. Ng, Global nutrition transition and the pandemic of obesity in developing countries, *Nutrition Reviews* 70 (2012): 3–21; M. H. Fernstrom and coauthors, Communication strategies to help reduce the prevalence of non-communicable diseases: Proceedings from the inaugural IFIC Foundation Global Diet and Physical Activity Communications Summit, *Nutrition Reviews* 70 (2012): 301–310; K. M. V. Narayan, M. K. Ali, and J. P. Koplan, Global noncommunicable diseases: Where worlds meet, *New England Journal of Medicine* 363 (2010): 1196–1198.
23. A. H. Mokdad and P. L. Remington, Measuring health behaviors in populations, *Preventing Chronic Diseases* 7 (2010): A75.
24. C. A. Schoenborn and P. F. Adams, Health behaviors of adults: United States, 2005–2007, National Center for Health Statistics, *Vital and Health Statistics*, 2010, www.cdc.gov/nchs/data/series/sr_10/sr10_245.pdf

HIGHLIGHT > 1
Nutrition Information and Misinformation

> **LEARN IT** Recognize misinformation and describe how to identify reliable nutrition information.

How can people distinguish valid nutrition information from misinformation? One excellent approach is to notice *who* is providing the information. The "who" behind the information is not always evident, though, especially in the world of electronic media. Keep in mind that *people* create websites on the Internet, just as people write books and report the news. In all cases, consumers need to determine whether the person is qualified to provide nutrition information.

This highlight begins by examining the unique potential as well as the problems of relying on the Internet and the media for nutrition information. It continues with a discussion of how to identify reliable nutrition information that applies to all resources, including the Internet and the news. (The accompanying glossary defines related terms.)

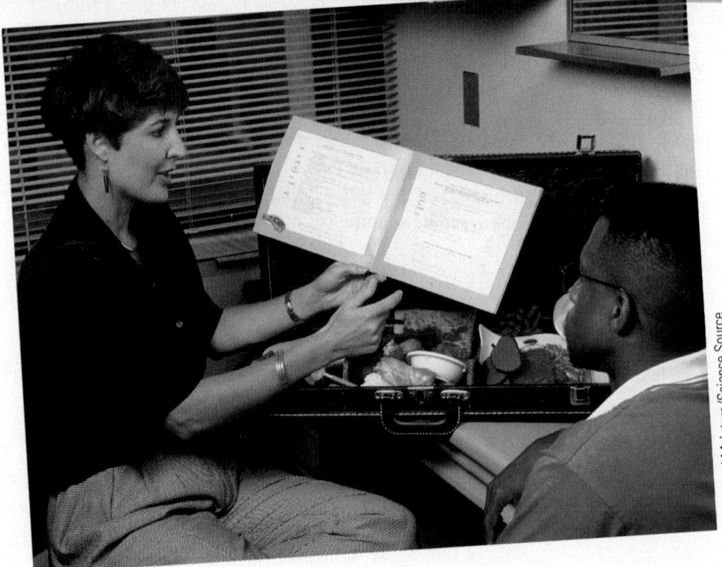

Will & Deni McIntyre/Science Source

Nutrition on the Internet

Got a question? The **Internet** has an answer. An estimated two out of three US adults use the Internet to look up health information or learn about health topics in online chat groups.[1] The Internet offers endless opportunities to obtain high-quality information, but it also delivers an abundance of incomplete, misleading, and inaccurate information.[2] Simply put: anyone can publish anything.

With hundreds of millions of **websites,** searching for nutrition information can be an overwhelming experience, with no guarantees of finding accurate information. When using the Internet, keep in mind that the quality of health-related information available covers a broad range. You must evaluate websites for their accuracy, just as you would any other source. The accompanying "How To" provides tips for determining whether a website is reliable.

One of the most trustworthy sites used by scientists and others is the US National Library of Medicine's PubMed, which provides free access to more than 23 million abstracts of research papers published in scientific journals around the world. Many abstracts provide links to the full articles. Figure H1-1 (p. 32) introduces this valuable resource.

Did you receive an e-mail warning of the health dangers associated with reusing or freezing plastic water bottles? If so, you've

GLOSSARY

Academy of Nutrition and Dietetics: the professional organization of dietitians in the United States; formerly the American Dietetic Association.

accredited: approved; in the case of medical centers or universities, certified by an agency recognized by the US Department of Education.

certified nutritionist or **certified nutritional consultant** or **certified nutrition therapist:** a person who has been granted a document declaring his or her authority as a nutrition professional.

dietetic technician: a person who has completed a minimum of an associate's degree from an accredited university or college and an approved dietetic technician program that includes a supervised practice experience. See also *dietetic technician, registered.*

dietetic technician, registered (DTR): a dietetic technician who has passed a national examination and maintains registration through continuing professional education.

dietitian: a person trained in nutrition, food science, and diet planning. See also *registered dietitian nutritionist.*

diploma mills: entities without valid accreditation that provide worthless degrees.

DTR: see *dietetic technician, registered.*

fraudulent: the promotion, for financial gain, of devices, treatments, services, plans, or products (including diets and supplements) that alter or claim to alter a human condition without proof of safety or effectiveness.

Internet (the Net): a worldwide network of millions of computers linked together to share information.

license to practice: permission under state or federal law, granted on meeting specified criteria, to use a certain title (such as dietitian) and offer certain services. *Licensed dietitians* may use the initials *LD* after their names.

misinformation: false or misleading information.

public health dietitians: dietitians who specialize in providing nutrition services through organized community efforts.

RDN: see *registered dietitian nutritionist.*

registered dietitian nutritionist (RDN): a person who has completed a minimum of a bachelor's degree from an accredited university or college, has completed approved course work and a supervised practice program, has passed a national examination, and maintains registration through continuing professional education; also called *registered dietitian (RD).*

registered dietitian (RD): an alternative term for an RDN.

registration: listing; with respect to health professionals, listing with a professional organization that requires specific course work, experience, and passing of an examination.

websites: Internet resources composed of text and graphic files, each with a unique URL (Uniform Resource Locator) that names the site (for example, www .usda.gov).

been a victim of urban scarelore. When nutrition information arrives in unsolicited e-mails, be suspicious if:

- The person sending it to you didn't write it and you cannot determine who did or if that person is a nutrition expert
- The phrase "Forward this to everyone you know" appears
- The phrase "This is not a hoax" appears because chances are good that it is
- The news is sensational and you've never heard about it from legitimate sources
- The language is emphatic and the text is sprinkled with capitalized words and exclamation marks
- No references are given or, if present, are of questionable validity when examined
- The message has been debunked on websites such as **www.quackwatch.org, www.snopes.com,** or **www.urbanlegends.about.com**

> **How To**
>
> ### Determine Whether a Website Is Reliable
>
> To determine whether a website offers reliable nutrition information, ask the following questions:
>
> - **Who?** Who is responsible for the site? Is it staffed by qualified professionals? Look for the authors' names and credentials. Have experts reviewed the content for accuracy?
> - **When?** When was the site last updated? Because nutrition is an ever-changing science, sites need to be dated and updated frequently.
> - **Where?** Where is the information coming from? The three letters following the dot in a Web address identify the site's affiliation. Addresses ending in "gov" (government), "edu" (educational institute), and "org" (organization) generally provide reliable information; "com" (commercial) sites represent businesses and, depending on their qualifications and integrity, may or may not offer dependable information.
> - **Why?** Why is the site giving you this information? Is the site providing a public service or selling a product? Many commercial sites provide accurate information, but some do not. When money is the prime motivation, be aware that the information may be biased.
>
> If you are satisfied with the answers to all of the previous questions, then ask this final question:
>
> - **What?** What is the message, and is it in line with other reliable sources? Information that contradicts common knowledge should be questioned. Many reliable sites provide links to other sites to facilitate your quest for knowledge, but this provision alone does not guarantee a reputable intention. Be aware that any site can link to any other site without permission.
>
> **› TRY IT** Visit a nutrition website and answer the five "W" questions to determine whether it is a reliable resource.

Nutrition in the News

Consumers get much of their nutrition information from Internet websites, television news, and magazine articles, which have heightened awareness of how diet influences the development of diseases. Consumers benefit from news coverage of nutrition when they learn to make lifestyle changes that will improve their health. Sometimes, however, popular reports mislead consumers and create confusion. They often tell a lopsided story quickly instead of presenting the integrated results of research studies or a balance of expert opinions.

Tight deadlines and limited understanding sometimes make it difficult to provide a thorough report. Hungry for the latest news, the media often report scientific findings quickly and prematurely—without benefit of careful interpretation, replication, or peer review. Usually, the reports present findings from a single, recently released study, making the news current and controversial. Consequently, the public receives diet and health news fast, but not always in perspective. Reporters may twist inconclusive findings into "meaningful discoveries" when pressured to write catchy headlines and sensational stories.

As a result "surprising new findings" sometimes seem to contradict one another, and consumers may feel frustrated and betrayed. Occasionally, the reports are downright false, but more often the apparent contradictions are simply the normal result of science at work. A single study contributes to the big picture, but when viewed alone, it can easily distort the image. To be meaningful the conclusions of any study must be presented cautiously within the context of other research findings.

Identifying Nutrition Experts

Regardless of whether the medium is electronic, print, or video, consumers need to ask whether the person behind the information is qualified to speak on nutrition. If the creator of an Internet website recommends eating three pineapples a day to lose weight, a trainer at the gym praises a high-protein diet, or a health-food store clerk suggests an herbal supplement, should you believe these people? Can you distinguish between accurate news reports and infomercials on television? Have you noticed that many televised nutrition messages are presented by celebrities, athletes, psychologists, food editors, and chefs—that is, almost anyone except a **dietitian**? When you are confused or need sound dietary advice, whom should you ask?

Physicians and Other Health-Care Professionals

Many people turn to physicians or other health-care professionals for dietary advice, expecting them to know about all health-related matters. But are they the best sources of accurate and current information on nutrition? Only about 30 percent of all medical schools in the

> FIGURE H1-1 PubMed: Internet Resource for Scientific Nutrition References

The US National Library of Medicine's PubMed website (www.pubmed.gov) offers tutorials to help teach beginners to use the search system effectively. Often, simply visiting the site, typing a query in the "Search for" box, and clicking "Go" will yield satisfactory results.

For example, to find research concerning calcium and bone health, typing "calcium bone" yields almost 50,000 results. Try setting limits on dates, types of articles, languages, and other criteria to obtain a more manageable number of abstracts to peruse.

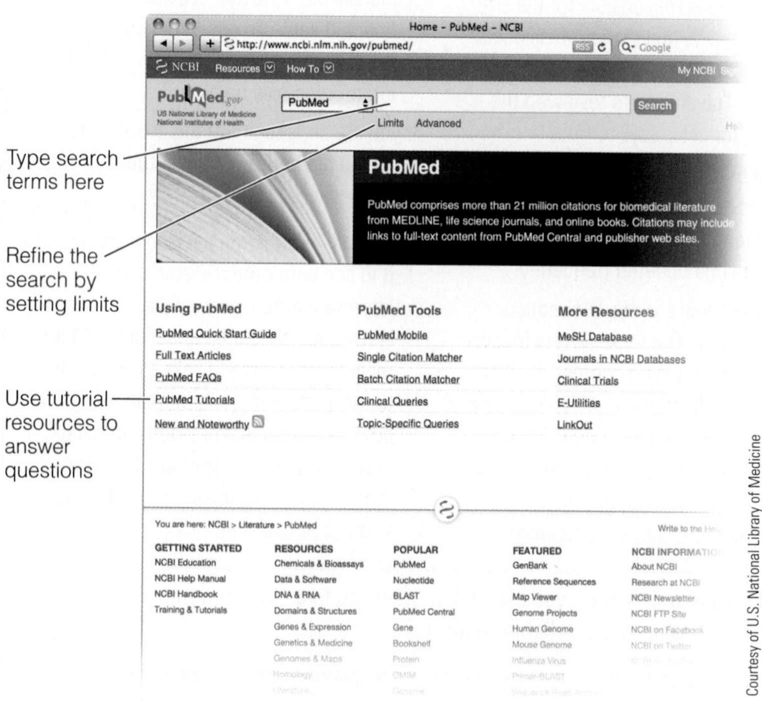

Courtesy of U.S. National Library of Medicine

United States require students to take a separate nutrition course; less than half require the minimum 25 hours of nutrition instruction recommended by the National Academy of Sciences. By comparison, most students reading this text are taking a nutrition class that provides an average of 45 hours of instruction.

The **Academy of Nutrition and Dietetics** (formerly the American Dietetic Association) asserts that standardized nutrition education should be included in the curricula for all health-care professionals: physicians, nurses, physician's assistants, dental hygienists, physical and occupational therapists, social workers, psychologists, and all others who provide services directly to clients. When these professionals understand the relevance of nutrition in the treatment and prevention of diseases and have command of reliable nutrition information, then all the people they serve will also be better informed.

Most health-care professionals appreciate the connections between health and nutrition. Those who have specialized in clinical nutrition are especially well qualified to speak on the subject. Few, however, have the time or experience to develop diet plans and provide detailed diet instructions for clients. Often they wisely refer clients to a qualified nutrition expert—a **registered dietitian nutritionist (RDN).**

Registered Dietitian Nutritionist (RDN)

To help consumers recognize credentialed dietitians and nutritionists, the Academy of Nutrition and Dietetics recently approved the optional use of both terms—registered dietitian nutritionist (RDN) and **registered dietitian (RD).** The meanings of RDN and RD are identical. A registered dietitian nutritionist (RDN) has the educational background necessary to deliver reliable nutrition advice and care.[3] To become an RDN, a person must earn an undergraduate degree requiring about 60 credit hours in nutrition, food science, and other related subjects; complete a year's clinical internship or the equivalent; pass a national examination administered by the Academy of Nutrition and Dietetics; and maintain up-to-date knowledge and **registration** by participating in required continuing education activities, such as attending seminars, taking courses, or conducting research.

Some states allow anyone to use the title dietitian or nutritionist, but others allow only an RDN or people with specified qualifications to call themselves dietitians. Many states provide a further guarantee: a state registration, certification, or **license to practice.** In this way, states identify people who have met minimal standards of education and experience. Still, these state standards may fall short of those defining an RDN. Similarly, some alternative educational programs qualify a graduate as a **certified nutritionist, certified nutritional consultant,** or **certified nutrition therapist**—terms that sound authoritative but lack the credentials of an RDN.

Dietitians perform a multitude of duties in many settings in most communities.[4] They work in the food industry, pharmaceutical companies, home health agencies, long-term care institutions, private practice, public health departments, research centers, education settings, fitness centers, and hospitals. Depending on their work settings, dietitians can assume a number of different job responsibilities and positions. In hospitals, administrative dietitians manage the foodservice system; clinical dietitians provide client care; and nutrition support team dietitians coordinate nutrition care with other health-care professionals. In the food industry, dietitians conduct research, develop products, and market services.

Public health dietitians who work in government-funded agencies such as health departments or clinics play a key role in delivering nutrition services to people in the community. Among their many roles, public health dietitians help plan, coordinate, and evaluate food assistance programs; act as consultants to other agencies; manage finances; and much more.

Dietetic Technician, Registered (DTR)

In some facilities, a **dietetic technician** assists an RDN in both administrative and clinical responsibilities. A dietetic technician has been educated and trained to work under the guidance of an RDN; upon passing a national examination, the title changes to **dietetic technician, registered (DTR).**

Other Dietary Employees

In addition to the dietetic technician, other dietary employees may include clerks, aides, cooks, porters, and assistants. These dietary employees do not have extensive formal training in nutrition, and their ability to provide accurate information may be limited.

Identifying Fake Credentials

In contrast to an RDN, thousands of people obtain fake nutrition degrees and claim to be nutrition consultants or doctors of "nutrimedicine." These and other such titles may sound meaningful, but most of these people lack the established credentials and training of an RDN. If you look closely, you can see signs of their fake expertise.

Consider educational background, for example. The minimum standards of education for an RDN specify a bachelor of science (BS) degree in food science and human nutrition or related fields from an **accredited** college or university.* Such a degree generally requires 4 to 5 years of study. Similarly, minimum standards of education for a dietetic technician specify an associate degree that typically requires 2 years of study. In contrast, a fake nutritionist may display a degree from a 6-month course. Such a degree simply falls short. In some cases, businesses posing as schools offer even less—they sell certificates to anyone who pays the fees. To obtain these "degrees," a candidate need not attend any classes, read any books, or pass any examinations.

To safeguard educational quality, an accrediting agency recognized by the US Department of Education (DOE) certifies that certain schools meet criteria established to ensure that an institution provides complete and accurate schooling. Unfortunately, fake nutrition degrees are available from schools "accredited" by phony accrediting agencies. Acquiring false degrees and credentials is especially easy today, with **diploma mills** and **fraudulent** businesses operating via the Internet.[5]

Knowing the qualifications of someone who provides nutrition information can help you determine whether that person's advice might be harmful or helpful. Don't be afraid to ask for credentials. Table H1-1 lists credible sources of nutrition information.

TABLE H1-1 Credible Sources of Nutrition Information

Government agencies, volunteer associations, consumer groups, and professional organizations provide consumers with reliable health and nutrition information. Credible sources of nutrition information include:

- Nutrition and food science departments at a university or community college
- Local agencies such as the health department or County Cooperative Extension Service
- Government resources such as:

Centers for Disease Control and Prevention (CDC)	**www.cdc.gov**
Department of Agriculture (USDA)	**www.usda.gov**
Department of Health and Human Services (DHHS)	**www.hhs.gov**
Dietary Guidelines for Americans	**fnic.nal.usda.gov/dietary-guidance**
Food and Drug Administration (FDA)	**www.fda.gov**
Health Canada	**www.hc-sc.gc.ca/index-eng.php**
Healthy People	**www.healthypeople.gov**
Let's Move!	**www.letsmove.gov**
MyPlate	**www.choosemyplate.gov**
National Institutes of Health	**www.nih.gov**
Physical Activity Guidelines for Americans	**www.health.gov/paguidelines**

- Volunteer health agencies such as:

American Cancer Society	**www.cancer.org**
American Diabetes Association	**www.diabetes.org**
American Heart Association	**www.americanheart.org**

- Reputable consumer groups such as:

American Council on Science and Health	**www.acsh.org**
International Food Information Council	**www.foodinsight.org**

- Professional health organizations such as:

Academy of Nutrition and Dietetics	**www.eatright.org**
American Medical Association	**www.ama-assn.org**
Dietitians of Canada	**www.dietitians.ca**

- Journals such as:

American Journal of Clinical Nutrition	**www.ajcn.org**
Journal of the Academy of Nutrition and Dietetics	**www.andjrnl.org**
New England Journal of Medicine	**www.nejm.org**
Nutrition Reviews	**www.ilsi.org**

*To ensure the quality and continued improvement of nutrition and dietetics education programs, an agency of the Academy of Nutrition and Dietetics known as the Accreditation Council for Education in Nutrition and Dietetics (ACEND) establishes and enforces eligibility requirements and accreditation standards for programs preparing students for careers as registered dietitian nutritionists or dietetics technicians. Programs meeting those standards are accredited by ACEND.

> FIGURE H1-2 **Red Flags of Nutrition Quackery**

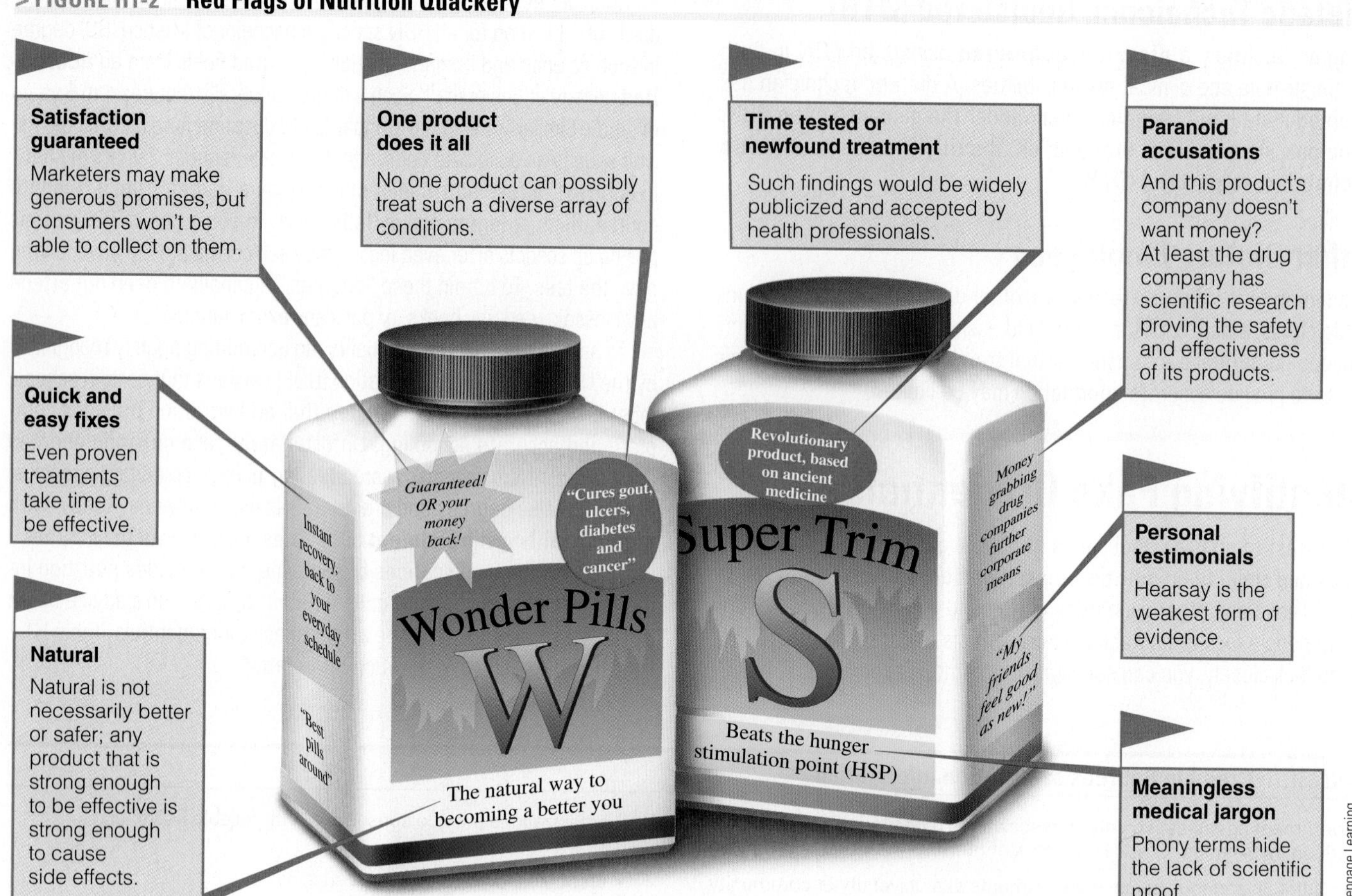

Satisfaction guaranteed
Marketers may make generous promises, but consumers won't be able to collect on them.
One product does it all
No one product can possibly treat such a diverse array of conditions.
Time tested or newfound treatment
Such findings would be widely publicized and accepted by health professionals.
Paranoid accusations
And this product's company doesn't want money? At least the drug company has scientific research proving the safety and effectiveness of its products.
Quick and easy fixes
Even proven treatments take time to be effective.
Natural
Natural is not necessarily better or safer; any product that is strong enough to be effective is strong enough to cause side effects.
Personal testimonials
Hearsay is the weakest form of evidence.
Meaningless medical jargon
Phony terms hide the lack of scientific proof.
Guaranteed! OR your money back!
"Cures gout, ulcers, diabetes and cancer"
Instant recovery, back to your everyday schedule
"Best pills around"
Wonder Pills
W
The natural way to becoming a better you
Revolutionary product, based on ancient medicine
Super Trim
S
Money grabbing drug companies further corporate means
"My friends feel good as new!"
Beats the hunger stimulation point (HSP)

Red Flags of Nutrition Quackery

Figure H1-2 features eight red flags consumers can use to identify nutrition **misinformation.** Sales of unproven and dangerous products have always been a concern, but the Internet now provides merchants with an easy and inexpensive way to reach millions of customers around the world. Because of the difficulty in regulating the Internet, fraudulent and illegal sales of medical products have hit a bonanza. As is the case with the air, no one owns the Internet, and similarly, no one has control over the pollution. Countries have different laws regarding sales of drugs, dietary supplements, and other health products, but applying these laws to the Internet marketplace is almost impossible. Even if illegal activities could be defined and identified, finding the person responsible for a particular website is not always possible. Websites can appear and disappear in a blink of a cursor. Now, more than ever, consumers must heed the caution "Buyer beware."

In summary, when you hear nutrition news, consider its source. Ask yourself these two questions: Is the person providing the information qualified to speak on nutrition? Is the information based on valid scientific research? If not, find a better source. After all, your health depends on it.

CRITICAL THINKING QUESTIONS

A. How would you judge the accuracy or validity of nutrition information?
B. You have just received a forwarded e-mail from a friend warning that the artificial sweetener aspartame is a TOXIN that causes muscle spasms, leg numbness, stomach cramps, vertigo, dizziness, headaches, tinnitus, joint pain, depression, anxiety, slurred speech, blurred vision, and memory loss. It goes on to say that this DEADLY POISON causes blindness, multiple sclerosis, brain tumors, and cancer! The message alleges that aspartame remains on the market because of a conspiracy between the FDA and the manufacturer to keep these dangers hidden from the public. How can you determine whether these claims are legitimate warnings or an irresponsible hoax?

REFERENCES

1. R. A. Cohen and P. F. Adams, Use of the Internet for health information: United States, 2009, *NCHS Data Brief*, July 2011.
2. Practice paper of the Academy of Nutrition and Dietetics abstract: Communicating accurate food and nutrition information, *Journal of the Academy of Nutrition and Dietetics* 112 (2012): 759.
3. Position of the Academy of Nutrition and Dietetics: The role of nutrition in health promotion and chronic disease prevention, *Journal of the Academy of Nutrition and Dietetics* 113 (2013): 972–979.
4. Comprehensive scope of practice resources for the registered dietitian or registered dietitian nutritionist, *Journal of the Academy of Nutrition and Dietetics*, June 2013, Supplement 2.
5. E. B. Cohen and R. Winch, Diploma and accreditation mills: New trends in credential abuse, March 2011, www.accredibase.com.

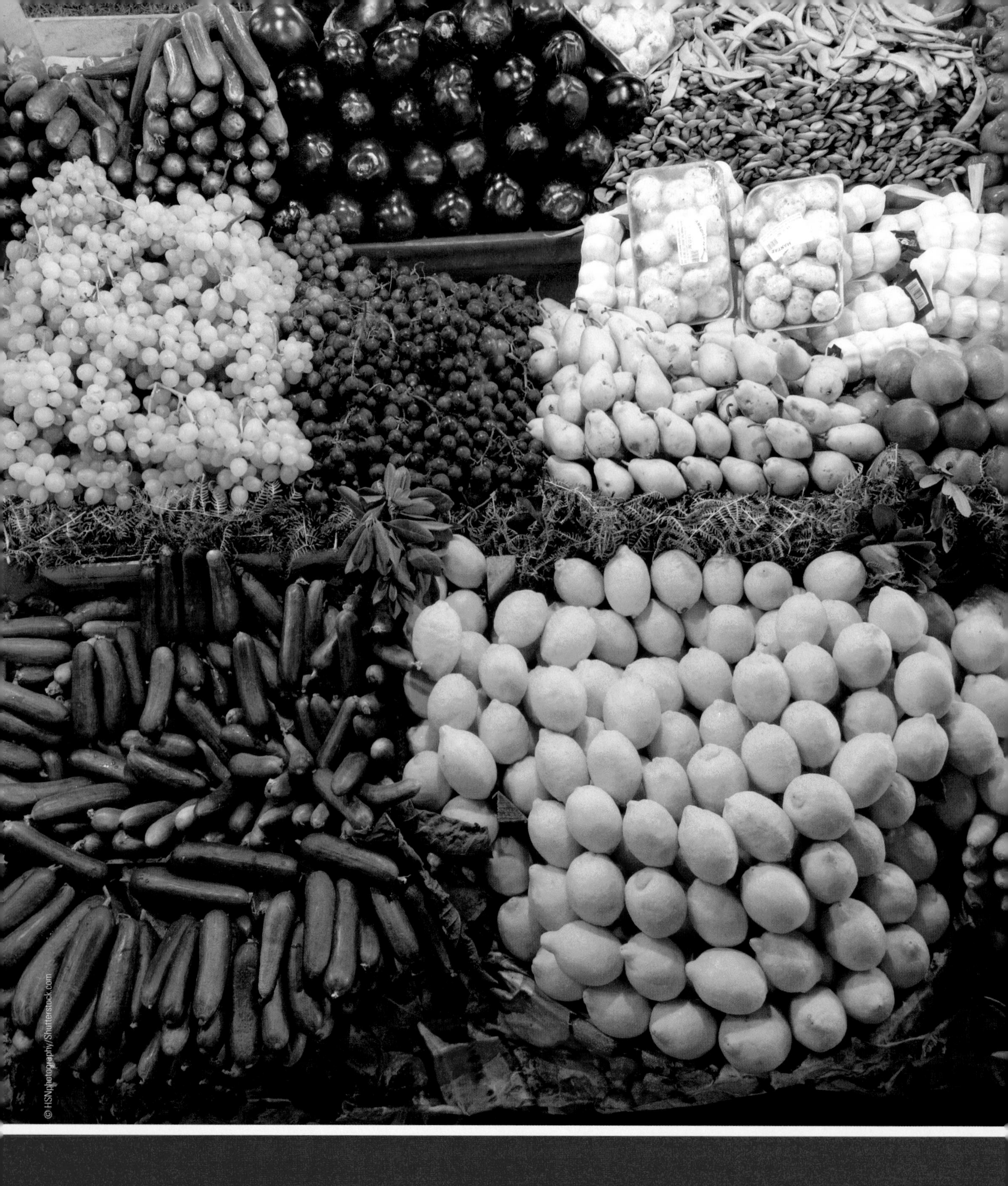

2

Planning a Healthy Diet

Nutrition in Your Life

You make food choices—deciding what to eat and how much to eat—more than 1000 times every year. We eat so frequently that it's easy to choose a meal without giving any thought to its nutrient contributions or health consequences. Even when we want to make healthy choices, we may not know which foods to select or how much to consume. With a few tools and tips, you can learn to plan a healthy diet. In the Nutrition Portfolio at the end of this chapter, you can compare your current diet against a healthy eating plan.

LEARNING GPS

Chapter 1 explained that the nutrients delivered by the foods people eat support the body's many activities. Food choices made over years and decades influence the body's health, and consistently poor choices increase the risks of developing chronic diseases. Stated positively, optimal nourishment supports a robust life of vigorous activity and good health. This chapter shows how a person can select from the tens of thousands of available foods to create a nutritionally balanced diet that meets the body's nutrient and energy needs. Fortunately, most foods provide several nutrients, so one trick for wise diet planning is to select a combination of foods that deliver a full array of nutrients.

This chapter begins by introducing the diet-planning principles and dietary guidelines that promote good health and reduce disease risks. It continues by showing how people can use diet-planning guides to create meal patterns that will deliver sufficient nutrients without excess energy (kcalories). Learning how to read food labels eases the task of making healthy selections at the market.

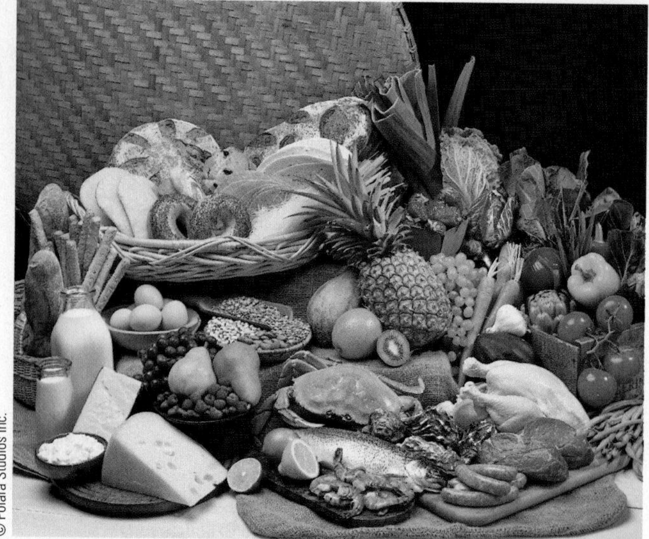

© Polara Studios Inc.

To ensure an adequate and balanced diet, eat a variety of foods daily, choosing different foods from each group.

2.1 Principles and Guidelines

› LEARN IT Explain how each of the diet-planning principles can be used to plan a healthy diet.

How well you nourish yourself does not depend on the selection of any one food. Instead, it depends on the overall **eating pattern**—the combination of many different foods and beverages at numerous meals over days, months, and years.[1] Diet-planning principles and dietary guidelines are key concepts to keep in mind whenever you are selecting foods—whether shopping at the grocery store, choosing from a restaurant menu, or preparing a home-cooked meal.

Diet-Planning Principles Diet planners have developed several ways to select foods. Whatever plan or combination of plans they use, though, they keep in mind these basic diet-planning principles:

- Adequacy
- Balance
- kCalorie (energy) control
- Nutrient density
- Moderation
- Variety

Adequacy **Adequacy** reflects a diet that provides sufficient energy and enough of all the nutrients to meet the needs of healthy people. Take the essential nutrient iron, for example. Because the body loses some iron each day, people have to replace it by eating foods that contain iron. A person whose diet fails to provide enough iron-rich foods may develop the symptoms of iron-deficiency anemia: the person may feel weak, tired, and listless; have frequent headaches; and find that even the smallest amount of muscular work brings disabling fatigue. To prevent these deficiency symptoms, a person must include foods that supply adequate iron. The same is true for all the other essential nutrients introduced in Chapter 1.

Balance **Balance** in the diet helps to ensure adequacy. The art of balancing the diet involves consuming enough—but not too much—of different types of foods in proportion to one another. In a balanced diet, foods rich in some nutrients do not crowd out foods that are rich in other nutrients. The essential minerals calcium and iron, taken together, illustrate the importance of dietary **balance**. Meat is rich in iron but poor in calcium. Conversely, milk is rich in calcium but poor in iron. Use some meat for iron; use some milk for calcium; and save some space for other foods, too, because a diet consisting of milk and meat alone would not be adequate. For the other nutrients, people need to eat other protein foods, whole grains, vegetables, and fruits.

kCalorie (Energy) Control Designing an adequate diet within a reasonable kcalorie allowance requires careful planning. Once again, balance plays a key role. The amount of energy coming into the body from foods should balance with the amount of energy being used by the body to sustain its metabolic and physical activities. Upsetting this balance leads to gains or losses in body weight. The discussion of energy balance and weight control in Chapters 8 and 9 examines this issue in more detail, but one key to **kcalorie control** is to select foods of high nutrient density.

Nutrient Density **Nutrient density** promotes adequacy and kcalorie control. To eat well without overeating, select nutrient-dense foods—that is, foods that deliver the most nutrients for the least food energy.[2] Consider foods containing calcium, for example. You can get about 300 milligrams of calcium from either 1½ ounces of cheddar cheese or 1 cup of fat-free milk, but the cheese delivers about twice as much food energy (kcalories) as the milk. The fat-free milk, then, is twice as calcium dense as the cheddar cheese; it offers the same amount of calcium

eating pattern: customary intake of foods and beverages over time.

adequacy (dietary): providing all the essential nutrients, fiber, and energy in amounts sufficient to maintain health.

balance (dietary): providing foods in proportion to one another and in proportion to the body's needs.

kcalorie (energy) **control:** management of food energy intake.

nutrient density: a measure of the nutrients a food provides relative to the energy it provides. The more nutrients and the fewer kcalories, the higher the nutrient density.

>How To

Compare Foods Based on Nutrient Density

One way to evaluate foods is simply to notice their nutrient contribution *per serving:* 1 cup of milk provides about 300 milligrams of calcium, and ½ cup of fresh, cooked turnip greens provides about 100 milligrams. Thus a serving of milk offers three times as much calcium as a serving of turnip greens. To get 300 milligrams of calcium, a person could choose either 1 cup of milk or 1½ cups of turnip greens.

Another valuable way to evaluate foods is to consider their nutrient density—their nutrient contribution *per kcalorie.* Fat-free milk delivers about 85 kcalories with its 300 milligrams of calcium. To calculate the nutrient density, divide milligrams by kcalories:

$$\frac{300 \text{ mg calcium}}{85 \text{ kcal}} = 3.5 \text{ mg per kcal}$$

Do the same for the fresh turnip greens, which provide 15 kcalories with the 100 milligrams of calcium:

$$\frac{100 \text{ mg calcium}}{15 \text{ kcal}} = 6.7 \text{ mg per kcal}$$

The more milligrams per kcalorie, the greater the nutrient density. Turnip greens are more calcium dense than milk. They provide more calcium *per kcalorie* than milk, but milk offers more calcium *per serving.* Both approaches offer valuable information, especially when combined with a realistic appraisal. What matters most is which are you more likely to consume—1½ cups of turnip greens or 1 cup of milk? You can get 300 milligrams of calcium from either, but the greens will save you about 40 kcalories (the savings would be even greater if you usually use whole milk).

Keep in mind, too, that calcium is only one of the many nutrients that foods provide. Similar calculations for protein, for example, would show that fat-free milk provides more protein both *per kcalorie* and *per serving* than turnip greens—that is, milk is more protein dense. Combining variety with nutrient density helps to ensure the adequacy of all nutrients.

› TRY IT Compare the thiamin density of 3 ounces of lean T-bone steak (174 kcalories, 0.09 milligrams thiamin) with ½ cup of fresh cooked broccoli (27 kcalories, 0.05 milligrams thiamin).

for half the kcalories. Both foods are excellent choices for adequacy's sake alone, but to achieve adequacy while controlling kcalories, the fat-free milk is the better choice. (Alternatively, a person could select a low-fat cheddar cheese with its kcalories comparable to fat-free milk.) The accompanying "How To" describes how to compare foods based on nutrient density.

Just as a financially responsible person pays for rent, food, clothes, and tuition on a limited budget, healthy people obtain iron, calcium, and all the other essential nutrients on a limited energy (kcalorie) allowance. Success depends on getting many nutrients for each kcalorie "dollar." As Figure 2-1 illustrates on p. 40, a breakfast of cereal, fruit, egg, and sausage delivers many more nutrients than a couple of doughnuts—even though they both provide about the same number of kcalories. A person who makes nutrient-dense choices can meet daily nutrient needs on a lower energy budget. Such choices support good health.

Foods that are notably low in nutrient density—such as potato chips, candy, and colas—are called **empty-kcalorie foods.** The kcalories these foods provide are called "empty" because they deliver a lot of energy (from added sugars, solid fats, or both) but little, or no, protein, vitamins, or minerals.

The concept of nutrient density is relatively simple when examining the contributions of one nutrient to a food or diet. With respect to calcium, milk ranks high and meats rank low. With respect to iron, meats rank high and milk ranks low. But it is a more complex task to answer the question, which food is more

empty-kcalorie foods: a popular term used to denote foods that contribute energy but lack protein, vitamins, and minerals.

> FIGURE 2-1 Nutrient Density of Two Breakfast Options Compared

Chapter 1 presented these two breakfasts to illustrate energy density—that for the same number of kcalories, the breakfast on the left delivered less energy per gram of food, which benefits weight management. These two breakfasts also illustrate nutrient density—that for the same number of kcalories, the breakfast on the left delivers more nutrients per kcalorie.

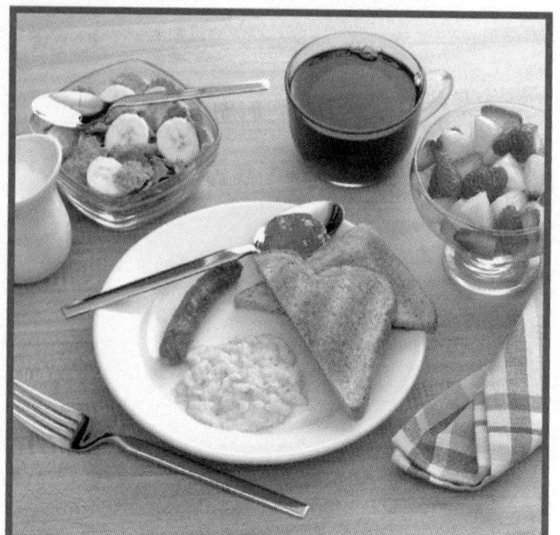

NUTRIENT-DENSE BREAKFAST

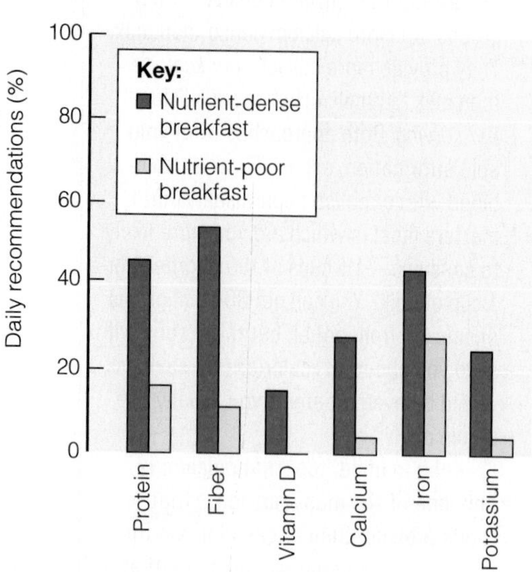

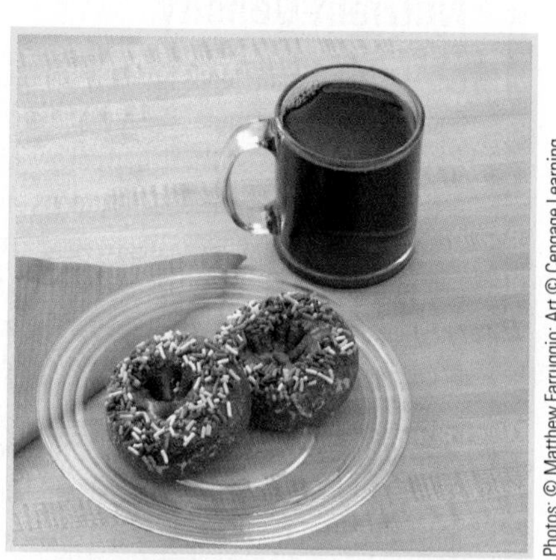

NUTRIENT-POOR BREAKFAST

Photos: © Matthew Farruggio; Art © Cengage Learning

nutritious? To answer that question, we need to consider several nutrients—including both nutrients that may harm health as well as those that may be beneficial. Ranking foods based on their overall nutrient composition is known as **nutrient profiling.** Researchers have yet to agree on an ideal way to rate foods based on the nutrient profile, but when they do, nutrient profiling will be quite useful in helping consumers identify nutritious foods and plan healthy diets.[3]

Moderation **Moderation** contributes to adequacy, balance, and kcalorie control. Foods rich in fat and sugar often provide enjoyment and energy but relatively few nutrients; in addition, they promote weight gain when eaten in excess. A person practicing moderation eats such foods only on occasion and regularly selects foods low in **solid fats** and **added sugars**, a practice that automatically improves nutrient density. Returning to the example of cheddar cheese versus fat-free milk, the fat-free milk not only offers the same amount of calcium for less energy, but it also contains much less fat than the cheese.

Variety **Variety** improves nutrient adequacy. A diet may have all of the virtues just described and still lack variety, if a person eats the same foods day after day. People should select foods from each of the food groups daily and vary their choices within each food group from day to day for several reasons. First, different foods within the same group contain different arrays of nutrients. Among the fruits, for example, strawberries are especially rich in vitamin C while apricots are rich in vitamin A. Second, no food is guaranteed entirely free of substances that, in excess, could be harmful. The strawberries might contain trace amounts of one contaminant, the apricots another. By alternating fruit choices, a person will ingest very little of either contaminant. (Contamination of foods is discussed in Chapter 19.) Third, as the adage goes, variety is the spice of life. A person who eats beans frequently can enjoy pinto beans in Mexican burritos today, garbanzo beans in a Greek salad tomorrow, and baked beans with barbecued chicken on the weekend. Eating nutritious meals need never be boring.

Dietary Guidelines for Americans

What should a person eat to stay healthy? The answers can be found in the *Dietary Guidelines for Americans*. These guidelines translate the *nutrient* recommendations of the DRI (presented in Chapter 1) into *food* recommendations.[4] The result is evidence-based advice designed to help people attain and maintain a healthy weight, reduce the risk of chronic diseases, and promote overall health through diet and physical activity.[5] In general, a healthy diet:

nutrient profiling: ranking foods based on their nutrient composition.

moderation (dietary): providing enough but not too much of a substance.

solid fats: fats that are not usually liquid at room temperature; commonly found in most foods derived from animals and vegetable oils that have been hydrogenated. Solid fats typically contain more saturated and *trans* fats than most oils (Chapter 5 provides more details).

added sugars: sugars and other kcaloric sweeteners that are added to foods during processing, preparation, or at the table. Added sugars do not include the naturally occurring sugars found in fruits and milk products.

variety (dietary): eating a wide selection of foods within and among the major food groups.

- Emphasizes a variety of fruits, vegetables, whole grains, and fat-free and low-fat milk products.
- Includes lean meats, poultry, seafood, legumes, eggs, seeds, and nuts.
- Is low in saturated and *trans* fats, cholesterol, salt (sodium), and added sugars.
- Stays within your daily energy needs for your recommended body weight.

Table 2-1 presents the key recommendations of the *Dietary Guidelines for Americans*, clustered into four major topic areas. The first area focuses on

TABLE 2-1 Key Recommendations of the *Dietary Guidelines for Americans*

Balancing kCalories to Manage Weight

- Prevent and/or reduce overweight and obesity through improved eating and physical activity behaviors (see Chapter 9).
- Control total kcalorie intake to manage body weight. For people who are overweight or obese, this will mean consuming fewer kcalories from foods and beverages (see Chapter 9).
- Increase physical activity and reduce time spent in sedentary behaviors (see Chapter 14).
- Maintain appropriate kcalorie balance during each stage of life—childhood, adolescence, adulthood, pregnancy and breastfeeding, and older age (see Chapters 15–17).

Foods and Food Components to Reduce

- Reduce daily sodium intake to less than 2300 milligrams and further reduce intake to 1500 milligrams among persons who are 51 and older and those of any age who are African American or have hypertension, diabetes, or chronic kidney disease (see Chapter 12).
- Consume less than 10 percent of kcalories from saturated fatty acids by replacing them with monounsaturated and polyunsaturated fatty acids (see Chapter 5).
- Consume less than 300 milligrams per day of dietary cholesterol (see Chapter 5).
- Keep *trans*-fatty acid consumption as low as possible by limiting foods that contain synthetic sources of *trans* fats, such as partially hydrogenated oils, and by limiting other solid fats (see Chapter 5).
- Reduce the intake of kcalories from solid fats and added sugars (see Chapters 4 and 5).
- Limit the consumption of foods that contain refined grains, especially refined grain foods that contain solid fats, added sugars, and sodium (see Chapters 4, 5, and 12).
- If alcohol is consumed it should be consumed in moderation—up to one drink per day for women and two drinks per day for men—and only by adults of legal drinking age (see Highlight 7).

Foods and Nutrients to Increase

- Increase vegetable and fruit intake.
- Eat a variety of vegetables, especially dark-green and red and orange vegetables and beans and peas.
- Consume at least half of all grains as whole grains. Increase whole-grain intake by replacing refined grains with whole grains.
- Increase intake of fat-free or low-fat milk and milk products, such as milk, yogurt, cheese, or fortified soy beverages.
- Choose a variety of protein foods, which include seafood, lean meat and poultry, eggs, beans and peas, soy products, and unsalted nuts and seeds.
- Increase the amount and variety of seafood consumed by choosing seafood in place of some meat and poultry.
- Replace protein foods that are higher in solid fats with choices that are lower in solid fats and kcalories and/or are sources of oils.
- Use oils to replace solid fats where possible (see Highlight 5).
- Choose foods that provide more potassium, dietary fiber, calcium, and vitamin D, which are nutrients of concern in American diets (see Chapters 4, 11, and 12). These foods include vegetables, fruits, whole grains, and milk and milk products.

Building Healthy Eating Patterns

- Select an eating pattern that meets nutrient needs over time at an appropriate kcalorie level.
- Account for all foods and beverages consumed and assess how they fit within a total healthy eating pattern.
- Follow food safety recommendations when preparing and eating foods to reduce the risk of foodborne illnesses (see Chapter 19).

NOTE: These guidelines are intended for adults and healthy children ages 2 and older.
SOURCE: The *Dietary Guidelines for Americans*, available at www.healthierus.gov/dietaryguidelines.

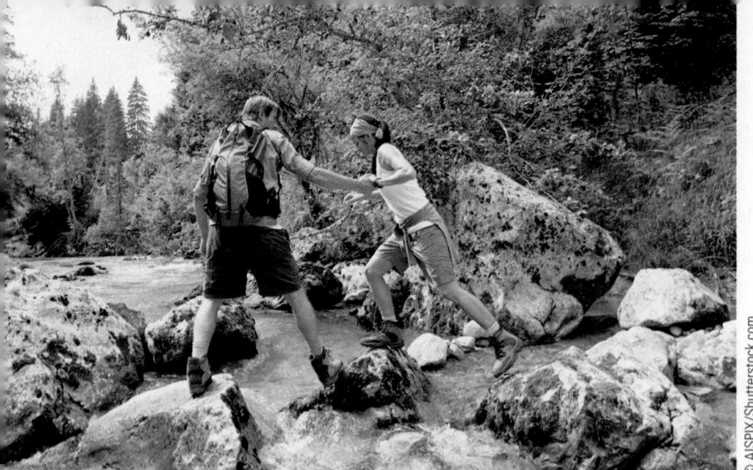
© AISPIX/Shutterstock.com

The *Dietary Guidelines* encourage Americans to increase the energy (kcalories) they expend through physical activity.

balancing kcalories to manage a healthy body weight by improving eating habits and engaging in regular physical activity. The second area advises people to reduce their intakes of such foods and food components as sodium, solid fats (with their saturated fats, *trans* fats, and cholesterol), added sugars, refined grain products, and alcoholic beverages (for those who partake). The third area encourages people to consume a variety of fruits and vegetables, whole grains, and low-fat milk products and protein foods (including seafood). The fourth area helps consumers build healthy eating patterns that meet energy and nutrient needs while reducing the risk of foodborne illnesses. Together, the *Dietary Guidelines for Americans* point the way toward longer, healthier, and more active lives. These key recommendations, along with additional recommendations for specific population groups, appear throughout the text as their subjects are discussed.

By law, the *Dietary Guidelines for Americans* are reviewed and revised as needed every five years. Each edition shares some similarities with previous editions but also sets precedent in new ways.[6] Perhaps most noteworthy to the current edition is the overarching focus on curbing the obesity epidemic and improving the health of the American population.[7]

Some people might wonder why *dietary* guidelines include recommendations for physical activity. The simple answer is that most people who maintain a healthy body weight do more than eat right. They also exercise—the equivalent of 30 to 60 minutes or more of moderately intense physical activity on most days.[8] As you will see repeatedly throughout this text, food and physical activity choices are integral partners in supporting good health.

› REVIEW IT Explain how each of the diet-planning principles can be used to plan a healthy diet.

A well-planned diet delivers adequate nutrients, a balanced array of nutrients, and an appropriate amount of energy. It is based on nutrient-dense foods, moderate in substances that can be detrimental to health, and varied in its selections. The *Dietary Guidelines* apply these principles, offering practical advice on how to eat for good health.

2.2 Diet-Planning Guides

› LEARN IT Use the USDA Food Patterns to develop a meal plan within a specified energy allowance.

To plan a diet that achieves all of the dietary ideals just outlined, a person needs tools as well as knowledge. Among the most widely used tools for diet planning are **food group plans** that build a diet from clusters of foods that are similar in nutrient content. Thus each food group represents a set of nutrients that differs somewhat from the nutrients supplied by the other groups. Selecting foods from each of the groups eases the task of creating an adequate and balanced diet.

USDA Food Patterns The *Dietary Guidelines* encourage consumers to adopt a balanced eating pattern, using the USDA's Food Patterns. The USDA Food Patterns assign foods to five major groups—fruits, vegetables, grains, protein foods, and milk and milk products—and recommend daily amounts of foods from each group to meet nutrient needs. Figure 2-2 (pp. 44–45) presents the food groups, the most notable nutrients of each group, the serving equivalents, and the foods within each group. Chapter 16 provides a food guide for young children.

Recommended Amounts All food groups offer valuable nutrients, and people should make selections from each group daily. The amounts from each food group needed daily to create a healthful diet differ depending on a person's

food group plans: diet-planning tools that sort foods into groups based on nutrient content and then specify that people should eat certain amounts of foods from each group.

energy (kcalorie) needs. Table 2-2 presents estimated daily energy needs for sedentary adults. As Table 2-3 shows, a person needing 2000 kcalories a day, for example, would select 2 cups of fruit; 2½ cups of vegetables; 6 ounces of grain foods; 5½ ounces of protein foods; and 3 cups of milk or milk products.* Additionally, a small amount of unsaturated oil, such as vegetable oil, or the oils of nuts, olives, or fatty fish, is required to supply needed nutrients.

> **DIETARY GUIDELINES FOR AMERICANS**
> Select an eating pattern that meets nutrient needs over time at an appropriate kcalorie level.

All vegetables provide an array of nutrients, but some vegetables are especially good sources of certain vitamins, minerals, and beneficial phytochemicals. For this reason, the vegetable group is sorted into five subgroups. The dark-green vegetables deliver the B vitamin folate; the red and orange vegetables provide vitamin A; legumes supply iron and protein; the starchy vegetables contribute carbohydrate energy; and the other vegetables fill in the gaps and add more of these same nutrients.

In a 2000-kcalorie diet, then, the recommended 2½ cups of daily vegetables should be varied among the subgroups over a week's time. In other words, consuming 2½ cups of potatoes or even nutrient-rich spinach every day for seven days does *not* meet the recommended amounts for vegetables. Potatoes and spinach make excellent choices when consumed in balance with vegetables from the other subgroups. One way to help ensure selections for all of the subgroups is to eat vegetables of various colors—for example, green broccoli, orange sweet potatoes, black beans, yellow corn, and white cauliflower. Intakes of vegetables are appropriately averaged over a week's time—it is not necessary to include every subgroup every day.

For similar reasons, the protein foods group is sorted into three subgroups. Perhaps most notably, each of these subgroups contributes a different assortment of fats. Table 2-4 on p. 46 presents the recommended *weekly* amounts for each of the subgroups for vegetables and protein foods.

Notable Nutrients As Figure 2-2 notes, each food group contributes key nutrients. This feature provides flexibility in diet planning because a person can select any food from a food group (or its subgroup) and receive similar nutrients. For example, a person can choose milk, cheese, or yogurt and receive the same key nutrients. Importantly, foods provide not only these key nutrients, but small amounts of other nutrients and phytochemicals as well.

Legumes contribute the same key nutrients—notably, protein, iron, and zinc—as meats, poultry, and seafood. They are also excellent sources of fiber, folate, and potassium, which are commonly found in vegetables. To encourage frequent consumption of these nutrient-rich foods, legumes are included as a subgroup of both the vegetable group and the protein foods group. Thus legumes can be counted in either the vegetable group or the protein foods group.[9]

*Milk and milk products also can be referred to as dairy products.

TABLE 2-2 Estimated Energy Needs for Sedentary Adults

	Energy (kcal/day)
Women	
19–30 yr	2000
31–50 yr	1800
51+ yr	1600
Men	
19–30 yr	2400
31–50 yr	2200
51+ yr	2000

NOTE: Sedentary describes a lifestyle that includes the activities typical of daily living with less than 30 minutes of moderate activity on most days. Because physical activity increases energy needs, people who are more physically active need more kcalories per day. Chapter 8 and Appendix F provide more details.

legumes (lay-GYOOMS or LEG-yooms): plants of the bean and pea family, with seeds that are rich in protein compared with other plant-derived foods.

TABLE 2-3 USDA Food Patterns: Recommended Daily Amounts from Each Food Group

	1600 kcal	1800 kcal	2000 kcal	2200 kcal	2400 kcal	2600 kcal	2800 kcal	3000 kcal
Fruits	1½ c	1½ c	2 c	2 c	2 c	2 c	2½ c	2½ c
Vegetables	2 c	2½ c	2½ c	3 c	3 c	3½ c	3½ c	4 c
Grains	5 oz	6 oz	6 oz	7 oz	8 oz	9 oz	10 oz	10 oz
Protein foods	5 oz	5 oz	5½ oz	6 oz	6½ oz	6½ oz	7 oz	7 oz
Milk and milk products	3 c	3 c	3 c	3 c	3 c	3 c	3 c	3 c
Oils	5 tsp	5 tsp	6 tsp	6 tsp	7 tsp	8 tsp	8 tsp	10 tsp
Discretionary kcalories	121 kcal	161 kcal	258 kcal	266 kcal	330 kcal	362 kcal	395 kcal	459 kcal

> FIGURE 2-2 **USDA Food Patterns: Food Groups and Subgroups**

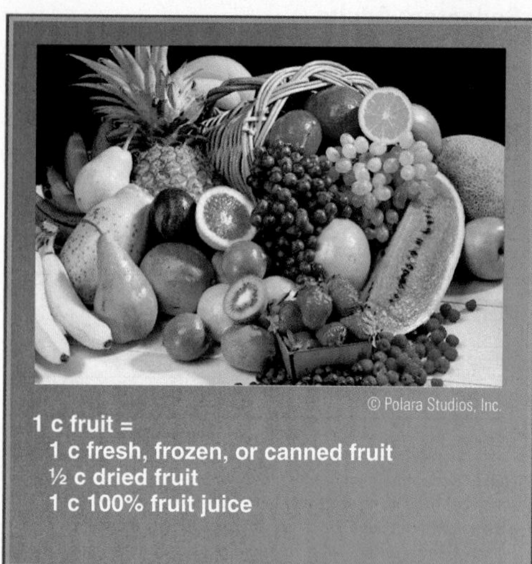

© Polara Studios, Inc.

1 c fruit =
1 c fresh, frozen, or canned fruit
½ c dried fruit
1 c 100% fruit juice

Fruits contribute folate, vitamin A, vitamin C, potassium, and fiber.

Consume a variety of fruits, and choose whole or cut-up fruits more often than fruit juice.

Apples, apricots, avocados, bananas, blueberries, cantaloupe, cherries, grapefruit, grapes, guava, honeydew, kiwi, mango, nectarines, oranges, papaya, peaches, pears, pineapples, plums, raspberries, strawberries, tangerines, watermelon; dried fruit (dates, figs, prunes, raisins); 100% fruit juices

Limit these fruits that contain solid fats and/or added sugars:
Canned or frozen fruit in syrup; juices, punches, ades, and fruit drinks with added sugars; fried plantains

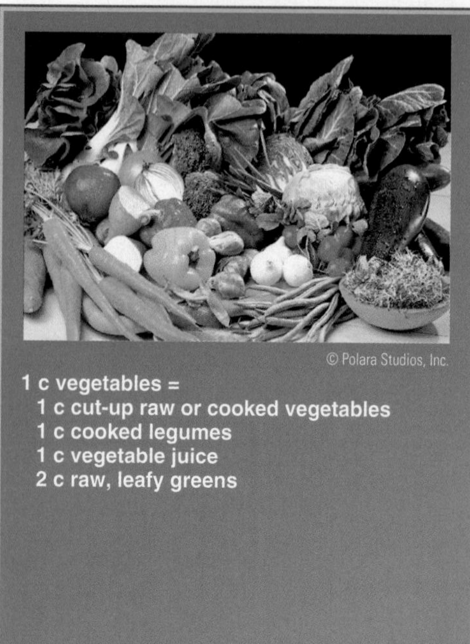

© Polara Studios, Inc.

1 c vegetables =
1 c cut-up raw or cooked vegetables
1 c cooked legumes
1 c vegetable juice
2 c raw, leafy greens

Vegetables contribute folate, vitamin A, vitamin C, vitamin K, vitamin E, magnesium, potassium, and fiber.

Consume a variety of vegetables each day, and choose from all five subgroups several times a week.

Dark-green vegetables: Broccoli and leafy greens such as arugula, beet greens, bok choy, collard greens, kale, mustard greens, romaine lettuce, spinach, turnip greens, watercress

Red and orange vegetables: Carrots, carrot juice, pumpkin, red bell peppers, sweet potatoes, tomatoes, tomato juice, vegetable juice, winter squash (acorn, butternut)

Legumes: Black beans, black-eyed peas, garbanzo beans (chickpeas), kidney beans, lentils, navy beans, pinto beans, soybeans and soy products such as tofu, split peas, white beans

Starchy vegetables: Cassava, corn, green peas, hominy, lima beans, potatoes

Other vegetables: Artichokes, asparagus, bamboo shoots, bean sprouts, beets, brussels sprouts, cabbages, cactus, cauliflower, celery, cucumbers, eggplant, green beans, green bell peppers, iceberg lettuce, mushrooms, okra, onions, seaweed, snow peas, zucchini

Limit these vegetables that contain solid fats and/or added sugars:
Baked beans, candied sweet potatoes, coleslaw, french fries, potato salad, refried beans, scalloped potatoes, tempura vegetables

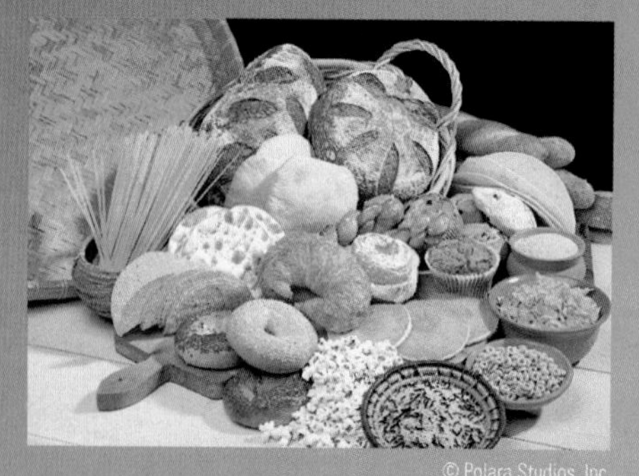

© Polara Studios, Inc.

1 oz grains =
1 slice bread
½ c cooked rice, pasta, or cereal
1 oz dry pasta or rice
1 c ready-to-eat cereal
3 c popped popcorn

Grains contribute folate, niacin, riboflavin, thiamin, iron, magnesium, selenium, and fiber.

Make most (at least half) of the grain selections whole grains.

Whole grains: amaranth, barley, brown rice, buckwheat, bulgur, cornmeal, millet, oats, quinoa, rye, wheat, wild rice and whole-grain products such as breads, cereals, crackers, and pastas; popcorn

Enriched refined products: bagels, breads, cereals, pastas (couscous, macaroni, spaghetti), pretzels, white rice, rolls, tortillas

Limit these grains that contain solid fats and/or added sugars:
Biscuits, cakes, cookies, cornbread, crackers, croissants, doughnuts, fried rice, granola, muffins, pastries, pies, presweetened cereals, taco shells

Art © Cengage Learning

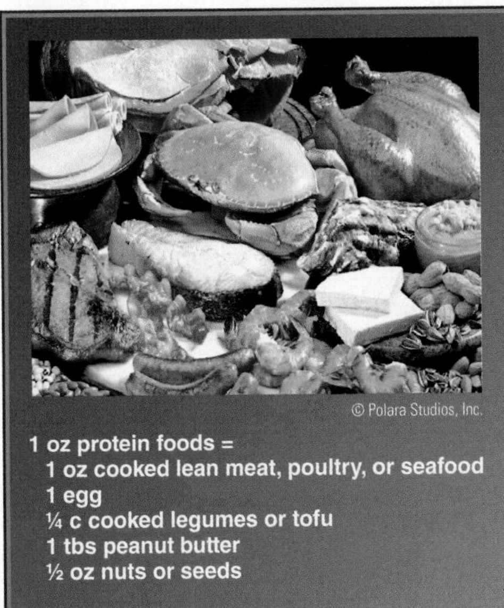
© Polara Studios, Inc.

1 oz protein foods =
1 oz cooked lean meat, poultry, or seafood
1 egg
¼ c cooked legumes or tofu
1 tbs peanut butter
½ oz nuts or seeds

Protein foods contribute protein, essential fatty acids, niacin, thiamin, vitamin B_6, vitamin B_{12}, iron, magnesium, potassium, and zinc.

Choose a variety of protein foods from the three subgroups, including seafood in place of meat or poultry twice a week.

Seafood: Fish (catfish, cod, flounder, haddock, halibut, herring, mackerel, pollock, salmon, sardines, sea bass, snapper, trout, tuna), shellfish (clams, crab, lobster, mussels, oysters, scallops, shrimp)

Meats, poultry, eggs: Lean or low-fat meats (fat-trimmed beef, game, ham, lamb, pork, veal), poultry (no skin), eggs

Nuts, seeds, soy products: Unsalted nuts (almonds, cashews, filberts, pecans, pistachios, walnuts), seeds (flaxseeds, pumpkin seeds, sesame seeds, sunflower seeds), legumes, soy products (textured vegetable protein, tofu, tempeh), peanut butter, peanuts

Limit these protein foods that contain solid fats and/or added sugars:
Bacon; baked beans; fried meat, seafood, poultry, eggs, or tofu; refried beans; ground beef; hot dogs; luncheon meats; marbled steaks; poultry with skin; sausages; spare ribs

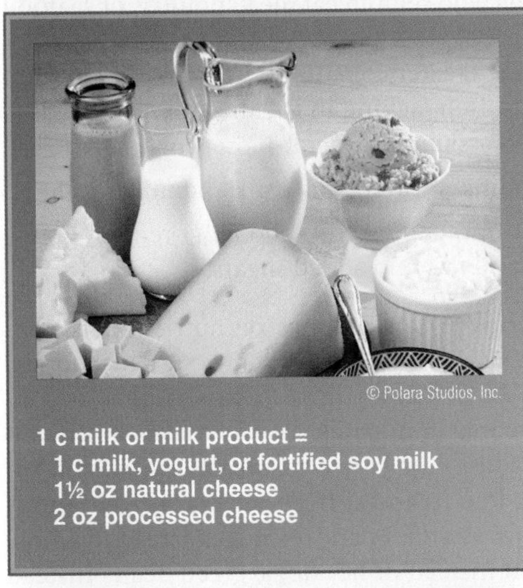
© Polara Studios, Inc.

1 c milk or milk product =
1 c milk, yogurt, or fortified soy milk
1½ oz natural cheese
2 oz processed cheese

Milk and milk products contribute protein, riboflavin, vitamin B_{12}, calcium, potassium, and, when fortified, vitamin A and vitamin D.

Make fat-free or low-fat choices. Choose other calcium-rich foods if you don't consume milk.

Fat-free or 1% low-fat milk and fat-free or 1% low-fat milk products such as buttermilk, cheeses, cottage cheese, yogurt; fat-free fortified soy milk

Limit these milk products that contain solid fats and/or added sugars:
2% reduced-fat milk and whole milk; 2% reduced-fat and whole-milk products such as cheeses, cottage cheese, and yogurt; flavored milk with added sugars such as chocolate milk, custard, frozen yogurt, ice cream, milk shakes, pudding, sherbet; fortified soy milk

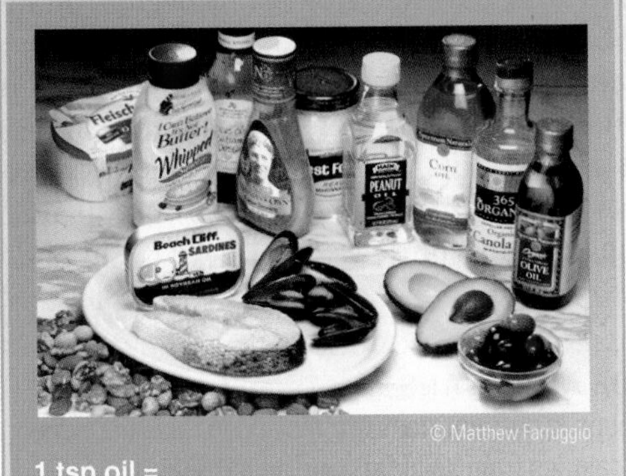

© Matthew Farruggio

1 tsp oil =
1 tsp vegetable oil
1 tsp soft margarine
1 tbs low-fat mayonnaise
2 tbs light salad dressing

Oils are not a food group, but are featured here because they contribute vitamin E and essential fatty acids.

Use oils instead of solid fats, when possible.

Liquid vegetable oils such as canola, corn, flaxseed, nut, olive, peanut, safflower, sesame, soybean, sunflower oils; mayonnaise, oil-based salad dressing, soft *trans*-fat-free margarine; unsaturated oils that occur naturally in foods such as avocados, fatty fish, nuts, olives, seeds (flaxseeds, sesame seeds), shellfish

Limit these solid fats:
Butter, animal fats, stick margarine, shortening

Art © Cengage Learning

TABLE 2-4 USDA Food Patterns: Recommended Weekly Amounts from the Vegetable and Protein Foods Subgroups

Table 2-3 specifies the recommended amounts of total vegetables and protein foods per *day*. This table shows those amounts dispersed among five vegetable and three protein foods subgroups per *week*.

	1600 kcal	1800 kcal	2000 kcal	2200 kcal	2400 kcal	2600 kcal	2800 kcal	3000 kcal
Vegetable Subgroups								
Dark green	1½ c	1½ c	1½ c	2 c	2 c	2½ c	2½ c	2½ c
Red and orange	4 c	5½ c	5½ c	6 c	6 c	7 c	7 c	7½ c
Legumes	1 c	1½ c	1½ c	2 c	2 c	2½ c	2½ c	3 c
Starchy	4 c	5 c	5 c	6 c	6 c	7 c	7 c	8 c
Other	3½ c	4 c	4 c	5 c	5 c	5½ c	5½ c	7 c
Protein Foods Subgroups								
Seafood	8 oz	8 oz	8 oz	9 oz	10 oz	10 oz	11 oz	11 oz
Meats, poultry, eggs	24 oz	24 oz	26 oz	29 oz	31 oz	31 oz	34 oz	34 oz
Nuts, seeds, soy products	4 oz	4 oz	4 oz	4 oz	5 oz	5 oz	5 oz	5 oz

In general, people who regularly eat meat, poultry, and seafood count legumes as a vegetable, and vegetarians and others who seldom eat meat, poultry, or seafood count legumes in the protein foods group.

The USDA Food Patterns encourage greater consumption from certain food groups to provide the nutrients most often lacking in the diets of Americans—dietary fiber, vitamin D, calcium, and potassium. In general, most people need to eat:

- *More* vegetables, fruits, whole grains, seafood, and milk and milk products.
- *Less* sodium, saturated fat, *trans* fat, cholesterol, and *fewer* refined grains and foods and beverages with solid fats and added sugars.

Nutrient-Dense Choices A healthy eating pattern emphasizes nutrient-dense options within each food group.[10] By consistently selecting nutrient-dense foods, a person can obtain all the nutrients needed and still keep kcalories under control. In contrast, eating foods that are low in nutrient density makes it difficult to get enough nutrients without exceeding energy needs and gaining weight. For this reason, consumers should select low-fat foods from each group and foods without solid fats or added sugars—for example, fat-free milk instead of whole milk, baked chicken without the skin instead of hot dogs, green beans instead of french fries, orange juice instead of fruit punch, and whole-wheat bread instead of biscuits. Notice that Figure 2-2 indicates which foods *within each group* contain solid fats and/or added sugars and therefore should be limited. Oil is a notable exception: even though oil is pure fat and therefore rich in kcalories, a small amount of oil from sources such as nuts, fish, or vegetable oils is necessary every day to provide nutrients lacking from other foods. Consequently, these high-fat foods are listed among the nutrient-dense foods (see Highlight 5 to learn why).

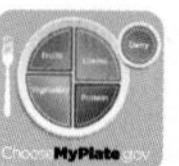

> DIETARY GUIDELINES FOR AMERICANS

Consume foods from all food groups in nutrient-dense forms and in recommended amounts. Reduce the intake of kcalories from solid fats and added sugars.

Discretionary kCalories People who consistently choose nutrient-dense foods may be able to meet most of their nutrient needs without consuming their full allowance of kcalories. The difference between the kcalories needed to supply nutrients and those needed to maintain weight might be considered **discretionary kcalories** (see Figure 2-3). Table 2-3 (p. 43) includes discretionary kcalories for each kcalorie level.

discretionary kcalories: the kcalories remaining in a person's energy allowance after consuming enough nutrient-dense foods to meet all nutrient needs for a day.

Discretionary kcalories allow a person to choose whether to:

- Eat additional nutrient-dense foods, such as an extra serving of skinless chicken or a second ear of corn.
- Select a few foods with fats or added sugars, such as reduced-fat milk or sweetened cereal.
- Add a little fat or sugar to foods, such as butter or jelly on toast.
- Consume some alcohol. (Highlight 7 explains why this may not be a good choice for some individuals.)

Alternatively, a person wanting to lose weight might choose to:

- *Not* use discretionary kcalories.

> FIGURE 2-3 **Discretionary kCalories in a 2000-kCalorie Diet**

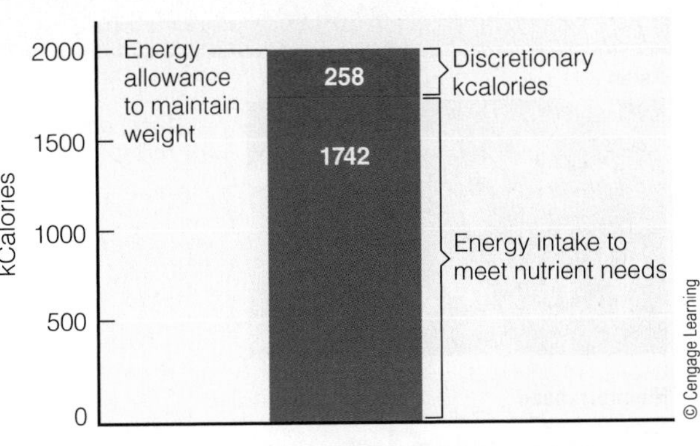

> **DIETARY GUIDELINES FOR AMERICANS**

For most people, no more than about 5 to 15 percent of kcalories from solid fats and added sugars (empty kcalories) can be reasonably accommodated in the USDA Food Patterns, which are designed to meet nutrient needs within kcalorie limits.

Serving Equivalents Recommended serving amounts for fruits, vegetables, and milk are measured in cups, and those for grains and protein foods, in ounces. Figure 2-2 (pp. 44–45) provides the **serving sizes** and equivalent measures for foods in each group specifying, for example, that 1 ounce of grains is equivalent to 1 slice of bread or ½ cup of cooked rice.

Consumers using the USDA Food Patterns can learn how standard serving sizes compare with their personal **portion sizes** by determining the answers to questions such as these: What portion of a cup is a small handful of raisins? Is a "helping" of mashed potatoes more or less than a half cup? How many ounces of cereal do you typically pour into the bowl? How many ounces is the steak at your favorite restaurant? How many cups of milk does your glass hold?

Ethnic Food Choices People can use the USDA Food Patterns and still enjoy a diverse array of culinary styles by sorting ethnic foods into their appropriate food groups. For example, a person eating Mexican foods would find tortillas in the grains group, jicama in the vegetable group, and guava in the fruit group. Table 2-5 (p. 48) features some ethnic food choices.

Vegetarian Food Guide Vegetarian diets are plant-based eating patterns that rely mainly on grains, vegetables, legumes, fruits, seeds, and nuts. Some vegetarian diets include eggs, milk products, or both. People who do not eat meats or milk products can still use the USDA Food Patterns to create an adequate diet.[11] The subgroups for protein foods have been reorganized to eliminate meats, poultry, and seafood (see Table H2-1 on p. 66). The other food groups and the recommended daily amounts for each food group remain the same. Highlight 2 defines vegetarian terms and provides details on planning healthy vegetarian diets.

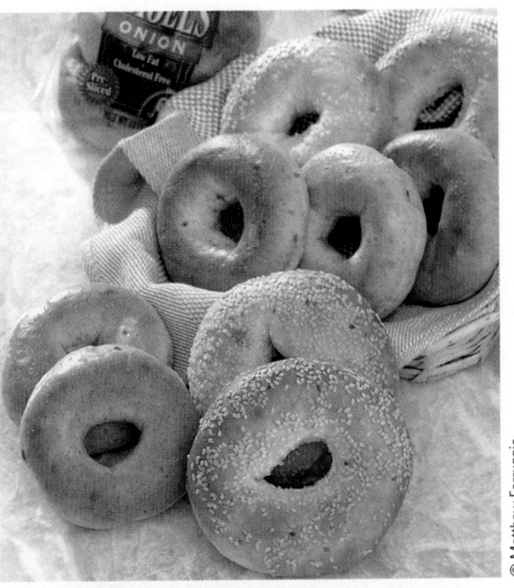

Most bagels today weigh in at 4 ounces or more—meaning that a person eating one of these large bagels for breakfast is actually getting four or more grain servings, not one.

Mixtures of Foods Some foods—such as casseroles, soups, and sandwiches—fall into two or more food groups. With a little practice, consumers can learn to see these mixtures of foods as items from various food groups. For example, from the USDA Food Patterns point of view, a taco represents four different food groups: the taco shell from the grains group; the onions, lettuce, and tomatoes from the vegetables group; the ground beef from the protein foods group; and the cheese from the milk group.

MyPlate The USDA created an educational tool called MyPlate to illustrate the five food groups. Figure 2-4 (p. 48) shows the MyPlate icon, which was designed to remind consumers to make healthy food choices.

serving sizes: the standardized quantity of a food; such information allows comparisons when reading food labels and consistency when following the *Dietary Guidelines*.

portion sizes: the quantity of a food served or eaten at one meal or snack; *not* a standard amount.

TABLE 2-5 Ethnic Food Choices

	Grains	Vegetables	Fruits	Protein Foods	Milk and Milk Products
Asian (© Josh Resnick/Shutterstock.com)	Rice, noodles, millet	Amaranth, baby corn, bamboo shoots, chayote, bok choy, mung bean sprouts, sugar peas, straw mushrooms, water chestnuts, kelp	Carambola, guava, kumquat, lychee, persimmon, melons, mandarin orange	Soybeans and soy products such as soy milk and tofu, squid, duck eggs, pork, poultry, fish and other seafood, peanuts, cashews	Usually excluded
Mediterranean (© PhotoDisc/Getty Images)	Pita pocket bread, pastas, rice, couscous, polenta, bulgur, focaccia, Italian bread	Eggplant, tomatoes, peppers, cucumbers, grape leaves	Olives, grapes, figs	Fish and other seafood, gyros, lamb, chicken, beef, pork, sausage, lentils, fava beans	Ricotta, provolone, parmesan, feta, mozzarella, and goat cheeses; yogurt
Mexican (© PhotoDisc/Getty Images)	Tortillas (corn or flour), taco shells, rice	Chayote, corn, jicama, tomato salsa, cactus, cassava, tomatoes, yams, chilies	Guava, mango, papaya, avocado, plantain, bananas, oranges	Refried beans, fish, chicken, chorizo, beef, eggs	Cheese, custard

© Cengage Learning

> **FIGURE 2-4 MyPlate**

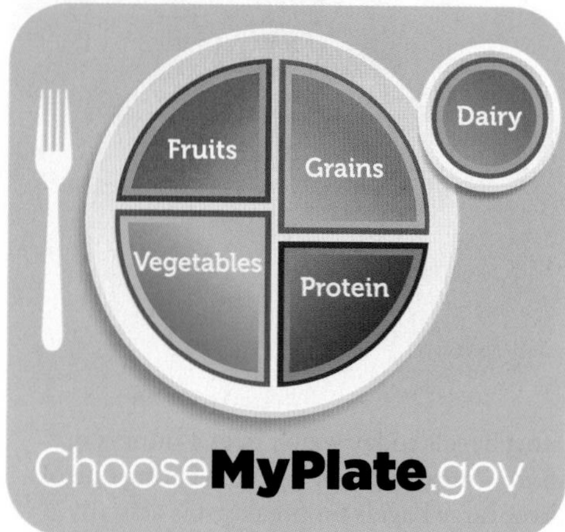

source: USDA, www.choosemyplate.gov.

The MyPlate icon divides a plate into four sections, each representing a food group—fruits, vegetables, grains, and protein foods. The sections vary in size, indicating the relative proportion each food group contributes to a healthy diet. A circle next to the plate represents the milk group (dairy).

The MyPlate icon does not stand alone as an educational tool. A wealth of information can be found at the website **(www.choosemyplate.gov)**. Consumers can choose the kinds and amounts of foods they need to eat each day based on their height, weight, age, gender, and activity level. Information is also available for children, pregnant and breastfeeding women, and college students. In addition to creating a personal plan, consumers can find daily tips to help them improve their diet and increase physical activity. A key message of the website is to enjoy food, but eat less by avoiding oversized portions.

Recommendations versus Actual Intakes The USDA Food Patterns and MyPlate were developed to help people choose a balanced and healthful diet. Are consumers actually eating according to these recommendations? The short answer is "not really." In general, consumers are not selecting the most nutrient-dense items from the food groups.[12] Instead, they are consuming too many foods high in solid fats and added sugars—soft drinks, desserts, whole milk products, and fatty meats. They are also not selecting the suggested quantities from each of the food groups, typically eating too few fruits, vegetables, whole grains, and milk products (see Figure 2-5).

An assessment tool, called the **Healthy Eating Index,** can be used to measure how well a diet meets the recommendations of the *Dietary Guidelines*.[13] Various components of the diet are given scores that reflect the quantities consumed. For most components, higher intakes result in higher scores. For example, selecting at least 3 ounces of whole grains (per 2000 kcalories) gives a score of 10 points,

Healthy Eating Index: a measure that assesses how well a diet meets the recommendations of the *Dietary Guidelines for Americans*.

> FIGURE 2-5 **Recommended and Actual Intakes Compared**

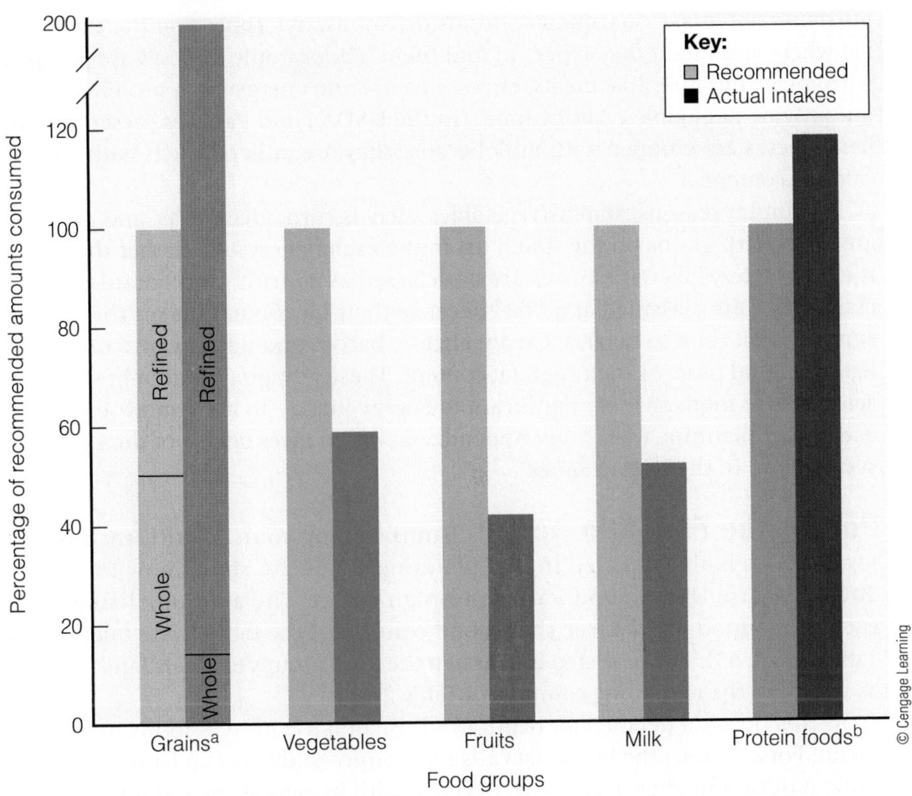

[a]At least half of the grain selections should be whole grains.
[b]On average, actual intakes of all protein foods is close to recommended levels, but actual intakes of the seafood subgroup is only 44 percent of recommended levels.

whereas selecting no whole grains gives a score of 0 points. For a few components, lower intakes provide higher scores. For example, less than 2.2 grams of sodium (per 2000 kcalories) receives 10 points, but more than 4 grams gets 0 points. An assessment of recent nutrition surveys using the Healthy Eating Index reports that the American diet scores 54 out of a possible 100 points.[14] To improve this score, the American diet needs to decrease kcalories from solid fats and added sugars by about 60 percent; increase fruits by 100 percent and vegetables and milk products by 70 percent; maintain the quantity of grains but shift the quality to four times as many whole grains; and reduce salt by more than half.[15]

MyPlate Shortcomings MyPlate is not perfect and critics are quick to point out its flaws.[16] The first main criticism is that MyPlate fails to convey enough information to help consumers choose a healthy diet. MyPlate contains few words and depends on its website to provide key information—which is helpful for those who have Internet access and are willing to take the time to become familiar with its teachings. The second main criticism is that MyPlate fails to recognize that some foods within a food group are healthier choices than others. For example, MyPlate does not distinguish between fish sticks and salmon or between broccoli and french fries. Many of the upcoming chapters examine the links between diet and health, and Chapter 18 presents a complete summary, including a look at an alternative Healthy Eating Plate created by the faculty members in the Harvard School of Public Health.

Exchange Lists Food group plans are particularly well suited to help a person achieve dietary adequacy, balance, and variety. **Exchange lists** provide additional help in achieving kcalorie control and moderation. Originally developed as a meal planning guide for people with diabetes, exchange lists have proved useful for general diet planning as well.

exchange lists: diet-planning tools that organize foods by their proportions of carbohydrate, fat, and protein. Foods on any single list can be used interchangeably.

Unlike the USDA Food Patterns, which sort foods primarily by their vitamin and mineral contents, the exchange system sorts foods according to their energy-nutrient contents. Consequently, foods do not always appear on the exchange list where you might first expect to find them. For example, cheeses are grouped with meats because, like meats, cheeses contribute energy from protein and fat but provide negligible carbohydrate. (In the USDA Food Patterns presented earlier, cheeses are grouped with milk because they are milk products with similar calcium contents.)

For similar reasons, starchy vegetables such as corn, green peas, and potatoes are listed with grains on the starch list in the exchange system, rather than with the vegetables. Likewise, olives are not classed as a "fruit" as a botanist would claim; they are classified as a "fat" because their fat content makes them more similar to oil than to berries. Cream cheese, bacon, and nuts are also on the fat list to remind users of their high fat content. These groupings highlight the characteristics of foods that are significant to energy intake. To learn more about this useful diet-planning tool, study Appendix G, which gives details of the exchange system used in the United States.

Putting the Plan into Action Familiarizing yourself with each of the food groups is the first step in diet planning. Table 2-6 shows how to use the 2000-kcalorie USDA Food Pattern to plan a diet. The amounts listed from each of the food groups (see the second column of the table) were taken from Table 2-3 (p. 43). The next step is to assign the food groups to meals (and snacks), as shown in the remaining columns of Table 2-6.

At this point, a person can begin to fill in a plan with real foods to create a menu. For example, the breakfast calls for 1 ounce grain, ½ cup fruit, and 1 cup milk. A person might select a bowl of cereal with banana slices and milk:

1 cup cereal = 1 ounce grain

½ large banana = ½ cup fruit

1 cup fat-free milk = 1 cup milk

Or ½ English muffin and a bowl of strawberries topped with yogurt:

½ English muffin = 1 ounce grain

½ cup strawberries = ½ cup fruit

1 cup fat-free plain yogurt = 1 cup milk

Then the person can continue to create a diet plan by creating menus for lunch, dinner, and snacks. The final menu might look like the one presented in Table 2-7.

As you can see, we all make countless food-related decisions daily—whether we have a plan or not. Following an eating pattern that incorporates health recommendations and diet-planning principles helps a person make wise nutrition decisions.

TABLE 2-6 Diet Planning Using the 2000-kCalorie USDA Food Pattern

This diet plan is one of many possibilities. It follows the amounts of foods suggested for a 2000-kcalorie diet as shown in Table 2-3 (p. 43), with a little less oil.

Food Group	Amounts	Breakfast	Lunch	Snack	Dinner	Snack
Fruits	2 c	½ c		½ c	1 c	
Vegetables	2½ c		1 c		1½ c	
Grains	6 oz	1 oz	2 oz	½ oz	2 oz	½ oz
Protein foods	5½ oz		2 oz		3½ oz	
Milk and milk products	3 c	1 c		1 c		1 c
Oils	6 tsp		1½ tsp		4 tsp	

TABLE 2-7 A Sample Menu

This sample menu provides about 1850 kcalories and meets the recommendations to provide 45 to 65 percent of kcalories from carbohydrate, 20 to 35 percent from fat, and 10 to 35 percent from protein.

Amounts	Sample Menu	Energy (kcal)
	Breakfast	
1 oz whole grains	1 c whole-grain cereal	108
1 c milk	1 c fat-free milk	100
½ c fruit	1 medium banana (sliced)	105
	Lunch	
2 oz meats, 2 oz whole grains	1 turkey sandwich on whole-wheat roll	272
1½ tsp oils	1½ tbs low-fat mayonnaise	71
1 c vegetables	1 c vegetable juice	50
	Snack	
½ oz whole grains	4 whole-wheat reduced-fat crackers	86
1 c milk	1½ oz low-fat cheddar cheese	74
½ c fruit	1 medium apple	72
	Dinner	
½ c vegetables	1 c raw spinach leaves	8
¼ c vegetables	¼ c shredded carrots	11
1 oz meats	¼ c garbanzo beans	71
2 tsp oils	2 tbs oil-based salad dressing and olives	76
¾ c vegetables, 2½ oz meat, 2 oz enriched grains	Spaghetti with meat and tomato sauce	425
½ c vegetables	½ c green beans	22
2 tsp oils	2 tsp soft margarine	67
1 c fruit	1 c strawberries	49
	Snack	
½ oz whole grains	3 graham crackers	90
1 c milk	1 c fat-free milk	100

From Guidelines to Groceries Dietary recommendations emphasize nutrient-rich foods such as whole grains, fruits, vegetables, lean meats, poultry, seafood, and low-fat milk products. You can design such a diet for yourself, but how do you begin? Start with the foods you regularly enjoy eating and then try to make a few improvements.[17] For most people that will mean eating less red meat, cheeses, and salted snacks and more fruits, vegetables, whole grains, legumes, nuts, milk products, and seafood. Such small changes can dramatically improve the diet. When shopping, think of the food groups, and choose nutrient-dense foods within each group.

Be aware that many of the tens of thousands of food options available today are **processed foods** that have lost valuable nutrients and gained sugar, fat, and salt as they were transformed from farm-fresh foods to those found in the bags, boxes, and cans that line grocery-store shelves. Their value in the diet depends on the original food and how it was prepared or processed. By eating more fresh foods and fewer processed foods, consumers can reduce their intakes of added sugars, solid fats, and sodium for relatively little effort. Sometimes processed foods have been **fortified** to improve their nutrient contents, which can be helpful in increasing dietary intake of specific vitamins and minerals.

Grains When shopping for grain products, you will find them described as *refined, enriched,* or *whole grain*. These terms refer to the milling process and the making of grain products, and they have different nutrition implications (see Figure 2-6, p. 52). **Refined** grains have lost many nutrients during processing; **enriched** grains have had some nutrients added back; and **whole-grain** products have all the nutrients and fiber found in the original grain. As such, whole-grain

processed foods: foods that have been treated to change their physical, chemical, microbiological, or sensory properties.

fortified: the addition to a food of nutrients that were either not originally present or present in insignificant amounts. Fortification can be used to correct or prevent a widespread nutrient deficiency or to balance the total nutrient profile of a food.

refined: the process by which the coarse parts of a food are removed. When wheat is refined into flour, the bran, germ, and husk are removed, leaving only the endosperm.

enriched: the addition to a food of specific nutrients to replace losses that occur during processing so that the food will meet a specified standard.

whole grain: a grain that maintains the same relative proportions of starchy endosperm, germ, and bran as the original (all but the husk); not refined.

> **FIGURE 2-6 A Wheat Plant**

The protective coating of **bran** around the kernel of grain is rich in nutrients and fiber.

The **endosperm** contains starch and proteins.

The **germ** is the seed that grows into a wheat plant, so it is especially rich in vitamins and minerals to support new life.

The outer **husk** (or **chaff**) is the inedible part of a grain.

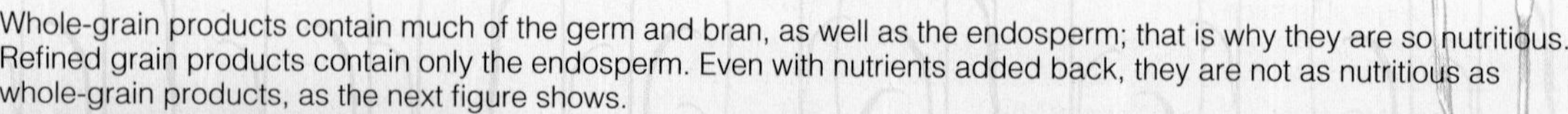

Whole-grain products contain much of the germ and bran, as well as the endosperm; that is why they are so nutritious. Refined grain products contain only the endosperm. Even with nutrients added back, they are not as nutritious as whole-grain products, as the next figure shows.

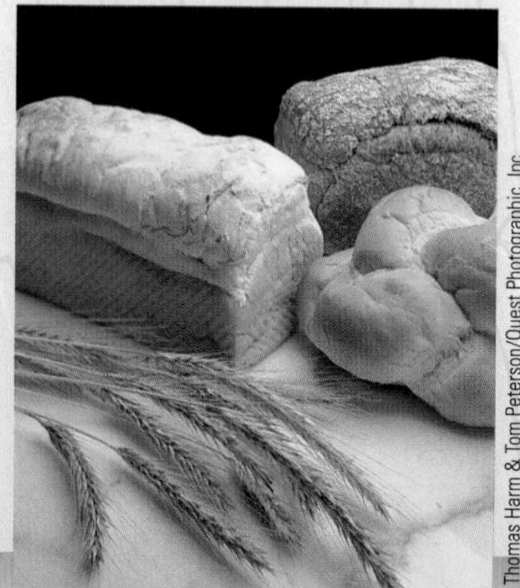

© Thomas Harm & Tom Peterson/Quest Photographic, Inc.

Common types of flour:

- **Refined flour:** finely ground endosperm that is usually enriched with nutrients and bleached for whiteness; sometimes called *white flour.*
- **Wheat flour:** any flour made from the endosperm of the wheat kernel.
- **Whole-wheat flour:** any flour made from the entire wheat kernel.

The difference between *white flour* and *white wheat* is noteworthy. Typically, *white flour* refers to refined flour (as defined above). Most flour—whether refined, white, or whole wheat—is made from red wheat. Whole-grain products made from red wheat are typically brown and full flavored.

To capture the health benefits of whole grains for consumers who prefer white bread, manufacturers use an albino variety of wheat called *white wheat.* Whole-grain products made from white wheat provide the nutrients and fiber of a whole grain with a light color and natural sweetness. Read labels carefully—white bread is a whole-grain product only if it is made from whole white wheat.

© Cengage Learning

products support good health and should account for at least half of the grains daily. Adding more whole grains to the diet can be as easy as eating oatmeal for breakfast and popcorn for a snack or substituting brown rice for white rice and whole-wheat bread for enriched white bread. To find whole-grain products, read food labels and select those that name a whole-grain first in the ingredient list. Examples of whole grains include:

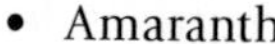

- Amaranth
- Barley
- Buckwheat
- Bulgur
- Corn (and popcorn)
- Millet
- Oats (and oatmeal)
- Quinoa
- Rice (brown or wild)
- Whole rye
- Whole wheat

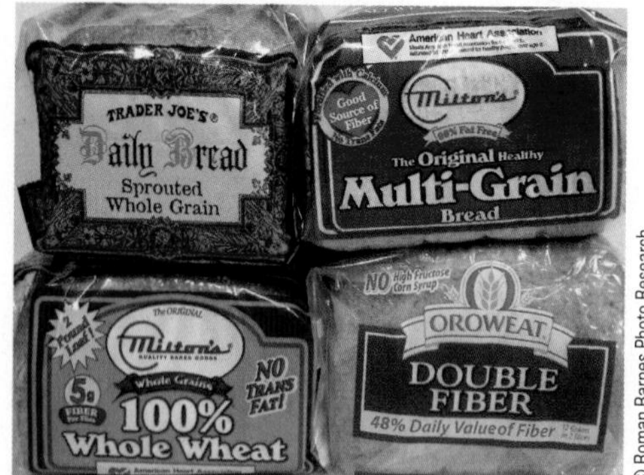

© Roman Barnes Photo Research

When shopping for bread, look for the descriptive words *whole grain* or *whole wheat* and check the fiber content on the Nutrition Facts panel of the label—the more fiber, the more likely the bread is a whole-grain product.

Products described as "multi-grain," "stone-ground," or "100% wheat" are usually *not* whole-grain products. Brown color is also not a useful hint, but fiber content often is.

When it became a common practice to refine the wheat flour used for bread by milling it and throwing away the bran and the germ, consumers suffered a tragic loss of many nutrients. As a consequence, in the early 1940s Congress passed legislation requiring that all grain products that cross state lines be enriched with iron, thiamin, riboflavin, and niacin. In 1996 this legislation was amended to include folate, a vitamin considered essential in the prevention of some birth defects. Most grain products that have been refined, such as rice, pastas such as macaroni and spaghetti, and cereals (both cooked and ready-to-eat types), have subsequently been enriched. Food labels must specify that products have been enriched and include the enrichment nutrients in the ingredients list.

Enrichment doesn't make a slice of bread rich in these added nutrients, but people who eat several slices a day obtain significantly more of these nutrients than they would from unenriched bread. Even though the enrichment of flour helps to prevent deficiencies of these nutrients, it fails to compensate for losses of many other nutrients and fiber. As Figure 2-7 shows, whole-grain items deliver many more nutrients than the enriched ones. Only *whole-grain* flour contains all of the nutritive portions of the grain. Whole-grain products, such as brown rice and oatmeal, provide more nutrients and fiber and contain less salt, sugar, and fat than refined grain products. This helps to explain why diet quality tends to be better for consumers who eat more whole grains.[18]

> DIETARY GUIDELINES FOR AMERICANS

Increase whole-grain intake. Consume at least half of all grains as whole grains. Whenever possible, replace refined grains with whole grains.

Speaking of processed foods, ready-to-eat breakfast cereals are the most highly fortified foods on the market. Like an enriched food, a *fortified* food has had nutrients added during processing, but in a fortified food, the added nutrients may not have been present in the original product. (The terms *fortified* and *enriched* may be used interchangeably.[19]) Some breakfast cereals made from refined flour and fortified with high doses of vitamins and minerals are actually more like dietary supplements disguised as cereals than they are like whole grains. They may be nutritious—with respect to the nutrients added—but they still may fail to convey the full spectrum of nutrients that a whole-grain food or a mixture of such foods might provide. Still, fortified foods help people meet their vitamin and mineral needs.

> FIGURE 2-7 Nutrients in Bread

Whole-grain bread is more nutritious than other breads, even enriched bread. For iron, thiamin, riboflavin, niacin, and folate, enriched bread provides about the same quantities as whole-grain bread and significantly more than unenriched bread. For fiber and the other nutrients (those shown here as well as those not shown), enriched bread provides less than whole-grain bread.

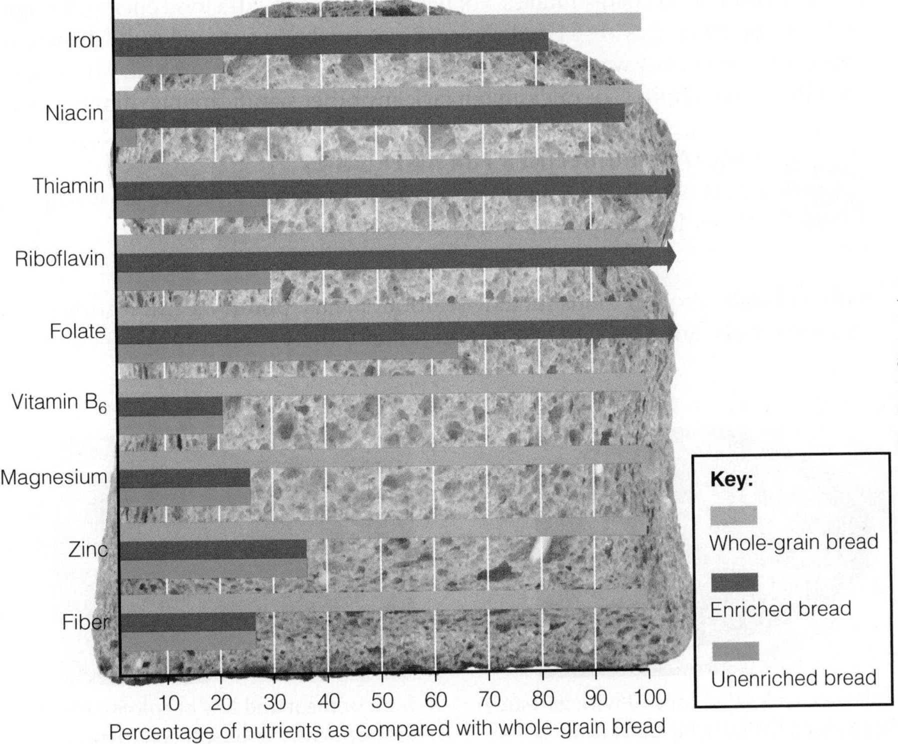

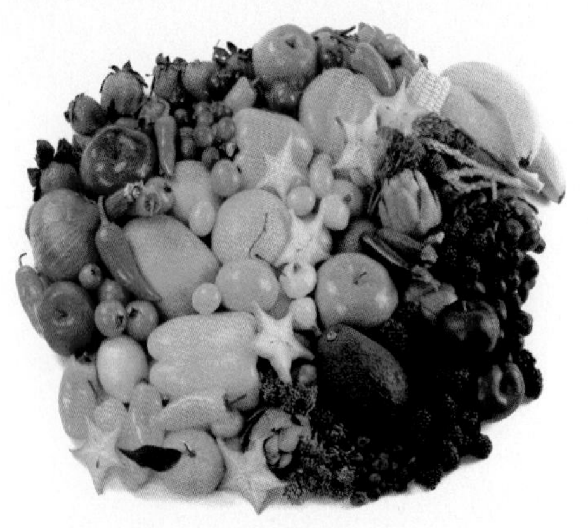

© iStockphoto.com/Kelly Cline

Consumers can remember to eat a variety of fruits and vegetables every day by selecting from each of five colors.

Vegetables Posters in the produce section of grocery stores encourage consumers to "think variety, think color." Such efforts are part of a national educational campaign to increase fruit and vegetable consumption. Easy ways to effectively increase vegetable consumption include serving a variety of vegetables at meals, increasing the portion sizes, and adding pureed vegetables to recipes such as muffins or casseroles.[20]

Choose fresh vegetables often, especially dark-green leafy and red and orange vegetables such as spinach, broccoli, tomatoes, and sweet potatoes. Cooked or raw, vegetables are good sources of vitamins, minerals, and fiber. Frozen and canned vegetables without added salt are acceptable alternatives to fresh. To control fat, energy, and sodium intakes, limit butter and salt on vegetables.

Choose often from the variety of legumes available:

- Adzuki beans
- Black beans
- Black-eyed peas
- Fava beans
- Garbanzo beans
- Great northern beans
- Kidney beans
- Lentils
- Lima beans
- Navy beans
- Peanuts
- Pinto beans
- Soybeans
- Split peas

Legumes are an economical, low-fat, nutrient- and fiber-rich food choice. Combining legumes with foods from other food groups creates delicious meals (see Figure 2-8).

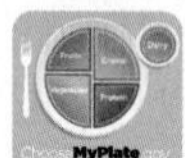

> DIETARY GUIDELINES FOR AMERICANS

Increase vegetable intake. Eat recommended amounts of vegetables and include a variety of vegetables, especially dark-green vegetables, red and orange vegetables, and legumes.

Fruit Choose fresh fruits often. Frozen, dried, and canned fruits without added sugar are acceptable alternatives to fresh. Fruits supply valuable vitamins, minerals, fibers, and phytochemicals. They add flavors, colors, and textures to meals, and their natural sweetness makes them enjoyable as snacks or desserts.

Fruit juices are healthy beverages but contain little dietary fiber compared with whole fruits. Whole fruits satisfy the appetite better than juices, thereby helping people to limit food energy intakes. For people who need extra food energy, though, 100 percent fruit juices are a good choice. Be aware that sweetened fruit "drinks" or "ades" contain mostly water, sugar, and a little juice for flavor. Some may have been fortified with vitamin C or calcium but lack any other significant nutritional value.

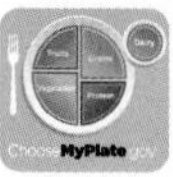

> DIETARY GUIDELINES FOR AMERICANS

Increase fruit intake. Eat recommended amounts of fruits and choose a variety of fruits. Choose whole or cut-up fruits more often than fruit juice.

Protein Foods Protein foods include seafood, meats, poultry, eggs, legumes, soy products, nuts, and seeds. In addition to protein, these foods provide B vitamins,

> FIGURE 2-8 Meals Featuring Legumes

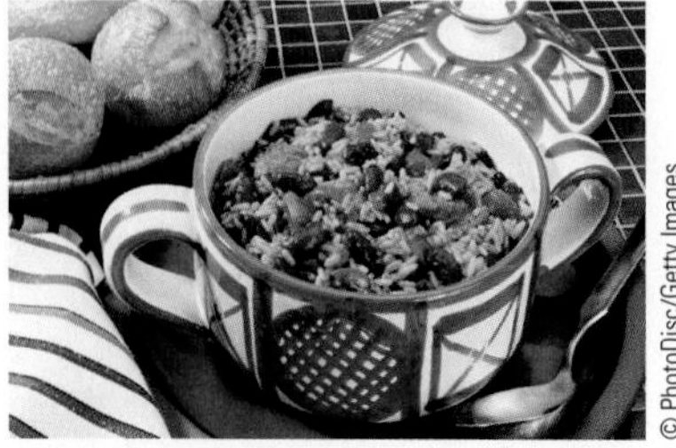

© PhotoDisc/Getty Images

Add rice to red beans for a hearty meal.

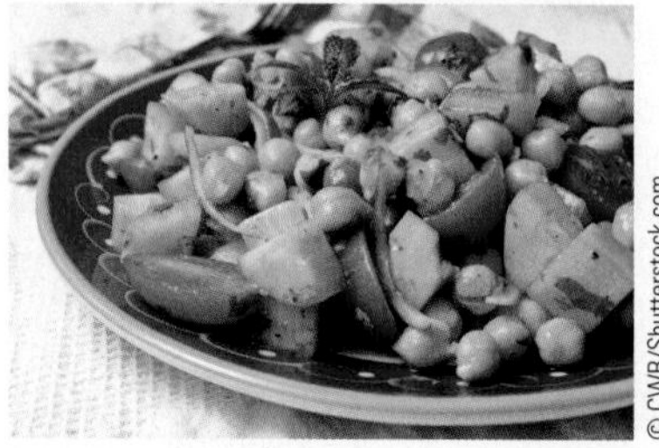

© CWB/Shutterstock.com

Enjoy a Greek salad topped with garbanzo beans for a little ethnic diversity.

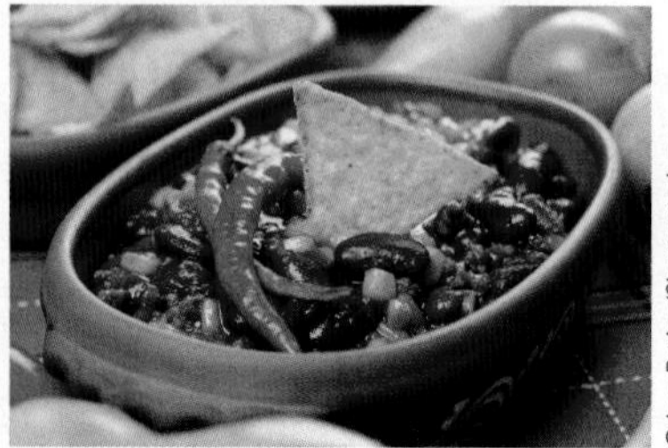

© Igor Dutina/Shutterstock.com

A bit of meat and lots of spices turn kidney beans into chili con carne.

vitamin E, iron, zinc, and magnesium. To buy and prepare these foods without adding excess energy, fat, and sodium takes a little knowledge and planning.

When shopping in the meat department, choose lean cuts of beef and pork named "round" or "loin" (as in top round or pork tenderloin). As a guide, "prime" and "choice" cuts generally have more fat than "select" cuts. Restaurants usually serve prime cuts. Ground beef, even "lean" ground beef, derives most of its food energy from fat. Have the butcher trim and grind a lean round steak instead. Alternatively, soy products such as **textured vegetable protein** can be used instead of ground beef in a casserole, spaghetti sauce, or chili, saving fat kcalories. Because nuts and seeds are energy dense, they need to be consumed in small quantities and in place of—not in addition to—other protein foods. To lower sodium intake, choose unsalted nuts and seeds.

Serving sizes for meats, poultry, and seafood reflect weight after cooking and without bones. In general, 4 ounces of raw meat is equal to about 3 ounces of cooked meat. Some examples of 3-ounce portions include 1 medium pork chop, ½ chicken breast, or 1 steak or fish filet about the size of a deck of cards. To keep fat intake moderate, bake, roast, broil, grill, or braise meats, poultry, and seafood (but do not fry them in fat); remove the skin from poultry after cooking; trim visible fat before cooking; and drain fat after cooking. Chapter 5 offers many additional strategies for moderating fat intake.

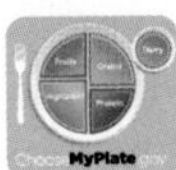

> DIETARY GUIDELINES FOR AMERICANS

Choose a variety of protein foods, which include seafood, lean meats and poultry, eggs, legumes, soy products, and unsalted nuts and seeds. Increase the amount and variety of seafood consumed by choosing seafood in place of some meat and poultry.

Milk and Milk Products Shoppers find a variety of fortified foods in the dairy case. Examples are milk, to which vitamins A and D have been added, and soy milk, to which calcium, vitamin D, and vitamin B_{12} have been added. Be aware that not all soy beverages have been fortified. Read labels carefully.

In addition, shoppers may find **imitation foods** (such as cheese products), **food substitutes** (such as egg substitutes), and functional foods (such as margarine with added plant sterols). As food technology advances, many such foods offer alternatives to traditional choices that may help people reduce their saturated fat and cholesterol intakes. Chapter 5 provides other examples.

Milk is often described by its fat contents:

- Fat-free milk (also called nonfat, skim, zero-fat, or no-fat)
- Low-fat milk (also called 1% milk)
- Reduced-fat milk (also called 2% milk)
- Whole milk

When shopping, choose fat-free or low-fat milk, yogurt, and cheeses. Such selections help consumers meet their vitamin and mineral needs within their energy and fat allowances. Milk products are important sources of calcium but can provide too much sodium and fat if not selected with care.

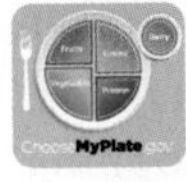

> DIETARY GUIDELINES FOR AMERICANS

Increase intake of fat-free or low-fat milk and milk products—such as milk, yogurt, cheese, or fortified soy milk—and replace whole milk products with fat-free or low-fat options.

› REVIEW IT Use the USDA Food Patterns to develop a meal plan within a specified energy allowance.

Food group plans such as the USDA Food Patterns help consumers select the types and amounts of foods to provide adequacy, balance, and variety in the diet. They make it easier to plan a diet that includes a balance of grains, vegetables, fruits, protein foods, and milk and milk products. In making any food choice, remember to view the food in the context of the total diet. The combination of many different foods provides the array of nutrients that is so essential to a healthy diet.

textured vegetable protein: processed soybean protein used in vegetarian products such as soy burgers.

2.3 Food Labels

› LEARN IT Compare the information on food labels to make selections that meet specific dietary and health goals.

Many consumers, especially those interested in preventing chronic diseases, read food labels to help them make healthy choices.[21] Food labels appear on virtually all packaged foods, and posters or brochures provide similar nutrition information for fresh fish, fruits, and vegetables. A few foods need not carry nutrition labels: those contributing few nutrients, such as plain coffee, tea, and spices; those produced by small businesses; and those prepared and sold in the same establishment. Markets selling nonpackaged items may voluntarily present nutrient information, either in brochures or on signs posted at the point of purchase.

Restaurants with 20 or more locations must provide menu listings of an item's kcalories, grams of saturated fat, and milligrams of sodium.[22] Other restaurants need not supply nutrition information for menu items unless claims such as "low-fat" or "heart healthy" have been made. When ordering such items, keep in mind that restaurants tend to serve extra-large portions—two to three times standard serving sizes.

The Ingredient List

All packaged foods must list *all* ingredients—including additives used to preserve or enhance foods, such as vitamins and minerals added to enrich or fortify products. The ingredients are listed on the label in descending order of predominance by weight. Knowing that the first ingredient predominates by weight, consumers can glean much information. Compare these products, for example:

- A beverage powder that contains "sugar, citric acid, natural flavors . . ." versus a juice that contains "water, tomato concentrate, concentrated juices of carrots, celery . . ."
- A cereal that contains "puffed milled corn, sugar, corn syrup, molasses, salt . . ." versus one that contains "100 percent rolled oats"
- A canned fruit that contains "sugar, apples, water" versus one that contains simply "apples, water"

In each of these comparisons, consumers can see that the second product is more nutrient dense.

Nutrition Facts Panel

The Nutrition Facts panel provides valuable nutrition information such as serving sizes, nutrient quantities, and Daily Values. Recent revisions to the nutrition facts panel reflect current nutrition science, updated serving sizes, and an improved design (see Figure 2-9).

Serving Sizes

Because labels present nutrient information based on one serving, they must identify the size of the serving. The Food and Drug Administration (FDA) has established serving sizes for various foods and requires that all labels for a given product use the same serving size. For example, the new standard serving size for all ice creams is 1 cup. This facilitates comparison shopping. Consumers can see at a glance which brand has more or fewer kcalories or grams of added sugars, for example.

When examining the nutrition facts on a food label, consumers need to compare the serving size on the label with how much they actually eat and adjust their calculations accordingly. For example, if the serving size is four cookies and you eat only two, then you need to cut the nutrient and kcalorie values in half; similarly, if you eat eight cookies, then you need to double the values. Packages, such as a 15-ounce can of soup, that contain more than one but less than two servings and are commonly eaten in one sitting are labeled as one serving. For

imitation foods: foods that substitute for and resemble another food, but are nutritionally inferior to it with respect to vitamin, mineral, or protein content. If the substitute is not inferior to the food it resembles and if its name provides an accurate description of the product, it need not be labeled "imitation."

food substitutes: foods that are designed to replace other foods.

> FIGURE 2-9 Example of a Food Label

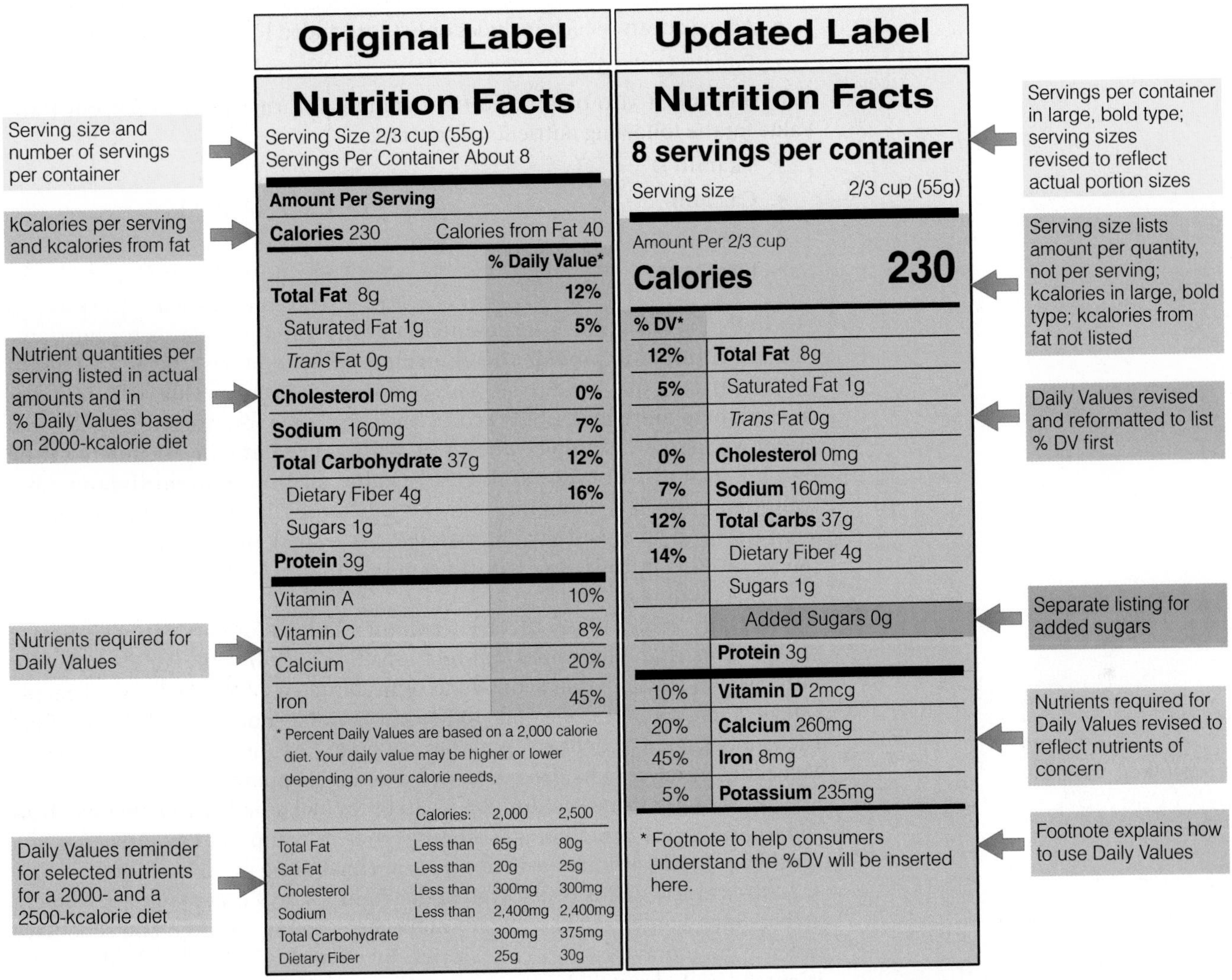

Original Label

Serving size and number of servings per container

kCalories per serving and kcalories from fat

Nutrient quantities per serving listed in actual amounts and in % Daily Values based on 2000-kcalorie diet

Nutrients required for Daily Values

Daily Values reminder for selected nutrients for a 2000- and a 2500-kcalorie diet

Nutrition Facts

Serving Size 2/3 cup (55g)
Servings Per Container About 8

Amount Per Serving	
Calories 230	Calories from Fat 40
	% Daily Value*
Total Fat 8g	**12%**
Saturated Fat 1g	**5%**
Trans Fat 0g	
Cholesterol 0mg	**0%**
Sodium 160mg	**7%**
Total Carbohydrate 37g	**12%**
Dietary Fiber 4g	**16%**
Sugars 1g	
Protein 3g	
Vitamin A	10%
Vitamin C	8%
Calcium	20%
Iron	45%

* Percent Daily Values are based on a 2,000 calorie diet. Your daily value may be higher or lower depending on your calorie needs,

	Calories:	2,000	2,500
Total Fat	Less than	65g	80g
Sat Fat	Less than	20g	25g
Cholesterol	Less than	300mg	300mg
Sodium	Less than	2,400mg	2,400mg
Total Carbohydrate		300mg	375mg
Dietary Fiber		25g	30g

Updated Label

Nutrition Facts

8 servings per container

Serving size 2/3 cup (55g)

Amount Per 2/3 cup

Calories 230

% DV*	
12%	**Total Fat** 8g
5%	Saturated Fat 1g
	Trans Fat 0g
0%	**Cholesterol** 0mg
7%	**Sodium** 160mg
12%	**Total Carbs** 37g
14%	Dietary Fiber 4g
	Sugars 1g
	Added Sugars 0g
	Protein 3g
10%	**Vitamin D** 2mcg
20%	**Calcium** 260mg
45%	**Iron** 8mg
5%	**Potassium** 235mg

* Footnote to help consumers understand the %DV will be inserted here.

Servings per container in large, bold type; serving sizes revised to reflect actual portion sizes

Serving size lists amount per quantity, not per serving; kcalories in large, bold type; kcalories from fat not listed

Daily Values revised and reformatted to list % DV first

Separate listing for added sugars

Nutrients required for Daily Values revised to reflect nutrients of concern

Footnote explains how to use Daily Values

packages that contain two to four servings, food labels present two columns, listing information both "per serving" and "per package." Such dual listings are particularly helpful for people who may consume the entire package in a single sitting. Examples include pints of ice cream and 20-ounce sodas.

Nutrient Quantities In addition to the serving size and the servings per container, the FDA requires that the Nutrition Facts panel on food labels present nutrient information in two ways—in quantities (such as grams) and as percentages of standards called the **Daily Values.** The Nutrition Facts panel must provide the nutrient amount, **percent Daily Value,** or both for the following:

- Total food energy (kcalories)
- Total fat (grams and percent Daily Value)
- Saturated fat (grams and percent Daily Value)
- *Trans* fat (grams)
- Cholesterol (milligrams and percent Daily Value)
- Sodium (milligrams and percent Daily Value)
- Total carbohydrate, which includes starch, sugar, and fiber (grams and percent Daily Value)
- Dietary fiber (grams and percent Daily Value)

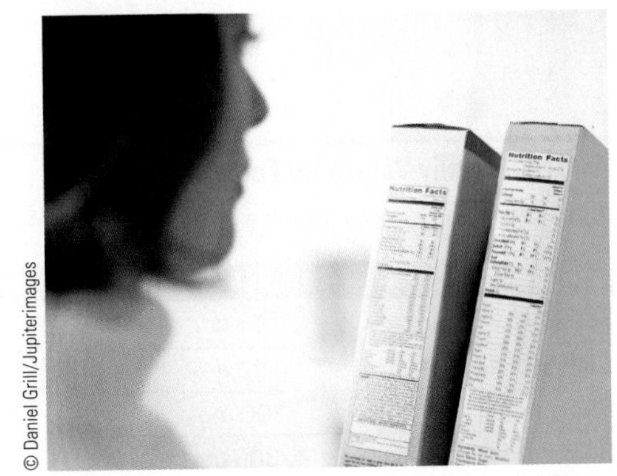

Consumers read food labels to learn about the nutrient contents of a food or to compare similar foods.

Daily Values (DV): reference values developed by the FDA specifically for use on food labels.

percent Daily Value (%DV): the percentage of a Daily Value recommendation found in a specified serving of food for key nutrients based on a 2000-kcalorie diet.

- Sugars, which includes both those naturally present in and those added to the food (grams)
- Added sugars, which includes only those added to the food (grams)
- Protein (grams)

The labels must also present nutrient content information as a percent Daily Value for the following nutrients of concern:

- Vitamin D
- Calcium
- Iron
- Potassium

The Daily Values Table 2-8 presents the Daily Value standards for nutrients that are required to provide this information. Food labels list the amount of some nutrients in a product as a percentage of its Daily Value, which makes the numbers more meaningful to consumers. A person reading a food label might wonder, for example, whether 1 milligram of iron or calcium is a little or a lot. As Table 2-8 shows, the Daily Value for iron is 18 milligrams, so 1 milligram of iron is enough to notice—it is more than 5 percent, and that is what the food label will say. But because the Daily Value for calcium on food labels is 1300 milligrams, 1 milligram of calcium is insignificant, and the food label will read "0%."

The Daily Values reflect dietary recommendations for nutrients and dietary components that have important relationships with health. For example, for heart health, consumers are advised to limit saturated fat to 10 percent of energy intake. For a 2000-kcalorie diet, 10 percent is 200 kcalories, or 22 grams of fat. (Remember that fats deliver 9 kcalories per gram.) As Table 2-8 shows, the Daily Value for saturated fat has been rounded down to 20 grams.

The "% Daily Value" column on a label provides a ballpark estimate of how individual foods contribute to the total diet. It compares key nutrients in a serving of food with the goals of a person consuming 2000 kcalories per day. A 2000-kcalorie diet is considered about right for sedentary younger women, active older women, and sedentary older men. Young children and sedentary older women may need fewer kcalories. By comparison, a 2500-kcalorie diet is considered about right for many men, teenage boys, and active younger women. People who are exceptionally active may have still higher energy needs.

People who consume 2000 kcalories a day can simply add up all of the "% Daily Values" for a particular nutrient to see if their diet for the day fits recommendations. People who require more or less than 2000 kcalories daily must do some calculations to see how foods compare with their personal nutrition goals. Those interested can use the Calculation Factors column in Table 2-8 or the suggestions presented in the "How To" feature.

Daily Values help consumers readily see whether a food contributes "a little" or "a lot" of a nutrient. For example, the "% Daily Value" column on a package of frozen macaroni and cheese may say 20 percent for saturated fat. This tells the consumer that each serving of this food contains about 20 percent of the day's allotted 20 grams of saturated fat. Be aware that for some nutrients (such as saturated fat and sodium) you will want to select foods with a low "% Daily Value" and for others (such as calcium and fiber) you will want a high "% Daily Value." To determine whether a particular food is a wise choice, a consumer needs to consider its place in the diet among all the other foods eaten during the day.

TABLE 2-8 Daily Values for Food Labels

Food labels must present the "% Daily Value" for these nutrients.

Nutrient	Daily Value	Calculation Factors
Fat (total)	65 g	30% of kcalories
Saturated fat	20 g	10% of kcalories
Cholesterol	300 mg	—
Sodium	2300 mg	—
Carbohydrate (total)	300 g	60% of kcalories
Fiber	28 g	14 g per 1000 kcalories
Vitamin D	20 µg	—
Calcium	1300 mg	—
Iron	18 mg	—
Potassium	4700 mg	—

NOTE: Daily Values were established for adults and children aged 4 years and older and are based on an energy intake of 2000 kcalories a day.

>How To

Calculate Personal Daily Values

The Daily Values on food labels are designed for a 2000-kcalorie intake, but you can calculate a personal set of Daily Values based on your energy allowance. Consider a 1500-kcalorie intake, for example. To calculate a daily goal for fat, multiply energy intake by 30 percent:

$$1500 \text{ kcal} \times 0.30 \text{ kcal from fat} = 450 \text{ kcal from fat}$$

$$450 \text{ kcal from fat} \div 9 \text{ kcal/g} = 50 \text{ g fat}$$

Alternatively, a person can calculate that 1500 kcalories is 75 percent of the 2000-kcalorie intake used for Daily Values:

$$1500 \text{ kcal} \div 2000 \text{ kcal} = 0.75$$
$$0.75 \times 100 = 75\%$$

Then, instead of using 100 percent of the Daily Value, a person consuming 1500 kcalories will aim for 75 percent (or less, in this example). Similarly, a person consuming 2800 kcalories would use 140 percent:

$$2800 \text{ kcal} \div 2000 \text{ kcal} = 1.40 \text{ or } 140\%$$

Table 2-8 includes a calculation column that can help you estimate your personal daily value for several nutrients.

› TRY IT Calculate the Daily Values for a 1800-kcalorie diet and revise the Daily Value percentages on the cereal label found on p. 57.

Daily Values also make it easy to compare foods. For example, a consumer might discover that frozen macaroni and cheese has a Daily Value for saturated fat of 20 percent, whereas macaroni and cheese prepared from a boxed mix has a Daily Value of 15 percent. By comparing labels, consumers who are concerned about their saturated fat intakes can make informed decisions.

Front-of-Package Labels Some consumers find the many numbers on Nutrition Facts panels overwhelming. They want an easier and quicker way to interpret information and select products. Food manufacturers responded by creating front-of-package labels that incorporate text, color, and icons to present key nutrient facts.[23] Without any regulations or oversight, however, different companies used a variety of different symbols to describe how healthful their products were. To calm the chaos and maintain the voluntary status of front-of-package labels, major food industry associations created a standardized presentation of nutrient information called Facts Up Front (see Figure 2-10). Whether consumers find this approach to be more helpful remains to be seen.[24] The FDA is currently evaluating the program and reviewing recommendations from the Institute of Medicine to determine the best way to present front-of-package information.[25]

> FIGURE 2-10 Facts Up Front

This example of front-of-package labeling (created by Grocery Manufacturers Association and the Food Marketing Institute) presents key nutrient facts.

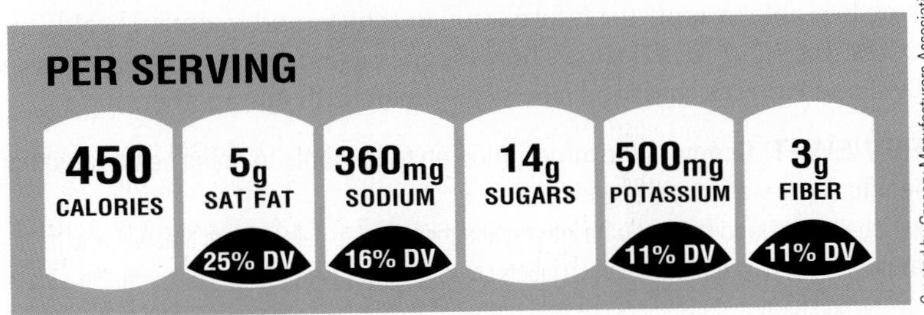

Created by Grocery Manufacturers Association and the Food Marketing Institute

Claims on Labels

In addition to the Nutrition Facts panel, consumers may find various claims on labels. These claims include nutrient claims, health claims, and structure-function claims.

Nutrient Claims Have you noticed phrases such as "good source of fiber" on a box of cereal or "rich in calcium" on a package of cheese? These and other **nutrient claims** may be used on labels so long as they meet FDA definitions, which include the conditions under which each term can be used. For example, in addition to having less than 2 milligrams of cholesterol, a "cholesterol-free" product may not contain more than 2 grams of saturated fat and *trans* fat combined per serving. The accompanying glossary defines nutrient terms on food labels, including criteria for foods described as "low," "reduced," and "free." When nutrients have been added to enriched or fortified products, they must appear in the ingredients list.

Some descriptions *imply* that a food contains, or does not contain, a nutrient. Implied claims are prohibited unless they meet specified criteria. For example, a claim that a product "contains no oil" *implies* that the food contains no fat. If the product is truly fat-free, then it may make the no-oil claim, but if it contains another source of fat, such as butter, it may not.

Health Claims **Health claims** describe a relationship between a food (or food component) and a disease or health-related condition. In some cases, the FDA authorizes health claims based on an extensive review of the scientific literature. For example, the health claim that "Diets low in sodium may reduce the risk of high blood pressure" is based on enough scientific evidence to establish a clear link between diet and health. In cases where there is emerging—but not established—evidence for a relationship between a food or food component and disease, the FDA allows the use of *qualified* health claims that must use specific language indicating that the evidence supporting the claim is limited. A qualified health claim might claim that "Very limited and preliminary research suggests that eating one-half to one cup of tomatoes and/or tomato sauce a week may reduce the risk of prostate cancer. The FDA concludes that there is little scientific evidence supporting the claim."

Structure-Function Claims Unlike health claims, which require food manufacturers to collect scientific evidence and petition the FDA, **structure-function claims** can be made without any FDA approval. Product labels can claim to "slow aging," "improve memory," and "build strong bones" without any proof. The only criterion for a structure-function claim is that it must not mention a disease or symptom. Unfortunately, structure-function claims can be deceptively similar to health claims, and most consumers do not distinguish between different types of claims.[26] Consider these statements:

- "May reduce the risk of heart disease"
- "Promotes a healthy heart"

The first is a health claim that requires FDA approval and the second is an unproven, but legal, structure-function claim. Figure 2-11 compares label claims.

Consumer Education

Food labels are a primary source of information for consumers trying to make healthy diet choices, which is why FDA recently updated labels to place a bigger emphasis on total kcalories, added sugars, and nutrients of concern, such as vitamin D and potassium. In addition, the FDA has designed several programs to educate consumers. Consumers who understand how to read labels are best able to apply the information to achieve and maintain healthful dietary practices. Table 2-9 (p. 62) shows how the messages from the *Dietary Guidelines*, the USDA Food Patterns, and food labels coordinate with one another.

› REVIEW IT Compare the information on food labels to make selections that meet specific dietary and health goals.

Food labels provide consumers with information they need to select foods that will help them meet their nutrition and health goals. When labels contain relevant information presented in a standardized, easy-to-read format, consumers are well prepared to plan and create healthful diets.

nutrient claims: statements that characterize the quantity of a nutrient in a food.

health claims: statements that characterize the relationship between a nutrient or other substance in a food and a disease or health-related condition.

structure-function claims: statements that characterize the relationship between a nutrient or other substance in a food and its role in the body.

> FIGURE 2-11 **Label Claims**

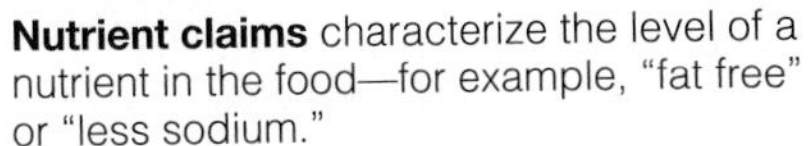

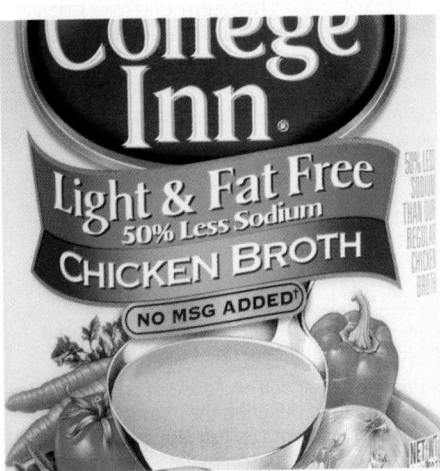

Nutrient claims characterize the level of a nutrient in the food—for example, "fat free" or "less sodium."

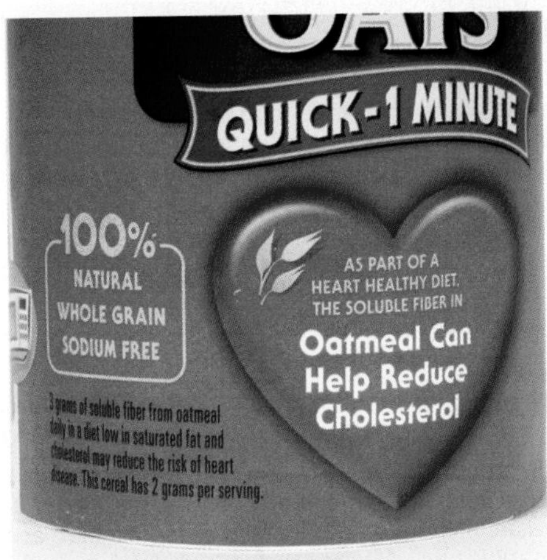

Health claims characterize the relationship of a food or food component to a disease or health-related condition—for example, "soluble fiber from oatmeal daily in a diet low in saturated fat and cholesterol may reduce the risk of heart disease" or "a diet low in total fat may reduce the risk of some cancers."

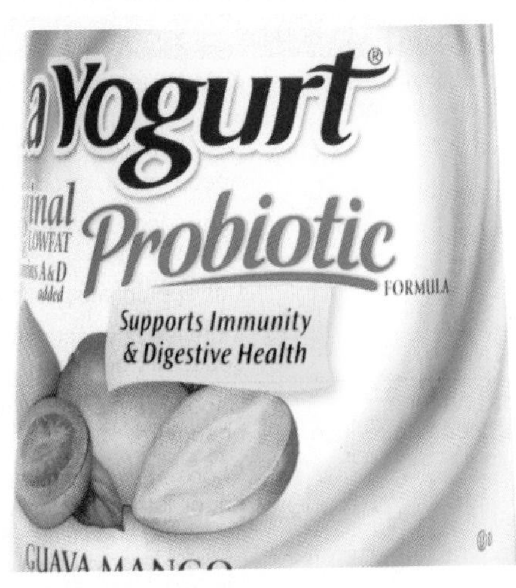

Structure/function claims describe the effect that a substance has on the structure or function of the body and do not make reference to a disease—for example, "supports immunity and digestive health" or "calcium builds strong bones."

GLOSSARY OF TERMS ON FOOD LABELS

GENERAL TERMS

free: "nutritionally trivial" and unlikely to have a physiological consequence; synonyms include *without, no,* and *zero.* A food that does not contain a nutrient naturally may make such a claim, but only as it applies to all similar foods (for example, "applesauce, a fat-free food").

gluten-free: a food that contains less that 20 parts per million of gluten from any source; synonyms include *no gluten, free of gluten,* or *without gluten.*

good source of: the product provides between 10 and 19 percent of the Daily Value for a given nutrient per serving.

healthy: a food that is low in fat, saturated fat, cholesterol, and sodium and that contains at least 10 percent of the Daily Values for vitamin D, potassium, iron, calcium, protein, or fiber.

high: 20 percent or more of the Daily Value for a given nutrient per serving; synonyms include *rich in* or *excellent source.*

less: at least 25 percent less of a given nutrient or kcalories than the comparison food (see individual nutrients); synonyms include *fewer* and *reduced.*

light or **lite:** one-third fewer kcalories than the comparison food; 50 percent or less of the fat or sodium than the comparison food; any use of the term other than as defined must specify what it is referring to (for example, "light in color" or "light in texture").

low: an amount that would allow frequent consumption of a food without exceeding the Daily Value for the nutrient. A food that is naturally low in a nutrient may make such a claim, but only as it applies to all similar foods (for example, "fresh cauliflower, a low-sodium food"); synonyms include *little, few,* and *low source of.*

more: at least 10 percent more of the Daily Value for a given nutrient than the comparison food; synonyms include *added* and *extra.*

organic: on food labels, that at least 95 percent of the product's ingredients have been grown and processed according to USDA regulations defining the use of fertilizers, herbicides, insecticides, fungicides, preservatives, and other chemical ingredients (see Chapter 19).

ENERGY

kcalorie-free: fewer than 5 kcalories per serving.

low kcalorie: 40 kcalories or less per serving.

reduced kcalorie: at least 25 percent fewer kcalories per serving than the comparison food.

FAT AND CHOLESTEROL[a]

percent fat-free: may be used only if the product meets the definition of *low fat* or *fat-free* and must reflect the amount of fat in 100 grams (for example, a food that contains 2.5 grams of fat per 50 grams can claim to be "95 percent fat-free").

fat-free: less than 0.5 gram of fat per serving (and no added fat or oil); synonyms include *zero-fat, no-fat,* and *nonfat.*

low fat: 3 grams or less of fat per serving.

less fat: 25 percent or less fat than the comparison food.

saturated fat-free: less than 0.5 gram of saturated fat and 0.5 gram of *trans* fat per serving.

low saturated fat: 1 gram or less of saturated fat and less than 0.5 gram of *trans* fat per serving.

less saturated fat: 25 percent or less of saturated fat and *trans* fat combined than the comparison food.

***trans* fat-free:** less than 0.5 gram of *trans* fat and less than 0.5 gram of saturated fat per serving.

cholesterol-free: less than 2 milligrams of cholesterol per serving and 2 grams or less of saturated fat and *trans* fat combined per serving.

low cholesterol: 20 milligrams or less of cholesterol per serving and 2 grams or less of saturated fat and *trans* fat combined per serving.

less cholesterol: 25 percent or less cholesterol than the comparison food (reflecting a reduction of at least 20 milligrams per serving), and 2 grams or less of saturated fat and *trans* fat combined per serving.

extra lean: less than 5 grams of fat, 2 grams of saturated fat and *trans* fat combined, and 95 milligrams of cholesterol per serving and per 100 grams of meat, poultry, and seafood.

lean: less than 10 grams of fat, 4.5 grams of saturated fat and *trans* fat combined, and 95 milligrams of cholesterol per serving and per 100 grams of meat, poultry, and seafood. For mixed dishes such as burritos and sandwiches, less than 8 grams of fat, 3.5 grams of saturated fat, and 80 milligrams of cholesterol per reference amount customarily consumed.

CARBOHYDRATES: FIBER AND SUGAR

high fiber: 5 grams or more of fiber per serving. A high-fiber claim made on a food that contains more than 3 grams of fat per serving and per 100 grams of food must also declare total fat.

sugar-free: less than 0.5 gram of sugar per serving.

SODIUM

sodium-free and **salt-free:** less than 5 milligrams of sodium per serving.

low sodium: 140 milligrams or less per serving.

very low sodium: 35 milligrams or less per serving.

[a]Foods containing more than 13 grams total fat per serving or per 50 grams of food must indicate those contents immediately after a cholesterol claim. As you can see, all cholesterol claims are prohibited when the food contains more than 2 grams saturated fat and *trans* fat combined per serving.

TABLE 2-9 From Guidelines to Groceries

Dietary Guidelines	USDA Food Patterns/MyPlate	Food Labels
Balancing kcalories to manage weight	Enjoy your food, but eat less. Select the recommended amounts from each food group at the energy level appropriate for your energy needs; meet, but do not exceed, energy needs. Limit foods and beverages with solid fats and added sugars. Use appropriate portion sizes; avoid oversized portions. Increase physical activity and reduce time spent in sedentary behaviors.	Read the Nutrition Facts to see how many kcalories are in a serving and the number of servings that are in a package. Look for foods that describe their kcalorie contents as *free, low, reduced, light,* or *less.*
Foods and food components to reduce	Choose foods within each group that are low in salt or sodium. Choose foods within each group that are lean, low fat, or fat free and have little solid fat (sources of saturated and *trans* fats); use unsaturated oils instead of solid fats whenever possible. Choose foods and beverages within each group that have little added sugars; drink water instead of sugary beverages. If alcohol is consumed by adults, use in moderation (no more than one drink a day for women and two drinks a day for men).	Read the Nutrition Facts to see how much sodium, saturated fat, *trans* fat, and cholesterol is in a serving of food. Look for foods that describe their salt and sodium contents as *free, low,* or *reduced*; foods that describe their saturated fat, *trans* fat, and cholesterol contents as *free, less, low, light, reduced, lean,* or *extra lean*; foods that describe their added sugar contents as *free* or *reduced.* Look for foods that provide no more than 5 percent of the Daily Value for sodium, saturated fat, and cholesterol. A food may be high in solid fats if its ingredients list begins with or contains several of the following: *beef fat (tallow, suet), butter, chicken fat, coconut oil, cream, hydrogenated oils, palm kernel oil, palm oil, partially hydrogenated oils, pork fat (lard), shortening,* or *stick margarine.* A food most likely contains *trans* fats if its ingredients list includes: *partially hydrogenated oils.* A food may be high in added sugars if its ingredients list begins with or contains several of the following: *brown sugar, confectioner's powdered sugar, corn syrup, dextrin, fructose, high-fructose corn syrup, honey, invert sugar, lactose, malt syrup, maltose, molasses, nectars, sucrose, sugar,* or *syrup.* Light beverages contain fewer kcalories and less alcohol than regular versions.
Foods and nutrients to increase	Make half your plate fruits and vegetables. Choose a variety of vegetables from all five subgroups (dark green, red and orange, legumes, starchy vegetables, and other vegetables) several times a week. Choose a variety of fruits; consume whole or cut-up fruits more often than fruit juice. Choose potassium-rich foods such as fruits and vegetables often. Choose fiber-rich fruits, vegetables, and whole grains often. Choose whole grains; make at least half of the grain selections whole grains by replacing refined grains with whole grains whenever possible. Choose fat-free or low-fat milk and milk products. Choose a variety of protein foods; increase the amount and variety of seafood by choosing seafood in place of some meat and poultry.	Look for foods that describe their fiber, calcium, potassium, iron, and vitamin D contents as *good, high,* or *excellent.* Look for foods that provide at least 10 percent of the Daily Value for fiber, calcium, potassium, iron, and vitamin D from a variety of sources. A food may be a good source of whole grains if its ingredients list begins with or contains several of the following: *barley, brown rice, buckwheat, bulgur, corn, millet, oatmeal, popcorn, quinoa, rolled oats, rye, sorghum, triticale, whole wheat,* or *wild rice.*
Building healthy eating patterns	Select nutrient-dense foods and beverages within and among the food groups. Keep foods safe.	Look for foods that describe their vitamin, mineral, or fiber contents as a *good source* or *high.* Follow the *safe handling instructions* on packages of meat and other safety instructions, such as *keep refrigerated,* on packages of perishable foods.

This chapter provides the links to go from dietary guidelines to buying groceries and offers helpful tips for selecting nutritious foods. For additional information on foods, including organic foods, irradiated foods, genetically modified foods, and more, turn to Chapter 19.

Nutrition Portfolio

The secret to making healthy food choices is learning to incorporate the *Dietary Guidelines for Americans* and the USDA Food Patterns into your decision-making process.

Go to Diet & Wellness Plus and choose one of the days on which you have tracked your diet for the entire day. Choose the MyPlate Report and, looking at it, record in your journal the answers to the following:

- How do the foods you consumed on the day you have chosen stack up with the daily goals (the percentages) in the MyPlate breakdown? Which food groups are over- or under-represented?
- Think about your choices within each food group for the day you recorded. Are they typical of the foods you choose from day to day? Are there simple and realistic ways to enhance the variety in your diet?
- Write yourself a letter describing the dietary changes you can make to improve your chances of enjoying good health.

DIET & WELLNESS **PLUS** To complete this exercise, go to your Diet & Wellness Plus at **www.cengagebrain.com.**

› STUDY IT To review the key points of this chapter and take a practice quiz, go to the study cards at the end of the book.

REFERENCES

1. Position of the Academy of Nutrition and Dietetics: Total diet approach to healthy eating, *Journal of the Academy of Nutrition and Dietetics* 113 (2013): 307–317.
2. Practice paper of the American Dietetic Association, Nutrient density: Meeting nutrient goals within calorie needs, *Journal of the American Dietetic Association* 107 (2007): 860–869.
3. The science behind current nutrition profiling systems to promote consumer intake of nutrient-dense foods, *American Journal of Clinical Nutrition* 91 (2010): entire supplement.
4. D. Mozaffarian and D. S. Ludwig, Dietary Guidelines in the 21st century: A time for food, *Journal of the American Medical Association* 304 (2010): 681–682.
5. J. M. Spahn and coauthors, The systematic review methodology used to support the 2010 Dietary Guidelines advisory committee, *Journal of the American Dietetic Association* 111 (2011): 520–523.
6. M. L. Watts and coauthors, The art of translating nutritional science into dietary guidance: History and evolution of the Dietary Guidelines for Americans, *Nutrition Reviews* 69 (2011): 404–412.
7. L. V. Horn, Development of the 2010 US Dietary Guidelines Advisory Committee Report: Perspectives from a registered dietitian, *Journal of the American Dietetic Association* 110 (2010): 1638–1645.
8. US Department of Health and Human Services, *2008 Physical Activity Guidelines for Americans*, www.health.gov/paguidelines; US Department of Agriculture and US Department of Health and Human Services, *Dietary Guidelines for Americans, 2010*, www.dietaryguidelines.gov.
9. www.choosemyplate.gov/food-groups/vegetables-beans-peas.html, accessed August 22, 2013.
10. P. Britten and coauthors, Updated US Department of Agriculture food patterns meet goals of the 2010 Dietary Guidelines, *Journal of the Academy of Nutrition and Dietetics* 112 (2012): 1648–1655.
11. Position of the American Dietetic Association: Vegetarian diets, *Journal of the American Dietetic Association* 109 (2009): 1266–1282.
12. P. Britten and coauthors, Impact of typical rather than nutrient-dense food choices in the US Department of Agriculture food patterns, *Journal of the Academy of Nutrition and Dietetics* 112 (2012): 1560–1569.
13. P. M. Guenther and coauthors, Update of the Healthy Eating Index: HEI-2010, *Journal of the Academy of Nutrition and Dietetics* 113 (2013): 569–580.
14. Center for Nutrition Policy and Promotion, Diet quality of Americans in 2001–02 and 2007–2008 as measured by the Healthy Eating Index—2010, www.cnpp.usda.gov, April 2013.
15. S. M. Krebs-Smith, J. Reedy, and C. Bosire, Healthfulness of the US food supply: Little improvement despite decades of dietary guidance, *American Journal of Preventive Medicine* 38 (2010): 472–477.
16. Harvard School of Public Health, *The Nutrition Source: Healthy Eating Plate vs. USDA's MyPlate*, www.hsph.harvard.edu, accessed October 4, 2011.
17. M. Maillot and coauthors, Individual diet modeling translates nutrient recommendations into realistic and individual-specific food choices, *American Journal of Clinical Nutrition* 91 (2010): 421–430.
18. C. E. O'Neil and coauthors, Whole-grain consumption is associated with diet quality and nutrient intake in adults: The National Health and Nutrition Examination Survey, 1999–2004, *Journal of the American Dietetic Association* 110 (2010): 1461–1468.
19. As cited in 21 Code of Federal Regulations—Food and Drugs, Section 104.20, 45 *Federal Register* 6323, January 25, 1980, as amended in 58 *Federal Register* 2228, January 6, 1993.
20. J. S. Meengs, L. S. Roe, and B. J. Rolls, Vegetable variety: An effective strategy to increase vegetable intake in adults, *Journal of the Academy of Nutrition and Dietetics* 112 (2012): 1211–1215; A. D. Blatt, L. S. Roes, and B. J. Rolls, Hidden vegetables: An effective strategy to reduce energy intake and increase vegetable intake in adults, *American Journal of Clinical Nutrition* 93 (2011): 756–763; B. J. Rolls, L. S. Roe, and J. S. Meengs, Portion size can be used strategically to increase vegetable consumption in adults, *American Journal of Clinical Nutrition* 91 (2010): 913–922.
21. N. J. Ollberding, R. L. Wolf, and I. Contento, Food label use and its relation to dietary intake among US adults, *Journal of the American Dietetic Association* 111 (2011): S47–S51.
22. L. Marr, National restaurant menu labeling legislation: Public nutrition education and professional opportunities, *Journal of the American Dietetic Association* 111 (2011): S7; K. Stein, A national approach to restaurant menu labeling: The Patient Protection and Affordable Health Care Act, section 4205, *Journal of the American Dietetic Association* 110 (2010): 1280–1286.
23. J. C. Hersey and coauthors, Effects of front-of-package and shelf nutrition labeling systems on consumers, *Nutrition Reviews* 71 (2013): 1–14.
24. K. D. Brownell and J. P. Koplan, Front-of-package nutrition labeling—An abuse of trust by the food industry? *New England Journal of Medicine* 364 (2011): 2373–2375.
25. E. A. Wartella and coauthors, *Front-of-Package Nutrition Rating Systems and Symbols: Promoting Healthier Choices* (Washington, D.C.: National Academies Press, 2011), available at www.iom.edu/Reports/2011/Front-of-Package-Nutrition-Rating-Systems-and-Symbols-Promoting-Healthier-Choices.aspx.
26. C. L. Wong and coauthors, Consumer attitudes and understanding of low-sodium claims on food: An analysis of healthy and hypertensive individuals, *American Journal of Clinical Nutrition* 97 (2013): 1288–1298.

HIGHLIGHT > 2
Vegetarian Diets

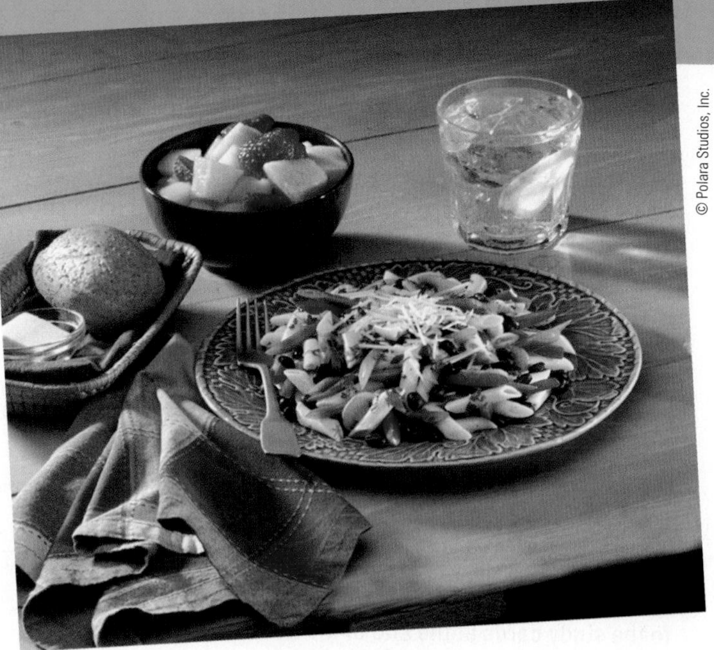

> LEARN IT Develop a well-balanced vegetarian meal plan.

The waiter presents this evening's specials: a fresh spinach salad topped with mandarin oranges, raisins, and sunflower seeds, served with a bowl of pasta smothered in a mushroom and tomato sauce and topped with grated parmesan cheese. Then this one: a salad made of chopped parsley, scallions, celery, and tomatoes mixed with bulgur wheat and dressed with olive oil and lemon juice, served with a spinach and feta cheese pie. Do these meals sound good to you? Or is something missing . . . a pork chop or chicken breast, perhaps?

Would vegetarian fare be acceptable to you some of the time? Most of the time? Ever? The health benefits of a primarily **vegetarian diet** seem to have encouraged many people to eat more plant-based meals. The popular press sometimes refers to individuals who eat small amounts of meat, seafood, or poultry from time to time as "flexitarians."

People who choose to exclude meat and other animal-derived foods from their diets today do so for many of the same reasons the Greek philosopher Pythagoras cited in the sixth century B.C.: physical health, ecological responsibility, and philosophical concerns. They might also cite world hunger issues, economic reasons, ethical concerns, or religious beliefs as motivating factors. Whatever their reasons—and even if they don't have a particular reason—people who exclude meat will be better prepared to plan well-balanced meals if they understand the nutrition and health implications of their choices.

Vegetarian diets generally are categorized, not by a person's motivations but by the foods that are excluded (see the accompanying glossary). Some diets exclude red meat only; some also exclude poultry or seafood; others also exclude eggs; and still others exclude milk and milk products as well. In contrast, **omnivorous** diets do not exclude foods, but include many foods derived from both animals and plants.

As you will see, though, the foods a person *excludes* are not nearly as important as the foods a person *includes* in the diet. **Plant-based diets** that include a variety of whole grains, vegetables, legumes, fruits, and nuts and seeds offer abundant complex carbohydrates and fibers, an assortment of vitamins and minerals, a mixture of phytochemicals, and little saturated fat—characteristics that reflect current dietary recommendations aimed at maintaining good health and an appropriate body weight. Each of these foods—whole grains, vegetables, legumes, fruits, and nuts and seeds—independently reduces the risk for several chronic diseases. This highlight examines the health benefits and potential problems of vegetarian diets and shows how to plan a well-balanced vegetarian diet. Highlight 20 includes a discussion of the environmental benefits of a plant-based diet.

Health Benefits of Vegetarian Diets

Research findings suggest that well-planned vegetarian diets offer sound nutrition and health benefits to adults.[1] Eating patterns that include very little, if any, meat are associated with a lower rate of death from all causes.[2] Some researchers estimate that for the general population, the risk of dying could be lowered by 7 to 19 percent by eliminating just one serving of meat a day.[3]

GLOSSARY

lactovegetarian diet: an eating pattern that includes milk and milk products, but excludes meat, poultry, seafood, and eggs from the diet.
- **lacto** = milk

lacto-ovo-vegetarian diet: an eating pattern that includes milk, milk products, and eggs, but excludes meat, poultry, and seafood from the diet.
- **ovo** = egg

macrobiotic diet: a philosophical eating pattern based on mostly plant foods such as whole grains, legumes, and vegetables, with small amounts of fish, fruits, nuts, and seeds.
- **macro** = large, great
- **biotic** = life

meat replacements: products formulated to look and taste like meat, seafood, or poultry; usually made of textured vegetable protein.

omnivorous: an eating pattern that includes foods derived from both animals and plants.
- **omni** = all
- **vores** = to eat

plant-based diets: an eating pattern that derives most of its protein from plant products (although some animal products may be included).

tempeh (TEM-pay): a fermented-soybean food, rich in protein and fiber.

tofu (TOE-foo): a curd made from soybeans, rich in protein and often fortified with calcium; used in many Asian and vegetarian dishes in place of meat.

vegan (VEE-gan) **diet:** an eating pattern that excludes all animal-derived foods (including meat, poultry, fish, eggs, and dairy products); also called *pure vegetarian, strict vegetarian*, or *total vegetarian.*

vegetarian diet: a general term used to describe an eating pattern that excludes meat, poultry, fish, or other animal-derived foods from the diet.

Obesity

Vegetarians tend to maintain a lower and healthier body weight than nonvegetarians. In general, those who eat meat have higher energy intakes and body weights. Vegetarians' lower body weights correlate with their high intakes of fiber and low intakes of fat. In general, their diets tend to be nutrient-dense and consistent with the *Dietary Guidelines*' recommendations for weight management.[4] Because obesity impairs health in a number of ways, vegetarian diets offer several health advantages.

Diabetes

Obesity and weight gains are strong risk factors for diabetes, which partially explains why nonvegetarian diets are more often associated with diabetes than vegetarian diets. Even when body weight and lifestyle factors are taken into account, vegetarian eating patterns seem to protect against diabetes.[5]

Hypertension

Vegetarians tend to have lower blood pressure and lower rates of hypertension than nonvegetarians.[6] Appropriate body weight helps to maintain a healthy blood pressure, as does a diet low in saturated fat and cholesterol and high in fiber, fruits, vegetables, whole grains, low-fat milk products, and protein from plant sources.[7] Lifestyle factors also influence blood pressure: smoking and alcohol intake raise blood pressure, and physical activity lowers it.

Heart Disease

Meat is associated with an increased risk of heart disease and stroke.[8] The incidence of heart disease and related deaths and the concentrations of blood cholesterol are lower for vegetarians than for nonvegetarians, which can partly be explained by their avoidance of meat.The dietary factor most directly related to heart disease is saturated animal fat, and in general, vegetarian diets are lower in total fat, saturated fat, and cholesterol than typical meat-based diets. The fats common in plant-based diets—the monounsaturated fats of olives, seeds, and nuts and the polyunsaturated fats of vegetable oils—are associated with a decreased risk of heart disease. Furthermore, vegetarian diets are generally higher in dietary fiber, antioxidant vitamins, and phytochemicals—all factors that help control blood lipids and protect against heart disease.

Many vegetarians include soy products such as **tofu** in their diets. Soy products—with their polyunsaturated fats, fibers, vitamins, and minerals, and little saturated fat—may help to protect against heart disease.[9]

Cancer

Vegetarians have a lower overall cancer incidence than the general population.[10] Their low cancer rates may be due to their high intakes of fruits and vegetables (as Highlight 11 explains). In fact, the ratio of vegetables to meat may be the most relevant dietary factor responsible for cancer prevention.

Some scientific findings indicate that vegetarian diets are associated not only with lower cancer mortality in general, but also with lower incidence of cancer at specific sites as well, most notably, colon cancer. People with colon cancer seem to eat more meat. Some cancer experts recommend limiting consumption of red meat to no more than 11 ounces a week, with very little (if any) processed meat.

Other Diseases

In addition to obesity, diabetes, hypertension, heart disease, and some cancers, vegetarian diets may help prevent osteoporosis, diverticular disease, gallstones, cataracts, and rheumatoid arthritis. Health benefits of a vegetarian diet depend on wise diet planning.

Vegetarian Diet Planning

The vegetarian has the same meal-planning task as everyone else—using a variety of foods to deliver all the needed nutrients within an energy allowance that maintains a healthy body weight (as discussed in Chapter 2). Vegetarians who include milk, milk products, and eggs can meet recommendations for most nutrients about as easily as nonvegetarians. Such eating patterns may rely on some fortified foods, but generally provide enough energy, protein, and other nutrients to support the health of adults and the growth of children and adolescents. The USDA Food Patterns for vegetarians are flexible enough that a variety of people can use them: people who have adopted various vegetarian diets, those who want to make the transition to a vegetarian diet, and those who simply want to reduce their meat intake and include more plant-based meals in their diets.

Vegan diets exclude milk, milk products, and eggs and include protein foods such as legumes, nuts, and seeds as well as foods made from them, such as peanut butter, **tempeh,** and tofu. Vegans who do not use milk can use soy "milk"—a product made from soybeans that provides similar nutrients if fortified with calcium, vitamin D, and vitamin B_{12} (see Figure H2-1 on p. 66). Similarly, "milks" made from rice, almonds, and oats are reasonable alternatives, if adequately fortified. Vegan eating patterns must include fortified foods or supplements to provide adequate intakes of all essential nutrients.

MyPlate includes tips for planning vegetarian diets using an adaptation of the USDA Food Patterns. The recommended daily amounts from the food groups is the same for both vegetarians and nonvegetarians (see Table 2-3, p. 43). Selections from within the food groups may differ, of course. For example, the milk group features fortified soy milks for those who do not use milk, cheese, or yogurt. When selecting from the vegetable and fruit groups, vegetarians may want to emphasize particularly good sources of calcium and iron. Green leafy vegetables provide almost five times as much calcium per serving as other vegetables. Similarly, dried fruits deserve special notice in the fruit group because they deliver six times as much iron as other fruits. The protein foods group includes eggs (for those who use them),

> **FIGURE H2-1 Low-Fat Milk and Soy Milk Compared**

A comparison of low-fat milk and enriched soy milk shows that they provide similar amounts of key nutrients.

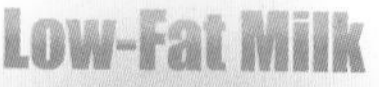

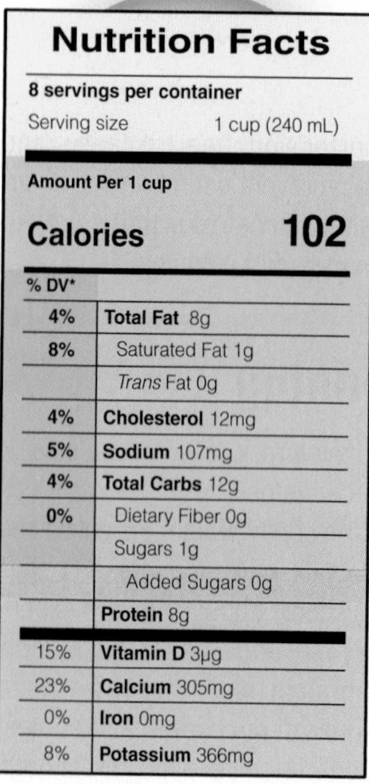

Nutrition Facts

8 servings per container
Serving size 1 cup (240 mL)

Amount Per 1 cup
Calories 102

% DV*	
4%	**Total Fat** 8g
8%	Saturated Fat 1g
	Trans Fat 0g
4%	**Cholesterol** 12mg
5%	**Sodium** 107mg
4%	**Total Carbs** 12g
0%	Dietary Fiber 0g
	Sugars 1g
	Added Sugars 0g
	Protein 8g
15%	**Vitamin D** 3µg
23%	**Calcium** 305mg
0%	**Iron** 0mg
8%	**Potassium** 366mg

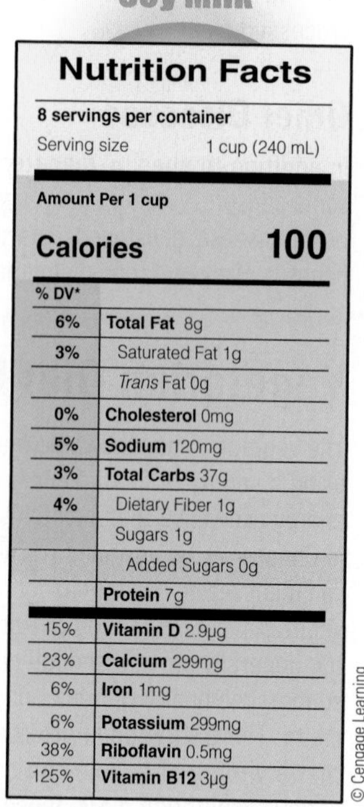

Nutrition Facts

8 servings per container
Serving size 1 cup (240 mL)

Amount Per 1 cup
Calories 100

% DV*	
6%	**Total Fat** 8g
3%	Saturated Fat 1g
	Trans Fat 0g
0%	**Cholesterol** 0mg
5%	**Sodium** 120mg
3%	**Total Carbs** 37g
4%	Dietary Fiber 1g
	Sugars 1g
	Added Sugars 0g
	Protein 7g
15%	**Vitamin D** 2.9µg
23%	**Calcium** 299mg
6%	**Iron** 1mg
6%	**Potassium** 299mg
38%	**Riboflavin** 0.5mg
125%	**Vitamin B12** 3µg

legumes, soy products, and nuts and seeds. Table H2-1 provides recommended *weekly* amounts of protein food subgroups for both vegetarians and vegans.

Most vegetarians easily obtain large quantities of the nutrients that are abundant in plant foods, including carbohydrate, fiber, thiamin, folate, vitamin B_6, vitamin C, vitamin A, and vitamin E. Well-planned vegetarian eating patterns help to ensure adequate intakes of the nutrients vegetarian diets might otherwise lack, including protein, iron, zinc, calcium, vitamin B_{12}, vitamin D, and omega-3 fatty acids. Table H2-2 presents good vegetarian sources of these key nutrients.

Protein

The protein RDA for vegetarians is the same as for others, although some have suggested that it should be higher because plant proteins are not digested as completely. **Lacto-ovo-vegetarian diets** that include animal-derived foods such as milk and eggs, deliver high-quality proteins and are likely to meet protein needs. Even vegetarians who adopt only plant-based diets are likely to meet protein needs provided that their energy intakes are adequate and the protein sources varied.[11] The proteins of whole grains, vegetables, legumes, and nuts and seeds can provide adequate amounts of all the amino acids. An advantage of many vegetarian sources of protein is that they are generally lower in saturated fat than meats and are often higher in fiber and richer in some vitamins and minerals.

Vegetarians sometimes use **meat replacements** made of textured vegetable protein (soy protein). These foods are formulated to look and taste like meat, seafood, or poultry. Many of these products are fortified to provide the vitamins and minerals found in animal sources of protein. Some may be high in salt, sugars, and saturated fats. A wise vegetarian learns to read labels and use a variety of whole, unrefined foods often and commercially prepared foods less frequently. Vegetarians may also use soy products such as tofu to bolster protein intake.

TABLE H2-1 USDA Food Patterns: Recommended Weekly Amounts of Protein Foods for Vegetarians and Vegans

The daily amounts for protein foods (listed in the top row) are the same for both vegetarians and nonvegetarians, but the subgroups and weekly amounts for protein foods differ (listed in the body of the table). The recommended daily amounts from each of the other food groups—fruits, vegetables, grains, and milk products—are the same (see Table 2-3, p. 43).

Protein Foods	1600 kcal	1800 kcal	2000 kcal	2200 kcal	2400 kcal	2600 kcal	2800 kcal	3000 kcal
Daily Amounts	5 oz	5 oz	5½ oz	6 oz	6½ oz	6½ oz	7 oz	7 oz
Vegetarian Subgroups								
Eggs	4 oz	4 oz	4 oz	4 oz	5 oz	5 oz	5 oz	5 oz
Legumes	9 oz	9 oz	10 oz	10 oz	11 oz	11 oz	12 oz	12 oz
Soy products	11 oz	11 oz	12 oz	13 oz	14 oz	14 oz	15 oz	15 oz
Nuts and seeds	12 oz	12 oz	13 oz	15 oz	16 oz	16 oz	17 oz	17 oz
Vegan Subgroups								
Legumes	12 oz	12 oz	13 oz	15 oz	16 oz	16 oz	17 oz	17 oz
Soy products	9 oz	9 oz	10 oz	11 oz	11 oz	11 oz	12 oz	12 oz
Nuts and seeds	14 oz	14 oz	15 oz	17 oz	18 oz	18 oz	20 oz	20 oz

NOTE: Total recommended amounts for legumes include the sum of both the vegetables and protein foods. An ounce-equivalent of legumes in the protein foods group is ¼ cup. For a 2000-kcal vegan diet, that's 3¼ cups of legumes for protein foods plus 1½ cups of legumes for vegetables (see Table 2-4, p. 46), or about almost 5 cups of legumes weekly.

TABLE H2-2 **Good Vegetarian Sources of Key Nutrients**

Nutrients	Grains	Vegetables	Fruits	Protein Foods	Milk	Oils
Protein[a]	Whole grains			Legumes, seeds, nuts, soy products (tempeh, tofu, veggie burgers) Eggs (for ovo-vegetarians)	Milk, cheese, yogurt (for lactovegetarians)	
Iron	Fortified cereals, enriched and whole grains	Dark green leafy vegetables (spinach, turnip greens)	Dried fruits (apricots, prunes, raisins)	Legumes (black-eyed peas, kidney beans, lentils)		
Zinc	Fortified cereals, whole grains			Legumes (garbanzo beans, kidney beans, navy beans), nuts, seeds (pumpkin seeds)	Milk, cheese, yogurt (for lactovegetarians)	
Calcium	Fortified cereals	Dark-green leafy vegetables (bok choy, broccoli, collard greens, kale, mustard greens, turnip greens, watercress)	Fortified juices, figs	Fortified soy products, nuts (almonds), seeds (sesame seeds)	Milk, cheese, yogurt (for lactovegetarians) Fortified soy milk	
Vitamin B_{12}	Fortified cereals			Eggs (for ovo-vegetarians) Fortified soy products	Milk, cheese, yogurt (for lactovegetarians) Fortified soy milk	
Vitamin D					Milk, cheese, yogurt (for lactovegetarians) Fortified soy milk	
Omega-3 fatty acids				Flaxseed, walnuts, soybeans		Flaxseed oil, walnut oil, soybean oil

[a]As Chapter 6 explains, many plant proteins do not contain all the essential amino acids in the amounts and proportions needed by human beings. To improve protein quality, vegetarians can eat grains and legumes together, for example, although it is not necessary if protein intake is varied and energy intake is sufficient.

Iron

Getting enough iron can be a problem even for meat eaters, and those who eat no meat must pay special attention to their iron intake. The iron in plant foods such as legumes, dark-green leafy vegetables, iron-fortified cereals, and whole-grain breads and cereals is poorly absorbed. Because iron absorption from a vegetarian diet is low, the iron RDA for vegetarians is higher than for others (see Chapter 13 for more details).

Fortunately, the body seems to adapt to a low-iron vegetarian diet by increasing iron absorption and decreasing iron losses. Furthermore, iron absorption is enhanced by vitamin C, and vegetarians typically eat many vitamin C–rich fruits and vegetables. Consequently, vegetarians are no more iron deficient than other people.

Zinc

Zinc is similar to iron in that meat is its richest food source, and zinc from plant sources is not well absorbed. In addition, phytates, fiber, and calcium, which are common in vegetarian diets, interfere with zinc absorption. Nevertheless, most vegetarian adults are not zinc deficient. Perhaps the best advice to vegetarians regarding zinc is to eat a variety of nutrient-dense foods; include whole grains, nuts, and legumes such as black-eyed peas, pinto beans, and kidney beans; and maintain an adequate energy intake. For those who include seafood in their diets, oysters, crabmeat, and shrimp are rich in zinc.

Calcium

The calcium intakes of those following a **lactovegetarian diet** are similar to those of the general population, but vegans who use no milk or milk products may risk inadequate intakes. To ensure adequate intakes, vegans can select calcium-rich foods, such as calcium-fortified juices, soy milk, and breakfast cereals, in ample quantities regularly. This advice is especially important for children and adolescents. Soy formulas for infants are fortified with calcium and can be used in cooking, even for adults. Other good calcium sources include figs, some legumes, some green vegetables such as broccoli and turnip greens, some nuts such as almonds, certain seeds such as sesame seeds, and calcium-set tofu.* The choices should be varied because calcium absorption from some plant foods may be limited (as Chapter 12 explains).

Vitamin B_{12}

The requirement for vitamin B_{12} is small, but this vitamin is found only in animal-derived foods. Consequently, vegetarians, in general, and vegans who eat no foods of animal original, in particular, may not get enough vitamin B_{12} in their diets.[12] Fermented soy products such as tempeh may contain some vitamin B_{12} from the bacteria, but unfortunately, much of the vitamin B_{12} found in these products may be an inactive form. Seaweeds such as nori and chlorella supply some vitamin B_{12}, but not much, and excessive intakes of these foods can lead to iodine toxicity. To defend against vitamin B_{12} deficiency, vegans must rely on vitamin B_{12}–fortified sources (such as soy milk or breakfast cereals) or supplements. Without vitamin B_{12}, the nerves suffer damage, leading to such health consequences as loss of vision.

Vitamin D

The vitamin D status of vegetarians is similar to that of nonvegetarians. People who do not use vitamin D–fortified foods and do not receive enough exposure to sunlight to synthesize adequate vitamin D may need supplements to defend against bone loss. This is particularly important for infants, children, and older adults. In northern climates during winter months, young children on vegan diets can readily develop rickets, the vitamin D–deficiency disease.

Omega-3 Fatty Acids

Both Chapter 5 and Highlight 5 describe the health benefits of unsaturated fats, most notably the omega-3 fatty acids commonly found in fatty fish. A diet that includes some meat, fish, and eggs provides much more omega-3 fatty acids than a vegetarian diet, but the *blood* differences between those eating fish and others is relatively small.[13] Researchers speculate that the smaller-than-expected differences may reflect a more efficient conversion of plant-derived fats to omega-3 fats in non-fish eaters. Vegetarians can obtain sufficient amounts of the essential omega-3 fatty acids from plant sources such as flaxseed, walnuts, soy, and canola oil. Supplements derived from marine algae that contain omega-3 fatty acids may also be beneficial.[14]

Healthy Food Choices

Later chapters provide details on how vegetarian diets can meet nutrient needs for various stages of the life cycle, including pregnancy, lactation, infancy, childhood, and adolescence. In general, well-planned vegetarian eating patterns may lower the risk of mortality and several chronic diseases, including obesity, diabetes, high blood pressure, heart disease, and some cancers.[15] But there is nothing mysterious or magical about a vegetarian eating pattern. A dietary pattern that includes small amounts of meat can be equally healthy.[16] The quality of the diet depends not on whether it includes meat but on whether the other food choices are nutritionally sound. A plant-based eating pattern that includes ample fruits, vegetables, whole grains, legumes, nuts, and seeds is higher in fiber, antioxidant vitamins, and phytochemicals and lower in saturated fats and cholesterol than meat-based diets. Variety is key to nutritional adequacy in a vegetarian diet. Restrictive plans that limit selections to a few grains and vegetables cannot possibly deliver a full array of nutrients.

Vegetarianism is not a religion like Buddhism or Hinduism, but merely an eating pattern that selects plant foods to deliver needed nutrients. That said, some vegetarians choose to follow a **macrobiotic diet.** Those following a macrobiotic diet select natural, organic foods and embrace a Zen-like spirituality. In other words, a macrobiotic diet represents a way of life, not just an eating pattern. Such a diet emphasizes whole grains, legumes, and vegetables, with small amounts of fish, fruits, nuts, and seeds. Practices include selecting locally grown foods, eating foods in their most natural state, and balancing cold, sweet, and passive foods with hot, salty, and aggressive ones. Some items, such as processed foods, alcohol, hot spices, and potatoes are excluded from the diet. Early versions of the macrobiotic diet followed a progression that ended with the "ultimate" diet of brown rice and water—a less than nutritionally balanced diet. Today's version reflects a modified vegetarian approach with an appreciation of how foods can enhance health. With careful planning, a macrobiotic diet can provide an array of nutrients that support good health.

If not properly balanced, any diet—vegetarian, macrobiotic, or otherwise—can lack nutrients. Poorly planned vegetarian diets typically lack iron, zinc, calcium, vitamin B_{12}, and vitamin D; without planning, meat-based diets may lack vitamin A, vitamin C, folate, and fiber, among others. Quite simply, the negative health aspects of any diet, including vegetarian diets, reflect poor diet planning. Careful attention to energy intake and specific nutrients of concern can ensure adequacy.

Keep in mind, too, that diet is only one factor influencing health. Whatever a diet consists of, its context is also important: no smoking, alcohol consumption in moderation (if at all), regular physical activity, adequate rest, and medical attention when needed all contribute to good health. Establishing these healthy habits early in life seems to be the most important step one can take to reduce the risks of chronic diseases later in life (as Highlight 16 explains).

*Calcium salts are often added during processing to coagulate the tofu.

CRITICAL THINKING QUESTIONS

A. What are the strengths and weaknesses of vegetarian diets?

B. Your interest in nutrition has been piqued by the concept of a vegetarian diet, and you wisely recognize that a well-planned diet involves more than simply replacing a turkey sandwich with peanut butter crackers. Design and follow a vegetarian meal plan for 3 days, including at least 1 vegan day. Outline the social, personal, and nutritional challenges you faced and describe how you might partially or fully integrate vegetarian meals into your current meal plan.

REFERENCES

1. Position of the American Dietetic Association: Vegetarian diets, *Journal of the American Dietetic Association* 109 (2009): 1266–1282.
2. M. J. Orlich and coauthors, Vegetarian dietary patterns and mortality in Adventist Health Study 2, *JAMA Internal Medicine* 173 (2013): 1230–1238.
3. A. Pan and coauthors, Red meat consumption and mortality, *Archives of Internal Medicine* 172 (2012): 555–563.
4. B. Farmer and coauthors, A vegetarian dietary pattern as a nutrient-dense approach to weight management: An analysis of the National health and Nutrition Examination Survey 1999–2004, *Journal of the American Dietetic Association* 111 (2011): 819–827.
5. S. Tonstad and coauthors, Vegetarian diets and incidence of diabetes in the Adventist Health Study-2, *Nutrition, Metabolism, and Cardiovascular Diseases* 23 (2013): 292–299.
6. B. J. Pettersen and coauthors, Vegetarian diets and blood pressure among white subjects: Results from the Adventist Health Study-2 (AHS-2), *Public Health Nutrition* 15 (2012): 1909–1916.
7. D. G. Hackam and coauthors, The 2010 Canadian Hypertension Education Program recommendations for the management of hypertension: Part 2, therapy, *Canadian Journal of Cardiology* 26 (2010): 249–258.
8. J. Kaluza, A. Wolk, and S. C. Larsson, Red meat consumption and risk of stroke: A meta-analysis of prospective studies, Stroke 43 (2012): 2556–2560; P. M. Clifton, Protein and coronary heart disease: The role of different protein sources, *Current Atherosclerosis Reports* 13 (2011): 493–498.
9. M. Messina, Insights gained from 20 years of soy research, *Journal of Nutrition* 140 (2010): 2289S–2295S.
10. T. Huang and coauthors, Cardiovascular disease mortality and cancer incidence in vegetarians: A meta-analysis and systematic review, *Annals of Nutrition and Metabolism* 60 (2012): 233–240.
11. Position of the American Dietetic Association, 2009.
12. R. Pawlak and coauthors, How prevalent is vitamin B_{12} deficiency among vegetarians? *Nutrition Reviews* 71 (2013): 110–117.
13. A. A. Welch and coauthors, Dietary intake and status of n-3 polyunsaturated fatty acids in a population of fish-eating and non-fish-eating meat-eaters, vegetarians, and vegans and the precursor product ratio of α-linolenic acid to long-chain n 3 polyunsaturated fatty acids: Results from the EPIC-Norfolk cohort, *American Journal of Clinical Nutrition* 92 (2010): 1040–1051.
14. A. M. Bernstein and coauthors, A meta-analysis shows that docosahexaenoic acid from algal oil reduces serum triglycerides and increases HDL-cholesterol and LDL-cholesterol in persons without coronary heart disease, *Journal of Nutrition* 142 (2012): 99–104.
15. W. J. Craig, Nutrition concerns and health effects of vegetarian diets, *Nutrition in Clinical Practice* 25 (2010): 613–620.
16. C. T. McEvoy, N. Temple, and J. V. Woodside, Vegetarian diets, low-meat diets and health: A review, *Public Health Nutrition* 15 (2012): 2287–2294.

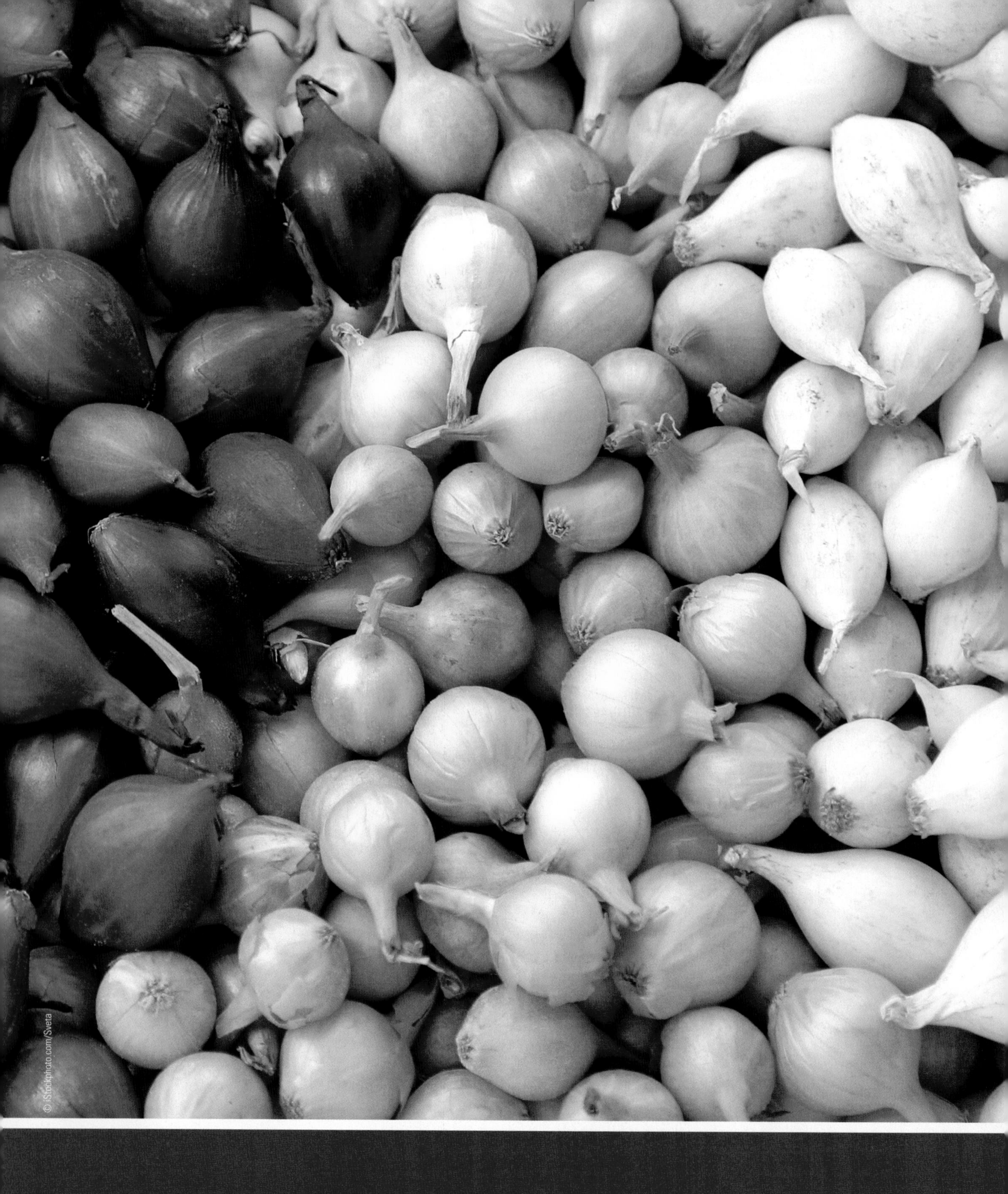

3

Digestion, Absorption, and Transport

LEARNING GPS

Nutrition in Your Life

Have you ever wondered what happens to the food you eat after you swallow it? Or how your body extracts nutrients from food? Have you ever marveled at how it all just seems to happen? Follow foods as they travel through the digestive system. Learn how a healthy digestive system takes whatever food you give it—whether sirloin steak and potatoes or tofu and brussels sprouts—and extracts the nutrients that will nourish the cells of your body. In the Nutrition Portfolio at the end of the chapter, you can determine whether your current eating habits are supporting a healthy digestive system.

Each cell in the body needs a continuous supply of many specific nutrients to maintain itself and carry out its work. These nutrients derive from the foods a person eats, but before the body's cells can use the nutrients, foods must first be broken down mechanically and chemically. This chapter follows the journey that breaks down foods into the nutrients featured in the later chapters. Then it follows the nutrients as they travel through the intestinal cells and into the body to do their work.

As you read about the complexities and intricacies of these processes, take a moment to appreciate the beauty and wisdom of the body. Recognize that the activities of the digestive system are finely coordinated and fully integrated with those of the circulatory, nervous, and hormonal systems. Then be thankful that your body can efficiently take care of its business without any direction from you, but know that it performs its best when you have given it optimal nourishment. This introduction presents a general overview of the processes common to all nutrients; later chapters discuss the specifics of digesting and absorbing individual nutrients.

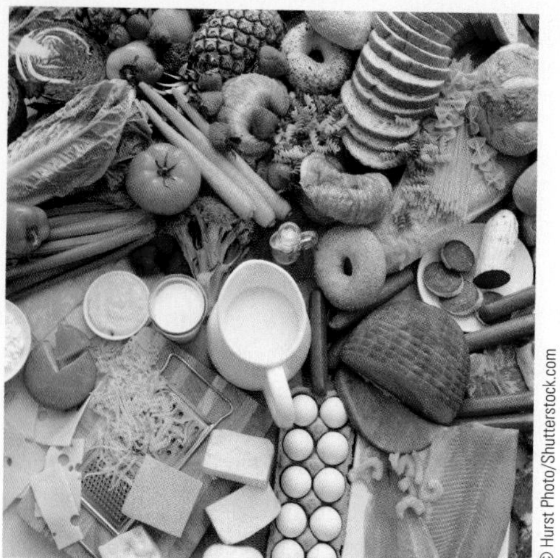
© Hurst Photo/Shutterstock.com

The process of digestion breaks down all kinds of *foods* into *nutrients*.

3.1 Digestion

› LEARN IT Explain how foods move through the digestive system, describing the actions of the organs, muscles, and digestive secretions along the way.

Digestion is the body's ingenious way of breaking down foods into nutrients in preparation for **absorption.** In the process, the body overcomes many challenges without any conscious effort. Consider these challenges:

1. Human beings breathe, eat, and drink through their mouths. Air taken in through the mouth must go to the lungs; food and liquid must go to the stomach. The throat must be arranged so that swallowing and breathing don't interfere with each other.
2. Below the lungs lies the diaphragm, a dome of muscle that separates the upper half of the major body cavity from the lower half. The body needs a passageway that will allow food from the mouth to pass through the diaphragm to reach the stomach below.
3. The contents of the digestive tract should be kept moving forward, slowly but steadily, at a pace that permits all reactions to reach completion.
4. To move through the system, food must be lubricated with fluids. Too much would form a liquid that would flow too rapidly; too little would form a paste too dry and compact to move at all. The amount of fluids must be regulated to keep the intestinal contents at the right consistency to move along smoothly.
5. For digestive enzymes to work, foods must be broken down into small particles and suspended in enough liquid so that every particle is accessible. Once digestion is complete and nutrients have been absorbed from the GI tract into the body, the remaining waste must be excreted. Excreting all the water along with the solid residue, however, would be both wasteful and messy. Some water must be withdrawn, leaving a solid waste product that is easy to pass.
6. The digestive enzymes are designed to digest carbohydrate, fat, and protein. The cells of the GI tract are also made of carbohydrate, fat, and protein. These cells must be protected against the powerful digestive juices that they secrete.
7. Once waste matter has reached the end of the GI tract, it must be excreted, but it would be inconvenient and embarrassing if this function occurred continuously. Evacuation needs to occur periodically.

The following sections show how the body elegantly and efficiently handles these challenges. Each section follows the GI tract from one end to the other—first describing its anatomy, then its muscular actions, and finally its secretions.

Anatomy of the Digestive Tract The **gastrointestinal (GI) tract** is a flexible muscular tube that extends from the mouth, through the esophagus, stomach, small intestine, large intestine, and rectum to the anus. Figure 3-1 on p. 74 traces the path followed by food from one end to the other. In a sense, the human body surrounds the GI tract. The inner space within the GI tract, called the **lumen,** is continuous from one end to the other. (GI anatomy terms appear in boldface type and are defined in the accompanying glossary.) Only when a nutrient or other substance finally penetrates the GI tract's wall does it enter the body proper; many materials pass through the GI tract without being digested or absorbed.

Mouth The process of digestion begins in the **mouth.** During chewing, teeth crush large pieces of food into smaller ones, and fluids from foods, beverages, and salivary glands blend with these pieces to ease swallowing.* Fluids also help dissolve the food so that the tongue can taste it; only particles in solution can react with taste buds. When stimulated, the taste buds detect one, or a combination, of the five basic

*The process of chewing is called *mastication* (mass-tih-KAY-shun).

digestion: the process by which food is broken down into absorbable units.
- **digest** = take apart

absorption: the uptake of nutrients by the cells of the small intestine for transport into either the blood or the lymph.
- **absorb** = suck in

gastrointestinal (GI) tract: the digestive tract. The principal organs are the stomach and intestines.
- **gastro** = stomach
- **intestinalis** = intestine

GLOSSARY OF GI ANATOMY TERMS

anus (AY-nus): the terminal outlet of the GI tract.

appendix: a narrow blind sac extending from the beginning of the colon that contains bacteria and lymph cells.

duodenum (doo-oh-DEEN-um or doo-ODD-num): the top portion of the small intestine (about "12 fingers' breadth" long in ancient terminology).

- **duodecim** = twelve

epiglottis (epp-ih-GLOTT-iss): cartilage in the throat that guards the entrance to the trachea and prevents fluid or food from entering it when a person swallows.

- **epi** = upon (over)
- **glottis** = back of tongue

esophageal (ee -SOFF-ah-GEE-al) **sphincter:** a sphincter muscle at the upper or lower end of the esophagus. The *lower esophageal sphincter* is also called the *cardiac sphincter* because of its proximity to the heart.

esophagus (ee-SOFF-ah-gus): the food pipe; the conduit from the mouth to the stomach.

gallbladder: the organ that stores and concentrates bile. When it receives the signal that fat is present in the duodenum, the gallbladder contracts and squirts bile through the bile duct into the duodenum.

ileocecal (ill-ee-oh-SEEK-ul) **valve:** the sphincter separating the small and large intestines.

ileum (ILL-ee-um): the last segment of the small intestine.

jejunum (je-JOON-um): the first two-fifths of the small intestine beyond the duodenum.

large intestine or **colon** (COAL-un): the lower portion of intestine that completes the digestive process. Its segments are the *ascending colon*, the *transverse colon*, the *descending colon*, and the *sigmoid colon*.

- **sigmoid** = shaped like the letter S (sigma in Greek)

lumen (LOO-men): the space within a vessel such as the intestine.

mouth: the oral cavity containing the tongue and teeth.

pancreas: a gland that secretes digestive enzymes and juices into the duodenum. (The pancreas also secretes hormones into the blood that help to maintain glucose homeostasis.)

pharynx (FAIR-inks): the passageway leading from the nose and mouth to the larynx and esophagus, respectively.

pyloric (pie-LORE-ic) **sphincter:** the circular muscle that separates the stomach from the small intestine and regulates the flow of partially digested food into the small intestine; also called *pylorus* or *pyloric valve*.

- **pylorus** = gatekeeper

rectum: the muscular terminal part of the intestine, extending from the sigmoid colon to the anus.

small intestine: a 10-foot length of small-diameter intestine that is the major site of digestion of food and absorption of nutrients. Its segments are the *duodenum*, *jejunum*, and *ileum*.

sphincter (SFINK-ter): a circular muscle surrounding, and able to close, a body opening. Sphincters are found at specific points along the GI tract and regulate the flow of food particles.

- **sphincter** = band (binder)

stomach: a muscular, elastic, saclike portion of the digestive tract that grinds and churns swallowed food, mixing it with acid and enzymes to form chyme.

taste sensations: sweet, sour, bitter, salty and umami (oo-MOM-ee), a savory flavor commonly associated with monosodium glutamate.[1] In addition to these chemical triggers, aroma, appearance, texture, and temperature also affect a food's flavor.

The tongue provides taste sensations and moves food around the mouth, facilitating chewing and swallowing. When a mouthful of food is swallowed, it passes through the **pharynx,** a short tube that is shared by both the **digestive system** and the respiratory system. To bypass the entrance to the lungs, the **epiglottis** closes off the airway so that choking doesn't occur when swallowing, thus resolving the first challenge. (Choking is discussed on pp. 90–91.) After a mouthful of food has been chewed and swallowed, it is called a **bolus.**

Esophagus The **esophagus** has a **sphincter** muscle at each end. During a swallow, the upper **esophageal sphincter** opens. The bolus then slides down the esophagus, which passes through a hole in the diaphragm (challenge 2) to the stomach. The lower esophageal sphincter at the entrance to the stomach closes behind the bolus so that it proceeds forward and doesn't slip back into the esophagus (challenge 3).

Stomach The **stomach** retains the bolus for a while in its upper portion. Little by little, the stomach transfers the food to its lower portion, adds juices to it, and grinds it to a semiliquid mass called **chyme.** Then, bit by bit, the stomach releases the chyme through the **pyloric sphincter,** which opens into the **small intestine** and then closes behind the chyme.

Small Intestine At the beginning of the small intestine, the chyme bypasses the opening from the common bile duct, which is dripping fluids (challenge 4) into the small intestine from two organs outside the GI tract—the **gallbladder** and the **pancreas.** The chyme travels on down the small intestine through its three segments—the **duodenum,** the **jejunum,** and the **ileum**—almost 10 feet of tubing coiled within the abdomen.*

Large Intestine (Colon) Having traveled the length of the small intestine, the remaining contents arrive at another sphincter (challenge 3 again): the **ileocecal valve,** located at the beginning of the **large intestine (colon)** in the lower right side of the abdomen. Upon entering the colon, the contents pass another opening. Should

*The small intestine is almost two and a half times shorter in living adults than it is at death, when muscles are relaxed and elongated.

digestive system: all the organs and glands associated with the ingestion and digestion of food.

bolus (BOH-lus): a portion; with respect to food, the amount swallowed at one time.

- **bolos** = lump

chyme (KIME): the semiliquid mass of partly digested food expelled by the stomach into the duodenum.

- **chymos** = juice

> **FIGURE 3-1** **The Gastrointestinal Tract**

INGESTION

↓

Mouth
Chews and mixes food with saliva

Pharynx
Directs food from mouth to esophagus

Salivary glands
Secrete saliva

Epiglottis
Protects airways during swallowing

Trachea
Allows air to pass to and from lungs

Esophagus
Passes food from the mouth to the stomach

Esophageal sphincters
Allow passage from mouth to esophagus and from esophagus to stomach; prevent backflow from stomach to esophagus and from esophagus to mouth

Diaphragm
Separates the abdomen from the thoracic cavity

Stomach
Churns, mixes, and grinds food to a liquid mass; adds acid, enzymes, and fluid

Pyloric sphincter
Allows passage from stomach to small intestine; prevents backflow from small intestine

Liver
Manufactures bile salts, detergent-like substances, to help digest fats

Gallbladder
Stores bile until needed

Bile duct
Conducts bile from the gallbladder to the small intestine

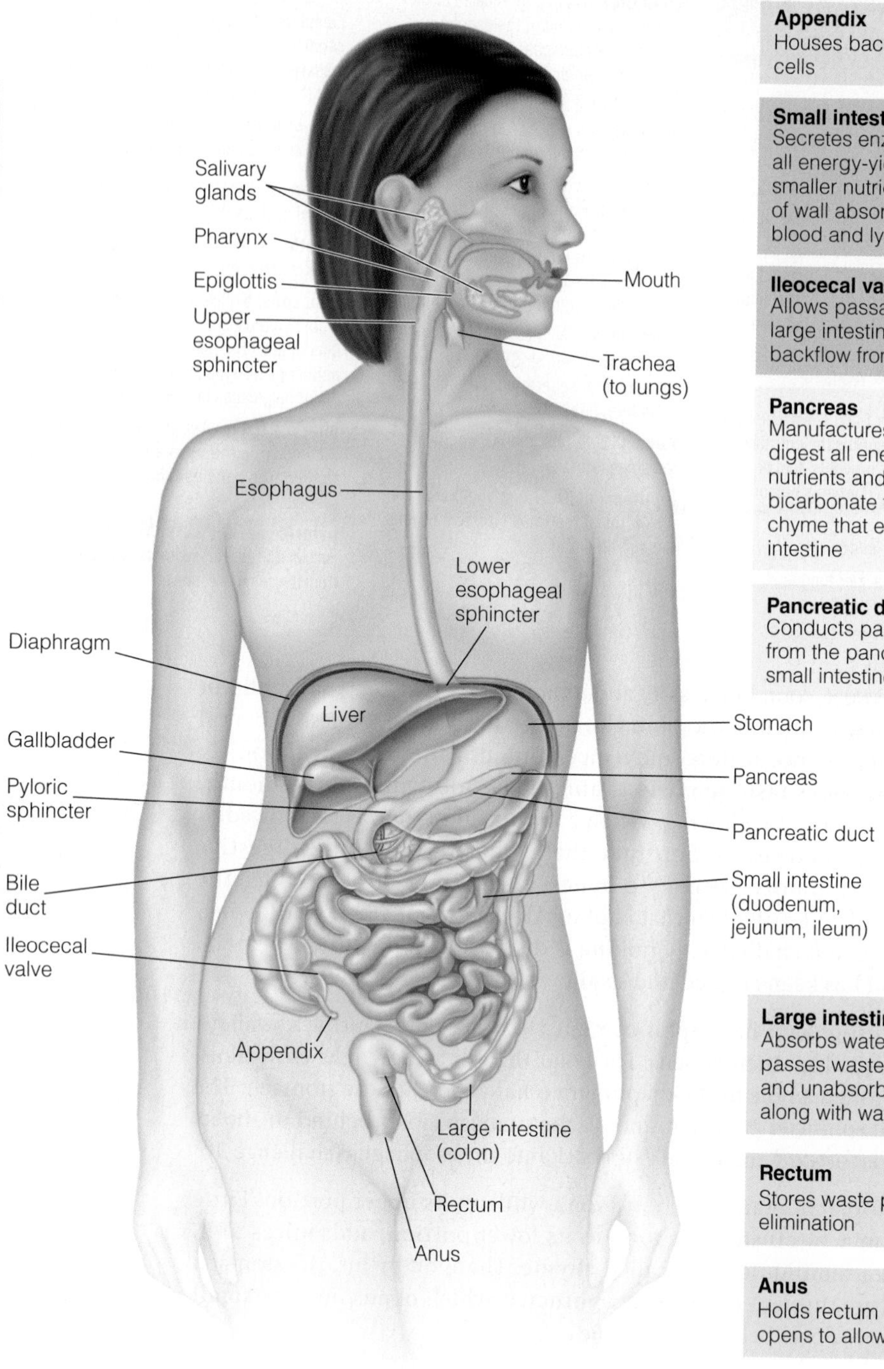

Salivary glands
Pharynx
Epiglottis
Upper esophageal sphincter
Mouth
Trachea (to lungs)
Esophagus
Lower esophageal sphincter
Diaphragm
Liver
Gallbladder
Stomach
Pyloric sphincter
Pancreas
Pancreatic duct
Bile duct
Small intestine (duodenum, jejunum, ileum)
Ileocecal valve
Appendix
Large intestine (colon)
Rectum
Anus

Appendix
Houses bacteria and lymph cells

Small intestine
Secretes enzymes that digest all energy-yielding nutrients to smaller nutrient particles; cells of wall absorb nutrients into blood and lymph

Ileocecal valve (sphincter)
Allows passage from small to large intestine; prevents backflow from large intestine

Pancreas
Manufactures enzymes to digest all energy-yielding nutrients and releases bicarbonate to neutralize acid chyme that enters the small intestine

Pancreatic duct
Conducts pancreatic juice from the pancreas to the small intestine

Large intestine (colon)
Absorbs water and minerals; passes waste (fiber, bacteria, and unabsorbed nutrients) along with water to the rectum

Rectum
Stores waste prior to elimination

Anus
Holds rectum closed; opens to allow elimination

ELIMINATION

↓

any intestinal contents slip into this opening, it would end up in the **appendix,** a blind sac about the size of your little finger. Normally, the contents bypass this opening, however, and travel along the large intestine up the right side of the abdomen, across the front to the left side, down to the lower left side, and finally below the other folds of the intestines to the back of the body, above the **rectum** (see Figure 3-2).

As the intestinal contents pass to the rectum, the colon withdraws water, leaving semisolid waste (challenge 5). The strong muscles of the rectum and anal canal hold back this waste until it is time to defecate. Then the rectal muscles relax (challenge 7), and the two sphincters of the **anus** open to allow passage of the waste.

The Muscular Action of Digestion

In the mouth, chewing, the addition of saliva, and the action of the tongue transform food into a coarse mash that can be swallowed. After swallowing, all the activity that follows occurs without much conscience thought. As is the case with so much else that happens in the body, the muscles of the digestive tract meet internal needs without any concerted effort on your part. They keep things moving at just the right pace, slow enough to get the job done and fast enough to make progress.*

Peristalsis The entire GI tract is ringed with circular muscles. Surrounding these rings of muscle are longitudinal muscles. When the rings tighten and the long muscles relax, the tube is constricted. When the rings relax and the long muscles tighten, the tube bulges. This action—called **peristalsis**—occurs continuously and pushes the intestinal contents along (challenge 3 again). (If you have ever watched a lump of food pass along the body of a snake, you have a good picture of how these muscles work.)

The waves of contraction normally ripple along the GI tract at varying rates and intensities depending on the part of the GI tract and on whether food is present. Factors such as stress, medicines, and medical conditions may interfere with normal GI tract contractions.

> FIGURE 3-2 **The Colon**

The colon begins with the ascending colon rising upward toward the liver. It becomes the transverse colon as it turns and crosses the body toward the spleen. The descending colon turns downward and becomes the sigmoid colon, which extends to the rectum. Along the way, the colon mixes the intestinal contents, absorbs water and salts, and forms stools.

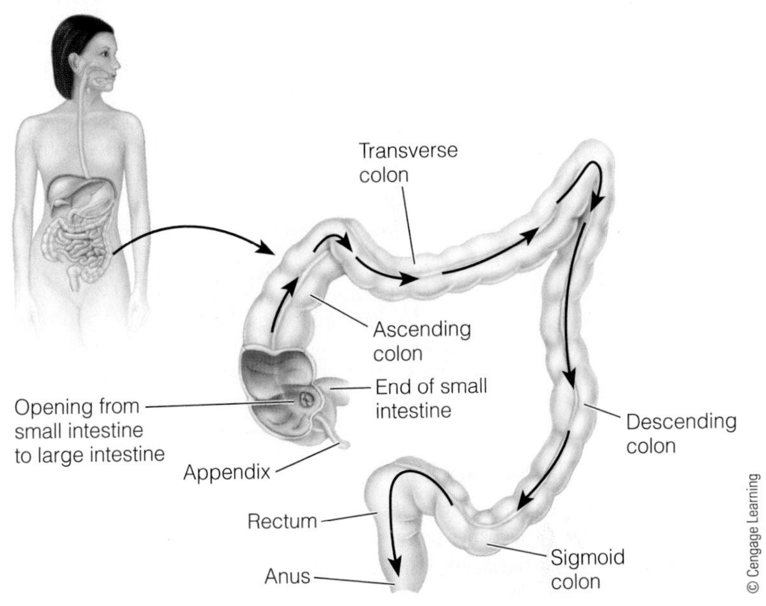

Stomach Action The stomach has the thickest walls and strongest muscles of all the GI tract organs. In addition to the circular and longitudinal muscles, it has a third layer of diagonal muscles that also alternately contract and relax (see Figure 3-3). These three sets of muscles work to force the chyme downward, but the pyloric sphincter usually remains tightly closed, preventing the chyme from passing into the duodenum of the small intestine. As a result, the chyme is churned and forced down, hits the pyloric sphincter, and remains in the stomach. Meanwhile, the stomach wall releases gastric juices. When the chyme is completely liquefied with gastric juices, the pyloric sphincter opens briefly, about three times a minute, to allow small portions of chyme to pass through. At this point, the chyme no longer resembles food in the least.

> FIGURE 3-3 **Stomach Muscles**

The stomach has three layers of muscles.

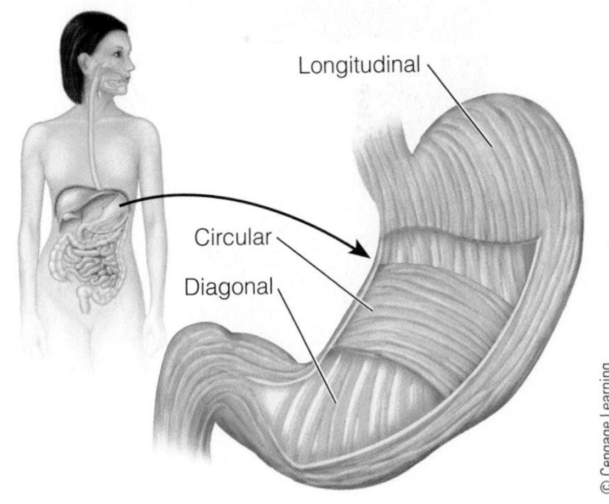

Segmentation The circular muscles of the intestines rhythmically contract and squeeze their contents. These contractions, called **segmentation,** mix the chyme and promote close contact with the digestive juices and the absorbing cells of the intestinal walls before letting the contents move slowly along.

Sphincter Contractions Sphincter muscles periodically open and close, allowing the contents of the GI tract to move along at a controlled pace (challenge 3 again). At the top of the esophagus, the upper esophageal sphincter opens in response to swallowing. At the bottom of the esophagus, the lower esophageal sphincter (sometimes called the cardiac sphincter because of its proximity to the heart) prevents **reflux** of the stomach contents. At the bottom of the stomach, the pyloric sphincter, which stays closed most of the time, holds the chyme in the stomach long enough for it to be thoroughly mixed with gastric juice and liquefied. The pyloric sphincter also prevents the intestinal contents from backing up into the stomach. At the end of the small intestine, the ileocecal valve performs a similar function, allowing

*The spontaneous movement of the GI tract muscles is called *motility* (moh-TIL-ih-tee).

peristalsis (per-ih-STALL-sis): wavelike muscular contractions of the GI tract that push its contents along.
- **peri** = around
- **stellein** = wrap

segmentation (SEG-men-TAY-shun): a periodic squeezing or partitioning of the intestine at intervals along its length by its circular muscles.

reflux: a backward flow.
- **re** = back
- **flux** = flow

> **FIGURE 3-4 An Example of a Sphincter Muscle**

When the circular muscles of a sphincter contract, the passage closes; when they relax, the passage opens.

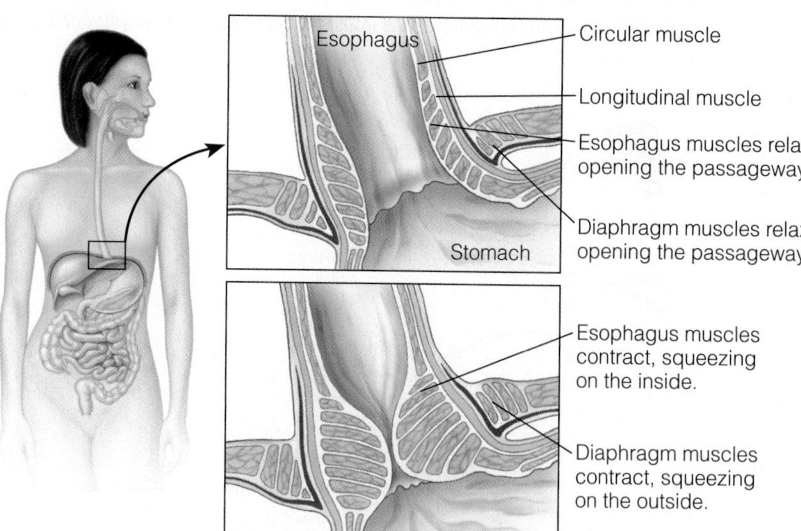

Esophagus
Circular muscle
Longitudinal muscle
Esophagus muscles relax, opening the passageway.
Diaphragm muscles relax, opening the passageway.
Stomach
Esophagus muscles contract, squeezing on the inside.
Diaphragm muscles contract, squeezing on the outside.

the contents of the small intestine to empty into the large intestine. Finally, the tightness of the rectal muscle acts as a kind of safety device; together with the two sphincters of the anus, it prevents continuous elimination (challenge 7). Figure 3-4 illustrates how sphincter muscles contract and relax to close and open passageways.

The Secretions of Digestion The breakdown of food into nutrients requires secretions from five different organs: the salivary glands, the stomach, the pancreas, the liver (via the gallbladder), and the small intestine. These secretions enter the GI tract at various points along the way, bringing an abundance of water (challenge 4) and a variety of enzymes.

Enzymes are formally introduced in Chapter 6, but for now a simple definition will suffice. An enzyme is a protein that facilitates a chemical reaction—making a molecule, breaking a molecule apart, changing the arrangement of a molecule, or exchanging parts of molecules. As a **catalyst,** the enzyme itself remains unchanged. The enzymes involved in digestion facilitate a chemical reaction known as **hydrolysis**—the addition of water *(hydro)* to break *(lysis)* a molecule into smaller pieces. The glossary below describes how to identify some of the common **digestive enzymes** and related terms; later chapters introduce specific enzymes. When learning about enzymes, it helps to know that the word ending ***-ase*** denotes an enzyme. Enzymes are often identified by the organ they come from and the compounds they work on. *Gastric lipase,* for example, is a stomach enzyme that acts on lipids, whereas *pancreatic lipase* comes from the pancreas (and also works on lipids).

> **FIGURE 3-5 The Salivary Glands**

The salivary glands secrete enzyme-rich saliva into the mouth and begin the digestive process. Given the short time food is in the mouth, salivary enzymes contribute little to digestion.

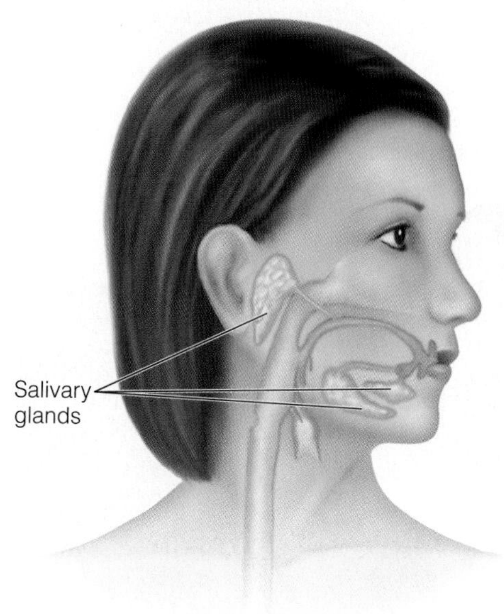

Saliva The **salivary glands,** shown in Figure 3-5, squirt just enough **saliva** to moisten each mouthful of food so that it can pass easily down the esophagus (challenge 4). (Digestive **glands** and their secretions are defined in the glossary on p. 77.) The saliva contains water, salts, mucus, and enzymes that initiate the digestion of carbohydrates. Saliva also protects the teeth and the linings of the mouth, esophagus, and stomach from substances that might cause damage.

Gastric Juice In the stomach, **gastric glands** secrete **gastric juice,** a mixture of water, enzymes, and **hydrochloric acid,** which acts primarily in protein digestion. The acid is so strong that it causes the sensation of heartburn if it happens to reflux into the esophagus. Highlight 3, following this chapter, discusses heartburn, ulcers, and other common digestive problems.

The strong acidity of the stomach prevents bacterial growth and kills most bacteria that enter the body with food. It would destroy the cells of the stomach as well, but for their natural defenses. To protect themselves from gastric juice, the cells of the stomach wall (in fact, of the entire gastrointestinal lining) secrete **mucus,** a

catalyst (CAT-uh-list): a compound that facilitates chemical reactions without itself being changed in the process.

GLOSSARY OF DIGESTIVE ENZYMES

-ase (ACE): suffix denoting an enzyme. The root of the word often identifies the compound the enzyme works on. Examples include:

- *carbohydrase* (KAR-boe-HIGH-drase), an enzyme that hydrolyzes carbohydrates.
- *lipase* (LYE-pase), an enzyme that hydrolyzes lipids (fats).
- *protease* (PRO-tee-ase), an enzyme that hydrolyzes proteins.

digestive enzymes: proteins found in digestive juices that act on food substances, causing them to break down into simpler compounds.

hydrolysis (high-DROL-ih-sis): a chemical reaction in which one molecule is split into two molecules, with hydrogen (H) added to one and a hydroxyl group (OH) added to the other (from water, H_2O). (The noun is *hydrolysis*; the verb is *hydrolyze.*)

- **hydro** = water
- **lysis** = breaking

thick, slippery, white substance that coats the cells, protecting them from the acid, enzymes, and disease-causing bacteria that might otherwise cause harm (challenge 6).

Figure 3-6 shows how the strength of acids is measured—in **pH** units. Note that the acidity of gastric juice registers below 2 on the pH scale—stronger than vinegar. The stomach enzymes work most efficiently in the stomach's strong acid, but the salivary enzymes, which are swallowed with food, do not work in acid this strong. Consequently, the salivary digestion of carbohydrates gradually ceases when the stomach acid penetrates each newly swallowed bolus of food. Once in the stomach, salivary enzymes simply become other proteins to be digested.

Pancreatic Juice and Intestinal Enzymes By the time food leaves the stomach, digestion of all three energy nutrients (carbohydrates, fats, and proteins) has begun, and the action gains momentum in the small intestine. There the pancreas contributes digestive juices by way of ducts leading into the duodenum. The **pancreatic juice** contains enzymes that act on all three energy nutrients, and the cells of the intestinal wall also possess digestive enzymes on their surfaces.

In addition to enzymes, the pancreatic juice contains sodium **bicarbonate,** which is basic or alkaline—the opposite of the stomach's acid (review Figure 3-6). The pancreatic juice thus neutralizes the acidic chyme arriving in the small intestine from the stomach. From this point on, the chyme remains at a neutral or slightly alkaline pH. The enzymes of both the intestine and the pancreas work best in this environment.

Bile **Bile** also flows into the duodenum. The **liver** continuously produces bile, which is then concentrated and stored in the gallbladder. The gallbladder squirts bile into the duodenum of the small intestine when fat arrives there. Bile is not an enzyme; it is an **emulsifier** that brings fats into suspension in water so that enzymes can break them down into their component parts. A summary of digestive secretions and their actions is presented in Table 3-1 on p. 78.

The Final Stage At this point, the three energy-yielding nutrients—carbohydrate, fat, and protein—have been digested and are ready to be absorbed. Some vitamins and minerals are altered slightly during digestion, but most are absorbed as they are. Undigested residues, such as some fibers, are not absorbed. Instead, they continue through the digestive tract, carrying some minerals, bile acids, additives, and contaminants out of the body. This semisolid mass helps exercise the GI muscles and keep them strong enough to perform peristalsis efficiently. Fiber also retains water, accounting for the consistency of **stools.**

By the time the contents of the GI tract reach the end of the small intestine, little remains but water, a few dissolved salts and body secretions, and undigested materials such as fiber (with some fat, cholesterol, and a few minerals bound to it). All of this remaining matter enters the large intestine (colon).

> FIGURE 3-6 **The pH Scale**

A substance's acidity or alkalinity is measured in pH units. The pH is the negative logarithm of the hydrogen ion concentration. Each increment represents a tenfold increase in concentration of hydrogen ions, meaning, for example, that a pH of 2 is 1000 times stronger than a pH of 5.

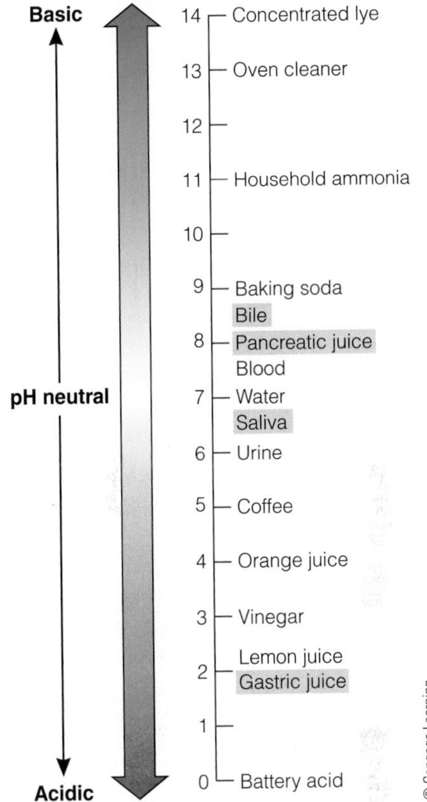

pH: the unit of measure expressing a substance's acidity or alkalinity. The lower the pH, the higher the H^+ ion concentration and the stronger the acid. A pH above 7 is alkaline, or base (a solution in which OH^- ions predominate).

stools: waste matter discharged from the colon; also called *feces* (FEE-seez).

GLOSSARY OF DIGESTIVE GLANDS AND THEIR SECRETIONS

bicarbonate: an alkaline compound with the formula HCO_3 that is secreted from the pancreas as part of the pancreatic juice. (Bicarbonate is also produced in all cell fluids from the dissociation of carbonic acid to help maintain the body's acid-base balance.)

bile: an emulsifier that prepares fats and oils for digestion; an exocrine secretion made by the liver, stored in the gallbladder, and released into the small intestine when needed.

emulsifier (ee-MUL-sih-fire): a substance with both water-soluble and fat-soluble portions that promotes the mixing of oils and fats in a watery solution.

gastric glands: exocrine glands in the stomach wall that secrete gastric juice into the stomach.

- **gastro** = stomach

gastric juice: the digestive secretion of the gastric glands of the stomach.

glands: cells or groups of cells that secrete materials for special uses in the body. Glands may be *exocrine* (EKS-oh-crin) *glands*, secreting their materials "out" (into the digestive tract or onto the surface of the skin), or *endocrine* (EN-doe-crin) *glands*, secreting their materials "in" (into the blood).

- **exo** = outside
- **endo** = inside
- **krine** = to separate

hydrochloric acid: an acid composed of hydrogen and chloride atoms (HCl) that is normally produced by the gastric glands.

liver: the organ that manufactures bile, among many other functions (described in Chapter 7).

mucus (MYOO-kus): a slippery substance secreted by cells of the GI lining (and other body linings) that protects the cells from exposure to digestive juices (and other destructive agents). The lining of the GI tract with its coat of mucus is a *mucous membrane.* (The noun is *mucus;* the adjective is *mucous.*)

pancreatic (pank-ree-AT-ic) **juice:** the exocrine secretion of the pancreas that contains both enzymes for the digestion of carbohydrate, fat, and protein as well as bicarbonate, a neutralizing agent. The juice flows from the pancreas into the small intestine through the pancreatic duct. (The pancreas also has an endocrine function, the secretion of insulin and other hormones.)

saliva: the secretion of the salivary glands. Its principal enzyme begins carbohydrate digestion.

salivary glands: exocrine glands that secrete saliva into the mouth.

TABLE 3-1 Summary of Digestive Secretions and Their Major Actions

Organ or Gland	Target Organ	Secretion	Action
Salivary glands	Mouth	Saliva	Fluid eases swallowing; salivary enzyme breaks down some **carbohydrate.***
Gastric glands	Stomach	Gastric juice	Fluid mixes with bolus; hydrochloric acid uncoils **proteins;** enzymes break down proteins; mucus protects stomach cells.*
Pancreas	Small intestine	Pancreatic juice	Bicarbonate neutralizes acidic gastric juices; pancreatic enzymes break down **carbohydrates, fats,** and **proteins.**
Liver	Gallbladder	Bile	Bile is stored until needed.
Gallbladder	Small intestine	Bile	Bile emulsifies **fat** so that enzymes can have access to break it down.
Intestinal glands	Small intestine	Intestinal juice	Intestinal enzymes break down **carbohydrate, fat,** and **protein** fragments; mucus protects the intestinal wall.

*Saliva and gastric juice also contain lipases, but most fat breakdown occurs in the small intestine.

In the colon, intestinal bacteria ferment some fibers, producing water, gas, and small fragments of fat that provide energy for the cells of the colon. The colon itself retrieves all materials that the body can recycle—water and dissolved salts. The waste that is finally excreted has little or nothing of value left in it. The body has extracted all that it can use from the food. Figure 3-7 summarizes digestion by following a sandwich through the GI tract and into the body.

› REVIEW IT Explain how foods move through the digestive system, describing the actions of the organs, muscles, and digestive secretions along the way.
As Figure 3-1 shows, food enters the mouth and travels down the esophagus and through the upper and lower esophageal sphincters to the stomach, then through the pyloric sphincter to the small intestine, on through the ileocecal valve to the large intestine, past the appendix to the rectum, ending at the anus. The wavelike contractions of peristalsis and the periodic squeezing of segmentation keep things moving at a reasonable pace. Along the way, secretions from the salivary glands, stomach, pancreas, liver (via the gallbladder), and small intestine deliver fluids and digestive enzymes.

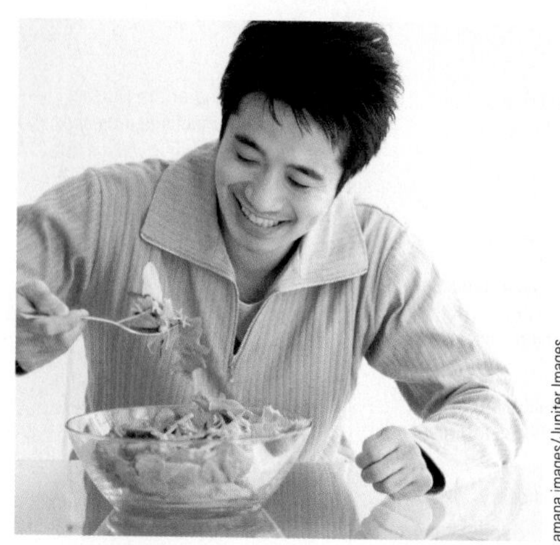

Foods must first be digested and nutrients must be absorbed before the body can use them.

3.2 Absorption

› LEARN IT Describe the anatomical details of the intestinal cells that facilitate nutrient absorption.

Within three or four hours after a person has eaten a dinner of beans and rice (or spinach lasagna, or steak and potatoes) with vegetable, salad, beverage, and dessert, the body must find a way to absorb the molecules derived from carbohydrate, protein, and fat digestion—and the vitamin and mineral molecules as well. Most absorption takes place in the small intestine, one of the most elegantly designed organ systems in the body. Within its 10-foot length, which provides a surface area equivalent to a tennis court, the small intestine traps and absorbs the nutrient molecules. To remove the absorbed molecules rapidly and provide room for more to be absorbed, a rush of circulating blood continuously washes the underside of this surface, carrying the absorbed nutrients away to the liver and other parts of the body. Figure 3-8 on p. 80 describes how most nutrients are absorbed by simple diffusion, facilitated diffusion, or active transport. Later

> FIGURE 3-7 **The Digestive Fate of a Sandwich**

To review the digestive processes, follow a peanut butter and banana sandwich on whole-wheat, sesame seed bread through the GI tract. As the graph on the right illustrates, digestion of the energy nutrients begins in different parts of the GI tract, but all are ready for absorption by the time they reach the end of the small intestine.

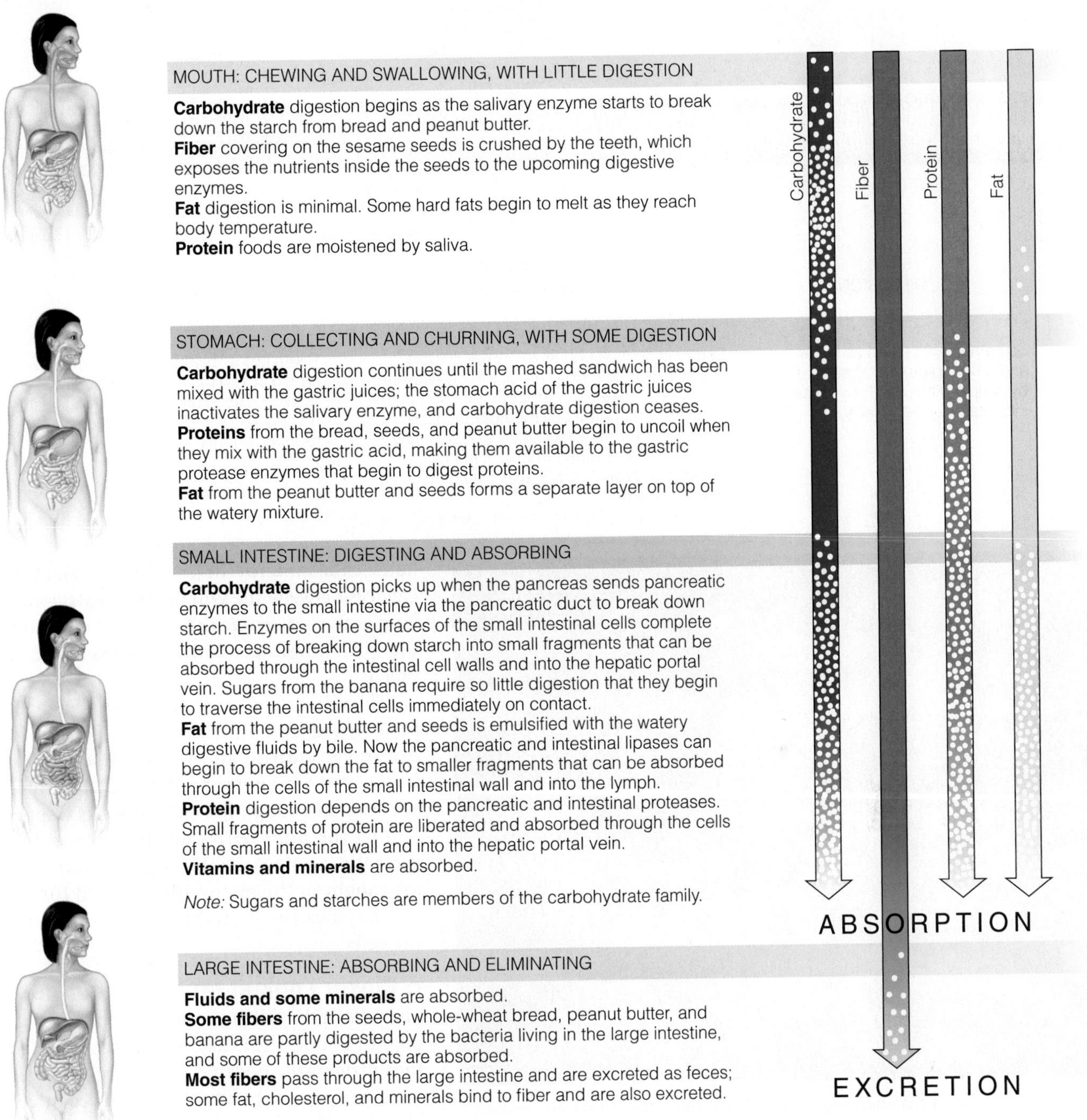

chapters provide details on specific nutrients. Before following nutrients through the body, we must look more closely at the anatomy of the absorptive system.

MOUTH: CHEWING AND SWALLOWING, WITH LITTLE DIGESTION
Carbohydrate digestion begins as the salivary enzyme starts to break down the starch from bread and peanut butter.
Fiber covering on the sesame seeds is crushed by the teeth, which exposes the nutrients inside the seeds to the upcoming digestive enzymes.
Fat digestion is minimal. Some hard fats begin to melt as they reach body temperature.
Protein foods are moistened by saliva.
STOMACH: COLLECTING AND CHURNING, WITH SOME DIGESTION
Carbohydrate digestion continues until the mashed sandwich has been mixed with the gastric juices; the stomach acid of the gastric juices inactivates the salivary enzyme, and carbohydrate digestion ceases.
Proteins from the bread, seeds, and peanut butter begin to uncoil when they mix with the gastric acid, making them available to the gastric protease enzymes that begin to digest proteins.
Fat from the peanut butter and seeds forms a separate layer on top of the watery mixture.
SMALL INTESTINE: DIGESTING AND ABSORBING
Carbohydrate digestion picks up when the pancreas sends pancreatic enzymes to the small intestine via the pancreatic duct to break down starch. Enzymes on the surfaces of the small intestinal cells complete the process of breaking down starch into small fragments that can be absorbed through the intestinal cell walls and into the hepatic portal vein. Sugars from the banana require so little digestion that they begin to traverse the intestinal cells immediately on contact.
Fat from the peanut butter and seeds is emulsified with the watery digestive fluids by bile. Now the pancreatic and intestinal lipases can begin to break down the fat to smaller fragments that can be absorbed through the cells of the small intestinal wall and into the lymph.
Protein digestion depends on the pancreatic and intestinal proteases. Small fragments of protein are liberated and absorbed through the cells of the small intestinal wall and into the hepatic portal vein.
Vitamins and minerals are absorbed.
Note: Sugars and starches are members of the carbohydrate family.
LARGE INTESTINE: ABSORBING AND ELIMINATING
Fluids and some minerals are absorbed.
Some fibers from the seeds, whole-wheat bread, peanut butter, and banana are partly digested by the bacteria living in the large intestine, and some of these products are absorbed.
Most fibers pass through the large intestine and are excreted as feces; some fat, cholesterol, and minerals bind to fiber and are also excreted.
Carbohydrate
Fiber
Protein
Fat
ABSORPTION
EXCRETION

Anatomy of the Absorptive System The inner surface of the small intestine looks smooth and slippery, but when viewed through a microscope, it turns out to be wrinkled into hundreds of folds. Each fold is contoured into thousands of fingerlike projections, as numerous as the hairs on velvet fabric. These small intestinal projections are called **villi**. A single villus, magnified still more, turns out to be composed of hundreds of cells, each covered with its own microscopic

villi (VILL-ee or VILL-eye): fingerlike projections from the folds of the small intestine; singular *villus*.

> FIGURE 3-8 **Absorption of Nutrients**

Absorption of nutrients into intestinal cells typically occurs by simple diffusion, facilitated diffusion, or active transport. Occasionally, a large molecule is absorbed by *endocytosis*—a process in which the cell membrane engulfs the molecule, forming a sac that separates from the membrane and moves into the cell.

Outside cell

Cell membrane

Inside cell

SIMPLE DIFFUSION

Carrier loads nutrient on outside of cell . . .

. . . and then releases it on inside of cell.

FACILITATED DIFFUSION

Carrier loads nutrient on outside of cell . . .

Energy

. . . and then releases it on inside of cell.

ACTIVE TRANSPORT

Some nutrients (such as water and small lipids) are absorbed by simple diffusion. They cross into intestinal cells freely.

Some nutrients (such as the water-soluble vitamins) are absorbed by facilitated diffusion. They need a specific carrier to transport them from one side of the cell membrane to the other. (Alternatively, facilitated diffusion may occur when the carrier changes the cell membrane in such a way that the nutrients can pass through.)

Some nutrients (such as glucose and amino acids) must be absorbed actively. These nutrients move against a concentration gradient, which requires energy.

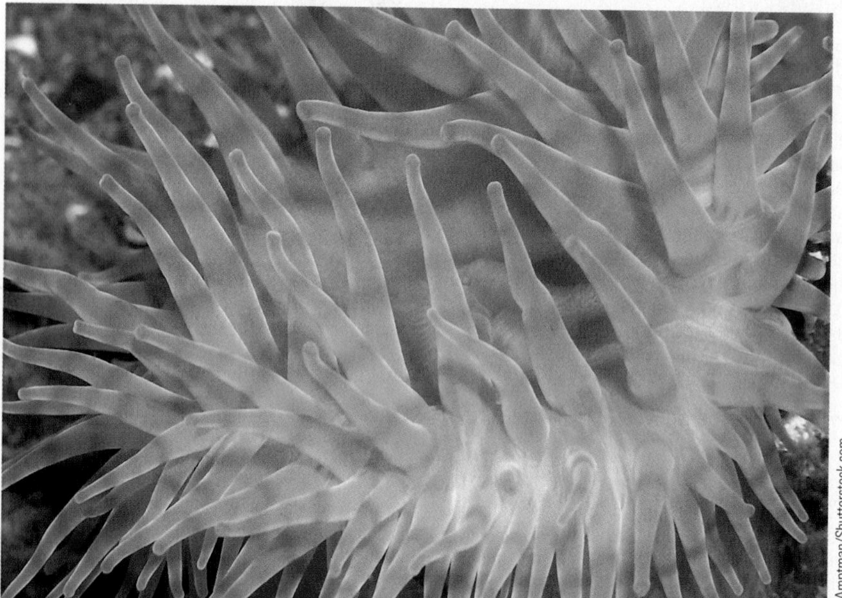

If you have ever watched a sea anemone with its fingerlike projections in constant motion, you have a good picture of how the intestinal villi move.

hairs, called **microvilli** (see Figure 3-9). In the crevices between the villi lie the **crypts**—tubular glands that secrete the intestinal juices into the small intestine. Nearby **goblet cells** secrete mucus.

The villi are in constant motion. Each villus is lined by a thin sheet of muscle, so it can wave, squirm, and wriggle like the tentacles of a sea anemone. Any nutrient molecule small enough to be absorbed is trapped among the microvilli and then drawn into the cells. Some partially digested nutrients are caught in the microvilli, digested further by enzymes there, and then absorbed into the cells.

A Closer Look at the Intestinal Cells

The cells of the villi are among the most amazing in the body, for they recognize and select the nutrients the body needs and regulate their absorption. As already described, each cell of a villus is coated with thousands of microvilli, which project from the cell's membrane (review Figure 3-9). In these microvilli, and in the membrane, lie hundreds of different kinds of enzymes and "pumps," which recognize and act on different nutrients. Descriptions of specific enzymes and pumps for each nutrient are presented in later chapters where appropriate; the point here is that the cells are equipped to handle all kinds and combinations of foods and their nutrients.

Specialized Cells A further refinement of the system is that the cells of successive portions of the intestinal tract are specialized to absorb different nutrients. The nutrients that are ready for absorption early are absorbed near the top of the GI

microvilli (MY-cro-VILL-ee or MY-cro-VILL-eye): tiny, hairlike projections on each cell of every villus that can trap nutrient particles and transport them into the cells; singular *microvillus*.

crypts (KRIPTS): tubular glands that lie between the intestinal villi and secrete intestinal juices into the small intestine.

goblet cells: cells of the GI tract (and lungs) that secrete mucus.

> **FIGURE 3-9 The Small Intestinal Villi**

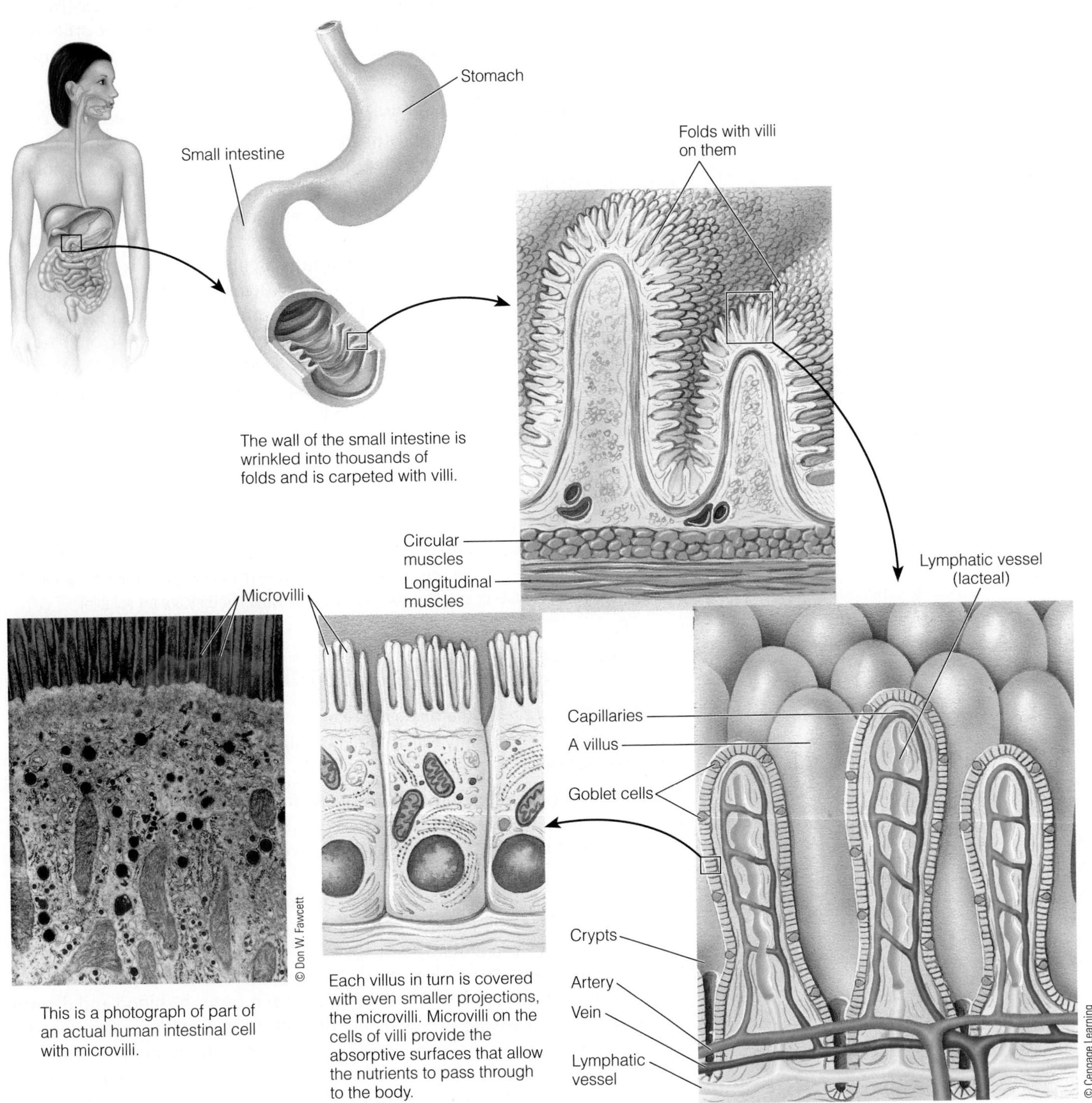

tract; those that take longer to be digested are absorbed farther down. Healthcare professionals who treat digestive disorders learn the specialized absorptive functions of different parts of the GI tract so that if one part becomes dysfunctional, the diet can be adjusted accordingly.

Food Combining The idea that people should not eat certain food combinations (for example, fruit and meat) at the same meal, because the digestive system cannot handle more than one task at a time, is a myth. The art of "food combining"—which actually emphasizes "food separating"—is based on this myth, and it represents faulty logic and a gross underestimation of the body's capabilities. In fact, the contrary is often true; foods eaten together can enhance each other's use by the body. For example, vitamin C in a pineapple or other citrus fruit can enhance the absorption of iron from a meal of chicken and rice or other iron-containing foods. Many other instances of mutually beneficial interactions are presented in later chapters.

Preparing Nutrients for Transport When a nutrient molecule has crossed the cell of a villus, it enters either the bloodstream or the lymphatic system. Both transport systems supply vessels to each villus, as shown in Figure 3-9. The water-soluble nutrients and the smaller products of fat digestion are released directly into the bloodstream and guided directly to the liver, where their fate and destination will be determined.

The larger fats and the fat-soluble vitamins are insoluble in water, however, and blood is mostly water. The intestinal cells assemble many of the products of fat digestion into larger molecules. These larger molecules cluster together with special proteins, forming chylomicrons. Chylomicrons (kye-lo-MY-cronz) are defined and described in more detail in Chapter 5. For now, keep in mind that because chylomicrons carry fats, they are released into the lymphatic system. They move through the lymph until they can enter the bloodstream at a point near the heart. Consequently, chylomicrons bypass the liver at first. Details follow.

› REVIEW IT Describe the anatomical details of the intestinal cells that facilitate nutrient absorption.

The many folds and villi of the small intestine dramatically increase its surface area, facilitating nutrient absorption. Nutrients pass through the cells of the villi and enter either the blood (if they are water soluble or small fat fragments) or the lymph (if they are fat soluble).

3.3 The Circulatory Systems

› LEARN IT Explain how nutrients are routed in the circulatory systems from the GI tract into the body and identify which nutrients enter the blood directly and which must first enter the lymph.

Once a nutrient has entered the bloodstream, it may be transported to any of the cells in the body, from the tips of the toes to the roots of the hair. The circulatory systems deliver nutrients wherever they are needed.

The Vascular System The vascular, or blood circulatory, system is a closed system of vessels through which blood flows continuously, with the heart serving as the pump (see Figure 3-10). As the blood circulates through this system, it picks up and delivers materials as needed.

All the body tissues derive nutrients and oxygen from the blood and deposit carbon dioxide and other wastes back into the blood. The digestive system supplies the nutrients. The lungs exchange oxygen (which enters the blood to be delivered to all cells) and carbon dioxide (which leaves the blood to be exhaled). The kidneys filter wastes other than carbon dioxide out of the blood to be excreted in the urine.

Blood leaving the right side of the heart circulates through the lungs and then back to the left side of the heart. The left side of the heart then pumps the blood out of the **aorta** through **arteries** to all systems of the body. The blood circulates in the **capillaries,** where it exchanges material with the cells and then collects into **veins,** which return it again to the right side of the heart. In short, blood travels this simple route:

Heart to arteries to capillaries to veins to heart

The routing of the blood leaving the digestive system has a special feature. The blood is carried to the digestive system (as to all organs) by way of an artery, which (as in all organs) branches into capillaries to reach every cell. Blood leaving the digestive system, however, goes by way of a vein. The **hepatic portal vein** directs blood not back to the heart but to another organ, the liver. This

aorta (ay-OR-tuh): the large, primary artery that conducts blood from the heart to the body's smaller arteries.

arteries: vessels that carry blood from the heart to the tissues.

capillaries (CAP-ill-aries): small vessels that branch from an artery. Capillaries connect arteries to veins. Exchange of oxygen, nutrients, and waste materials takes place across capillary walls.

veins (VANES): vessels that carry blood to the heart.

hepatic portal vein: the vein that collects blood from the GI tract and conducts it to the liver.

- **portal** = gateway

> **FIGURE 3-10 The Vascular System**

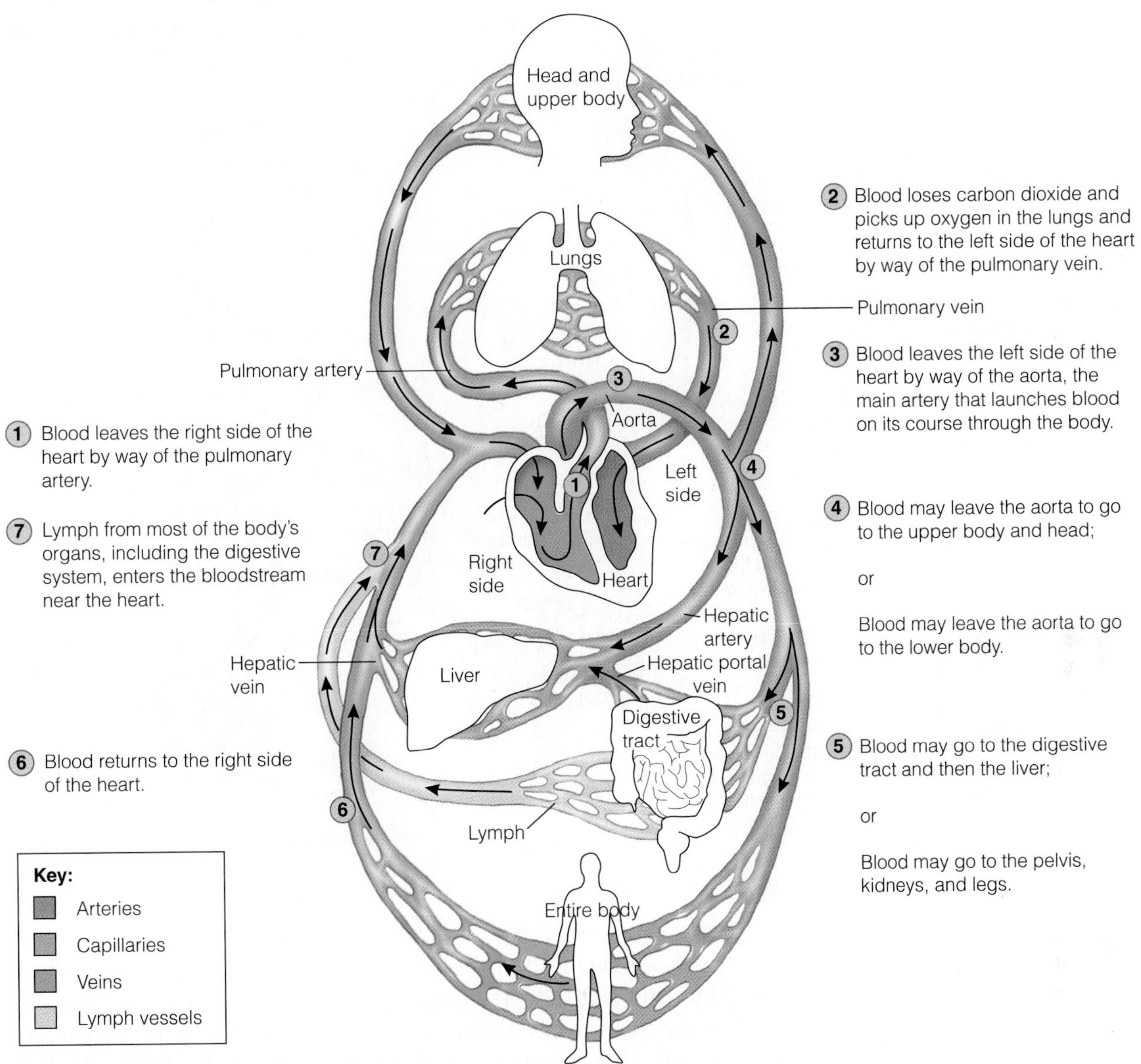

Head and upper body
Lungs
Pulmonary artery
Pulmonary vein
Aorta
Left side
Right side
Heart
Hepatic artery
Hepatic portal vein
Hepatic vein
Liver
Digestive tract
Lymph
Entire body
1 Blood leaves the right side of the heart by way of the pulmonary artery.
2 Blood loses carbon dioxide and picks up oxygen in the lungs and returns to the left side of the heart by way of the pulmonary vein.
3 Blood leaves the left side of the heart by way of the aorta, the main artery that launches blood on its course through the body.
4 Blood may leave the aorta to go to the upper body and head;
or
Blood may leave the aorta to go to the lower body.
5 Blood may go to the digestive tract and then the liver;
or
Blood may go to the pelvis, kidneys, and legs.
6 Blood returns to the right side of the heart.
7 Lymph from most of the body's organs, including the digestive system, enters the bloodstream near the heart.
Key:
Arteries
Capillaries
Veins
Lymph vessels

vein branches into a network of large capillaries so that every cell of the liver has access to the blood. Blood leaving the liver then collects into the **hepatic vein,** which returns blood to the heart. The route is:

Heart to arteries to capillaries (in intestines) to hepatic portal vein to capillaries (in liver) to hepatic vein to heart

Figure 3-11 on p. 84 shows the liver's key position in nutrient transport. An anatomist studying this system knows there must be a reason for this special arrangement. The liver's placement ensures that it will be first to receive the nutrients absorbed from the GI tract. In fact, the liver has many jobs to do in preparing the absorbed nutrients for use by the body. Of all the body's organs, the liver is the most metabolically active.

In addition, the liver defends the body by detoxifying substances that might cause harm and preparing waste products for excretion. This is why, when people ingest poisons that succeed in passing the first barrier (the intestinal cells), the liver quite often suffers the damage—from viruses such as hepatitis, from drugs such as barbiturates or alcohol, from toxins such as pesticide residues, and from contaminants such as mercury. Perhaps, in fact, you have been undervaluing your liver, not knowing what heroic tasks it quietly performs for you.

hepatic vein: the vein that collects blood from the liver and returns it to the heart.

- **hepatic** = liver

> **FIGURE 3-11 The Liver**

1 Vessels gather up nutrients from the digestive tract.

Not shown here:
Parallel to these vessels (veins) are other vessels (arteries) that carry oxygen-rich blood from the heart to the intestines.

2 The vessels merge into the hepatic portal vein, which conducts all absorbed materials to the liver.

3 The hepatic artery brings a supply of freshly oxygenated blood (not loaded with nutrients) from the lungs to supply oxygen to the liver's own cells.

4 A network of large capillaries branch all over the liver, making nutrients and oxygen available to all its cells and giving the cells access to blood from the digestive system.

5 The hepatic vein gathers up blood in the liver and returns it to the heart.

In contrast, nutrients absorbed into lymph do not go to the liver first. They go to the heart, which pumps them to all the body's cells. The cells remove the nutrients they need, and the liver then has to deal only with the remnants.

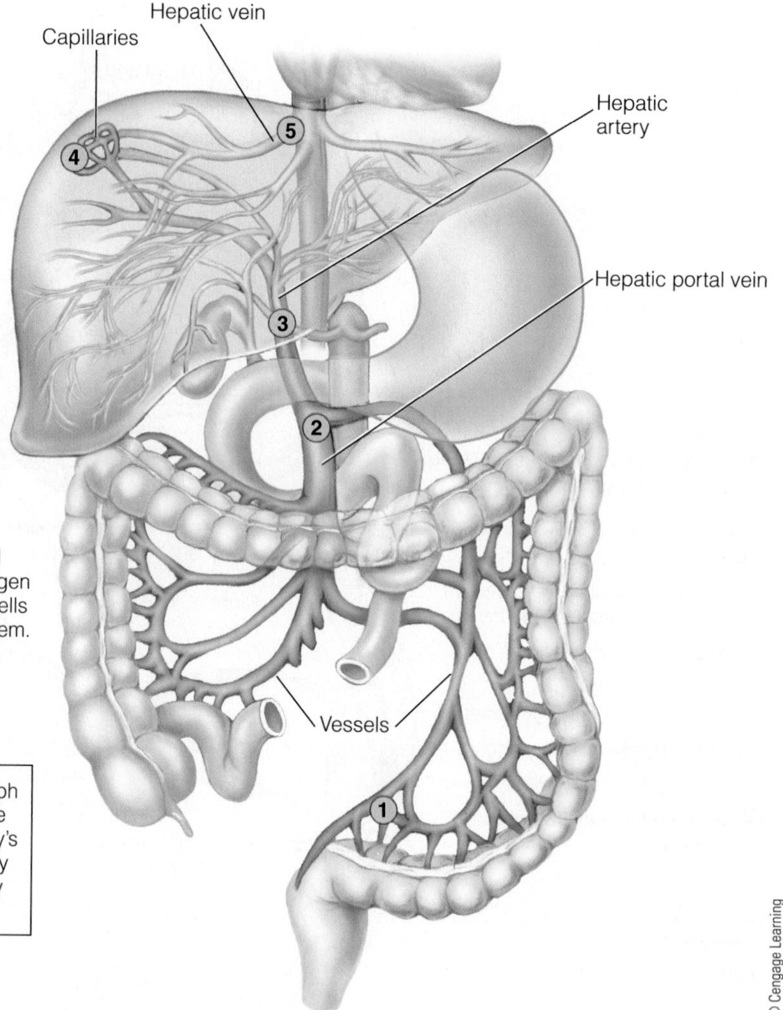

The Lymphatic System The **lymphatic system** provides a one-way route for fluid from the tissue spaces to enter the blood. Unlike the vascular system, the lymphatic system has no pump; instead, **lymph** circulates *between* the cells of the body and collects into tiny vessels. The fluid moves from one portion of the body to another as muscles contract and create pressure here and there. Ultimately, much of the lymph collects in the **thoracic duct** behind the heart. The thoracic duct opens into the **subclavian vein,** where the lymph enters the bloodstream. Thus nutrients from the GI tract that enter lymphatic vessels (large fats and fat-soluble vitamins) ultimately enter the bloodstream, circulating through arteries, capillaries, and veins like the other nutrients, with a notable exception—they bypass the liver at first.*

Once inside the vascular system, the nutrients can travel all over the body, where they can be taken into cells and used as needed. What becomes of them is described in later chapters.

> **REVIEW IT** Explain how nutrients are routed in the circulatory systems from the GI tract into the body and identify which nutrients enter the blood directly and which must first enter the lymph.

Nutrients leaving the digestive system via the blood are routed directly to the liver before being transported to the body's cells. Those leaving via the lymphatic system (large fats and fat-soluble vitamins) eventually enter the vascular system but bypass the liver at first.

lymphatic (lim-FAT-ic) **system:** a loosely organized system of vessels and ducts that convey fluids toward the heart. The GI part of the lymphatic system carries the products of fat digestion into the bloodstream.

lymph (LIMF): a clear yellowish fluid that is similar to blood except that it contains no red blood cells or platelets. Lymph from the GI tract transports fat and fat-soluble vitamins to the bloodstream via lymphatic vessels.

thoracic (thor-ASS-ic) **duct:** the main lymphatic vessel that collects lymph and drains into the left subclavian vein.

subclavian (sub-KLAY-vee-an) **vein:** the vein that provides passageway from the lymphatic system to the vascular system.

*The lymphatic vessels of the intestine that take up nutrients and pass them to the lymph circulation are called *lacteals* (LACK-tee-als).

3.4 The Health and Regulation of the GI Tract

› LEARN IT Describe how bacteria, hormones, and nerves influence the health and activities of the GI tract.

This section describes the bacterial conditions and hormonal regulation of a healthy GI tract, but many factors can influence normal GI function. For example, peristalsis and sphincter action are poorly coordinated in newborns, so infants tend to "spit up" during the first several months of life. Older adults often experience constipation, in part because the intestinal wall loses strength and elasticity with age, which slows GI motility. Diseases can also interfere with digestion and absorption and often lead to malnutrition. Lack of nourishment, in general, and lack of certain dietary constituents such as fiber, in particular, alter the structure and function of GI cells. Quite simply, GI tract health depends on adequate nutrition.

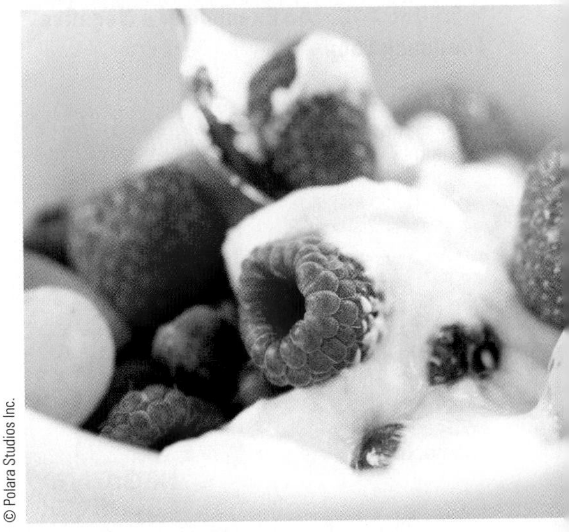

Eaten regularly, yogurt can alleviate common digestive problems.

Gastrointestinal Microbiome A healthy GI tract is home to a vibrant community of some 100 trillion **microbes**—bacteria, viruses, fungi, protozoa, and other microorganisms, collectively known as the **human microbiome.** Weighing less than a pound in total, these microbial cells outnumber the body's cells tenfold. The bacteria alone represent more than 400 different species and subspecies. The prevalence of different microbes in various parts of the GI tract depends on such factors as pH, peristalsis, diet, and other microbes. Relatively few microbes can live in the low pH of the stomach with its somewhat rapid peristalsis, whereas the neutral pH and slow peristalsis of the lower small intestine and the large intestine permit the growth of a diverse and abundant population.

Recent research has revealed that a person's health reflects the relative stability, disturbance, and resilience of the microbiome.[2] Its composition and activity may contribute to dozens of common diseases, including inflammatory bowel disease and obesity.[3]

The microbiome population and environment change dramatically in response to diet—both in the short term (daily meals) and in the long term (habitual diet patterns).[4] Consider, for example, that fibers that cannot be digested by the human body provide a major source of energy for bacteria, fostering their growth. As GI bacteria digest and metabolize fibers and other nutrients, they produce compounds such as short fragments of fat, which can influence energy metabolism and immunity.[5] Fibers and some other food components are called **prebiotics** because they encourage the growth and activity of bacteria. Research suggests that prebiotics may reduce the risk of GI infections, inflammation, and disorders; increase the bioavailability of nutrients; and regulate appetite and satiety.[6]

Some foods contain **probiotics,** live microbes that change the conditions in the GI tract in ways that seem to benefit health.[7] For example, **yogurt** contains *Lactobacillus* and other living bacteria. The potential GI health benefits of probiotics or products of their metabolism include helping to alleviate diarrhea, constipation, inflammatory bowel disease, ulcers, allergies, lactose intolerance, and infant colic; enhance immune function; and protect against colon cancer.[8] Research studies continue to explore how diet influences GI bacteria and which foods—with their prebiotics and probiotics—affect GI health. In addition, research studies are beginning to reveal several health benefits beyond the GI tract—such as improving blood pressure and immune responses.

Bacteria in the GI tract also produce several vitamins, including biotin, folate, pantothenic acid, riboflavin, thiamin, vitamin B_6, vitamin B_{12}, and vitamin K. Because the amount produced is insufficient to meet the body's needs, these vitamins are considered essential nutrients that must be provided by the diet.

Gastrointestinal Hormones and Nerve Pathways The ability of the digestive tract to handle its ever-changing contents illustrates an important physiological principle that governs the way all living things function—the principle of **homeostasis.** Simply stated, survival depends on body conditions staying about the same; if they deviate too far from the norm, the body must

microbes (MY-krobes): microscopically small organisms including bacteria, viruses, fungi, and protozoa; also called *microorganisms.*
- **mikros** = small

human microbiome: the collection of microbes found in or on the human body.

prebiotics: food components (such as fibers) that are not digested by the human body but are used as food by the GI bacteria to promote their growth and activity.

probiotics: living microorganisms found in foods and dietary supplements that, when consumed in sufficient quantities, are beneficial to health.
- **pro** = for
- **bios** = life

yogurt: milk product that results from the fermentation of lactic acid in milk by *Lactobacillus bulgaricus* and *Streptococcus thermophilus.*

homeostasis (HOME-ee-oh-STAY-sis): the maintenance of constant internal conditions (such as blood chemistry, temperature, and blood pressure) by the body's control systems. A homeostatic system is constantly reacting to external forces to maintain limits set by the body's needs.
- **homeo** = like, similar
- **stasis** = staying

> **FIGURE 3-12 An Example of a Negative Feedback Loop**

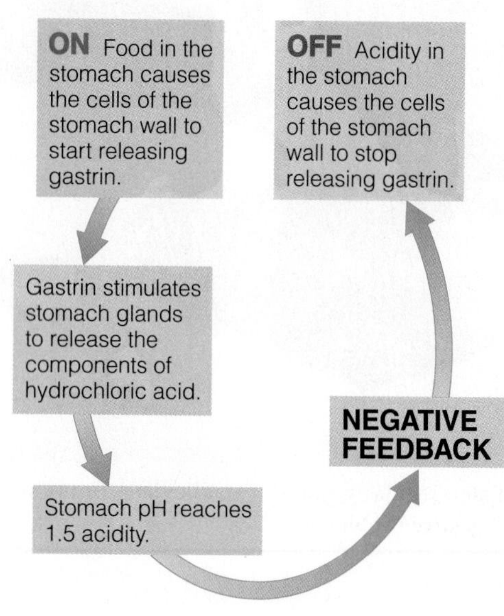
ON Food in the stomach causes the cells of the stomach wall to start releasing gastrin.
OFF Acidity in the stomach causes the cells of the stomach wall to stop releasing gastrin.
Gastrin stimulates stomach glands to release the components of hydrochloric acid.
NEGATIVE FEEDBACK
Stomach pH reaches 1.5 acidity.

"do something" to bring them back to normal. The body's regulation of digestion is one example of homeostatic regulation. The body also regulates its temperature, its blood pressure, and all other aspects of its blood chemistry in similar ways.

Two intricate and sensitive systems coordinate all the digestive and absorptive processes: the hormonal (or endocrine) system and the nervous system. Even before the first bite of food is taken, the mere thought, sight, or smell of food can trigger a response from these systems. Then, as food travels through the GI tract, it either stimulates or inhibits digestive secretions by way of messages that are carried from one section of the GI tract to another by both **hormones** and nerve pathways. (Appendix A presents a brief summary of the body's hormonal system and nervous system.)

Notice that the kinds of regulation described below are all examples of *feedback* mechanisms. A certain condition demands a response. The response changes that condition, and the change then cuts off the response. Thus the system is self-correcting.

- *The stomach normally maintains a pH between 1.5 and 1.7. How does it stay that way?* Food entering the stomach stimulates cells in the stomach wall to release the hormone **gastrin.** Gastrin, in turn, stimulates the stomach glands to secrete the components of hydrochloric acid. When pH 1.5 is reached, the acid itself turns off the gastrin-producing cells; they stop releasing gastrin, and the glands stop producing hydrochloric acid. Thus the system adjusts itself, as Figure 3-12 shows.

Nerve receptors in the stomach wall also respond to the presence of food and stimulate the gastric glands to secrete juices and the muscles to contract. As the stomach empties, the receptors are no longer stimulated, the flow of juices slows, and the stomach quiets down.

- *The pyloric sphincter opens to let out a little chyme, then closes again. How does it know when to open and close?* When the pyloric sphincter relaxes, acidic chyme slips through. The cells of the pyloric muscle on the intestinal side sense the acid, causing the pyloric sphincter to close tightly. Only after the chyme has been neutralized by pancreatic bicarbonate and the juices surrounding the pyloric sphincter have become alkaline can the muscle relax again. This process ensures that the chyme will be released slowly enough to be neutralized as it flows through the small intestine. This is important because the small intestine has less of a mucous coating than the stomach does and so is not as well protected from acid.

- *As the chyme enters the small intestine, the pancreas adds bicarbonate to it so that the intestinal contents always remain at a slightly alkaline pH. How does the pancreas know how much to add?* The presence of chyme stimulates the cells of the duodenual wall to release the hormone **secretin** into the blood. When secretin reaches the pancreas, it stimulates the pancreas to release its bicarbonate-rich juices. Thus, whenever the duodenum signals that acidic chyme is present, the pancreas responds by sending bicarbonate to neutralize it. When the need has been met, the cells of the duodenal wall are no longer stimulated to release secretin, the hormone no longer flows through the blood, and the pancreas no longer receives the message and stops sending pancreatic juice. Nerves also regulate pancreatic secretions.

- *Pancreatic secretions contain a mixture of enzymes to digest carbohydrate, fat, and protein. How does the pancreas know how much of each type of enzyme to provide?* This is one of the most interesting questions physiologists have asked. Clearly, the pancreas does know what its owner has been eating, and it secretes enzyme mixtures tailored to handle the food mixtures that have been arriving recently (over the past several days). Enzyme activity changes proportionately in response to the amounts of carbohydrate, fat, and protein in the diet. If a person has been eating mostly carbohydrates, the pancreas makes and secretes mostly carbohydrases; if the person's diet has been high in fat, the pancreas produces more lipases; and so forth. Hormones from the GI tract, secreted in response to meals, keep the pancreas informed as to its digestive tasks. The day or two lag between the time a person's diet changes dramatically

hormones: chemical messengers. Hormones are secreted by a variety of glands in response to altered conditions in the body. Each hormone travels to one or more specific target tissues or organs, where it elicits a specific response to maintain homeostasis.

gastrin: a hormone secreted by cells in the stomach wall. Target organ: the glands of the stomach. Response: secretion of gastric acid.

secretin (see-CREET-in): a hormone produced by cells in the duodenum wall. Target organ: the pancreas. Response: secretion of bicarbonate-rich pancreatic juice.

and the time digestion of the new diet becomes efficient explains why dietary changes can "upset digestion" and should be made gradually.

- *Why don't the digestive enzymes damage the pancreas?* The pancreas protects itself from harm by producing an inactive form of the enzymes.* It releases these proteins into the small intestine, where they are activated to become enzymes. In pancreatitis, the digestive enzymes become active within the infected pancreas, causing inflammation and damaging the delicate pancreatic tissues.

- *When fat is present in the intestine, the gallbladder contracts to squirt bile into the intestine to emulsify the fat. How does the gallbladder get the message that fat is present?* Fat in the intestine stimulates cells of the intestinal wall to release the hormone **cholecystokinin (CCK)**. This hormone travels by way of the blood to the gallbladder and stimulates it to contract, which releases bile into the small intestine. Cholecystokinin also travels to the pancreas and stimulates it to secrete its juices, which releases bicarbonate and enzymes into the small intestine. Once the fat in the intestine is emulsified and enzymes have begun to work on it, the fat no longer provokes release of the hormone, and the message to contract is canceled. (By the way, fat emulsification can continue even after a diseased gallbladder has been surgically removed because the liver can deliver bile directly to the small intestine.)

- *Fat and protein take longer to digest than carbohydrate does. When fat or protein is present, intestinal motility slows to allow time for its digestion. How does the intestine know when to slow down?* Cholecystokinin is released in response to fat or protein in the small intestine. In addition to its role in fat emulsification and digestion, cholecystokinin slows GI tract motility. Slowing the digestive process helps to maintain a pace that allows all reactions to reach completion. Hormonal and nervous mechanisms like these account for much of the body's ability to adapt to changing conditions.

Table 3-2 summarizes the actions of these three GI hormones. Gastrin, secretin, and cholecystokinin are among the most studied GI hormones, but the GI tract releases more than 20 hormones. In addition to assisting with digestion and absorption, many of these hormones regulate food intake and influence satiation—the feeling of satisfaction and fullness that occurs during a meal and halts eating. Current research is focusing on the roles these hormones may play in the development of obesity and its treatments (more details provided in Chapter 8).

Discovering the answers to questions like these has led some people to devote their whole lives to the study of physiology. For now, however, these few examples illustrate how all the processes throughout the digestive system are precisely and automatically regulated without any conscious effort.

The System at Its Best This chapter describes the anatomy of the digestive tract on several levels: the sequence of digestive organs, the cells and structures of the villi, and the selective machinery of the cell membranes. The intricate architecture of the digestive system makes it sensitive and responsive to conditions in

cholecystokinin (COAL-ee-SIS-toe-KINE-in), or **CCK:** a hormone produced by cells of the intestinal wall. Target organ: the gallbladder. Response: release of bile and slowing of GI motility.

*The inactive precursor of an enzyme is called a *zymogen* (ZYE-mo-jen).

TABLE 3-2 The Primary Actions of Selected GI Hormones

Hormone	Responds to	Secreted from	Stimulates	Response
Gastrin	Food in the stomach	Stomach wall	Stomach glands	Hydrochloric acid secreted into the stomach to maintain an acidic pH
Secretin	Acidic chyme in the small intestine	Duodenal wall	Pancreas	Bicarbonate-rich juices secreted into the small intestine to maintain a slightly alkaline pH
Cholecystokinin	Fat or protein in the small intestine	Intestinal wall	Gallbladder	Bile secreted into the duodenum to emulsify fats
			Pancreas	Bicarbonate- and enzyme-rich juices secreted into the small intestine to maintain a slightly alkaline pH, digest fats and proteins, and slow GI tract motility

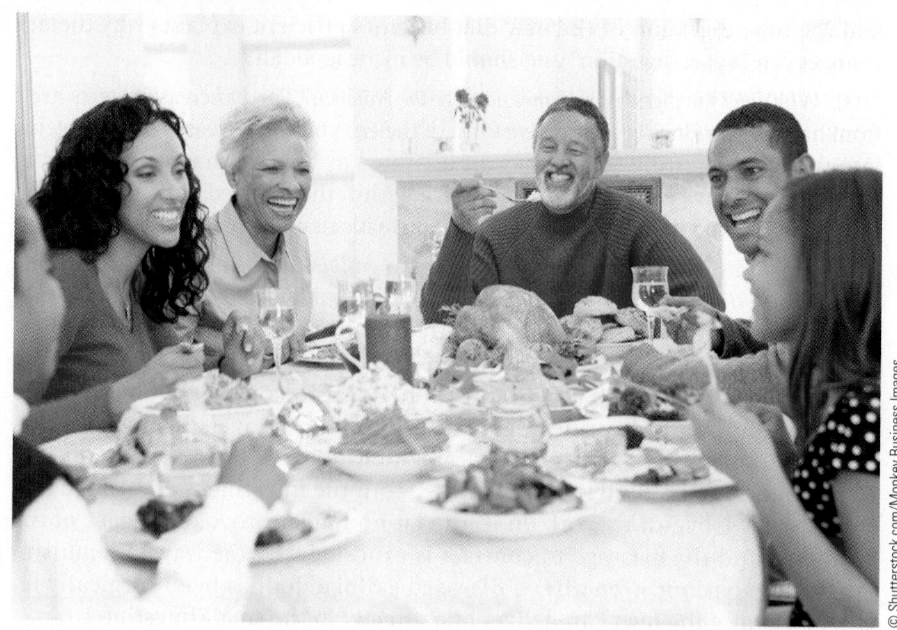

Nourishing foods and pleasant conversations support a healthy digestive system.

its environment. Several different kinds of GI tract cells confer specific immunity against intestinal diseases such as inflammatory bowel disease. In addition, secretions from the GI tract—saliva, mucus, gastric acid, and digestive enzymes—not only help with digestion, but also defend against foreign invaders. Together the GI's team of bacteria, cells, and secretions defend the body against many illnesses.

One indispensable condition is good health of the digestive system itself. Like all the other organs of the body, the GI tract depends on a healthy supply of blood. The cells of the GI tract become weak and inflamed when blood flow is diminished, as may occur in heart disease when arteries become clogged or blood clots form. Just as a diminished blood flow to the heart or brain can cause a heart attack or stroke, respectively, too little blood to the intestines can also be damaging—or even fatal. A diminished blood flow to the intestines—called **intestinal ischemia**—is characterized by abdominal pain, forceful bowel movements, and blood in the stool.

The health of the digestive system is also affected by such lifestyle factors as sleep, physical activity, and state of mind. Adequate sleep allows for repair and maintenance of tissue and removal of wastes that might impair efficient functioning. Activity promotes healthy muscle tone. Stress alters GI motility, secretions, permeability, blood flow, and bacteria.[9] For healthy digestion, mealtimes should be relaxed and tranquil. Pleasant conversations and peaceful environments during meals ease the digestive process.

Another factor in GI health is the kind of foods eaten. Among the characteristics of meals that promote optimal absorption of nutrients are those mentioned in Chapter 2: balance, moderation, variety, and adequacy. Balance and moderation require having neither too much nor too little of anything. For example, too much fat can be harmful, but some fat is beneficial in slowing down intestinal motility and providing time for absorption of some of the nutrients that are slow to be absorbed.

Variety is important for many reasons, but one is that some food constituents interfere with nutrient absorption. For example, some compounds common in high-fiber foods such as whole-grain cereals, certain leafy green vegetables, and legumes bind with minerals. To some extent, then, the minerals in those foods may become unavailable for absorption. These high-fiber foods are still valuable, but they need to be balanced with a variety of other foods that can provide the minerals.

As for adequacy—in a sense, this entire book is about dietary adequacy. A diet must provide all the essential nutrients, fiber, and energy in amounts sufficient to maintain health. But here, at the end of this chapter, is a good place

intestinal ischemia (is-KEY-me-ah): a diminished blood flow to the intestines that is characterized by abdominal pain, forceful bowel movements, and blood in the stool.

to emphasize the interdependence of the nutrients. It could almost be said that every nutrient depends on every other. All the nutrients work together, and all are present in the cells of a healthy digestive tract. To maintain health and promote the functions of the GI tract, make balance, moderation, variety, and adequacy features of every day's meals.

> **REVIEW IT** Describe how bacteria, hormones, and nerves influence the health and activities of the GI tract.
>
> A diverse and abundant bacteria population supports GI health. The regulation of GI processes depends on the coordinated efforts of the hormonal system and the nervous system. Together, digestion and absorption break down foods into nutrients for the body's use. To function optimally, a healthy GI tract needs a balanced diet, adequate rest, and regular physical activity.

Nutrition Portfolio

A digestive system that is well cared for most of the time can adjust to handle almost any diet or combination of foods with ease on occasion. Go to Diet & Wellness Plus and choose one of the days on which you have tracked your diet for the entire day. Choose the day you thought you ate most poorly, and looking at it, record in your journal answers to the following:

- Describe the physical and emotional environment that typically surrounds your meals, including how it affects you and how it might be improved.
- Did you experience any GI discomfort on that day? Do you experience any GI discomfort regularly? If so, which of the foods that you ate might have contributed to your discomfort? What can you do to prevent or alleviate GI problems in the future? Use Table H3-1 (p. 95) as a guide.
- List any changes you can make in your eating habits to promote overall GI health.

DIET & WELLNESS **PLUS** To complete this exercise, go to your Diet & Wellness Plus at **www.cengagebrain.com.**

> **STUDY IT** To review the key points of this chapter and take a practice quiz, go to the study cards at the end of the book.

REFERENCES

1. X. Chen and coauthors, A gustotopic map of taste qualities in the mammalian brain, *Science* 333 (2011): 1262-1266; N. Chaudhari and S. D. Roper, The cell biology of taste, *Journal of Cell Biology* 190 (2010): 285–296.
2. D. A. Relman, The human microbiome: Ecosystem resilience and health, *Nutrition Reviews* 70 (2012): S2–S9.
3. E. LeChatelier and coauthors, Richness of human gut microbiome correlates with metabolic markers, *Nature* 500 (2013): 541–546; F. Bäckhed, Host responses to the human microbiome, *Nutrition Reviews* 70 (2012): S14–S17; W. M. deVos and E. A. J. deVos, Role of the intestinal microbiome in health and disease: From correlation to causation, *Nutrition Reviews* 70 (2012): S45–S56.
4. H. J. Flint, The impact of nutrition on the human microbiome, *Nutrition Reviews* 70 (2012): S10–S13; G. D. Wu and coauthors, Linking long-term dietary patterns with gut microbial enterotypes, *Science* 334 (2011): 105–108; R. Jumpertz and coauthors, Energy-balance studies reveal associations between gut microbes, caloric load, and nutrient absorption in humans, *American Journal of Clinical Nutrition* 94 (2011): 58–65.
5. N. M. Delzenne and P. D. Cani, Interaction between obesity and the gut microbiota: Relevance in nutrition, *Annual Review of Nutrition* 31 (2011): 15–31.
6. A. M. Brownawell and coauthors, Prebiotics and the health benefits of fiber: Current regulatory status, future research, and goals, *Journal of Nutrition* 142 (2012): 962–974.
7. T. C. Wallace and coauthors, Human gut microbiota and its relationship to health and disease, *Nutrition Reviews* 69 (2011): 392–403; S. C. Bischoff and M. Zeitz, Scientific evidence for the medical use of probiotics, *Annals of Nutrition and Metabolism* 57 (2010): S1–S5; N. T. Williams, Probiotics, *American Journal of Health System Pharmacy* 15 (2010): 449–458.
8. S. Hempel and coauthors, Probiotics for the prevention and treatment of antibiotic-associated diarrhea: A systematic review and meta-analysis, *Journal of the American Medical Association* 307 (2012): 1959–1969; B. C. Johnston and coauthors, Probiotics for the prevention of *Clostridium difficile*–associated diarrhea: A systematic review and meta-analysis, *Annals of Internal Medicine* 157 (2012): 878–888; M. Kumar and coauthors, Probiotic metabolites as epigenetic targets in the prevention of colon cancer, *Nutrition Reviews* 71 (2012): 23–34.
9. P. C. Konturek, T. Brzozowski, and S. J. Donturek, Stress and the gut: Pathophysiology, clinical consequences, diagnostic approach and treatment options, *Journal of Physiology and Pharmacology* 62 (2011): 591–599; C. Hughes and coauthors, Galactooligosaccharide supplementation reduces stress-induced gastrointestinal dysfunction and days of cold or flu: A randomized double-blind, controlled trial in healthy university students, *American Journal of Clinical Nutrition* 93 (2011): 1305–1311.

HIGHLIGHT > 3
Common Digestive Problems

> LEARN IT Outline strategies to prevent or alleviate common GI problems.

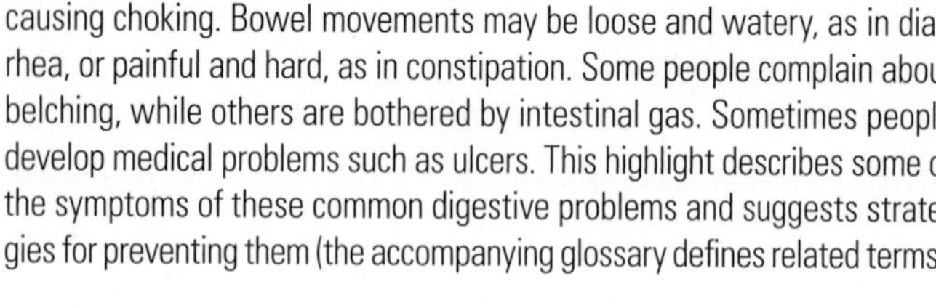

The facts of anatomy and physiology presented in Chapter 3 permit easy understanding of some common problems that occasionally arise in the digestive tract. Food may slip into the airways instead of the esophagus, causing choking. Bowel movements may be loose and watery, as in diarrhea, or painful and hard, as in constipation. Some people complain about belching, while others are bothered by intestinal gas. Sometimes people develop medical problems such as ulcers. This highlight describes some of the symptoms of these common digestive problems and suggests strategies for preventing them (the accompanying glossary defines related terms).

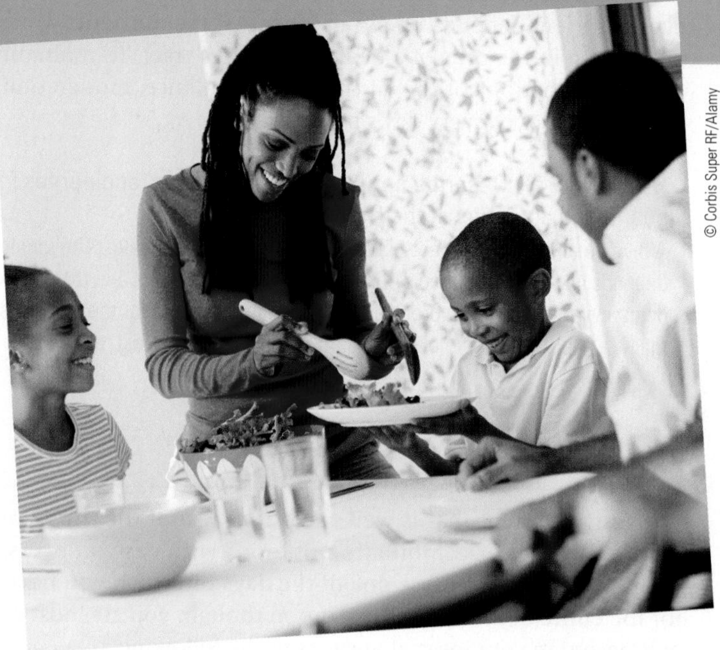

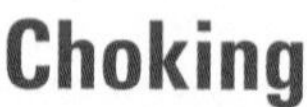

Choking

Sometimes a sip of a beverage or a tiny bit of food "slips down the wrong pipe." The body's first response is to cough, and quite often coughing clears the passage. When someone is truly choking, however, food has slipped into the **trachea** and completely blocked the air passageways (see Figure H3-1). Thus the person cannot cough—or even breathe. Without oxygen, the person may suffer permanent brain damage within 5 minutes or may even die. For this reason, it is imperative that everyone learn to recognize the universal distress signal for choking (shown in Figure H3-2) and act promptly.

Because the **larynx** is in the trachea and makes sounds only when air is pushed across it, a person choking will be unable to speak. For this reason, to help a person who is choking, first ask "Can you speak?" If the person is coughing, breathing adequately, or able to speak, do not interfere. Whatever you do, do not hit him on the back as the particle may become lodged more firmly in his air passageway. If the person cannot speak or cough, shout for help and perform the **Heimlich maneuver** (described in Figure H3-2). Almost any food can cause choking, although some are cited more often than others: chunks of meat, hot dogs, nuts,

GLOSSARY

acid controllers: medications used to prevent or relieve indigestion by suppressing production of acid in the stomach; also called *H2 blockers.* Common brands include Pepcid AC, Tagamet HB, Zantac 75, and Axid AR.

antacids: medications used to relieve indigestion by neutralizing acid in the stomach. Common brands include Alka-Seltzer, Maalox, Rolaids, and Tums.

belching: the release of air or gas from the stomach through the mouth.

bloating: uncomfortable abdominal fullness or distention.

celiac disease: an intestinal disorder in which the inability to absorb the protein portion of gluten results in an immune response that damages intestinal cells; also called *celiac sprue* or *gluten-sensitive enteropathy.*

colitis (ko-LYE-tis): inflammation of the colon.

colonic irrigation: the popular, but potentially harmful practice of "washing" the large intestine with a powerful enema machine; also called *colonic hydrotherapy.*

constipation: the condition of having infrequent or difficult bowel movements.

defecate (DEF-uh-cate): to move the bowels and eliminate waste.

- **defaecare** = to remove dregs

diarrhea: the frequent passage of watery bowel movements.

diverticula (dye-ver-TIC-you-la): sacs or pouches that develop in the weakened areas of the intestinal wall (like bulges in an inner tube where the tire wall is weak).

- **divertir** = to turn aside

diverticulitis (DYE-ver-tic-you-LYE-tis): infected or inflamed diverticula.

- **itis** = infection or inflammation

diverticulosis (DYE-ver-tic-you-LOH-sis): the condition of having diverticula. Diverticulosis affects more than 50 percent of adults in later life.

- **osis** = condition

enema: solution inserted into the rectum and colon to stimulate a bowel movement and empty the lower large intestine.

flatulence: passage of excessive amounts of intestinal gas.

gastroesophageal reflux: the backflow of stomach acid into the esophagus, causing damage to the cells of the esophagus and the sensation of heartburn; commonly known as *heartburn* or *acid indigestion. Gastroesophageal reflux disease (GERD)* is characterized by symptoms of reflux occurring two or more times a week.

Heimlich (HIME-lick) **maneuver (abdominal thrusts):** a technique for dislodging an object from the trachea of a choking person (see Figure H3-2); named for the physician who developed it.

hemorrhoids (HEM-oh-royds): painful swelling of the veins surrounding the rectum.

indigestion: incomplete or uncomfortable digestion, usually accompanied by pain, nausea, vomiting, heartburn, intestinal gas, or belching.

- **in** = not

irritable bowel syndrome: an intestinal disorder of unknown cause. Symptoms include abdominal discomfort and cramping, diarrhea, constipation, or alternating diarrhea and constipation.

larynx (LAIR-inks): the entryway to the trachea that contains the vocal cords; also called the *voice box* (see Figure H3-1).

laxatives: substances that loosen the bowels and thereby prevent or treat constipation.

mineral oil: a purified liquid derived from petroleum and used to treat constipation.

peptic ulcer: a lesion in the mucous membrane of either the stomach (a *gastric ulcer*) or the duodenum (a *duodenal ulcer*).

- **peptic** = concerning digestion

trachea (TRAKE-ee-uh): the air passageway from the larynx to the lungs; also called the *windpipe.*

ulcer: a lesion of the skin or mucous membranes characterized by inflammation and damaged tissues. See also *peptic ulcer.*

vomiting: expulsion of the contents of the stomach up through the esophagus to the mouth.

whole grapes, raw carrots, marshmallows, hard or sticky candies, gum, popcorn, and peanut butter. These foods are particularly difficult for young children (especially those 4 years of age and younger) to safely chew and swallow. Each year more than 10,000 children (14 years old or younger) in the United States choke; more than half choke on food. Every 5 days, a child in the United States chokes to death on food.[1] An adult should be present and alert to the dangers of choking whenever young children are eating. To prevent choking, cut food into small pieces, chew thoroughly before swallowing, don't talk or laugh with food in your mouth, and don't eat when breathing hard.

Vomiting

Vomiting can be a symptom of many different diseases or may arise in situations that upset the body's equilibrium, such as air or sea travel. For whatever reason, the contents of the stomach are propelled up through the esophagus to the mouth and expelled. Sometimes the muscular contractions will extend

> FIGURE H3-1 **Normal Swallowing and Choking**

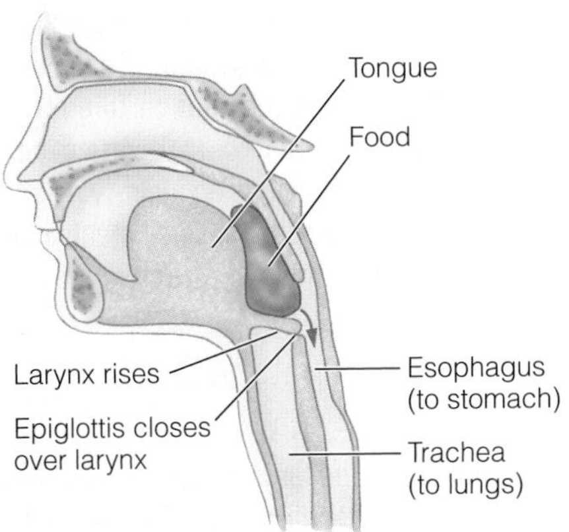

Swallowing. The epiglottis closes over the larynx, blocking entrance to the lungs via the trachea. The red arrow shows that food is heading down the esophagus normally.

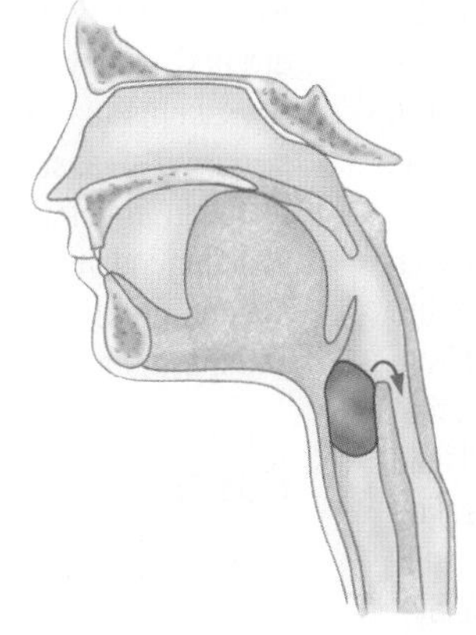

Choking. A choking person cannot speak or gasp because food lodged in the trachea blocks the passage of air. The red arrow points to where the food should have gone to prevent choking.

> FIGURE H3-2 **First Aid for Choking**

First aid for choking relies on abdominal thrusts, sometimes called the Heimlich maneuver. If abdominal thrusts are not successful and the person loses consciousness, lower him to the floor, call 911, remove the object blocking the airway if possible, and begin CPR. Because there is no time for hesitation when called upon to perform this death-defying act, you would do well to take a life-saving course to learn these techniques.

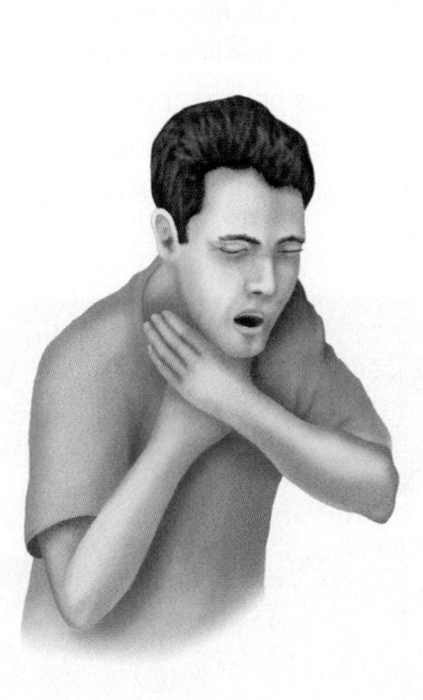

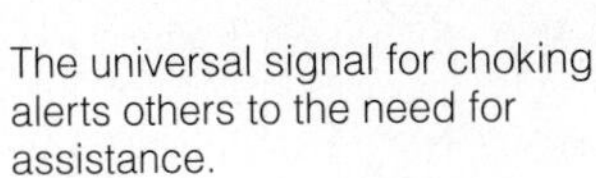

The universal signal for choking alerts others to the need for assistance.

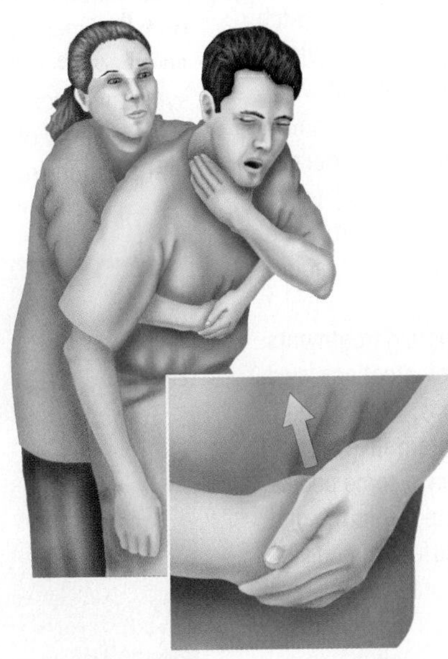

Stand behind the person with your arms wrapped around him. Make a fist with one hand and place the thumb side snugly against the body, slightly above the navel and below the breastbone.

Grasp the fist with your other hand and make a quick upward and inward thrust. Repeat thrusts until the object is dislodged.

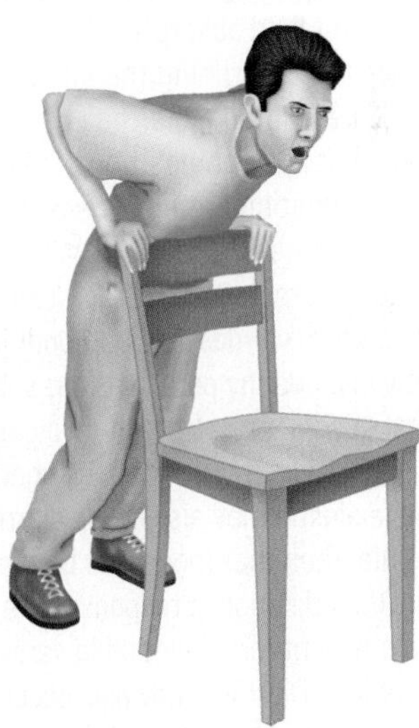

To perform abdominal thrusts on yourself, make a fist and place the thumb below your breastbone and above your navel. Grasp your fist with your other hand and press inward with a quick upward thrust. Alternatively, quickly thrust your upper body against a table edge, chair, or railing.

beyond the stomach and carry the contents of the duodenum, with its green bile, into the stomach and then up the esophagus. Although certainly unpleasant and wearying for the nauseated person, vomiting is often not a cause for alarm. Vomiting is one of the body's adaptive mechanisms to rid itself of something irritating. The best advice is to rest and drink small amounts of liquids as tolerated until the nausea subsides.

A physician's care may be needed, however, if vomiting causes such large losses of fluid as to threaten dehydration. As fluid is lost from the GI tract, the body's other fluids redistribute themselves, taking fluid from every cell of the body. Fluid leaving the cells is accompanied by salts that are absolutely essential to the life of the cells. Replacing salts and fluid is difficult if the vomiting continues, and intravenous feedings of saline and glucose may be necessary. Vomiting and dehydration are especially serious in an infant, and a physician should be contacted without delay.

Self-induced vomiting, such as occurs in bulimia nervosa, also has serious consequences. In addition to fluid and salt imbalances, repeated vomiting can cause irritation and infection of the pharynx, esophagus, and salivary glands; erosion of the teeth and gums; and dental caries. The esophagus may rupture or tear, as may the stomach. Sometimes the eyes become red from pressure during vomiting. Bulimic behavior reflects underlying psychological problems that require intervention. (Bulimia nervosa is discussed fully in Highlight 8.)

Diarrhea

Diarrhea is characterized by frequent, loose, watery stools. Such stools indicate that the intestinal contents have moved too quickly through the intestines for fluid absorption to take place or that water has been drawn from the cells lining the intestinal tract and added to the food residue. Like vomiting, diarrhea can lead to considerable fluid and salt losses, but the composition of the fluids is different. Stomach fluids lost in vomiting are highly acidic, whereas intestinal fluids lost in diarrhea are nearly neutral. When fluid losses require medical attention, correct replacement is crucial.

Diarrhea is a symptom of various medical conditions and treatments. It may occur abruptly in a healthy person as a result of infections (such as foodborne illness) or as a side effect of medications. When used in large quantities, food ingredients such as the sugar alternative sorbitol and the fat alternative olestra may also cause diarrhea in some people. If a food is responsible, then that food must be omitted from the diet, at least temporarily. If medication is responsible, a different medicine, when possible, or a different form (injectable versus oral, for example) may alleviate the problem. Diarrhea may also occur as a result of disorders of the GI tract, such as irritable bowel syndrome or colitis.

Irritable Bowel Syndrome

Irritable bowel syndrome is one of the most common GI disorders and is characterized by frequent or severe abdominal discomfort and a disturbance in the motility of the GI tract.[2] In most cases, GI contractions are stronger and last longer than normal, forcing intestinal contents through quickly and causing gas, **bloating,** and diarrhea. In some cases, however, GI contractions are weaker than normal, slowing the passage of intestinal contents and causing constipation. The exact cause of irritable bowel syndrome is not known, but researchers are actively investigating the role of the nervous system.[3] The condition seems to worsen for some people when they eat certain foods or during stressful events. These triggers seem to aggravate symptoms but not cause them. Dietary treatment hinges on identifying and avoiding individual foods that aggravate symptoms; small meals may also be beneficial. Other treatments that may be effective include antispasmodic drugs and peppermint oil.

Colitis

People with **colitis,** an inflammation of the large intestine, may also suffer from severe diarrhea. They often benefit from complete bowel rest and medication. If treatment fails, surgery to remove the colon and rectum may be necessary.

Celiac Disease

Celiac disease is an autoimmune disease characterized by inflammation of the small intestine that occurs in response to foods that contain gluten, a protein commonly found in wheat, barley, rye, and possibly oats. The prevalence of celiac disease in the United States is estimated at 1 in 141.[4] In people with celiac disease, gluten triggers an immune system reaction in the small intestine that causes inflammation, which damages the villi and decreases nutrient absorption. Common symptoms include abdominal pains, bloating and gas, and diarrhea—making it commonly misdiagnosed as irritable bowel syndrome. Treatment focuses on a gluten-free diet.[5] Despite the growing popularity of gluten-free products, there is no evidence to suggest that a gluten-free diet is beneficial for the general population.[6]

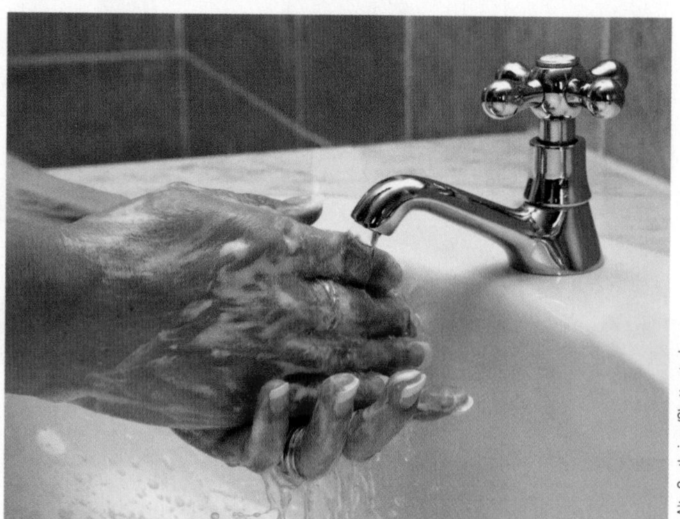

Personal hygiene (such as regular hand washing with soap and water) and safe food preparation (as described in Chapter 19) are easy and effective steps to take in preventing diarrheal diseases.

Treatment

Treatment for diarrhea depends on cause and severity, but it always begins with rehydration. Mild diarrhea may subside with simple rest and extra liquids (such as clear juices and soups) to replace fluid losses. If diarrhea is bloody or if it worsens or persists—especially in an infant, young child, elderly person, or person with a compromised immune system—call a physician. Severe diarrhea can be life threatening.

Constipation

Like diarrhea, **constipation** describes a symptom, not a disease. Each person's GI tract has its own cycle of waste elimination, which depends on its owner's health, the type of food eaten, when it was eaten, and when the person takes time to **defecate.** What's normal for some people may not be normal for others. Some people have bowel movements three times a day; others may have them three times a week. The symptoms of constipation include straining during bowel movements, hard stools, and infrequent bowel movements (fewer than three per week). Abdominal discomfort, headaches, backaches, and the passing of gas sometimes accompany constipation.

Often a person's lifestyle may cause constipation. Being too busy to respond to the defecation signal is a common complaint. If a person receives the signal to defecate and ignores it, the signal may not return for several hours. In the meantime, fluids continue to be withdrawn from the fecal matter, so when the person does defecate, the stools are dry and hard. In such a case, a person's daily regimen may need to be revised to allow time to have a bowel movement when the body sends its signal.

Although constipation usually reflects lifestyle habits, in some cases it may be a side effect of medication or a medical problem such as bowel obstruction. If discomfort is associated with passing fecal matter, seek medical advice to rule out disease. Once this has been done, simple treatments, such as increased fiber, fluids, and exercise, are recommended before the use of medications.

One dietary measure that may be appropriate is to increase dietary fiber to 25 to 28 grams per day gradually over the course of a week or two. Fibers found in fruits, vegetables, and whole grains help to prevent constipation by increasing fecal mass. In the GI tract, fiber attracts water, creating soft, bulky stools that stimulate bowel contractions to push the contents along. These contractions strengthen the intestinal muscles. The improved muscle tone, together with the water content of the stools, eases elimination, reducing the pressure in the rectal veins and helping to prevent **hemorrhoids.** Chapter 4 provides more information on fiber's role in maintaining a healthy colon and reducing the risks of colon cancer and diverticulosis. **Diverticulosis** is a condition in which the intestinal walls develop bulges in weakened areas, most commonly in the colon (see Figure H3-3). These bulging pockets, known as **diverticula,** can worsen constipation, entrap feces, and become painfully infected and inflamed **(diverticulitis).** Treatment may require hospitalization, antibiotics, or surgery.

Drinking plenty of water in conjunction with eating high-fiber foods also helps to prevent constipation. The increased bulk physically stimulates the upper GI tract, promoting peristalsis throughout. Similarly, physical activity improves the muscle tone and motility of the digestive tract. As little as 30 minutes of physical activity a day can help prevent or alleviate constipation.

> **FIGURE H3-3 Diverticula in the Colon**
> Diverticula may develop anywhere along the GI tract, but they are most common in the colon.

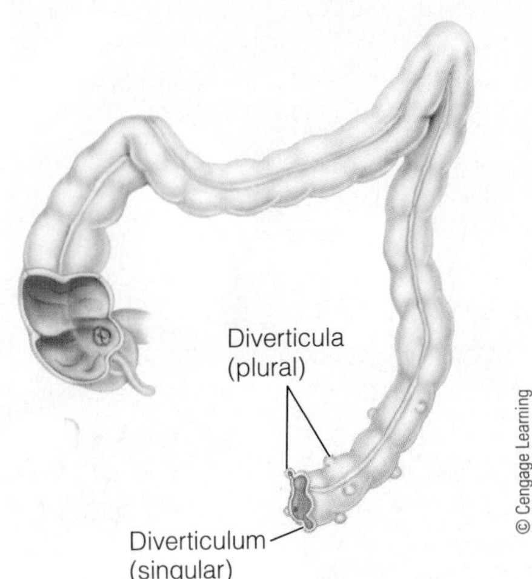

Eating prunes—or "dried plums" as some have renamed them—can also be helpful. Prunes are high in fiber and also contain a laxative substance.* If a morning defecation is desired, a person can drink prune juice at bedtime; if the evening is preferred, the person can drink prune juice with breakfast.

If these suggested changes in lifestyle or diet do not correct constipation, then a physician might recommend the use of stool softeners, **laxatives,** or **mineral oil.** These products are best used for brief periods. If needed for extended times, they should be used under physician supervision. Frequent use of laxatives can lead to dependency and upset the body's fluid, salt, and mineral balances. Mineral oil interferes with the absorption of fat-soluble vitamins.

One potentially harmful but currently popular practice is **colonic irrigation**—the internal washing of the large intestine with a powerful **enema** machine. Such an extreme cleansing is not only unnecessary, but it can be hazardous, especially for those with a history of digestive diseases. Side effects may be relatively minor (cramping, abdominal pain, bloating, nausea, and vomiting) or quite severe (infections, kidney failure, pancreatitis, and heart failure), sometimes leading to death.[7] Common problems include equipment contamination, electrolyte abnormalities, and intestinal perforation. Less extreme practices can cause problems, too.

Belching and Gas

Many people complain of problems that they attribute to excessive gas. For some, belching is the complaint. Others blame intestinal gas for abdominal discomforts and embarrassment.

*This laxative substance is *dihydroxyphenyl isatin.*

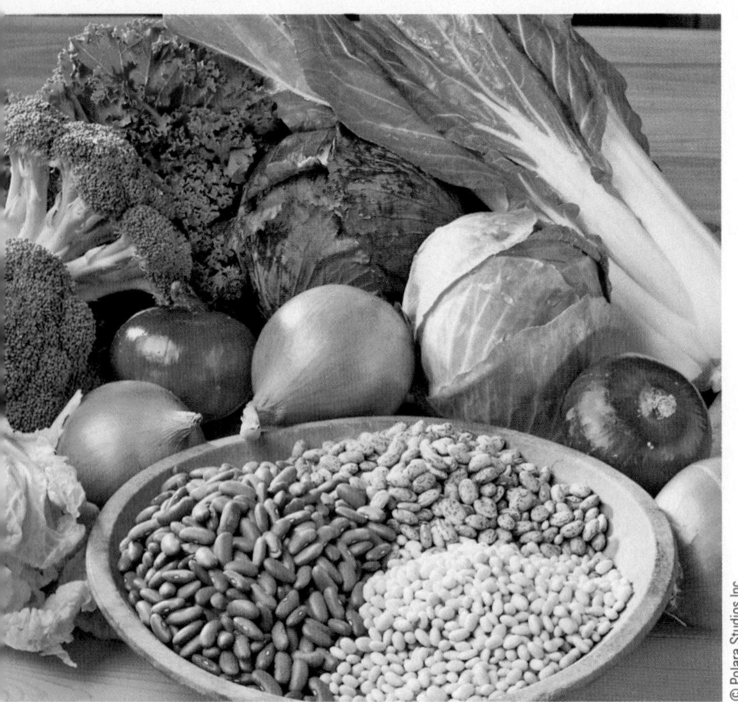

People troubled by intestinal gas need to determine which foods bother them and then eat those foods in moderation.

© Polara Studios Inc.

Belching

Belching results from swallowing air. Everyone swallows a little bit of air with each mouthful of food, but people who eat too fast may swallow too much air. Ill-fitting dentures, carbonated beverages, and chewing gum can also contribute to the swallowing of air with resultant belching. The best advice for belching seems to be to eat slowly, chew thoroughly, and relax while eating.

Intestinal Gas

Although **flatulence** can be an embarrassing experience, it is quite normal. (People who experience painful bloating from malabsorption diseases, however, require medical treatment.) Healthy people expel several hundred milliliters of intestinal gas several times a day. Almost all (99 percent) of the gases expelled—nitrogen, oxygen, hydrogen, methane, and carbon dioxide—are odorless. The remaining "volatile" gases are the infamous ones.

Foods that produce gas usually must be determined individually. The most common offenders are foods rich in the carbohydrates—sugars, starches, and fibers. When partially digested carbohydrates reach the large intestine, bacteria digest them, giving off gas as a by-product. People can test foods suspected of forming gas by omitting them individually for a trial period to see if there is any improvement.

Gastroesophageal Reflux

Almost everyone has experienced heartburn at one time or another, usually soon after eating a meal. Medically known as **gastroesophageal reflux,** heartburn is the painful sensation a person feels behind the breastbone when the lower esophageal sphincter allows the stomach contents to reflux into the esophagus (see Figure H3-4). This may happen if a person eats or drinks too much (or both). Tight clothing and even changes of position (lying down, bending over) can cause it, too, as can some medications and smoking. Weight gain and overweight increase the frequency, severity, and duration of heartburn symptoms. A defect of the sphincter muscle itself is a possible, but less common, cause.

If heartburn is not caused by an anatomical defect, treatment is fairly simple. To avoid such misery in the future, the person needs to learn to eat less at a sitting, chew food more thoroughly, and eat more slowly. Additional strategies are presented in Table H3-1.

People who overeat or eat too quickly are likely to suffer from **indigestion.** The muscular reaction of the stomach to unchewed lumps or to being overfilled may be so intense that it upsets normal peristalsis. When this happens, overeaters may taste the stomach acid and feel pain. Over-the-counter **antacids** and **acid controllers**

> FIGURE H3-4 **Gastroesophageal Reflux**

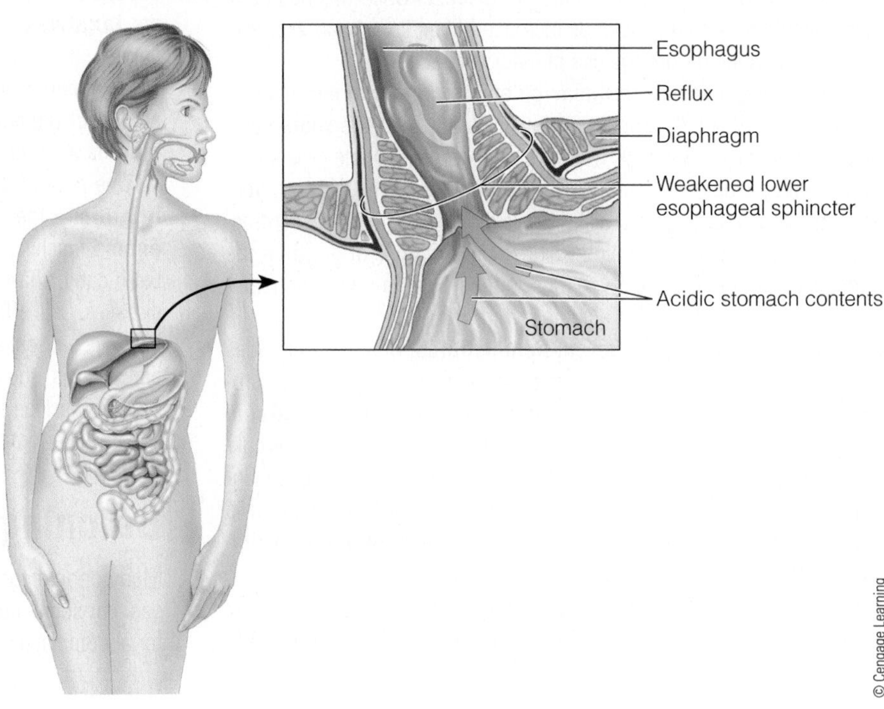

© Cengage Learning

TABLE H3-1 **Strategies to Prevent or Alleviate Common GI Problems**

GI Problem	Strategies	GI Problem	Strategies
Choking	• Take small bites of food. • Chew thoroughly before swallowing. • Don't talk or laugh with food in your mouth. • Don't eat when breathing hard.	**Heartburn**	• Eat small meals. • Drink liquids between meals. • Sit up while eating; elevate your head when lying down. • Wait 3 hours after eating before lying down. • Wait 2 hours after eating before exercising. • Refrain from wearing tight-fitting clothing. • Avoid foods, beverages, and medications that aggravate your heartburn. Common irritants include foods that are fried or high in fat; chocolate and peppermint; coffee, alcoholic beverages, and carbonated beverages; mustard, ketchup, and tomato sauces; acidic substances such as vinegar, citrus juices, and citrus fruits. • Refrain from smoking cigarettes or using tobacco products. • Lose weight if overweight. • Take medicine as prescribed by your physician.
Diarrhea	• Avoid strenuous activity. • Rest. • Drink fluids to replace losses. • Call for medical help if diarrhea persists.		
Constipation	• Eat a high-fiber diet. • Drink plenty of fluids. • Exercise regularly. • Respond promptly to the urge to defecate.		
Belching	• Eat slowly. • Chew thoroughly. • Relax while eating.	**Ulcer**	• Avoid coffee and caffeine- and alcohol-containing beverages. • Avoid foods that aggravate your ulcer. • Minimize aspirin, ibuprofen, and naproxen use. • Refrain from smoking cigarettes.
Intestinal gas	• Eat bothersome foods in moderation.		

may provide relief but should be used only infrequently for occasional heartburn; they may mask or cause problems if used regularly. If problems continue, people who suffer from frequent and regular bouts of heartburn and indigestion may need to see a physician, who can prescribe specific medication to control gastroesophageal reflux. Without treatment, the repeated splashes of acid can severely damage the cells of the esophagus, creating a condition known as Barrett's esophagus. At that stage, the risk of cancer in the esophagus increases dramatically.[8] To repeat, if symptoms persist, see a doctor—don't self-medicate.

Ulcers

Ulcers are another common digestive problem, affecting an estimated 1 out of every 12 adults in the United States. An **ulcer** is a lesion (a sore), and a **peptic ulcer** is a lesion in the lining of the stomach (gastric ulcers) or the duodenum of the small intestine (duodenal ulcers). The compromised lining is left unprotected and exposed to gastric juices, which can be painful. In some cases, ulcers can cause internal bleeding. If GI bleeding is excessive, iron deficiency may develop. Ulcers that perforate the GI lining can pose life-threatening complications.

Many people naively believe that an ulcer is caused by stress or spicy foods, but this is not the case. The stomach lining in a healthy person is well protected by its mucous coat. What, then, causes ulcers to form?

Three major causes of ulcers have been identified: bacterial infection with *Helicobacter pylori* (commonly abbreviated *H. pylori*); the use of certain anti-inflammatory drugs such as aspirin, ibuprofen, and naproxen; and disorders that cause excessive gastric acid secretion. Most commonly, ulcers develop in response to *H. pylori* infection. The cause of the ulcer dictates the type of medication used in treatment. For example, people with ulcers caused by infection receive antibiotics, whereas those with ulcers caused by medicines discontinue their use. In addition, all treatment plans aim to relieve pain, heal the ulcer, and prevent recurrence.

The regimen for ulcer treatment is to treat for infection, eliminate any food that routinely causes indigestion or pain, and avoid coffee and caffeine- and alcohol-containing beverages. Both regular and decaffeinated coffee stimulate acid secretion and so aggravate *existing* ulcers.

Ulcers and their treatments highlight the importance of not self-medicating when symptoms persist. People with *H. pylori* infection often take over-the-counter acid controllers to relieve the pain of their ulcers when, instead, they need physician-prescribed antibiotics. Suppressing gastric acidity not only fails to heal the ulcer, but it also actually worsens inflammation during an *H. pylori* infection. Furthermore, *H. pylori* infection has been linked with stomach cancer, making prompt diagnosis and appropriate treatment essential.

Table H3-1 summarizes strategies to prevent or alleviate common GI problems. Many of these problems reflect hurried lifestyles. For this reason, many of their remedies require that people slow down and take the time to eat at a leisurely pace; chew food thoroughly to prevent choking, heartburn, and acid indigestion; rest until vomiting and diarrhea subside; and heed the urge to defecate. In addition, people must learn how to handle life's day-to-day problems and challenges without overreacting and becoming upset; learn how to relax, get enough sleep, and enjoy life. Remember, "what's eating you" may cause more GI distress than what you eat.

CRITICAL THINKING QUESTIONS

A. What strategies would be most helpful in preventing common digestive problems?

B. You've noticed the abundance of gluten-free foods on the grocery store shelves. The demand for gluten-free products has increased dramatically over the past decade as gluten-free diets have gained in popularity. Although a gluten-free diet is the best treatment for people with celiac disease, it has been adopted by millions of other people for a variety of other reasons. Compare the kcalories, fiber, added sugars, and saturated fat on the labels of two similar products—one whole grain and the other gluten free—and determine what benefits and risks might accompany a gluten-free diet for those with celiac disease and for others. Which product would you now be more likely to buy? Why?

REFERENCES

1. American Academy of Pediatrics, Policy statement: Prevention of choking among children, *Pediatrics* 125 (2010): 601–607.
2. D. Keszthelyi, F. J. Troost, and A. A. Masclee, Irritable bowel syndrome: Methods, mechanisms, and pathophysiology. Methods to assess visceral hypersensitivity in irritable bowel syndrome, *American Journal of Physiology: Gastrointestinal and Liver Physiology* 303 (2012): G141-G154; M. Camilleri, Peripheral mechanisms in irritable bowel syndrome, *New England Journal of Medicine* 367 (2012): 1626–1635.
3. C. M. Surawicz, Mechanisms of diarrhea, *Current Gastroenterology Reports* 12 (2010): 236–241.
4. A. Rubio-Tapia and coauthors, The prevalence of celiac disease in the United States, *American Journal of Gastroenterology* 107 (2012): 1538–1544.
5. P. Fric, D. Gabrovska, and J. Nevoral, Celiac disease, gluten-free diet, and oats, *Nutrition Reviews* 69 (2011): 107–115.
6. G. A. Gaesser and S. S. Angadi, Gluten-free diet: Imprudent dietary advice for the general population? *Journal of the Academy of Nutrition and Dietetics* 112 (2012): 1330–1333.
7. R. Mishori, A. Otubu, A. A. Jones, The dangers of colon cleansing, *Journal of Family Practice* 60 (2011): 454–457.
8. S. J. Spechler, Barrett esophagus and risk of esophageal cancer: A clinical review, *Journal of the American Medical Association* 310 (2013): 627–636; F. Hvid-Jensen and coauthors, Incidence of adenocarcinoma among patients with Barrett's esophagus, *New England Journal of Medicine* 365 (2011): 1375–1383.

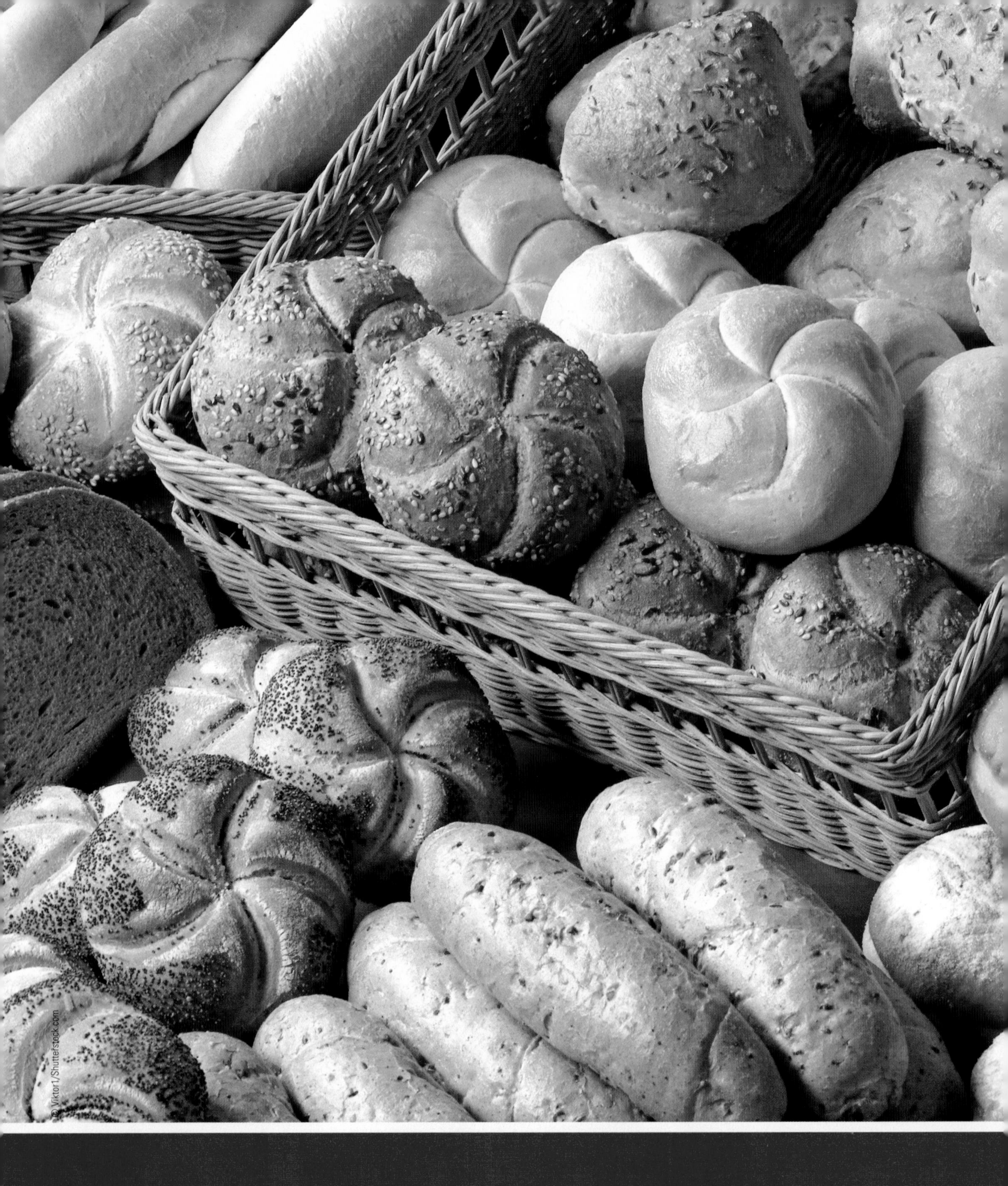

4

The Carbohydrates: Sugars, Starches, and Fibers

LEARNING GPS

Nutrition in Your Life

Whether you are studying for an exam or daydreaming about your next vacation, your brain needs carbohydrate to power its activities. Your muscles need carbohydrate to fuel their work, too, whether you are racing up the stairs to class or moving on the dance floor to your favorite music. Where can you get carbohydrate? Are some foods healthier choices than others? As you will learn from this chapter, whole grains, vegetables, legumes, and fruits naturally deliver ample carbohydrate and fiber with valuable vitamins and minerals and little or no fat. Milk products typically lack fiber, but they also provide carbohydrate along with an assortment of vitamins and minerals. In the Nutrition Portfolio at the end of this chapter, you can examine whether your current carbohydrate choices are meeting dietary goals.

A student, quietly studying, is seldom aware of the billions of glucose molecules in his brain cells that provide the energy to learn. Yet glucose fuels nearly all of the brain's activities. Similarly, a marathon runner, triumphantly crossing the finish line, seldom gives credit to the glycogen her muscles have used to fuel the race. Yet, together, these two **carbohydrates**—glucose and its storage form glycogen—provide about half of all the energy muscles and other body tissues use. The other half comes mostly from fat.

People don't eat glucose and glycogen. When they eat foods rich in carbohydrates, their bodies receive glucose for immediate energy and convert some glucose into glycogen for reserve energy. All plant foods—whole grains, vegetables, legumes, and fruits—provide carbohydrate. Milk also contains carbohydrate.

Some people mistakenly think of carbohydrates as "fattening" and avoid them when trying to lose weight. This strategy may help if the carbohydrates are the added sugars of soft drinks, candies, and cookies, but it is counterproductive if the carbohydrates are from whole grains, vegetables, and legumes. As the next section explains, not all carbohydrates are created equal.

carbohydrates: compounds composed of carbon, oxygen, and hydrogen arranged as monosaccharides or multiples of monosaccharides. Most, but not all, carbohydrates have a ratio of one carbon molecule to one water molecule: $(CH_2O)_n$.

- **carbo** = carbon (C)
- **hydrate** = with water (H_2O)

4.1 The Chemist's View of Carbohydrates

› LEARN IT Identify the monosaccharides, disaccharides, and polysaccharides common in nutrition by their chemical structures and major food sources.

The dietary carbohydrate family includes:

- Monosaccharides: single sugars
- Disaccharides: sugars composed of pairs of monosaccharides
- Polysaccharides: large molecules composed of chains of monosaccharides

Monosaccharides and disaccharides (the sugars) are sometimes called *simple carbohydrates,* and polysaccharides (starches and fibers) are sometimes called *complex carbohydrates.*

To understand the structure of carbohydrates, look at the atoms within them. Each atom can form a certain number of chemical bonds with other atoms:

- Hydrogen atoms, one
- Oxygen atoms, two
- Nitrogen atoms, three
- Carbon atoms, four

Chemists represent the bonds as lines between the chemical symbols (such as H, O, N, and C) that stand for the atoms (see Figure 4-1).

Atoms form molecules in ways that satisfy the bonding requirements of each atom. Figure 4-1 includes the structure of ethyl alcohol, the active ingredient of alcoholic beverages, as an example. The two carbons each have four bonds represented by lines; the oxygen has two; and each hydrogen has one bond connecting it to other atoms. Chemical structures always bond according to these rules.

The following list of the most important **sugars** in nutrition symbolizes them as hexagons and pentagons of different colors.* Three are monosaccharides:

- Glucose
- Fructose
- Galactose

Three are disaccharides:

- Maltose (glucose + glucose) 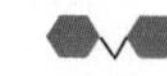
- Sucrose (glucose + fructose)
- Lactose (glucose + galactose)

> FIGURE 4-1 Atoms and Their Bonds

The four main types of atoms found in nutrients are hydrogen (H), oxygen (O), nitrogen (N), and carbon (C).

H— (1) —O— (2) —N— (3) —C— (4)

Each atom has a characteristic number of bonds it can form with other atoms.

H–C(H)(H)–C(H)(H)–O–H

Notice that in this simple molecule of ethyl alcohol, each H has one bond, O has two, and each C has four.

Monosaccharides The three **monosaccharides** most important in nutrition all have the same numbers and kinds of atoms—each contains 6 carbon atoms, 12 hydrogens, and 6 oxygens (written in shorthand as $C_6H_{12}O_6$). The monosaccharides differ in their arrangements of the atoms. These chemical differences account for the differing sweetness of the monosaccharides. A pinch of purified glucose on the tongue gives only a mild sweet flavor, and galactose hardly tastes sweet at all. Fructose, however, is as intensely sweet as honey and, in fact, is the sugar primarily responsible for honey's sweetness.

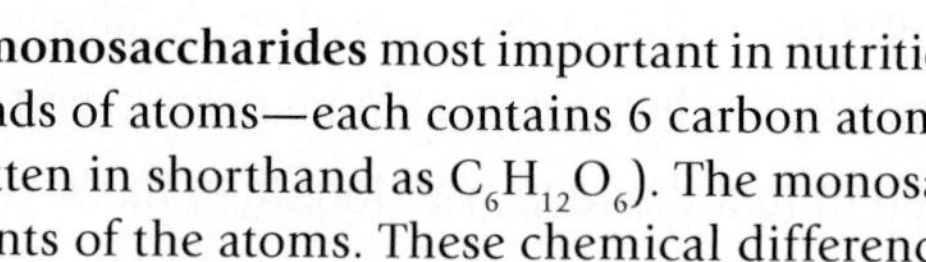

Glucose Chemically, **glucose** is a larger and more complicated molecule than the ethyl alcohol shown in Figure 4-1, but it obeys the same rules of chemistry: each carbon atom has four bonds; each oxygen, two bonds; and each hydrogen, one bond. Figure 4-2 illustrates the chemical structure of a glucose molecule.

Commonly known as blood sugar, glucose serves as an essential energy source for all the body's activities. Its significance to nutrition is tremendous.

sugars: simple carbohydrates composed of monosaccharides, disaccharides, or both.

monosaccharides (mon-oh-SACK-uh-rides): carbohydrates of the general formula $C_nH_{2n}O_n$ that typically form a single ring. The monosaccharides important in nutrition are *hexoses,* sugars with six atoms of carbon and the formula $C_6H_{12}O_6$. See Appendix C for the chemical structures of the monosaccharides.

- **mono** = one
- **saccharide** = sugar
- **hex** = six

glucose (GLOO-kose): a monosaccharide; sometimes known as *blood sugar* in the body or *dextrose* in foods.

- **ose** = carbohydrate
- (hexagon) = glucose

*Fructose is shown as a pentagon, but like the other monosaccharides, it has six carbons (as you will see in Figure 4-3). The disaccharides are illustrated with a simple bond, but actual linkages differ (as shown in Appendix C).

> **FIGURE 4-2 Chemical Structure of Glucose**

The diagram of a glucose molecule on the left shows all the bonds between the 6 carbon (C), 12 hydrogen (H), and 6 oxygen (O) atoms. It proves simple on examination, but chemists have adopted shortcuts to depict chemical structures. The middle and right diagrams also present the chemical structure of glucose, but as simplified versions with fewer symbols and bonds showing.

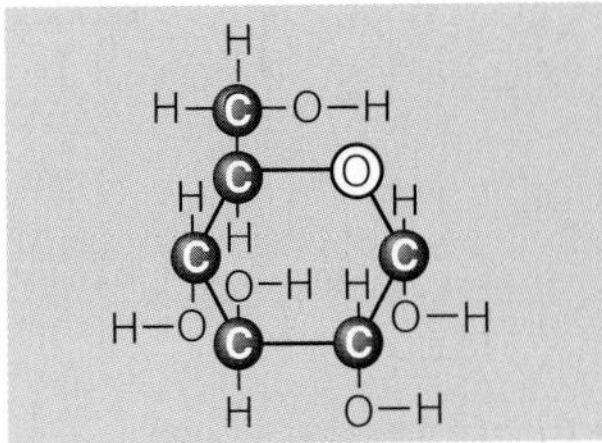

On paper, the structure of glucose has to be drawn flat, but in nature the five carbons and oxygen are roughly in a plane. The atoms attached to the ring carbons extend above and below the plane.

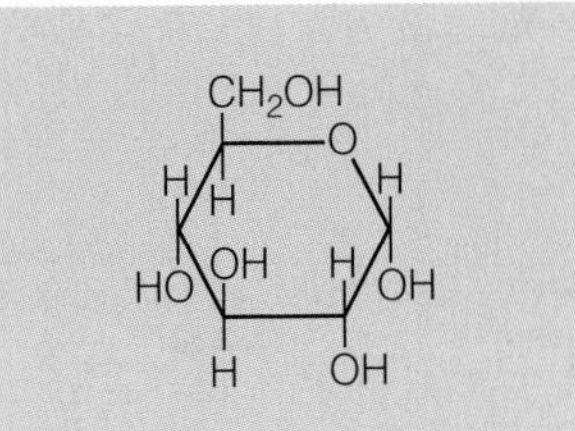

The lines representing some of the bonds and the carbons at the corners are not shown.

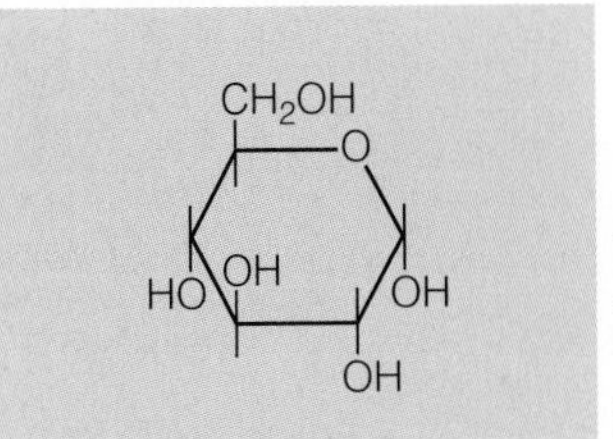

Now the single hydrogens are not shown, but lines still extend upward or downward from the ring to show where they belong.

Later sections explain that glucose is one of the two sugars in every disaccharide and the unit from which the polysaccharides are made almost exclusively. One of these polysaccharides, starch, is the chief food source of energy for all the world's people; another, glycogen, is an important storage form of energy in the body. Glucose reappears frequently throughout this chapter and all those that follow.

Fructose **Fructose** is the sweetest of the sugars. Curiously, fructose has exactly the same chemical *formula* as glucose—$C_6H_{12}O_6$—but its *structure* differs (see Figure 4-3). The arrangement of the atoms in fructose stimulates the taste buds on the tongue to produce the sweet sensation. Fructose occurs naturally in fruits and honey; other sources include products such as soft drinks, ready-to-eat cereals, and desserts that have been sweetened with high-fructose corn syrup (defined on p. 114).

Galactose The monosaccharide **galactose** occurs naturally in foods as a single sugar only in very small amounts. Galactose has the same numbers and kinds of atoms as glucose and fructose in yet another arrangement. Figure 4-3 shows galactose beside a molecule of glucose for comparison.

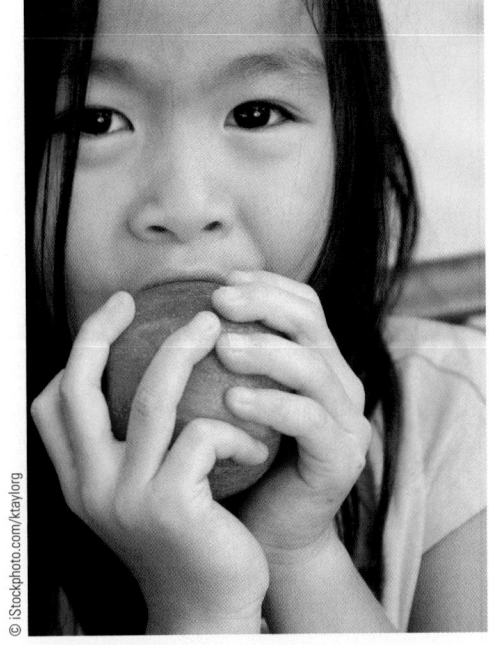

Fruits package their sugars with fibers, vitamins, and minerals, making them a sweet and healthy snack.

> **FIGURE 4-3 The Monosaccharides**

Notice the similarities—all three monosaccharides have 6 carbons (those shown plus one in each corner), 12 hydrogens (those shown plus one at the end of each single line), and 6 oxygens (all shown). Also notice the differences compared with glucose—in fructose, the ring is five-sided and in galactose, the position of one OH group differs slightly.

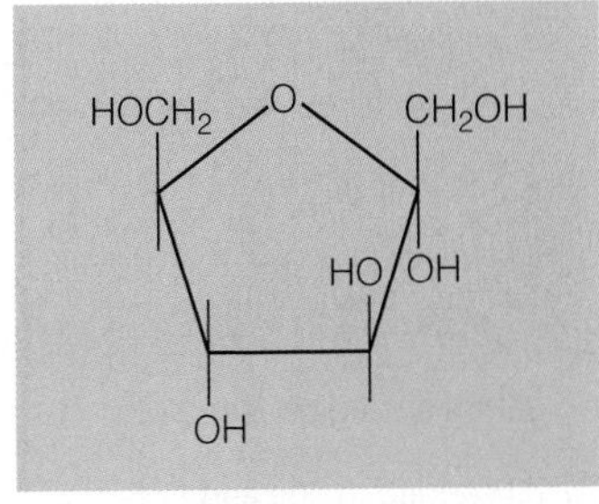

Fructose

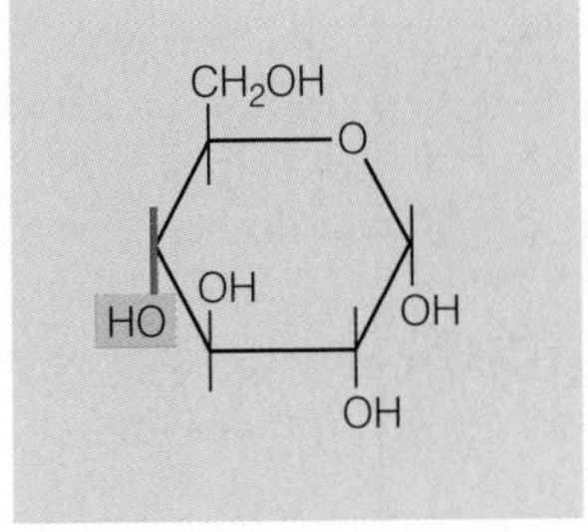

Glucose

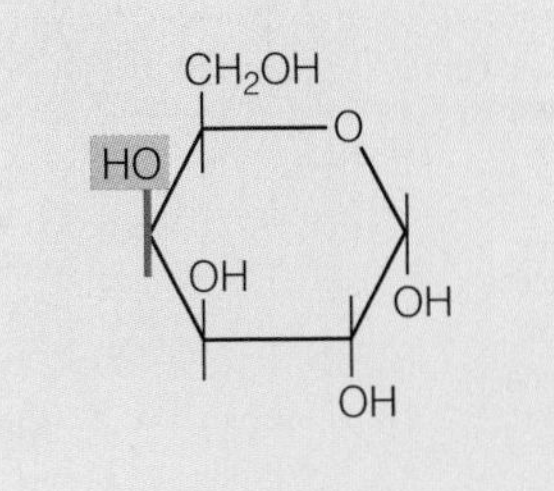

Galactose

fructose (FRUK-tose or FROOK-tose): a monosaccharide; sometimes known as *fruit sugar* or *levulose.* Fructose is found abundantly in fruits, honey, and saps.

- **fruct** = fruit
- = fructose

galactose (ga-LAK-tose): a monosaccharide; part of the disaccharide lactose.

- = galactose

> FIGURE 4-4 **Condensation of Two Monosaccharides to Form a Disaccharide**

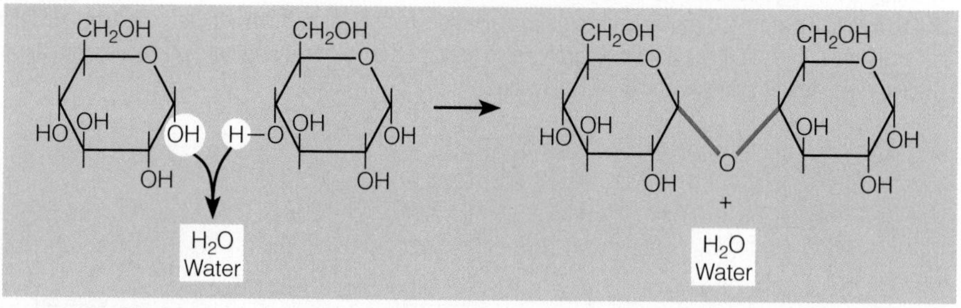

H_2O Water

H_2O Water

Glucose + glucose → Maltose

An OH group from one glucose and an H atom from another glucose combine to create a molecule of H_2O.

The two glucose molecules bond together with a single O atom to form the disaccharide maltose.

© Cengage Learning

Disaccharides The **disaccharides** are pairs of the three monosaccharides just described. Glucose occurs in all three; the second member of the pair is fructose, galactose, or another glucose. These carbohydrates—and all the other energy nutrients—are put together and taken apart by similar chemical reactions: condensation and hydrolysis.

Condensation To make a disaccharide, a chemical reaction known as **condensation** links two monosaccharides together (see Figure 4-4). A hydroxyl (OH) group from one monosaccharide and a hydrogen atom (H) from the other combine to create a molecule of water (H_2O). The two originally separate monosaccharides link together with a single oxygen (O).

Hydrolysis To break a disaccharide in two, a chemical reaction known as **hydrolysis** occurs (see Figure 4-5). A molecule of water (H_2O) splits to provide the H and OH needed to complete the resulting monosaccharides. Hydrolysis reactions commonly occur during digestion.

Maltose The disaccharide **maltose** consists of two glucose units. Maltose is produced whenever starch breaks down—as happens in human beings during carbohydrate digestion. It also occurs during the fermentation process that yields alcohol. Maltose is only a minor constituent of a few foods, most notably barley.

Sucrose Fructose and glucose together form the disaccharide **sucrose.** Sucrose is the sweetest of the disaccharides because it contains fructose, the sweetest of the monosaccharides. These sugars account for the natural sweetness of fruits, vegetables, and grains. To make table sugar, sucrose is refined from the juices of sugarcane and sugar beets, then granulated. Depending on the extent to which it

> FIGURE 4-5 **Hydrolysis of a Disaccharide**

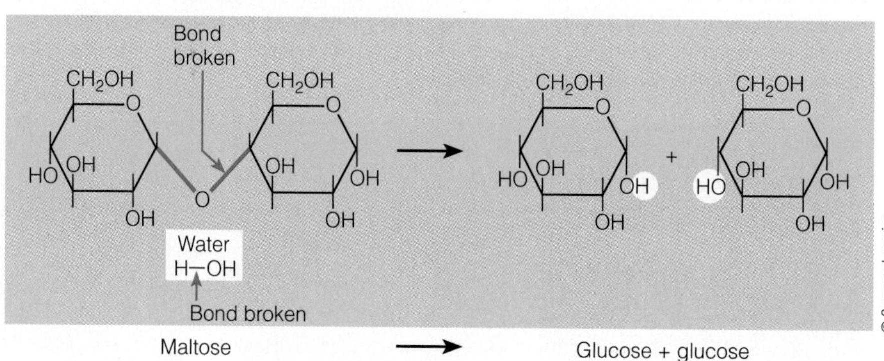

The disaccharide maltose splits into two glucose molecules with H added to one and OH to the other (from the water molecule).

disaccharides (dye-SACK-uh-rides): pairs of monosaccharides linked together. See Appendix C for the chemical structures of the disaccharides.

- **di** = two

condensation: a chemical reaction in which water is released as two molecules combine to form one larger product.

hydrolysis (high-DROL-ih-sis): a chemical reaction in which one molecule is split into two molecules, with hydrogen (H) added to one and a hydroxyl group (OH) to the other (from water, H_2O). (The noun is *hydrolysis*; the verb is *hydrolyze*.)

- **hydro** = water
- **lysis** = breaking

maltose (MAWL-tose): a disaccharide composed of two glucose units; sometimes known as *malt sugar.*

- 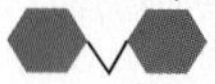  = maltose

sucrose (SUE-krose): a disaccharide composed of glucose and fructose; commonly known as *table sugar, beet sugar,* or *cane sugar.* Sucrose also occurs in many fruits and some vegetables and grains.

- **sucro** = sugar
- 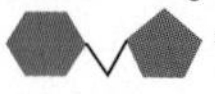  = sucrose

is refined, the product becomes the familiar brown, white, and powdered sugars available at grocery stores.

Lactose The combination of galactose and glucose makes the disaccharide **lactose,** the principal carbohydrate of milk. Known as milk sugar, lactose contributes half of the energy (kcalories) provided by fat-free milk.

Polysaccharides

In contrast to the simple carbohydrates just mentioned—the monosaccharides glucose, fructose, and galactose and the disaccharides maltose, sucrose, and lactose—the **polysaccharides** are slightly more complex, containing many glucose units and, in some cases, a few other monosaccharides strung together. Three types of polysaccharides are important in nutrition: glycogen, starches, and fibers.

Glycogen is a storage form of energy in the body; starch is the storage form of energy in plants; and fibers provide structure in stems, trunks, roots, leaves, and skins of plants. Both glycogen and starch are built of glucose units; fibers are composed of a variety of monosaccharides and other carbohydrate derivatives.

Glycogen **Glycogen** is found to only a limited extent in meats and not at all in plants.* For this reason, food is not a significant source of glycogen. Glycogen performs an important role in the body, however: it stores glucose for future use. Glycogen is made of many glucose molecules linked together in highly branched chains (see the left side of Figure 4-6). When the hormonal message "release energy" arrives at a liver or muscle cell, enzymes respond by attacking the many branches of glycogen simultaneously, making a surge of glucose available.**

Starches The human body stores glucose as glycogen, but plant cells store glucose as **starches**—long, branched or unbranched chains of hundreds or thousands of glucose molecules linked together (see the middle and right side of Figure 4-6). These giant starch molecules are packed side by side in grains such as wheat or rice, in root crops and tubers such as yams and potatoes, and in legumes such as peas and beans. When you eat the plant, your body hydrolyzes the starch to glucose and uses the glucose for its own energy purposes.

All starchy foods come from plants. Grains are the richest food source of starch, providing much of the food energy for people all over the world—rice in Asia; wheat in Canada, the United States, and Europe; corn in much of Central

*Glycogen in animal muscles rapidly breaks down after slaughter.

**Normally, liver cells produce glucose from glycogen to be sent directly to the blood; muscle cells can also produce glucose from glycogen, but must use it themselves. Muscle cells can restore the blood glucose level indirectly, however, as Chapter 7 explains.

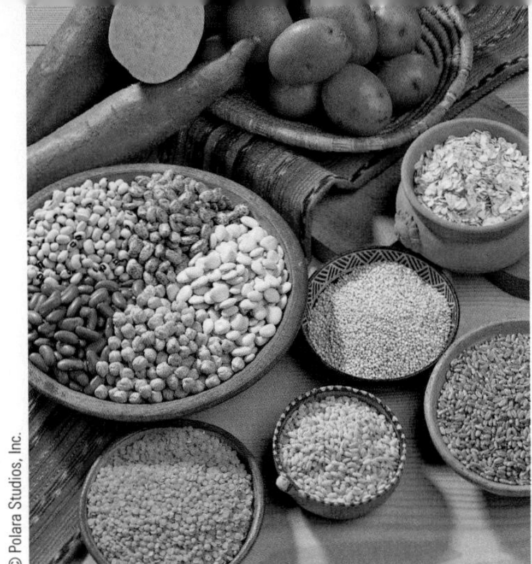

Major sources of starch include grains (such as rice, wheat, millet, rye, barley, and oats), legumes (such as kidney beans, black-eyed peas, pinto beans, navy beans, and garbanzo beans), tubers (such as potatoes), and root crops (such as yams and cassava).

lactose (LAK-tose): a disaccharide composed of glucose and galactose; commonly known as *milk sugar.*
- **lac** = milk

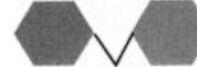 = lactose

polysaccharides: compounds composed of many monosaccharides linked together. An intermediate string of 3 to 10 monosaccharides is an *oligosaccharide.*
- **poly** = many
- **oligo** = few

glycogen (GLY-ko-jen): an animal polysaccharide composed of glucose; a storage form of glucose manufactured and stored in the liver and muscles. Glycogen is not a significant food source of carbohydrate and is not counted as a dietary carbohydrate in foods.
- **glyco** = glucose
- **gen** = gives rise to

starches: plant polysaccharides composed of many glucose molecules.

> **FIGURE 4-6 Glycogen and Starch Compared**

For details of the chemical structures, see Appendix C.

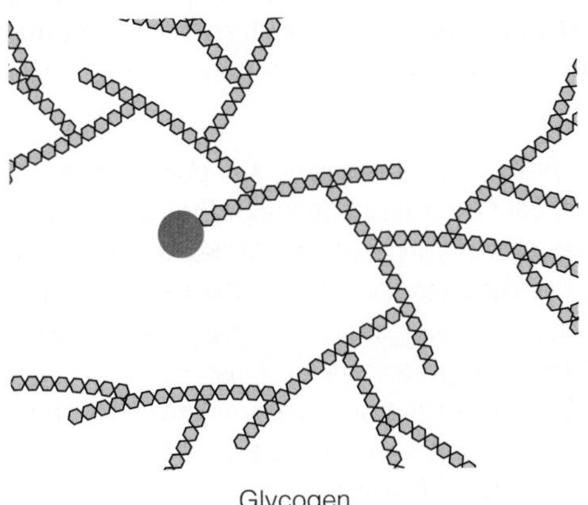

Glycogen

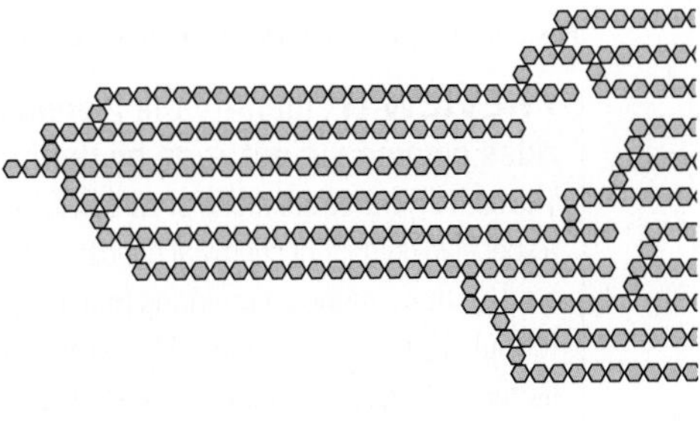

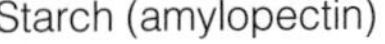

Starch (amylopectin)

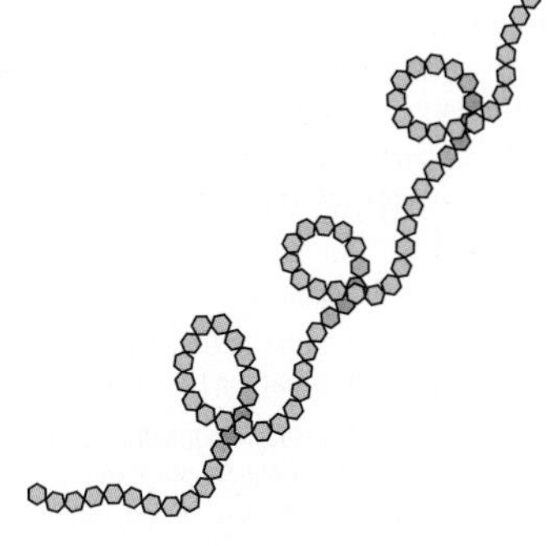

Starch (amylose)

A glycogen molecule contains hundreds of glucose units in highly branched chains. Each new glycogen molecule needs a special protein (shown here in red) for the attachment of the first glucose.

A starch molecule contains hundreds of glucose molecules in either occasionally branched chains (amylopectin) or unbranched chains (amylose).

> FIGURE 4-7 The Bonds of Starch and Cellulose Compared

Human enzymes can digest starch but they cannot digest cellulose because the bonds that link the glucose molecules together are different. See Appendix C for chemical structures and descriptions of linkages.

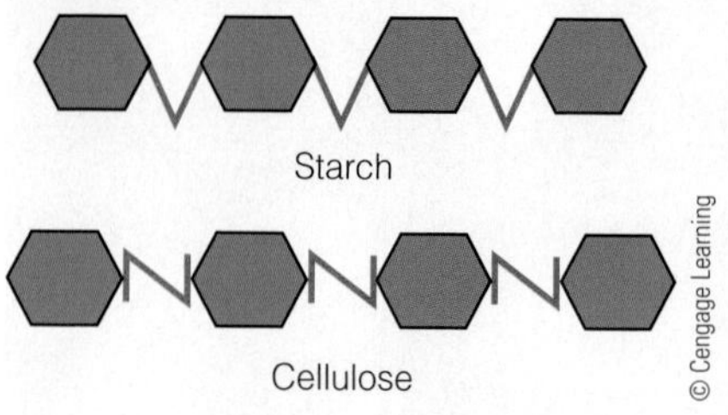

and South America; and millet, rye, barley, and oats elsewhere. Legumes and tubers are also important sources of starch.

Fibers **Dietary fibers** are the structural parts of plants and thus are found in all plant-derived foods—vegetables, fruits, whole grains, and legumes. Most dietary fibers are polysaccharides. As mentioned earlier, starches are also polysaccharides, but dietary fibers differ from starches in that the bonds between their monosaccharides cannot be broken down by digestive enzymes in the body. For this reason, dietary fibers are often described as *nonstarch polysaccharides.** Figure 4-7 illustrates the difference in the bonds that link glucose molecules together in starch with those found in the fiber cellulose. Because dietary fibers pass through the body undigested, they contribute no monosaccharides, and therefore little or no energy.

Even though most foods contain a variety of fibers, researchers often sort dietary fibers into two groups according to their solubility. Such distinctions help to explain their actions in the body.

Some dietary fibers dissolve in water (**soluble fibers**), form gels (**viscous**), and are easily digested by bacteria in the colon (**fermentable**).** Commonly found in oats, barley, legumes, and citrus fruits, soluble fibers are most often associated with protecting against heart disease and diabetes by lowering blood cholesterol and glucose levels, respectively.

Other fibers do not dissolve in water (**insoluble fibers**), do not form gels (nonviscous), and are less readily fermented. Found mostly in whole grains (bran) and vegetables, insoluble fibers promote bowel movements, alleviate constipation, and prevent diverticular disease.

As mentioned, *dietary fibers* occur naturally in plants. When these fibers have been extracted from plants or are manufactured and then added to foods or used in supplements, they are called *functional fibers*—if they have beneficial health effects. Cellulose in cereals, for example, is a dietary fiber, but when consumed as a supplement to alleviate constipation, cellulose is considered a functional fiber. *Total fiber* refers to the sum of dietary fibers and functional fibers.

A few starches are classified as dietary fibers. Known as **resistant starches,** these starches escape digestion and absorption in the small intestine. Starch may resist digestion for several reasons, including the body's digestive activities and the food's physical properties. Resistant starch is common in whole or partially milled grains, legumes, and just-ripened bananas. Cooked potatoes, pasta, and rice that have been chilled also contain resistant starch. Similar to insoluble fibers, resistant starch may support a healthy colon.

Phytic acid is not a dietary fiber, but it is often found in fiber-rich foods. Because of this close association, researchers have been unable to determine whether it is the dietary fiber, the phytic acid, or both, that binds with minerals, preventing their absorption. This binding presents a risk of mineral deficiencies, but the risk is minimal when total fiber intake is reasonable (less than 40 grams a day) and mineral intake is adequate. The nutrition consequences of mineral losses are described further in Chapters 12 and 13.

> REVIEW IT Identify the monosaccharides, disaccharides, and polysaccharides common in nutrition by their chemical structures and major food sources.

The carbohydrates are made of carbon (C), oxygen (O), and hydrogen (H). Each of these atoms can form a specified number of chemical bonds: carbon forms four, oxygen forms two, and hydrogen forms one.

The three monosaccharides (glucose, fructose, and galactose) all have the same chemical formula ($C_6H_{12}O_6$), but their structures differ. The three disaccharides (maltose, sucrose, and lactose) are pairs of monosaccharides, each containing a glucose paired with one of the three monosaccharides. The sugars derive primarily from plants, except for lactose and its component galactose, which come from milk and milk products. Two monosaccharides can be linked together by a condensation reaction to form a disaccharide and water. A disaccharide, in turn, can be broken into its two monosaccharides by a hydrolysis reaction using water.

*The nonstarch polysaccharide fibers include cellulose, hemicelluloses, pectins, gums, and mucilages. Fibers also include some *nonpolysaccharides* such as lignins, cutins, and tannins.

**Dietary fibers are fermented by bacteria in the colon to short-chain fatty acids, which are absorbed and metabolized by cells in the GI tract and liver (Chapter 5 describes fatty acids).

dietary fibers: in plant foods, the *nonstarch polysaccharides* that are not digested by human digestive enzymes, although some are digested by GI tract bacteria.

soluble fibers: nonstarch polysaccharides that dissolve in water to form a gel. An example is pectin from fruit, which is used to thicken jellies.

viscous: a gel-like consistency.

fermentable: the extent to which bacteria in the GI tract can break down fibers to fragments that the body can use.

insoluble fibers: nonstarch polysaccharides that do not dissolve in water. Examples include the tough, fibrous structures found in the strings of celery and the skins of corn kernels.

resistant starches: starches that escape digestion and absorption in the small intestine of healthy people.

phytic (FYE-tick) acid: a nonnutrient component of plant seeds; also called *phytate* (FYE-tate). Phytic acid occurs in the husks of grains, legumes, and seeds and is capable of binding minerals such as zinc, iron, calcium, magnesium, and copper in insoluble complexes in the intestine, which the body excretes unused.

The polysaccharides are chains of monosaccharides and include glycogen, starches, and dietary fibers. Both glycogen and starch are storage forms of glucose—glycogen in the body, and starch in plants—and both yield energy for human use. The dietary fibers also contain glucose (and other monosaccharides), but their bonds cannot be broken by human digestive enzymes, so they yield little, if any, energy. Table 4-1 summarizes the carbohydrate family of compounds.

TABLE 4-1 The Carbohydrate Family

Monosaccharides
Glucose
Fructose
Galactose
Disaccharides
Maltose (glucose + glucose)
Sucrose (glucose + fructose)
Lactose (glucose + galactose)
Polysaccharides
Glycogen[a]
Starches (amylose and amylopectin)
Fibers (soluble and insoluble)

[a]Glycogen is a polysaccharide, but not a common dietary source of carbohydrate.

4.2 Digestion and Absorption of Carbohydrates

› LEARN IT Summarize carbohydrate digestion and absorption.

The ultimate goal of digestion and absorption of sugars and starches is to break them into small molecules—chiefly glucose—that the body can absorb and use. The large starch molecules require extensive breakdown; the disaccharides need be broken only once and the monosaccharides not at all. The details follow.

Carbohydrate Digestion Figure 4-8 (p. 106) traces the digestion of carbohydrates through the GI tract. When a person eats foods containing starch, enzymes hydrolyze the long chains to shorter chains, the short chains to disaccharides, and, finally, the disaccharides to monosaccharides.* This process begins in the mouth.

In the Mouth In the mouth, thoroughly chewing high-fiber foods slows eating and stimulates the flow of saliva. The salivary enzyme **amylase** starts to work, hydrolyzing starch to shorter polysaccharides and to the disaccharide maltose. In fact, you can taste the change if you chew a piece of starchy food like a cracker and hold it in your mouth for a few minutes without swallowing it—the cracker begins tasting sweeter as the enzyme acts on it. Because food is in the mouth for a relatively short time, very little carbohydrate digestion takes place there; it begins again in the small intestine.

In the Stomach Carbohydrate digestion ceases in the stomach. The activity of salivary amylase diminishes as the stomach's acid and protein-digesting enzymes inactivate the enzyme. The stomach's digestive juices contain no enzymes to break down carbohydrates. Fibers are not digested, but because they linger in the stomach, they delay gastric emptying, thereby providing a feeling of fullness and **satiety.**

In the Small Intestine The small intestine performs most of the work of carbohydrate digestion. A major carbohydrate-digesting enzyme, pancreatic amylase, enters the intestine via the pancreatic duct and continues breaking down the polysaccharides to shorter glucose chains and maltose. The final step takes place on the outer membranes of the intestinal cells. There specific enzymes break down specific disaccharides:

- **Maltase** breaks maltose into two glucose molecules.
- **Sucrase** breaks sucrose into one glucose and one fructose molecule.
- **Lactase** breaks lactose into one glucose and one galactose molecule.

At this point, all polysaccharides and disaccharides have been broken down to monosaccharides—mostly glucose molecules, with some fructose and galactose molecules as well.

In the Large Intestine Within 1 to 4 hours after a meal, all the sugars and most of the starches have been digested. Only the fibers remain in the digestive tract. Fibers in the large intestine attract water, which softens the stools for passage without straining. Also, bacteria in the GI tract ferment some fibers. This process

*The short chains of glucose units that result from the breakdown of starch are known as *dextrins*. The word sometimes appears on food labels because dextrins can be used as thickening agents in processed foods.

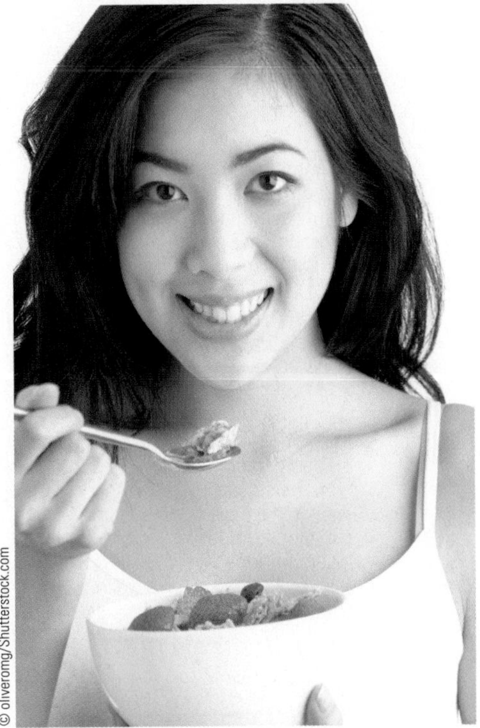

When a person eats carbohydrate-rich foods, the body receives a valuable commodity—glucose.

amylase (AM-ih-lace): an enzyme that hydrolyzes amylose (a form of starch). Amylase is a *carbohydrase*, an enzyme that breaks down carbohydrates.

satiety (sah-TIE-eh-tee): the feeling of fullness and satisfaction that occurs after a meal and inhibits eating until the next meal. Satiety determines how much time passes between meals.

- **sate** = to fill

maltase: an enzyme that hydrolyzes maltose.

sucrase: an enzyme that hydrolyzes sucrose.

lactase: an enzyme that hydrolyzes lactose.

> FIGURE 4-8 Carbohydrate Digestion in the GI Tract

STARCH

Mouth and salivary glands
The salivary glands secrete saliva into the mouth to moisten the food. The salivary enzyme amylase begins digestion:

Starch —Amylase→ Small polysaccharides, maltose

Stomach
Stomach acid inactivates salivary enzymes, halting starch digestion.

Small intestine and pancreas
The pancreas produces an amylase that is released through the pancreatic duct into the small intestine:

Starch —Pancreatic amylase→ Small polysaccharides, maltose

Then disaccharidase enzymes on the surface of the small intestinal cells hydrolyze the disaccharides into monosaccharides:

Maltose —Maltase→ Glucose + Glucose

Sucrose —Sucrase→ Fructose + Glucose

Lactose —Lactase→ Galactose + Glucose

Intestinal cells absorb these monosaccharides.

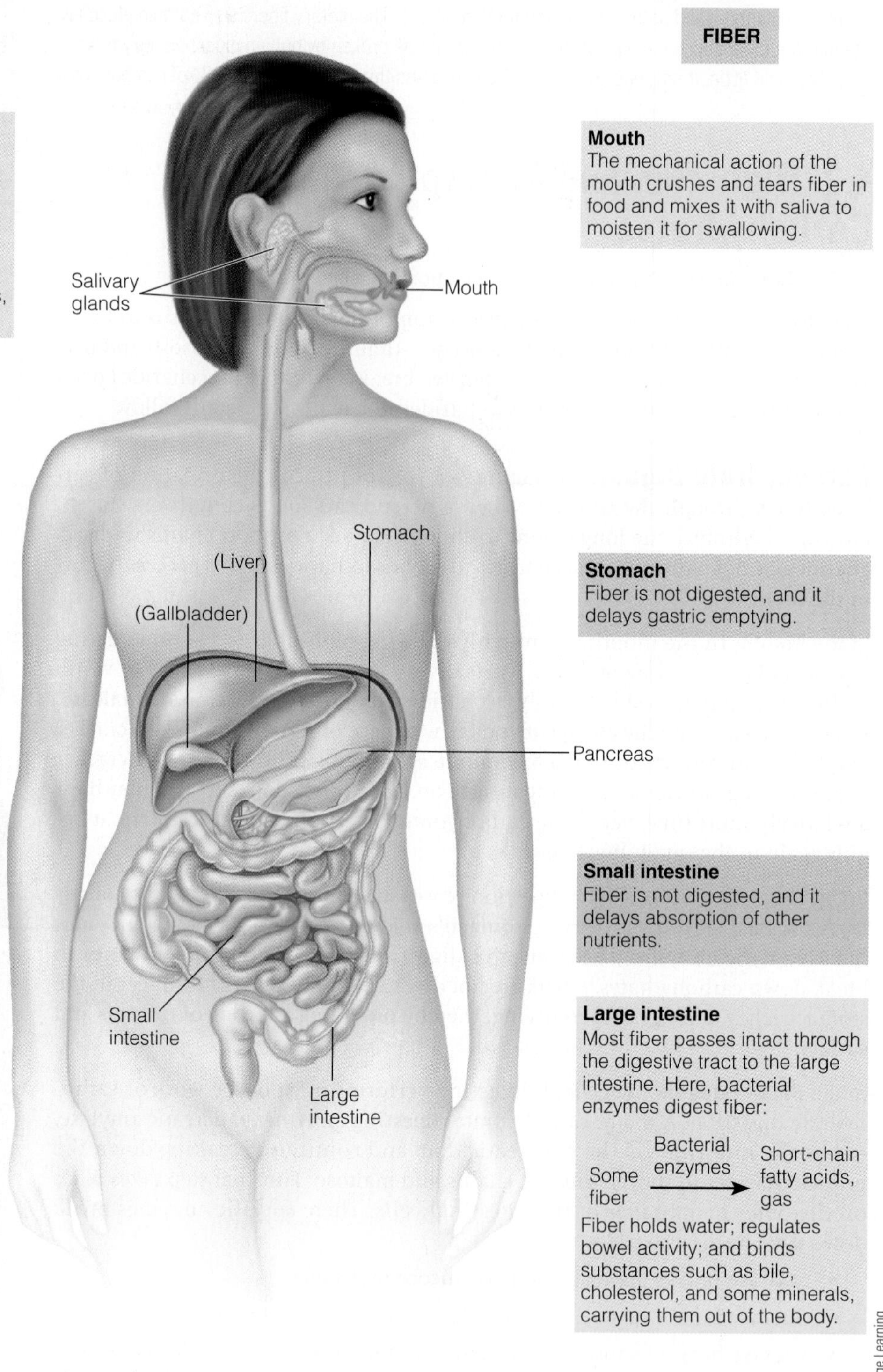

FIBER

Mouth
The mechanical action of the mouth crushes and tears fiber in food and mixes it with saliva to moisten it for swallowing.

Stomach
Fiber is not digested, and it delays gastric emptying.

Small intestine
Fiber is not digested, and it delays absorption of other nutrients.

Large intestine
Most fiber passes intact through the digestive tract to the large intestine. Here, bacterial enzymes digest fiber:

Some fiber —Bacterial enzymes→ Short-chain fatty acids, gas

Fiber holds water; regulates bowel activity; and binds substances such as bile, cholesterol, and some minerals, carrying them out of the body.

generates water, gas, and short-chain fatty acids (described in Chapter 5).* The cells of the colon use these small fat molecules for energy. Metabolism of short-chain fatty acids also occurs in the cells of the liver. Fibers, therefore, can contribute some energy (1.5 to 2.5 kcalories per gram), depending on the extent to which they are broken down by bacteria and the fatty acids are absorbed. How much energy fiber contributes to a person's daily intake remains unclear.

*The short-chain fatty acids produced by GI bacteria are primarily acetic acid, propionic acid, and butyric acid.

Carbohydrate Absorption Glucose is unique in that it can be absorbed to some extent through the lining of the mouth, but for the most part, nutrient absorption takes place in the small intestine. Glucose and galactose enter the cells lining the small intestine by active transport; fructose is absorbed by facilitated diffusion.

As the blood from the small intestine circulates through the liver, cells there take up fructose and galactose and most often convert them to compounds within the same metabolic pathways as glucose. Figure 4-9 shows that fructose and galactose are mostly metabolized in the liver, whereas glucose is sent out to the body's cells for energy. In the end, all disaccharides provide at least one glucose molecule directly, and they can provide the equivalent of another one indirectly—through the metabolism of fructose and galactose in the liver.

Lactose Intolerance Normally, the intestinal cells produce enough of the enzyme lactase to ensure that the disaccharide lactose found in milk is both digested and absorbed efficiently. Lactase activity is highest immediately after birth, as befits an infant whose first and only food for a while will be breast milk or infant formula. In the great majority of the world's populations, lactase activity declines dramatically during childhood and adolescence to about 5 to 10 percent of the activity at birth. Only a relatively small percentage (about 30 percent) of the people in the world retain enough lactase to digest and absorb lactose efficiently throughout adult life.

Symptoms When more lactose is consumed than the available lactase can handle, lactose molecules remain in the intestine undigested, attracting water and causing bloating, abdominal discomfort, and diarrhea—the symptoms of **lactose intolerance.** The undigested lactose becomes food for intestinal bacteria, which multiply and produce irritating acid and gas, further contributing to the discomfort and diarrhea.

Causes As mentioned, lactase activity commonly declines with age. **Lactase deficiency** may also develop when the intestinal villi are damaged by disease, certain medicines, prolonged diarrhea, or malnutrition. Depending on the extent of the intestinal damage, lactose malabsorption may be temporary or permanent. In extremely rare cases, an infant is born with a lactase deficiency, making feeding a challenge.

Prevalence The prevalence of lactose intolerance varies widely among ethnic groups, indicating that the trait has a genetic component. The prevalence of

lactose intolerance: a condition that results from the inability to digest the milk sugar lactose; characterized by bloating, gas, abdominal discomfort, and diarrhea. Lactose intolerance differs from milk allergy, which is caused by an immune reaction to the protein in milk.

lactase deficiency: a lack of the enzyme required to digest the disaccharide lactose into its component monosaccharides (glucose and galactose).

> FIGURE 4-9 **Absorption of Monosaccharides**

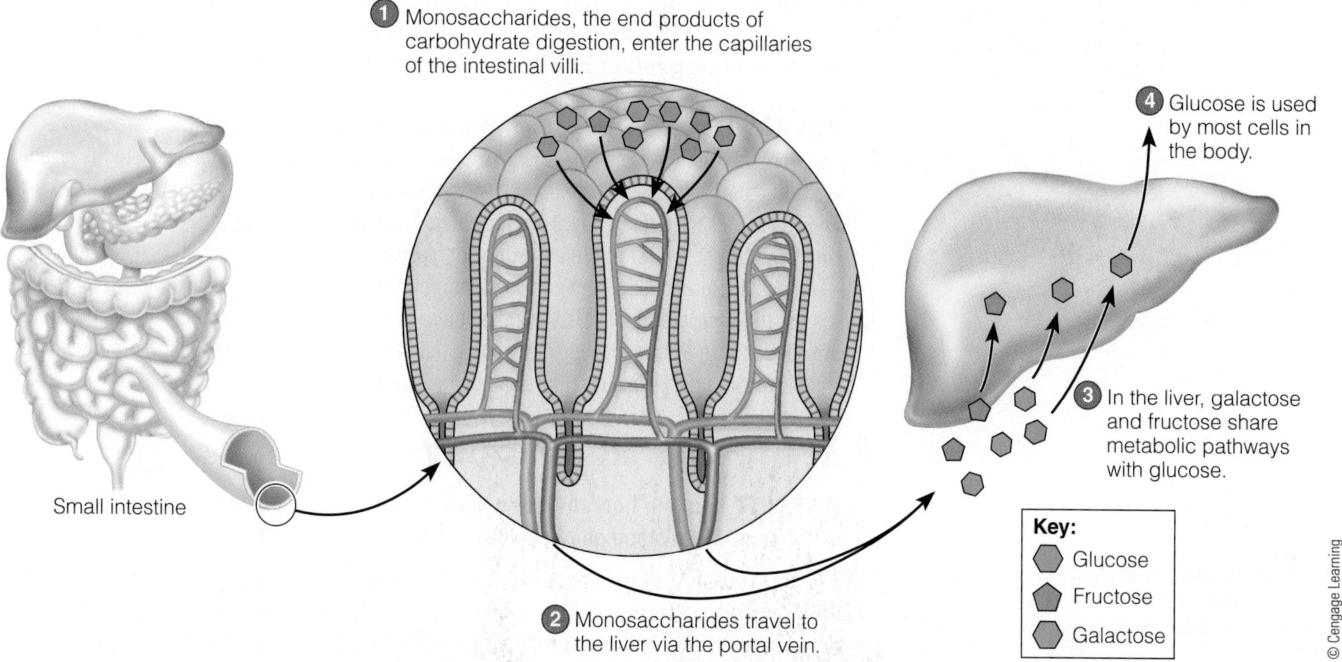

1 Monosaccharides, the end products of carbohydrate digestion, enter the capillaries of the intestinal villi.
Small intestine
2 Monosaccharides travel to the liver via the portal vein.
3 In the liver, galactose and fructose share metabolic pathways with glucose.
4 Glucose is used by most cells in the body.
Key:
Glucose
Fructose
Galactose

lactose intolerance is lowest among Scandinavians and other northern Europeans and highest among native North Americans and Southeast Asians. An estimated 30 million to 50 million people in the United States are lactose intolerant.

Dietary Changes Managing lactose intolerance requires some dietary changes, although total elimination of milk products usually is not necessary.[1] Excluding all milk products from the diet can lead to nutrient deficiencies because these foods are a major source of several nutrients, notably the mineral calcium, vitamin D, and the B vitamin riboflavin. Fortunately, many people with lactose intolerance can consume foods containing up to 6 grams of lactose (½ cup milk) without symptoms. The most successful strategies are to increase intake of milk products gradually, consume them with other foods in meals, and spread their intake throughout the day. In addition, yogurt containing live bacteria seems to improve lactose intolerance. A change in the type, number, and activity of GI bacteria—not the reappearance of the missing enzyme—accounts for the ability to adapt to milk products. Importantly, most lactose-intolerant individuals need to *manage* their dairy consumption rather than *restrict* it.

In many cases, lactose-intolerant people can tolerate fermented milk products such as yogurt and **kefir.** The bacteria in these products digest lactose for their own use, thus reducing the lactose content. Even when the lactose content is equivalent to milk's, yogurt produces fewer symptoms. Hard cheeses, such as cheddar, and cottage cheese are often well tolerated because most of the lactose is removed with the whey during manufacturing. Lactose continues to diminish as cheese ages.

Many lactose-intolerant people use commercially prepared milk products (such as Lactaid) that have been treated with an enzyme that breaks down the lactose. Alternatively, they take enzyme tablets with meals or add enzyme drops to their milk. The enzyme hydrolyzes much of the lactose in milk to glucose and galactose, which lactose-intolerant people can absorb without ill effects.

Because people's tolerance to lactose varies widely, lactose-restricted diets must be highly individualized. A completely lactose-free diet can be difficult because lactose appears not only in milk and milk products but also as an ingredient in many nondairy foods such as breads, cereals, breakfast drinks, salad dressings, and cake mixes (see Table 4-2). People on strict lactose-free diets need to read labels and avoid foods that include milk, milk solids, whey (milk liquid), and casein (milk protein, which may contain traces of lactose). They also need to check all medications with the pharmacist because 20 percent of prescription drugs and 5 percent of over-the-counter drugs contain lactose as a filler.

People who consume few milk products must take care to meet riboflavin, vitamin D, and calcium needs. Later chapters on the vitamins and minerals offer help with finding good nonmilk sources of these nutrients.

TABLE 4-2 Lactose in Selected Foods

Foods	Lactose (g)
Whole-wheat bread, 1 slice	0.5
Dinner roll, 1	0.5
Cheese, 1 oz	
Cheddar or American	0.5
Parmesan or cream	0.8
Doughnut (cake type), 1	1.2
Chocolate candy, 1 oz	2.3
Sherbet, 1 c	4.0
Cottage cheese (low-fat), 1 c	7.5
Ice cream, 1 c	9.0
Milk, 1 c	12.0
Yogurt (low-fat), 1 c	15.0

NOTE: Yogurt is often enriched with nonfat milk solids, which increase its lactose content to a level higher than milk's.

› REVIEW IT Summarize carbohydrate digestion and absorption.

In the digestion and absorption of carbohydrates, the body breaks down starches into the disaccharide maltose. Maltose and the other disaccharides (lactose and sucrose) from foods are broken down into monosaccharides, which are absorbed. The fibers help to regulate the passage of food through the GI tract and slow the absorption of glucose, but they contribute little, if any, energy.

Lactose intolerance is a common condition that occurs when there is insufficient lactase to digest the disaccharide lactose found in milk and milk products. Symptoms are limited to GI distress. Because treatment requires limiting milk and milk products in the diet, other sources of riboflavin, vitamin D, and calcium must be included.

4.3 Glucose in the Body

› LEARN IT Explain how the body maintains its blood glucose concentration and what happens when blood glucose rises too high or falls too low.

The primary role of carbohydrates in the body is to supply the cells with glucose for energy. Scientists have long known that providing energy is glucose's primary role in the body, but they have recently uncovered additional roles that

kefir (keh-FUR): a fermented milk created by adding *Lactobacillus acidophilus* and other bacteria that break down lactose to glucose and galactose, producing a sweet, lactose-free product.

glucose and other sugars perform in the body.* When sugar molecules adhere to the body's protein and fat molecules, the consequences can be dramatic. Sugars attached to a protein change the protein's shape and function; when they bind to lipids in a cell's membranes, sugars alter the way cells recognize one another.**

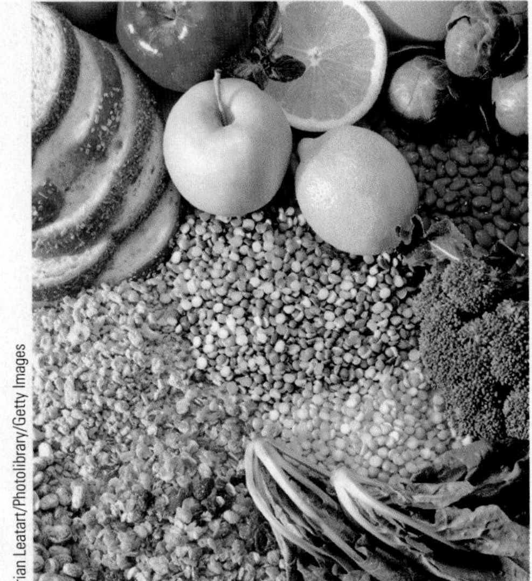

The carbohydrates of grains, vegetables, fruits, and legumes supply most of the energy in a healthful diet.

A Preview of Carbohydrate Metabolism

Glucose plays the central role in carbohydrate metabolism. This brief discussion provides just enough information about carbohydrate metabolism to illustrate that the body needs and uses glucose as a chief energy nutrient. Chapter 7 provides a full description of energy metabolism.

Storing Glucose as Glycogen

After a meal, blood glucose rises, and liver cells link excess glucose molecules by condensation reactions into long, branching chains of glycogen (review Figure 4-6, p.103). When blood glucose falls, the liver cells break down glycogen by hydrolysis reactions into single molecules of glucose and release them into the bloodstream. Thus glucose becomes available to supply energy to the brain and other tissues regardless of whether the person has eaten recently.

The liver stores about one-third of the body's total glycogen and releases glucose into the bloodstream as needed. Muscle cells can also store glucose as glycogen (the other two-thirds), but muscles hoard most of their supply, using it just for themselves during exercise. The brain maintains a small amount of glycogen, which is thought to provide an emergency energy reserve during times of severe glucose deprivation.

Glycogen holds water and, therefore, is rather bulky. The body can store only enough glycogen to provide energy for relatively short periods of time—less than a day during rest and a few hours at most during exercise. For its long-term energy reserves, for use over days or weeks of food deprivation, the body uses its abundant, water-free fuel, fat, as Chapter 5 describes.

Using Glucose for Energy

Glucose fuels the work of most of the body's cells and is the preferred energy source for brain cells, other nerve cells, and developing red blood cells. Inside a cell, a series of reactions can break glucose into smaller compounds that yield energy when broken down completely to carbon dioxide and water (see Chapter 7).

Making Glucose from Protein

As mentioned, the liver's glycogen stores are limited, and the brain needs glucose to fuel its activities. To keep providing glucose to meet energy needs, a person has to eat carbohydrate-rich foods frequently. Yet people who do not always attend faithfully to their bodies' carbohydrate needs still survive. How do they manage without glucose from dietary carbohydrate? Do they simply draw energy from the other two energy-yielding nutrients, fat and protein? They do draw energy from them, but not simply.

Fat cannot make glucose to any significant extent. The amino acids of protein can be used to make glucose to some extent, but amino acids and proteins have jobs of their own that no other nutrient can perform. Still, when a person does not replenish glucose by eating carbohydrate, body proteins are broken down to make glucose to fuel the brain and other special cells. These body proteins derive primarily from the liver and skeletal muscles.

The conversion of protein to glucose is called **gluconeogenesis**—literally, the making of new glucose. Only adequate dietary carbohydrate can prevent this use of protein for energy, and this role of carbohydrate is known as its **protein-sparing action.**

Making Ketone Bodies from Fat Fragments

An inadequate supply of carbohydrate can shift the body's energy metabolism in a precarious direction. With less carbohydrate providing glucose to meet the brain's energy needs, fat takes an alternative

gluconeogenesis (gloo-ko-nee-oh-JEN-ih-sis): the making of glucose from a noncarbohydrate source such as amino acids or glycerol (described in more detail in Chapter 7).
- **gluco** = glucose
- **neo** = new
- **genesis** = making

protein-sparing action: the action of carbohydrate (and fat) in providing energy that allows protein to be used for other purposes.

*The study of sugars and their derivatives is known as *glycobiology*.
**These combination molecules are known as *glycoproteins* and *glycolipids*, respectively.

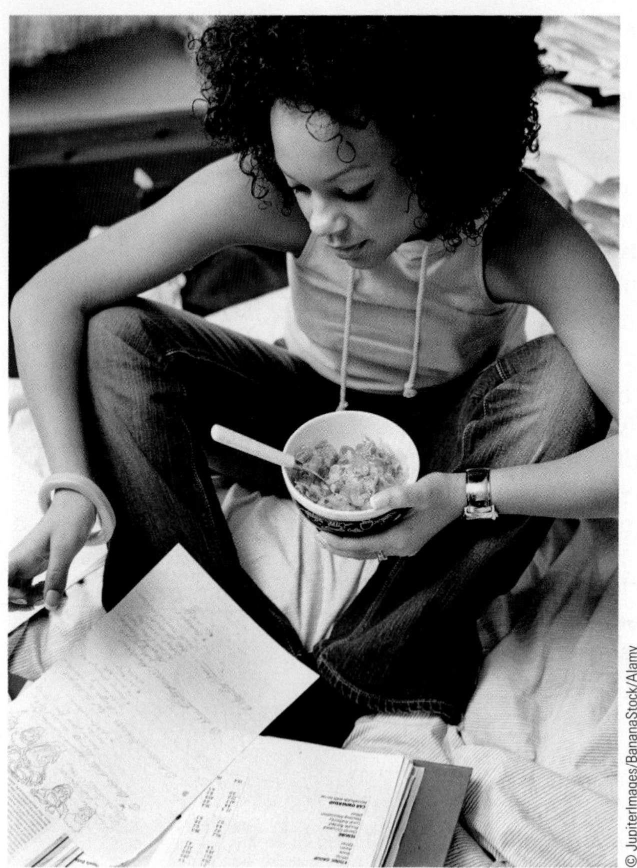
© JupiterImages/BananaStock/Alamy

The brain uses glucose as its primary fuel for energy.

metabolic pathway; instead of entering the main energy pathway, fat fragments combine with one another, forming **ketone bodies.** Ketone bodies provide an alternative fuel source during starvation, but when their production exceeds their use, they accumulate in the blood, causing **ketosis.** Because most ketone bodies are acidic, ketosis disturbs the body's normal **acid-base balance.** (Chapter 7 explores ketosis and the metabolic consequences of low-carbohydrate diets further.)

To spare body protein and prevent ketosis, the body needs at least 50 to 100 grams of carbohydrate a day. Dietary recommendations urge people to select abundantly from carbohydrate-rich foods to provide for considerably more.

Using Glucose to Make Fat After meeting its immediate energy needs and filling its glycogen stores to capacity, the body must find a way to handle any extra glucose. When glucose is abundant, energy metabolism shifts to use more glucose instead of fat. If that isn't enough to restore glucose balance, the liver breaks glucose into smaller molecules and puts them together into the more permanent energy-storage compound—fat. Thus when carbohydrate is abundant, fat is either conserved (by using more carbohydrate in the fuel mix) or created (by using excess carbohydrate to make body fat). The fat then travels to the fatty tissues of the body for storage. Unlike the liver cells, which can store only enough glycogen to meet less than a day's energy needs, fat cells can store seemingly unlimited quantities of fat.

The Constancy of Blood Glucose

Every body cell depends on glucose for its fuel to some extent, and the cells of the brain and the rest of the nervous system depend almost exclusively on glucose for their energy. The activities of these cells never cease, and they have limited ability to store glucose. Day and night, they continually draw on the supply of glucose in the fluid surrounding them. To maintain the supply, a steady stream of blood moves past these cells bringing more glucose from either the small intestine (food) or the liver (via glycogen breakdown or gluconeogenesis).

Maintaining Glucose Homeostasis To function optimally, the body must maintain blood glucose within limits that permit the cells to nourish themselves. If blood glucose falls below normal, a person may become dizzy and weak; if it rises above normal, a person may become fatigued. Left untreated, fluctuations to the extremes—either high or low—can be fatal.

The Regulating Hormones Blood glucose homeostasis is regulated primarily by two hormones: *insulin,* which moves glucose from the blood into the cells, and *glucagon,* which brings glucose out of storage when necessary. Figure 4-10 depicts these hormonal regulators at work.

After a meal, as blood glucose rises, special cells of the pancreas respond by secreting **insulin** into the blood.* In general, the amount of insulin secreted corresponds with the rise in glucose. As the circulating insulin contacts the body's cells, receptors respond by ushering glucose from the blood into the cells. Most of the cells take only the glucose they can use for energy right away, but the liver and muscle cells can assemble the small glucose units into long, branching chains of glycogen for storage. The liver cells also convert extra glucose to fat.[2] Thus elevated blood glucose returns to normal levels as excess glucose is stored as glycogen and fat.

When blood glucose falls (as occurs between meals), other special cells of the pancreas respond by secreting **glucagon** into the blood.** Glucagon raises blood glucose by signaling the liver to break down its glycogen stores and release glucose into the blood for use by all the other body cells.

*The *beta* (BAY-tuh) *cells,* one of several types of cells in the pancreas, secrete insulin in response to elevated blood glucose concentration.

**The *alpha cells* of the pancreas secrete glucagon in response to low blood glucose concentration.

ketone (KEE-tone) **bodies:** acidic compounds produced by the liver during the breakdown of fat when carbohydrate is not available.

ketosis (kee-TOE-sis): an undesirably high concentration of ketone bodies in the blood and urine.

acid-base balance: the equilibrium in the body between acid and base concentrations (see Chapter 12).

insulin (IN-suh-lin): a hormone secreted by special cells in the pancreas in response to (among other things) elevated blood glucose concentration. Insulin controls the transport of glucose from the bloodstream into the muscle and fat cells.

glucagon (GLOO-ka-gon): a hormone secreted by special cells in the pancreas in response to low blood glucose concentration. Glucagon elicits release of glucose from liver glycogen stores.

> **FIGURE 4-10 Maintaining Blood Glucose Homeostasis**

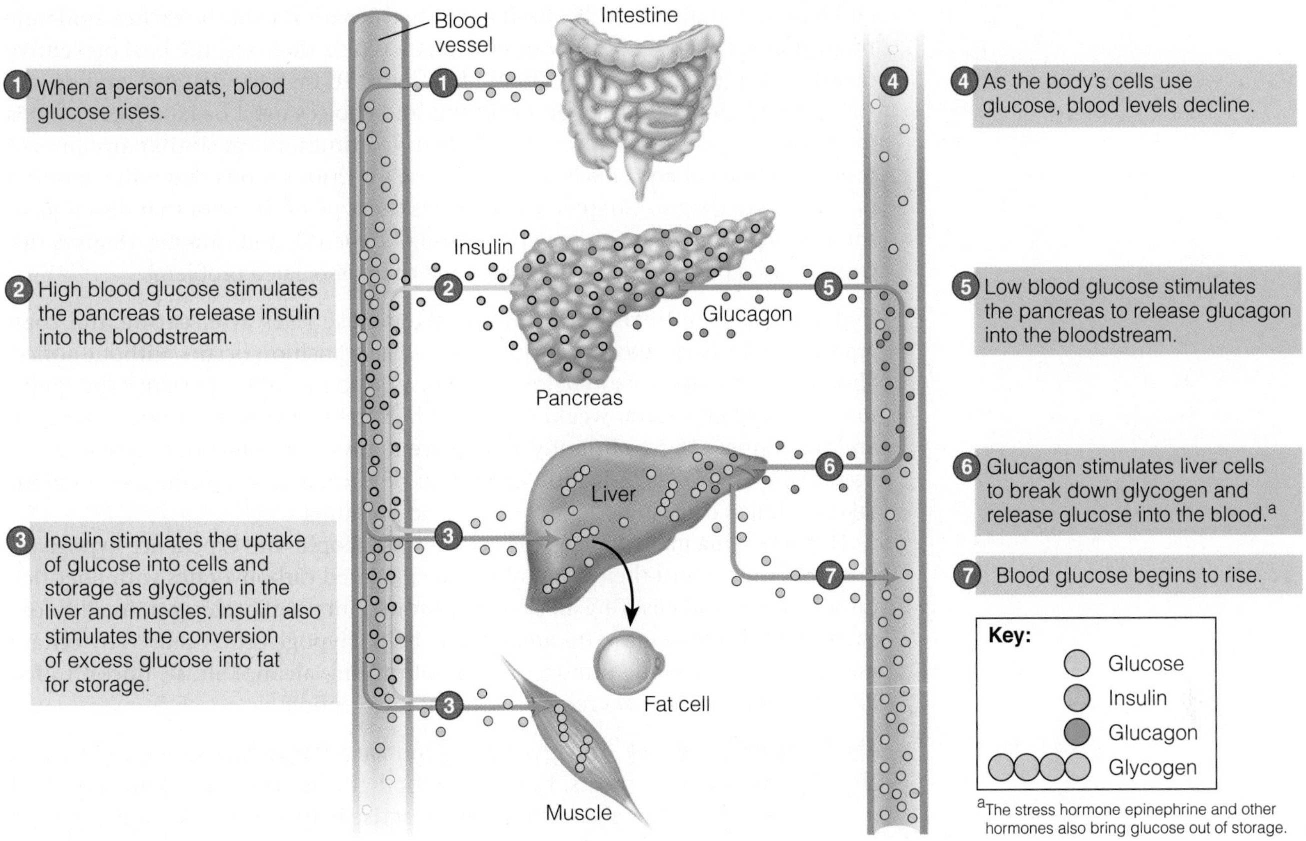

1. When a person eats, blood glucose rises.
2. High blood glucose stimulates the pancreas to release insulin into the bloodstream.
3. Insulin stimulates the uptake of glucose into cells and storage as glycogen in the liver and muscles. Insulin also stimulates the conversion of excess glucose into fat for storage.
4. As the body's cells use glucose, blood levels decline.
5. Low blood glucose stimulates the pancreas to release glucagon into the bloodstream.
6. Glucagon stimulates liver cells to break down glycogen and release glucose into the blood.[a]
7. Blood glucose begins to rise.

Blood vessel
Intestine
Insulin
Glucagon
Pancreas
Liver
Fat cell
Muscle

Key:
Glucose
Insulin
Glucagon
Glycogen

[a]The stress hormone epinephrine and other hormones also bring glucose out of storage.

Another hormone that signals the liver cells to release glucose is the "fight-or-flight" hormone, **epinephrine.** When a person experiences stress, epinephrine acts quickly to ensure that all the body cells have energy fuel in emergencies. Among its many roles in the body, epinephrine works to release glucose from liver glycogen to the blood.

Balancing within the Normal Range The maintenance of normal blood glucose depends on foods and hormones. When blood glucose falls below normal, food can replenish it, or in the absence of food, glucagon can signal the liver to break down glycogen stores. When blood glucose rises above normal, insulin can signal the cells to take in glucose for energy. Eating balanced meals that provide abundant carbohydrates, including fibers, and a little fat help to slow down the digestion and absorption of carbohydrate so that glucose enters the blood gradually. Eating at regular intervals also helps the body maintain a balance between the extremes.

Falling outside the Normal Range In some people, blood glucose regulation fails. When this happens, either of two conditions can result: diabetes or hypoglycemia. People with these conditions need to plan their diets and physical activities to help maintain their blood glucose within a normal range. Table 4-3 presents the blood glucose levels defining normal, prediabetes, and diabetes.

Diabetes In **diabetes,** blood glucose rises after a meal and remains above normal levels because insulin is either inadequate or ineffective. Elevated blood glucose is a characteristic of two main types of diabetes. In **type 1 diabetes,** the less common type, the pancreas fails to produce insulin. Although the exact cause is unclear, some research suggests that in genetically susceptible people, certain viruses activate the immune system to attack and destroy cells in the pancreas as if they were foreign cells. In **type 2 diabetes,** the more common type of diabetes, the cells fail to respond to insulin. This condition tends to occur as a consequence

TABLE 4-3 Fasting Blood Glucose

Normal	70–99 mg/dL
Prediabetes	100–125 mg/dL
Diabetes	≥126 mg/dL

epinephrine (EP-ih-NEFF-rin): a hormone of the adrenal gland that modulates the stress response; formerly called *adrenaline.* When administered by injection, epinephrine counteracts anaphylactic shock by opening the airways and maintaining heartbeat and blood pressure.

diabetes (DYE-ah-BEE-teez): metabolic disorder characterized by elevated blood glucose resulting from insufficient insulin, ineffective insulin, or both; the complete medical term is *diabetes mellitus* (meh-LIE-tus). When blood glucose levels are higher than normal, but below the diagnosis of diabetes, the condition is called *prediabetes.*

type 1 diabetes: the less common type of diabetes in which the pancreas produces little or no insulin. Type 1 diabetes usually results from autoimmune destruction of pancreatic beta cells.

type 2 diabetes: the more common type of diabetes in which the cells fail to respond to insulin. Type 2 diabetes usually accompanies obesity and results from insulin resistance coupled with insufficient insulin secretion.

of obesity. As the incidence of obesity in the United States has risen in recent decades, so too has the incidence of diabetes. This trend is most notable among children and adolescents as obesity among the nation's youth reaches epidemic proportions. Because obesity can precipitate type 2 diabetes, the best preventive measure is to maintain a healthy body weight. To manage diabetes and ensure stable blood glucose levels, food portions and choices must be balanced. It helps to eat meals and snacks at regularly scheduled times, to eat similar amounts of food at each meal and snack, and to choose nutritious foods that will support a healthy body weight. Chapter 15 describes the type of diabetes that develops in some women during pregnancy (gestational diabetes), and Chapter 18 gives full coverage to type 1 and type 2 diabetes and their associated problems.

Hypoglycemia In healthy people, blood glucose rises after eating and then gradually falls back into the normal range. The transition occurs without notice. Should blood glucose drop below normal, a person would experience the symptoms of **hypoglycemia:** weakness, rapid heartbeat, sweating, anxiety, hunger, and trembling. Most commonly, hypoglycemia is a consequence of poorly managed diabetes: too much insulin, strenuous physical activity, inadequate food intake, or illness cause blood glucose levels to plummet.

Hypoglycemia in healthy people is rare. Most people who experience hypoglycemia need only adjust their diets by replacing refined carbohydrates with fiber-rich carbohydrates and ensuring an adequate protein intake at each meal. In addition, smaller meals eaten more frequently may help. Hypoglycemia caused by certain medications, pancreatic tumors, overuse of insulin, alcohol abuse, uncontrolled diabetes, or other illnesses requires medical intervention.

The Glycemic Response The **glycemic response** refers to how quickly glucose is absorbed after a person eats, how high blood glucose rises, and how quickly it returns to normal. Slow absorption, a modest rise in blood glucose, and a smooth return to normal are desirable (a low glycemic response). Fast absorption, a surge in blood glucose, and an overreaction that plunges glucose below normal are less desirable (a high glycemic response). The glycemic response may be particularly important to people with diabetes, who may benefit from limiting foods that produce too great a rise, or too sudden a fall, in blood glucose.

Different foods elicit different glycemic responses; the **glycemic index** classifies foods accordingly (see Table 4-4). Some studies have shown that selecting

TABLE 4-4 Glycemic Index of Selected Common Foods

Glycemic Index	Grains	Fruits	Vegetables	Milk Products	Protein Foods[a]	Other
Low	Barley, chapati, corn tortilla, rice noodles, rolled oats, udon noodles, spaghetti	Apple, apple juice, banana, dates, mango, orange, orange juice, peaches (canned), strawberry jam	Carrots, corn	Ice cream, milk, soy milk, yogurt	Legumes	Chocolate
Medium	Brown rice, couscous	Pineapple	Potatoes (french fries), sweet potatoes			Popcorn, potato chips, soft drinks
High	Breads, breakfast cereals, white rice	Watermelon	Potatoes (boiled)			Rice crackers

NOTE: Using the glucose reference scale, foods are classified as low (55 or less), medium (56 to 69), or high (70 or greater).

[a]Protein foods that contain little or no carbohydrate (such as meats, poultry, fish, and eggs) do not raise blood glucose, and therefore do not have a glycemic index.

SOURCE: Adapted from F. S. Atkinson, K. Foster-Powell, and J. C. Brand-Miller, International tables of glycemic index and glycemic load values: 2008, *Diabetes Care* 31 (2008): 2281–2283.

hypoglycemia (HIGH-po-gly-SEE-me-ah): an abnormally low blood glucose concentration.

glycemic (gly-SEEM-ic) **response:** the extent to which a food raises the blood glucose concentration and elicits an insulin response.

glycemic index: a method of classifying foods according to their potential for raising blood glucose.

foods with a low glycemic index is a practical way to improve dietary adequacy and glucose control.[3] Lowering the glycemic index of the diet may improve blood lipids, reduce inflammation, and lower the risk of heart disease as well.[4] A low glycemic diet may also help with appetite regulation and weight management, although research findings are mixed.[5]

Researchers debate whether selecting foods based on the glycemic index is practical or offers any real health benefits. Those opposing the use of the glycemic index argue that it is not sufficiently supported by scientific research. The glycemic index has been determined for relatively few foods, and when the glycemic index has been established, it is based on an average of multiple tests with wide variations in their results. Values vary because of differences in the physical and chemical characteristics of foods, testing methods of laboratories, and digestive processes of individuals. Calculating the glycemic index for meals or diets based on individual foods greatly overestimates the values.[6]

Furthermore, the practical utility of the glycemic index is limited because this information is neither provided on food labels nor intuitively apparent. Indeed, a food's glycemic index is not always what one might expect. Ice cream, for example, is a high-sugar food but produces less of a glycemic response than baked potatoes, a high-starch food. Perhaps most relevant to real life, a food's glycemic effect differs depending on plant variety, food processing, cooking method, and whether it is eaten alone or with other foods. Most people eat a variety of foods, cooked and raw, that provide different amounts of carbohydrate, fat, and protein—all of which influence the glycemic index of a meal.

Paying attention to the glycemic index may be unnecessary because current guidelines already suggest many low and moderate glycemic index choices: whole grains, legumes, vegetables, fruits, and milk and milk products. In addition, eating frequent, small meals spreads glucose absorption across the day and thus offers similar metabolic advantages to eating foods with a low glycemic response. People wanting to follow a low glycemic diet should be careful not to adopt a low-carbohydrate diet as well. Highlight 4 explores the controversies surrounding low-carbohydrate diets.

› REVIEW IT Explain how the body maintains its blood glucose concentration and what happens when blood glucose rises too high or falls too low.

Dietary carbohydrates provide glucose that can be used by the cells for energy, stored by the liver and muscles as glycogen, or converted into fat if intakes exceed needs. All of the body's cells depend on glucose; those of the brain and central nervous system are especially dependent on it. Without glucose, the body is forced to break down its protein tissues to make glucose and to alter energy metabolism to make ketone bodies from fats. Blood glucose regulation depends primarily on two pancreatic hormones: insulin to move glucose from the blood into the cells when levels are high and glucagon to free glucose from glycogen stores and release it into the blood when levels are low.

4.4 Health Effects and Recommended Intakes of Sugars

› LEARN IT Describe how added sugars can contribute to health problems.

Almost everyone finds pleasure in sweet foods—after all, the taste preference for sweets is inborn. To a child, the sweeter the food, the better. In adults, this preference is somewhat diminished, but most adults still enjoy at least an occasional sweet food or beverage.

In the United States, the natural sugars of milk, fruits, vegetables, and grains account for about half of the sugar intake; the other half consists of concentrated sugars that have been refined and added to foods for a variety of purposes (see Table 4-5 on p.114). The use of added sugars has risen steadily over the past several decades, both in the United States and around the world, with soft drinks and sugared fruit drinks accounting for most of the increase. An estimated 75 percent of the packaged foods in the United States contain sweeteners, mostly added

TABLE 4-5 Functions of Sugar in Foods

- Acts as a bulking agent in ice cream and baked goods
- Adds texture and color to baked goods
- Balances the acidity of tomato- and vinegar-based products such as sauces, salad dressings, and other condiments
- Enhances flavor
- Imparts a creamy consistency in frozen desserts
- Inhibits microbial growth by binding with water in jams and jellies
- Maintains the natural color and texture of preserved fruits
- Provides fuel for yeast fermentation, causing bread to rise or producing alcohol

sugars.[7] On average, US adults consume almost 15 percent of their daily energy intake from added sugars.[8] These added sugars assume various names on food labels: sucrose, invert sugar, corn sugar, corn syrups and solids, high-fructose corn syrup, and honey. A food is likely to be high in added sugars if its ingredient list starts with any of the monosaccharides or disaccharides already defined or any of the sugars named in the accompanying glossary, or if it includes several of them.

Health Effects of Sugars In moderate amounts, sugars add pleasure to meals without harming health.[9] In excess, however, sugars can be detrimental, and the average American diet currently delivers excessive amounts. The *Dietary Guidelines* caution that added sugars may increase the risk of certain chronic diseases—even in the absence of overweight or obesity.[10]

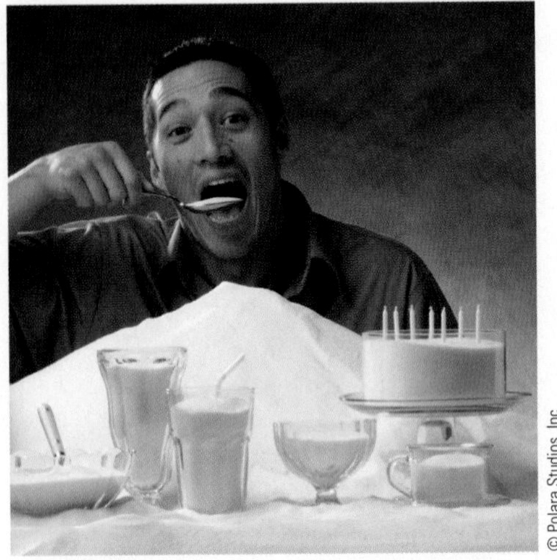

Almost half of the added sugars in our diet come from sugar-sweetened beverages, but baked goods, ice cream, candy, and breakfast cereals also make substantial contributions.

Obesity and Chronic Diseases Over the past several decades, as obesity rates increased sharply, consumption of added sugars reached an all-time high—much of it because of the surge in high-fructose corn syrup use, especially in beverages.[11] High-fructose corn syrup is composed of fructose and glucose in a ratio of roughly 50:50. Compared with sucrose, high-fructose corn syrup is less expensive, easier to use, and more soluble. Manufacturers prefer high-fructose corn syrup because it retains moisture, resists drying out, controls crystallization, prevents microbial growth and blends easily with other sweeteners, acids, and flavorings. In addition to being used in beverages, high-fructose corn syrup sweetens candies, baked goods, and hundreds of other foods.

In general, the energy intake of people who drink soft drinks, fruit punches, and other sugary beverages is greater than those who choose differently. Adolescents, for example, who drink as much as 26 ounces or more (about two cans) of sugar-sweetened soft drinks daily, consume 400 more kcalories a day than teens who don't. Not too surprisingly, they also tend to weigh more. Overweight

GLOSSARY OF ADDED SUGARS

brown sugar: refined white sugar crystals to which manufacturers have added molasses syrup with natural flavor and color; 91 to 96 percent pure sucrose.

confectioners' sugar: finely powdered sucrose, 99.9 percent pure.

corn sweeteners: corn syrup and sugars derived from corn.

corn syrup: a syrup made from cornstarch that has been treated with acid, high temperatures, and enzymes to produce glucose, maltose, and dextrins. It may be dried and used as *corn syrup solids.* See also *high-fructose corn syrup (HFCS).*

dextrose: the name food manufacturers use for the sugar that is chemically the same as glucose; *anhydrous dextrose* is similar, differing primarily in the temperature of crystallization.

high-fructose corn syrup (HFCS): a syrup made from cornstarch that has been treated with an enzyme that converts some of the glucose to the sweeter fructose; made especially for use in processed foods and beverages, where it is the predominant sweetener. With a chemical structure similar to sucrose, most HFCS has a fructose content of 42 or 55 percent, with glucose making up the remainder.

honey: sugar (mostly sucrose) formed from nectar gathered by bees. Composition and flavor vary, but honey always contains a mixture of sucrose, fructose, and glucose.

invert sugar: a mixture of glucose and fructose formed by the hydrolysis of sucrose in a chemical process; sold only in liquid form and sweeter than sucrose. Invert sugar is used as a food additive to help preserve freshness and prevent shrinkage.

levulose: an older name for fructose.

malt syrup: a sweetener made from sprouted barley and containing mostly maltose.

maple sugar: a sugar (mostly sucrose) purified from the concentrated sap of the sugar maple tree.

molasses: the thick brown syrup produced during sugar refining. Molasses retains residual sugar and other by-products and a few minerals; blackstrap molasses contains significant amounts of calcium and iron.

nectar: a sugary fluid secreted by plants to encourage pollination by insects.

raw sugar: the first crop of crystals harvested during sugar processing. Raw sugar cannot be sold in the United States because it contains too much filth (dirt, insect fragments, and the like). Sugar sold as "raw sugar" domestically has actually gone through more than half of the refining steps.

tagatose (TAG-ah-tose): poorly absorbed monosaccharide similar in structure to fructose; naturally occurring or derived from lactose.

turbinado (ter-bih-NOD-oh) **sugar**: sugar produced using the same refining process as white sugar, but without the bleaching and anticaking treatment. Traces of molasses give turbinado its sandy color.

white sugar: granulated sucrose or "table sugar," produced by dissolving, concentrating, and recrystallizing raw sugar.

children and adolescents consume more sweet desserts and soft drinks than their normal-weight peers. Research confirms that consuming sugary beverages correlates with increases in energy intake, body weight, and associated diseases.[12]

Some research suggests that added sugars in general, and fructose in particular, favor the fat-making pathways and impair the fat-clearing pathways in the liver.[13] The resulting blood lipid profile increases the risk of heart disease.[14] As the liver busily makes lipids, its handling of glucose becomes unbalanced and insulin resistance develops—an indicator of prediabetes. All in all, research is finding links between added sugars and the risk of diabetes, inflammation, hypertension, and heart disease.[15] Importantly, moderate intakes of sugars do not cause these health problems.[16] For this reason, researchers suggest replacing sugar-sweetened beverages with water, and the American Heart Association recommends limiting added sugars to no more than 100 kcalories per day for women and 150 kcalories per day for men (which is about 5 percent of a 2000- and 2500-kcalorie diet, respectively).[17]

Nutrient Deficiencies Foods such as whole grains, vegetables, legumes, and fruits that contain some natural sugars and lots of starches and fibers provide vitamins and minerals as well. By comparison, foods and beverages that contain lots of added sugars such as cakes, candies, and sodas provide the body with glucose and energy, but few, if any, other essential nutrients or fiber. The more added sugars (and solid fats) in the diet, the more difficult it is to meet recommendations for dietary fiber, vitamins, and minerals and still stay within kcalorie limits.

A person spending 200 kcalories of a day's energy allowance on a 16-ounce soda gets little of value for those kcalories. In contrast, a person using 200 kcalories on three slices of whole-wheat bread gets 9 grams of protein, 6 grams of fiber, plus several of the B vitamins with those kcalories. For the person who wants something sweet, a reasonable compromise might be two slices of bread with a teaspoon of jam on each. The amount of sugar a person can afford to eat depends on how many discretionary kcalories are available beyond those needed to deliver indispensable vitamins and minerals.

By following the USDA Food Pattern and making careful food selections, a typical adult can obtain all the needed nutrients within an allowance of about 1500 kcalories. An inactive older woman who is limited to fewer than 1500 kcalories a day can afford to eat only the most nutrient-dense foods—with few, or no, discretionary kcalories available. In contrast, an active teenage boy may need as many as 3000 kcalories a day. If he chooses wisely, then he may use discretionary kcalories for nutrient-dense foods that contain added sugars—or even an occasional empty kcalorie choice such as a cola beverage. Examples of nutrient-dense foods containing some added sugars include whole-grain breakfast cereals and vanilla yogurt.

Some people believe that because honey is a natural food, it is nutritious—or, at least, more nutritious than sugar.* A look at their chemical structures reveals the truth. Honey, like table sugar, contains glucose and fructose. The primary difference is that in table sugar the two monosaccharides are bonded together as the disaccharide sucrose, whereas in honey some of the monosaccharides are free. Whether a person eats monosaccharides individually, as in honey, or linked together, as in table sugar, they end up the same way in the body: as glucose and fructose.

Honey does contain a few vitamins and minerals, but not many. Honey is denser than crystalline sugar, too, so it provides more energy per spoonful. Table 4-6 on p. 116 shows that honey and white sugar are similar nutritionally—and both fall short of milk, legumes, fruits, grains, and vegetables.

Although the body cannot distinguish whether fructose and glucose derive from honey or table sugar, this is not to say that all sugar sources are alike. Some sugar sources are more nutritious than others. Consider a fruit, say, an orange. The fruit may give you the same amounts of fructose and glucose and the same number of kcalories as a spoonful of sugar or honey, but the packaging is more valuable nutritionally. The fruit's sugars arrive in the body diluted in a large

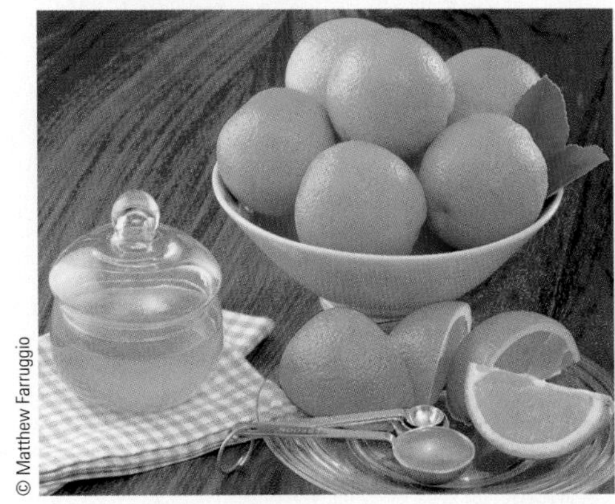

You receive about the same amount and kinds of sugars from an orange as from a tablespoon of honey, but the packaging makes a big nutrition difference.

*Honey should never be fed to infants because of the risk of botulism. Chapters 16 and 19 provide more details.

TABLE 4-6 Sample Nutrients in Sugar and Other Foods

The indicated portion of any of these foods provides approximately 100 kcalories. Notice that for a similar number of kcalories and grams of carbohydrate, foods such as milk, legumes, fruits, grains, and vegetables offer more of the other nutrients than do the sugars.

	Size of 100 kcal Portion	Carbohydrate (g)	Protein (g)	Calcium (mg)	Iron (mg)	Potassium (mg)	Vitamin D (µg)
Foods							
Milk, 1% low-fat	1 c	12	8	300	0.1	397	2
Kidney beans	½ c	20	7	45	1.6	303	0
Apricots	6	24	3	30	0.8	544	0
Bread, whole-wheat	1½ slices	20	4	77	1.2	122	0
Broccoli, cooked	2 c	20	7	125	2.1	914	0
Sugars							
Sugar, white	2 tbs	24	0	0	trace	0	0
Molasses	2 tbs	28	0	82	1.9	586	0
Cola beverage	1 c	26	0	6	trace	7	0
Honey	1½ tbs	26	trace	2	0.1	16	0

volume of water, packaged in fiber, and mixed with essential vitamins, minerals, and phytochemicals.

As these comparisons illustrate, the significant difference between sugar sources is not between "natural" honey and "purified" sugar but between concentrated added sugars and the dilute, naturally occurring sugars that sweeten foods. You can suspect an exaggerated nutrition claim when someone asserts that one product is more nutritious than another because it contains honey.

Added sugars contribute to nutrient deficiencies by displacing nutrients. For nutrition's sake, the appropriate attitude to take is not that sugar is "bad" and must be avoided, but that nutritious foods must come first. If nutritious foods crowd sugar out of the diet, that is fine—but not the other way around. As always, balance, variety, and moderation guide healthy food choices.

> **FIGURE 4-11 Dental Caries**

Dental caries begins when acid dissolves the enamel that covers the tooth. If not repaired, the decay may penetrate the dentin and spread into the pulp of the tooth, causing inflammation, abscess, and possible loss of the tooth.

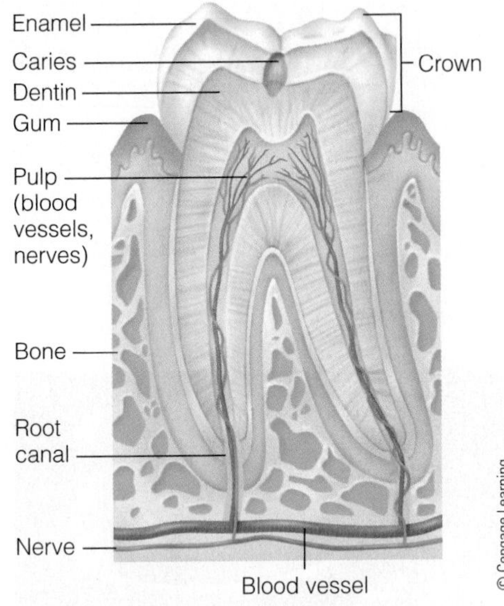

Dental Caries Both naturally occurring and added sugars from foods and from the breakdown of starches in the mouth can contribute to tooth decay. Bacteria in the mouth ferment the sugars and, in the process, produce an acid that erodes tooth enamel (see Figure 4-11), causing **dental caries,** or tooth decay. People can eat sugar without this happening, though. Much depends on how long foods stay in the mouth. Sticky foods stay on the teeth longer and continue to yield acid longer than foods that are readily cleared from the mouth. For that reason, sugar in a juice consumed quickly, for example, is less likely to cause dental caries than sugar in a pastry. By the same token, the sugar in sticky foods such as raisins can be more detrimental than the quantity alone would suggest.

Another concern is how often people eat sugar. Bacteria produce acid for 20 to 30 minutes after each exposure. If a person eats three pieces of candy at one time, the teeth will be exposed to approximately 30 minutes of acid destruction. But, if the person eats three pieces at half-hour intervals, the time of exposure increases to 90 minutes. Likewise, slowly sipping a sugary sports beverage may be more harmful than drinking quickly and clearing the mouth of sugar. Nonsugary foods can help remove sugar from tooth surfaces; hence, it is better to eat sugar with meals than between meals. Foods such as milk and cheese may be particularly helpful in protecting against dental caries by neutralizing acids, stimulating salivary flow, inhibiting bacterial activity, and promoting remineralization of damaged enamel.

Beverages such as soft drinks, orange juice, and sports drinks not only contain sugar but also have a low pH. These acidic drinks can erode tooth enamel and may explain why the prevalence of dental erosion is growing steadily.

dental caries: decay of teeth.
- **caries** = rottenness

The development of caries depends on several factors: the bacteria that reside in **dental plaque,** the saliva that cleanses the mouth, the minerals that form the teeth, and the foods that remain after swallowing. For most people, good oral hygiene will prevent dental caries (see Table 4-7). In fact, regular brushing (twice a day, with a fluoride toothpaste) and flossing may be more effective in preventing dental caries than restricting sugary foods. Still, nutrition is a key component of dental health.[18] *The Dietary Guidelines for Americans* recommend a combined approach to prevent dental caries—practicing good oral hygiene, drinking fluoridated water, and consuming sugar- and starch-containing foods and beverages less frequently.

TABLE 4-7 Behaviors to Prevent Dental Caries

- Limit between meal sugar-sweetened beverages (such as carbonated beverages and fruit drinks), sticky foods (such as raisins and caramels), slow-dissolving candies (such as lollipops and jaw breakers), and snacks containing sugars and starches (such as cookies and cakes).
- Brush with a fluoride toothpaste and floss teeth regularly.
- If brushing and flossing are not possible, drink some milk, rinse with water, or chew sugarless gum immediately after a meal or snack.
- Get a dental checkup regularly.
- Drink fluoridated water.

Recommended Intakes of Sugars Estimates indicate that, on average, each person in the United States consumes about 30 teaspoons (about 120 grams) of sugars a day.[19] Most of the sugars in the average American diet are added to foods and beverages by manufacturers during processing; major sources of added sugars include sugar-sweetened beverages (sodas, energy drinks, sports drinks, fruit drinks), desserts, and candy. Some sugars are also added by consumers during food preparation and at the table. Because added sugars deliver kcalories, but few or no nutrients or fiber, the *Dietary Guidelines for Americans* urge consumers to "reduce the intake of kcalories from added sugars." These added sugar kcalories (and those from solid fats and alcohol) are considered discretionary kcalories—and most people need to limit their intake. By reducing the intake of foods and beverages with added sugars, consumers can lower the kcalorie content of the diet without compromising the nutrient content. The "How To" on p. 118 provides strategies for reducing the intake of added sugars.

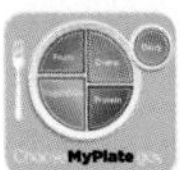

> DIETARY GUIDELINES FOR AMERICANS

Reduce the intake of kcalories from added sugars.

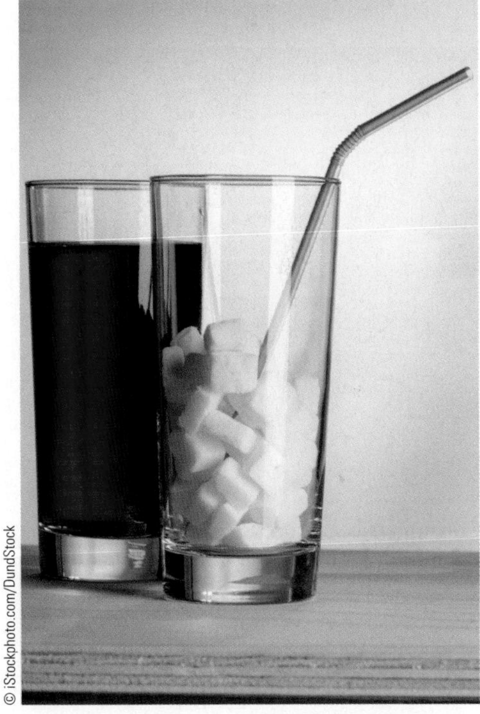

Soft drinks deliver a startling amount of sugar.

To help consumers make healthier choices, food labels include the amounts of *added sugars* in a serving. Food labels also list the *total* grams of sugar a food provides, which reflects both added sugars and those occurring naturally in foods. To help estimate sugar and energy intakes accurately, keep in mind that 1 teaspoon of sugar—whether white sugar, brown sugar, corn syrup, honey, nectar, jam, jelly, maple syrup, or molasses—provides about 5 grams of carbohydrate and *about* 20 kcalories per teaspoon. Some are lower (16 kcalories for table sugar) and others are higher (22 kcalories for honey), but a 20-kcalorie average is an acceptable approximation. For a person who uses ketchup liberally, it may help to remember that 1 tablespoon of ketchup supplies about 1 teaspoon of sugar. And those who drink soft drinks regularly should keep in mind that a 12-ounce can of soda delivers about 10 teaspoons of sugar.

The Dietary Reference Intakes (DRI) committee did not publish a Tolerable Upper Intake Level (UL) for sugar, but as mentioned, excessive intakes can interfere with sound nutrition and good health. Few people can eat lots of sugary treats and still meet all of their nutrient needs without exceeding their kcalorie allowance. Specifically, the DRI suggests that added sugars should account for no more than 25 percent of the day's total energy intake.[20] One out of eight in the US population exceeds this maximum intake.[21] When added sugars occupy this much of a diet, intakes from the five food groups usually fall below recommendations. For a person consuming 2000 kcalories a day, 25 percent represents 500 kcalories (that is, 125 grams, or 31 teaspoons) from concentrated sugars—and that's a lot of sugar. Consider that 500 kcalories of sugar is 40 ounces of cola, 1/2 cup of honey, 125 jelly beans, 23 marshmallows, or 30 teaspoons of sugar. Perhaps an athlete in training whose energy needs are high can afford the added sugars from sports drinks without compromising nutrient intake, but most people do better by limiting their use of added sugars. Added sugars contribute an average of 16 percent of the total energy in the typical American diet. The World Health Organization (WHO) suggests limiting added sugars to less than 10 percent of energy intake,

dental plaque: a gummy mass of bacteria that grows on teeth and can lead to dental caries and gum disease.

>How To

Reduce the Intake of Added Sugars

- Use less table sugar when preparing meals and at the table.
- Use your sugar kcalories to sweeten nutrient-dense foods (such as oatmeal) instead of consuming empty kcalorie foods and beverages (such as candy and soda).
- Drink fewer regular sodas, sports drinks, energy drinks, and fruit drinks; choose water, fat-free milk, 100 percent fruit juice, or unsweetened tea or coffee instead. If you do drink sugar-sweetened beverages, have a small portion.
- Select fruit for dessert. Eat less cake, cookies, ice cream, other desserts, and candy. If you do eat these foods, have a small portion.
- Read the Nutrition Facts on a label to choose foods with fewer added sugars. Select the unsweetened version of a food (such as cornflakes) instead of the sweetened version (such as frosted cornflakes) to reduce the quantity of added sugars in the diet.
- The ingredients list also helps to identify foods with added sugars. A food is likely to be high in added sugars if its ingredient list starts with any of the sugars named in the glossary on p. 114, or if it includes several of them.

> TRY IT Compare the energy contents, added sugars, and ingredients lists of 1 cup of the following foods: fruit-flavored yogurt and plain yogurt, sugar-frosted cornflakes and plain cornflakes, orange soda and orange juice.

Consumers use artificial sweeteners to help them limit kcalories and minimize sugar intake.

and notes that 5 percent or less provides additional benefits, which is in line with American Heart Association recommendations mentioned earlier.

Alternative Sweeteners To control weight gain, blood glucose, and dental caries, many consumers turn to alternative sweeteners to help them limit kcalories and minimize added sugars in the diet.[22] In doing so, they encounter three sets of alternative sweeteners: artificial sweeteners, an herbal sweetener, and sugar alcohols.

Artificial Sweeteners **Artificial sweeteners** are sometimes called **nonnutritive sweeteners** because they provide virtually no energy. Table 4-8 provides general details about each of the sweeteners approved for use in the United States, including their **Acceptable Daily Intakes (ADI).** (The table does not include the nonnutritive sweeteners alitame, cyclamate, neohesperidine, and thaumatin, which are approved in other countries, but not in the United States.) Chapter 9 includes a discussion of their use in weight control and Chapter 19 focuses on some of the safety issues surrounding their use. Considering that all substances are toxic at some dose, it is little surprise that large doses of artificial sweeteners (or their components or metabolic by-products) may have adverse effects. The question to ask is whether their ingestion is safe for human beings in quantities people normally use (and potentially abuse).

Other High-Intensity Sweeteners Stevia leaves and monk fruit have long been used by the people of South America and China, respectively, to sweeten their foods and beverages. The FDA has granted these sweeteners the status of "generally recognized as safe," and they can be used as additives in a variety of foods and beverages.

Sugar Alcohols Some "sugar-free" or reduced-kcalorie products contain **sugar alcohols.** The sugar alcohols (or polyols) occur naturally in fruits and vegetables; manufacturers also use sugar alcohols in many processed foods to add bulk and texture, to provide a cooling effect or sweet taste, to inhibit browning from heat, and to retain moisture. These products may claim to be "sugar-free" on their labels, but in this case, "sugar-free" does not mean free of kcalories. Sugar alcohols do

artificial sweeteners: sugar substitutes that provide negligible, if any, energy; sometimes called *nonnutritive sweeteners*.

nonnutritive sweeteners: sweeteners that yield no energy (or insignificant energy in the case of aspartame).

Acceptable Daily Intake (ADI): the estimated amount of a sweetener that individuals can safely consume each day over the course of a lifetime without adverse effect.

sugar alcohols: sugarlike compounds that can be derived from fruits or commercially produced from dextrose; also called *polyols*. Examples include *erythritol, isomalt, lactitol, maltitol, mannitol, sorbitol,* and *xylitol*.

TABLE 4-8 **Nonnutritive Alternative Sweeteners**

Sweetener	Chemical Composition	Body's Response	Relative Sweetness[a]	Energy (kcal/g)	ADI and (Estimated Equivalent)[b]	Comments
Acesulfame potassium or Acesulfame K[c] (AY-sul-fame)	Potassium salt	Not digested or absorbed	200	0	15 mg/kg body weight[d] (30 cans diet soda)	Approved for general use (except in meats and poultry); combines well with other sweeteners; heat stable at baking temperatures
Advantame (ad-VAN-tame)	Aspartame derivative, similar to neotame	Rapidly, but poorly absorbed	20,000	0	32.8 mg/kg body weight (4000 packets of sweetener)	Approved for general use (except in meat and poultry); heat stable at baking temperatures
Aspartame[e] (ah-SPAR-tame or ASS-par-tame)	Amino acids (phenylalanine and aspartic acid) and a methyl group	Digested and absorbed	200	4[f]	50 mg/kg body weight[g] (18 cans diet soda)	Approved for general use; degrades at high temperatures
Luo han guo[h]	Cucurbitane glycosides extracts from *Siraitia grosvenorii* swingle fruit (also known as monk fruit)	Digested and absorbed	225	1	Not determined	GRAS;[i] general use as a tabletop sweetener and food ingredient
Neotame (NEE-oh-tame)	Aspartame with an additional side group attached	Not digested or absorbed	10,000	0	18 mg/day	Approved for general use (except in meats and poultry); used minimally in food processing
Saccharin[j] (SAK-ah-ren)	Benzoic sulfimide	Rapidly absorbed and excreted	300	0	5 mg/kg body weight (10 packets of sweetener)	Restricted use in beverages, in individual packages, and in processed foods
Stevia[k] (STEE-vee-ah)	Glycosides found in the leaves of the *Stevia rebaudiana* herb	Digested and absorbed	300	0	4 mg/kg body weight	GRAS
Sucralose[l] (SUE-kra-lose)	Sucrose with Cl atoms instead of OH groups	Not digested or absorbed	600	0	5 mg/kg body weight (6 cans diet soda)	Approved for general use; heat stable at baking temperatures

[a]Relative sweetness is determined by comparing the approximate sweetness of a sugar substitute with the sweetness of pure sucrose, which has been defined as 1.0. Chemical structure, temperature, acidity, and other flavors of the foods in which the substance occurs all influence relative sweetness.
[b]The Acceptable Daily Intake (ADI) is the estimated amount of a sweetener that individuals can safely consume each day over the course of a lifetime without adverse effects. The Estimated Equivalent is based on a person weighing 70 kg (154 lb).
[c]Marketed under the trade names Sunett and Sweet One.
[d]Recommendations from the World Health Organization limit acesulfame K intake to 9 mg per kilogram of body weight per day.
[e]Marketed under the trade names NutraSweet, Equal, and Sugar Twin.
[f]Aspartame provides 4 kcal per gram, as does protein, but because so little is used, its energy contribution is negligible. In powdered form, it is sometimes mixed with lactose, however, so a 1-g packet may provide 4 kcal.
[g]Recommendations from the World Health Organization and in Europe and Canada limit aspartame intake to 40 mg per kilogram of body weight per day.
[h]Marketed under the trade name Fruit-Sweetness.
[i]GRAS = generally recognized as safe. The GRAS list is subject to revision as new facts become known.
[j]Marketed under the trade names Sweet'N Low, Sweet Twin, and Necta Sweet.
[k]Marketed under the trade names SweetLeaf, Purevia, Truvia, and Honey Leaf.
[l]Marketed under the trade name Splenda.

provide kcalories (0.2 to 2.6 kcalories per gram), but fewer than the sugars. Because sugar alcohols yield energy, they are sometimes referred to as **nutritive sweeteners.**

Sugar alcohols evoke a low glycemic response. The body partially absorbs some sugar alcohols and absorbs others slowly; consequently, they are slower to enter the bloodstream than other sugars. Unabsorbed sugar alcohols may be metabolized by bacteria in the GI tract, producing side effects such as intestinal gas, abdominal discomfort, and diarrhea. For this reason, regulations require food labels to state "Excess consumption may have a laxative effect" if reasonable consumption of that food could result in the daily ingestion of 50 grams of a sugar alcohol. For perspective, a low-carbohydrate energy bar or shake may contain 10 to 15 grams of a sugar alcohol.

The real benefit of using sugar alcohols is that they do not contribute to dental caries. Bacteria in the mouth cannot metabolize sugar alcohols as rapidly as sugar. Sugar alcohols are therefore valuable in chewing gums, breath mints, and other products that people keep in their mouths for a while. Figure 4-12 presents labeling information for products using sugar alternatives.

nutritive sweeteners: sweeteners that yield energy, including both sugars and sugar alcohols.

> **FIGURE 4-12 Sugar Alternatives on Food Labels**

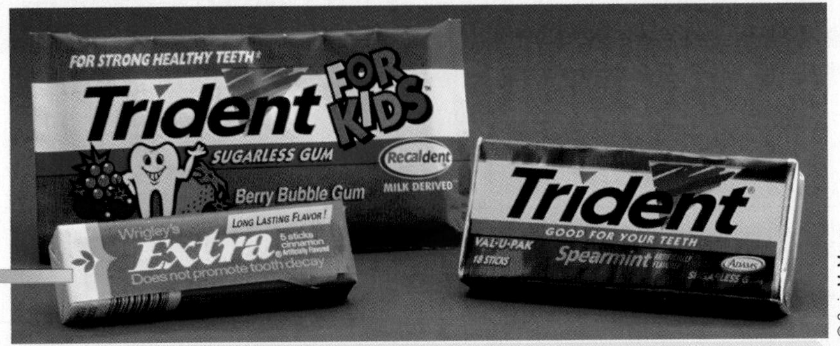

Products containing sugar replacers may claim to "not promote tooth decay" if they meet FDA criteria for dental plaque activity.

INGREDIENTS: SORBITOL, MALTITOL, GUM BASE, MANNITOL, ARTIFICIAL AND NATURAL FLAVORING, ACACIA, SOFTENERS, TITANIUM DIOXIDE (COLOR), ASPARTAME, ACESULFAME POTASSIUM AND CANDELILLA WAX.
PHENYLKETONURICS: CONTAINS PHENYLALANINE.

This ingredient list includes both sugar alcohols and artificial sweetenters.

Products containing aspartame must carry a warning for people with phenylketonuria.

35% FEWER CALORIES THAN SUGARED GUM.

Products that claim to be "reduced kcalories" must provide at least 25% fewer kcalories per serving than the comparison item.

Nutrition Facts

6 servings per container

Serving size 2 pieces (3g)

Amount Per 2 pieces

Calories 5

% DV	
0%	**Total Fat** 0g
0%	**Sodium** 0mg
1%	**Total Carbs** 2g
	Sugars 0g
	Added Sugars 0g
	Sugar Alcohol 2g
	Protein 0g

Not a significant source of other nutrients.

Products containing less than 0.5 g of sugar per serving can claim to be "sugarless" or "sugar-free."

For consumers choosing to use alternative sweeteners, the Academy of Nutrition and Dietetics wisely advises that they be used in moderation and only as part of a well-balanced nutritious diet.[23] When used in moderation, these sweeteners will do no harm. In fact, they may even help, by providing an alternative to sugar for people with diabetes, by inhibiting caries-causing bacteria, and by limiting energy intake. People may find it appropriate to choose from among any of the sweeteners at times: artificial sweeteners, an herbal sweetener, sugar alcohols, and sugar itself.

> **REVIEW IT** Describe how added sugars can contribute to health problems.
> Sugars increase the risk of dental caries; excessive intakes displace needed nutrients and fiber and contribute to obesity when energy intake exceeds needs. A person deciding to limit daily sugar intake should recognize that not all sugars need to be restricted, just concentrated sweets, which are relatively empty of other nutrients and high in kcalories. Sugars that occur naturally in fruits, vegetables, and milk are acceptable. Alternative sweeteners may help to limit kcalories and sugar intake.

4.5 Health Effects and Recommended Intakes of Starch and Fibers

> **LEARN IT** Identify the health benefits of, and recommendations for, starches and fibers.

Carbohydrates and fats are the two major sources of energy in the diet. When one is high, the other is usually low—and vice versa. A diet that provides abundant carbohydrate (45 to 65 percent of energy intake) and some fat (20 to 35 percent of energy intake) within a reasonable energy allowance best supports good health.

To increase carbohydrates in the diet, focus on whole grains, vegetables, legumes, and fruits—foods noted for their starch, fibers, and naturally occurring sugars.

Health Effects of Starch and Fibers

In addition to starch, fibers, and natural sugars, remember that whole grains, vegetables, legumes, and fruits supply valuable vitamins and minerals and little or no fat. The following paragraphs describe some of the health benefits of diets that include a variety of these foods daily.

Heart Disease Unlike high-carbohydrate diets rich in added sugars that can alter blood lipids to favor heart disease, those rich in whole grains, legumes, vegetables, and fruits may protect against heart attack and stroke by lowering blood pressure, improving blood lipids, and reducing inflammation.[24] Such diets are low in animal fat and cholesterol and high in dietary fibers, vegetable proteins, and phytochemicals—all factors associated with a lower risk of heart disease. (The role of animal fat and cholesterol in heart disease is discussed in Chapter 5. The role of vegetable proteins in heart disease is presented in Chapter 6. The benefits of phytochemicals in disease prevention are featured in Highlight 13.)

Oatmeal was one of the first foods recognized for its ability to reduce cholesterol and the risk of heart disease. Foods rich in soluble fibers (such as oat bran, barley, and legumes) lower blood cholesterol by binding with bile acids in the GI tract and thereby increasing their excretion. Consequently, the liver must use its cholesterol to make new bile acids. In addition, the bacterial by-products of fiber fermentation in the colon also inhibit cholesterol synthesis in the liver. The net result is that soluble fibers such as those found in oats lower blood cholesterol.[25]

Several researchers have speculated that fiber may also exert its effect by displacing fats in the diet. Although this is certainly helpful, even when dietary fat is low, fibers exert a separate and significant cholesterol-lowering effect. In other words, a high-fiber diet helps to decrease the risk of heart disease independent of fat intake.

Diabetes High-fiber foods—especially whole grains—play a key role managing and preventing type 2 diabetes. When soluble fibers trap nutrients and delay their transit through the GI tract, glucose absorption is slowed, which helps to prevent glucose surge and rebound.

GI Health Dietary fibers also enhance the health of the large intestine. The healthier the intestinal walls, the better they can block absorption of unwanted constituents. Taken with ample fluids, insoluble fibers such as cellulose (as in cereal brans, fruits, and vegetables) increase stool weight, ease passage, and reduce transit time.

Large, soft stools ease elimination for the rectal muscles and reduce pressure in the lower bowel, preventing constipation and making it less likely that rectal veins will swell (hemorrhoids). Fiber prevents compaction of the intestinal contents, which could obstruct the appendix and permit bacteria to invade and infect it (appendicitis). In addition, fiber stimulates the GI tract muscles so that they retain their strength and resist bulging out into pouches known as diverticula (illustrated in Figure H3-3 on p. 93).[26] Recommendations typically suggest increasing fiber to protect against diverticular disease, although research findings are inconsistent.[27]

Cancer Research studies suggest that a high-fiber diet protects against colon cancer. When a large study of diet and cancer examined the diets of more than a half million people in ten countries for several years, the researchers found an inverse association between dietary fiber and colon cancer. People who ate the most dietary fiber (35 grams per day) reduced their risk of colon cancer by 40 percent compared with those who ate the least fiber (15 grams per day). Importantly, the study focused on dietary fiber, not fiber supplements or additives, which lack valuable nutrients and phytochemicals that also help protect against cancer. Plant foods—vegetables, fruits, and whole-grain products—reduce the risks of colon and rectal cancers.

Fibers may help prevent colon cancer by diluting, binding, and rapidly removing potential cancer-causing agents from the colon. In addition, soluble fibers stimulate bacterial fermentation of resistant starch and fiber in the colon, a process

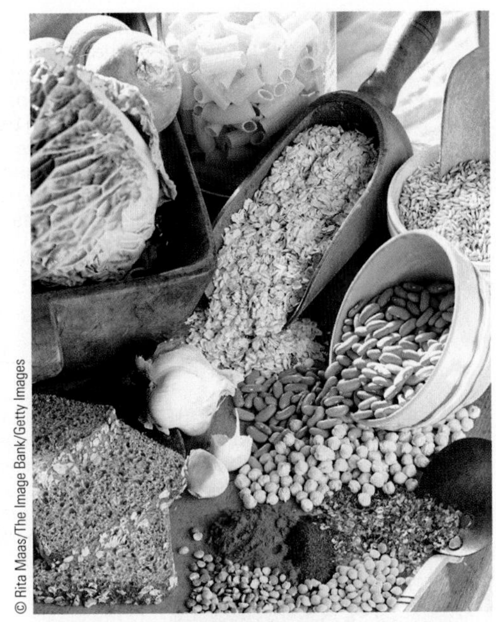

Foods rich in starch and fiber offer many health benefits.

that produces short-chain fatty acids that lower the pH. These small fat molecules activate cancer-killing enzymes and inhibit inflammation in the colon.[28]

Weight Management High-fiber and whole-grain foods may help a person to maintain a healthy body weight.[29] Foods rich in fiber tend to be low in solid fats and added sugars and therefore prevent weight gain and promote weight loss by delivering less energy per bite. In addition, as fibers absorb water from the digestive juices, they swell, creating feelings of fullness, lowering food intake, and delaying hunger.

Many weight-loss products on the market today contain bulk-inducing fibers such as methylcellulose, but buying pure fiber compounds like this is neither necessary nor advisable. Instead of fiber supplements, consumers should select whole grains, legumes, fruits, and vegetables. High-fiber foods not only add bulk to the diet but are economical and nutritious as well.

Dietary fiber provides numerous health benefits. Table 4-9 summarizes fiber characteristics, food sources, actions in the body, and their health benefits.

Harmful Effects of Excessive Fiber Intake Despite fibers' benefits to health, a diet excessively high in fiber also has a few drawbacks. A person who has a small capacity and eats mostly high-fiber foods may not be able to eat enough food to meet energy or nutrient needs. The malnourished, the elderly, and young children adhering to all-plant (vegan) diets are especially vulnerable to this problem.

Switching from a low-fiber diet to a high-fiber diet suddenly can cause temporary bouts of abdominal discomfort, gas, and diarrhea and, more seriously, can obstruct the GI tract. To prevent such complications, a person adopting a high-fiber diet can take the following precautions:

- Increase fiber intake gradually over several weeks to give the GI tract time to adapt.
- Drink plenty of liquids to soften the fiber as it moves through the GI tract.
- Select fiber-rich foods from a variety of sources—fruits, vegetables, legumes, and whole-grain breads and cereals.

TABLE 4-9 Characteristics, Sources, and Health Effects of Fibers

	Major Food Sources	Types of Fibers	Actions in the Body	Probable Health Benefits
			Viscous, Soluble, More Fermentable	
Brian Leatart/Photolibrary/Getty Images	Barley, oats, oat bran, rye, fruits (apples, citrus), legumes (especially young green peas and black-eyed peas), seaweeds, seeds and husks, many vegetables, fibers used as food additives	Gums Pectins Psyllium[a] Some hemicellulose	Lower blood cholesterol by binding bile Slow glucose absorption Slow transit of food through upper GI tract Hold moisture in stools, softening them Yield small fat molecules after fermentation that the colon can use for energy Increase satiety	Lower risk of heart disease Lower risk of diabetes Lower risk of colon and rectal cancer Increased satiety, and may help with weight management
			Nonviscous, Insoluble, Less Fermentable	
© Stockbyte/Getty Images	Brown rice, fruits, legumes, seeds, vegetables (cabbage, carrots, brussels sprouts), wheat bran, whole grains, extracted fibers used as food additives	Cellulose Lignins Resistant starch Hemicellulose	Increase fecal weight and speed fecal passage through colon Provide bulk and feelings of fullness	Alleviate constipation May lower risk of diverticulosis, hemorrhoids, and appendicitis Lower risk of colon and rectal cancer

[a]Psyllium, a soluble fiber derived from seeds, is used as a laxative and food additive.

Some fibers can limit the absorption of nutrients by speeding the transit of foods through the GI tract and by binding to minerals. When mineral intake is adequate, however, a *reasonable* intake of high-fiber foods (less than 40 grams a day) does not compromise mineral balance.

Clearly, fiber is like all nutrients in that "more" is "better" only up to a point. Again, the key dietary goals are balance, moderation, and variety. Table 4-10 presents a list of fiber sources and tips to increase fiber intake.

Recommended Intakes of Starch and Fibers The DRI suggest that carbohydrates provide about half (45 to 65 percent) of the energy requirement. (The remainder comes from fat, with 20 to 35 percent, and protein, with 10 to 35 percent.) A person consuming 2000 kcalories a day should therefore have 900 to 1300 kcalories of carbohydrate, or about 225 to 325 grams. (Appendix K explains how to calculate such math problems.) This amount is more than adequate to meet the RDA for carbohydrate, which is set at 130 grams per day, based on the average minimum amount of glucose used by the brain.

On food labels, the Food and Drug Administration (FDA) uses the guideline of 60 percent of a 2000-kcalorie diet in setting the Daily Value for carbohydrate at 300 grams per day. To meet this goal, the *Dietary Guidelines* encourage people to choose a variety of whole grains, vegetables, fruits, and legumes daily.

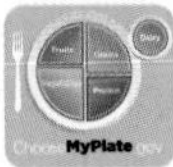

> DIETARY GUIDELINES FOR AMERICANS
Choose foods that provide more dietary fiber, a nutrient of concern in American diets. Dietary fiber is found in plants, notably legumes, vegetables, fruits, whole grains, and nuts.

TABLE 4-10 Fiber in Selected Foods

Grains		Tips to Increase Fiber Intake
Whole-grain products provide about 1 to 2 g (or more) of fiber per serving: • 1 slice whole-wheat, pumpernickel, rye bread • 1 oz ready-to-eat cereal (100% bran cereals contain 10 g or more) • ½ c cooked barley, bulgur, grits, oatmeal	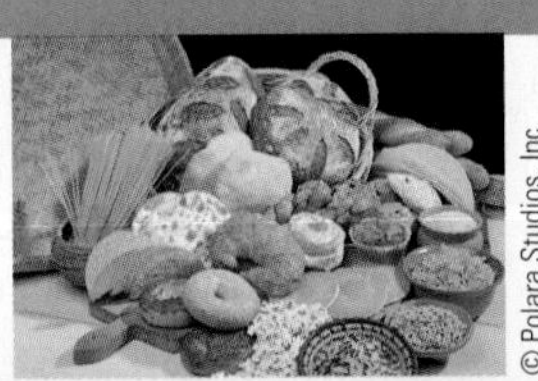 © Polara Studios, Inc.	Eat whole-grain breads that contain ≥3 g fiber per serving. Eat whole-grain cereals that contain ≥5 g fiber per serving.
Vegetables		**Tips to Increase Fiber Intake**
Most vegetables contain about 2 to 3 g of fiber per serving: • 1 c raw bean sprouts • ½ c cooked broccoli, brussels sprouts, cabbage, carrots, cauliflower, collards, corn, eggplant, green beans, green peas, kale, mushrooms, okra, parsnips, potatoes, pumpkin, spinach, sweet potatoes, swiss chard, winter squash • ½ c chopped raw carrots, peppers	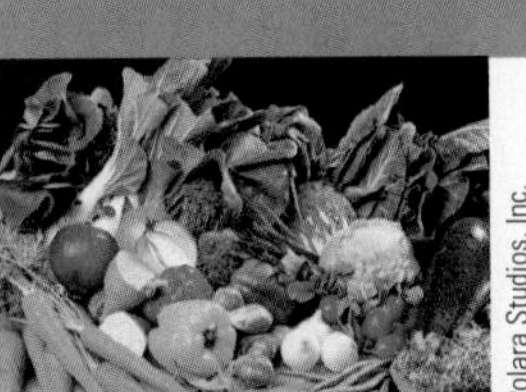 © Polara Studios, Inc.	Eat raw vegetables. Eat vegetables (such as potatoes and zucchini) with their skins.
Fruit		**Tips to Increase Fiber Intake**
Fresh, frozen, and dried fruits have about 2 g of fiber per serving: • 1 medium apple, banana, kiwi, nectarine, orange, pear • ½ c applesauce, blackberries, blueberries, raspberries, strawberries • Fruit juices contain very little fiber	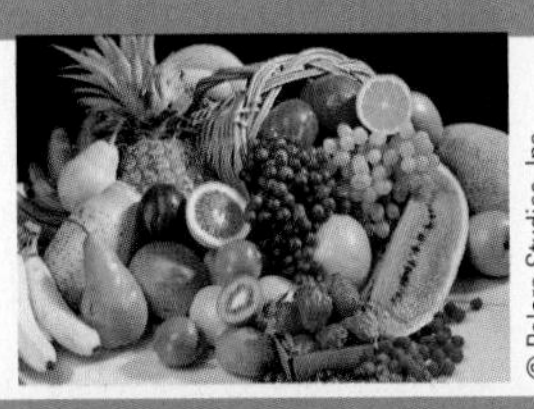 © Polara Studios, Inc.	Eat fresh and dried fruit for snacks. Eat fruits (such as apples and pears) with their skins.
Legumes		**Tips to Increase Fiber Intake**
Many legumes provide about 6 to 8 g of fiber per serving: • ½ c cooked baked beans, black beans, black-eyed peas, kidney beans, navy beans, pinto beans Some legumes provide about 5 g of fiber per serving: • ½ c cooked garbanzo beans, great northern beans, lentils, lima beans, split peas	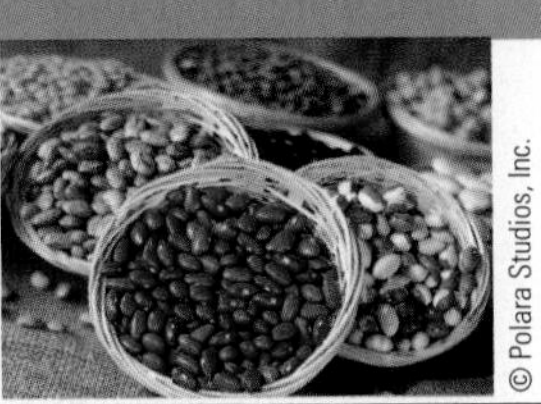 © Polara Studios, Inc.	Add legumes to soups, salads, and casseroles.

NOTE: Appendix H provides fiber grams for more than 2000 foods.

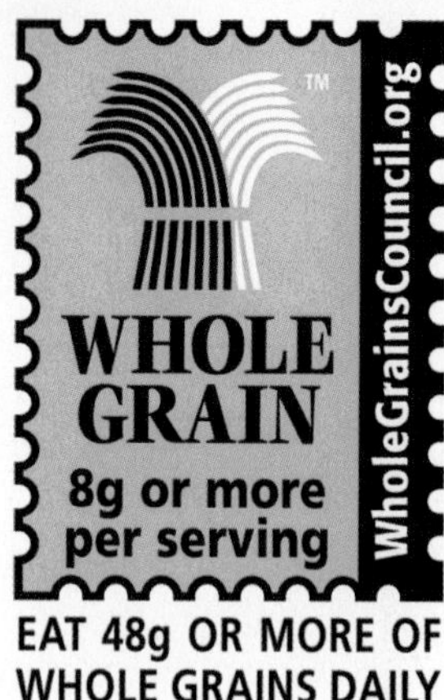

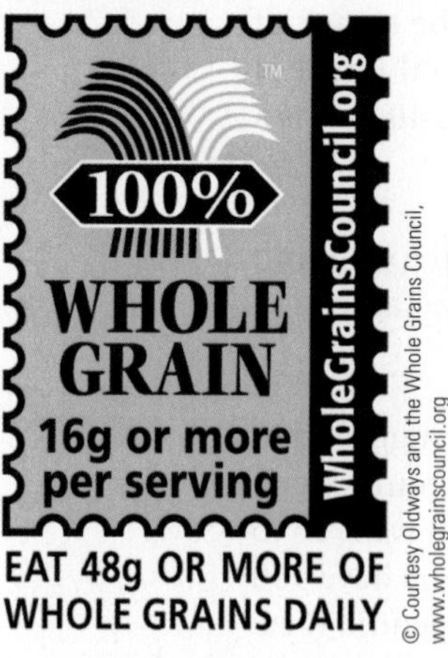

Some food labels use a "whole-grain stamp" to help consumers identify whole-grain foods.

Recommendations for fiber suggest the same foods just mentioned: whole grains, vegetables, fruits, and legumes, which also provide minerals and vitamins. The FDA sets the Daily Value for fiber at 28 grams for a 2000-kcalorie intake. The DRI recommendation is in agreement at 14 grams per 1000-kcalorie intake. These recommendations are almost two times higher than the usual intake in the United States.[30] An effective way to add fiber while lowering fat is to substitute plant sources of proteins (legumes) for animal sources (meats).

Because high-fiber foods are so filling, they are not likely to be eaten in excess. Too much fiber can cause GI problems for some people, but it generally does not have adverse effects in most healthy people. For these reasons, the DRI committee did not set an Upper Level for fiber.

From Guidelines to Groceries A diet following the USDA Food Patterns, which include several servings of fruits, vegetables, and whole grains daily, can easily supply the recommended amount of carbohydrates and fiber. In selecting high-fiber foods, keep in mind the principle of variety. The fibers in oats lower cholesterol, whereas those in bran help promote GI tract health. (Review Table 4-9 to see the diverse health effects of various fibers.)

Grains An ounce-equivalent of most foods in the grain group (for example, one slice of bread) provides about 15 grams of carbohydrate, mostly as starch. Be aware that some foods in this group, especially snack crackers and baked goods such as biscuits, croissants, and muffins, contain added sugars, solid fats, and sodium. When selecting from the grain group, limit refined grains and be sure to include at least half as whole-grain products (see Figure 4-13). The "three are key" message may help consumers to remember to choose a whole-grain cereal for breakfast, a whole-grain bread for lunch, and a whole-grain pasta or rice for dinner. Because whole grains are typically high in fiber, nutrients, and antioxidants, consumers who eat more whole grains tend to have healthier diets and reduced risks for heart disease, diabetes, and certain cancers.[31]

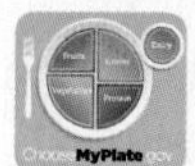

> DIETARY GUIDELINES FOR AMERICANS

Limit the consumption of foods that contain refined grains, especially refined-grain foods that contain solid fats, added sugars, and sodium. Replace refined grains with whole grains.

Vegetables The amount of carbohydrate a serving of vegetables provides depends primarily on its starch content. Starchy vegetables—corn, peas, or potatoes—provide about 15 grams of carbohydrate per half-cup serving. A serving of most other *nonstarchy* vegetables—such as a half-cup of broccoli, green beans, or tomatoes—provides about 5 grams.

Fruits A typical fruit serving—a small banana, apple, or orange or a half-cup of most canned or fresh fruit—contains an average of about 15 grams of carbohydrate, mostly as sugars, including the fruit sugar fructose. Fruits vary greatly in their water and fiber contents and, therefore, in their sugar concentrations.

Milks and Milk Products A serving (a cup) of milk or yogurt provides about 12 grams of carbohydrate. Cottage cheese provides about 6 grams of carbohydrate per cup, but most other cheeses contain little, if any, carbohydrate.

Protein Foods With two exceptions, protein foods deliver almost no carbohydrate to the diet. The exceptions are nuts, which provide a little starch and fiber along with their abundant fat, and legumes, which provide an abundance of

> **FIGURE 4-13 Bread Labels Compared**

Although breads may appear similar, their ingredients vary widely. Breads made mostly from whole-grain flours provide more benefits to the body than breads made of enriched, refined, wheat flours.

Some "high-fiber" breads may contain purified cellulose or more nutritious whole grains. "Low-carbohydrate" breads may be regular white bread, thinly sliced to reduce carbohydrates per serving, or may contain soy flour, barley flour, or flaxseed to reduce starch content.

A trick for estimating a bread's content of a nutritious ingredient, such as whole-grain flour, is to read the ingredients list (ingredients are listed in order of predominance). Bread recipes generally include one teaspoon of salt per loaf. Therefore, when a bulky nutritious ingredient, such as whole grain, is listed after the salt, you'll know that less than a teaspoonful of the nutritious ingredient was added to the loaf—not enough to significantly improve the nutrient value of one slice of bread.

Whole Grain WHOLE WHEAT

Nutrition Facts
18 servings per container
Serving size 1 slice (30g)
Amount per 1 slice
Calories 90

% DV	
2%	Total Fat 1.5g
	Trans Fat 0g
6%	Sodium 135mg
5%	Total Carbohydrate 15g
7%	Dietary Fiber 2g
	Sugars 2g
	Added Sugars 2g
	Protein 4g

MADE FROM: UNBROMATED STONE GROUND 100% WHOLE WHEAT FLOUR, WATER, CRUSHED WHEAT, HIGH-FRUCTOSE CORN SYRUP, PARTIALLY HYDROGENATED VEGETABLE SHORTENING (SOYBEAN AND COTTONSEED OILS), RAISIN JUICE CONCENTRATE, WHEAT GLUTEN, YEAST, WHOLE WHEAT FLAKES, UNSULPHURED MOLASSES, SALT, HONEY, VINEGAR, ENZYME MODIFIED SOY LECITHIN, CULTURED WHEY, UNBLEACHED WHEAT FLOUR AND SOY LECITHIN.

Natural Wheat Bread

Nutrition Facts
15 servings per container
Serving size 1 slice (30g)
Amount per 1 slice
Calories 90

% DV	
2%	Total Fat 1.5g
	Trans Fat 0g
10%	Sodium 220mg
5%	Total Carbohydrate 15g
2%	Dietary Fiber Less than 1g
	Sugars 2g
	Added Sugars 2g
	Protein 4g

INGREDIENTS: UNBLEACHED ENRICHED WHEAT FLOUR [MALTED BARLEY FLOUR, NIACIN, REDUCED IRON, THIAMIN MONONITRATE (VITAMIN B1), RIBOFLAVIN (VITAMIN B2), FOLIC ACID], WATER, HIGH-FRUCTOSE CORN SYRUP, MOLASSES, PARTIALLY HYDROGENATED SOYBEAN OIL, YEAST, CORN FLOUR, SALT, GROUND CARAWAY, WHEAT GLUTEN, CALCIUM PROPIONATE (PRESERVATIVE), MONOGLYCERIDES, SOY LECITHIN.

Multi-fiber Low carb

Nutrition Facts
21 servings per container
Serving size 1 slice (30g)
Amount per 1 slice
Calories 60

% DV	
2%	Total Fat 1.5g
	Trans Fat 0g
6%	Sodium 135mg
3%	Total Carbohydrate 9g
11%	Dietary Fiber 3g
	Sugars 0g
	Added Sugars 0g
	Protein 5g

INGREDIENTS: UNBLEACHED ENRICHED WHEAT FLOUR, WATER, WHEAT GLUTEN, CELLULOSE, YEAST, SOYBEAN OIL, CRACKED WHEAT, SALT, BARLEY, NATURAL FLAVOR PRESERVATIVES, MONOCALCIUM PHOSPHATE, MILLET, CORN, OATS, SOYBEANS, BROWN RICE, FLAXSEED, SUCRALOSE.

both starch and fiber. Just a half-cup serving of legumes provides about 20 grams of carbohydrate, a third from fiber.

Read Food Labels Food labels list the amount, in grams, of *total* carbohydrate—including starch, fibers, and sugars—per serving (review Figure 4-13). Fiber grams are also listed separately, as are the grams of sugars and added sugars. With this information, you can calculate starch grams by subtracting the grams of fibers and sugars from the total carbohydrate. Using the first label in Figure 4-13 as an example, subtracting the 4 grams of fibers and sugars from the 15 grams of total carbohydrate leaves 11 grams of starch. Total carbohydrate and dietary fiber are also expressed as "% Daily Values" for a person consuming 2000 kcalories; there is no Daily Value for sugars or added sugars.

> **REVIEW IT** Identify the health benefits of, and recommendations for, starches and fibers.

Clearly, a diet rich in starches and fibers supports efforts to control body weight and prevent heart disease, some cancers, diabetes, and GI disorders. For these reasons, recommendations urge people to eat plenty of whole grains, vegetables, legumes, and fruits—enough to provide 45 to 65 percent of the daily energy intake from carbohydrate.

In today's world, there is one other reason why plant foods rich in complex carbohydrates and natural sugars are a better choice than animal foods or foods high in concentrated sugars: in general, less energy and fewer resources are required to grow and process plant foods than to produce sugar or foods derived from animals. Chapter 20 takes a closer look at the environmental impacts of food production and use.

Nutrition Portfolio

Foods that derive from plants—whole grains, vegetables, legumes, and fruits—naturally provide ample carbohydrates and fiber with little or no fat. Refined foods often contain added sugars and solid fats.

Go to Diet & Wellness Plus and choose one of the days on which you have tracked your diet for the entire day. Go to the Intake Spreadsheet report. Scroll down until you see: carb (g).

- Which of your foods for this day were highest in carbohydrate? Which of these foods also contain added sugars and solid fats? List better alternatives.
- List the types and amounts of grain products you ate on that day, making note of which are whole-grain or refined foods and how your choices could include more whole-grain options.
- List the types and amounts of fruits and vegetables you ate on that day, making note of how many are dark green, red and orange, or deep yellow, how many are starchy or legumes, and how your choices could include more of these options.
- Describe choices you can make in selecting and preparing foods and beverages to lower your intake of added sugars.

DIET & WELLNESS PLUS To complete this exercise, go to your Diet & Wellness Plus at **www.cengagebrain.com.**

› **STUDY IT** To review the key points of this chapter and take a practice quiz, go to the study cards at the end of the book.

REFERENCES

1. NIH Consensus Development Conference: Lactose intolerance and health, http://consensus.nih.gov/2010/lactosestatement.htm.
2. K. Sevastianova and coauthors, Effect of short-term carbohydrate overfeeding and long-term weight loss on liver fat in overweight humans, *American Journal of Clinical Nutrition* 96 (2012): 727–734.
3. G. Livesey and coauthors, Is there a dose-response relation of dietary glycemic load to risk of type 2 diabetes? Meta-analysis of prospective cohort studies, *American Journal of Clinical Nutrition* 97 (2013): 584–596; A. Pande, G. Krishnamoorthy, and N. D. Moulickm, Hypoglycaemic and hypolipidaemic effects of low GI and medium GL Indian diets in type 2 diabetics for a period of 4 weeks: A prospective study, *International Journal of Food Sciences and Nutrition* 63 (2012): 649–658; J. C. Y. Louie and coauthors, The link between dietary glycemic index and nutrient adequacy, *American Journal of Clinical Nutrition* 95 (2012): 694–702; A. N. Fabricatore and coauthors, Continuous glucose monitoring to assess the ecologic validity of dietary glycemic index and glycemic load, *American Journal of Clinical Nutrition* 94 (2011): 1519–1524.
4. L. M. Goff and coauthors, Low glycaemic index diets and blood lipids: A systematic review and meta-analysis of randomised controlled trials, *Nutrition, Metabolism, and Cardiovascular Diseases* 23 (2013): 1–10; Pande, Krishnamoorthy, and Moulickm, 2012; M. L. Neuhouser and coauthors, A low-glycemic load diet reduces serum C-reactive protein and modestly increases adiponectin in overweight and obese adults, *Journal of Nutrition* 142 (2012): 369–374; J. Brand-Miller and A. E. Buyken, The glycemic index issue, *Current Opinion in Lipidology* 23 (2012): 62–67; O. Gögebakan and coauthors, Effects of weight loss and long-term weight maintenance with diets varying in protein and glycemic index on cardiovascular risk factors: The Diet, Obesity, and Genes (DiOGenes) study: A randomized, controlled trial, *Circulation* 124 (2011): 2829–2838; E. Denova-Gutiérrez and coauthors, Dietary glycemic index, dietary glycemic load, blood lipids, and coronary heart disease, *Journal of Nutrition and Metabolism* (2010): doi:10.1155/2010/170680. Epub February 28, 2010.
5. G. M. Turner-McGrievy and coauthors, Decreases in dietary glycemic index are related to weight loss among individuals following therapeutic diets for type 2 diabetes, *Journal of Nutrition* 141 (2011): 1469–1474.
6. H. Dodd and coauthors, Calculating meal glycemic index by using measured and published food values compared with directly measured meal glycemic index, *American Journal of Clinical Nutrition* 94 (2011): 992–996.
7. S. W. Ng, M. M. Slining, and B. M. Popkin, Use of caloric and noncaloric sweeteners in US consumer packaged foods, 2005-2009, *Journal of the Academy of Nutrition and Dietetics* 112 (2012): 1828–1834.
8. Position of the Academy of Nutrition and Dietetics: Use of nutritive and nonnutritive sweeteners, *Journal of the Academy of Nutrition and Dietetics* 112 (2012): 739–758.
9. S. W. Rizkalla, Health implications of fructose consumption: A review of recent data, *Nutrition and Metabolism* 4 (2010): 82–98.
10. US Department of Agriculture and US Department of Health and Human Services, *Dietary Guidelines for Americans, 2010*, www.dietaryguidelines .gov; R. E. Kavey, How sweet it is: Sugar sweetened beverage consumption, obesity, and cardiovascular risk in childhood, *Journal of the American Dietetic Association* 110 (2010): 1456–1460.

11. O. I. Bermudez and X. Gao, Greater consumption of sweetened beverages and added sugars is associated with obesity among US young adults, *Annals of Nutrition and Metabolism* 57 (2010): 211–218.
12. V. S. Malik and coauthors, Sugar-sweetened beverages and weight gain in children and adults: A systematic review and meta-analysis, *American Journal of Clinical Nutrition* 98 (2013): 1084-1102; C. A. Grimes and coauthors, Dietary salt intake, sugar-sweetened beverage consumption, and obesity risk, *Pediatrics* 131 (2013): 14–21; D. I. Jalal and coauthors, Increased fructose associates with elevated blood pressure, *Journal of the American Society of Nephrology* 21 (2010): 1543–1549; R. K. Johnson and B. A. Yon, Weighing in on added sugars and health, *Journal of the American Dietetic Association* 110 (2010): 1296–1299; V. S. Malik and coauthors, Sugar-sweetened beverages and risk of metabolic syndrome and type 2 diabetes: A meta-analysis, *Diabetes Care* 33 (2010): 2477–2483; L. Tappy and coauthors, Fructose and metabolic diseases: New findings, new questions, *Nutrition* 26 (2010): 1044–1049.
13. M. Maersk and coauthors, Sucrose-sweetener beverages increase fat storage in the liver, muscle, and visceral fat depot: A 6-mo randomized intervention study, *American Journal of Clinical Nutrition* 95 (2012): 283–289; K. Sevastianova and coauthors, Effect of short-term carbohydrate overfeeding and long-term weight loss on liver fat in overweight humans, *American Journal of Clinical Nutrition* 96 (2012): 727–734; M. J. Dekker and coauthors, Fructose: A highly lipogenic nutrient implicated in insulin resistance, hepatic steatosis, and the metabolic syndrome, *American Journal of Physiology, Endocrinology and Metabolism* 299 (2010): E685–E694; M. E. Bocarsly and coauthors, High-fructose corn syrup causes characteristics of obesity in rats: Increased body weight, body fat and triglyceride levels, *Pharmacology Biochemistry and Behavior* 97 (2010): 101–106.
14. K. L. Stanhope, Role of fructose-containing sugars in the epidemics of obesity and metabolic syndrome, *Annual Review of Medicine* 63 (2012): 19.1–19.15; K. L. Stanhope and coauthors, Consumption of fructose and high fructose corn syrup increase postprandial triglycerides, LDL-cholesterol, and apolipoprotein-B in young men and women, *Journal of Clinical Endocrinology and Metabolism* 96 (2011): 1596–1605; J. A. Welsh and coauthors, Consumption of added sugars and indicators of cardiovascular disease risk among US adolescents, *Circulation* 123 (2011): 249–257; J. A. Welsh and coauthors, Caloric sweetener consumption and dyslipidemia among US adults, *Journal of the American Medical Association* 303 (2010): 1490–1497; N. Wiernsperger, A. Geloen, and J. R. Rapin, Fructose and cardiometabolic disorders: The controversy will, and must, continue, *Clinics* 65 (2010): 729–738.
15. E. S. Eshak and coauthors, Soft drink intake in relation to incident ischemic heart disease, stroke, and stroke subtypes in Japanese men and women: The Japan Public Health Centre-based study cohort I, *American Journal of Clinical Nutrition* 96 (2012): 1390–1397; L. de Koning and coauthors, Sweetened beverage consumption, incident coronary heart disease and biomarkers of risk in men, *Circulation* 125 (2012): 1735–1741; L. de Koning and coauthors, Sugar-sweetened and artificially sweetened beverage consumption and risk of type 2 diabetes in men, *American Journal of Clinical Nutrition* 93 (2011): 1321–1327; L. Tappy and coauthors, Fructose and metabolic diseases: New findings, new questions, *Nutrition* 26 (2010): 1044–1049; K. J. Duffey and coauthors, Drinking caloric beverages increases the risk of adverse cardiometabolic outcomes in the Coronary Artery Risk Development in Young Adults (CARDIA) Study, *American Journal of Clinical Nutrition* 92 (2010): 954–959; F. B. Hu and V. S. Malik, Sugar-sweetened beverages and risk of obesity and type 2 diabetes: Epidemiologic evidence, *Physiology and Behavior* 100 (2010): 47–54.
16. L. C. Dolan, S. M. Potter, and G. A. Burdock, Evidence-based review on the effect of normal dietary consumption of fructose on blood lipids and body weight of overweight and obese individuals, *Critical Reviews in Food Science and Nutrition* 50 (2010): 889–918.
17. F. B. Hu and V. S. Malik, Sugar-sweetened beverages and risk of obesity and type 2 diabetes: Epidemiologic evidence, *Physiology and Behavior* 100 (2010): 47–54; R. K. Johnson and coauthors, Dietary sugars intake and cardiovascular health: A scientific statement from the American Heart Association, *Circulation* 120 (2009): 1011–1020.
18. Position of the Academy of Nutrition and Dietetics: Oral health and nutrition, *Journal of the Academy of Nutrition and Dietetics* 113 (2013): 693–701.
19. US Department of Agriculture, Agricultural Research Service, Beltsville Human Nutrition Research Center, Food Surveys Research Group (Beltsville, MD) and US Department of Health and Human Services, Centers for Disease Control and Prevention, National Center for Health Statistics (Hyattsville, MD), *What We Eat in America*, NHANES 2007–2008, www.ars.usda.gov/ba/bhnrc/fsrg, published 2010.
20. Committee on Dietary Reference Intakes, *Dietary Reference Intakes: Energy, Carbohydrate, Fiber, Fat, Fatty Acids, Cholesterol, Protein, and Amino Acids*, Washington, D.C.: National Academies Press, 2005.
21. B. P. Marriott and coauthors, Intake of added sugars and selected nutrients in the United States, National Health and Nutrition Examination Survey (NHANES) 2003–2006, *Critical Reviews in Food Science and Nutrition* 50 (2010): 228–258.
22. C. Gardner and coauthors, Nonnutritive sweeteners: Current use and health perspectives, A scientific statement from the American Heart Association and the American Diabetes Association, *Diabetes Care* 35 (2012): 1798–1808.
23. Position of the Academy of Nutrition and Dietetics: Use of nutritive and nonnutritive sweeteners, *Journal of the Academy of Nutrition and Dietetics* 112 (2012): 739–758.
24. M. U. Jakobsen and coauthors, Intake of carbohydrates compared with intake of saturated fatty acids and risk of myocardial infarction: Importance of the glycemic index, *American Journal of Clinical Nutrition* 91 (2010): 1764–1768.
25. R. A. Othman, M. H. Moghadasian, and P. J. H. Jones, Cholesterol lowering effects of oat β-glucan, *Nutrition Reviews* 69 (2011): 299–309.
26. S. Tarleton and J. K. Dibaise, Low-residue diet in diverticular disease: Putting an end to a myth, *Nutrition in Clinical Practice* 26 (2011): 137–142.
27. C. Ünlü and coauthors, A systematic review of high-fibre dietary therapy in diverticular disease, International Journal of Colorectal Disease 27 (2012): 419–427; L. L. Strate, Lifestyle factors and the course of diverticular disease, *Digestive Diseases* 30 (2012): 35–45; A. F. Peery and coauthors, A high-fiber diet does not protect against asymptomatic diverticulosis, *Gastroenterology* 142 (2012): 266–272; F. L. Crowe and coauthors, Diet and risk of diverticular disease in Oxford cohort of European Prospective Investigation into Cancer and Nutrition (EPIC): Prospective study of British vegetarians and non-vegetarians, *British Medical Journal* 343 (2011): d4131; J. E. Ravikoff and J. R. Korzenik, The role of fiber in diverticular disease, *Journal of Clinical Gastroenterology* 45 (2011): S7–S11.
28. M. H. Pan and coauthors, Molecular mechanisms for chemoprevention of colorectal cancer by natural dietary compounds, *Molecular Nutrition and Food Research* 55 (2011): 32–45.
29. H. Du and coauthors, Dietary fiber and subsequent changes in body weight and waist circumference in European men and women, *American Journal of Clinical Nutrition* 91 (2010): 329–336.
30. D. E. King, A. G. Mainous, and C. A. Lambourne, Trends in dietary fiber intake in the United States, 1999–2008, *Journal of the Academy of Nutrition and Dietetics* 112 (2012): 642–648.
31. T. Wirström and coauthors, Consumption of whole grain reduces risk of deteriorating glucose tolerance, including progression to prediabetes, *American Journal of Clinical Nutrition* 97 (2013): 179–187; E. Q. Ye and coauthors, Greater whole-grain intake is associated with lower risk of type 2 diabetes, cardiovascular disease, and weight gain, *Journal of Nutrition* 142 (2012): 1304–1313; M. Lefevre and S. Jonnalagadda, Effect of whole grains on markers of subclinical inflammation, *Nutrition Reviews* 70 (2012): 387–396; I. Y. Hur and M. Reicks, Relationship between whole-grain intake, chronic disease risk indicators, and weight status among adolescents in the National Health and Nutrition Examination Survey, 1999–2004, *Journal of the Academy of Nutrition and Dietetics* 112 (2012): 46–55; S. S. Jonnalagadda and coauthors, Putting the whole grain puzzle together: Health benefits associated with whole grains—Summary of American Society for Nutrition 2010 Satellite Symposium, *Journal of Nutrition* 141 (2011): 1011S–1022S; C. E. O'Neil and coauthors, Consumption of whole grains is associated with improved diet quality and nutrient intake in children and adolescents: The National Health and Nutrition Examination Survey 1999–2004, *Public Health Nutrition* 14 (2011): 347–355; C. E. O'Neil and coauthors, Whole-grain consumption is associated with diet quality and nutrient intake in adults: The National Health and Nutrition Examination Survey, 1999–2004, *Journal of the American Dietetic Association* 110 (2010): 1461–1468.

HIGHLIGHT > 4

Carbs, kCalories, and Controversies

> **LEARN IT** Summarize the key scientific evidence behind some of the current controversies surrounding carbohydrates and their kcalories.

Carbohydrate-rich foods are easy to like. Mashed potatoes, warm muffins, blueberry pancakes, freshly baked bread, and tasty rice and pasta dishes tempt most people's palates. In recent years, such homey foods have been blamed for causing weight gain and harming health. Popular writers have persuaded consumers that carbohydrates are "bad." In contrast, the *Dietary Guidelines* urge people to consume plenty of fruits, vegetables, legumes, and whole grains—all carbohydrate-rich foods.

Do carbohydrate-rich foods cause obesity and related health problems? Should people "cut carbs" to lose weight and protect their health? Many popular diet books espouse a carbohydrate-restricted or carbohydrate-modified diet. Some claim that all or some types of carbohydrates are bad. Some go so far as to equate carbohydrates with toxic poisons or addictive drugs. "Bad" carbohydrates—such as sugar, white flour, and potatoes—are considered evil because they are absorbed easily and raise blood glucose. The pancreas then responds by secreting insulin—and insulin is touted as the real villain responsible for our nation's obesity epidemic. Whether restricting overall carbohydrate intake or replacing certain "bad" carbohydrates with "good" carbohydrates, many of these popular diets tend to distort the facts. This highlight examines the scientific evidence behind some of the current controversies surrounding carbohydrates and their kcalories.

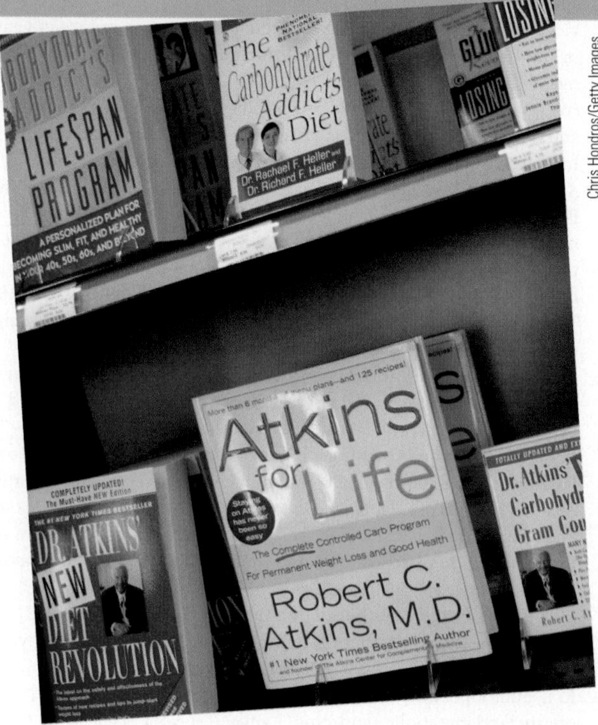

Chris Hondros/Getty Images

Carbohydrates' kCalorie Contributions

The incidence of obesity in the United States has risen dramatically over the past several decades.[1] Popular diet books often blame carbohydrates for this increase in obesity. One way researchers can explore whether the amount of carbohydrate in the diet contributes to increases in body weight over time is by reviewing national food intake survey records, such as NHANES (introduced in Chapter 1). Figure H4-1 presents a summary of energy nutrient data over the past three decades. Since the 1970s, kcalories from carbohydrates increased from 42 percent to 51 percent today.[2] At the same time, kcalories from fat dropped from 41 percent to 34 percent. The percentage of protein intake stayed about the same.

A closer look at the data reveals that, as the percentage of kcalories from the three energy nutrients shifted slightly, total daily energy intake increased significantly. In general, as food became more readily available in this nation, consumers began to eat more than they had in the past. Since the 1970s, total energy intakes have increased by about 200 to 300 kcalories a day (see Figure H4-2).[3] All of the increase in kcalories came from an increase in carbohydrate kcalories. At the same time, most people were not active enough to use up those extra kcalories; in fact, activity levels declined.[4] Consequently, the average body weight for adults increased over these decades by about 25 to 30 pounds (see Figure H4-3).

Might too many carbohydrates in the diet be to blame for weight gains? Interestingly, epidemiological studies find an *inverse* relationship between carbohydrate intake and body weight. Those with the highest carbohydrate intake have the lowest body weight and vice versa. Dietary fiber, which favors a healthy body weight, explains some but not all of this relationship.

Might a low-carbohydrate diet support weight losses? For the most part, weight loss is similar for people following either a low-carbohydrate

> FIGURE H4-1 **Energy Nutrients over Time**

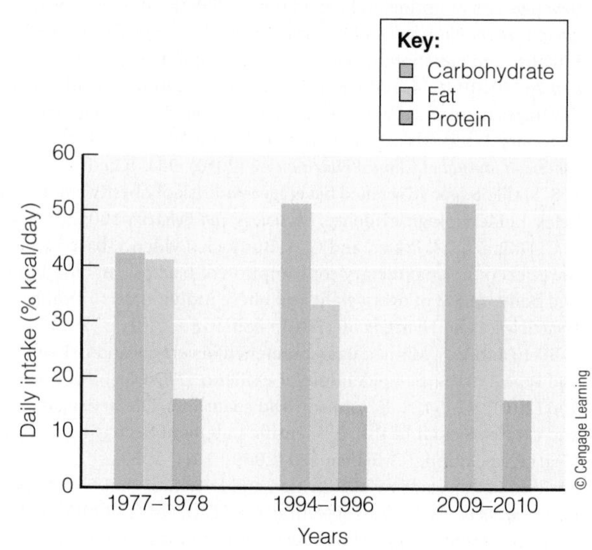

© Cengage Learning

> FIGURE H4-2 **Daily Energy Intake over Time**

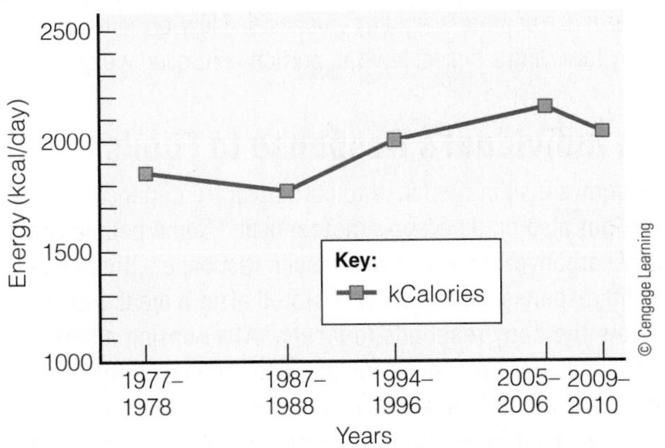

> FIGURE H4-3 **Increases in Adult Body Weight over Time**

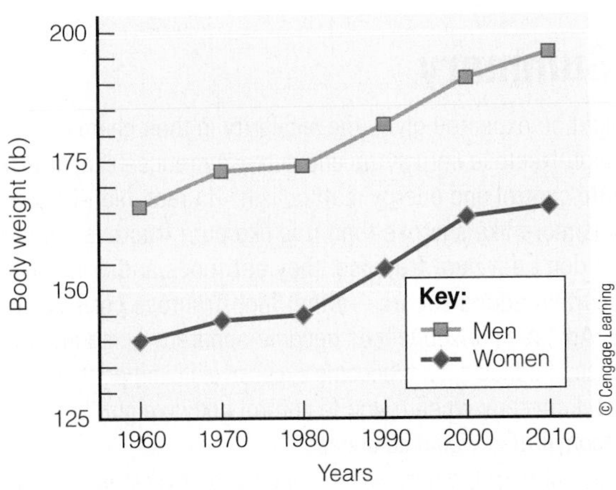

diet or a low-fat diet.[5] This is an important point. Weight losses reflect restricted kcalories—not the proportion of energy nutrients in the diet. Any diet can produce weight loss, at least temporarily, if energy intake is restricted. And most weight-loss diets also restrict sugars.

Sugars' Share in the Problem

As the chapter mentioned, the use of high-fructose corn syrup sweetener parallels unprecedented increases in the incidence of obesity, but does it mean that the increasing sugar intakes are responsible for the increase in body fat and its associated health problems?[6] Excess sugar in the diet is associated with more fat on the body. When eaten in excess of need, energy from added sugars contributes to body fat stores, just as excess energy from other sources does. Added sugars provide excess energy, raising the risk of weight gain. When total energy intake is controlled, however, *moderate* amounts of sugar do not *cause* obesity.[7] In other words, foods containing added sugars are no more likely to contribute to weight gain than any other foods.[8] Yet moderating sugar intake can be a challenge.

The liquid form of sugar in soft drinks makes it especially easy to overconsume kcalories. Swallowing liquid kcalories requires little effort. The sugar kcalories of sweet beverages also cost less than many other energy sources, and they are widely available. Also, beverages are energy-dense, providing more than 150 kcalories per 12-ounce can, and many people drink several cans a day. Drinking these beverages seems to correlate with a higher energy intake from foods as well, thus raising energy intake in two ways.[9] The convenience, economy, availability, and flavors of sugary foods and beverages make overconsumption especially likely.

Limiting selections of foods and beverages high in added sugars can be an effective weight-loss strategy, especially for people whose excess kcalories come primarily from added sugars. Replacing sodas with water every day, for example, can help a person lose a pound (or at least not gain a pound) in 1 month.[10] That may not sound like much, but it adds up to more than 10 pounds a year, for very little effort.

Cravings and Addictions

Some people describe themselves as having "carbohydrate cravings" or being "sugar addicts." One frequently noted theory is that people seek carbohydrates as a way to increase their levels of the brain neurotransmitter serotonin, which elevates mood. Interestingly, when those with self-described carbohydrate cravings indulge, they tend to eat more of everything; the percentage of energy from carbohydrates remains unchanged.

One reasonable explanation for the carbohydrate cravings that some people experience involves the self-imposed labeling of a food as both "good" and "bad"—that is, one that is desirable but should be eaten with restraint. Restricting intake heightens the desire further (a "craving"). Then "addiction" is used to explain why resisting the food is so difficult and, sometimes, even impossible. Carbohydrates, and sugars more specifically, are not addictive in the same ways that drugs are, but they share some of the same biological and psychological systems that are involved in rewards and self-control. Highlight 8 includes more details on the concept of food addictions.

Fructose Metabolism

Unlike glucose, which is metabolized by all the body's cells, fructose is metabolized primarily in the liver. When the diet delivers high intakes of added sugars (which is half fructose), the liver handles the excess by making fat. This fat is either retained in the liver or transported out, raising blood lipids and increasing fat stores—all risk factors for chronic diseases.

Appetite Control

Recall from Chapter 4 that glucose stimulates the release of insulin from the pancreas. Insulin, in turn, sets off a sequence of hormonal actions that suppress the appetite. Fructose, in contrast, does not stimulate the release of insulin, and therefore does not suppress appetite.

Whether the meal or snack is liquid or solid may also affect appetite. Even when kcaloric intake is the same, a fresh apple suppresses appetite more than apple juice. Consequently, beverages can influence weight gains both by providing energy and by not satisfying hunger.

Insulin's Response

Several popular diet books hold insulin responsible for the obesity problem and a low-glycemic diet as the weight-loss solution. Yet, among nutrition researchers, controversy continues to surround the questions of whether insulin promotes weight gain or a low-glycemic diet fosters weight loss.

Recall that just after a meal, blood glucose rises and insulin responds. How high insulin levels surge may influence whether the body stores or uses its glucose and fat supplies. What does insulin do? Among its roles, insulin facilitates the transport of glucose into the cells, the storage of fatty acids as fat, and the synthesis of protein. It is an anabolic hormone that builds and stores. True—but there's more to the story. Insulin is only one of many factors involved in the body's metabolism of nutrients and regulation of body weight.

Most importantly, insulin is critical to maintaining health, as any person with type 1 diabetes can attest. Insulin causes problems only when a person develops insulin resistance—that is, when the body's cells do not respond to the large quantities of insulin that the pancreas continues to pump out in an effort to get a response. Insulin resistance is a major health problem—but it is not caused by carbohydrate, or by protein, or by fat. It most often results from being obese. Importantly, when a person loses weight, insulin response usually improves.

The Glycemic Index and Body Weight

As Chapter 4's discussion of the glycemic index explained, the glycemic effect of a particular food varies. The glycemic effect of a food depends on how the food is ripened, processed, and cooked; the time of day the food is eaten; the other foods eaten with it; and the presence or absence of certain diseases such as type 2 diabetes in the person eating the food. All these factors influence a food's glycemic index, yet diet books often mislead people by claiming that each food has a specific glycemic index.

Even if a true glycemic index is known, what is the relationship between a diet's glycemic index and body weight? In general, studies find that diets with a high glycemic index are positively associated with body weight.

Might a low-glycemic diet foster weight loss? In general, research examining the use of low glycemic diets for weight loss finds inconsistent results.[11] Still, a low-glycemic diet may offer other advantages. A low-glycemic meal seems to curb appetite and limit energy intake of the next meal. Low-glycemic diets are also more likely to be rich in nutrients and fiber than high-glycemic diets.

Clearly, if kcalories are low, obese people on either a low-glycemic diet or a traditional low-fat diet can lose weight. Overweight people can lose as much or more weight by emphasizing low-glycemic foods as they can by following a typical low-fat, portion-controlled weight-loss diet.

The Individual's Response to Foods

The body's insulin response to carbohydrate depends not only on a food, but also on a person's metabolism.[12] Some people react to dietary carbohydrate with a low insulin response. Others have a high insulin response. How energy is stored after a meal depends in part on how the body responds to insulin. After eating a high-carbohydrate meal, normal-weight people who are insulin resistant tend to synthesize about half as much glycogen in muscles and make about twice as much fat in the liver as people who are insulin sensitive. Some research suggests that restricting carbohydrate intake may improve glucose control, insulin response, and blood lipids.

In Summary

As might be expected given the similarity in their chemical composition, high-fructose corn syrup and sucrose produce similar effects in appetite control and energy metabolism.[13] In fact, high-fructose corn syrup is more like sucrose than it is like pure fructose. Importantly, people don't eat pure fructose; they eat foods and drink beverages that contain added sugars—either high-fructose corn syrup or sucrose. Adverse consequences become apparent when intakes of either type of added sugars become excessive.[14] Limiting these sugars is a helpful strategy when trying to control body weight, but restricting all carbohydrates would be unwise.

The quality of the diet suffers when carbohydrates are restricted. Without fruits, vegetables, and whole grains, low-carbohydrate diets lack not only carbohydrate, but fiber, vitamins, minerals, and phytochemicals as well—all dietary factors protective against disease. The DRI recommends that carbohydrates contribute between 45 and 65 percent of daily energy intake. Intakes within this range can support healthy body weight and do not contribute to obesity—when added sugar intake is moderate and total energy intake is appropriate. Similarly, added sugars increase energy intake, but need not contribute to obesity—when added sugar intake is moderate and total energy intake is appropriate. When choosing carbohydrates, emphasize a variety of naturally occurring carbohydrates—such as whole grains, legumes, vegetables, and fruits—and limit foods and beverages with added sugars.

CRITICAL THINKING QUESTIONS

A. How are sugars, starches, and fibers related to weight gains and losses?

B. Your mom wants to lose 20 pounds before her high school reunion next month. She has done some research on the Internet, and has discovered an easy diet that seems to offer great success. The basis of the diet is that a person needs to eat "slow carb" foods and avoid sweets (including fruits) and starches. All white foods—such as potatoes, rice, pastas, tofu, breads, cereals, and milk—are banned and two to three workouts each week are encouraged. What evidence supports or contradicts a "slow carb" diet for weight loss?

REFERENCES

1. K. M. Flegal and coauthors, Prevalence and trends in obesity among US adults, 1999–2008, *Journal of the American Medical Association* 303 (2010): 235–241.
2. US Department of Agriculture, Agricultural Research Service, Beltsville Human Nutrition Research Center, Food Surveys Research Group (Beltsville, MD) and US Department of Health and Human Services, Centers for Disease Control and Prevention, National Center for Health Statistics (Hyattsville, MD), *What We Eat in America,* NHANES 2009–2010, www.ars.usda.gov/, published July 2012.
3. *What We Eat in America,* 2012.
4. US Department of Health and Human Services, *2008 Physical Activity Guidelines for Americans* Summary, www.health.gov/PAGuidelines /guidelines/summary.aspx.
5. G. D. Foster and coauthors, Weight and metabolic outcomes after 2 years on a low-carbohydrate versus low-fat diet: A randomized trial, *Annals of Internal Medicine* 153 (2010): 147–157.
6. R. D. Mattes and coauthors, Nutritively sweetened beverage consumption and body weight: A systematic review and meta-analysis of randomized experiments, *Obesity Reviews* 12 (2011): 346–365.
7. L. T. Morenga, S. Mallard, J. Mann, Dietary sugars and body weight: Systematic review and meta-analyses of randomised controlled trials and cohort studies, *British Medical Journal* 346 (2013): e7492; J. L. Sievenpiper and coauthors, Effect of fructose on body weight in controlled feeding trials: A systematic review and meta-analysis, *Annals of Internal Medicine* 156 (2012): 291–304.
8. R. D. Mattes and coauthors, Nutritively sweetened beverage consumption and body weight: A systematic review and meta-analysis of randomized experiments, *Obesity Reviews* 12 (2011): 346–365.
9. A. K. Kant, B. I. Graubard, and R. D. Mattes, Association of food form with self-reported 24-h energy intake and meal patterns in US adults: NHANES 2003–2008, *American Journal of Clinical Nutrition* 96 (2012): 1369–1378.
10. D. F. Tate and coauthors, Replacing caloric beverages with water or diet beverages for weight loss in adults: Main results of the Choose Healthy Options Consciously Everyday (CHOICE) randomized clinical trial, *American Journal of Clinical Nutrition* 95 (2012): 555–563.
11. A. Esfahani and coauthors, The application of the glycemic index and glycemic load in weight loss: A review of the clinical evidence, *International Union of Biochemistry and Molecular Biology* 63 (2011): 7–13.
12. W. J. Whelan and coauthors, The glycemic response is a personal attribute, *International Union of Biochemistry and Molecular Biology* 62 (2010): 637–641.
13. K. L. Stanhope and P. J. Havel, Fructose consumption: Recent results and their potential implications, *Annals of the New York Academy of Sciences* 1190 (2010): 15–24.
14. L. Tappy and K. Lê, Metabolic effects of fructose and the worldwide increase in obesity, *Physiology Reviews* 90 (2010): 23–46.

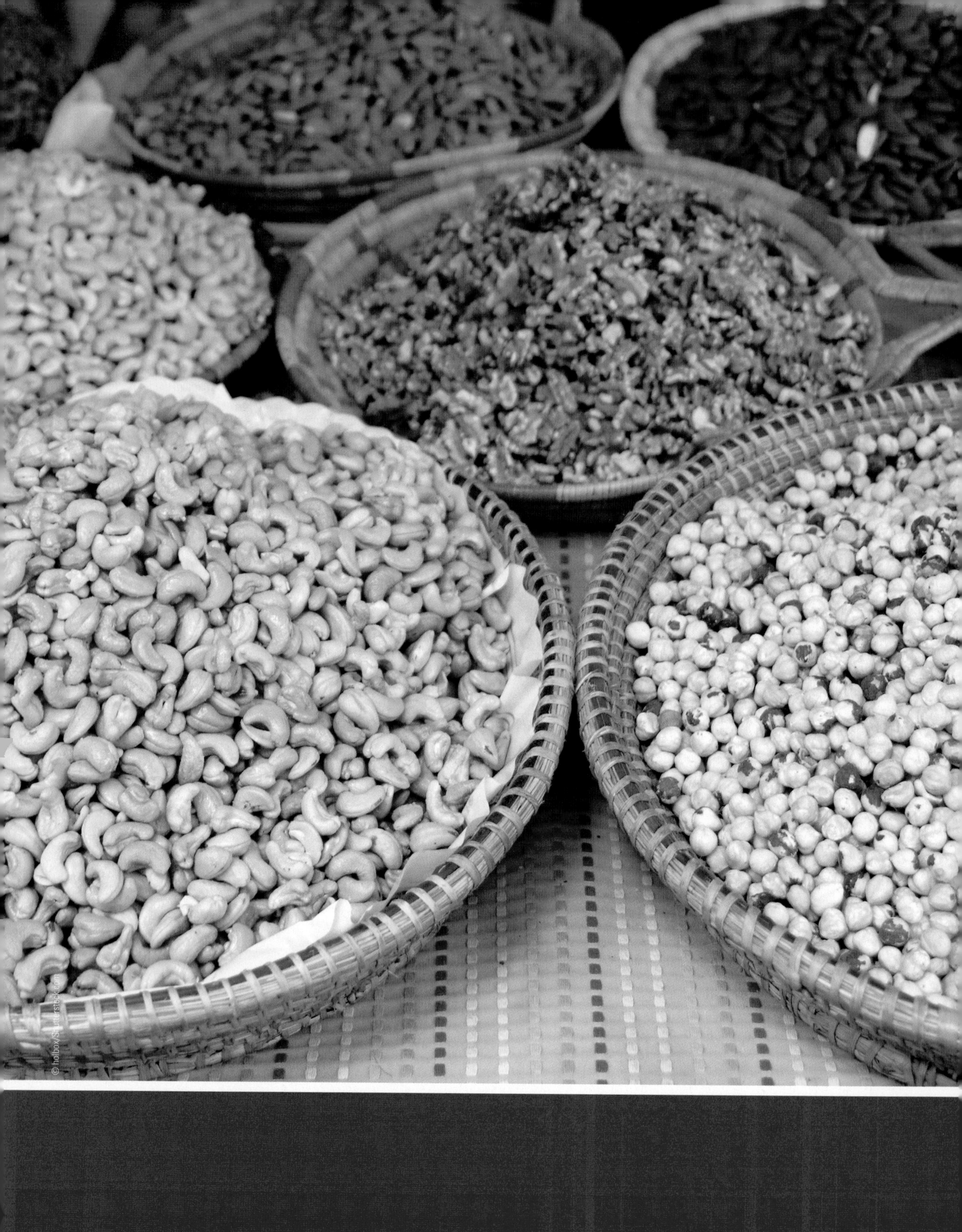

5

The Lipids: Triglycerides, Phospholipids, and Sterols

Nutrition in Your Life

Most likely, you know what you don't like about body fat, but do you appreciate how it insulates you against the cold or powers your hike around a lake? And what about food fat? You're right to credit fat for providing the delicious flavors and aromas of buttered popcorn and fried chicken—and to criticize it for contributing to the weight gain and heart disease so common today. The challenge is to strike a healthy balance of enjoying some fat, but not too much. Learning which kinds of fats are beneficial and which are most harmful will also help you make wise decisions. In the Nutrition Portfolio at the end of this chapter, you can examine whether your current fat choices are meeting dietary goals.

No doubt you have heard that fats can contribute to the development of several chronic diseases, but did you realize that some fats are also essential to good health? Most people are surprised to learn that fat has virtues and that a well-balanced diet needs at least a little fat. Getting enough fat is rarely a problem. At least traces of fat can be found in almost all foods. In our society of abundance, people are more likely to consume too much fat, or too much of some kinds of fat—with consequent health problems. Learning which kinds of fats are harmful or helpful is key to healthy diet planning.

Fat refers to the class of nutrients known as lipids. The lipid family includes triglycerides (fats and oils), phospholipids, and sterols. Triglycerides are most abundant, both in foods and in the body. The following sections describe the similarities and differences among the remarkably diverse members of the lipid family.[1]

LEARNING GPS

5.1 The Chemist's View of Fatty Acids and Triglycerides

› LEARN IT Recognize the chemistry of fatty acids and triglycerides and differences between saturated and unsaturated fats.

Like carbohydrates, **lipids** are composed of carbon (C), hydrogen (H), and oxygen (O). Because lipids have many more carbons and hydrogens in proportion to their oxygens, they can supply more energy per gram than carbohydrates can (Chapter 7 provides details).

The many names and relationships in the lipid family can seem overwhelming—like meeting a friend's extended family for the first time. To ease the introductions, this chapter first presents each of the lipids from a chemist's point of view using both words and diagrams. Then the chapter follows the lipids through digestion and absorption and into the body to examine their roles in health and disease. For people who think more easily in words than in chemical symbols, this *preview* of the upcoming chemistry may be helpful:

1. Every triglyceride contains one molecule of glycerol and three fatty acids (basically, chains of carbon atoms).
2. Fatty acids may be 4 to 24 (even numbers of) carbons long, the 18-carbon ones being the most common in foods and especially noteworthy in nutrition.
3. Fatty acids may be saturated or unsaturated. Unsaturated fatty acids may have one or more points of unsaturation—that is, they may be *mono*unsaturated or *poly*unsaturated.
4. Of special importance in nutrition are the polyunsaturated fatty acids known as omega-3 fatty acids and omega-6 fatty acids.
5. The 18-carbon polyunsaturated fatty acids are linolenic acid (omega-3) and linoleic acid (omega-6). Both are essential fatty acids that the body cannot make. Each is the primary member of a family of longer-chain fatty acids that help to regulate blood pressure, blood clotting, and other body functions important to health.

The paragraphs, definitions, and diagrams that follow present this information again in much more detail.

Fatty Acids

All **fatty acids** have the same basic structure—a chain of carbon and hydrogen atoms with an acid group (COOH) at one end and a methyl group (CH_3) at the other end. Fatty acids may differ from one another, however, in the length of their carbon chains and in the number and location of their double bonds, as the following paragraphs describe. (Fatty acids and related terms are defined in the accompanying glossary.)

The Length of the Carbon Chain Most naturally occurring fatty acids contain even numbers of carbons in their chains—up to 24 carbons in length. This discussion begins with the 18-carbon fatty acids, which are abundant in our food supply. Stearic acid is the simplest of the 18-carbon fatty acids; the bonds between its carbons are all alike:

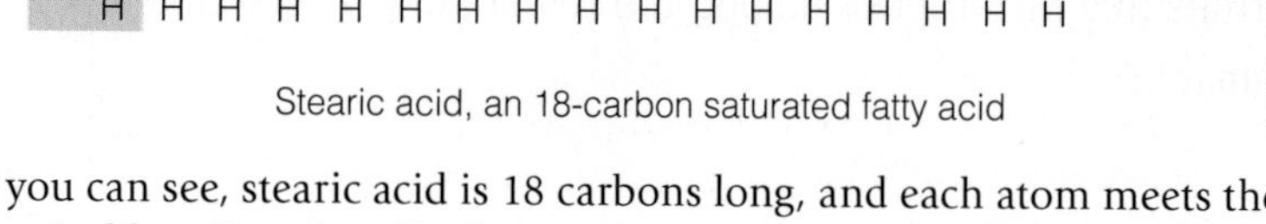

Stearic acid, an 18-carbon saturated fatty acid

© Cengage Learning

As you can see, stearic acid is 18 carbons long, and each atom meets the rules of chemical bonding described in Figure 4-1 on p. 100. The following structure

lipids: a family of compounds that includes triglycerides, phospholipids, and sterols. Lipids are characterized by their insolubility in water. (Lipids also include the fat-soluble vitamins, described in Chapter 11.)

GLOSSARY OF FATTY ACID TERMS

fatty acids: organic compounds composed of a carbon chain with hydrogens attached and an acid group (COOH) at one end and a methyl group (CH_3) at the other end.

monounsaturated fatty acid: a fatty acid that lacks two hydrogen atoms and has one double bond between carbons; abbreviated *MUFA*. Examples include palmitoleic acid and oleic acid. A *monounsaturated fat* is composed of triglycerides in which most of the fatty acids are monounsaturated.

- **mono** = one

point of unsaturation: the double bond of a fatty acid, where hydrogen atoms can easily be added to the structure.

polyunsaturated fatty acid: a fatty acid that lacks four or more hydrogen atoms and has two or more double bonds between carbons; abbreviated *PUFA*. Examples include linoleic acid (two double bonds) and linolenic acid (three double bonds). A *polyunsaturated fat* is composed of triglycerides in which most of the fatty acids are polyunsaturated.

- **poly** = many

saturated fatty acid: a fatty acid carrying the maximum possible number of hydrogen atoms—for example, stearic acid. A *saturated fat* is composed of triglycerides in which most of the fatty acids are saturated.

unsaturated fatty acid: a fatty acid that lacks hydrogen atoms and has at least one double bond between carbons (includes monounsaturated and polyunsaturated fatty acids). An *unsaturated fat* is composed of triglycerides in which most of the fatty acids are unsaturated.

also depicts stearic acid, but in a simpler way, with each "corner" on the zigzag line representing a carbon atom with two attached hydrogens:

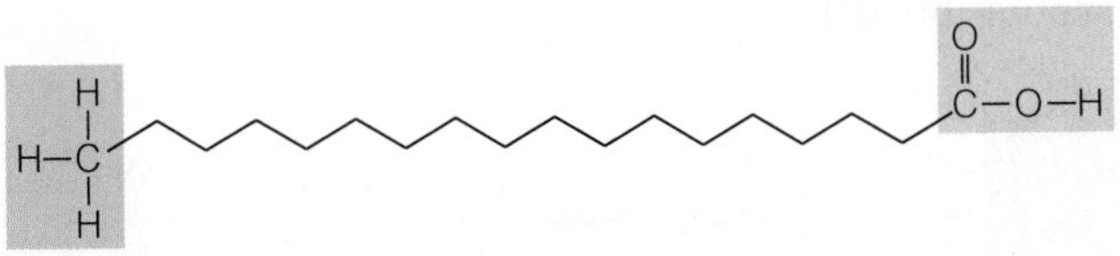

Stearic acid (simplified structure)

© Cengage Learning

As mentioned, the carbon chains of fatty acids vary in length. The long-chain (12 to 24 carbons) fatty acids of meats, seafood, and vegetable oils are most common in the diet. Smaller amounts of medium-chain (6 to 10 carbons) and short-chain (fewer than 6 carbons) fatty acids also occur, primarily in dairy products. (Tables C-1 and C-2 in Appendix C provide the names, chain lengths, and sources of fatty acids commonly found in foods.)

The Number of Double Bonds Stearic acid (described and shown previously) is a **saturated fatty acid.** A saturated fatty acid is fully loaded with all its hydrogen atoms and contains only single bonds between its carbon atoms. If two hydrogens were missing from the middle of the carbon chain, the remaining structure might be:

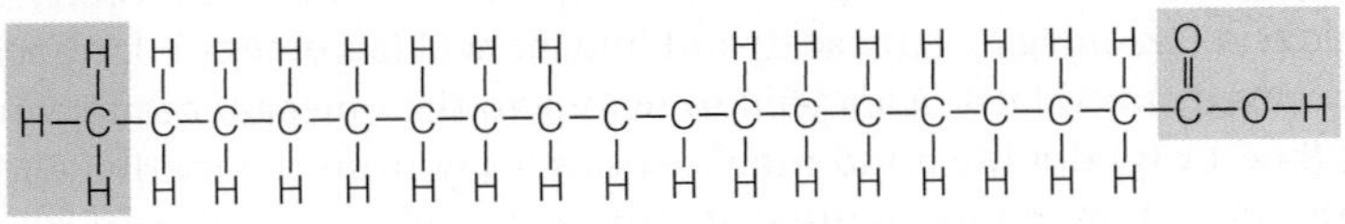

An impossible chemical structure

© Cengage Learning

Notice that in the impossible chemical structure shown above, two of the carbons have only three bonds each. Such a compound cannot exist because every carbon must have four bonds. To satisfy this rule, the two carbons form a double bond:

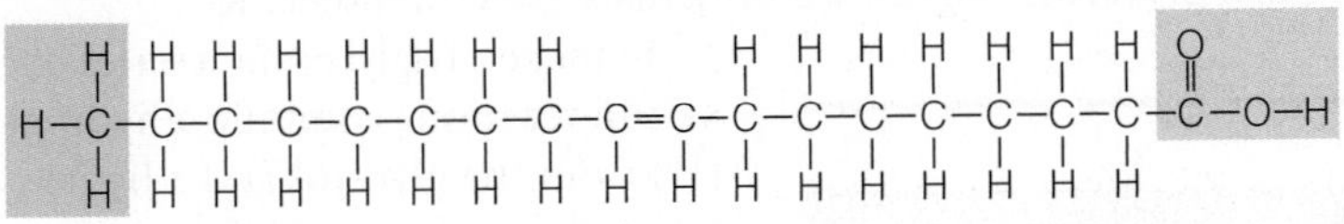

Oleic acid, an 18-carbon monounsaturated fatty acid

© Cengage Learning

The same structure drawn more simply looks like this:*

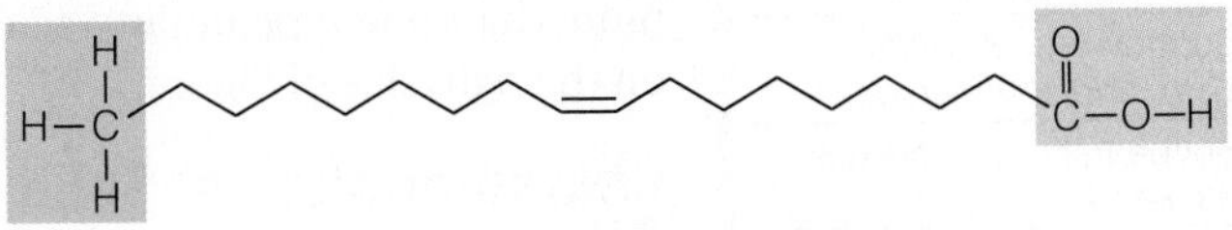

Oleic acid (simplified structure)

© Cengage Learning

*Remember that each "corner" on the zigzag line represents a carbon atom with two attached hydrogens.

Although drawn straight here, the actual shape bends at the double bond. The double bond is a **point of unsaturation.** A fatty acid like this—with two hydrogens missing and a double bond—is an **unsaturated fatty acid.** This one is the 18-carbon **monounsaturated fatty acid** oleic acid, which is abundant in olive oil and canola oil.

A **polyunsaturated fatty acid** has two or more carbon-to-carbon double bonds. **Linoleic acid,** the 18-carbon fatty acid common in vegetable oils, lacks four hydrogens and has two double bonds:

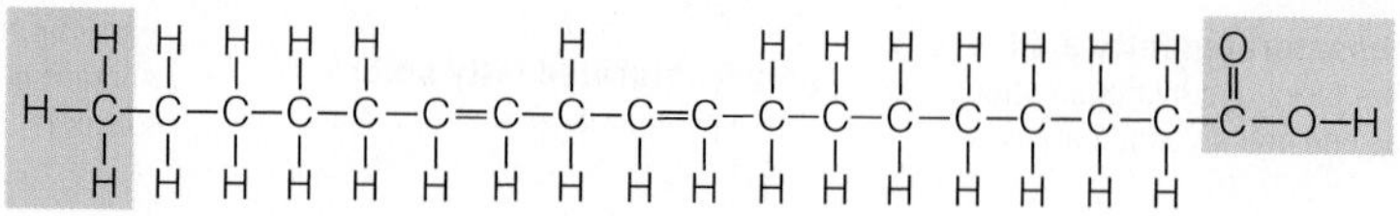

Linoleic acid, an 18-carbon polyunsaturated fatty acid

© Cengage Learning

Drawn more simply, linoleic acid looks like this (though the actual shape would bend at the double bonds):

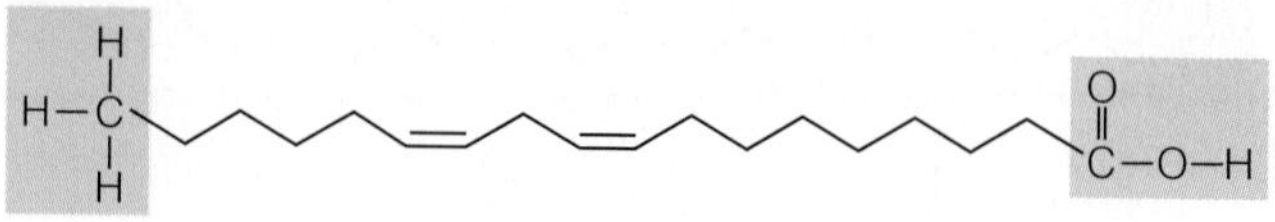

Linoleic acid (simplified structure)

© Cengage Learning

A fourth 18-carbon fatty acid is **linolenic acid,** which has three double bonds. Table 5-1 presents the 18-carbon fatty acids.

The Location of Double Bonds Fatty acids differ not only in the length of their chains and their degree of saturation, but also in the locations of their double bonds. Chemists identify polyunsaturated fatty acids by the position of the double bond closest to the methyl (CH_3) end of the carbon chain, which is described by an **omega** number. A polyunsaturated fatty acid with its closest double bond three carbons away from the methyl end is an **omega-3 fatty acid.** Similarly, an **omega-6 fatty acid** is a polyunsaturated fatty acid with its closest double bond six carbons away from the methyl end. Figure 5-1 compares two 18-carbon fatty acids—linolenic acid (an omega-3 fatty acid) and linoleic acid (an omega-6 fatty acid).

Monounsaturated fatty acids tend to belong to the omega-9 group, with their closest (and only) double bond nine carbons away from the methyl end. Oleic acid—the 18 carbon monounsaturated fatty acid common in olive oil mentioned earlier—is an omega-9 fatty acid. It is also the most predominant monounsaturated fatty acid in the diet.

Triglycerides

Few fatty acids occur free in foods or in the body. Most often, they are incorporated into **triglycerides**—lipids composed of three fatty acids attached to a **glycerol.*** Figure 5-2 presents a glycerol molecule.

To make a triglyceride, a series of **condensation** reactions combine a hydrogen atom (H) from the glycerol and a hydroxyl (OH) group from a fatty acid, forming a molecule of water (H_2O) and leaving a bond between the two molecules (see the left side of Figure 5-3). Most triglycerides contain a mixture of more than one type of fatty acid (as shown on the right side of Figure 5-3).

Characteristics of Solid Fats and Oils

The chemistry of a fatty acid—whether it is short or long, saturated or

linoleic (lin-oh-LAY-ick) **acid:** an essential fatty acid with 18 carbons and two double bonds.

linolenic (lin-oh-LEN-ick) **acid:** an essential fatty acid with 18 carbons and three double bonds.

omega: the last letter of the Greek alphabet (ω), used by chemists to refer to the position of the closest double bond to the methyl (CH_3) end of a fatty acid.

omega-3 fatty acid: a polyunsaturated fatty acid in which the closest double bond to the methyl (CH_3) end of the carbon chain is three carbons away.

omega-6 fatty acid: a polyunsaturated fatty acid in which the closest double bond to the methyl (CH_3) end of the carbon chain is six carbons away.

triglycerides (try-GLISS-er-rides): the chief form of fat in the diet and the major storage form of fat in the body; composed of a molecule of glycerol with three fatty acids attached; also called *triacylglycerols* (try-ay-seel-GLISS-er-ols).
- **tri** = three
- **glyceride** = of glycerol

glycerol (GLISS-er-ol): an alcohol composed of a three-carbon chain, which can serve as the backbone for a triglyceride.

condensation: a chemical reaction in which water is released as two molecules combine to form one larger product.

TABLE 5-1 18-Carbon Fatty Acids

Name	Number of Carbon Atoms	Number of Double Bonds	Saturation	Common Food Sources
Stearic acid	18	0	Saturated	Most animal fats
Oleic acid	18	1	Monounsaturated	Olive and canola oils
Linoleic acid	18	2	Polyunsaturated	Sunflower, safflower, corn, and soybean oils
Linolenic acid	18	3	Polyunsaturated	Soybean and canola oils, flaxseed, walnuts

NOTE: Chemists use a shorthand notation to describe fatty acids. The first number indicates the number of carbon atoms; the second, the number of the double bonds. For example, the notation for stearic acid is 18:0.

© Cengage Learning 2013

*Research scientists commonly use the term *triacylglycerols;* this book continues to use the more familiar term *triglycerides,* as do many other health and nutrition books and journals.

> FIGURE 5-1 Omega-3 and Omega-6 Fatty Acids Compared

The omega number indicates the position of the double bond closest to the methyl (CH_3) end. The fatty acids of an omega family may have different lengths and different numbers of double bonds, but the location of the double bond closest to the methyl end is the same in all of them. These structures are drawn linearly here to ease counting carbons and locating double bonds, but their shapes actually bend at the double bonds.

Linolenic acid, an 18-carbon, omega-3 fatty acid

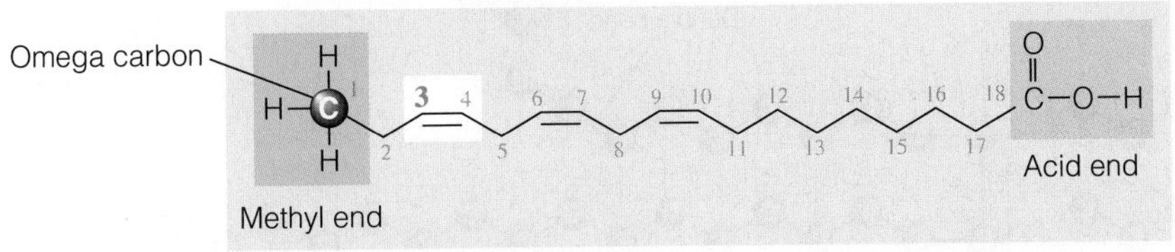

Linoleic acid, an 18-carbon, omega-6 fatty acid

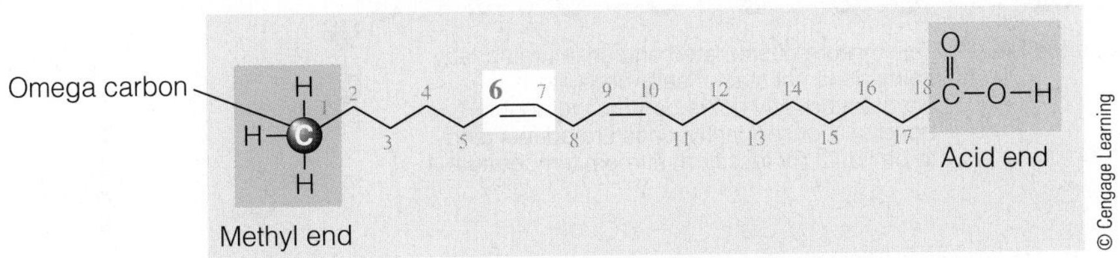

unsaturated, with its closest double bond at carbon 3 or carbon 6—influences the characteristics of foods and the health of the body. A section later in this chapter explains how these features affect health; this section describes how the chemistry influences the **fats** and **oils** in foods.

Firmness The degree of unsaturation influences the firmness of fats at room temperature (see Figure 5-4 on p. 138). Generally speaking, most polyunsaturated vegetable oils are liquid at room temperature, and the more saturated animal fats are solid. Some oils—notably, cocoa butter, palm oil, palm kernel oil, and coconut oil—are saturated; they are firmer than most vegetable oils because of their saturation, but softer than most animal fats because of their shorter carbon chains (8 to 14 carbons long). Generally, the shorter the carbon chain, the softer the fat is at room temperature. Fatty acid compositions of selected fats and oils are shown in Figure 5-5 (p. 138), and Appendix H provides the fat and fatty acid contents of many other foods.

> FIGURE 5-2 Glycerol

When glycerol is free, an OH group is attached to each carbon. When glycerol is part of a triglyceride, each carbon is attached to a fatty acid (as shown in the next figure).

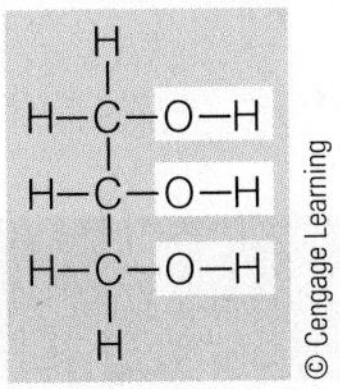

fats: lipids that are solid at room temperature (77°F, or 25°C).

oils: lipids that are liquid at room temperature (77°F, or 25°C).

> FIGURE 5-3 Condensation of Glycerol and Fatty Acids to Form a Triglyceride

To make a triglyceride, three fatty acids attach to glycerol in condensation reactions.

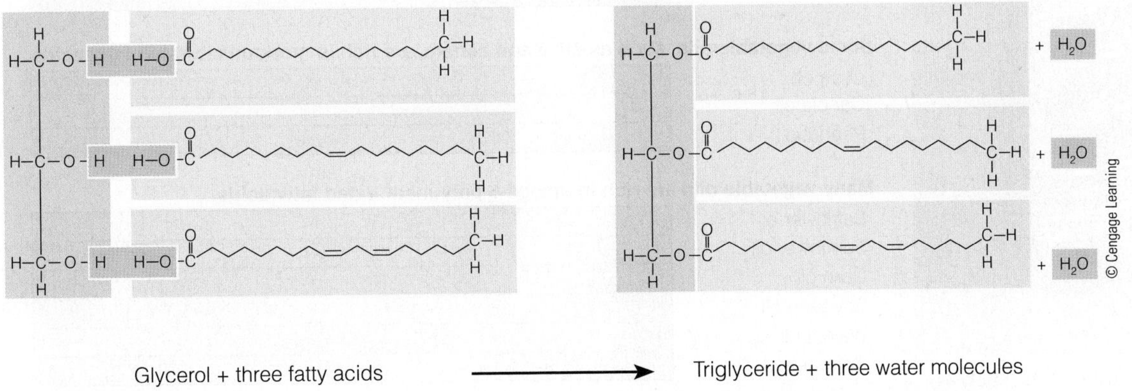

An H atom from glycerol and an OH group from a fatty acid combine to create water, leaving the O on the glycerol and the C at the acid end of each fatty acid to form a bond.

Three fatty acids attached to a glycerol form a triglyceride and yield water. In this example, the triglyceride includes (from top to bottom) a saturated fatty acid, a monounsaturated fatty acid, and a polyunsaturated fatty acid.

> FIGURE 5-4 Diagram of Saturated and Unsaturated Fatty Acids Compared

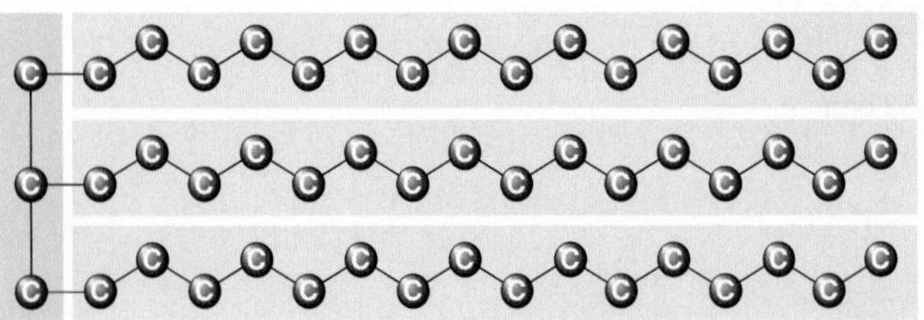

Saturated fatty acids tend to stack together. Consequently, saturated fats tend to be solid (or more firm) at room temperature.

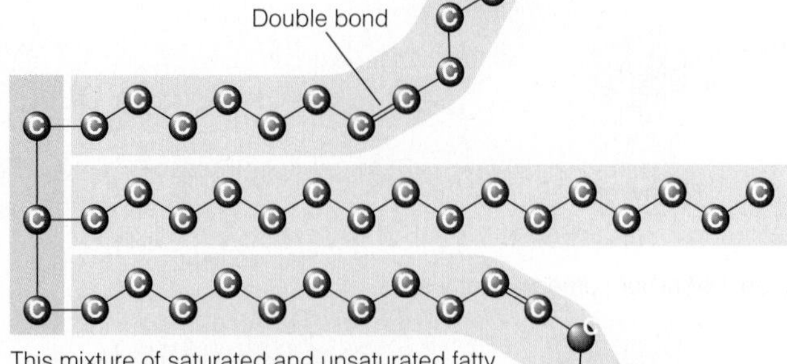

This mixture of saturated and unsaturated fatty acids does not stack neatly because unsaturated fatty acids bend at the double bond(s). Consequently, unsaturated fats tend to be liquid (or less firm) at room temperature.

© Cengage Learning

oxidation (OKS-ee-day-shun): the process of a substance combining with oxygen; oxidation reactions involve the loss of electrons.

Stability The degree of unsaturation also influences stability. All fats become spoiled when exposed to oxygen. The **oxidation** of fats produces a variety of compounds that smell and taste rancid. (Other types of spoilage can occur due to microbial growth.) Polyunsaturated fats spoil most readily because their double

> FIGURE 5-5 Fatty Acid Composition of Common Food Fats

Most fats are a mixture of saturated, monounsaturated, and polyunsaturated fatty acids.

Key:
Saturated fatty acids
Polyunsaturated, omega-6 fatty acids
Monounsaturated fatty acids
Polyunsaturated, omega-3 fatty acids

Animal fats and the tropical oils of coconut and palm contain mostly saturated fatty acids.

Coconut oil
Butter
Beef tallow (beef fat)
Palm oil
Lard (pork fat)
Chicken fat

Some vegetable oils, such as olive and canola, are rich in monounsaturated fatty acids.

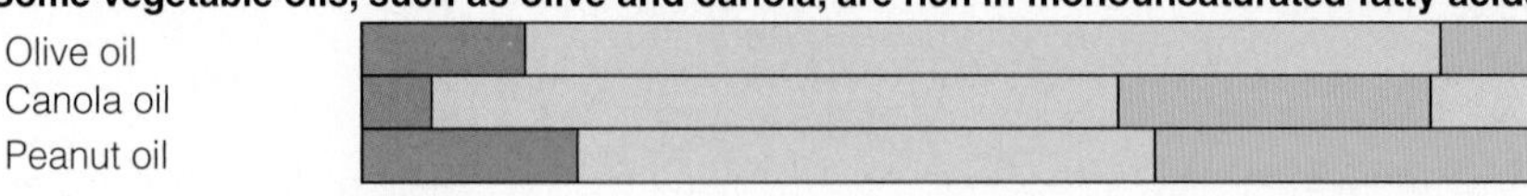

Many vegetable oils are rich in omega-6 polyunsaturated fatty acids.

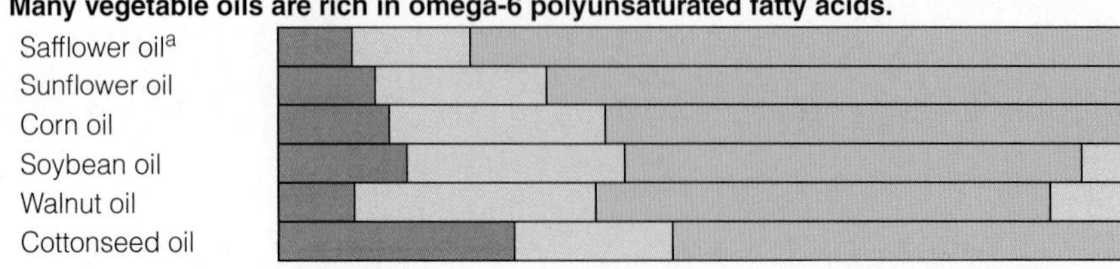

Only a few oils provide significant omega-3 polyunsaturated fatty acids.

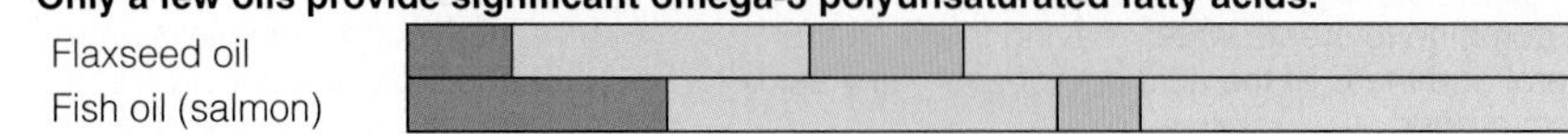

[a]*Salad or cooking type over 70% linoleic acid.*

© Cengage Learning

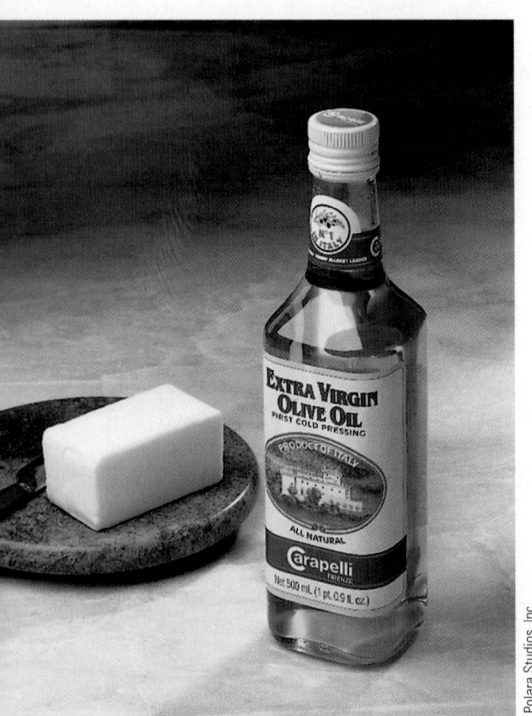

© Polara Studios, Inc.

At room temperature, saturated fats (such as those commonly found in butter and other animal fats) are solid, whereas unsaturated fats (such as those found in vegetable oils) are usually liquid.

> **FIGURE 5-6 Hydrogenation**

Double bonds carry a slightly negative charge and readily accept positively charged hydrogen atoms, creating a saturated fatty acid. Most often, fat is *partially* hydrogenated, creating a *trans*-fatty acid (shown in the next figure).

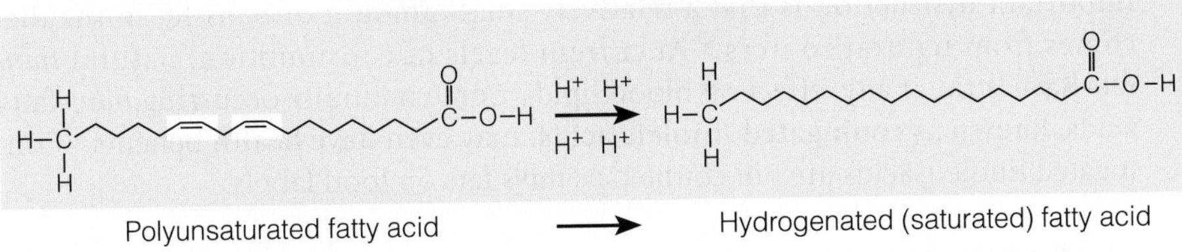

bonds are unstable; monounsaturated fats are slightly less susceptible. Saturated fats are most resistant to oxidation and thus least likely to become rancid.

Manufacturers can protect fat-containing products against rancidity in three ways—none of which are perfect. First, products may be sealed in air-tight, nonmetallic containers, protected from light, and refrigerated—an expensive and inconvenient storage system. Second, manufacturers may add **antioxidants** to compete for the oxygen and thus protect the oil (examples are the additives BHA and BHT and vitamin E).* The advantages and disadvantages of antioxidant additives in food processing are presented in Chapter 19. Third, products may undergo a process known as hydrogenation.

Hydrogenation During **hydrogenation,** some or all of the points of unsaturation are saturated by adding hydrogen molecules. Hydrogenation offers two advantages. First, it protects against oxidation (thereby prolonging shelf life) by making polyunsaturated fats more saturated. Second, it alters the texture of foods by making liquid vegetable oils more solid (as in margarine and shortening). Hydrogenated fats improve the texture of foods, making margarines spreadable, pie crusts flaky, and puddings creamy.

Figure 5-6 illustrates the *total* hydrogenation of a polyunsaturated fatty acid to a saturated fatty acid. Total hydrogenation rarely occurs during food processing. Most often, a fat is *partially* hydrogenated, and some of the double bonds that remain after processing change their configuration from ***cis*** to ***trans.***

***Trans*-Fatty Acids** In nature, most double bonds are *cis*—meaning that the hydrogens next to the double bonds are on the same side of the carbon chain. Only a few fatty acids (notably a small percentage of those found in milk and meat products) naturally occur as ***trans*-fatty acids**—meaning that the hydrogens next to the double bonds are on opposite sides of the carbon chain (see Figure 5-7). In the body, *trans*-fatty acids behave more like saturated fats, increasing blood cholesterol and the risk of heart disease (as a later section describes).[2]

> **FIGURE 5-7 *Cis*- and *Trans*-Fatty Acids Compared**

This example compares the *cis* configuration for an 18-carbon monounsaturated fatty acid (oleic acid) with its corresponding *trans* configuration (elaidic acid).

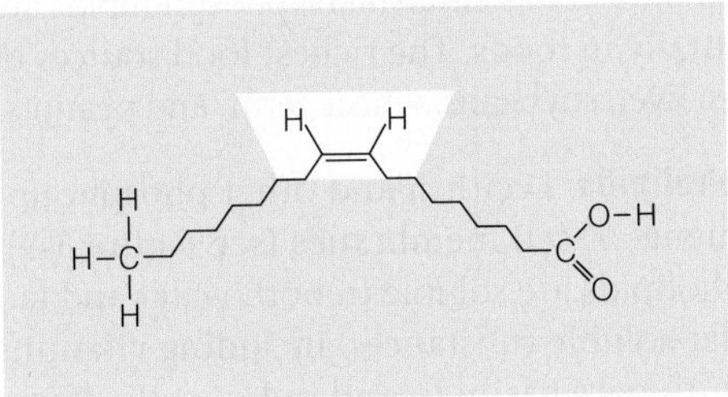

A *cis*-fatty acid has its hydrogens on the same side of the double bond; *cis* molecules bend into a U-like formation. Most naturally occuring unsaturated fatty acids in foods are *cis*.

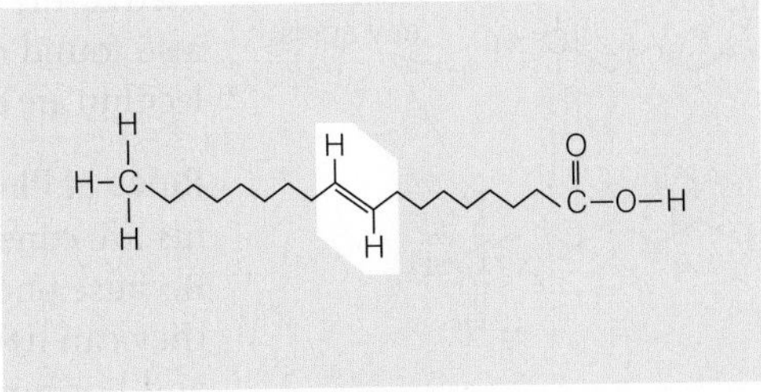

A *trans*-fatty acid has its hydrogens on the opposite sides of the double bond; *trans* molecules are more linear. The *trans* form typically occurs in partially hydrogenated foods when hydrogen atoms shift around some double bonds and change the configuration from *cis* to *trans*.

antioxidants: as a food additive, preservatives that delay or prevent rancidity of fats in foods and other damage to food caused by oxygen.

hydrogenation (HIGH-dro-jen-AY-shun or high-DROJ-eh-NAY-shun): a chemical process by which hydrogens are added to monounsaturated or polyunsaturated fatty acids to reduce the number of double bonds, making the fats more saturated (solid) and more resistant to oxidation (protecting against rancidity). Hydrogenation produces *trans*-fatty acids.

cis: on the near side of; refers to a chemical configuration in which the hydrogen atoms are located on the same side of a double bond.

trans: on the other side of; refers to a chemical configuration in which the hydrogen atoms are located on opposite sides of a double bond.

***trans*-fatty acids:** fatty acids with hydrogens on opposite sides of the double bond.

*BHA is butylated hydroxyanisole; BHT is butylated hydroxytoluene.

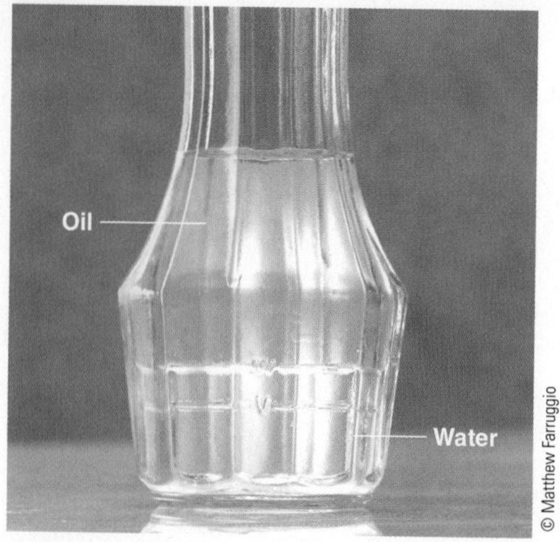

© Matthew Farruggio

Without help from emulsifiers, fats and water don't mix.

Some research suggests that both naturally occurring and commercially created *trans* fats change blood lipids similarly; other research suggests that the negative effects are specific to only the commercial *trans* fats.[3] In any case, the important distinction is that a relatively small amount of *trans*-fat in the diet comes from natural sources.* At current levels of consumption, natural *trans* fats have little, if any, effect on blood lipids. Some naturally occurring *trans*-fatty acids, known as **conjugated linoleic acids,** may even have health benefits.[4] Conjugated linoleic acids are not counted as *trans* fats on food labels.

› REVIEW IT Recognize the chemistry of fatty acids and triglycerides and differences between saturated and unsaturated fats.
The predominant lipids both in foods and in the body are triglycerides: a molecule of glycerol with three fatty acids attached. Fatty acids vary in the length of their carbon chains, their degrees of unsaturation (number of double bonds), and the location of their double bond(s). Those that are fully loaded with hydrogens are saturated; those that are missing hydrogens and therefore have double bonds are unsaturated (monounsaturated or polyunsaturated). The vast majority of triglycerides contain more than one type of fatty acid. Fatty acid saturation affects fats' physical characteristics and storage properties. Hydrogenation, which converts polyunsaturated fats to saturated fats, protects fats from oxidation and alters the texture by making liquid vegetable oils more solid. In the process, hydrogenation creates *trans*-fatty acids that damage health in ways similar to those of saturated fatty acids.

5.2 The Chemist's View of Phospholipids and Sterols

› LEARN IT Describe the chemistry, food sources, and roles of phospholipids and sterols.

The preceding pages have been devoted to one of the classes of lipids, the triglycerides, and their component parts, glycerol and the fatty acids. The other lipids, the phospholipids and sterols, make up only 5 percent of the lipids in the diet.

Phospholipids The best-known **phospholipid** is **lecithin** (see Figure 5-8). Notice that lecithin has one glycerol with two of its three attachment sites occupied by fatty acids like those in triglycerides. The third site is occupied by a phosphate group and a molecule of **choline.** The **hydrophobic** fatty acids make phospholipids soluble in fat; the **hydrophilic** phosphate group allows them to dissolve in water. Such versatility enables the food industry to use phospholipids as an **emulsifier** to mix fats with water in such products as mayonnaise, salad dressings, and candy bars.

Phospholipids in Foods In addition to the phospholipids used by the food industry as emulsifiers, phospholipids are also found naturally in foods. The richest food sources of lecithin are eggs, liver, soybeans, wheat germ, and peanuts.

Roles of Phospholipids Lecithin and other phospholipids are constituents of cell membranes (see Figure 5-9). Because phospholipids are soluble in both water and fat, they can help fat-soluble substances, including vitamins and hormones, to pass easily in and out of cells. Phospholipids also act as emulsifiers in the body, helping to keep fats suspended in the blood and body fluids.

Sterols In addition to triglycerides and phospholipids, the lipids include the **sterols,** compounds with a

conjugated linoleic acids: several fatty acids that have the same chemical formula as linoleic acid (18 carbons, two double bonds) but with different configurations (the double bonds occur on adjacent carbons).

phospholipid (FOS-foe-LIP-id): a compound similar to a triglyceride but having a phosphate and choline (or another nitrogen-containing compound) in place of one of the fatty acids.

lecithin (LESS-uh-thin): one of the phospholipids. Lecithin acts as an emulsifier to combine water-soluble and fat-soluble ingredients that do not ordinarily mix, such as water and oil.

choline (KOH-leen): a nitrogen-containing compound found in foods and made in the body from the amino acid methionine. Choline is part of the phospholipid lecithin and the neurotransmitter acetylcholine.

hydrophobic (high-dro-FOE-bick): water-fearing, or non-water-soluble, substances; also known as *lipophilic* (fat loving).

hydrophilic (high-dro-FIL-ick): water-loving, or water-soluble, substances.

emulsifier: a substance with both water-soluble and fat-soluble portions that promote the mixing of oils and fats in watery solutions.

sterols (STARE-ols or STEER-ols): compounds containing a four-ring carbon structure with side chains attached.

› FIGURE 5-8 Lecithin

Lecithin is similar to a triglyceride but contains only two fatty acids. The third position is occupied by a phosphate group and a molecule of choline. Other phospholipids have different fatty acids and different groups attached to phosphate.

From 2 fatty acids

The plus charge on the N is balanced by a negative ion—usually chloride.

From choline

From glycerol

From phosphate

© Cengage Learning

*For example, most dairy products contain less than 0.5 gram of naturally occurring *trans* fat per serving.

multiple-ring structure.* The most well-known sterol is **cholesterol;** Figure 5-10 shows its chemical structure.

Sterols in Foods Foods derived from both plants and animals contain sterols, but only those from animals contain significant amounts of cholesterol—meats, eggs, seafood, poultry, and dairy products. Some people, confused about the distinction between dietary cholesterol and blood cholesterol, have asked which foods contain the "good" cholesterol. "Good" cholesterol is not a type of cholesterol found in foods, but it refers to the way the body transports cholesterol in the blood, as explained in a later section of this chapter.

Sterols other than cholesterol are naturally found in plants. Being structurally similar to cholesterol, plant sterols interfere with cholesterol absorption. By inhibiting cholesterol absorption, a diet rich in plant sterols lowers blood cholesterol levels. Food manufacturers have fortified foods such as margarine with plant sterols, creating a functional food that helps to reduce blood cholesterol.

Roles of Sterols Many vitally important body compounds are sterols. Among them are bile acids, the sex hormones (such as testosterone, androgen, and estrogen), the adrenal hormones (such as cortisol, cortisone, and aldosterone), and vitamin D, as well as cholesterol itself. Cholesterol in the body can serve as the starting material for the synthesis of these compounds or as a structural component of cell membranes; more than 90 percent of all the body's cholesterol is found in the cells. Despite common misconceptions, cholesterol is not a villain lurking in some evil foods—it is a compound the body makes and uses. The chemical structure is the same, but cholesterol that is made in the body is referred to as **endogenous,** whereas cholesterol from outside the body (from foods) is referred to as **exogenous.** Right now, as you read, your liver is manufacturing cholesterol from fragments of carbohydrate, protein, and fat. In fact, the liver makes about 800 to 1500 milligrams of cholesterol per day, thus contributing much more to the body's total than does the diet. For perspective, the Daily Value on food labels for cholesterol is 300 milligrams per day.

Cholesterol's harmful effects in the body occur when it accumulates in the artery walls and contributes to the formation of **plaque.** These plaque deposits lead to **atherosclerosis,** a disease that causes heart attacks and strokes. Chapter 18 provides many more details.

› REVIEW IT Describe the chemistry, food sources, and roles of phospholipids and sterols.

Phospholipids, including lecithin, have a unique chemical structure that allows them to be soluble in both water and fat. The food industry uses phospholipids as emulsifiers, and in the body, phospholipids are part of cell membranes. Sterols have a multiple-ring structure that differs from the structure of other lipids. In the body, sterols include cholesterol, bile, vitamin D, and some hormones. Animal-derived foods are rich sources of cholesterol. Table 5-2 summarizes the lipid family of compounds.

TABLE 5-2 The Lipid Family

Triglycerides

- 1 Glycerol (per triglyceride) and
- 3 Fatty acids (per triglyceride); depending on the number of double bonds, fatty acids may be:
  - *Saturated* (no double bonds)
  - *Monounsaturated* (one double bond)
  - *Polyunsaturated* (more than one double bond); depending on the location of the double bonds, polyunsaturated fatty acids may be:
    - *Omega-3* (double bond closest to methyl end is 3 carbons away)
    - *Omega-6* (double bond closest to methyl end is 6 carbons away)

Phospholipids (such as lecithin)

Sterols (such as cholesterol)

*The four-ring core structure identifies a steroid; sterols are alcohol derivatives with a steroid ring structure.

> FIGURE 5-9 Phospholipids of a Cell Membrane

A cell membrane is made of phospholipids assembled into an orderly formation called a bilayer. The fatty acid "tails" orient themselves away from the watery fluid inside and outside of the cell. The glycerol and phosphate "heads" are attracted to the watery fluid.

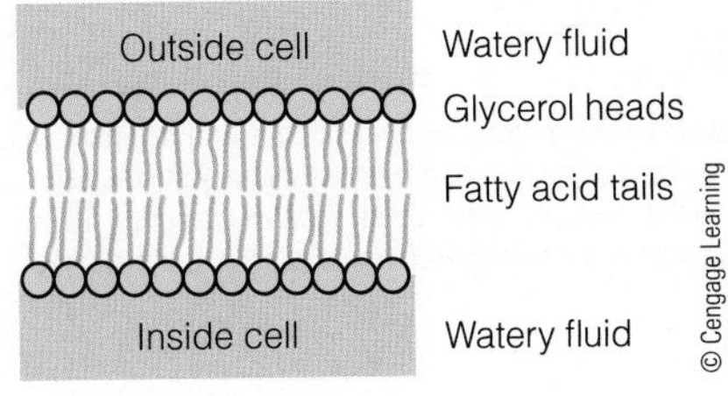

> FIGURE 5-10 Cholesterol

Notice how different cholesterol is from the triglycerides and phospholipids. The fat-soluble vitamin D is synthesized from cholesterol; notice the many structural similarities. The only difference is that cholesterol has a closed ring (highlighted in red), whereas vitamin D's is open, accounting for its vitamin activity.

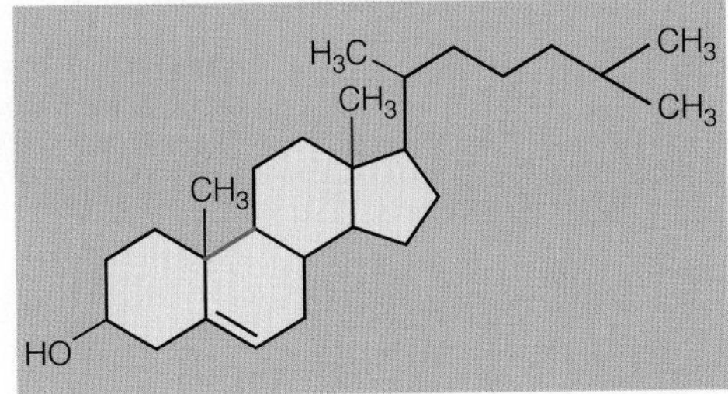

Cholesterol

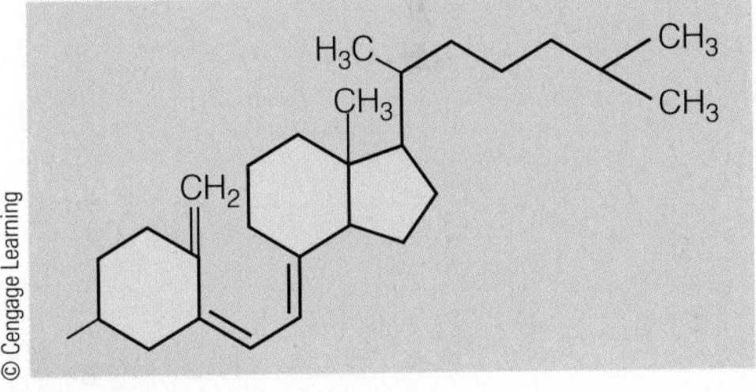

Vitamin D_3

cholesterol (koh-LESS-ter-ol): one of the sterols containing a four-ring carbon structure with a carbon side chain.

endogenous (en-DODGE-eh-nus): from within the body.
- **endo** = within

exogenous (eks-ODGE-eh-nus): from outside the body.
- **exo** = outside

plaque (PLACK): an accumulation of fatty deposits, smooth muscle cells, and fibrous connective tissue that develops in the artery walls in atherosclerosis; also known as *atheromatous* (ATH-er-OH-ma-tus) *plaque.*

atherosclerosis (ATH-er-oh-scler-OH-sis): a type of artery disease characterized by plaques (accumulations of lipid-containing material) on the inner walls of the arteries.

5.3 Digestion, Absorption, and Transport of Lipids

› LEARN IT Summarize fat digestion, absorption, and transport.

Each day, the GI tract receives, on average from the food we eat, 50 to 100 grams of triglycerides, 4 to 8 grams of phospholipids, and 200 to 350 milligrams of cholesterol. These lipids are hydrophobic, whereas the digestive enzymes are hydrophilic. As you read, notice how the body elegantly meets the challenges of keeping the lipids mixed in the watery fluids of the GI tract and facilitating the work of the **lipases.**

lipases (LYE-pasez): enzymes that hydrolyze lipids. *Lingual lipase* is a fat-digesting enzyme secreted from the salivary gland at the base of the tongue; *gastric lipase* is a fat-digesting enzyme secreted from the cells of the stomach.

Lipid Digestion Figure 5-11 traces the digestion of fat through the GI tract. The goal of fat digestion is to dismantle triglycerides into small molecules that

> FIGURE 5-11 **Fat Digestion in the GI Tract**

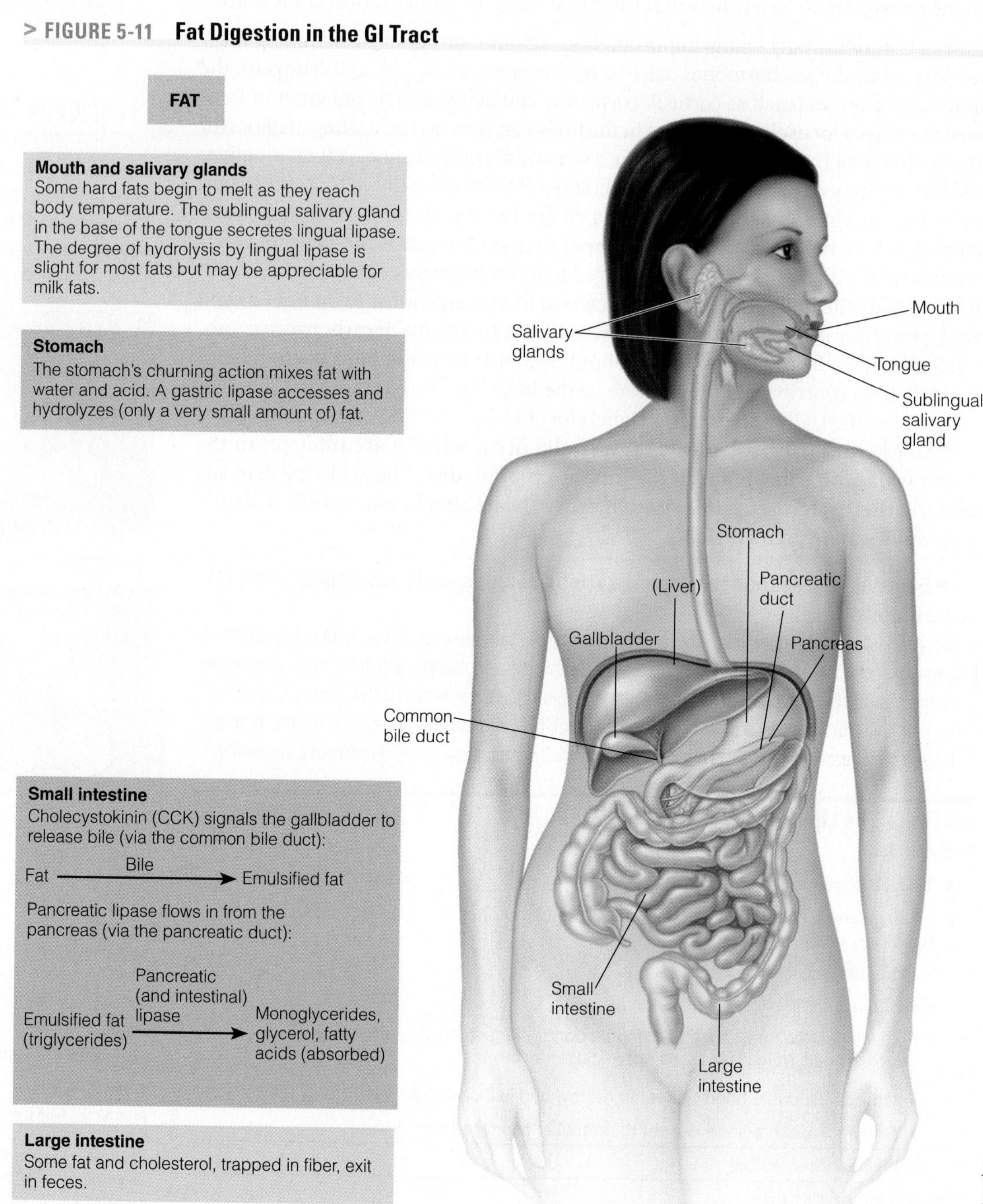

FAT
Mouth and salivary glands
Some hard fats begin to melt as they reach body temperature. The sublingual salivary gland in the base of the tongue secretes lingual lipase. The degree of hydrolysis by lingual lipase is slight for most fats but may be appreciable for milk fats.
Stomach
The stomach's churning action mixes fat with water and acid. A gastric lipase accesses and hydrolyzes (only a very small amount of) fat.
Small intestine
Cholecystokinin (CCK) signals the gallbladder to release bile (via the common bile duct):
Fat —Bile→ Emulsified fat
Pancreatic lipase flows in from the pancreas (via the pancreatic duct):
Emulsified fat (triglycerides) —Pancreatic (and intestinal) lipase→ Monoglycerides, glycerol, fatty acids (absorbed)
Large intestine
Some fat and cholesterol, trapped in fiber, exit in feces.
Salivary glands
Mouth
Tongue
Sublingual salivary gland
Stomach
(Liver)
Pancreatic duct
Gallbladder
Pancreas
Common bile duct
Small intestine
Large intestine

the body can absorb and use—namely, **monoglycerides,** fatty acids, and glycerol. The following paragraphs provide the details.

In the Mouth Fat digestion starts off slowly in the mouth, with some hard fats beginning to melt when they reach body temperature. A salivary gland at the base of the tongue releases an enzyme (lingual lipase) that plays an active role in fat digestion in infants, but a relatively minor role in adults. In infants, this enzyme efficiently digests the short- and medium-chain fatty acids found in milk.

In the Stomach In a quiet stomach, fat would float as a layer above the watery components of swallowed food. But whenever food is present, the stomach becomes active. The strong muscle contractions of the stomach propel its contents toward the pyloric sphincter. Some chyme passes through the pyloric sphincter periodically, but the remaining partially digested food is propelled back into the body of the stomach. This churning grinds the solid pieces to finer particles, mixes the chyme, and disperses the fat into small droplets. These actions help to expose the fat for attack by the gastric lipase enzyme—an enzyme that performs best in the acidic environment of the stomach. Still, little fat digestion takes place in the stomach; most of the action occurs in the small intestine.

In the Small Intestine When fat enters the small intestine, it triggers the release of the hormone cholecystokinin (CCK), which signals the gallbladder to release its stores of bile. (Remember that the liver makes bile, and the gallbladder stores bile until it is needed.) Among bile's many ingredients are bile acids, which are made in the liver from cholesterol and have a similar structure. In addition, bile acids often pair up with an amino acid (a building block of protein). The amino acid end is hydrophilic, and the sterol end is hydrophobic. This structure enables bile to act as an emulsifier, drawing fat molecules into the surrounding watery fluids. There, the fats are fully digested as they encounter lipase enzymes from the pancreas and small intestine. The process of emulsification is diagrammed in Figure 5-12.

Most of the hydrolysis of triglycerides occurs in the small intestine. The major fat-digesting enzymes are pancreatic lipases; some intestinal lipases are also active. These enzymes remove each of a triglyceride's outer fatty acids one at a time, leaving a monoglyceride. Occasionally, enzymes remove all three fatty acids, leaving a free molecule of glycerol. Hydrolysis of a triglyceride is shown in Figure 5-13 (p. 144).

Phospholipids are digested similarly—that is, their fatty acids are removed by hydrolysis. The two fatty acids and the remaining glycerol and phosphate fragments are then absorbed. Most sterols can be absorbed as is; if any fatty acids are attached, they are first hydrolyzed off.

monoglycerides: molecules of glycerol with one fatty acid attached. A molecule of glycerol with two fatty acids attached is a *diglyceride.*
- **mono** = one
- **di** = two

> **FIGURE 5-12 Emulsification of Fat by Bile**

Like bile, detergents are emulsifiers and work the same way, which is why they are effective in removing grease spots from clothes. Molecule by molecule, the grease is dissolved out of the spot and suspended in the water, where it can be rinsed away.

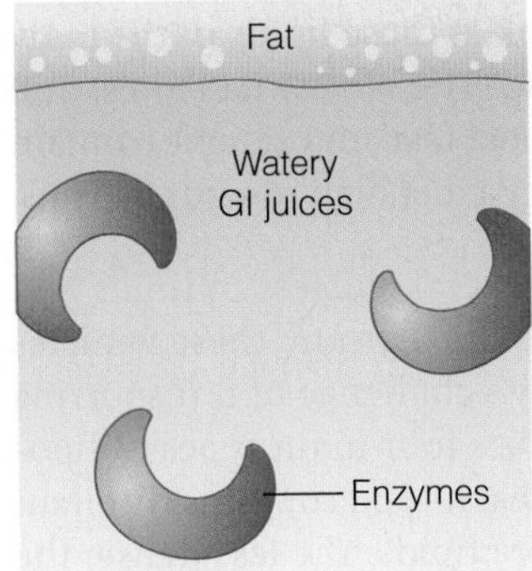

In the stomach, the fat and watery GI juices tend to separate. The enzymes in the GI juices can't get at the fat.

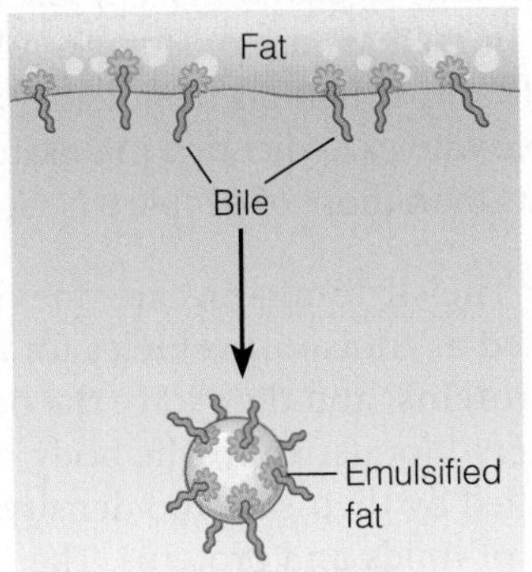

When fat enters the small intestine, the gallbladder secretes bile. Bile has an affinity for both fat and water, so it can bring the fat into the water.

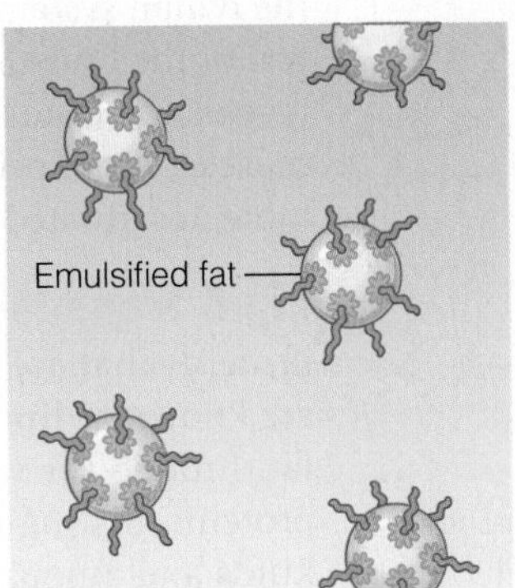

Bile's emulsifying action converts large fat globules into small droplets that repel one another.

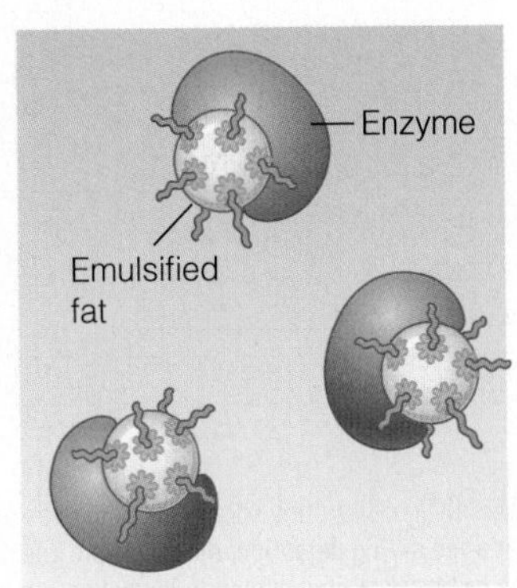

After emulsification, more fat is exposed to the enzymes, making fat digestion more efficient.

> **FIGURE 5-13 Digestion (Hydrolysis) of a Triglyceride**

H–O–H

Bonds break

H–O–H

Bonds break

Triglyceride

The triglyceride and two molecules of water are split. The H and OH from water complete the structures of two fatty acids and leave a monoglyceride.

Monoglyceride + two fatty acids

These products may pass into the intestinal cells, but sometimes the monoglyceride is split with another molecule of water to give a third fatty acid and glycerol. Fatty acids, monoglycerides, and glycerol are absorbed into intestinal cells.

> **FIGURE 5-14 Enterohepatic Circulation**

Most of the bile released into the small intestine is reabsorbed and sent back to the liver to be reused. This cycle is called the *enterohepatic circulation* of bile. Some bile is excreted.

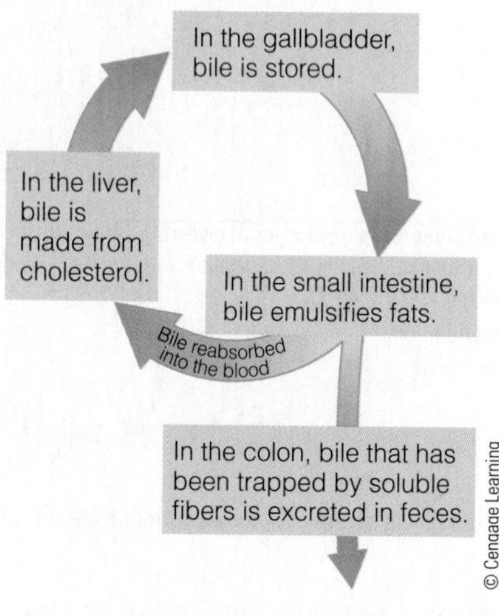

In the gallbladder, bile is stored.
In the liver, bile is made from cholesterol.
In the small intestine, bile emulsifies fats.
Bile reabsorbed into the blood
In the colon, bile that has been trapped by soluble fibers is excreted in feces.
© Cengage Learning

Bile's Routes After bile enters the small intestine and emulsifies fat, it has two possible destinations, illustrated in Figure 5-14. Most of the bile is reabsorbed from the small intestine and recycled. The other possibility is that some of the bile can be trapped by dietary fibers in the large intestine and excreted. Because cholesterol is needed to make bile, the excretion of bile effectively reduces blood cholesterol. As Chapter 4 explains, the dietary fibers most effective at lowering blood cholesterol this way are the soluble fibers commonly found in fruits, whole grains, and legumes.

Lipid Absorption

Figure 5-15 illustrates the absorption of lipids. Small molecules (glycerol and short- and medium-chain fatty acids) can diffuse easily into the intestinal cells; they are absorbed directly into the bloodstream. Larger molecules (monoglycerides and long-chain fatty acids) are emulsified by bile, forming spherical complexes known as **micelles.** The micelles diffuse into the intestinal cells, where the monoglycerides and long-chain fatty acids are reassembled into new triglycerides.

Within the intestinal cells, the newly made triglycerides and other lipids (cholesterol and phospholipids) are packed with protein into transport vehicles known as chylomicrons. The intestinal cells then release the chylomicrons into the lymphatic system. The chylomicrons glide through the lymph until they reach a point of entry into the bloodstream at the thoracic duct near the heart. (Recall from Chapter 3 that nutrients from the GI tract that enter the lymph system initially bypass the liver.) The blood carries these lipids to the rest of the body for immediate use or storage. A look at these lipids in the body reveals the kinds of fat the diet has been delivering. The blood, fat stores, and muscle cells of people who eat a diet rich in unsaturated fats, for example, contain more unsaturated fats than those of people who select a diet high in saturated fats.

Lipid Transport

The chylomicrons are one of several clusters of lipids and proteins that are used as transport vehicles for fats. As a group, these vehicles are known as **lipoproteins,** and they solve the body's challenge of transporting fat through the watery bloodstream. The body makes four main types of lipoproteins, distinguished by their size and density.* Each type contains different kinds and amounts of lipids and proteins. The more lipids, the less dense; the

micelles (MY-cells): tiny spherical complexes of emulsified fat that arise during digestion; most contain bile salts and the products of lipid digestion, including fatty acids, monoglycerides, and cholesterol.

lipoproteins (LIP-oh-PRO-teenz): clusters of lipids associated with proteins that serve as transport vehicles for lipids in the lymph and blood.

*Chemists can identify the various lipoproteins by their density. They place a blood sample below a thick fluid in a test tube and spin the tube in a centrifuge. The most buoyant particles (highest in lipids) rise to the top and have the lowest density; the densest particles (highest in proteins) remain at the bottom and have the highest density. Others distribute themselves in between.

> **FIGURE 5-15 Absorption of Fat**

The end products of fat digestion are mostly monoglycerides, some fatty acids, and very little glycerol. Their absorption differs depending on their size. (In reality, molecules of fatty acid are too small to see without a powerful microscope, whereas villi are visible to the naked eye.)

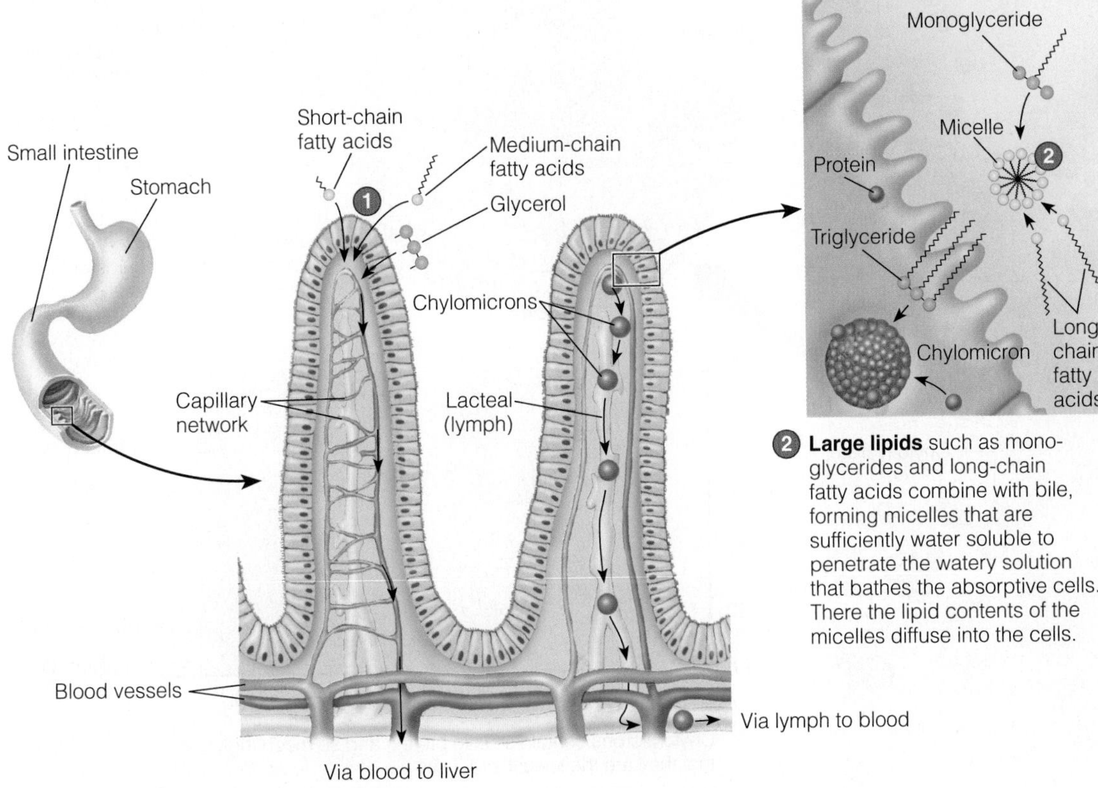

1 **Glycerol and small lipids** such as short- and medium-chain fatty acids can move directly into the bloodstream.

2 **Large lipids** such as monoglycerides and long-chain fatty acids combine with bile, forming micelles that are sufficiently water soluble to penetrate the watery solution that bathes the absorptive cells. There the lipid contents of the micelles diffuse into the cells.

more proteins, the more dense. Figure 5-16 (p. 146) shows the relative compositions and sizes of the lipoproteins.

Chylomicrons The **chylomicrons** are the largest and least dense of the lipoproteins. They transport *diet*-derived lipids (mostly triglycerides) from the small intestine (via the lymph system) to the rest of the body. Cells all over the body remove triglycerides from the chylomicrons as they pass by, so the chylomicrons get smaller and smaller. Within 14 hours after absorption, most of the triglycerides have been depleted, and only a few remnants of protein, cholesterol, and phospholipid remain. Special protein receptors on the membranes of the liver cells recognize and remove these chylomicron remnants from the blood.

VLDL (Very-Low-Density Lipoproteins) Meanwhile, in the liver—the most active site of lipid synthesis—cells are making cholesterol, fatty acids, and other lipid compounds. Ultimately, the lipids made in the liver and those collected from chylomicron remnants are packaged with proteins as a **VLDL (very-low-density lipoprotein)** and shipped to other parts of the body.

As the VLDL travel through the body, cells remove triglycerides. As they lose triglycerides, the VLDL shrink and the proportion of lipids shifts. Cholesterol becomes the predominant lipid, and the lipoprotein becomes smaller and more dense. As this occurs, the VLDL becomes an **LDL (low-density lipoprotein),** loaded with cholesterol, but containing relatively few triglycerides.*

*Before becoming LDL, the VLDL are first transformed into intermediate-density lipoproteins (IDL), sometimes called VLDL remnants. Some IDL may be picked up by the liver and rapidly broken down; those IDL that remain in circulation continue to deliver triglycerides to the cells and eventually become LDL. Researchers debate whether IDL are simply transitional particles or a separate class of lipoproteins; normally, IDL do not accumulate in the blood. Measures of blood lipids include IDL with LDL.

chylomicrons (kye-lo-MY-cronz): the class of lipoproteins that transport lipids from the intestinal cells to the rest of the body.

VLDL (very-low-density lipoprotein): the type of lipoprotein made primarily by liver cells to transport lipids to various tissues in the body; composed primarily of triglycerides.

LDL (low-density lipoprotein): the type of lipoprotein derived from very-low-density lipoproteins (VLDL) as triglycerides are removed and broken down; composed primarily of cholesterol.

> **FIGURE 5-16 Sizes and Compositions of the Lipoproteins**

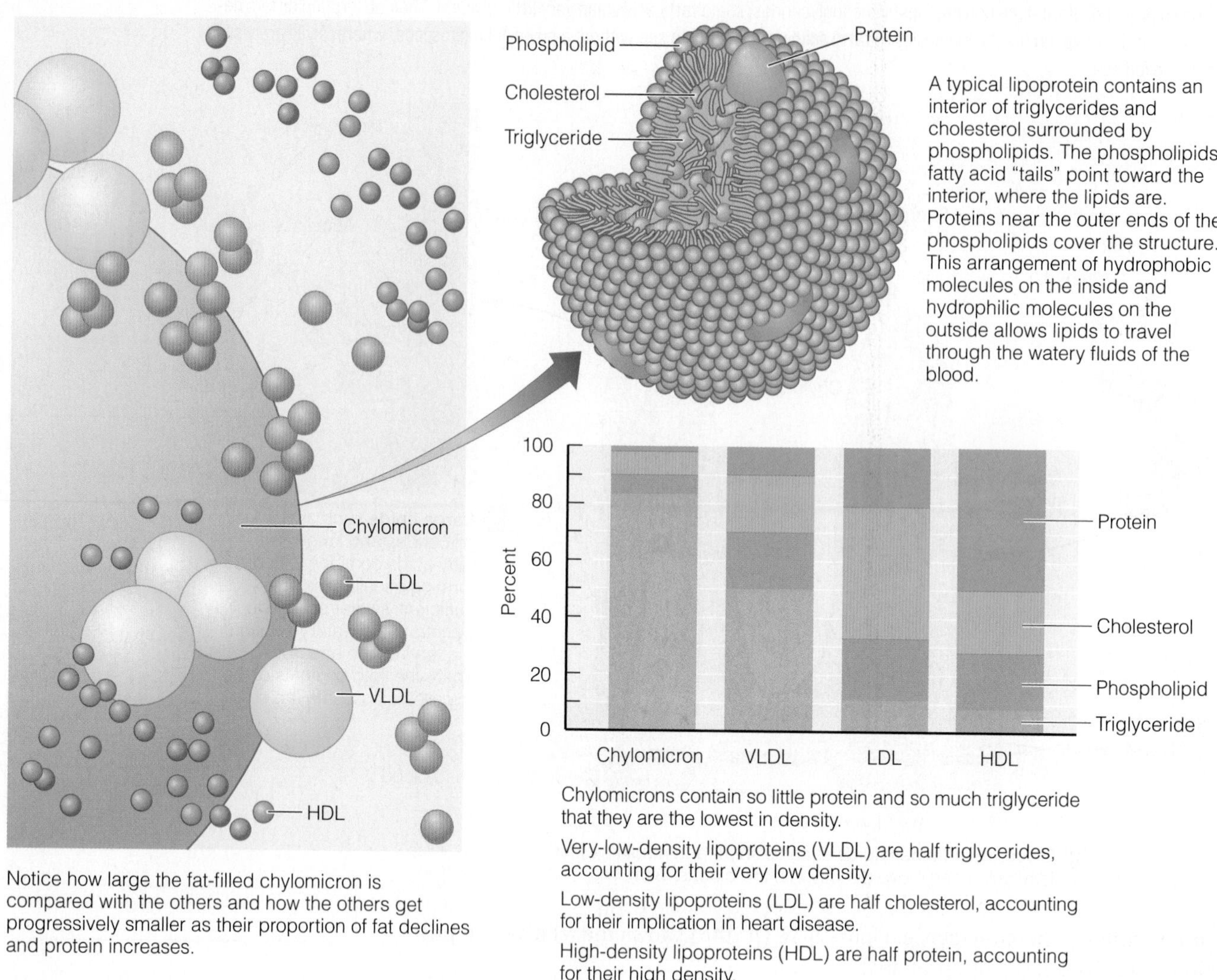

Phospholipid
Protein
Cholesterol
Triglyceride
A typical lipoprotein contains an interior of triglycerides and cholesterol surrounded by phospholipids. The phospholipids' fatty acid "tails" point toward the interior, where the lipids are. Proteins near the outer ends of the phospholipids cover the structure. This arrangement of hydrophobic molecules on the inside and hydrophilic molecules on the outside allows lipids to travel through the watery fluids of the blood.
Chylomicron
LDL
VLDL
HDL
Percent
100
80
60
40
20
0
Chylomicron
VLDL
LDL
HDL
Protein
Cholesterol
Phospholipid
Triglyceride

Notice how large the fat-filled chylomicron is compared with the others and how the others get progressively smaller as their proportion of fat declines and protein increases.

Chylomicrons contain so little protein and so much triglyceride that they are the lowest in density.

Very-low-density lipoproteins (VLDL) are half triglycerides, accounting for their very low density.

Low-density lipoproteins (LDL) are half cholesterol, accounting for their implication in heart disease.

High-density lipoproteins (HDL) are half protein, accounting for their high density.

LDL (Low-Density Lipoproteins) The LDL circulate throughout the body, making their contents available to the cells of all tissues—muscles (including the heart muscle), fat stores, the mammary glands, and others. The cells take triglycerides, cholesterol, and phospholipids to use for energy, make hormones or other compounds, or build new membranes. Special LDL receptors on the liver cells play a crucial role in the control of blood cholesterol concentrations by removing LDL from circulation.

HDL (High-Density Lipoproteins) The liver makes **HDL (high-density lipoprotein)** to remove cholesterol from the cells and carry it back to the liver for recycling or disposal. By efficiently clearing cholesterol, HDL lowers the risk of heart disease.[5] In addition, HDL have anti-inflammatory properties that seem to keep artery-clogging plaque from breaking apart and causing heart attacks.[6] Figure 5-17 summarizes lipid transport via the lipoproteins.

Health Implications The distinction between LDL and HDL has implications for the health of the heart and blood vessels. The blood lipid linked most directly to heart disease is LDL cholesterol. As mentioned, HDL also carry cholesterol, but elevated HDL represent cholesterol returning from the rest of the body to the liver for breakdown and excretion. The transport of cholesterol from the tissues back to the liver is sometimes called *reverse cholesterol transport* or the *scavenger pathway.*

High LDL and low HDL cholesterol are both associated with a high risk of heart disease. Having adequate HDL is beneficial, but having high HDL is not

HDL (high-density lipoprotein): the type of lipoprotein that transports cholesterol back to the liver from the cells; composed primarily of protein.

> **FIGURE 5-17 Lipid Transport via Lipoproteins**

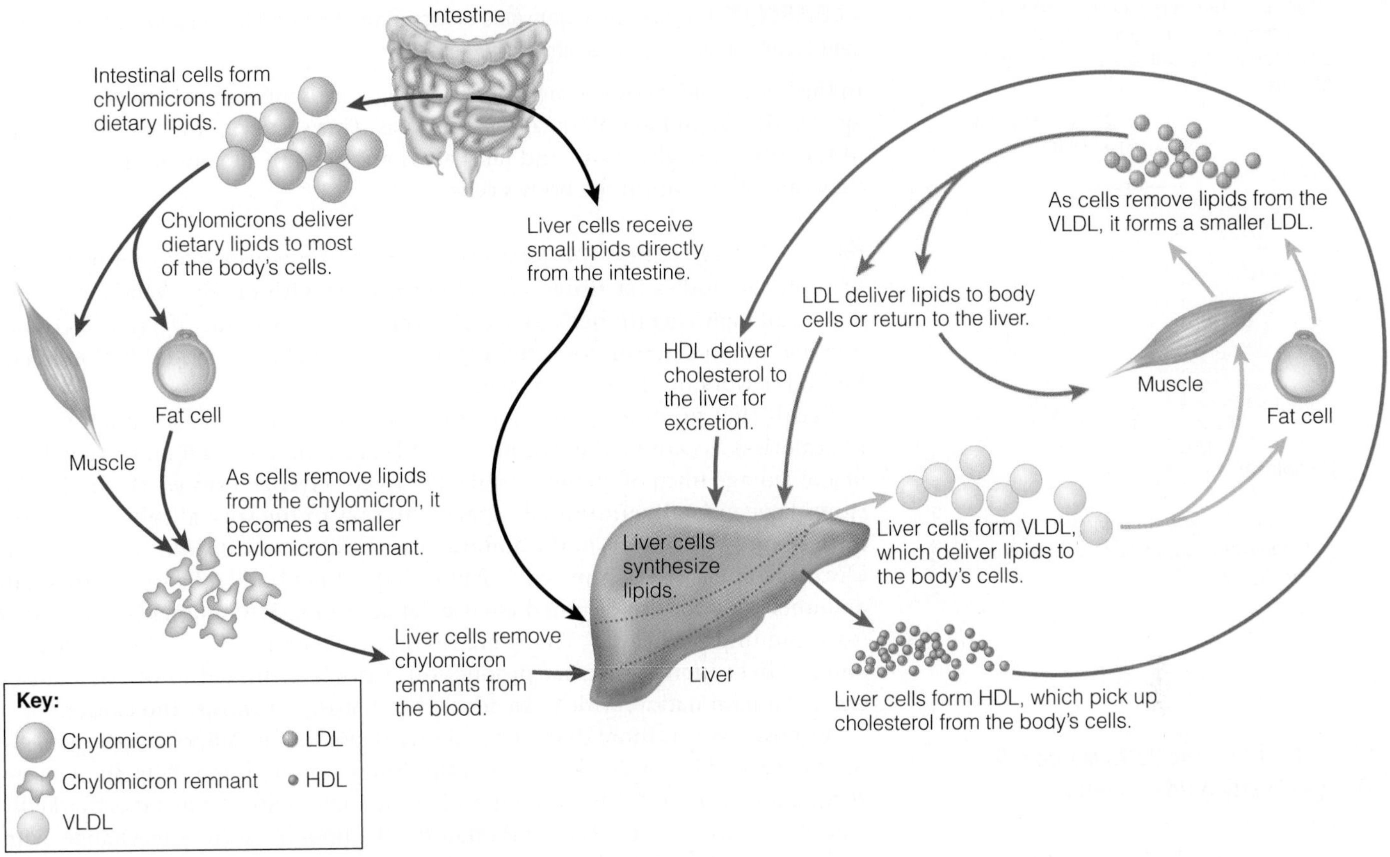

Intestine

Intestinal cells form chylomicrons from dietary lipids.

Chylomicrons deliver dietary lipids to most of the body's cells.

Liver cells receive small lipids directly from the intestine.

Muscle

Fat cell

As cells remove lipids from the chylomicron, it becomes a smaller chylomicron remnant.

Liver cells remove chylomicron remnants from the blood.

Liver cells synthesize lipids.

Liver

HDL deliver cholesterol to the liver for excretion.

LDL deliver lipids to body cells or return to the liver.

As cells remove lipids from the VLDL, it forms a smaller LDL.

Muscle

Fat cell

Liver cells form VLDL, which deliver lipids to the body's cells.

Liver cells form HDL, which pick up cholesterol from the body's cells.

Key:
Chylomicron
Chylomicron remnant
VLDL
LDL
HDL

necessarily more beneficial. Some people think of HDL as healthy and LDL as lousy, or refer to LDL as "bad," and HDL as "good," cholesterol. Keep in mind that the cholesterol itself is the same and that the differences between LDL and HDL reflect the *proportions* and *types* of lipids and proteins within them—not the type of cholesterol. The following factors help to lower LDL and/or raise HDL:

- Weight control
- Monounsaturated or polyunsaturated, instead of saturated, fat in the diet
- Soluble dietary fibers
- Phytochemicals
- *Moderate* alcohol consumption
- Physical activity

Chapter 18 provides many more details.

Not too surprisingly, numerous genes influence how the body handles the synthesis, transport, and degradation of lipids and lipoproteins. Much current research is focused on how nutrient-gene interactions may direct the progression of heart disease.

> **REVIEW IT** Summarize fat digestion, absorption, and transport.

The body makes special arrangements to digest and absorb lipids. It provides the emulsifier bile to make them accessible to the fat-digesting lipases that dismantle triglycerides, mostly to monoglycerides and fatty acids, for absorption by the intestinal cells. Four types of lipoproteins transport all classes of lipids (triglycerides, phospholipids, and cholesterol), but the chylomicrons are the largest and contain mostly triglycerides from the diet; VLDL are smaller and are about half triglycerides; LDL are smaller still and contain mostly cholesterol; and HDL are the densest and are rich in protein. High LDL cholesterol indicates increased risk of heart disease, whereas high HDL cholesterol has a protective effect.

> **FIGURE 5-18 An Adipose Cell**

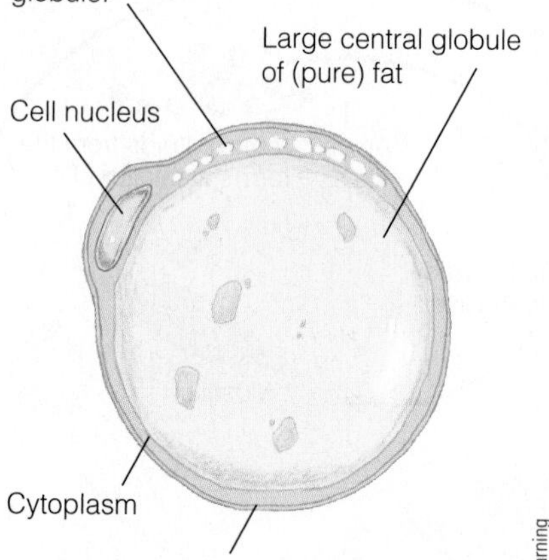

Newly imported triglycerides first form small droplets at the periphery of the cell, then merge with the large, central globule.
Large central globule of (pure) fat
Cell nucleus
Cytoplasm
As the central globule enlarges, the fat cell membrane expands to accommodate its swollen contents.
© Cengage Learning

> **FIGURE 5-19 The Pathway from One Omega-6 Fatty Acid to Another**

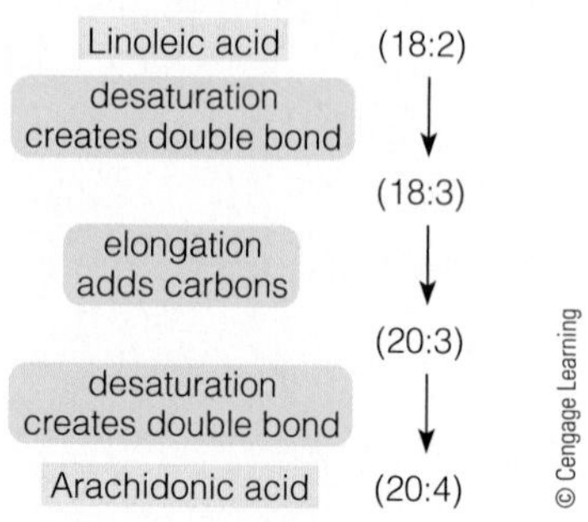

The first number indicates the number of carbons and the second, the number of double bonds. Similar reactions occur when the body makes the omega-3 fatty acids EPA and DHA from linolenic acid.

5.4 Lipids in the Body

> **LEARN IT** Outline the major roles of fats in the body, including a discussion of essential fatty acids and the omega fatty acids.

In the body, lipids provide energy, insulate against temperature extremes, protect against shock, and maintain cell membranes. This section provides an overview of the roles of triglycerides and fatty acids and then of the metabolic pathways they can follow within the body's cells.

Roles of Triglycerides First and foremost, triglycerides—either from food or from the body's fat stores—provide the cells with energy. When a person dances all night, her dinner's triglycerides provide some of the fuel that keeps her moving. When a person loses his appetite, his stored triglycerides fuel much of his body's work until he can eat again.

Recall that gram for gram, fat provides more than twice as much energy (9 kcalories) as carbohydrate or protein (4 kcalories), making it an extremely efficient storage form of energy. Unlike the liver's glycogen stores, the body's fat stores have virtually unlimited capacity, thanks to the special cells of the **adipose tissue.** The fat cells of the adipose tissue readily take up and store triglycerides. An adipose cell is depicted in Figure 5-18. Other body cells store only small amounts of fat for their immediate use; fat accumulation in nonadipose cells is toxic and impairs health.[7] This scenario occurs when the diet delivers excesses and the liver increases its fat production. Fatty liver linked to obesity causes chronic inflammation, which can advance to fibrosis, cirrhosis, and cancer.[8]

Adipose tissue is more than just a storage depot for fat. Adipose tissue actively secretes several hormones known as **adipokines**—proteins that help regulate energy balance and influence several body functions.[9] When body fat is markedly reduced or excessive, the type and quantity of adipokine secretions change, with consequences for the body's health. Researchers are currently exploring how adipokines influence the links between obesity and chronic diseases such as type 2 diabetes, hypertension, and heart disease.[10] Obesity, for example, increases the release of the adipokine **resistin** that promotes inflammation and insulin resistance—factors that predict heart disease and diabetes. Similarly, obesity decreases the release of the adipokine **adiponectin** that protects against inflammation, diabetes, and heart disease.

Fat serves other roles in the body as well. Because fat is a poor conductor of heat, the layer of fat beneath the skin insulates the body from temperature extremes. Fat pads also serve as natural shock absorbers, providing a cushion for the bones and vital organs. Fat provides the structural material for cell membranes and participates in cell signaling pathways.

Essential Fatty Acids The human body needs fatty acids, and it can make all but two of them—linoleic acid (the 18-carbon omega-6 fatty acid) and linolenic acid (the 18-carbon omega-3 fatty acid). These two fatty acids must be supplied by the diet and are therefore **essential fatty acids.** The cells do not possess the enzymes to make any of the omega-6 or omega-3 fatty acids from scratch, nor can they convert an omega-6 fatty acid to an omega-3 fatty acid or vice versa. Cells *can,* however, use the 18-carbon member of an omega family from the diet to make the longer fatty acids of that family by forming double bonds (desaturation) and lengthening the chain two carbons at a time (elongation), as shown in Figure 5-19. This is a slow process because the omega-3 and omega-6 families compete for the same enzymes. Too much of a fatty acid from one family can create a deficiency of the other family's longer fatty acids, which becomes critical only when the diet fails to deliver adequate supplies. Therefore, the most effective way to maintain body supplies of all the omega-6 and omega-3 fatty acids is to obtain them directly from foods—most notably, from vegetable oils, seeds, nuts, fish, and other seafoods.

adipose (ADD-ih-poce) **tissue:** the body's fat tissue; consists of masses of triglyceride-storing cells.

adipokines (ADD-ih-poe-kines): proteins synthesized and secreted by adipose cells.

resistin (ree-ZIS-tin): a protein produced by adipose cells that promotes inflammation and causes insulin resistance.

adiponectin: a protein produced by adipose cells that inhibits inflammation and protects against insulin resistance, type 2 diabetes, and cardiovascular disease.

essential fatty acids: fatty acids that the body requires but cannot make, and so must be obtained from the diet; both linoleic acid and linolenic acid are essential fatty acids.

Linoleic Acid and the Omega-6 Family Linoleic acid is an essential fatty acid and the primary member of the omega-6 fatty acid family. When the body receives linoleic acid from the diet, it can make other members of the omega-6 family—such as the 20-carbon polyunsaturated fatty acid, **arachidonic acid** (as shown in Figure 5-19). Should a linoleic acid deficiency develop, arachidonic acid, and all other omega-6 fatty acids that derive from linoleic acid, would also become essential and have to be obtained from the diet. A nonessential nutrient (such as arachidonic acid) that must be supplied by the diet in special circumstances (as in a linoleic acid deficiency) is considered a **conditionally essential nutrient.** Normally, vegetable oils and meats supply enough omega-6 fatty acids to meet the body's needs.

Linolenic Acid and the Omega-3 Family Linolenic acid is an essential fatty acid and the primary member of the omega-3 fatty acid family.* Like linoleic acid, linolenic acid cannot be made in the body and must be supplied by foods. Given the 18-carbon linolenic acid, the body can make small amounts of the 20- and 22-carbon members of the omega-3 family, **eicosapentaenoic acid (EPA)** and **docosahexaenoic acid (DHA),** respectively. These omega-3 fatty acids play critical roles in the optimal structure and function of cells.[11] Found abundantly in the eyes and brain, the omega-3 fatty acids are essential for normal growth, visual acuity, and cognitive development.[12] They may also play an important role in the prevention and treatment of heart disease, as later sections explain.

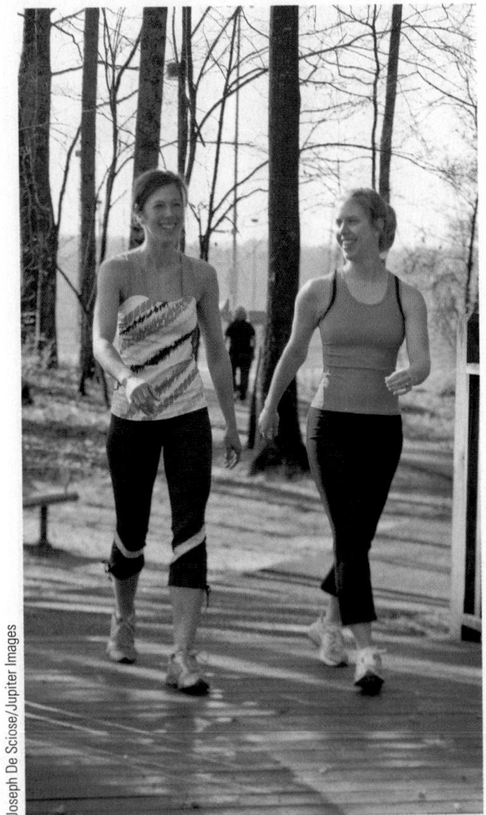
Joseph De Sciose/Jupiter Images

Double thanks: The body's fat stores provide energy for a walk, and fat pads on the heels provide cushion against the hard pavement.

Eicosanoids The body uses the longer omega-3 and omega-6 fatty acids to make substances known as **eicosanoids.** Eicosanoids are a diverse group of more than 100 compounds. Sometimes described as "hormonelike," eicosanoids differ from hormones in important ways. For one, hormones are secreted in one location and travel to affect cells all over the body, whereas eicosanoids appear to affect only the cells in which they are made or nearby cells in the same localized environment. For another, hormones elicit the same response from all their target cells, whereas eicosanoids often have different effects on different cells.

The actions of various eicosanoids sometimes oppose one another. For example, one causes muscles to relax and blood vessels to dilate, whereas another causes muscles to contract and blood vessels to constrict. Certain eicosanoids participate in the immune response to injury and infection, producing fever, inflammation, and pain. One of the ways aspirin relieves these symptoms is by slowing the synthesis of these eicosanoids.

Eicosanoids that derive from omega-3 fatty acids differ from those that derive from omega-6 fatty acids, with the omega-3 family providing greater health benefits. The omega-3 eicosanoids help lower blood pressure, prevent blood clot formation, protect against irregular heartbeats, and reduce inflammation, whereas the omega-6 eicosanoids tend to promote clot formation, inflammation, and blood vessel constriction.[13]

Omega-6 to Omega-3 Ratio Because omega-6 and omega-3 fatty acids compete for the same enzymes and their actions often oppose each other, researchers have studied whether there is an ideal ratio that best supports health.[14] Suggested ratios range from 4:1 to 10:1; while some researchers support such recommendations, others find the ratio of little value in improving health or predicting risk.[15] Increasing the amount of omega-3 fatty acids in the diet is clearly beneficial, but reducing the amount of omega-6 fatty acids in the diet to improve the ratio may not be helpful. Omega-6 fatty acids protect heart health by lowering LDL cholesterol and improving insulin resistance.[16]

Fatty Acid Deficiencies Most diets in the United States meet the minimum essential fatty acid requirement adequately. Historically, deficiencies have developed only in infants and young children who have been fed fat-free milk and low-fat diets or in hospital clients who have been mistakenly fed formulas

*This omega-3 linolenic acid is known as alpha-linolenic acid and is the fatty acid referred to in this chapter. Another fatty acid, also with 18 carbons and three double bonds, belongs to the omega-6 family and is known as gamma-linolenic acid.

arachidonic (a-RACK-ih-DON-ic) **acid:** an omega-6 polyunsaturated fatty acid with 20 carbons and four double bonds; present in small amounts in meat and other animal products and synthesized in the body from linoleic acid.

conditionally essential nutrient: a nutrient that is normally nonessential, but must be supplied by the diet in special circumstances when the need for it exceeds the body's ability to produce it.

eicosapentaenoic (EYE-cossa-PENTA-ee-NO-ick) **acid (EPA):** an omega-3 polyunsaturated fatty acid with 20 carbons and five double bonds; present in fatty fish and synthesized in limited amounts in the body from linolenic acid.

docosahexaenoic (DOE-cossa-HEXA-ee-NO-ick) **acid (DHA):** an omega-3 polyunsaturated fatty acid with 22 carbons and six double bonds; present in fatty fish and synthesized in limited amounts in the body from linolenic acid.

eicosanoids (eye-COSS-uh-noyds): derivatives of 20-carbon fatty acids; biologically active compounds that help to regulate blood pressure, blood clotting, and other body functions. They include *prostaglandins* (PROS-tah-GLAND-ins), *thromboxanes* (throm-BOX-ains), and *leukotrienes* (LOO-ko-TRY-eens).

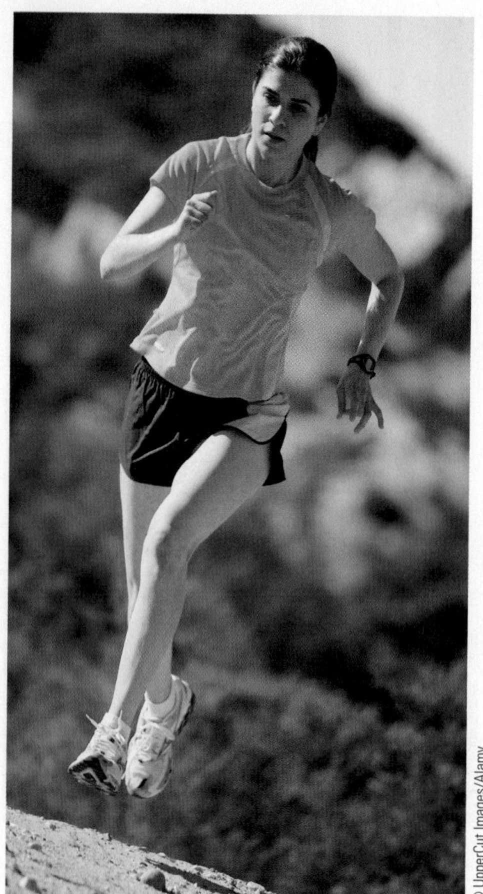

© UpperCut Images/Alamy

Fat supplies most of the energy during a long-distance run.

that provided no polyunsaturated fatty acids for long periods of time. Classic deficiency symptoms include growth retardation, reproductive failure, skin lesions, kidney and liver disorders, and subtle neurological and visual problems.

A Preview of Lipid Metabolism

This preview of fat metabolism describes how the cells store and release energy from fat. Chapter 7 provides details.

Storing Fat as Fat When meals deliver more energy than the body needs, the excess is stored as fat in the adipose cells for later use. An enzyme—**lipoprotein lipase (LPL)**—hydrolyzes triglycerides from circulating lipoproteins, releasing fatty acids, diglycerides, and monoglycerides into the adipose cells. Enzymes inside the adipose cells reassemble these fatty acids, diglycerides, and monoglycerides into triglycerides again for storage. As Figure 5-18 (p. 148) shows, triglycerides fill the adipose cells, storing a lot of energy in a relatively small space.

Using Fat for Energy After meals, the blood delivers chylomicrons and VLDL loaded with triglycerides to the body's cells for energy. Fat supplies about 60 percent of the body's ongoing energy needs during rest. During prolonged light to moderately intense exercise or extended periods of food deprivation, fat may make a slightly greater contribution to energy needs.

During energy deprivation, several lipase enzymes (most notably **hormone-sensitive lipase**) inside the adipose cells respond by dismantling stored triglycerides and releasing the glycerol and fatty acids directly into the blood. Energy-hungry cells anywhere in the body can then capture these compounds and take them through a series of chemical reactions to yield energy, carbon dioxide, and water.

A person who fasts (drinking only water) will rapidly metabolize body fat. Even with abundant body fat, the person has to obtain some energy from lean protein tissue because the brain, nerves, and red blood cells need glucose—and without carbohydrate, only protein and the small glycerol molecule of a triglyceride can be converted to glucose; fatty acids cannot be. Still, in times of severe hunger and starvation, a fatter person can survive longer than a thinner person thanks to this energy reserve. But as Chapter 7 explains, fasting for too long will eventually cause death, even if the person still has ample body fat.

› REVIEW IT Outline the major roles of fats in the body, including a discussion of essential fatty acids and the omega fatty acids.

In the body, triglycerides provide energy, insulate against temperature extremes, protect against shock, provide structural material for cell membranes, and participate in cell signaling pathways. Linoleic acid (18 carbons, omega-6) and linolenic acid (18 carbons, omega-3) are essential fatty acids. They serve as structural parts of cell membranes and as precursors to the longer fatty acids that can make eicosanoids—powerful compounds that participate in blood pressure regulation, blood clot formation, and the immune response to injury and infection. Because essential fatty acids are common in the diet and stored in the body, deficiencies are unlikely. The body can easily store unlimited amounts of fat if given excesses, and this body fat is used for energy when needed.

5.5 Health Effects and Recommended Intakes of Saturated Fats, *Trans* Fats, and Cholesterol

› LEARN IT Explain the relationships among saturated fats, *trans* fat, and cholesterol and chronic diseases, noting recommendations.

Some fats in the diet are essential for good health, but others can be harmful. The current American diet delivers excessive amounts of **solid fats,** representing an average of almost one-fifth of the day's total kcalories. Major sources of solid fats in the American diet include desserts, pizza, cheese, and processed and fatty meats (sausages, hot dogs, bacon, ribs). Because foods made with solid fats provide abundant energy, but few if any essential nutrients, they

lipoprotein lipase (LPL): an enzyme that hydrolyzes triglycerides passing by in the bloodstream and directs their parts into the cells, where they can be metabolized for energy or reassembled for storage.

hormone-sensitive lipase: an enzyme inside adipose cells that responds to the body's need for fuel by hydrolyzing triglycerides so that their parts (glycerol and fatty acids) escape into the general circulation and thus become available to other cells for fuel. The signals to which this enzyme responds include epinephrine and glucagon, which oppose insulin (see Chapter 4).

solid fats: fats that are not usually liquid at room temperature; commonly found in most foods derived from animals and vegetable oils that have been hydrogenated. Solid fats typically contain more saturated and *trans* fats than most oils.

contribute to weight gain and make it difficult to meet nutrient needs. Solid fats also provide abundant saturated fat, *trans* fat, and cholesterol. Even without overweight or obesity, high intakes of solid fats increase the risk of some chronic diseases. The easiest way to control saturated fat, *trans* fat, cholesterol, and kcalories is to limit solid fats in the diet.

Health Effects of Saturated Fats, *Trans* Fats, and Cholesterol

Hearing a physician say, "Your blood lipid profile looks fine," is reassuring (see Table 5-3). The **blood lipid profile** reveals the concentrations of various lipids in the blood, notably triglycerides and cholesterol, and their lipoprotein carriers (VLDL, LDL, and HDL). This information alerts people to possible disease risks and perhaps to a need for changing their physical activity and eating habits. Both the amounts and types of fat in the diet influence the risk for disease.

TABLE 5-3 Desirable Blood Lipid Profile

Total cholesterol	<200 mg/dL
LDL cholesterol	<100 mg/dL
HDL cholesterol	>60 mg/dL
Triglycerides	<100 mg/dL

Heart Disease As mentioned earlier, elevated LDL cholesterol is a major risk factor for **cardiovascular disease (CVD)**.[17] As LDL cholesterol accumulates in the arteries, blood flow becomes restricted and blood pressure rises. The consequences are deadly; in fact, heart disease is the nation's number-one killer of adults. LDL cholesterol is often used to predict the likelihood of a person's suffering a heart attack or stroke; the higher the LDL, the earlier and more likely the tragedy. Much of the effort to prevent and treat heart disease focuses on lowering LDL cholesterol.[18]

Saturated fats are most often implicated in raising LDL cholesterol. In general, the more saturated fat in the diet, the more LDL cholesterol in the blood. Not all saturated fats have the same cholesterol-raising effect, however. Most notable among the saturated fatty acids that raise blood cholesterol are lauric, myristic, and palmitic acids (12, 14, and 16 carbons, respectively). In contrast, stearic acid (18 carbons) seems to have little or no effect on blood cholesterol.[19] Making such distinctions may be impractical in diet planning, however, because these saturated fatty acids typically appear together in the same foods. In addition to raising blood cholesterol, saturated fatty acids contribute to heart disease by promoting blood clotting. Fats from animal sources (meats, milk, and milk products) are the main sources of saturated fats in most people's diets. Selecting lean cuts of meat, skinless poultry, and fat-free milk products helps to lower saturated fat intake and the risk of heart disease.

Research also suggests an association between dietary *trans* fats and heart disease.[20] In the body, *trans* fats alter blood cholesterol the same way some saturated fats do: they raise LDL cholesterol and lower HDL cholesterol.[21] Limiting the intake of *trans* fats can improve blood cholesterol and lower the risk of heart disease. To that end, many restaurants and manufacturers have taken steps to eliminate or greatly reduce *trans* fats in foods.[22] The decrease in *trans* fatty acids in the food supply is apparent in a decrease in plasma concentrations of *trans* fatty acids in consumers.[23]

Unlike saturated fat and *trans* fat, dietary cholesterol raises blood cholesterol very little, if at all.[24] Less clear is its role in heart disease.[25]

Cancer The links between dietary fats and cancer are not as evident as they are for heart disease. Dietary fat does not seem to *initiate* cancer development but, instead, may *promote* cancer once it has arisen. Stronger risk factors for cancer include smoking, alcohol, and environmental contaminants. (Chapter 18 provides many more details about these risk factors and the development of cancer.)

The relationship between dietary fat and the risk of cancer differs for various types of cancers. In the case of breast cancer, evidence has been weak and inconclusive. Some studies indicate an association between dietary fat and breast cancer; more convincing evidence indicates that body fatness contributes to the risk. In the case of colon cancer, limited evidence suggests a harmful association with foods containing animal fats.

blood lipid profile: results of blood tests that reveal a person's total cholesterol, triglycerides, and various lipoproteins.

cardiovascular disease (CVD): diseases of the heart and blood vessels throughout the body. Atherosclerosis is the main cause of CVD. When the arteries that carry blood to the heart muscle become blocked, the heart suffers damage known as *coronary heart disease (CHD)*.

- **cardio** = heart
- **vascular** = blood vessels

The relationship between dietary fat and the risk of cancer differs for various types and combinations of fats as well. The increased risk in cancer from fat appears to be due primarily to saturated fats or dietary fat from meats (which is mostly saturated). Fat from milk or fish has not been implicated in cancer risk. Olive oil seems to have a protective effect.[26]

Obesity Remember that fat contributes more than twice as many kcalories per gram as either carbohydrate or protein. Consequently, people who eat high-fat diets regularly may exceed their energy needs and gain weight, especially if they are inactive. Because fat boosts energy intake, cutting fat from the diet can be an effective strategy in cutting kcalories. In some cases, though, choosing a fat-free food offers no kcalorie savings. Fat-free frozen desserts, for example, often have so much sugar added that the kcalorie count can be as high as in the regular-fat product. In this case, cutting fat and adding carbohydrate offers no kcalorie savings or weight-loss advantage. In fact, it may even raise energy intake and exacerbate weight problems. Later chapters revisit the role of dietary fat in the development of obesity.

Recommended Intakes of Saturated Fat, *Trans* Fat, and Cholesterol

Defining the exact amount of saturated fat, *trans* fat, or cholesterol that begins to harm health is difficult.[27] For this reason, no RDA or Upper Level has been set. Instead, the DRI and *Dietary Guidelines* suggest a diet that provides 20 to 35 percent of the daily energy intake from fat, less than 10 percent of daily energy intake from saturated fat, as little *trans* fat as possible, and less than 300 milligrams of cholesterol. These recommendations recognize that diets with up to 35 percent of kcalories from fat can be compatible with good health if energy intake is reasonable and saturated fat, *trans* fat, and cholesterol intakes are low. When total fat exceeds 35 percent, however, saturated fat usually rises to unhealthy levels. For a 2000-kcalorie diet, 20 to 35 percent represents 400 to 700 kcalories from fat (roughly 45 to 75 grams).

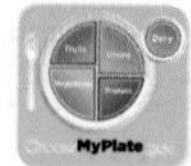

> DIETARY GUIDELINES FOR AMERICANS

Consume less than 10 percent of kcalories from saturated fat. Consume less than 300 milligrams per day of dietary cholesterol. Keep *trans*-fat consumption as low as possible by limiting foods that contain synthetic sources of *trans* fats, such as partially hydrogenated oils, and by limiting other solid fats.

According to surveys, diets in the United States provide about 34 percent of their total energy from fat, with saturated fat contributing about 11 percent of the total.[28] The average daily intake of *trans*-fatty acids in the United States is about 5 grams per day—mostly from products that have been hydrogenated. Cholesterol intakes in the United States average 224 milligrams a day for women and 333 for men.

Although it is very difficult to do, some people actually manage to eat too little fat—to their detriment. Among them are people with eating disorders, described in Highlight 8, and athletes. Athletes following a diet too low in fat (less than 20 percent of total kcalories) fall short on energy, vitamins, minerals, and essential fatty acids as well as on performance.[29] As a practical guideline, it is wise to include the equivalent of at least a teaspoon of fat in every meal—a little peanut butter on toast or mayonnaise in tuna salad, for example. Dietary recommendations that limit fat are designed for healthy people older than age 2; Chapter 16 discusses the fat needs of infants and young children.

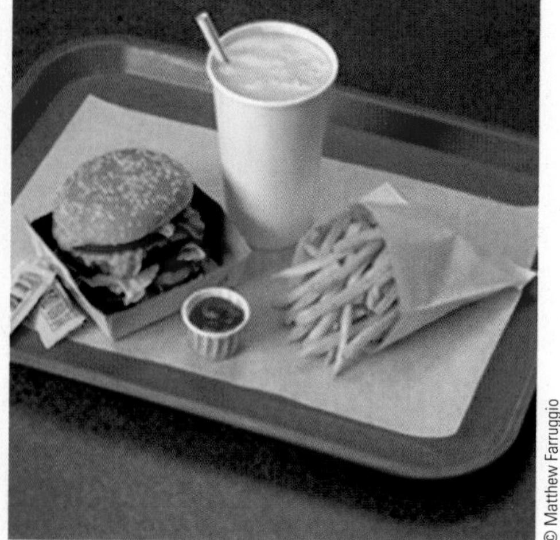

Beware of fast-food meals delivering too much fat, especially saturated fat. This double bacon cheeseburger, fries, and milkshake provide more than 1600 kcalories, with almost 90 grams of fat and more than 30 grams of saturated fat—far exceeding dietary fat guidelines for the entire day.

> REVIEW IT Explain the relationships among saturated fats, *trans* fat, and cholesterol and chronic diseases, noting recommendations.

Although some fat in the diet is necessary, too much fat adds kcalories without nutrients, which leads to obesity and nutrient inadequacies. Too much saturated fat, *trans* fat, and cholesterol increases the risk of heart disease and possibly cancer. For these reasons, health authorities recommend a diet moderate in total fat and low in saturated fat, *trans* fat, and cholesterol.

5.6 Health Effects and Recommended Intakes of Monounsaturated and Polyunsaturated Fats

› LEARN IT Explain the relationships between monounsaturated and polyunsaturated fats and health, noting recommendations.

Whereas saturated fats, *trans* fats, and cholesterol are implicated in chronic diseases, monounsaturated and polyunsaturated fats seem to offer health benefits. For this reason, dietary recommendations suggest replacing sources of saturated fats, *trans* fats, and cholesterol with foods rich in monounsaturated and polyunsaturated fats—foods such as seafood, nuts, seeds, and vegetable oils. Table 5-4 lists major food sources of these various lipids.

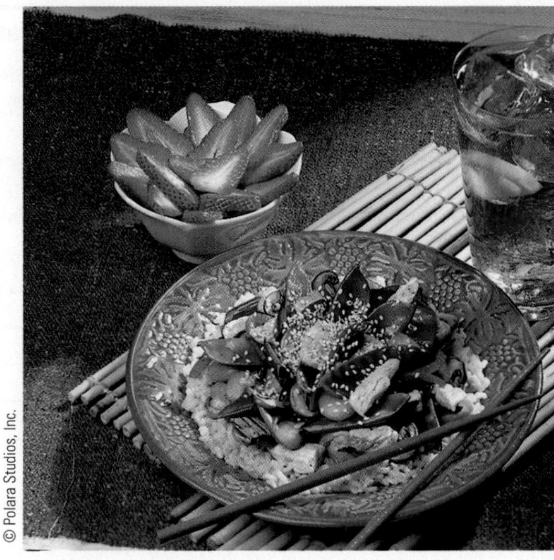

Well-balanced, healthy meals provide some fat with an emphasis on monounsaturated and polyunsaturated fats.

Health Effects of Monounsaturated and Polyunsaturated Fats

Researchers examining eating patterns from around the world have noted that some diets support good health despite being high in fat. As Highlight 5 explains, the *type* of fat may be more important than the *amount* of fat.

Heart Disease Replacing saturated fats with unsaturated fats reduces LDL cholesterol and lowers the risk of heart disease.[30] To replace saturated fats with unsaturated fats, sauté foods in olive oil instead of butter, garnish salads with sunflower seeds instead of bacon, snack on mixed nuts instead of potato chips, use avocado instead of cheese on a sandwich, and eat salmon instead of steak. Table 5-5 (p. 154) shows how these simple substitutions can lower the saturated fat and raise the unsaturated fat in a meal. Highlight 5 provides more details about the benefits of healthy fats in the diet.

TABLE 5-4 **Major Sources of Various Lipids**

Potentially Healthful Lipids Monounsaturated Fats	Omega-6 Polyunsaturated Fats	Omega-3 Polyunsaturated Fats
Avocado	Margarine (nonhydrogenated)	Fatty fish (herring, mackerel, salmon, sardines, tuna)
Nuts (almonds, cashews, filberts, hazelnuts, macadamia nuts, peanuts, pecans, pistachios)	Mayonnaise	Flaxseed, chia seed
Oils (canola, olive, peanut, sesame)	Nuts (pine nuts, walnuts)	Marine algae
Olives	Oils (corn, cottonseed, safflower, soybean)	Nuts (walnuts)
Peanut butter	Salad dressing	Oils (canola, flaxseed)
Seeds (sesame)	Seeds (pumpkin, sunflower)	Yeast
Potentially Harmful Lipids Saturated Fats	***Trans* Fats**	**Cholesterol**
Bacon	Commercial baked goods (including doughnuts, cakes, cookies, pastries)	Eggs
Butter	Fried foods (hydrogenated shortening)	Meat, poultry, shellfish
Cheese	Many fast foods	Milk and milk products
Chocolate	Many snack foods (including microwave popcorn, chips, crackers)	
Coconut	Margarine (hydrogenated or partially hydrogenated)	
Cream cheese	Nondairy creamers	
Cream, half-and-half	Shortening	
Ice cream		
Lard		
Meats (fatty cuts of pork and beef)		
Milk and milk products (whole)		
Oils (coconut, palm, palm kernel) and products containing them (such as candies, cookies, doughnuts, pastries, pies)		
Shortening		
Sour cream		

NOTE: Keep in mind that foods contain a mixture of fatty acids.

TABLE 5-5 Replacing Saturated Fat with Unsaturated Fat

Portion sizes have been adjusted so that each of these foods provides approximately 100 kcalories. Notice that for a similar number of kcalories and total grams of fat, the second choices offer less saturated fat and more unsaturated fat.

Replace these foods . . .

	Saturated Fat (g)	Unsaturated Fat (g)	Total Fat (g)
Butter (1 tbs)	7	4	11
Bacon (2 slices)	3	6	9
Potato chips (10 chips)	2	5	7
Cheese (1 slice)	4	4	8
Steak (1½ oz)	2	3	5
Totals	**18**	**22**	**40**

. . . with these foods.

	Saturated Fat (g)	Unsaturated Fat (g)	Total Fat (g)
Olive oil (1 tbs)	2	9	11
Sunflower seeds (2 tbs)	1	7	8
Mixed nuts (2 tbs)	1	8	9
Avocado (6 slices)	2	8	10
Salmon (2 oz)	1	3	4
Totals	**7**	**35**	**42**

Research on the different types of fats has spotlighted the many beneficial effects of the omega-3 polyunsaturated fatty acids. Regular consumption of omega-3 fatty acids may help to prevent blood clots, protect against irregular heartbeats, improve blood lipids, and lower blood pressure, especially in people with hypertension or atherosclerosis.[31] In addition, omega-3 fatty acids support a healthy immune system and suppress inflammation.

Cancer The omega-3 fatty acids of fatty fish may protect against some cancers as well, perhaps by suppressing inflammation.[32] Even when omega-3 fats do not protect against cancer development, there seems to be a significant reduction in cancer-related deaths.[33] Thus dietary advice to reduce cancer risks parallels that given to reduce heart disease risks: reduce saturated fats and increase omega-3 fatty acids. Evidence does not support omega-3 supplementation.

Other Diseases Limited research suggests that the omega-3 fatty acids of fish may protect against bone loss, asthma, periodontal diseases, and eye diseases.[34] Omega-3 fats also appear to play a role in improving memory and cognition, but not depression.[35] Evidence on associations between fish consumption, omega-3 fatty acids, and diabetes is inconsistent.[36]

Omega-3 Supplements Omega-3 fatty acids are available in capsules of fish oil supplements, although routine supplementation is not recommended. High intakes of omega-3 polyunsaturated fatty acids may increase bleeding time, interfere with wound healing, raise LDL cholesterol, and suppress immune function. Such findings reinforce the concept that too much of a good thing can sometimes be harmful. People with heart disease, however, may benefit from doses greater than can be achieved through diet alone. Because high intakes of omega-3 fatty acids can cause excessive bleeding, supplements should be used only under close medical supervision.[37] For those who decide to use fish oil supplements, Figure 5-20 explains how to read the label.

Recommended Intakes of Monounsaturated and Polyunsaturated Fats

The 20 to 35 percent of kcalories from fat recommendation provides for the essential fatty acids—linoleic acid and linolenic acid—and Adequate Intakes (AI) have been established for these two fatty acids (see the inside front cover for details). The DRI suggest that linoleic acid provide 5 to 10 percent of the daily energy intake and linolenic acid 0.6 to 1.2 percent.

From Guidelines to Groceries

Fats accompany protein in foods derived from animals such as meat, seafood, poultry, and eggs, and fats accompany carbohydrate in foods derived from some plants such as avocados and coconuts. Fats carry with them the four fat-soluble vitamins—A, D, E, and K—together with many of the compounds that give foods their flavor, texture, and palatability. Fat is responsible for the delicious aromas associated with sizzling bacon,

> FIGURE 5-20 **How to Read a Fish Oil Supplement Label**

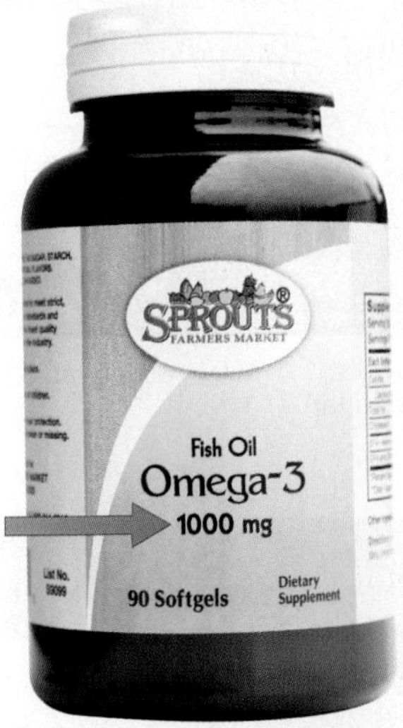

Supplement Facts

Serving Size: 1 Softgel
Servings Per Container: 120

	Amount Per Serving	% Daily Value
Calories	10	*
Total Fat	1	2%
Saturated Fat	0.5 g	3%
Trans Fat	0g	*
Polyunsaturated Fat	0.5g	*
Monounsaturated Fat	0 g	*
Cholesterol	5 mg	2%
Omega-3 Fatty Acids	300 mg	*
EPA (Eicosapentaenoic Acid)	180 mg	*
DHA (Docosahexaenoic Acid)	120 mg	*

* Daily Value not established.

Notice that this supplement offers 1000 mg of fish oil concentrate per capsule, but the oils offering the most health benefits are EPA and DHA. That information is in the Supplement Facts panel on the back.

Notice that one capsule of this supplement offers 180 mg of EPA and 120 mg of DHA, for a total of 300 mg of omega-3 oils—not 1000 mg. The recommended intake for omega-3 fatty acids is 500 mg per day. For heart health, consumers may need more, perhaps 2 to 4 grams (2000 to 4000 mg) per day.

hamburgers on the grill, onions being sautéed, and vegetables in a stir-fry. The essential oils of many spices are fat-soluble. Of course, these wonderful characteristics lure people into eating too much from time to time. With careful selections, a diet can support good health and still meet fat recommendations.

As the photos in Figure 5-21 (p. 156) show, fat accounts for much of the energy in foods, and removing the fat from foods cuts energy and saturated fat intakes dramatically. To reduce dietary fat, eliminate fat as a seasoning and in cooking; remove the fat from high-fat foods; replace high-fat foods with low-fat alternatives; and emphasize whole grains, fruits, and vegetables. The "How To" feature on p. 157 suggests additional heart-healthy choices by food group.

In general, except for seafood, animal fats tend to have a higher proportion of saturated fatty acids. Except for the tropical oils, plant foods tend to have a higher proportion of monounsaturated and polyunsaturated fatty acids. Consumers can find an abundant array of fresh, unprocessed foods that are naturally low in saturated fat, *trans* fat, cholesterol, and total fat. In addition, many familiar foods have been processed to provide less fat. For example, fat can be removed by skimming milk or trimming meats. Manufacturers can dilute fat by adding water or whipping in air. They can use fat-free milk in creamy desserts and lean meats in frozen entrées. Sometimes manufacturers simply prepare the products differently. For example, fat-free potato chips may be baked instead of fried. Such choices make healthy eating easy.

Protein Foods The fats in seafood, nuts, and seeds are considered oils, whereas the fats in meat, poultry, and eggs are considered solid fats because of their high fat, saturated fat, and cholesterol content. Because these meats provide high-quality protein and valuable vitamins and minerals, however, they can be included in a healthy diet if a person makes lean choices (see Table 5-6), prepares them using the suggestions

TABLE 5-6 **Fat Options among the Protein Foods**

Very lean options	Chicken (white meat, no skin) Cod, flounder, trout, tuna (canned in water) Legumes
Lean options	Beef or pork "round" or "loin" cuts Chicken (dark meat, no skin) Herring, salmon, tuna (canned in oil)
Medium-fat options	Ground beef Eggs Tofu
High-fat options	Bacon, hot dogs, luncheon meats, sausage Peanut butter Nuts

> FIGURE 5-21 **Cutting Fat Cuts kCalories—and Saturated Fat**

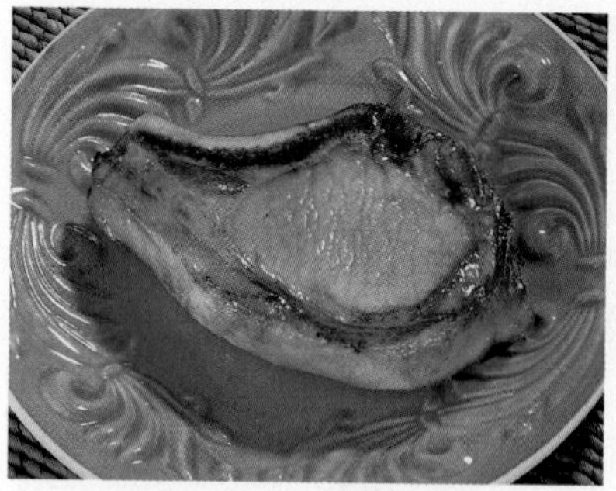

Pork chop with fat (340 kcal, 19 g fat, 7 g saturated fat)

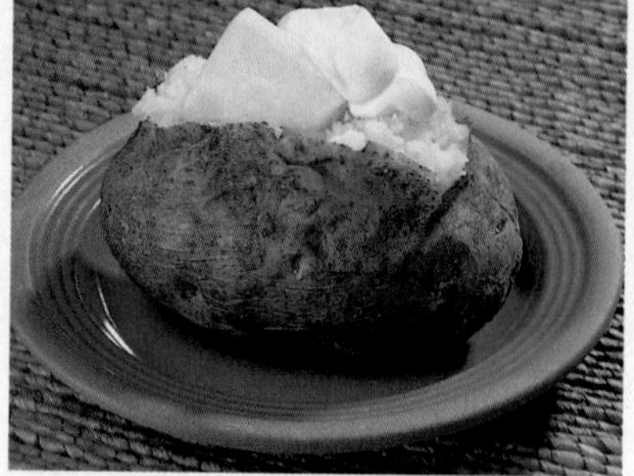

Potato with 1 tbs butter and 1 tbs sour cream (350 kcal, 14 g fat, 10 g saturated fat)

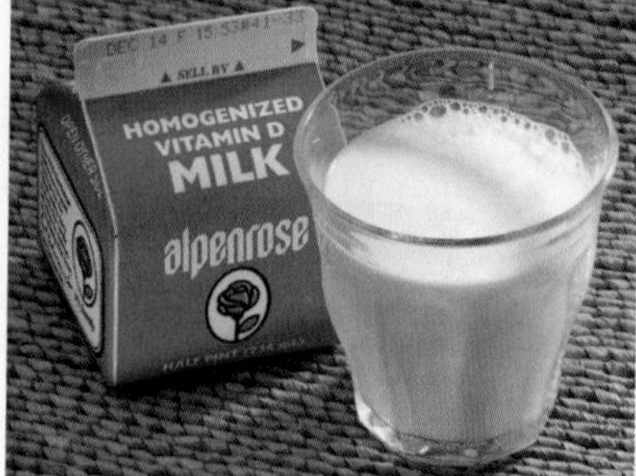

Whole milk, 1 c (150 kcal, 8 g fat, 5 g saturated fat)

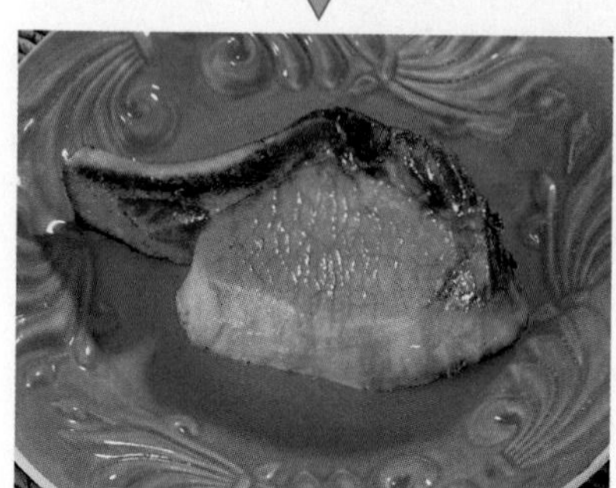

Pork chop with fat trimmed off (230 kcal, 9 g fat, 3 g saturated fat)

Savings:
110 kcal, 10 g fat, 4 g saturated fat

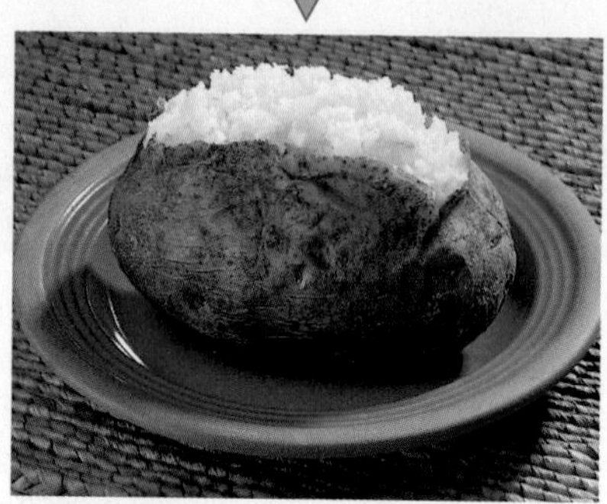

Plain potato (200 kcal, <1 g fat, 0 g saturated fat)

Savings:
150 kcal, 13 g fat, 10 g saturated fat

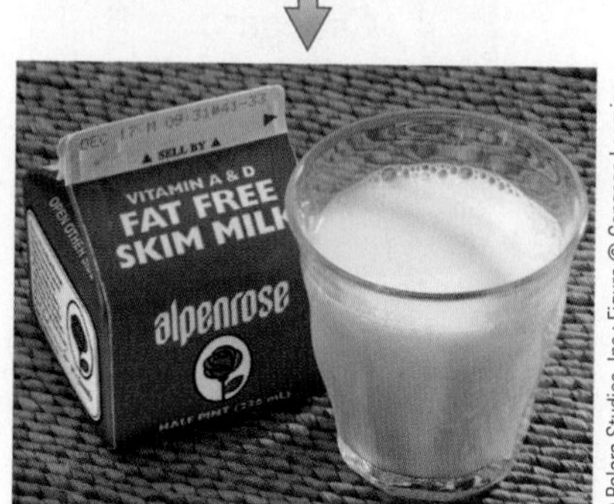

Fat-free milk, 1 c (90 kcal, <1 g fat, <1 g saturated fat)

Savings:
60 kcal, 7 g fat, 4 g saturated fat

outlined in the "How To" feature, and eats small portions. Selecting wild game or grass-fed cattle or bison instead of grain-fed livestock offers the nutrient advantages of being lower in fat and higher in omega-3 polyunsaturated fatty acids.[38] Another strategy to lower blood cholesterol is to prepare meals using soy protein instead of animal protein. When preparing meat, fish, or poultry, consider grilling, baking, or broiling, but not frying. Fried fish does not benefit heart disease.[39] Fried fish from fast-food restaurants and frozen fried fish products are often low in omega-3 fatty acids and high in *trans*- and saturated fatty acids.

Table 5-4 (p. 153) includes sources of omega-3 and omega-6 fatty acids, and Table 5-7 sorts fish and seafood by their quantity of omega 3 fatty acids. Fatty fish are among the best sources of omega-3 fatty acids, and Highlight 5 features their role in supporting heart health. The American Heart Association recommends eating at least two servings of fish a week, with an emphasis on fatty fish (salmon, herring, and mackerel, for example). Fish provides many minerals (except iron) and

TABLE 5-7 **Omega 3 Fatty Acids in Fish and Seafood**

3.5-oz serving	
500 mg	European sea bass (bronzini), herring (Atlantic and Pacific), mackerel, oysters (Pacific wild), salmon (wild and farmed), sardines, toothfish (includes Chilean sea bass), trout (wild and farmed)
150–500 mg	Black bass, catfish (wild and farmed), clams, cod (Atlantic), crab (Alaskan king), croakers, flounder, haddock, hake, halibut, oysters (eastern and farmed), perch, scallops, shrimp (mixed varieties), sole, swordfish, tilapia (farmed)
<150 mg	Cod (Pacific), grouper, lobster, mahi mahi, monkfish, red snapper, skate, triggerfish, tuna, wahoo

>How To

Make Heart-Healthy Choices—by Food Group

In General

- Select the most nutrient-dense foods from all food groups.
- Consume fewer and smaller portions of foods and beverages that contain solid fats.
- Check the Nutrition Facts label to choose foods with little or no saturated fat and no *trans* fat.

Grains

- Select breads, cereals, and crackers that are low in saturated and *trans* fat (for example, bagels instead of croissants).
- Prepare pasta with a tomato sauce instead of a cheese or cream sauce.
- Limit intake of cookies, doughnuts, pastries, and croissants.

Vegetables and Fruits

- Enjoy the natural flavor of steamed or roasted vegetables (without butter) for dinner and fruits for dessert.
- Eat at least two vegetables (in addition to a salad) with dinner.
- Snack on raw vegetables or fruits instead of high-fat items like potato chips.
- Buy frozen vegetables without sauce.

Milk and Milk Products

- Switch from whole milk to reduced-fat, from reduced-fat to low-fat, and from low-fat to fat-free (nonfat).
- Use fat-free and low-fat cheeses (such as part-skim ricotta and low-fat mozzarella) instead of regular cheeses.
- Use fat-free or low-fat yogurt or sour cream instead of regular sour cream.
- Use evaporated fat-free milk instead of cream.
- Enjoy fat-free frozen yogurt, sherbet, or ice milk instead of ice cream.

Protein Foods

- Fat adds up quickly, even with lean meat; limit intake to about 6 ounces (cooked weight) daily.
- Eat at least two servings of fish per week (particularly fish such as mackerel, lake trout, herring, sardines, and salmon).
- Choose fish, poultry, or lean cuts of pork or beef; look for unmarbled cuts named *round* or *loin* (eye of round, top round, bottom round, round tip, tenderloin, sirloin, center loin, and top loin).
- Choose processed meats such as lunch meats and hot dogs that are low in saturated fat and cholesterol.
- Trim the fat from pork and beef; remove the skin from poultry.
- Grill, roast, broil, bake, stir-fry, stew, or braise meats; don't fry. When possible, place food on a rack so that fat can drain.
- Use lean ground turkey or lean ground beef in recipes; brown ground meats without added fat, then drain off fat.
- Select tuna, sardines, and other canned meats packed in water; rinse oil-packed items with hot water to remove much of the fat.
- Fill kabob skewers with lots of vegetables and slivers of meat; create main dishes and casseroles by combining a little meat, fish, or poultry with a lot of pasta, rice, or vegetables.
- Use legumes often.
- Eat a meatless meal or two daily.
- Use egg substitutes in recipes instead of whole eggs or use two egg whites in place of each whole egg.

Fats and Oils

- Use small amounts of vegetable oils in place of solid fats.
- Use butter or stick margarine sparingly; select soft margarines instead of hard margarines.
- When selecting margarine, look for soft (liquid or tub) instead of hard (stick), $\leq$2 g saturated fat, liquid vegetable oil (not hydrogenated or partially hydrogenated) as the first ingredient, and "*trans*-fat free."
- Use fruit butters, reduced-kcalorie margarines, or butter replacers instead of butter.
- Use low-fat or fat-free mayonnaise and salad dressing instead of regular.
- Limit use of lard and meat fat.
- Limit use of products made with coconut oil, palm kernel oil, and palm oil (read labels on bakery goods, processed foods, popcorn oils, and nondairy creamers).
- Reduce use of hydrogenated shortenings and stick margarines and products that contain them (read labels on crackers, cookies, and other commercially prepared baked goods); use vegetable oils instead.

Miscellaneous

- Use a nonstick pan or coat the pan lightly with vegetable oil.
- Refrigerate soups and stews; when the fat solidifies, remove it before reheating.
- Use wine; lemon, orange, or tomato juice; herbs; spices; fruits; or broth instead of butter or margarine when cooking.
- Stir-fry in a small amount of oil; add moisture and flavor with broth, tomato juice, or wine.
- Use variety to enhance enjoyment of the meal: vary colors, textures, and temperatures—hot cooked versus cool raw foods—and use garnishes to complement food.
- Omit high-fat meat gravies and cheese sauces.
- Order pizzas with lots of vegetables, a little lean meat, and half the cheese.

> TRY IT Compare the total kcalories, grams of fat, and percent kcalories from fat for 1 cup of whole milk, reduced-fat milk, low-fat milk, and nonfat milk.

vitamins. Because fish is leaner than most other animal-protein sources it can help with weight-loss efforts. The combination of losing weight and eating fish improves blood lipids even more effectively than can be explained by either the weight loss or the omega-3 fats of the fish. Chapter 19 discusses the adverse consequences of mercury, an environmental contaminant common in some fish; in general, mercury is relatively high in tilefish (also called golden snapper or golden bass), swordfish, king mackerel, and shark and relatively low in cod, haddock, pollock, salmon, sole, tilapia, and most shellfish. Most healthy people who eat two servings of fish a week can maximize the health benefits while incurring minimal risks. Nonfish sources of omega-3 fatty acids such as flaxseed may have less benefit.[40]

Recall that cholesterol is found in all foods derived from animals. Consequently, eating fewer meats, eggs, and milk products helps lower dietary cholesterol intake (as well as total and saturated fat intakes). Most foods that are high in cholesterol are also high in saturated fat, but eggs are an exception. An egg contains only 1 gram of saturated fat but has a little more than 200 milligrams of cholesterol—roughly two-thirds of the recommended daily limit. Still, for the general population, eating eggs does not seem to increase the risk of heart disease.[41] For people with high blood cholesterol, however, limiting daily cholesterol intake to less than 200 milligrams may be beneficial. When eggs are included in the diet, other sources of cholesterol may need to be limited on that day. Eggs are a valuable part of the diet because they are inexpensive, useful in cooking, and a source of high-quality protein, other nutrients, and phytochemicals. To help consumers improve their omega-3 fatty acid intake, hens fed flaxseed, fish oil, or marine algae produce eggs rich in omega-3 fatty acids (up to 200 milligrams per egg).[42] Including even one enriched egg in the diet daily can significantly increase a person's intake of omega-3 fatty acids. Food manufacturers have produced several fat-free, cholesterol-free egg substitutes.

> **DIETARY GUIDELINES FOR AMERICANS**
>
> Replace protein foods that are higher in solid fats (meat, poultry, and eggs) with choices that are lower in solid fats and higher in oils (seafood, nuts, and seeds).

TABLE 5-8 Fat Options among Milk and Milk Products

Fat-free and low-fat options	Fat-free (skim) or 1% (low-fat) milk or yogurt (plain)
Reduced-fat options	2% milk or yogurt (plain)
High-fat options	Whole milk, yogurt Most cheeses

Milk and Milk Products Like meats, milk and milk products should also be selected with an awareness of their fat, saturated fat, and cholesterol contents (see Table 5-8). Keep in mind that the fat in milk is a solid fat; it is apparent as butter, but less so when suspended in homogenized milk. Fat-free and low-fat milk products provide as much or more protein, calcium, and other nutrients as their whole-milk versions—but with little or no saturated fat. Selecting fermented milk products, such as yogurt, may also help to lower blood cholesterol. These foods increase the population and activity of bacteria in the colon that use cholesterol. Interestingly, cheese does not seem to raise LDL cholesterol as its saturated fat content might predict, perhaps because its calcium promotes fat excretion in the GI tract.[43] Such findings suggest that specific foods or nutrients within them influence the actions of their associated saturated fats.[44]

Vegetables, Fruits, and Grains Most vegetables and fruits naturally contain little or no fat. Although avocados and olives are exceptions, most of their fat is unsaturated, which is not harmful to heart health. Most grains contain only small amounts of fat. Consumers need to read food labels carefully, though, because many refined grain products such as fried taco shells, croissants, and biscuits are high in saturated fat, and pastries, crackers, and cookies may contain *trans* fats. Similarly, many people add butter, margarine, or cheese sauce to grains and vegetables, which raises the saturated- and *trans*-fat contents. Because fruits are often eaten without added fat, a diet that includes several servings of fruit daily can help a person meet the dietary recommendations for fat.

A diet rich in vegetables, fruits, whole grains, and legumes also offers abundant vitamin C, folate, vitamin A, vitamin E, and dietary fiber—all important in supporting health. Consequently, such a diet protects against disease by reducing saturated fat, cholesterol, and total fat as well as by increasing nutrients. It also provides valuable phytochemicals, which help defend against heart disease.

Solid Fats and Oils Solid fats include the fats in meat and poultry (as in poultry skin, luncheon meats, and sausage); the fats in whole milk, cheeses, and butter; shortening (as in fried foods and baked goods); and hard margarines. Because solid fats deliver an abundance of saturated fatty acids, they are considered discretionary kcalories. The fats of fish, nuts, and vegetable oils are *not* counted as discretionary kcalories because they provide valuable omega-3 fatty acids, essential fatty acids, and vitamin E. When discretionary kcalories are available, they may be used to add fats in cooking or at the table or to select higher fat items from the food groups.

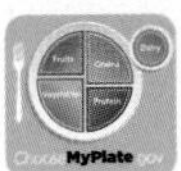

> DIETARY GUIDELINES FOR AMERICANS

Reduce intake of solid fats (major sources of saturated and *trans* fats). Replace solid fats with oils (major sources of polyunsaturated and monounsaturated fats) when possible.

Some solid fats, such as butter and the fat trimmed from meat, are easy to see. Others—such as the fat that "marbles" a steak or is hidden in foods such as cheese—are less apparent and can be present in foods in surprisingly high amounts. Any *fried* food contains abundant solid fats—potato chips, french fries, fried wontons, and fried fish. Many *baked* goods, too, are high in solid fats—pie crusts, pastries, crackers, biscuits, cornbread, doughnuts, sweet rolls, cookies, and cakes.

Reports on *trans*-fatty acids raise the question whether margarine or butter is a better choice for heart health. The American Heart Association has stated that because butter is rich in both saturated fat and cholesterol whereas margarine is made from vegetable fat with no dietary cholesterol, margarine is still preferable to butter. Be aware that soft margarines (liquid or tub) are less hydrogenated and relatively lower in *trans*-fatty acids; consequently, they do not raise blood cholesterol as much as the saturated fats of butter or the *trans* fats of hard (stick) margarines do. Many manufacturers are now offering nonhydrogenated margarines that are "*trans*-fat free." In addition, manufacturers have developed margarines fortified with plant sterols that lower blood cholesterol. (Highlight 13 explores these and other functional foods designed to support health.) Whichever you decide to use, remember to use them sparingly.

Read Food Labels Labels list total fat, saturated fat, *trans* fat, and cholesterol contents of foods. Because each package provides information for a single serving and because serving sizes are standardized, consumers can easily compare similar products.

Total fat, saturated fat, and cholesterol are also expressed as "% Daily Values" for a person consuming 2000 kcalories. Using 30 percent of energy intake as the guideline for fat, the Daily Value is 65 grams of fat; using 10 percent for saturated fat, the Daily Value is 20 grams of saturated fat. The Daily Value for cholesterol is 300 milligrams regardless of energy intake. There is no Daily Value for *trans* fat, but consumers should try to keep intakes as low as possible and within the 10 percent allotted for saturated fat. People who consume more or less than 2000 kcalories daily can calculate their personal Daily Value for fat as described in the "How To" feature (p. 160).

Be aware that the "% Daily Value" for fat is not the same as "% kcalories from fat." This important distinction is explained in the "How To" feature on p. 161. Because recommendations apply to average daily intakes rather than individual food items, food labels do not provide "% kcalories from fat." Still, you can get an idea of whether a particular food is high or low in fat.

>How To

Calculate a Personal Daily Value for Fat

The % Daily Value for fat on food labels is based on 65 grams. To know how your intake compares with this recommendation, you can either count grams until you reach 65 or add the "% Daily Values" until you reach 100 percent—if your energy intake is 2000 kcalories a day. If your energy intake is more or less, you can calculate your personal daily fat allowance in grams. Suppose your energy intake is 1800 kcalories per day and your goal is 30 percent kcalories from fat. Multiply your total energy intake by 30 percent, then divide by 9:

$$1800 \text{ total kcal} \times 0.30 \text{ from fat} = 540 \text{ fat kcal}$$
$$540 \text{ fat kcal} \div 9 \text{ kcal/g} = 60 \text{ g fat}$$

(In familiar measures, 60 grams of fat is about the same as ⅔ stick of butter or ¼ cup of oil.)

The accompanying table shows the numbers of grams of fat allowed per day for various energy intakes. With one of these numbers in mind, you can quickly evaluate the number of fat grams in foods you are considering eating.

Energy (kcal/day)	20% kCal from Fat	35% kCal from Fat	Fat (g/day)
1200	240	420	27–47
1400	280	490	31–54
1600	320	560	36–62
1800	360	630	40–70
2000	400	700	44–78
2200	440	770	49–86
2400	480	840	53–93
2600	520	910	58–101
2800	560	980	62–109
3000	600	1050	67–117

> TRY IT Calculate a personal daily fat allowance for a person with an energy intake of 2100 kcalories and a goal of 25 percent kcalories from fat.

Fat Replacers Some foods are made with **fat replacers**—ingredients that provide some of the taste and texture of fats, but with fewer kcalories. Because the body may digest and absorb some of these fat replacers, they may contribute energy, although significantly less energy than fat's 9 kcalories per gram.

Some fat replacers are derived from carbohydrate, protein, or fat. Carbohydrate-based fat replacers are used primarily as thickeners or stabilizers in foods such as soups and salad dressings. Protein-based fat replacers provide a creamy feeling in the mouth and are often used in foods such as ice creams and yogurts. Fat-based replacers act as emulsifiers and are heat stable, making them most versatile in shortenings used in cake mixes and cookies.

Fat replacers offering the sensory and cooking qualities of fats but none of the kcalories are called **artificial fats.** A familiar example of an artificial fat that has been approved for use in snack foods such as potato chips, crackers, and tortilla chips is **olestra.** Olestra's chemical structure is similar to that of a triglyceride but with important differences. A triglyceride is composed of a glycerol molecule with three fatty acids attached, whereas olestra is made of a sucrose molecule with six to eight fatty acids attached. Enzymes in the digestive tract cannot break the bonds of olestra, so unlike sucrose or fatty acids, olestra passes through the digestive system unabsorbed.

The FDA's evaluation of olestra's safety addressed two questions. First, is olestra toxic? Research on both animals and human beings supports the safety of olestra as a partial replacement for dietary fats and oils, with no reports of cancer or birth defects. Second, does olestra affect either nutrient absorption or the health of the digestive tract? When olestra passes through the digestive tract unabsorbed, it binds with some of the fat-soluble vitamins, A, D, E, and K, and carries them out of the body, robbing the person of these valuable nutrients. To compensate for these losses, the FDA requires manufacturers to fortify olestra

fat replacers: ingredients that replace some or all of the functions of fat and may or may not provide energy.

artificial fats: zero-energy fat replacers that are chemically synthesized to mimic the sensory and cooking qualities of naturally occurring fats but are totally or partially resistant to digestion.

olestra: a synthetic fat made from sucrose and fatty acids that provides 0 kcalories per gram; also known as *sucrose polyester.*

>How To

Understand "% Daily Value" and "% kCalories from Fat"

The "% Daily Value" that is used on food labels to describe the amount of fat in a food is not the same as the "% kcalories from fat" that is used in dietary recommendations to describe the amount of fat in the diet. They may appear similar, but their difference is worth understanding. Consider, for example, a piece of lemon meringue pie that provides 140 kcalories and 12 grams of fat. Because the Daily Value for fat is 65 grams for a 2000-kcalorie intake, 12 grams represent about 18 percent:

$$12 \text{ g} \div 65 \text{ g} = 0.18$$
$$0.18 \times 100 = 18\%$$

The pie's "% Daily Value" is 18 percent, or almost one-fifth, of the day's fat allowance.

Uninformed consumers may mistakenly believe that this food meets recommendations to limit fat to "20 to 35 percent kcalories," but it doesn't—for two reasons. First, the pie's 12 grams of fat contribute 108 of the 140 kcalories, for a total of 77 percent kcalories from fat:

$$12 \text{ g fat} \times 9 \text{ kcal/g} = 108 \text{ kcal}$$
$$108 \text{ kcal} \div 140 \text{ kcal} = 77\%$$

Second, the "percent kcalories from fat" guideline applies to a day's total intake, not to an individual food. Of course, if every selection throughout the day exceeds 35 percent kcalories from fat, you can be certain that the day's total intake will, too.

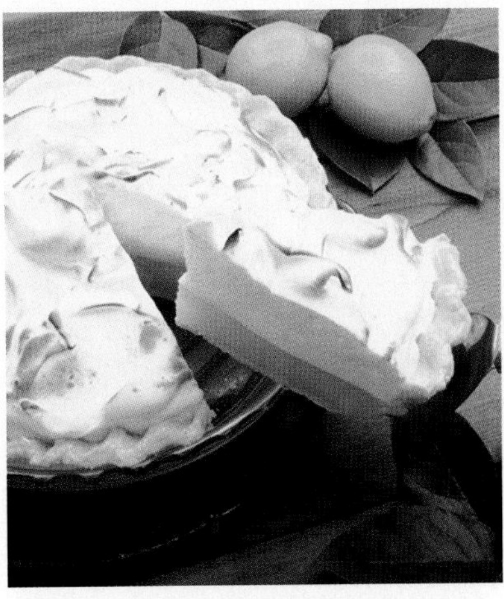

© PhotoDisc/Getty Images

Whether a person's energy and fat allowance can afford a piece of a lemon meringue pie depends on the other food and activity choices made that day.

> TRY IT Calculate the percent Daily Value and the percent kcalories from fat for ½ cup frozen yogurt that provides 115 kcalories and 4 grams of fat.

with vitamins A, D, E, and K. Saturating olestra with these vitamins does not make the product a good source of vitamins, but it does block olestra's ability to bind with the vitamins from other foods. An asterisk in the ingredients list informs consumers that these added vitamins are "dietarily insignificant."

Consumers need to keep in mind that low-fat and fat-free foods still deliver kcalories. Alternatives to fat can help to lower energy intake and support weight loss only when they actually *replace* fat and energy in the diet.[45]

> REVIEW IT Explain the relationships between monounsaturated and polyunsaturated fats and health, noting recommendations.

Some fat in the diet has health benefits, especially the monounsaturated and polyunsaturated fats that protect against heart disease and possibly cancer. For this reason, *Dietary Guidelines* recommend replacing saturated fats with monounsaturated and polyunsaturated fats, particularly omega-3 fatty acids from foods such as fatty fish, not from supplements. Many selection and preparation strategies can help bring these goals within reach, and food labels help to identify foods consistent with these guidelines.

Perhaps the best advice for consumers regarding fat in the diet would be to replace saturated fat with unsaturated fat. Sometimes these choices can be difficult, though, because fats make foods taste delicious. To maintain good health, must a person give up all high-fat foods forever—never again to eat marbled steak, hollandaise sauce, or gooey chocolate cake? Not at all. These foods bring pleasure to a meal and can be enjoyed as part of a healthy diet when eaten occasionally in small quantities; but they should not be everyday foods. The key dietary principle for fat is *moderation,* not *deprivation.* Appreciate the energy and enjoyment that fat provides, but take care not to exceed your needs.

Nutrition Portfolio

To maintain good health, eat enough, but not too much, fat and select the right kinds. Go to Diet & Wellness Plus and choose one of the days on which you have tracked your diet for the entire day. Go to the Intake Spreadsheet report. Scroll down until you see: fat (g), sat fat (g), mono fat (g), poly fat (g), and chol (g), which stand for grams of total fat, saturated fat, monounsaturated fat, polyunsaturated fat, and cholesterol, respectively. Use these columns to answer the following questions:

- List the types and amounts of fats and oils you ate on that day, making note of which are saturated, monounsaturated, or polyunsaturated and how your choices could include fewer saturated options.
- List the types and amounts of milk and milk products, meats, fish, and poultry you eat daily, noting how your choices could include more low-fat options.
- Describe choices you can make in selecting and preparing foods to lower your intake of solid fats.

DIET & WELLNESS **PLUS** To complete this exercise, go to your Diet & Wellness Plus at **www.cengagebrain.com.**

› STUDY IT To review the key points of this chapter and take a practice quiz, go to the study cards at the end of the book.

REFERENCES

1. O. Quehenberger and E. A. Dennis, The human plasma lipidome, *New England Journal of Medicine* 365 (2011): 1812–1823.
2. V. Remig and coauthors, *Trans* fats in America: A review of their use, consumption, health implications, and regulation, *Journal of the American Dietetic Association* 110 (2010): 585–592.
3. I. A. Brouwer, A. J. Wanders, and M. B. Katan, Effect of animal and industrial *trans* fatty acids on HDL and LDL cholesterol levels in humans—A quantitative review, *PLos One* 5 (2010): e9434.
4. S. W. Ing and M. A. Belury, Impact of conjugated linoleic acid on bone physiology: Proposed mechanism involving inhibition of adipogenesis, *Nutrition Reviews* 69 (2011): 123–131.
5. A. V. Khera and coauthors, Cholesterol efflux capacity, high-density lipoprotein function, and atherosclerosis, *New England Journal of Medicine* 364 (2011): 127–135.
6. X. Zhu and J. S. Parks, New roles of HDL in inflammation and hematopoiesis, *Annual Review of Nutrition* 32 (2012): 161–182.
7. D. M. Muoio, Metabolism and vascular fatty acid transport, *New England Journal of Medicine* 363 (2010): 291–293.
8. M. Krawczyk, L. Bonfrate, and P. Portincasa, Nonalcoholic fatty liver disease, *Best Practice and Research, Clinical Gastroenterology* 24 (2010): 695–708; G. Tarantino, S. Savastano, and A. Colao, Hepatic steatosis, low-grade chronic inflammation and hormone/growth factor/adipokine imbalance, *World Journal of Gastroenterology* 16 (2010): 4773–4783.
9. Y. Deng and P. E. Scherer, Adipokines as novel biomarkers and regulators of the metabolic syndrome, *Annals of the New York Academy of Sciences* 1212 (2010): E1–E19.
10. N. Ouchi and coauthors, Adipokines in inflammation and metabolic disease, *Nature Reviews, Immunology* 11 (2011): 85–97; C. Stryjecki and D. M. Mutch, Fatty acid-gene interactions, adipokines and obesity, *European Journal of Clinical Nutrition* 65 (2011): 285–297.
11. P. C. Calder, Mechanisms of action of (n-3) fatty acids, *Journal of Nutrition* 142 (2012): 592S–599S.
12. N. G. Bazan, M. F. Molina, and W. C. Gordon, Docosahexaenoic acid signalolipidomics in nutrition: Significance in aging, neuroinflammation, macular degeneration, Alzheimer's, and other neurodegenerative diseases, *Annual Review of Nutrition* 31 (2011): 321–351; E. E. Birch and coauthors, The DIAMOND (DHA Intake and Measurement of Neural Development) Study: A double-masked, randomized controlled clinical trial of the maturation of infant visual acuity as a function of the dietary level of docosahexaenoic acid, *American Journal of Clinical Nutrition* 91 (2010): 848–859; R. K. McNamara and coauthors, Docosahexaenoic acid supplementation increases prefrontal cortex activation during sustained attention in healthy boys: A placebo-controlled, dose-ranging, functional magnetic resonance imaging study, *American Journal of Clinical Nutrition* 91 (2010): 1060–1067.
13. R. Wall and coauthors, Fatty acids from fish: The anti-inflammatory potential of long-chain omega-3 fatty acids, *Nutrition Reviews* 68 (2010): 280–289.
14. A. P. Simopoulos, Evolutionary aspects of diet: The omega-6/omega-3 ratio and the brain, *Molecular Neurobiology* 44 (2011): 203–215.
15. K. Zelman, The great fat debate: A closer look at the controversy—Questioning the validity of age-old dietary guidance, *Journal of the American Dietetic Association* 111 (2011): 655–658.
16. P. Kris-Etherton, J. Fleming, and W. S. Harris, The debate about n-6 polyunsaturated fatty acid recommendations for cardiovascular health, *Journal of the American Dietetic Association* 110 (2010): 201–204.
17. L. H. Kuller, The great fat debate: Reducing cholesterol, *Journal of the American Dietetic Association* 111 (2011): 663–664.
18. Vital signs: Prevalence, treatment, and control of high levels of low-density lipoprotein cholesterol—United States, 1999–2002 and 2005–2008, *Morbidity and Mortality Weekly Report* 60 (2011): 109–114.
19. J. E. Hunter, J. Zhang, and P. M. Kris-Etherton, Cardiovascular disease risk of dietary stearic acid compared with *trans*, other saturated, and unsaturated fatty acids: A systematic review, *American Journal of Clinical Nutrition* 91 (2010): 46–63.
20. J. N. Kiage and coauthors, Intake of trans fat and all-cause mortality in the Reasons for Geographical and Racial Differences in Stroke (REGARDS) cohort, *American Journal of Clinical Nutrition* 97 (2013): 1121–1128; F. Imamura and coauthors, Novel circulating fatty acid patterns and risk of cardiovascular disease: The Cardiovascular Health Study, *American Journal of Clinical Nutrition* 96 (2012): 1252–1261.

21. I. A. Brouwer, A. J. Wanders, and M. B. Katan, Effect of animal and industrial trans fatty acids on HDL and LDL cholesterol levels in humans—A quantitative review, *PLos One* 5 (2010): e9434.
22. F. O. Otite and coauthors, Trends in trans fatty acids reformulations of US supermarket and brand-name foods from 2007 through 2011, *Preventing Chronic Disease* 10 (2013): 120198; W. H. Dietz and K. S. Scanlon, Eliminating the use of partially hydrogenated oil in food production and preparation, *Journal of the American Medical Association* 308 (2012): 143–144; I. Rahkovsky, S. Martinez, and F. Kuchler, *New Food Choices Free of Trans Fats Better Align US Diets with Health Recommendations*, EIB-95, US Department of Agriculture, Economic Research Service, April 2012.
23. A. Baylin, Secular trends in trans fatty acids: Decreased trans fatty acids in the food supply are reflected in decreased *trans* fatty acids in plasma, *American Journal of Clinical Nutrition* 97 (2013): 665–666.
24. J. M. Lecerf and M. deLorgeril, Dietary cholesterol: From physiology to cardiovascular risk, *British Journal of Nutrition* 106 (2011): 6–14.
25. A. M. Brownawell and M. C. Falk, Cholesterol: Where science and public health policy intersect, *Nutrition Reviews* 68 (2010): 355–364; M. L. Fernandez and M. Calle, Revisiting dietary cholesterol recommendations: Does the evidence support a limit of 300 mg/d? *Current Atherosclerosis Reports* 12 (2010): 377–383.
26. T. Psaltopoulou and coauthors, Olive oil intake is inversely related to cancer prevalence: A systematic review and a meta-analysis of 13800 patients and 23340 controls in 19 observational studies, *Lipids in Health and Disease* 10 (2011): 127.
27. P. R. Trumbo and T. Shimakawa, Tolerable upper intake levels for *trans* fat, saturated fat, and cholesterol, *Nutrition Reviews* 69 (2011): 270–278.
28. US Department of Agricultural Research Service, Nutrient intakes from food: Mean amounts consumed per individual, 2009–2010, www.ars.usda.gov/ba/bhnrc/fsrg, updated July 2012.
29. Position of the American Dietetic Association, Dietitians of Canada, and the American College of Sports Medicine: Nutrition and athletic performance, *Journal of the American Dietetic Association* 100 (2000): 1543–1556.
30. A. Astrup, The role of reducing intakes of saturated fats in the prevention of cardiovascular disease: Where does the evidence stand in 2010? *American Journal of Clinical Nutrition* 93 (2011): 684–688.
31. A. C. Skulas-Ray and coauthors, Dose-response effects of omega-3 fatty acids on triglycerides, inflammation, and endothelial function in healthy persons with moderate hypertriglyceridemia, *American Journal of Clinical Nutrition* 93 (2011): 243–252; K. Musa-Velosa and coauthors, Long-chain omega-3 fatty acids eicosapentaenoic acid and docosahexaenoic acid dose-dependently reduce fasting serum triglycerides, *Nutrition Reviews* 68 (2010): 155–167.
32. J. Zheng and coauthors, Intake of fish and marine n-3 polyunsaturated fatty acids and risk of breast cancer: Meta-analysis of data from 21 independent prospective cohort studies, *British Medical Journal* 346 (2013): f3706; K. He and coauthors, Types of fish consumed and fish preparation methods in relation to pancreatic cancer incidence: The VITAL Cohort Study, *American Journal of Epidemiology* 177 (2013): 152–160; S. Wu and coauthors, Fish consumption and colorectal cancer risk in humans: A systematic review and meta-analysis, *American Journal of Medicine* 125 (2012): 551–559; V. M. Heinze and A. B. Actis, Dietary conjugated linoleic acid and long-chain n-3 fatty acids in mammary and prostate cancer protection: A review, *International Journal of food Sciences and Nutrition* 63 (2012): 66–78; M. Touvier and coauthors, Modulation of the association between plasma intercellular adhesion molecule-1 and cancer risk by n-3 PUFA intake: A nested case-control study, *American Journal of Clinical Nutrition* 95 (2012): 944–950; T. M. Brasky and coauthors, Specialty supplements and breast cancer risk in the VITamins And Lifestyle (VITAL) Cohort, *Cancer Epidemiology, Biomarkers and Prevention* 19 (2010): 1696–1708.
33. K. M. Szymanski, D. C. Wheeler, and L. A. Mucci, Fish consumption and prostate cancer risk: A review and meta-analysis, *American Journal of Clinical Nutrition* 92 (2010): 1223–1233.
34. J. Li and coauthors, Intakes of long-chain omega-3 (n-3) PUFAs and fish in relation to incidence of asthma among American young adults: The CARDIA study, *American Journal of Clinical Nutrition* 97 (2013): 173–178; E. K. Farina and coauthors, Protective effects of fish intake and interactive effects of long-chain polyunsaturated fatty acid intakes on hip bone mineral density in older adults: The Framingham Osteoporosis Study, *American Journal of Clinical Nutrition* 93 (2011): 1142–1151; W. G. Christen and coauthors, Dietary v-3 fatty acid and fish intake and incident age-related macular degeneration in women, *Archives of Ophthalmology* 129 (2011): 921–929; E. Y. Chew, Fatty acids and retinopathy, *New England Journal of Medicine* 364 (2011): 1970–1971; A. Liu and coauthors, Long-chain and very long-chain polyunsaturated fatty acids in ocular aging and age-related macular degeneration, *Journal of Lipid Research* 51 (2010): 3217–3229; E. K. Kaye, n-3 Fatty acid intake and periodontal disease, *Journal of the American Dietetic Association* 110 (2010): 1650–1652.
35. W. Stonehouse, DHA supplementation improved both memory and reaction time in healthy young adults: A randomized controlled trial, *American Journal of Clinical Nutrition* 97 (2013): 1134–1143; L. J. Frensham, J. Bryan, and N. Parletta, Influences of micronutrient and omega-3 fatty acid supplementation on cognition, learning, and behavior: Methodical considerations and implications for children and adolescents in developed societies, *Nutrition Reviews* 70 (2012): 594–610; C. Chiu and coauthors, Associations between n-3 PUFA concentrations and cognitive function after recovery from late-life depression, *American Journal of Clinical Nutrition* 95 (2012): 420–427; M. Lucas and coauthors, Dietary intake of n-3 and n-6 fatty acids and the risk of clinical depression in women: A 10-y prospective follow-up study, *American Journal of Clinical Nutrition* 93 (2011): 1337–1343.
36. P. Xun and K. He, Meta-analysis of data from 438,000 individuals in 12 independent prospective cohorts with an average 11-year follow-up, *Diabetes Care* 35 (2012): 930–938; A. Wallin and coauthors, Fish consumption, dietary long-chain n-3 fatty acids, and risk of type 2 diabetes: Systematic review and meta-analysis of prospective studies, *Diabetes Care* 32 (2012): 918–929; A. Nanri and coauthors, Fish intake and type 2 diabetes in Japanese men and women: The Japan Public Health Center-based Prospective Study, *American Journal of Clinical Nutrition* 94 (2011): 884–891; R. Villegas and coauthors, Fish, shellfish, and long-chain n-3 fatty acid consumption and risk of incident type 2 diabetes in middle-aged Chinese men and women, *American Journal of Clinical Nutrition* 94 (2011): 543–551; D. P. Brostow and coauthors, Omega-3 fatty acids and incident type 2 diabetes: The Singapore Chinese Health Study, *American Journal of Clinical Nutrition* 94 (2011): 520-526; L. Djoussé and coauthors, Plasma omega-3 fatty acids and incident diabetes in older adults, *American Journal of Clinical Nutrition* 94 (2011): 527–533.
37. American Heart Association, Fish 101, www.heart.org, updated March 2013.
38. A. J. McAfee and coauthors, Red meat from animals offered a grass diet increases plasma and platelet n-3 PUFA in healthy consumers, *British Journal of Nutrition* 105 (2011): 80–89.
39. R. J. Belin and coauthors, Fish intake and risk of incident heart failure: The Women's Health Initiative, *Circulation: Heart Failure* 4 (2011): 404–413.
40. D. B. Jump, C. M. Depner, and S. Tripathy, Omega-3 fatty acid supplementation and cardiovascular disease, *Journal of Lipid Research* 53 (2012): 2525–2545.
41. J. Y. Shin and coauthors, Egg consumption in relation to risk of cardiovascular disease and diabetes: A systematic review and meta-analysis, *American Journal of Clinical Nutrition* 98 (2013): 146–159; Y. Rong and coauthors, Egg consumption and risk of coronary heart disease and stroke: Dose-response meta-analysis of prospective cohort studies, *British Medical Journal* 346 (2013): e8539.
42. I. Fraeye and coauthors, Dietary enrichment of eggs with omega-3 fatty acids: A review, *Food Research International* 48 (2012): 961–969.
43. J. Hjerpsted, E. Leedo, and T. Tholstrup, Cheese intake in large amounts lowers LDL-cholesterol concentrations compared with butter intake of equal fat content, *American Journal of Clinical Nutrition* 94 (2011): 1479–1484.
44. M. C. Otto and coauthors, Dietary intake of saturated fat by food source and incident cardiovascular disease: the Multi-Ethnic Study of Atherosclerosis, *American Journal of Clinical Nutrition* 96 (2012): 397–404.
45. Position of the American Dietetic Association: Fat replacers, *Journal of the American Dietetic Association* 105 (2005): 266–275.

HIGHLIGHT > 5

High-Fat Foods—Friend or Foe?

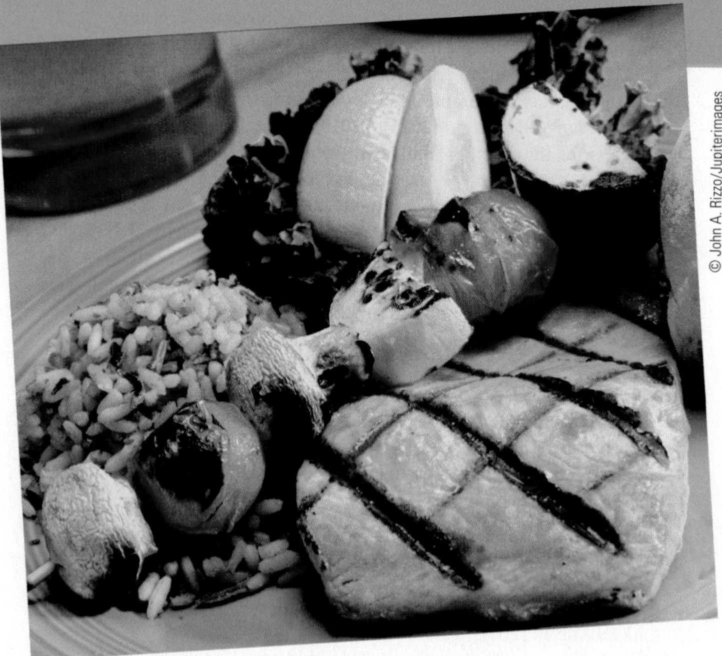
© John A. Rizzo/Jupiterimages

› LEARN IT Identify which fats support health and which impair it.

Eat less fat. Eat more fatty fish. Give up butter. Use margarine. Give up margarine. Use olive oil. Steer clear of saturated. Seek out omega-3. Stay away from *trans*. Stick with monounsaturated and polyunsaturated. Keep fat intake moderate. Today's fat messages seem to be forever multiplying and changing. No wonder some people feel confused about dietary fat. The confusion stems in part from the complexities of fat and in part from the nature of recommendations. As Chapter 5 explained, "dietary fat" refers to several kinds of fats. Some fats support health whereas others impair it, and foods typically provide a mixture of fats in varying proportions. Researchers have spent decades sorting through the relationships among the various kinds of fat and their roles in supporting or harming health. Translating these research findings into dietary recommendations is challenging. Too little information can mislead consumers, but too much detail can overwhelm them. As research findings accumulate, recommendations slowly evolve and become more refined. Fortunately, that's where we are with fat recommendations today—refining them from the general to the specific. Though they may seem to be "forever multiplying and changing," in fact, they are becoming more meaningful.

This highlight begins with a look at the dietary guidelines for fat intake. It continues by identifying which foods provide which fats and presenting the Mediterranean diet, an example of an eating pattern that embraces the heart-healthy fats. It closes with strategies to help consumers choose the right amounts of the right kinds of fats for a healthy diet.

Guidelines for Fat Intake

Dietary recommendations for fat have shifted emphasis from lowering total fat, in general, to limiting saturated and *trans* fat, specifically. Instead of urging people to cut back on all fats, recommendations suggest carefully replacing the "bad" saturated fats with the "good" unsaturated fats and enjoying them in moderation.[1] The goal is to create a diet moderate in kcalories that provides enough of the fats that support good health, but not too much of those that harm health. (Turn to pp. 150–154 for a review of the health consequences of each type of fat.)

With these findings and goals in mind, the Dietary Reference Intakes (DRI) committee suggests a healthy range of 20 to 35 percent of energy intake from fat. This range appears to be compatible with low rates of heart disease, diabetes, obesity, and cancer. Heart-healthy recommendations suggest that within this range, consumers should try to minimize their intakes of saturated fat, *trans* fat, and cholesterol and use monounsaturated and polyunsaturated fats instead.

Asking consumers to limit their total fat intake is less than perfect advice, but it is straightforward—find the fat and cut back. Asking consumers to keep their intakes of saturated fats, *trans* fats, and cholesterol low and to use monounsaturated and polyunsaturated fats instead is more on target with heart health, but it also makes diet planning a bit more challenging. To make appropriate selections, consumers must first learn which foods contain which fats.

High-Fat Foods and Heart Health

Avocados, bacon, walnuts, potato chips, and mackerel are all high-fat foods, yet some of these foods have detrimental effects on heart health when consumed in excess, whereas others seem neutral or even beneficial. This section presents some of the accumulating evidence that help distinguish which high-fat foods belong in a healthy diet and which ones need to be kept to a minimum. As you will see, fat in the diet can be compatible with heart health, but only if most of it is unsaturated.

Cook with Olive Oil

As it turns out, the traditional diets of Greece and other countries in the Mediterranean region offer an excellent example of eating patterns that use "good" fats liberally. The primary fat in these diets is olive oil, which seems to play a key role in providing health benefits.[2] A classic study of the world's people, the Seven Countries Study, found that death rates from heart disease were strongly associated with diets high in saturated fats but only weakly linked with total fat.[3] In fact, the two countries with the highest fat intakes, Finland and the Greek island of Crete, had the highest (Finland) and lowest (Crete) rates of heart disease deaths. In both countries, the people consumed 40 percent or more of their kcalories from fat. Clearly, a high-fat diet is not the primary problem.[4] When researchers refocused their attention on the *type* of fat, they began to notice the benefits of olive oil.

A diet that uses olive oil instead of other fats, especially butter, stick margarine, and meat fats, offers numerous health benefits. Olive oil, canola oil, and other oils rich in monounsaturated fatty acids help to protect against heart disease and stroke by:[5]

- Lowering total and LDL cholesterol and not lowering HDL cholesterol or raising triglycerides
- Lowering LDL cholesterol susceptibility to oxidation
- Lowering blood-clotting factors
- Providing phytochemicals that act as antioxidants (see Highlight 11)
- Lowering blood pressure
- Interfering with the inflammatory response

When compared with other fats, olive oil seems to be a wise choice, but controlled clinical trials are too scarce to support population-wide recommendations to switch to a high-fat diet rich in olive oil. Importantly, olive oil is not a magic potion; drizzling it on foods does not make them healthier. Like other fats, olive oil delivers 9 kcalories per gram, which can contribute to weight gain in people who fail to balance their energy intake with physical activity. Its role in a healthy diet is to *replace* the saturated fats. Other vegetable oils, such as canola or safflower oil, are also generally low in saturated fats and high in unsaturated fats. For this reason, heart-healthy diets use these unsaturated vegetable oils to replace the more saturated fats of butter, hydrogenated stick margarine, lard, or shortening. (Remember that the tropical oils—coconut, palm, and palm kernel—are too saturated to be included with the heart-healthy vegetable oils.)

Nibble on Nuts

Tree nuts and peanuts are traditionally excluded from low-fat diets, and for good reasons. Nuts provide up to 80 percent of their kcalories from fat, and a quarter cup (about an ounce) of mixed nuts provides more than 200 kcalories. Frequent nut consumption, however, correlates with lower risk of mortality and chronic diseases, such as diabetes and heart disease.[6]

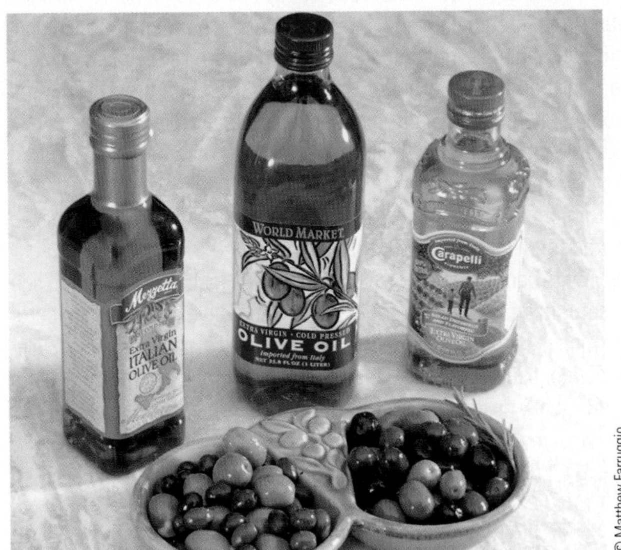

© Matthew Farruggio

Olives and their oil may benefit heart health.

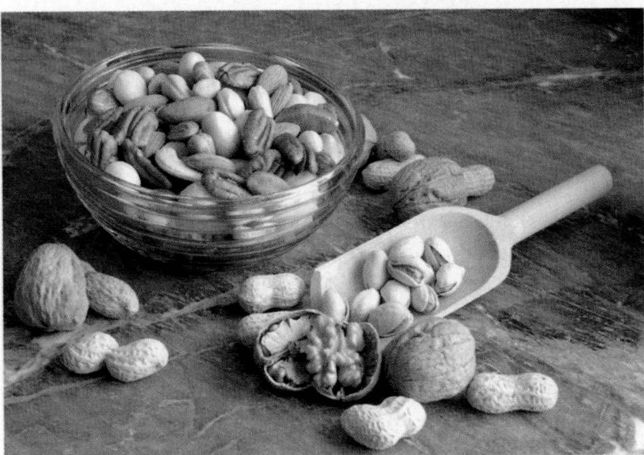
© Matthew Farruggio

For heart health, snack on a few nuts instead of potato chips. Because nuts are energy dense (high in kcalories per ounce), it is especially important to keep portion size in mind when eating them.

Benefits are seen for a variety of nuts commonly eaten in the United States: almonds, Brazil nuts, cashews, hazelnuts, macadamia nuts, pecans, pistachios, walnuts, and even peanuts. On average, these nuts contain mostly monounsaturated fat (59 percent), some polyunsaturated fat (27 percent), and little saturated fat (14 percent). Nuts also provide valuable fiber, vegetable protein, vitamin E, minerals, and phytochemicals.

Including nuts may be a wise diet strategy against heart disease. Nuts may protect against heart disease by:[7]

- Lowering blood cholesterol
- Lowering blood pressure
- Limiting oxidative stress and inflammation

Some research suggests that a diet that includes nuts may benefit other diseases as well.

Before advising consumers to include nuts in their diets, however, a caution is in order. As mentioned, most of the energy nuts provide comes from fats. Consequently, they deliver many kcalories per bite. Incorporating nuts in the diet, however, does not necessarily lead to weight gains and may even help with weight control.[8] Consumers can enjoy nuts without increasing total kcalories by using nuts *instead of, not in addition to,* other foods (such as meats, potato chips, oils, margarine, and butter).

Feast on Fish

Research into the health benefits of the long-chain omega-3 polyunsaturated fatty acids began with a simple observation: the native peoples of Alaska, northern Canada, and Greenland, who eat a traditional diet rich in omega-3 fatty acids, notably EPA (eicosapentaenoic acid) and DHA (docosaheaenoic acid), have a remarkably low rate of heart disease even though their diets are relatively high in fat. These omega-3 fatty acids help to protect against heart disease by:[9]

- Reducing blood triglycerides
- Stabilizing plaque

- Lowering blood pressure and resting heart rate
- Reducing inflammation
- Serving as precursors to eicosanoids

For people with hypertension or atherosclerosis, these actions can be life saving.

Research studies have provided strong evidence that increasing omega-3 fatty acids in the diet supports heart health and lowers the rate of deaths from heart disease.[10] For this reason, the American Heart Association recommends including fish in a heart-healthy diet. People who eat some fish each week can lower their risks of heart attack and stroke.

Fish is the best source of EPA and DHA in the diet, but it is also a source of mercury, an environmental contaminant. Most fish contain at least trace amounts of mercury, but some have especially high levels. For this reason, the FDA advises pregnant and lactating women, women of childbearing age who may become pregnant, and young children to include fish in their diets, but to avoid:

- Tilefish (also called golden snapper or golden bass), swordfish, king mackeral, marlin, and shark

And to limit average weekly consumption of:

- A variety of ocean fish and shellfish to 12 ounces (cooked or canned)
- White (albacore) tuna to 6 ounces (cooked or canned)

Commonly eaten seafood relatively low in mercury include shrimp, catfish, pollock, salmon, and canned light tuna.

In addition to the direct toxic effects of mercury, some research suggests that mercury may diminish the health benefits of omega-3 fatty acids. Such findings serve as a reminder that our health depends on the health of our planet. The protective effect of fish in the diet is available, provided that the fish and their surrounding waters are not heavily contaminated. (Chapter 19 discusses the adverse consequences of mercury, and Chapter 20 presents the relationships between diet and the environment in more detail.)

In an effort to limit exposure to pollutants, some consumers choose farm-raised fish. Compared with fish caught in the wild, farm-raised fish tend to be lower in mercury, but they are also lower in omega-3 fatty acids. When selecting fish, keep the diet strategies of variety and moderation in mind. Varying choices and eating moderate amounts helps to limit the intake of contaminants such as mercury.

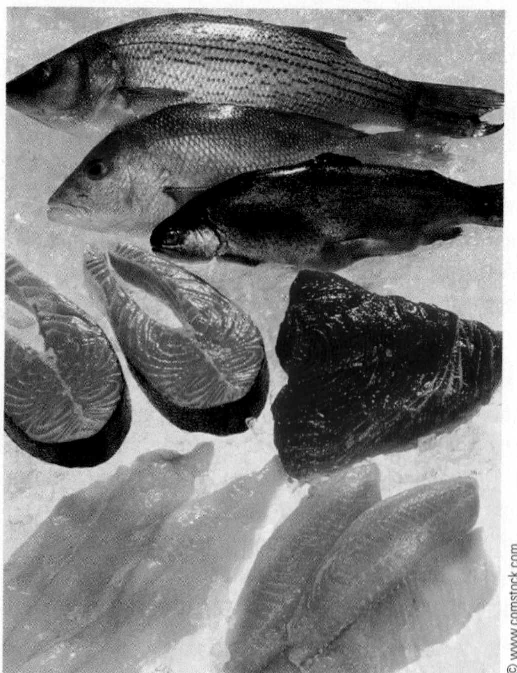

Fish is a good source of the omega-3 fatty acids.

High-Fat Foods and Heart Disease

The number-one dietary determinant of LDL cholesterol is saturated fat. Each 1 percent increase in energy from saturated fatty acids in the diet produces a 2 percent jump in heart disease risk by elevating LDL cholesterol. Conversely, reducing saturated fat intake by 1 percent can be expected to produce a 2 percent drop in heart disease risk by the same mechanism. Even a 2 percent drop in LDL represents a significant improvement for heart health. Like saturated fats, *trans* fats also raise heart disease risk by elevating LDL cholesterol. A heart-healthy diet limits foods rich in these two types of fat.

Limit Fatty Meats, Whole-Milk Products, and Tropical Oils

The major sources of saturated fats in the US diet are fatty meats, whole milk, tropical oils, and products made from any of these foods. To limit saturated fat intake, consumers must choose carefully among these high-fat foods. More than a third of the fat in most meats is saturated. Similarly, more than half of the fat is saturated in whole milk and other high-fat milk products, such as cheese, butter, cream, half-and-half, cream cheese, sour cream, and ice cream. The tropical oils of palm, palm kernel, and coconut, which are rarely used by consumers in the kitchen, are used heavily by food manufacturers, and are commonly found in many commercially prepared foods.

When choosing meats, milk products, and commercially prepared foods, look for those lowest in saturated fat. Labels provide a useful guide for comparing products in this regard, and Appendix H lists the saturated fat in several thousand foods.

Even with careful selections, a nutritionally adequate diet will provide some saturated fat. Zero saturated fat is not possible even when experts design menus with the mission to keep saturated fat as low as possible. Because most saturated fats come from animal foods, vegetarian diets can, and usually do, deliver fewer saturated fats than mixed diets.

Limit Hydrogenated Foods

Chapter 5 explained that solid shortening and margarine are made from vegetable oil that has been hardened through hydrogenation. This process both saturates some of the unsaturated fatty acids and introduces *trans*-fatty acids. Many convenience foods contain *trans* fats, including:

- Fried foods such as french fries, chicken, and other commercially fried foods
- Commercial baked goods such as cookies, doughnuts, pastries, breads, and crackers
- Snack foods such as chips
- Imitation cheeses

To keep *trans*-fat intake low, use these foods sparingly.

Table 5-4 (p. 153) summarizes which foods provide which fats. Substituting unsaturated fats for saturated fats at each meal and snack can help protect against heart disease. Figure H5-1 compares two meals and shows how such substitutions can lower saturated fat and raise unsaturated fat—even when total fat and kcalories remain unchanged.

The Mediterranean Diet

The links between good health and traditional Mediterranean eating patterns of the mid-1900s were introduced earlier with regard to olive oil. For people who eat these diets, the incidence of heart disease, some cancers, diabetes, and other chronic inflammatory diseases is low, and life expectancy is high.[11] Some research suggests that the health benefits of the Mediterranean eating pattern are partially due to its favorable effects on body weight.[12]

Although each of the many countries that border the Mediterranean Sea has its own culture, traditions, and dietary habits, their similarities are much greater than the use of olive oil alone. In fact, no one factor alone can be credited with reducing disease risks—the association holds true only when the overall eating pattern is present. Apparently, each of the foods contributes small benefits that harmonize to produce either a substantial cumulative or synergistic effect.

The Mediterranean eating pattern features fresh, whole foods. The people select crusty breads, whole grains, potatoes, and pastas; a variety of vegetables (including wild greens) and legumes; feta and mozzarella cheeses and yogurt; nuts; and fruits (especially grapes and figs). They eat some fish, other seafood, poultry, a few eggs, and little meat. Along with olives and olive oil, their principal sources of fat are nuts and fish; they rarely use butter or encounter hydrogenated fats. They commonly use herbs and spices instead of salt. Consequently, traditional Mediterranean diets are:

- Low in saturated fat
- Very low in *trans* fat

> **FIGURE H5-1 Two Meals Compared: Replacing Saturated Fat with Unsaturated Fat**

Examples of ways to replace saturated fats with unsaturated fats include sautéing vegetables in olive oil instead of butter, garnishing salads with avocado and sunflower seeds instead of bacon and blue cheese, and eating salmon instead of steak. Each of these meals provides roughly the same number of kcalories and grams of fat, but the one on the left has almost four times as much saturated fat and only half as many omega-3 fatty acids.

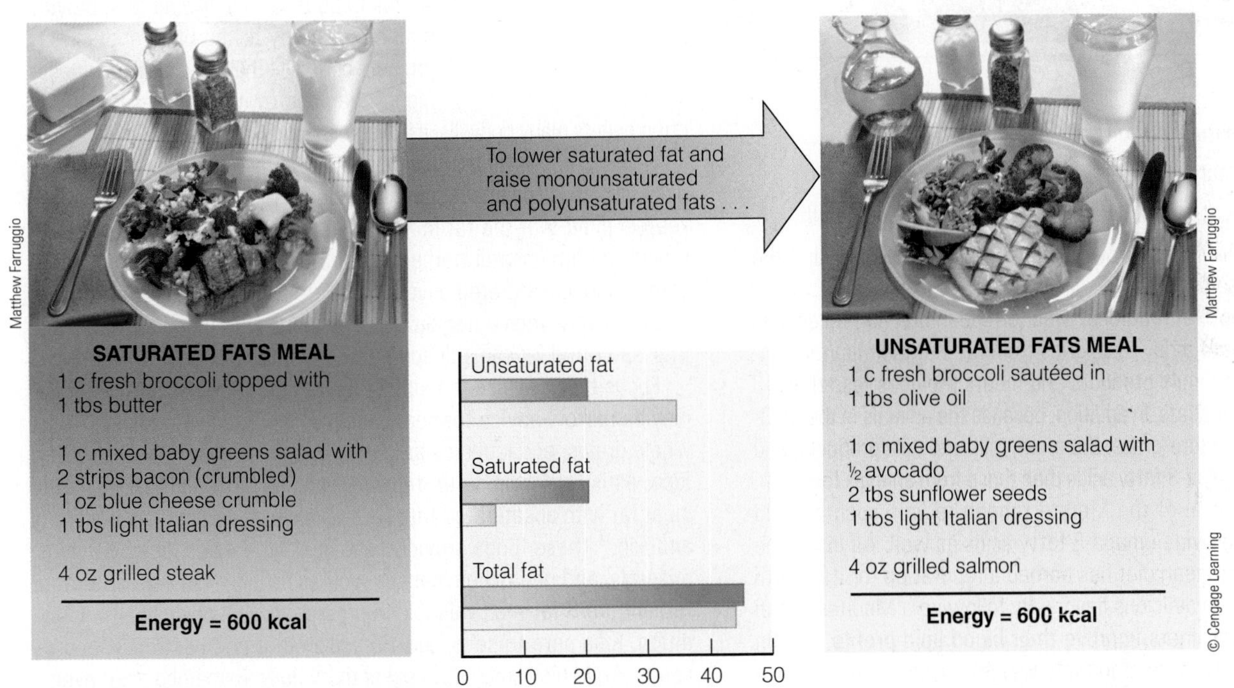

Matthew Farruggio
SATURATED FATS MEAL
1 c fresh broccoli topped with
1 tbs butter
1 c mixed baby greens salad with
2 strips bacon (crumbled)
1 oz blue cheese crumble
1 tbs light Italian dressing
4 oz grilled steak
Energy = 600 kcal
To lower saturated fat and raise monounsaturated and polyunsaturated fats . . .
Unsaturated fat
Saturated fat
Total fat
0
10
20
30
40
50
GRAMS
Matthew Farruggio
UNSATURATED FATS MEAL
1 c fresh broccoli sautéed in
1 tbs olive oil
1 c mixed baby greens salad with
½ avocado
2 tbs sunflower seeds
1 tbs light Italian dressing
4 oz grilled salmon
Energy = 600 kcal
© Cengage Learning

> FIGURE H5-2 **Mediterranean Diet Pyramid**

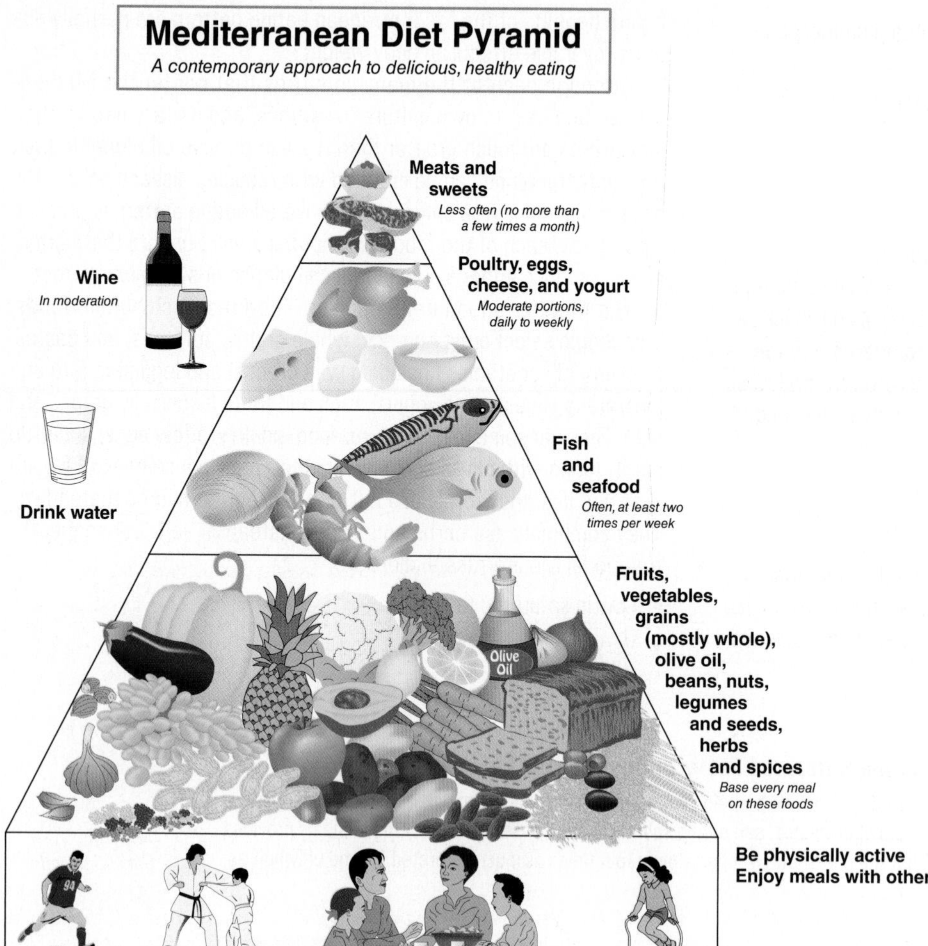

- Rich in monounsaturated and polyunsaturated fat
- Rich in complex carbohydrate and fiber
- Rich in nutrients and phytochemicals that support good health

As a result, lipid profiles improve, inflammation diminishes, and the risk of heart disease declines.

People following the traditional Mediterranean diet can receive as much as 40 percent of a day's kcalories from fat, but their limited consumption of milk and milk products and meats provides less than 10 percent from saturated fats. In addition, because the animals in the Mediterranean region pasture-graze, the meat, milk and milk products, and eggs are richer in omega-3 fatty acids than those from animals fed grain.

Other foods typical of the Mediterranean region, such as wild plants and snails, provide omega-3 fatty acids as well. All in all, the traditional Mediterranean diet has earned a reputation for its health benefits as well as its delicious flavors. By following a Mediterranean eating pattern, consumers improve their blood lipid profile, insulin resistance, blood pressure, and body weight.[13] Consumers need to beware that the typical Mediterranean-style cuisine available in US restaurants, however, has been adjusted to popular tastes. Quite often, these meals are much higher in saturated fats and meats—and much lower in the potentially beneficial constituents—than the traditional fare. Unfortunately, it appears that people in the Mediterranean region who are replacing some of their traditional dietary habits with those of the United States are losing the health benefits previously enjoyed. Figure H5-2 presents a Mediterranean Diet Pyramid. Notice the emphasis on abundant plant foods.

Conclusion

Are some fats "good," and others "bad" from the body's point of view? The saturated and *trans* fats indeed seem mostly bad for the health of the heart. Aside from providing energy, which unsaturated fats can do equally well, saturated and *trans* fats bring no indispensable benefits to the body. Furthermore, no harm can come from consuming diets low in them. Still, foods rich in these fats are often delicious, giving them an occasional place in the diet.

In contrast, the unsaturated fats are mostly good for heart health when consumed in moderation. To date, their one proven fault seems to be that they, like all fats, provide abundant energy to the body and so may promote obesity if they drive kcalorie intakes higher than energy needs. Obesity, in turn, often begets many body ills, as Chapters 8 and 9 describe.

Clearly, different fatty acids have different actions in the body and risks of chronic diseases.[14] When judging foods by their fatty acids, keep in mind that the fat in foods is a mixture of "good" and "bad," providing both unsaturated and saturated fatty acids. Even predominantly monounsaturated olive oil delivers some saturated fat. Consequently, even when a person chooses foods with mostly unsaturated fats, saturated fat can still add up if total fat is too high.

Focusing all efforts on simply lowering saturated fat in the diet may be narrow advice for heart health.[15] Including vegetables, fruits, whole grains, and legumes as part of a balanced daily diet is a good idea, as is *replacing* saturated fats such as butter, shortening, and meat fat with unsaturated fats such as olive oil and the oils from nuts and fish.[16] These foods provide beneficial fatty acids, fiber, vitamins, minerals, and phytochemicals as well as little (or no) salt, saturated fat, and *trans* fat—all valuable in protecting the body's health. In addition, take care to select portion sizes that will best meet energy needs. And enjoy some physical activity daily. Remember that even a healthy eating pattern can be detrimental if eaten in excess.[17]

CRITICAL THINKING QUESTIONS

A. What are the features of a healthy high-fat diet?

B. Heart disease is rare among the Inuit people of Alaska who continue to eat their traditional diet of seal meat and blubber. A traditional Nordic diet of game meats, berries, root vegetables, and legumes helps to lower blood cholesterol and reduce heart disease risk. People following the traditional Mediterranean diet that emphasizes fruits, vegetables, whole grains, beans, nuts and seeds, and olive oil also enjoy good heart health. How are dietary fats related to heart health? How is it that such diverse diets can have such similar health outcomes?

REFERENCES

1. D. Mozaffarian, R. Micha, and S. Wallace, Effects on coronary heart disease of increasing polyunsaturated fat in place of saturated fat: A systematic review and meta-analysis of randomized controlled trials, *PLoS Medicine* 7 (2010): e10000252.
2. B. Bendinelli and coauthors, Fruit, vegetables, and olive oil and risk of coronary heart disease in Italian women: The EPICOR Study, *American Journal of Clinical Nutrition* 93 (2011): 275–283.
3. A. Keys, *Seven Countries: A Multivariate Analysis of Death and Coronary Heart Disease* (Cambridge: Harvard University Press, 1980).
4. W. C. Willet, The great fat debate: Total fat and health, *Journal of the American Dietetic Association* 111 (2011): 660–662.
5. L. Lin, Evidence of health benefits of canola oil, *Nutrition Reviews* 71 (2013): 370–385; L. Lucas, A. Russell, and R. Keast, Molecular mechanisms of inflammation: Anti-inflammatory benefits of virgin olive oil and the phenolic compound oleocanthal, *Current Pharmaceutical Design* 17 (2011): 754–768; C. Samieri and coauthors, Olive oil consumption, plasma oleic acid, and stroke incidence: The Three-City Study, *Neurology* 77 (2011): 1–8; D. Bester and coauthors, Cardiovascular effects of edible oils: A comparison between four popular edible oils, *Nutrition Research Reviews* 23 (2010): 334–348.
6. Y. Bao and coauthors, Association of nut consumption with total and cause-specific mortality, *New England Journal of Medicine* 369 (2013): 2001–2011; J. Sabaté and M. Wien, Nuts, blood lipids and cardiovascular disease, *Asia Pacific Journal of Clinical Nutrition* 19 (2010): 131–136.
7. C. E. Berryman and coauthors, Effects of almond consumption on the reduction of LDL-cholesterol: A discussion of potential mechanisms and future research directions, *Nutrition Reviews* 69 (2011): 171–185; E. Ros, L. C. Tapsell, and J. Sabaté, Nuts and berries for heart health, *Current Atherosclerosis Reports* 12 (2010): 397–406; J. Sabaté, K. Oda, and E. Ros, Nut consumption and blood lipid levels: A pooled analysis of 25 intervention trials, *Archives of Internal Medicine* 170 (2010): 821–827.
8. G. Flores-Mateo and coauthors, Nut intake and adiposity: Meta-analysis of clinical trials, *American Journal of Clinical Nutrition* 97 (2013): 1346–1355; V. Vadivel, C. N. Kunyanga, and H. K. Biesalski, Health benefits of nut consumption with special reference to body weight control, *Nutrition* 28 (2012): 1089–1097; M. Fogelhom and coauthors, Dietary macronutrients and food consumption as determinants of long-term weight change in adult populations: A systematic literature review, *Food and Nutrition Research* 56 (2012): doi 10.3402.
9. A. C. Skulas-Ray and coauthors, Dose-response effects of omega-3 fatty acids on triglycerides, inflammation, and endothelial function in healthy persons with moderate hypertriglyceridemia, *American Journal of Clinical Nutrition* 93 (2011): 243–252; P. C. Calder and P. Yaqoob, Omega-3 (n-3) fatty acids, cardiovascular disease and stability of atherosclerotic plaques, *Journal of Molecular Cell Biology* 56 (2010): 28–37; F. Dangardt and coauthors, Omega-3 fatty acid supplementation improves vascular function and reduces inflammation in obese adolescents, *Atherosclerosis* 212 (2010): 580–585; M. N. DiMinno and coauthors, Exploring newer cardioprotective strategies: ω-3 Fatty acids in perspective, *Journal of Thrombosis and Haemostasis* 104 (2010): 664–680.
10. D. Mozaffarian and J. H. Y. Wu, Omega-3 fatty acids and cardiovascular disease: Effects on risk factors, molecular pathways, and clinical events, *Journal of the American College of Cardiology* 58 (2011): 2047–2067.
11. K. Esposito and coauthors, Prevention and control of type 2 diabetes by Mediterranean diet: A systematic review, *Diabetes Research and Clinical Practice* 89 (2010): 97–102; P. P. McKeown and coauthors, Session 4: CVD, diabetes and cancer: Evidence for the use of the Mediterranean diet in patients with CHD, *Proceedings of the Nutrition Society* 69 (2010): 45–60; F. Sofi and coauthors, Accruing evidence on benefits of adherence to the Mediterranean diet on health: An updated systematic review and meta-analysis, *American Journal of Clinical Nutrition* 92 (2010): 1189–1196; L. Verberne and coauthors, Association between the Mediterranean diet and cancer risk: A review of observational studies, *Nutrition and Cancer* 62 (2010): 860–870.
12. J. J. Beunza and coauthors, Adherence to the Mediterranean diet, long-term weight change, and incident overweight or obesity: The Seguimiento Universidad de Navarra (SUN) cohort, *American Journal of Clinical Nutrition* 92 (2010): 1484–1493.
13. R. Estruch, Anti-inflammatory effects of the Mediterranean diet: The experience of the PREDIMED study, *Proceedings of the Nutrition Society* 69 (2010): 333–340.
14. S. J. Baum and coauthors, Fatty acids in cardiovascular health and disease: A comprehensive update, *Journal of Clinical Lipidology* 6 (2012): 216–234.
15. D. J. A. Jenkins, Effect of a dietary portfolio of cholesterol-lowering foods given at 2 levels of intensity of dietary advice on serum lipids in hyperlipidemia: A randomized controlled trial, *Journal of the American Medical Association* 306 (2011): 831–839.
16. Position of the Academy of Nutrition and Dietetics: Dietary fatty acids for healthy adults, *Journal of the Academy of Nutrition and Dietetics* 114 (2014): 136–153; D. Kromhout and coauthors, The confusion about dietary fatty acids recommendations for CHD prevention, *British Journal of Nutrition* 106 (2011): 627–632; D. Mozaffarian, The great fat debate: Taking the focus off of saturated fat, *Journal of the American Dietetic Association* 111 (2011): 665–666.
17. A. H. Lichtenstein, The great fat debate: The importance of message translation, *Journal of the American Dietetic Association* 111 (2011): 667–670.

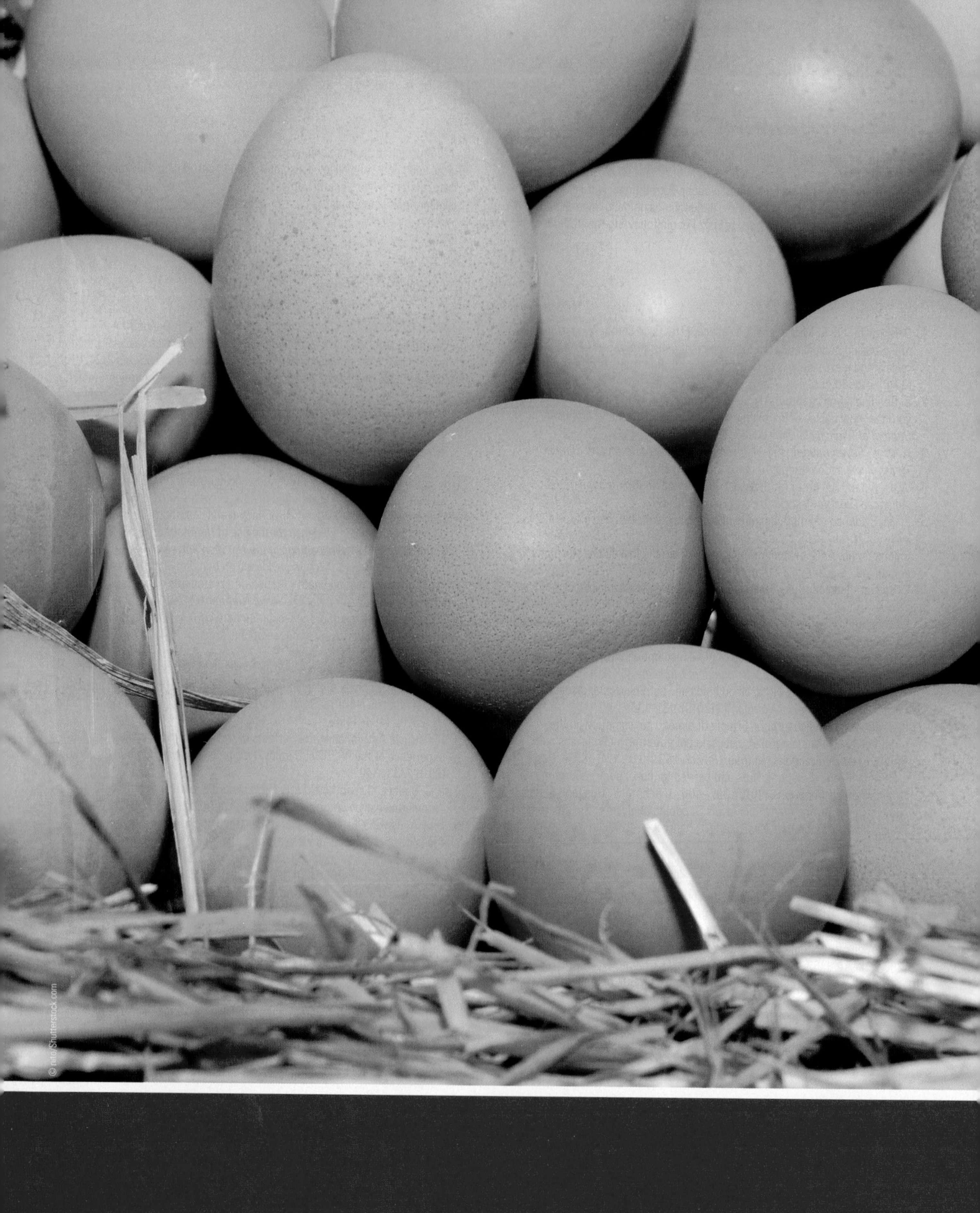

6

Protein: Amino Acids

Nutrition in Your Life

The versatility of proteins in the body is impressive. They help your muscles to contract, your blood to clot, and your eyes to see. They keep you alive and well by facilitating chemical reactions and defending against infections. Without them, your bones, skin, and hair would have no structure. No wonder they were named *proteins,* meaning "of prime importance." Does that mean proteins deserve top billing in your diet as well? Are the best sources of protein beef, beans, or broccoli? Learn which foods will supply you with enough, but not too much, high-quality protein. In the Nutrition Portfolio at the end of this chapter, you can determine whether your diet is meeting your protein needs.

A few misconceptions surround the roles of protein in the body and the importance of protein in the diet. For example, people who associate meat with protein and protein with strength may eat steak to build muscles. Their thinking is only partly correct, however. Protein is a vital structural and working substance in all cells—not just muscle cells. To build strength, muscle cells need physical activity and all the nutrients—not just protein. Furthermore, protein is found in milk, eggs, legumes, and many grains and vegetables—not just meat. By overvaluing protein and overemphasizing meat in the diet, a person may mistakenly crowd out other, equally important nutrients and foods. As this chapter describes the various roles of protein in the body and food sources in the diet, keep in mind that protein is one of many nutrients needed to maintain good health.

LEARNING GPS

6.1 The Chemist's View of Proteins

› LEARN IT Recognize the chemical structures of amino acids and proteins.

Chemically, **proteins** contain nitrogen (N) atoms in addition to the same atoms as carbohydrates and lipids—carbon (C), hydrogen (H), and oxygen (O). These nitrogen atoms give the name *amino* (nitrogen containing) to the amino acids that make the links in the chains of proteins.

Amino Acids All **amino acids** have the same basic structure—a central carbon (C) atom with a hydrogen atom (H), an amino group (NH_2), and an acid group (COOH) attached to it. Remember, however, that carbon atoms must have four bonds, so a fourth attachment is necessary. This fourth site distinguishes each amino acid from the others. Attached to the central carbon at the fourth bond is a distinct atom, or group of atoms, known as the *side group* or *side chain* (see Figure 6-1).

Unique Side Groups The side groups on the central carbon vary from one amino acid to the next, making proteins more complex than either carbohydrates or lipids. A polysaccharide (starch, for example) may be several thousand units long, but each unit is a glucose molecule just like all the others. A protein, on the other hand, is made up of about 20 different amino acids, each with a different side group. Table 6-1 lists the amino acids most common in proteins.*

The simplest amino acid, glycine, has a hydrogen atom as its side group. A slightly more complex amino acid, alanine, has an extra carbon with three hydrogen atoms. Other amino acids have more complex side groups (see Figure 6-2 for examples). Thus, although all amino acids share a common structure, they differ in size, shape, electrical charge, and other characteristics because of differences in these side groups.

Nonessential Amino Acids More than half of the amino acids are *nonessential,* meaning that the body can synthesize them for itself. Proteins in foods usually deliver these amino acids, but it is not essential that they do so. The body can make all **nonessential amino acids,** given nitrogen to form the amino group and fragments from carbohydrate or fat to form the rest of the structure.

› FIGURE 6-1 Amino Acid Structure

All amino acids have a central carbon with an amino group (NH_2), an acid group (COOH), a hydrogen (H), and a side group attached. The side group is a unique chemical structure that differentiates one amino acid from another.

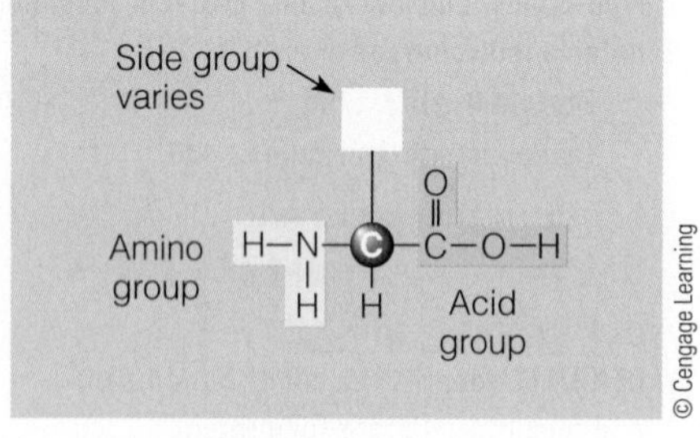

© Cengage Learning

TABLE 6-1 Amino Acids

Proteins are made up of about 20 common amino acids. The first column lists the *essential amino acids* for human beings (those the body cannot make—that must be provided in the diet). The second column lists the *nonessential amino acids.* In special cases, some nonessential amino acids may become *conditionally essential.* In a newborn, for example, only five amino acids are truly nonessential; the other nonessential amino acids are conditionally essential until the metabolic pathways are developed enough to make those amino acids in adequate amounts.

Essential Amino Acids		Nonessential Amino Acids	
Histidine	(HISS-tuh-deen)	Alanine	(AL-ah-neen)
Isoleucine	(eye-so-LOO-seen)	Arginine	(ARJ-ih-neen)
Leucine	(LOO-seen)	Asparagine	(ah-SPAR-ah-geen)
Lysine	(LYE-seen)	Aspartic acid	(ah-SPAR-tic acid)
Methionine	(meh-THIGH-oh-neen)	Cysteine	(SIS-teh-een)
Phenylalanine	(fen-il-AL-ah-neen)	Glutamic acid	(GLU-tam-ic acid)
Threonine	(THREE-oh-neen)	Glutamine	(GLU-tah-meen)
Tryptophan	(TRIP-toe-fan, TRIP-toe-fane)	Glycine	(GLY-seen)
Valine	(VAY-leen)	Proline	(PRO-leen)
		Serine	(SEER-een)
		Tyrosine	(TIE-roe-seen)

© Cengage Learning

*These 20 amino acids can all be commonly found in proteins. In addition, other amino acids do not occur in proteins but can be found individually (for example, taurine and ornithine). Some amino acids occur in related forms (for example, proline can acquire an OH group to become hydroxyproline).

proteins: compounds composed of carbon, hydrogen, oxygen, and nitrogen atoms, arranged into amino acids linked in a chain. Some amino acids also contain sulfur atoms.

amino (a-MEEN-oh) acids: building blocks of proteins. Each contains an amino group, an acid group, a hydrogen atom, and a distinctive side group, all attached to a central carbon atom.

- **amino** = containing nitrogen

nonessential amino acids: amino acids that the body can make (see Table 6-1); also called *dispensable amino acids.*

> FIGURE 6-2 Examples of Amino Acids

Note that all amino acids have a common chemical structure but that each has a different side group. Appendix C presents the chemical structures of the 20 amino acids most common in proteins.

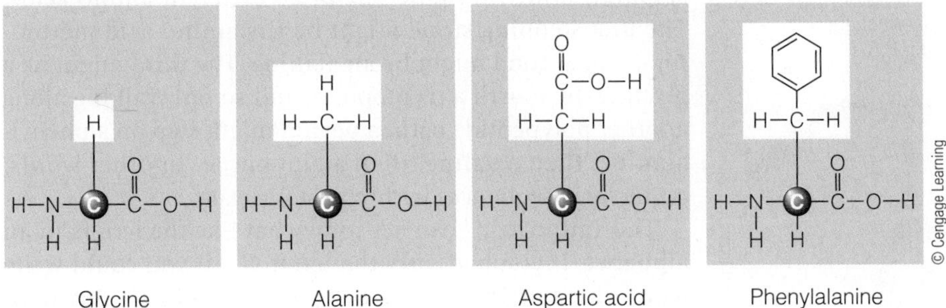

Essential Amino Acids There are nine amino acids that the human body either cannot make at all or cannot make in sufficient quantity to meet its needs. These nine amino acids must be supplied by the diet; they are *essential.* The first column in Table 6-1 presents the **essential amino acids.** Some researchers refer to essential amino acids as *indispensable* and to nonessential amino acids as *dispensable.*

Conditionally Essential Amino Acids Sometimes a nonessential amino acid becomes essential under special circumstances. For example, the body normally uses the essential amino acid phenylalanine to make tyrosine (a nonessential amino acid). But if the diet fails to supply enough phenylalanine, or if the body cannot make the conversion for some reason (as happens in the inherited disease phenylketonuria, described in Highlight 6), then tyrosine becomes a **conditionally essential amino acid.**

Proteins

Cells link amino acids end-to-end in a variety of sequences to form thousands of different proteins. A **peptide bond** unites each amino acid to the next.

Amino Acid Chains Condensation reactions connect amino acids, just as they combine two monosaccharides to form a disaccharide and three fatty acids with a glycerol to form a triglyceride. Two amino acids bonded together form a **dipeptide** (see Figure 6-3). By another such reaction, a third amino acid can be added to the chain to form a **tripeptide.** As additional amino acids join the chain, a **polypeptide** is formed. Most proteins are a few dozen to several hundred amino acids long. Figure 6-4 (p. 174) illustrates the protein insulin.

Primary Structure—Amino Acid Sequence The primary structure of a protein is determined by the sequence of amino acids. If a person could walk along a carbohydrate molecule like starch, the first stepping stone would be a glucose.

> FIGURE 6-3 Condensation of Two Amino Acids to Form a Dipeptide

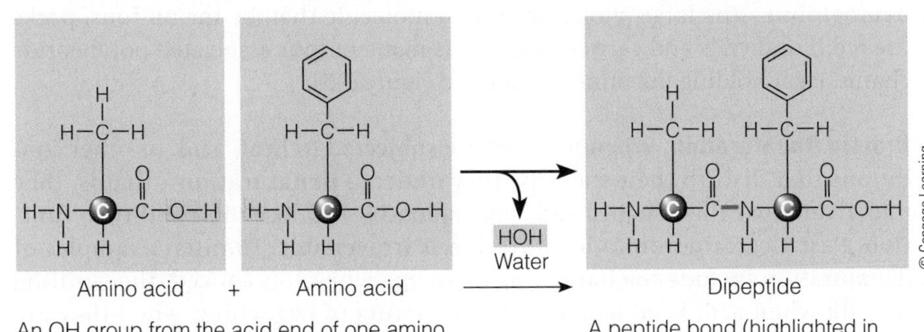

An OH group from the acid end of one amino acid and an H atom from the amino group of another join to form a molecule of water.

A peptide bond (highlighted in red) forms between the two amino acids, creating a dipeptide.

essential amino acids: amino acids that the body requires but cannot make, and so must be obtained from the diet (see Table 6-1); also called *indispensable amino acids.*

conditionally essential amino acid: an amino acid that is normally nonessential, but must be supplied by the diet in special circumstances when the need for it exceeds the body's ability to make it.

peptide bond: a bond that connects the acid end of one amino acid with the amino end of another, forming a link in a protein chain.

dipeptide (dye-PEP-tide)**:** two amino acids bonded together.

- **di** = two
- **peptide** = amino acid

tripeptide: three amino acids bonded together.

- **tri** = three

polypeptide: many (10 or more) amino acids bonded together.

- **poly** = many

> **FIGURE 6-4 Amino Acid Sequence of Human Insulin**

Human insulin is a relatively small protein that consists of 51 amino acids in two short polypeptide chains. (For amino acid abbreviations, see Appendix C.) Two bridges link the two chains. A third bridge spans a section within the short chain. Known as *disulfide bridges*, these links form between the cysteine (Cys) amino acids, whose side group contains sulfur (S).

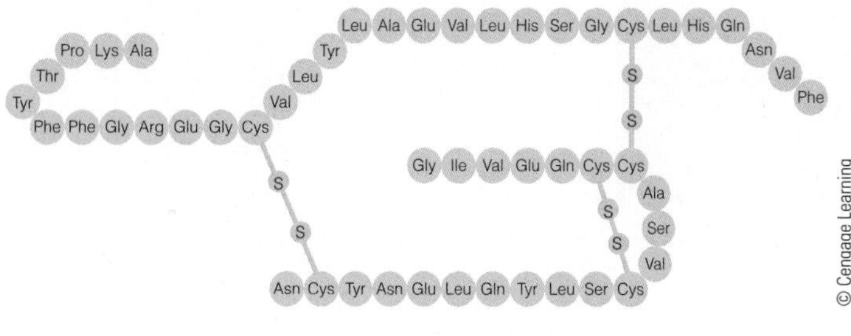

The next stepping stone would also be a glucose, and it would be followed by a glucose, and yet another glucose. But if a person were to walk along a polypeptide chain, each stepping stone would be one of 20 different amino acids. The first stepping stone might be the amino acid methionine. The second might be an alanine. The third might be a glycine, the fourth a tryptophan, and so on. Walking along another polypeptide path, a person might step on a phenylalanine, then a valine, then a glutamine. In other words, amino acid sequences within proteins vary.

The amino acids can act somewhat like the letters in an alphabet. If you had only the letter G, all you could write would be a string of Gs: G–G–G–G–G–G–G. But with 20 different letters available, you can create poems, songs, and novels. Similarly, the 20 amino acids can be linked together in a variety of sequences—even more than are possible for letters in a word or words in a sentence. Thus the variety of possible sequences for polypeptide chains is tremendous.

Secondary Structure—Polypeptide Shapes The secondary structure of proteins is determined not by chemical bonds as between the amino acids but by weak electrical attractions within the polypeptide chain. As positively charged hydrogens attract nearby negatively charged oxygens, sections of the polypeptide chain twist into a helix or fold into a pleated sheet, for example. These shapes give proteins strength and rigidity.

Tertiary Structure—Polypeptide Tangles The tertiary structure of proteins occurs as long polypeptide chains twist and fold into a variety of complex, tangled shapes. The unique side group of each amino acid gives it characteristics that attract it to, or repel it from, the surrounding fluids and other amino acids. Some amino acid side groups are attracted to water molecules; they are *hydrophilic*. Other side groups are repelled by water; they are *hydrophobic*. As amino acids are linked together to make a polypeptide, the chain folds so that its hydrophilic side groups are on the outer surface near water; the hydrophobic groups tuck themselves inside, away from water. Similarly, the disulfide bridges in insulin (see Figure 6-4) determine its tertiary structure. The extraordinary and unique shapes of proteins enable them to perform their various tasks in the body. Some form globular or spherical structures that can carry and store materials within them, and some, such as those of tendons, form linear structures that are more than 10 times as long as they are wide. The intricate shape a protein finally assumes gives it maximum stability.

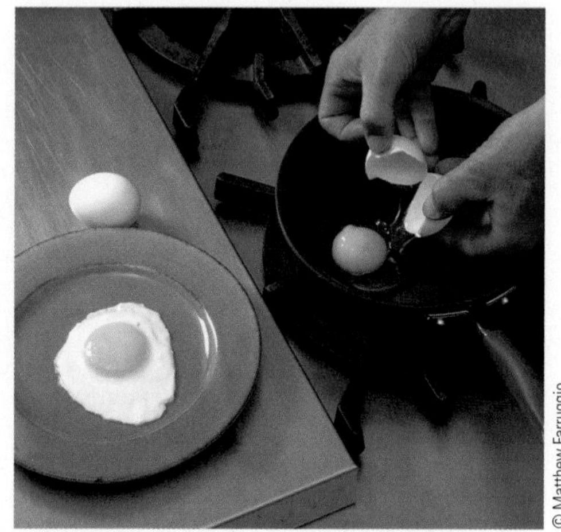

Cooking an egg denatures its proteins.

Quaternary Structure—Multiple Polypeptide Interactions Some polypeptides are functioning proteins just as they are; others need to associate with other polypeptides to form larger working complexes. The quaternary structure of proteins involves the interactions between two or more polypeptides. One molecule of **hemoglobin**—the large, globular protein molecule that, by the billions, packs the red blood cells and carries oxygen—is made of four associated polypeptide chains, each holding the mineral iron (see Figure 6-5).

Protein Denaturation When proteins are subjected to heat, acid, or other conditions that disturb their stability, they undergo **denaturation**—that is, they uncoil and lose their shapes and, consequently, also lose their ability to function. Past a certain point, denaturation is irreversible. Familiar examples of denaturation include the hardening of an egg when it is cooked, the curdling of milk when acid is added, and the stiffening of egg whites when they are whipped. In the body, proteins are denatured when they are exposed to stomach acid.

hemoglobin (HE-moh-GLO-bin): the globular protein of the red blood cells that transports oxygen from the lungs to tissues throughout the body; hemoglobin accounts for 80 percent of the body's iron.

- **hemo** = blood
- **globin** = globular protein

denaturation (dee-NAY-chur-AY-shun): the change in a protein's shape and consequent loss of its function brought about by heat, agitation, acid, base, alcohol, heavy metals, or other agents.

› REVIEW IT Recognize the chemical structures of amino acids and proteins.
Chemically speaking, proteins are more complex than carbohydrates or lipids; they are made of some 20 different amino acids, 9 of which the body cannot make (the essential amino acids). Each amino acid contains an amino group, an acid group, a hydrogen atom, and a distinctive side group, all attached to a central carbon atom. Peptide bonds link amino acids together in a series of condensation reactions to create proteins. The distinctive sequence of amino acids in each protein determines its unique shape and function.

6.2 Digestion and Absorption of Proteins

› LEARN IT Summarize protein digestion and absorption.

Proteins in foods do not become body proteins directly. Instead, dietary proteins supply the amino acids from which the body makes its own proteins. When a person eats foods containing protein, enzymes break the long polypeptides into short polypeptides, the short polypeptides into tripeptides and dipeptides, and, finally, the tripeptides and dipeptides into individual amino acids.

Protein Digestion Figure 6-6 (p. 176) illustrates the digestion of protein through the GI tract and includes the names and actions of protein's digestive enzymes. Proteins are crushed and moistened in the mouth, but the real action begins in the stomach.

In the Stomach The major event in the stomach is the partial breakdown (hydrolysis) of proteins. Hydrochloric acid uncoils (denatures) each protein's tangled strands so that digestive enzymes can attack the peptide bonds. The hydrochloric acid also converts the inactive form of the enzyme pepsinogen to its active form, **pepsin.*** Pepsin cleaves proteins—large polypeptides—into smaller polypeptides and some amino acids.

In the Small Intestine When polypeptides enter the small intestine, several pancreatic and intestinal **proteases** hydrolyze them further into short peptide chains, tripeptides, dipeptides, and amino acids.** Then **peptidase** enzymes on the membrane surfaces of the intestinal cells split most of the dipeptides and tripeptides into single amino acids. Only a few peptides escape digestion and enter the blood intact.

Protein Absorption A number of specific carriers transport amino acids (and some dipeptides and tripeptides) into the intestinal cells. Once inside the intestinal cells, amino acids may be used for energy or to synthesize needed compounds. Amino acids that are not used by the intestinal cells are transported across the cell membrane into the surrounding fluid where they enter the capillaries on their way to the liver.

Consumers lacking nutrition knowledge may fail to realize that most proteins are broken down to amino acids before absorption. They may be misled by advertisements urging them to "Take this enzyme supplement to help you digest your food." Or "Don't eat this food that contains these enzymes that will digest cells in your body." In reality, enzymes in supplements and foods are proteins that are digested to amino acids, just as all proteins are. Even the digestive enzymes—which function optimally at their specific pH—are denatured and digested when the pH of their environment changes. The enzyme pepsin, for example, which works best in the low pH of the stomach becomes inactive and digested when it enters the higher pH of the small intestine.

Another misconception is that eating predigested proteins (amino acid supplements) saves the body from having to digest proteins and keeps the digestive system from "overworking." Such a belief grossly underestimates the body's abilities. As a matter of fact, the digestive system handles whole proteins *better* than predigested ones because it dismantles and absorbs the amino acids at rates that are optimal for the body's use. (The last section of this chapter discusses protein and amino acid supplements further.)

*The inactive form of an enzyme is called a *proenzyme* or a *zymogen* (ZYE-moh-jen).
**A short peptide chain of four to nine amino acids is called an *oligopeptide* (OL-ee-go-PEP-tide); *oligo* means few.

› FIGURE 6-5 The Structure of Hemoglobin

The shape of each polypeptide chain is determined by an amino acid sequence (primary structure) that twists into a helix (secondary structure) and bends itself into a ball shape (tertiary structure). Together, the four polypeptide chains make the globular hemoglobin protein (quaternary structure).

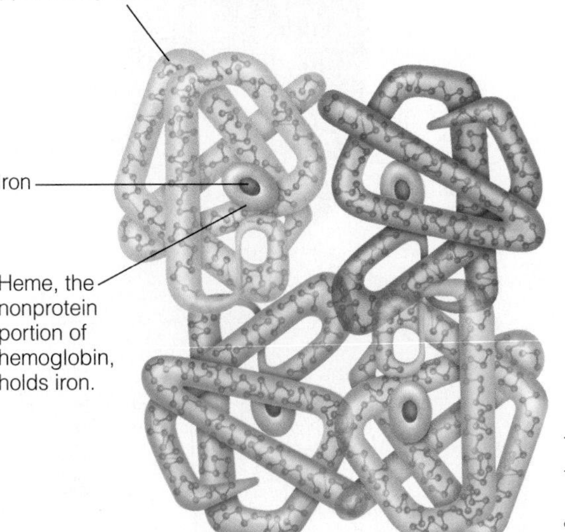

Iron
Heme, the nonprotein portion of hemoglobin, holds iron.

pepsin: a gastric enzyme that hydrolyzes protein. Pepsin is secreted in an inactive form, *pepsinogen*, which is activated by hydrochloric acid in the stomach.

proteases (PRO-tee-aces): enzymes that hydrolyze protein.

peptidase: a digestive enzyme that hydrolyzes peptide bonds. *Tripeptidases* cleave tripeptides; *dipeptidases* cleave dipeptides.

- **tri** = three
- **di** = two

> FIGURE 6-6 Protein Digestion in the GI Tract

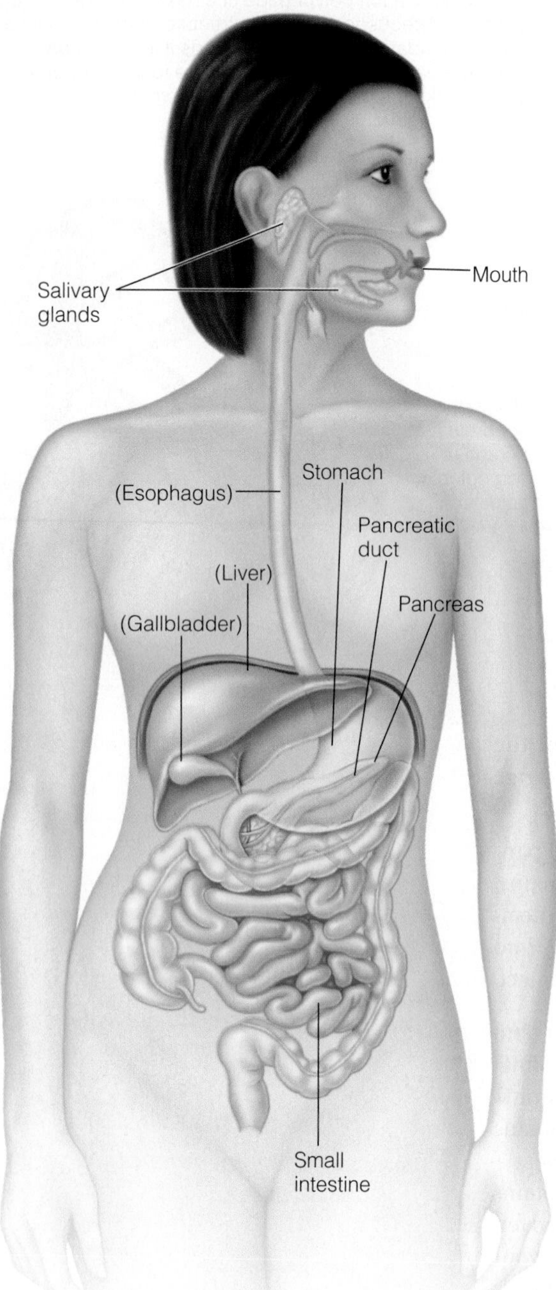

PROTEIN

Mouth and salivary glands

Chewing and crushing moisten protein-rich foods and mix them with saliva to be swallowed

Stomach

Hydrochloric acid (HCl) uncoils protein strands and activates stomach enzymes:

Protein —(Pepsin, HCl)→ Smaller polypeptides

Small intestine and pancreas

Pancreatic and small intestinal enzymes split polypeptides further:

Polypeptides —(Pancreatic and intestinal proteases)→ Tripeptides, dipeptides, amino acids

Then enzymes on the surface of the small intestinal cells hydrolyze these peptides and the cells absorb them:

Peptides —(Intestinal tripeptidases and dipeptidases)→ Amino acids (absorbed)

HYDROCHLORIC ACID AND THE DIGESTIVE ENZYMES

In the stomach:

Hydrochloric acid (HCl)
- Denatures protein structure
- Activates pepsinogen to pepsin

Pepsin
- Cleaves proteins to smaller polypeptides and some free amino acids
- Inhibits pepsinogen synthesis

In the small intestine:

Enteropeptidase
- Converts pancreatic trypsinogen to trypsin

Trypsin
- Inhibits trypsinogen synthesis
- Cleaves peptide bonds next to the amino acids lysine and arginine
- Converts pancreatic procarboxypeptidases to carboxypeptidases
- Converts pancreatic chymotrypsinogen to chymotrypsin

Chymotrypsin
- Cleaves peptide bonds next to the amino acids phenylalanine, tyrosine, tryptophan, methionine, asparagine, and histidine

Carboxypeptidases
- Cleave amino acids from the acid (carboxyl) ends of polypeptides

Elastase and collagenase
- Cleave polypeptides into smaller polypeptides and tripeptides

Intestinal tripeptidases
- Cleave tripeptides to dipeptides and amino acids

Intestinal dipeptidases
- Cleave dipeptides to amino acids

Intestinal aminopeptidases
- Cleave amino acids from the amino ends of small polypeptides (oligopeptides)

› REVIEW IT Summarize protein digestion and absorption.

Digestion is facilitated mostly by the stomach's acid and enzymes, which first denature dietary proteins, then cleave them into smaller polypeptides and some amino acids. Pancreatic and intestinal enzymes split these short polypeptides further, to tripeptides and dipeptides, and then split most of these to single amino acids. Then carriers in the membranes of intestinal cells transport the amino acids into the cells, where they are released into the bloodstream.

6.3 Proteins in the Body

› LEARN IT Describe how the body makes proteins and uses them to perform various roles.

The human body has an estimated 20,000 to 25,000 genes that code for hundreds of thousands of proteins. Relatively few proteins have been studied in detail, although this number is growing rapidly with the surge in knowledge gained from sequencing the human genome. The relatively few proteins described in this chapter illustrate the versatility, uniqueness, and importance of proteins. As you will see, each protein has a specific function, and that function is determined during protein synthesis.

Protein Synthesis

Each human being is unique because of small differences in the body's proteins. These differences are determined by the amino acid sequences of proteins, which, in turn, are determined by genes. The following paragraphs describe in words the ways cells synthesize proteins; Figure 6-7 (p. 178) provides a pictorial description. Protein synthesis depends on a diet that provides adequate protein and all the essential amino acids.

The instructions for making every protein in a person's body are transmitted by way of the genetic information received at conception. This body of knowledge, which is filed in the DNA (deoxyribonucleic acid) within the nucleus of every cell, never leaves the nucleus.

Delivering the Instructions Transforming the information in DNA into the appropriate sequence of amino acids needed to make a specific protein requires two major steps:

$$\text{DNA} \xrightarrow{\text{transcription}} \text{RNA} \xrightarrow{\text{translation}} \text{protein.}$$

In the first step, known as **transcription,** a stretch of DNA is used as a template to make messenger RNA. Messenger RNA then carries the code across the nuclear membrane into the body of the cell, where it seeks out and attaches itself to one of the ribosomes (a protein-making machine, which is itself composed of RNA and protein). There the second step, known as **translation,** takes place. Situated on a ribosome, messenger RNA specifies the sequence in which the amino acids line up for the synthesis of a protein.

Lining Up the Amino Acids Other forms of RNA, called transfer RNA, collect amino acids from the cell fluid and take them to messenger RNA. Each of the 20 amino acids has a specific transfer RNA. Thousands of transfer RNA, each carrying its amino acid, cluster around the ribosomes, awaiting their turn to unload. When the messenger RNA calls for a specific amino acid, the transfer RNA carrying that amino acid moves into position. Then the next loaded transfer RNA moves into place and then the next and the next. In this way, the amino acids line up in the sequence that is genetically determined, and enzymes bind them together. Finally, the completed protein strand is released, and the transfer RNA are freed to return for another load of amino acids.

Sequencing Errors The sequence of amino acids in each protein determines its shape, which supports a specific function. An error in the amino acid sequence results in an altered protein—sometimes with dramatic consequences. The protein hemoglobin offers one example of such a genetic variation. In a person with **sickle-cell anemia,** two of hemoglobin's four polypeptide chains (described earlier on pp. 174–175) have the normal sequence of amino acids, but the other two chains do not—they have the amino acid valine in a position that is normally occupied by glutamic acid (see Figure 6-8, p. 179). This single alteration in the amino acid sequence changes the characteristics and shape of hemoglobin so much that it loses its ability to carry oxygen effectively. The red blood cells filled with this abnormal hemoglobin stiffen into elongated sickle, or crescent, shapes instead of maintaining their normal pliable disc shape—hence the name, sickle-cell anemia. Sickle-cell anemia raises energy needs, causes many medical problems, and can be fatal.[1] Caring for people with sickle-cell anemia includes diligent attention to factors such as infection, stress, and dehydration, all of which can trigger a crisis.

transcription: the process of messenger RNA being made from a template of DNA.

translation: the process of messenger RNA directing the sequence of amino acids and synthesis of proteins.

sickle-cell anemia: a hereditary form of anemia characterized by abnormal sickle- or crescent-shaped red blood cells. Sickled cells interfere with oxygen transport and blood flow. Symptoms are precipitated by dehydration and insufficient oxygen (as may occur at high altitudes) and include hemolytic anemia (red blood cells burst), fever, and severe pain in the joints and abdomen.

> FIGURE 6-7 **Protein Synthesis**

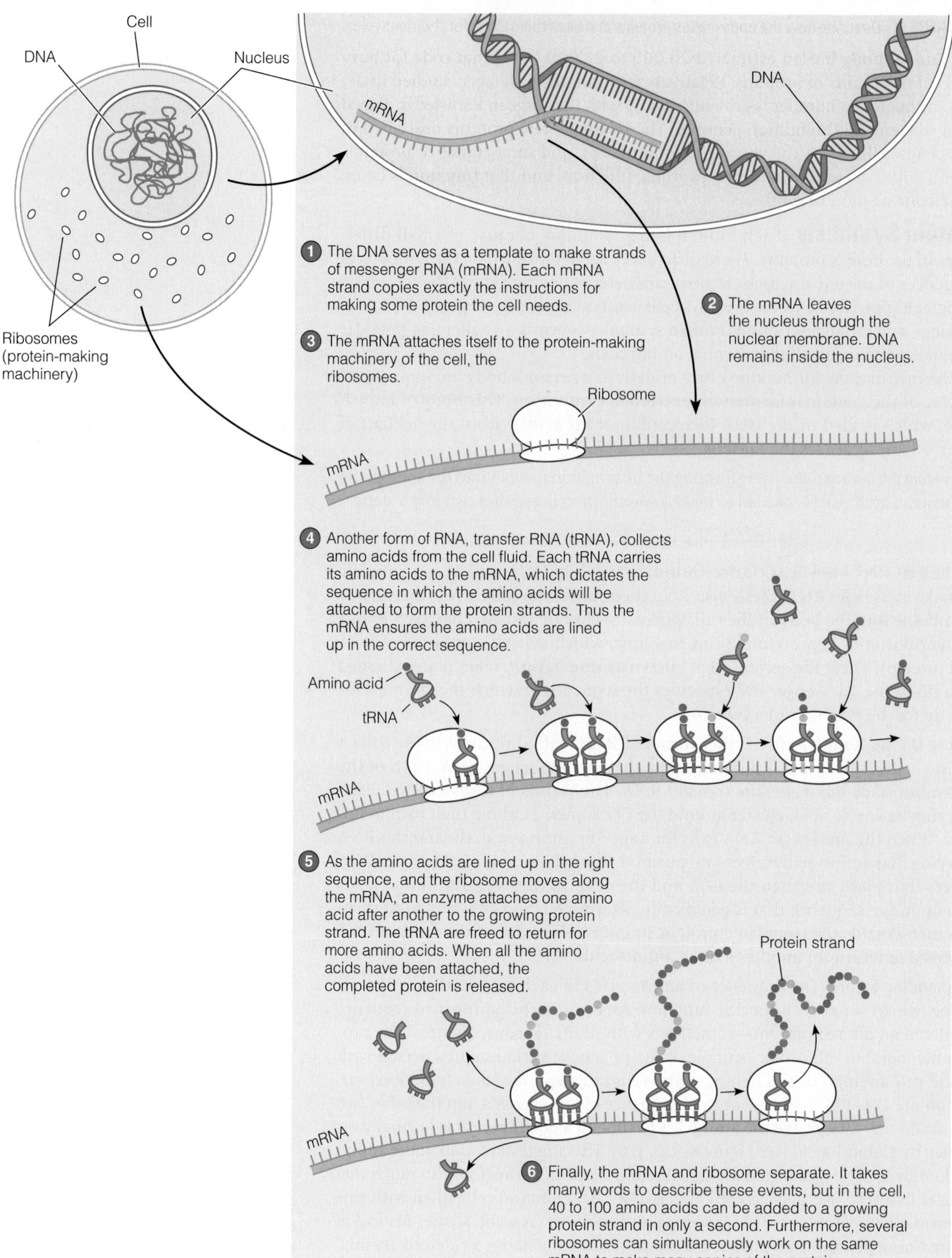

Cell
DNA
Nucleus
Ribosomes (protein-making machinery)
mRNA
DNA
1 The DNA serves as a template to make strands of messenger RNA (mRNA). Each mRNA strand copies exactly the instructions for making some protein the cell needs.
2 The mRNA leaves the nucleus through the nuclear membrane. DNA remains inside the nucleus.
3 The mRNA attaches itself to the protein-making machinery of the cell, the ribosomes.
Ribosome
mRNA
4 Another form of RNA, transfer RNA (tRNA), collects amino acids from the cell fluid. Each tRNA carries its amino acids to the mRNA, which dictates the sequence in which the amino acids will be attached to form the protein strands. Thus the mRNA ensures the amino acids are lined up in the correct sequence.
Amino acid
tRNA
mRNA
5 As the amino acids are lined up in the right sequence, and the ribosome moves along the mRNA, an enzyme attaches one amino acid after another to the growing protein strand. The tRNA are freed to return for more amino acids. When all the amino acids have been attached, the completed protein is released.
Protein strand
mRNA
6 Finally, the mRNA and ribosome separate. It takes many words to describe these events, but in the cell, 40 to 100 amino acids can be added to a growing protein strand in only a second. Furthermore, several ribosomes can simultaneously work on the same mRNA to make many copies of the protein.
© Cengage Learning

Gene Expression When a cell makes a protein as described earlier, scientists say that the gene for that protein has been "expressed." Cells can regulate **gene expression** to make the type of protein, in the amounts and at the rate, they need. Nearly all of the body's cells possess the genes for making all human proteins, but each type of cell makes only the proteins it needs. For example, cells of the pancreas express the gene for insulin; in other cells, that gene is idle. Similarly, the cells of the pancreas do not make the protein hemoglobin, which is needed only by the red blood cells.

Recent research has unveiled some of the fascinating ways nutrients regulate gene expression and protein synthesis (see Highlight 6). Because diet plays an ongoing role in our lives from conception to death, it has a major influence on gene expression and disease development. The benefits of polyunsaturated fatty acids in defending against heart disease, for example, are partially explained by their role in influencing gene expression for lipid enzymes. Later chapters provide additional examples of relationships among nutrients, genes, and disease development.

Roles of Proteins

Whenever the body is growing, repairing, or replacing tissue, proteins are involved. Sometimes their role is to facilitate or to regulate; other times it is to become part of a structure. Versatility is a key feature of proteins.

As Structural Materials From the moment of conception, proteins form the building blocks of muscles, blood, and skin—in fact, protein is the major structural component of all the body's cells. To build a bone or a tooth, for example, cells first lay down a **matrix** of the protein **collagen** and then fill it with crystals of calcium, phosphorus, magnesium, fluoride, and other minerals.

> **FIGURE 6-8 Sickle Cell Compared with Normal Red Blood Cell**

Normally, red blood cells are disc-shaped, but in the inherited disorder sickle-cell anemia, red blood cells are sickle- or crescent-shaped. This alteration in shape occurs because valine replaces glutamic acid in the amino acid sequence of two of hemoglobin's polypeptide chains. As a result of this one alteration, the hemoglobin has a diminished capacity to carry oxygen.

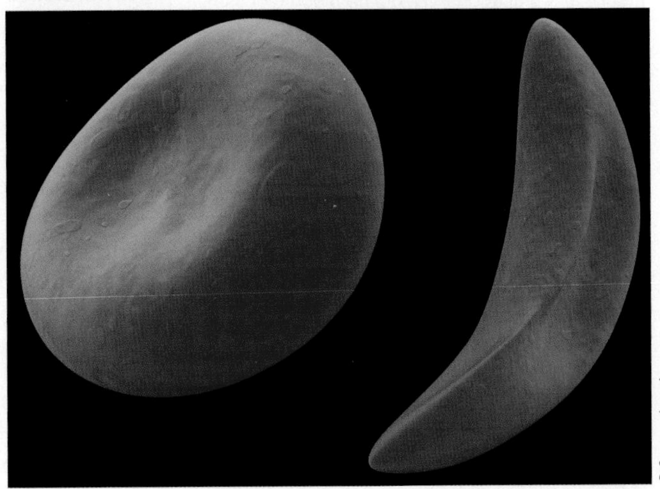

Normal red blood cell — Sickle-shaped blood cell

Amino acid sequence of normal hemoglobin:
Val—His—Leu—Thr—Pro—Glu—Glu

Amino acid sequence of sickle-cell hemoglobin:
Val—His—Leu—Thr—Pro—Val—Glu

Collagen also provides the material of ligaments and tendons and the strengthening "glue" between the cells of the artery walls that enables the arteries to withstand the pressure of the blood surging through them with each heartbeat. Also made of collagen are scars that knit the separated parts of torn tissues together.

Proteins are also needed for replacing dead or damaged cells. The average life span of a skin cell is only about 30 days. As old skin cells are shed, new cells made largely of protein grow from underneath to replace them. Cells in the deeper skin layers synthesize new proteins to form hair and fingernails. Muscle cells make new proteins to grow larger and stronger in response to exercise. Cells of the GI tract are replaced every few days. Both inside and outside, the body continuously uses protein to create new cells that replace those that have been lost.

gene expression: the process by which a cell converts the genetic code into RNA and protein.

matrix (MAY-tricks): the basic substance that gives form to a developing structure; in the body, the formative cells from which teeth and bones grow.

collagen (KOL-ah-jen): the structural protein from which connective tissues such as scars, tendons, ligaments, and the foundations of bones and teeth are made.

enzymes: proteins that facilitate chemical reactions without being changed in the process; protein catalysts.

As Enzymes Some proteins act as **enzymes.** Digestive enzymes have appeared in every chapter since Chapter 3, but digestion is only one of the many processes facilitated by enzymes. Enzymes not only break down substances, but they also build substances (such as bone) and transform one substance into another (amino acids into glucose, for example). Breaking down reactions are *catabolic,* whereas building up reactions are *anabolic.* (Chapter 7 provides more details.) Figure 6-9 diagrams a synthesis reaction.

An analogy may help to clarify the role of enzymes. Enzymes are comparable to the clergy and judges who make and dissolve marriages. When a minister marries two people, they become a couple, with a new bond between them. They are joined together—but the minister remains unchanged. The minister represents enzymes that synthesize large compounds from smaller ones. One minister can perform thousands of marriage ceremonies, just as one enzyme can expedite billions of reactions.

> **FIGURE 6-9 Enzyme Action**

Each enzyme facilitates a specific chemical reaction. In this diagram, an enzyme enables two compounds to make a more complex structure, but the enzyme itself remains unchanged.

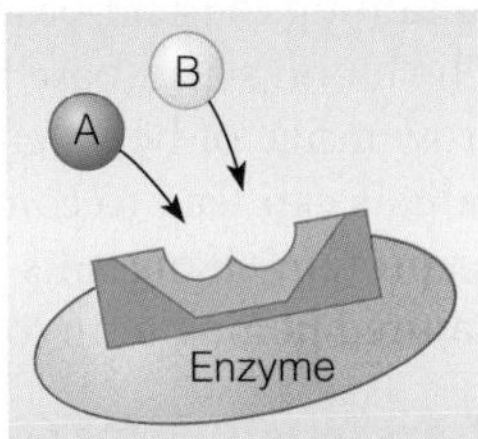

The separate compounds, A and B, are attracted to the enzyme's active site, making a reaction likely.

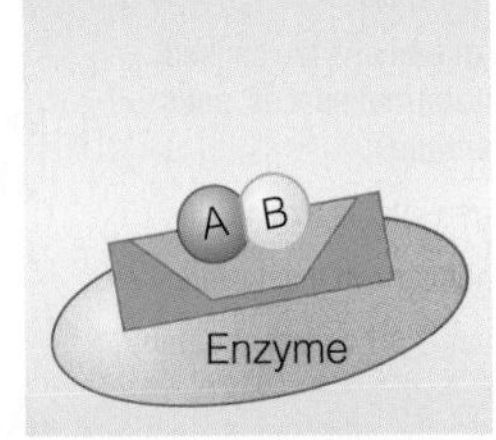

The enzyme forms a complex with A and B.

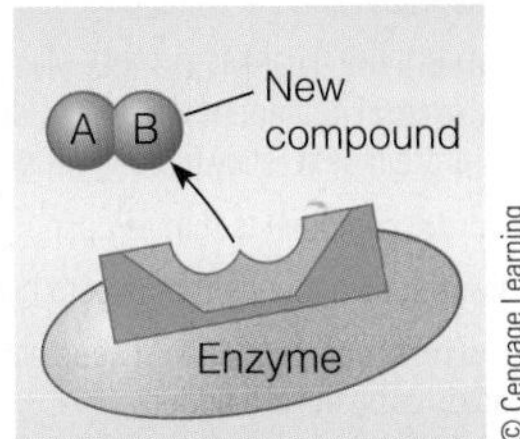

The enzyme is unchanged, but A and B have formed a new compound, AB.

TABLE 6-2 Examples of Hormones and Their Actions

Hormones	Actions
Oxytocin and prolactin	Support lactation (see Chapter 15)
Growth hormone	Promotes growth
Insulin and glucagon	Regulate blood glucose (see Chapter 4)
Thyroxin	Regulates the body's metabolic rate (see Chapter 8)
Calcitonin and parathyroid hormone	Regulate blood calcium (see Chapter 12)
Angiotensin, renin, and antidiuretic hormone	Regulate fluid and electrolyte balance (see Chapter 12)

Similarly, a judge who lets married couples separate may decree many divorces before retiring. The judge represents enzymes that hydrolyze larger compounds to smaller ones; for example, the digestive enzymes. The point is that, like the minister and the judge, enzymes themselves are not altered by the reactions they facilitate. They are catalysts, permitting reactions to occur more quickly and efficiently than if substances depended on chance encounters alone.

As Hormones The body's many hormones are messenger molecules, and *some* hormones are proteins. (Recall from Chapter 5 that some hormones, such as estrogen and testosterone, are made from the lipid cholesterol.) Various endocrine glands in the body release hormones in response to changes that challenge the body. The blood carries the hormones from these glands to their target tissues, where they elicit the appropriate responses to restore and maintain normal conditions.

The hormone insulin provides a familiar example. After a meal, when blood glucose rises, the pancreas releases insulin. Insulin stimulates the transport proteins of the muscles and adipose tissue to pump glucose into the cells faster than it can leak out. After acting on the message, the cells destroy the insulin. As blood glucose falls, the pancreas slows its release of insulin. Many other proteins act as hormones, regulating a variety of actions in the body (see Table 6-2 for examples).

As Regulators of Fluid Balance Proteins help to maintain the body's **fluid balance.** Normally, proteins are found primarily within the cells and in the plasma (essentially blood without its red blood cells). Being large, proteins do not normally cross the walls of the blood vessels. During times of critical illness or protein malnutrition, however, plasma proteins leak out of the blood vessels into the spaces between the cells. Because proteins attract water, fluid accumulates and causes swelling. Swelling due to an excess of fluid in the tissues is known as **edema.** The protein-related causes of edema include:

- Excessive protein losses caused by inflammation and critical illnesses
- Inadequate protein synthesis caused by liver disease
- Inadequate dietary intake of protein

Whatever the cause of edema, the result is the same: a diminished capacity to deliver nutrients and oxygen to the cells and to remove wastes from them. As a consequence, cells fail to function adequately.

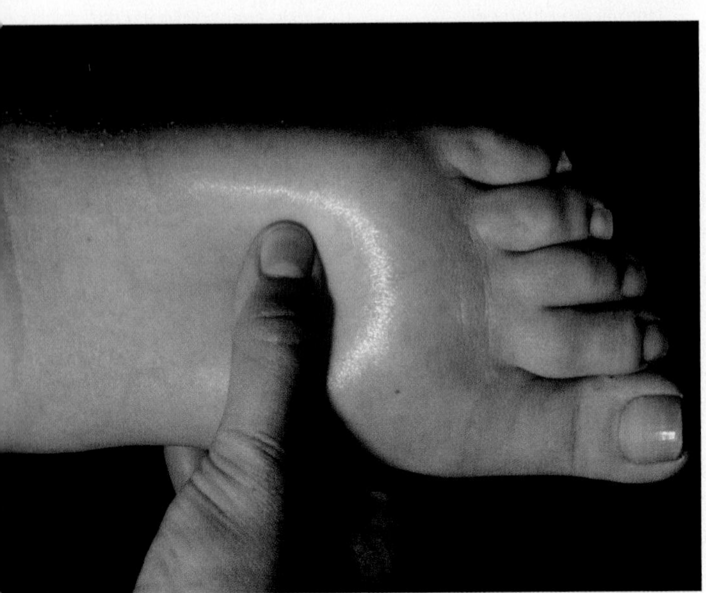

In critical illness and protein malnutrition, blood vessels become "leaky" and allow plasma proteins to move into the tissues. Because proteins attract water, the tissues swell, causing edema.

As Acid-Base Regulators Proteins also help to maintain the balance between **acids** and **bases** within the body fluids. Normal body processes continuously produce acids and bases, which the blood carries to the kidneys and lungs for excretion. The challenge is to maintain acid-base balance as conditions continually change.

An acid solution contains an abundance of hydrogen ions (H^+); the greater the concentration of hydrogen ions, the more acidic the solution and the lower the pH. Proteins, which have negative charges on their surfaces, attract hydrogen ions, which have positive charges. By accepting and releasing hydrogen ions, proteins act as **buffers,** maintaining the acid-base balance of the blood and body fluids.

The blood's acid-base balance is tightly controlled to maintain pH within the narrow range of between 7.35 and 7.45. Outside this range, either **acidosis** or **alkalosis** can lead to coma and death, largely by denaturing proteins. Denaturing a protein changes its shape and renders it useless. To give just one example, denatured hemoglobin loses its capacity to carry oxygen.

As Transporters Some proteins move about in the body fluids, carrying nutrients and other molecules. The protein hemoglobin carries oxygen from the lungs to the cells. The lipoproteins transport lipids around the body. Special transport proteins carry vitamins and minerals.

fluid balance: maintenance of the proper types and amounts of fluid in each compartment of the body fluids (see also Chapter 12).

edema (eh-DEEM-uh): the swelling of body tissue caused by excessive amounts of fluid in the interstitial spaces; seen in protein deficiency (among other conditions).

acids: compounds that release hydrogen ions in a solution.

bases: compounds that accept hydrogen ions in a solution.

buffers: compounds that keep a solution's pH constant when acids or bases are added.

acidosis (assi-DOE-sis): higher-than-normal acidity in the blood and body fluids.

alkalosis (alka-LOE-sis): higher-than-normal alkalinity (base) in the blood and body fluids.

The transport of the mineral iron provides an especially good illustration of these proteins' specificity and precision. When iron is absorbed, it is captured in an intestinal cell by a protein. Before leaving the intestinal cell, iron is attached to another protein that carries it through the bloodstream to the cells. Once iron enters a cell, it is attached to a storage protein that will hold the iron until it is needed. When it is needed, iron is incorporated into proteins in the red blood cells and muscles that assist in oxygen transport and use. (Chapter 13 provides more details on how these protein carriers transport and store iron.)

Some transport proteins reside in cell membranes and act as "pumps," picking up compounds on one side of the membrane and releasing them on the other as needed. Each transport protein is specific for a certain compound or group of related compounds. Figure 6-10 illustrates how a membrane-bound transport protein helps to maintain the sodium and potassium concentrations in the fluids inside and outside cells. The balance of these two minerals is critical to nerve transmissions and muscle contractions; imbalances can cause irregular heartbeats, muscular weakness, kidney failure, and even death.

As Antibodies Proteins also defend the body against disease. A virus—whether it is one that causes flu, smallpox, measles, or the common cold—enters the cells and multiplies there. One virus may produce 100 replicas of itself within an hour or so. Each replica can then burst out and invade 100 different cells, soon yielding 10,000 viruses, which invade 10,000 cells. Left free to do their worst, they will soon overwhelm the body with disease.

Fortunately, when the body detects these invading **antigens,** it manufactures **antibodies,** giant protein molecules designed specifically to combat them. The antibodies work so swiftly and efficiently that in a healthy individual, most diseases never get started. Without sufficient protein, though, the body cannot maintain its army of antibodies to resist infectious diseases.

Each antibody is designed to destroy a specific antigen. Once the body has manufactured antibodies against a particular antigen (such as the measles virus), it "remembers" how to make them. Consequently, the next time the body encounters that same antigen, it produces antibodies even more quickly. In other words, the body develops a molecular memory, known as **immunity.** (Chapter 16 describes food allergies—the immune system's response to food antigens.)

As a Source of Energy and Glucose Without energy, cells die; without glucose, the brain and nervous system falter. Even though proteins are needed to do the

antigens: substances that elicit the formation of antibodies or an inflammation reaction from the immune system. A bacterium, a virus, a toxin, and a protein in food that causes allergy are all examples of antigens.

antibodies: large proteins of the blood and body fluids, produced by the immune system in response to the invasion of the body by foreign molecules (usually proteins called *antigens*). Antibodies combine with and inactivate the foreign invaders, thus protecting the body.

immunity: the body's ability to defend itself against diseases (see also Chapter 18).

> FIGURE 6-10 **An Example of a Transport Protein**

This transport protein resides within a cell membrane and acts as a two-door passageway. Molecules enter on one side of the membrane and exit on the other, but the protein doesn't leave the membrane. This example shows how the transport protein moves sodium and potassium in opposite directions across the membrane to maintain a high concentration of potassium and a low concentration of sodium within the cell. This active transport system requires energy.

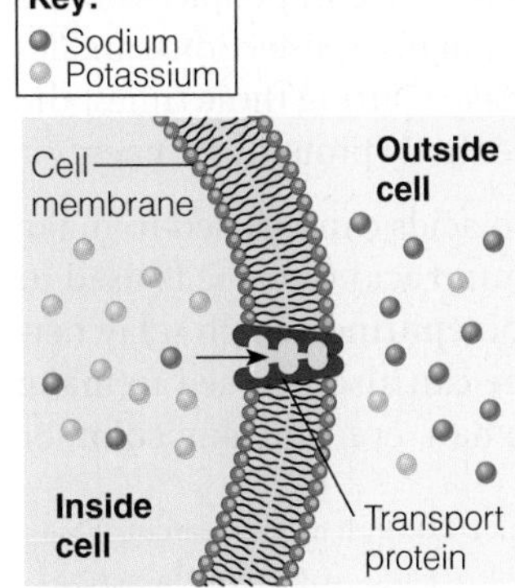

The transport protein picks up sodium from inside the cell.

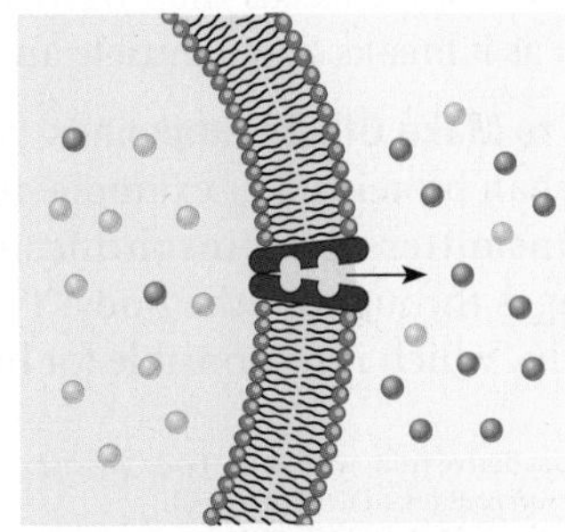

The protein changes shape and releases sodium outside the cell.

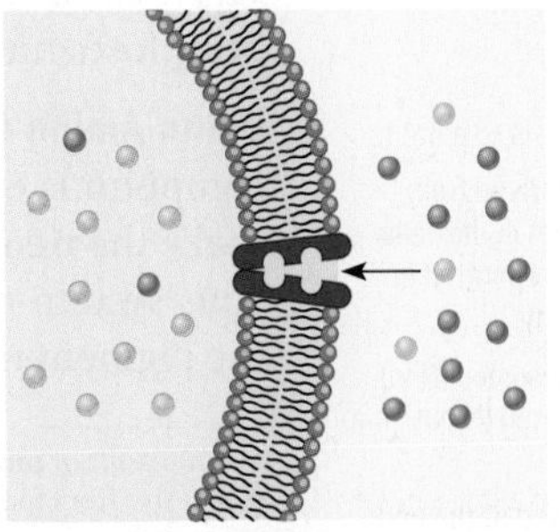

The transport protein picks up potassium from outside the cell.

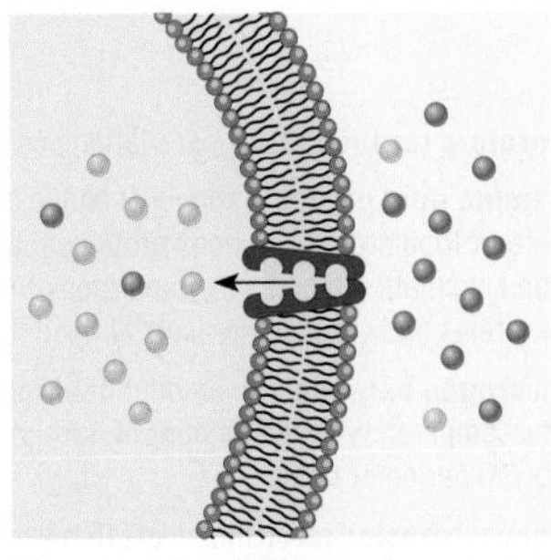

The protein changes shape and releases potassium inside the cell.

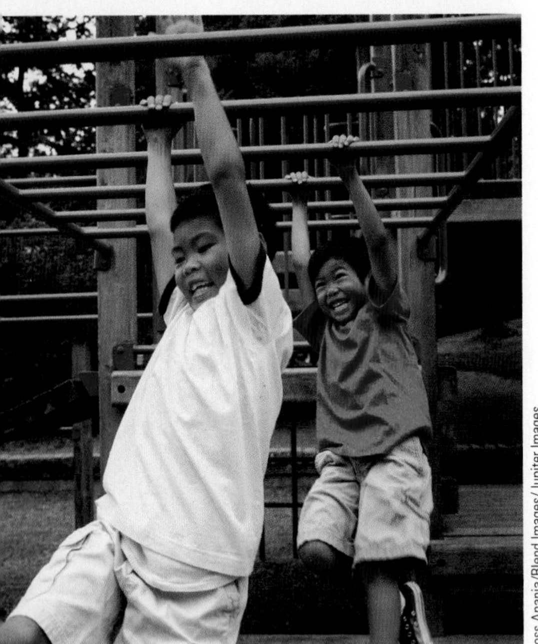
Ross Anania/Blend Images/Jupiter Images

Growing children end each day with more bone, blood, muscle, and skin cells than they had at the beginning of the day.

work that only they can perform, they will be sacrificed to provide energy and glucose during times of starvation or insufficient carbohydrate intake. The body will break down its tissue proteins to make amino acids available for energy or glucose production (a process known as *gluconeogenesis*). In this way, protein can maintain blood glucose levels, but at the expense of losing lean body tissue. Chapter 7 provides many more details on energy metabolism.

Other Roles As mentioned earlier, proteins form integral parts of most body structures such as skin, muscles, and bones. They also participate in some of the body's most amazing activities such as blood clotting and vision. When a tissue is injured, a rapid chain of events leads to the production of fibrin, a stringy, insoluble mass of protein fibers that forms a solid clot from liquid blood. Later, more slowly, the protein collagen forms a scar to replace the clot and permanently heal the wound. The light-sensitive pigments in the cells of the eye's retina are molecules of the protein opsin. Opsin responds to light by changing its shape, thus initiating the nerve impulses that convey the sense of sight to the brain.

The amino acids are as versatile as the proteins. In addition to serving as building blocks for proteins in the body, amino acids have multiple roles in regulating pathways that support growth, reproduction, metabolism, and immunity.

A Preview of Protein Metabolism

This section previews protein metabolism; Chapter 7 provides a full description. Cells have several metabolic options, depending on their protein and energy needs.

Protein Turnover and the Amino Acid Pool Within each cell, proteins are continually being made and broken down, a process known as **protein turnover.** Protein breakdown releases amino acids. These amino acids mix with amino acids from dietary protein to form an **"amino acid pool"** within the cells and circulating blood.* The rate of protein degradation and the amount of protein intake may vary, but the pattern of amino acids within the pool remains fairly constant. Regardless of their source, any of these amino acids can be used to make body proteins or other nitrogen-containing compounds, or they can be stripped of their nitrogen and used for energy (either immediately or stored as fat for later use).

Nitrogen Balance Protein turnover and **nitrogen balance** go hand in hand. In healthy adults, protein synthesis balances with degradation, and protein intake from food balances with nitrogen excretion in the urine, feces, and sweat. When nitrogen intake equals nitrogen output, the person is in nitrogen equilibrium, or zero nitrogen balance. Researchers use nitrogen balance studies to estimate protein requirements.**

If the body synthesizes more than it degrades, then protein is added and nitrogen status becomes positive. Nitrogen status is positive in growing infants, children, adolescents, pregnant women, and people recovering from protein deficiency or illness; their nitrogen intake exceeds their nitrogen excretion. They are retaining protein in new tissues as they add blood, bone, skin, and muscle cells to their bodies.

If the body degrades more than it synthesizes, then protein is being lost and nitrogen status becomes negative. Nitrogen status is negative in people who are starving or suffering other severe stresses such as burns, injuries, infections, and fever; their nitrogen excretion exceeds their nitrogen intake. During these times, the body loses nitrogen as it breaks down muscle and other body proteins for energy.

Using Amino Acids to Make Other Compounds Amino acids can be used to make compounds other than proteins. For example, the amino acid tyrosine is used to make the **neurotransmitters** norepinephrine and epinephrine, which relay nervous system messages throughout the body. Tyrosine can also be used to make the pigment melanin, which is responsible for brown hair, eye, and skin color, or

protein turnover: the degradation and synthesis of protein.

amino acid pool: the supply of amino acids derived from either food proteins or body proteins that collect in the cells and circulating blood and stand ready to be incorporated in proteins and other compounds or used for energy.

nitrogen balance: the amount of nitrogen consumed (N in) as compared with the amount of nitrogen excreted (N out) in a given period of time.

neurotransmitters: chemicals that are released at the end of a nerve cell when a nerve impulse arrives there. They diffuse across the gap to the next cell and alter the membrane of that second cell to either inhibit or excite it.

*Amino acids or proteins that derive from within the body are *endogenous* (en-DODGE-eh-nus). In contrast, those that derive from foods are *exogenous* (eks-ODGE-eh-nus).

**The genetic materials DNA and RNA contain nitrogen, but the quantity is insignificant compared with the amount in protein. Protein is 16 percent nitrogen. Said another way, the average protein weighs about 6.25 times as much as the nitrogen it contains, so scientists can estimate the amount of protein in a sample of food, body tissue, or other material by multiplying the weight of the nitrogen in it by 6.25.

the hormone thyroxine, which helps to regulate the metabolic rate. For another example, the amino acid tryptophan serves as a precursor for the vitamin niacin and for **serotonin,** a neurotransmitter important in sleep regulation, appetite control, and sensory perception.

Using Amino Acids for Energy and Glucose As mentioned earlier, when glucose or fatty acids are limited, cells are forced to use amino acids for energy and glucose. The body does not have a specialized storage site for protein as it does for carbohydrate and fat. Recall that glucose is stored as glycogen in the liver and fat as triglycerides in adipose tissue, but protein is not stored as such. When the need arises, the body breaks down its working and structural proteins and uses the amino acids for energy or glucose. Thus, over time, energy deprivation (fasting or starvation) always causes wasting of lean body tissue as well as fat loss. An adequate supply of carbohydrates and fats spares amino acids from being used for energy and allows proteins to perform their unique roles.

Using Amino Acids to Make Fat Amino acids may be converted to fat when energy and protein intakes exceed needs and carbohydrate intake is adequate. In this way, protein-rich foods can contribute to weight gain.

Deaminating Amino Acids When amino acids are broken down (as occurs when they are used for energy or to make glucose or fat), they are first deaminated—stripped of their nitrogen-containing amino groups (see Figure 6-11). Two products result from **deamination:** one is **ammonia** (NH_3); the other product is the carbon structure without its amino group—often a **keto acid.** Keto acids may enter a number of metabolic pathways—for example, they may be used for energy or for the production of glucose, ketones, cholesterol, or fat.* They may also be used to make nonessential amino acids.

Using Amino Acids to Make Proteins and Nonessential Amino Acids As mentioned, cells can assemble amino acids into the proteins they need to do their work. If an essential amino acid is missing, the body may break down some of its own proteins to obtain it. If a particular nonessential amino acid is not readily available, cells can make it from a keto acid—if a nitrogen source is available. Cells can also make a nonessential amino acid by transferring an amino group from one amino acid to its corresponding keto acid, as shown in Figure 6-12. Through many such **transamination** reactions, involving many different keto acids, the liver cells can synthesize the nonessential amino acids.

Converting Ammonia to Urea As mentioned earlier, deamination produces ammonia. Ammonia is a toxic compound chemically identical to the strong-smelling ammonia in bottled cleaning solutions. Because ammonia is a base, excessive

> **FIGURE 6-11 Deamination and Synthesis of a Nonessential Amino Acid**

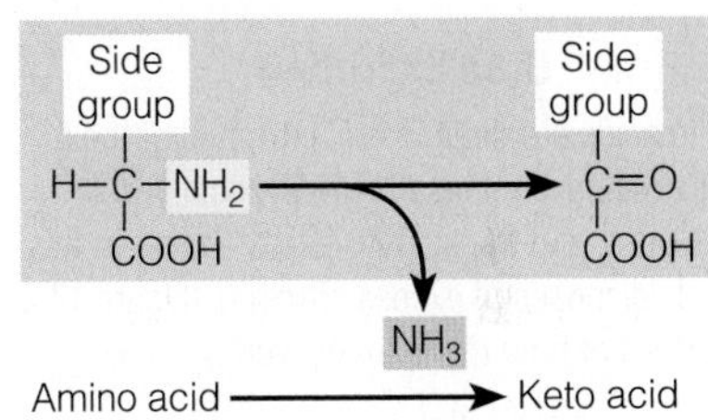

The deamination of an amino acid produces ammonia (NH_3) and a keto acid.

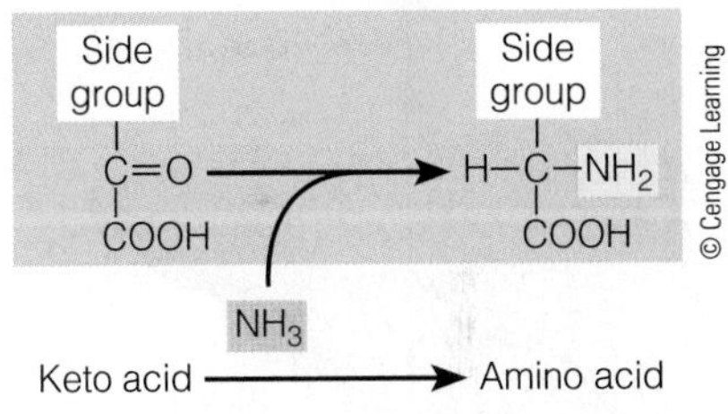

Given a source of NH_3, the body can make nonessential amino acids from keto acids.

> **FIGURE 6-12 Transamination and Synthesis of a Nonessential Amino Acid**

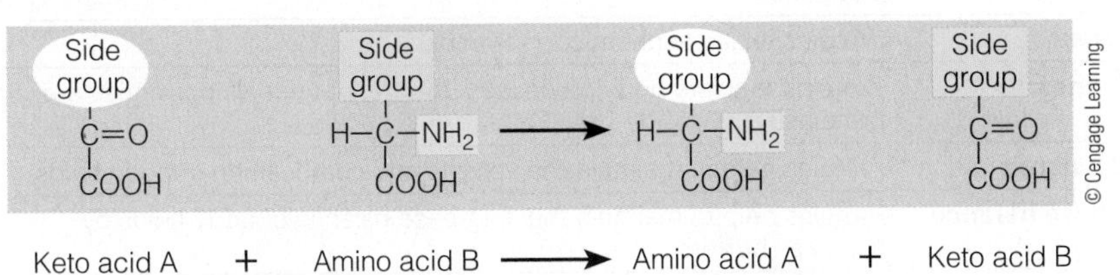

The body can transfer amino groups (NH_2) from an amino acid to a keto acid, forming a new *nonessential* amino acid and a new keto acid. Transamination reactions require the vitamin B_6 coenzyme.

*Chemists sometimes classify amino acids according to the destinations of their carbon fragments after deamination. If the fragment leads to the production of glucose, the amino acid is called *glucogenic;* if it leads to the formation of ketone bodies, fats, and sterols, the amino acid is called *ketogenic*. There is no sharp distinction between glucogenic and ketogenic amino acids, however. A few are both, most are considered glucogenic, only leucine and lysine are clearly ketogenic.

serotonin (SER-oh-TONE-in): a neurotransmitter important in sleep regulation, appetite control, and sensory perception, among other roles. Serotonin is synthesized in the body from the amino acid tryptophan with the help of vitamin B_6.

deamination (dee-AM-ih-NAY-shun): removal of the amino (NH_2) group from a compound such as an amino acid.

ammonia: a compound with the chemical formula NH_3, produced during the deamination of amino acids.

keto (KEY-toe) **acid:** an organic acid that contains a carbonyl group (C=O).

transamination (TRANS-am-ih-NAY-shun): the transfer of an amino group from one amino acid to a keto acid, producing a new nonessential amino acid and a new keto acid.

> **FIGURE 6-13 Urea Synthesis**

Ammonia is produced when amino acids are deaminated. The liver detoxifies ammonia by combining it with another waste product, carbon dioxide, to produce urea. See Appendix C for details.

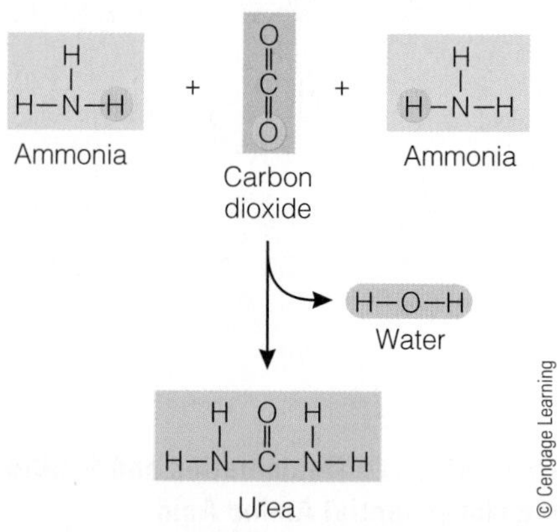

> **FIGURE 6-14 Urea Excretion**

When amino acids are deaminated (stripped of their nitrogen), ammonia is released. The liver converts ammonia to urea, and the kidneys excrete urea. In this way the body disposes of excess nitrogen. (Figure 12-2 provides details of how the kidneys work.)

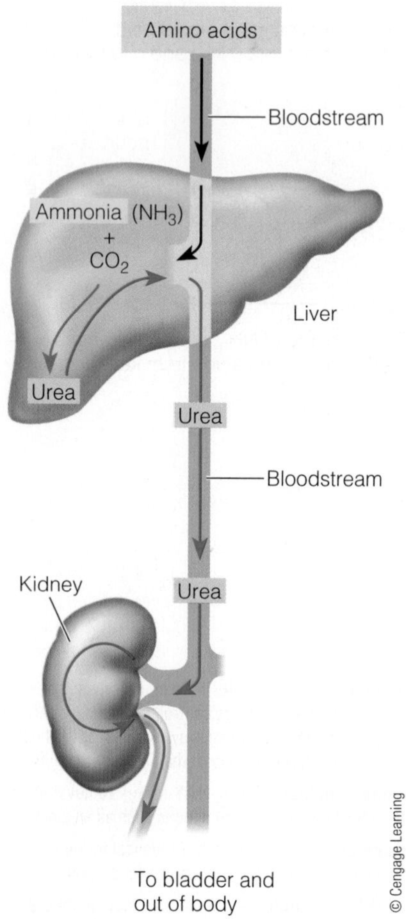

urea (you-REE-uh): the principal nitrogen-excretion product of protein metabolism. Two ammonia fragments are combined with carbon dioxide to form urea.

quantities upset the blood's critical acid-base balance. To prevent such a crisis, the liver combines ammonia with carbon dioxide to make **urea,** a much less toxic compound. Figure 6-13 provides a greatly oversimplified diagram of urea synthesis; details are shown in Appendix C. The production of urea increases as dietary protein increases, until production hits its maximum rate at intakes approaching 250 grams of protein per day. (For perspective, the average daily intake of protein in the United States is 80 grams.[2])

Excreting Urea Liver cells release urea into the blood, where it circulates until it passes through the kidneys (see Figure 6-14). The kidneys then filter urea out of the blood for excretion in the urine. Normally, the liver efficiently captures all the ammonia, makes urea from it, and releases the urea into the blood; then the kidneys clear all the urea from the blood. This division of labor allows easy diagnosis of diseases of both organs. In liver disease, blood ammonia is high; in kidney disease, blood urea is high.

Urea is the body's principal vehicle for excreting unused nitrogen, and the amount of urea produced increases with protein intake. To keep urea in solution, the body needs water. For this reason, a person who regularly consumes a high-protein diet (say, 100 grams a day or more) must drink plenty of water to dilute and excrete urea from the body. Without extra water, a person on a high-protein diet risks dehydration because the body uses its water to rid itself of urea. This explains some of the water loss that accompanies high-protein diets. Such losses may make high-protein diets *appear* to be effective, but water loss, of course, is of no value to the person who wants to lose body fat (as Highlight 9 explains).

› REVIEW IT Describe how the body makes proteins and uses them to perform various roles.

Cells synthesize proteins according to genetic information that dictates the sequence in which amino acids are linked together. Each protein plays a specific role. Table 6-3 summarizes some of the many roles proteins play and conveys a sense of the immense variety and importance of proteins in the body. Proteins are constantly being synthesized and broken down as needed. The body's assimilation of amino acids into proteins and its release of amino acids via protein breakdown and excretion can be tracked by measuring nitrogen balance, which should be positive during growth and steady in adulthood. An energy deficit or an inadequate protein intake may force the body to use amino acids as fuel, creating a negative nitrogen balance. Protein eaten in excess of need is broken down and stored as body fat.

TABLE 6-3 Protein Functions in the Body

Structural materials	Proteins form integral parts of most body tissues and provide strength and shape to skin, tendons, membranes, muscles, organs, and bones.
Enzymes	Proteins facilitate chemical reactions.
Hormones	Proteins regulate body processes. (Some, but not all, hormones are proteins.)
Fluid balance	Proteins help to maintain the volume and composition of body fluids.
Acid-base balance	Proteins help to maintain the acid-base balance of body fluids by acting as buffers.
Transportation	Proteins transport substances, such as lipids, vitamins, minerals, and oxygen, around the body.
Antibodies	Proteins inactivate foreign invaders, thus protecting the body against diseases.
Energy and glucose	Proteins provide some fuel, and glucose if needed, for the body's energy needs.
Other	The protein fibrin creates blood clots; the protein collagen forms scars; the protein opsin participates in vision.

© Cengage Learning

6.4 Protein in Foods

› LEARN IT Explain the differences between high-quality and low-quality proteins, including notable food sources of each.

In the United States and other countries where nutritious foods are abundant, most people eat protein in such large quantities that they receive all the amino acids they need. In countries where food is scarce and the people eat only marginal amounts of protein-rich foods, however, the *quality* of the protein becomes crucial.

Protein Quality

The protein quality of the diet determines, in large part, how well children grow and how well adults maintain their health. Put simply, **high-quality proteins** provide enough of all the essential amino acids needed to support the body's work, and low-quality proteins don't. Two factors influence protein quality—the protein's digestibility and its amino acid composition.

Digestibility As explained earlier, proteins must be digested before they can provide amino acids. **Protein digestibility** depends on such factors as the protein's source and the other foods eaten with it. The digestibility of most animal proteins is high (90 to 99 percent); plant proteins are less digestible (70 to 90 percent for most, but more than 90 percent for soy and other legumes).

Amino Acid Composition To make proteins, a cell must have all the needed amino acids available simultaneously. The liver can make any nonessential amino acid that may be in short supply so that the cells can continue linking amino acids into protein strands. If an essential amino acid is missing, though, a cell must dismantle its own proteins to obtain it. Therefore, to prevent protein breakdown in the body, dietary protein must supply at least the nine essential amino acids plus enough nitrogen-containing amino groups and energy for the synthesis of the nonessential ones. If the diet supplies too little of any essential amino acid, protein synthesis will be limited. The body makes whole proteins only; if one amino acid is missing, the others cannot form a "partial" protein. An essential amino acid supplied in less than the amount needed to support protein synthesis is called a **limiting amino acid.**

Reference Protein The quality of a food protein is determined by comparing its amino acid composition with the essential amino acid requirements of preschool-age children. Such a standard is called a **reference protein.** The rationale behind using the requirements of this age group is that if a protein will effectively support a young child's growth and development, then it will meet or exceed the requirements of older children and adults.

High-Quality Proteins As mentioned earlier, a high-quality protein contains all the essential amino acids in relatively the same amounts and proportions that human beings require; it may or may not contain all the nonessential amino acids. Proteins that are low in an essential amino acid cannot, by themselves, support protein synthesis. Generally, foods derived from animals (meat, seafood, poultry, eggs, and milk and milk products) provide high-quality proteins, although gelatin is an exception. Gelatin lacks tryptophan and cannot support growth and health as a diet's sole protein. Proteins from plants (vegetables, nuts, seeds, grains, and legumes) have more diverse amino acid patterns and tend to be limiting in one or more essential amino acids. Some plant proteins are notoriously low quality (for example, corn protein). A few others are high quality (for example, soy protein).

Researchers have developed several methods for evaluating the quality of food proteins and identifying high-quality proteins. Appendix D provides details.

Complementary Proteins

In general, plant proteins are lower quality than animal proteins, and plants also offer less protein (per weight or measure of food). For this reason, many vegetarians improve the quality of proteins in their diets by combining plant-protein foods that have different but complementary amino acid

high-quality proteins: dietary proteins containing all the essential amino acids in relatively the same amounts that human beings require. They may also contain nonessential amino acids.

protein digestibility: a measure of the amount of amino acids absorbed from a given protein intake.

limiting amino acid: the essential amino acid found in the shortest supply relative to the amounts needed for protein synthesis in the body. Four amino acids are most likely to be limiting:

- Lysine
- Methionine
- Threonine
- Tryptophan

reference protein: a standard against which to measure the quality of other proteins.

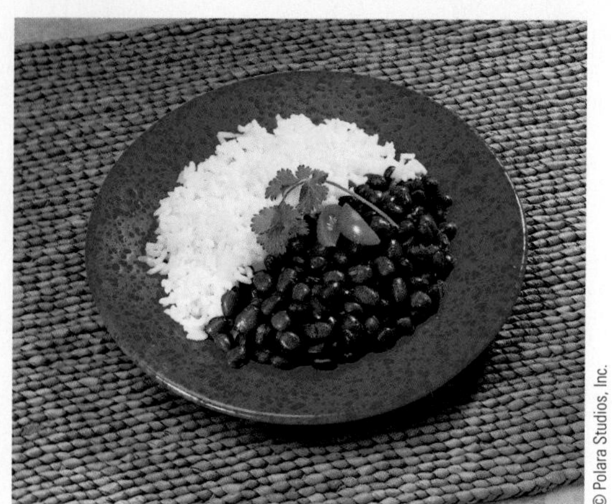

© Polara Studios, Inc.

Black beans and rice, a favorite Hispanic combination, together provide a balanced array of amino acids.

> **FIGURE 6-15 Complementary Proteins**

In general, legumes provide plenty of isoleucine (Ile) and lysine (Lys) but fall short in methionine (Met) and tryptophan (Trp). Grains have the opposite strengths and weaknesses, making them a perfect match for legumes.

	Ile	Lys	Met	Trp
Legumes	✓	✓		
Grains			✓	✓
Together	✓	✓	✓	✓

© Cengage Learning

patterns. This strategy yields **complementary proteins** that together contain all the essential amino acids in quantities sufficient to support health. The protein quality of the combination is greater than either food alone (see Figure 6-15).

Some people have long believed that combining plant proteins at every meal is critical to protein nutrition. For most healthy vegetarians, though, it is *not* necessary to balance amino acids at each meal if protein intake is varied and energy intake is sufficient.[3] Vegetarians can receive all the amino acids they need over the course of a day by eating a variety of whole grains, legumes, seeds, nuts, and vegetables. Protein deficiency will develop, however, when fruits and certain vegetables make up the core of the diet, severely limiting both the *quantity* and *quality* of protein. Highlight 2 describes how to plan a nutritious vegetarian diet.

> **REVIEW IT** Explain the differences between high-quality and low-quality proteins, including notable food sources of each.

A diet that supplies all of the essential amino acids in adequate amounts ensures protein synthesis. The best guarantee of amino acid adequacy is to eat foods containing high-quality proteins or mixtures of foods containing complementary proteins that can each supply the amino acids missing in the other. In addition to its amino acid content, the quality of protein is measured by its digestibility and its ability to support growth. Such measures are of great importance in dealing with malnutrition worldwide, but in countries where protein deficiency is not common, the protein quality of individual foods deserves little emphasis.

6.5 Health Effects and Recommended Intakes of Protein

> **LEARN IT** Identify the health benefits of, and recommendations for, protein.

As you know by now, protein is indispensable to life. This section examines the health effects and recommended intakes of protein.

Health Effects of Protein It should come as no surprise that protein deficiency can have devastating effects on people's health. But like the other nutrients, protein in excess can also be harmful. High-protein diets have been implicated in several chronic diseases, including heart disease, cancer, osteoporosis, obesity, and kidney stones, but evidence is insufficient to establish an Upper Level (UL).[4]

Protein Deficiency Protein deficiency develops when the diet consistently supplies too little protein or lacks essential amino acids. When this occurs, the synthesis of body proteins decreases and degradation increases to provide cells with the amino acids they need. Without proteins to perform their critical roles, many of the body's activities come to a halt. The consequences of protein deficiency include slowed growth, impaired brain and kidney functions, poor immunity, and inadequate nutrient absorption.

The term *protein-energy malnutrition* has traditionally been used to describe the condition that develops when the diet delivers too little protein, too little energy, or both. The causes and consequences are complex, but clearly, such malnutrition reflects insufficient food intake. Importantly, not only are protein and energy inadequate, but so are many, if not all, of the vitamins and minerals. For this reason, severe malnutrition and its clinical forms—marasmus and kwashiorkor—are included in Chapter 20's discussion of world hunger.

Heart Disease In the United States and other developed countries, protein is so abundant that problems of excess are more common than deficiency. Depending on the food source, a high-protein diet may contribute to the progression of heart disease. As Chapter 5 mentions, foods rich in animal protein also tend to be rich in saturated fats. Consequently, it is not surprising to find a correlation between animal-protein intake (red meats and milk products) and heart disease.[5] On the other hand, substituting vegetable protein (legumes and nuts) for animal protein

complementary proteins: two or more dietary proteins whose amino acid assortments complement each other in such a way that the essential amino acids missing from one are supplied by the other.

and using low-fat milk, poultry, and fish may improve blood pressure and blood lipids and decrease heart disease mortality.[6]

Many observational studies suggest that elevated levels of the amino acid homocysteine may be an independent risk factor for heart disease, heart attacks, and sudden death in patients with heart disease; findings from prospective studies, however, are far less conclusive.[7] Researchers do not yet fully understand the many factors—including a diet high in saturated fatty acids—that can raise homocysteine in the blood or whether elevated levels are a cause or an effect of heart disease.[8] Elevated homocysteine is associated with increased oxidative stress and inflammation.[9] Until researchers can determine the exact role homocysteine plays in heart disease, they are following several leads in pursuit of the answers. Coffee's role in heart disease has been controversial, but research suggests it is among the most influential factors in raising homocysteine, which may explain some of the adverse health effects of heavy consumption. Elevated homocysteine levels are among the many adverse health consequences of smoking cigarettes and drinking alcohol as well. Homocysteine is also elevated with inadequate intakes of B vitamins and can usually be lowered with fortified foods or supplements of vitamin B_{12}, vitamin B_6, and folate.[10] Lowering homocysteine, however, may not help in lowering risks or preventing heart attacks.[11] Supplements of the B vitamins do not always benefit those with heart disease and, in fact, may actually increase risks.[12]

In contrast to homocysteine, the amino acid arginine may help protect against heart disease by lowering blood pressure and homocysteine levels.[13] Additional research is needed to confirm the benefits of arginine. In the meantime, it is unwise for consumers to use supplements of arginine, or any other amino acid for that matter (as pp. 190–191 explain). Physicians, however, may consider the benefits of adding arginine supplements to their heart patients' treatment plan.

Cancer Protein does not seem to increase the risk of cancer, but some protein-rich foods do. For example, evidence suggests a correlation between high intakes of red meat and processed meats with cancer of the colon, pancreas, and ovaries.[14]* In contrast, protein-rich legumes, fish, and milk may lower the risk of some cancers. Chapter 18 discusses dietary links with cancer, and Chapter 19 presents food safety issues of processed meats and their additives.

Adult Bone Loss (Osteoporosis) Chapter 12 presents calcium metabolism, and Highlight 12 elaborates on the main factors that influence osteoporosis. This section briefly describes the relationships between protein intake and bone loss. When protein intake is high, calcium excretion increases. Whether excess protein depletes the bones of their chief mineral may depend upon the ratio of calcium intake to protein intake. After all, bones need both protein and calcium. An ideal ratio has not been determined, but a young woman whose intake meets recommendations for both nutrients has a calcium-to-protein ratio of more than 20 to 1 (milligrams to grams), which probably provides adequate protection for the bones. For most women in the United States, however, average calcium intakes are lower and protein intakes are higher, yielding a 13-to-1 ratio, which may produce calcium losses significant enough to compromise bone health. In other words, the problem may reflect too little calcium, not too much protein. In establishing recommendations, the DRI Committee considered protein's effect on calcium metabolism and bone health, but it did not find sufficient evidence to warrant an adjustment for calcium or a UL for protein.[15]

Importantly, adequate protein does not harm bones and may even improve bone mineral density, whereas *inadequate* intakes of protein may compromise bone health.[16] Osteoporosis is particularly common in elderly women and in adolescents with anorexia nervosa—groups who typically receive less protein than they need. For these people, a high-protein diet may be just what they need to protect their bones.[17]

---

*Processed meats include ham, bacon, pastrami, salami, sausage, bratwurst, and hot dogs that have been preserved by smoking, curing, salting, or adding preservatives.

Weight Control Research on the associations between protein intake and body weight has revealed some interesting, although often inconsistent, findings. One study suggests that inconsistent findings may reflect differences between animal and vegetable proteins, with animal proteins having a positive association with overweight and vegetable proteins having a negative one.[18] Another study examined people who were deliberately overfed by 1000 kcalories daily.[19] Not too surprisingly, they all gained weight, but those receiving a low-protein diet gained about half as much weight as those receiving an adequate- or high-protein diet. A look at their body composition revealed that the low-protein group stored almost all their excess kcalories as fat and lost a little lean body tissue. By comparison, the other protein groups stored about half the excess kcalories as fat and gained lean body tissue. Importantly, the excess kcalories increased total body fat similarly for all groups; the different amounts of dietary protein affected changes in lean body mass.[20] These findings highlight the importance of distinguishing between body weight and body fat—a point revisited in Chapters 8 and 9.

Fad weight-loss diets that encourage a high-protein, low-carbohydrate diet may be effective, but only because they are low-kcalorie diets. Diets that provide adequate protein (at least 65 to 70 grams a day), moderate fat, and sufficient energy from carbohydrates can better support weight loss and good health. Including protein at each meal may help with weight loss by providing satiety.[21] Selecting too many protein-rich foods may crowd out fruits, vegetables, and whole grains, making the diet inadequate in other nutrients.

Kidney Disease Excretion of the end products of protein metabolism depends, in part, on an adequate fluid intake and healthy kidneys. A high protein intake does not cause kidney disease, but it does increase the work of the kidneys. It may also accelerate kidney deterioration in people with chronic kidney disease. Restricting dietary protein may help to slow the progression of kidney disease in people who have this condition.

Recommended Intakes of Protein

As mentioned earlier, the body continuously breaks down and loses some protein and it cannot store proteins or amino acids. To replace protein, the body needs dietary protein for two reasons. First, dietary protein is the only source of the *essential* amino acids, and second, it is the only practical source of *nitrogen* with which to build the nonessential amino acids and other nitrogen-containing compounds the body needs.

Given recommendations that fat should contribute 20 to 35 percent of total food energy and carbohydrate should contribute 45 to 65 percent, that leaves 10 to 35 percent for protein. In a 2000-kcalorie diet, that represents 200 to 700 kcalories from protein, or 50 to 175 grams. The average intake in the United States is 80 grams per day.

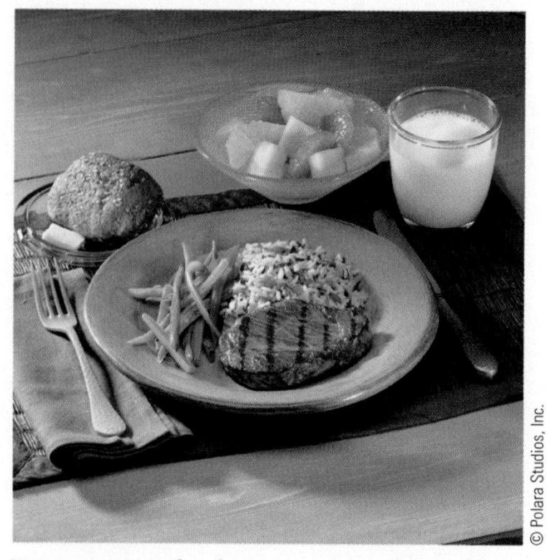

© Polara Studios, Inc.

For many people, this 5-ounce steak provides almost all of the meat and much of the protein recommended for a day's intake.

Protein RDA The protein RDA for adults is 0.8 grams per kilogram of healthy body weight per day. For infants and children, the RDA is slightly higher. The table on the inside front cover lists the RDA for males and females at various ages in two ways—grams per day based on reference body weights and grams per kilogram of body weight per day.

The RDA covers the needs for replacing worn-out tissue, so it increases for larger people; it also covers the needs for building new tissue during growth, so it increases for infants, children, adolescents, and pregnant and lactating women. The accompanying "How To" feature explains how to calculate your RDA for protein.

The protein RDA is the same for athletes as for others, even though athletes may need more protein and many fitness authorities recommend a higher range of protein intakes for athletes pursuing different activities (see Table 14-5 in Chapter 14 for details). Most athletes in training typically don't need to actually increase their protein intakes, however, because the additional foods they eat to meet their high energy needs deliver protein as well. Importantly, these higher recommendations still fall within the 10 to 35 percent Acceptable Macronutrient Distribution Range (AMDR).

In setting the RDA, the DRI Committee assumes that people are healthy and do not have unusual metabolic needs for protein, that the protein eaten will be of

>How To

Calculate Recommended Protein Intakes

To figure your protein RDA:

- Look up the healthy weight for a person of your height (inside back cover). If your present weight falls within that range, use it for the following calculations. If your present weight falls outside the range, use the midpoint of the healthy weight range as your reference weight.
- Convert pounds to kilograms, if necessary (pounds divided by 2.2 equals kilograms).
- Multiply kilograms by 0.8 to get your RDA in grams per day. (Teens 14 to 18 years old, multiply by 0.85.) Example:

Weight = 150 lb

150 lb ÷ 2.2 lb/kg = 68 kg (rounded off)

68 kg × 0.8 g/kg = 54 g protein (rounded off)

> TRY IT Calculate your protein RDA.

mixed quality (from both high- and low-quality sources), and that the body will use the protein efficiently. In addition, the committee assumes that the protein is consumed along with sufficient carbohydrate and fat to provide adequate energy and that other nutrients in the diet are also adequate.

Adequate Energy Note the qualification "adequate energy" in the preceding statement, and consider what happens if energy intake falls short of needs. An intake of 50 grams of protein provides 200 kcalories, which represents 10 percent of the total energy from protein, if the person receives 2000 kcalories a day. But if the person cuts energy intake drastically—to, say, 800 kcalories a day—then an intake of 200 kcalories from protein is suddenly 25 percent of the total; yet it's still the same amount of protein (number of grams). The protein intake is reasonable, but the energy intake is not. The low energy intake forces the body to use the protein to meet energy needs rather than to replace lost body protein. Similarly, if the person's energy intake is high—say, 4000 kcalories—the 50-gram protein intake represents only 5 percent of the total; yet it *still* is a reasonable protein intake. Again, the energy intake is unreasonable for most people, but in this case, it permits the protein to be used to meet the body's needs.

Be careful when judging protein (or carbohydrate or fat) intake as a percentage of energy. Always consider the number of grams as well, and compare it with the RDA or another standard stated in grams. A recommendation stated as a percentage of energy intake is useful only if the energy intake is within reason.

From Guidelines to Groceries

A diet following the USDA Food Patterns can easily supply the recommended amount of protein. In selecting foods for protein, keep in mind the principles of variety and moderation.

Protein Foods An ounce of most protein foods delivers about 7 grams of protein. The USDA Food Patterns encourage a variety by sorting protein foods into three subgroups (review Figure 2-2, p. 44 and Table 2-4, p. 46). Over a week's time, the total recommended intake of protein foods should be about 20 percent from seafood; almost 70 percent from meat, poultry, and eggs; and 10 percent from nuts, seeds, and legumes.

Either plant or animal sources of protein can support a healthy eating pattern, but some protein foods—notably those derived from animals—may be high in saturated fat. To minimize saturated fat intake, select lean meats and poultry. Trim fat from meats before cooking and drain fat from meat after cooking. Remove skin from poultry before eating. Include plant sources of protein as well. By selecting a variety of protein foods, consumers can improve their nutrient

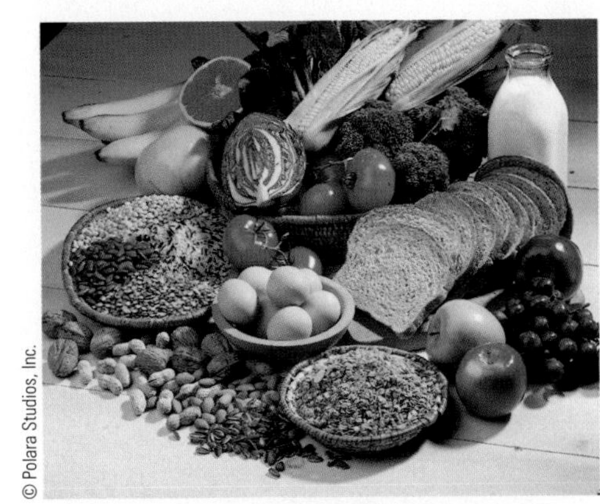

Vegetarians obtain their protein from whole grains, legumes, nuts, vegetables, and, in some cases, eggs and milk products.

intake and incur health benefits. Highlight 5 describes how nuts and fish can reduce the risks of heart disease when consumed in place of other protein foods.

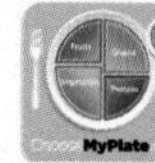

> **DIETARY GUIDELINES FOR AMERICANS**
> Choose a variety of foods from the protein foods group, which includes seafood, lean meat and poultry, eggs, beans and peas, soy products, and unsalted nuts and seeds. Increase the amount and variety of seafood consumed by choosing seafood in place of some meat and poultry. Replace protein foods that are higher in solid fats with choices that are lower in solid fats and kcalories.

Milk and Milk Products The only other food group to provide significant amounts of protein per serving is the milk and milk products group. A serving (a cup) of milk or yogurt provides about 8 grams of protein.

Fruits, Vegetables, and Grains Fruits do not contain protein. A serving of vegetables or grains provides 2 to 3 grams of protein, respectively.

Read Food Labels

Food labels state the quantity of protein in grams. The "% Daily Value" for protein is not mandatory on all labels but is required whenever a food makes a protein claim or is intended for consumption by children younger than 4 years old. Whenever the Daily Value percentage is declared, researchers must determine the *quality* of the protein. Thus, when a % Daily Value is stated for protein, it reflects both quantity and quality.

To illustrate how easy it is to get enough protein, consider the amounts recommended by the USDA Food Pattern for a 2000-kcalorie diet. Six ounces of grains provide about 18 grams of protein; 2½ cups of vegetables deliver about 10 grams; 3 cups of milk offer 24 grams; and 5½ ounces of protein foods supply 38 grams. This totals 90 grams of protein—higher than the protein RDA for most people.

People in the United States typically get more protein than they need. If they have an adequate *food* intake, they have a more-than-adequate protein intake. The key diet-planning principle to emphasize for protein is moderation. Even though most people receive plenty of protein, some feel compelled to take supplements as well, as the next section describes.

Protein and Amino Acid Supplements

Websites, health-food stores, and popular magazine articles advertise a wide variety of protein supplements, and consumers spend billions of dollars taking these supplements for many different reasons. Athletes take protein powders to build muscle. Dieters take them to spare their bodies' protein while losing weight. Women take them to strengthen their fingernails. People take individual amino acids, too—to cure herpes, to make themselves sleep better, to lose weight, and to relieve pain and depression. Like many other magic solutions to health problems, protein and amino acid supplements don't work these miracles.

Protein Powders Because the body builds muscle protein from amino acids, many athletes take protein powders with the false hope of stimulating muscle growth. Muscle work builds muscle; protein supplements do not, and most athletes do not need them. Getting enough protein to support protein synthesis in the muscles is certainly important, but ingesting "more than enough" protein does not further enhance muscle growth or function. (Highlight 14 presents more information on other supplements athletes commonly use.) Protein powders can supply amino acids to the body, but nature's protein sources—lean meat, milk, eggs, and legumes—supply all these amino acids and more.

Whey protein appears to be particularly popular among athletes hoping to achieve greater muscle gains. A waste product of cheese manufacturing, whey protein is a common ingredient in many low-cost protein powders. When

whey protein: a by-product of cheese production; falsely promoted as increasing muscle mass. Whey is the watery part of milk that separates from the curds.

combined with strength training, whey supplements may increase protein synthesis slightly, but they do not seem to enhance athletic performance. To build stronger muscles, athletes need to eat food with adequate energy and protein to support the weight-training work that does increase muscle mass. Those who still think they need more whey can drink a glass of milk; one cup provides 1.5 grams of whey.

Amino Acid Supplements Single amino acids do not occur naturally in foods and offer no benefit to the body; in fact, they may be harmful. The body was not designed to handle the high concentrations and unusual combinations of amino acids found in supplements. Large doses of amino acids cause diarrhea. An excess of one amino acid can create such a demand for a carrier that it limits the absorption of another amino acid, presenting the possibility of a deficiency. Those amino acids winning the competition enter in excess, creating the possibility of toxicity. Anyone considering taking amino acid supplements should be cautious not to exceed levels normally found in foods.[22]

Most healthy athletes eating well-balanced diets do not need amino acid supplements. Advertisers point to research that identifies the **branched-chain amino acids** as the main ones used as fuel by exercising muscles. What the ads leave out is that compared to glucose and fatty acids, branched-chain amino acids provide very little fuel and that ordinary foods provide them in abundance anyway. Large doses of branched-chain amino acids can raise plasma ammonia concentrations, which can be toxic to the brain. Branched-chain amino acid supplements may be beneficial in conditions such as liver disease, but otherwise, they are not routinely recommended.

In two cases, recommendations for single amino acid supplements have led to widespread public use—lysine to prevent or relieve the infections that cause herpes cold sores on the mouth or genital organs, and tryptophan to relieve depression and insomnia. In both cases, enthusiastic popular reports preceded careful scientific experiments and health recommendations. Research has not determined that lysine suppresses herpes infections, but it appears safe (up to 3 grams per day) when taken in divided doses with meals.

Tryptophan may be effective with respect to inducing drowsiness, but caution is still advised. About 25 years ago, more than 1500 people who had taken tryptophan supplements developed a rare blood disorder known as eosinophilia-myalgia syndrome (EMS). EMS is characterized by severe muscle and joint pain, extremely high fever, and, in more than three dozen cases, death. Treatment for EMS usually involves physical therapy and low doses of corticosteroids to relieve symptoms temporarily. The Food and Drug Administration implicated impurities in the supplements and issued a recall of all products containing manufactured tryptophan. A recent review of the effects and side effects of tryptophan supplements currently on the market found only modest, short-lived side effects at doses typical of use (up to 5 grams per day).[23] People taking serotonin reuptake inhibitor drugs should consult with their physicians before taking tryptophan supplements.

› REVIEW IT Identify the health benefits of, and recommendations for, protein.
Protein deficiency impairs the body's ability to grow and function optimally. Excesses of protein offer no advantage; in fact, overconsumption of protein-rich foods may incur health problems as well. The optimal diet is adequate in energy from carbohydrate and fat and delivers 0.8 grams of protein per kilogram of healthy body weight each day. US diets are typically more than adequate in this respect. Normal, healthy people do not need protein or amino acid supplements.

As is true for the other nutrients as well, it is safest to obtain amino acids and protein from foods, eaten with abundant carbohydrate and some fat to facilitate their use in the body. With all that we know about science, it is hard to improve on nature.

branched-chain amino acids: the essential amino acids leucine, isoleucine, and valine, which are present in large amounts in skeletal muscle tissue; falsely promoted as fuel for exercising muscles.

Nutrition Portfolio

Foods that derive from animals—meats, fish, poultry, eggs, and milk products—provide plenty of protein but are often accompanied by fat. Those that derive from plants—whole grains, vegetables, and legumes—may provide less protein but also less fat.

Go to Diet & Wellness Plus and choose one of the days on which you have tracked your diet for the entire day. Go to the Intake Spreadsheet report. Scroll down until you see: protein (g).

- Which of your food choices provided you with the most protein on that day? Does that food also have a lot of fat? Refer to the fat (g) column for this information.
- Describe your dietary sources of proteins and whether you use mostly plant-based or animal-based protein foods in your diet.

Now take a look at the Intake vs. Goals report.

- How do your protein needs compare with your protein intake? Consider whether you receive enough, but not too much, protein daily. Remember, 100 percent means your intake is meeting your needs based on your intake and profile information.
- If your protein intake exceeds 100 percent, consider the possible negative consequences of a high protein intake over many years.
- Debate the risks and benefits of taking protein or amino acid supplements.

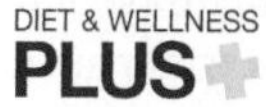

To complete this exercise, go to your Diet & Wellness Plus at **www.cengagebrain.com.**

› STUDY IT To review the key points of this chapter and take a practice quiz, go to the study cards at the end of the book.

REFERENCES

1. M. Brown, Managing the acutely ill adult with sickle cell disease, *British Journal of Nursing* 21 (2012): 90–96.
2. US Department of Agriculture, Agricultural Research Service, Nutrient Intakes from Food, *What We Eat in America,* NHANES 2009–2010, www. ars.usda.gov/ba/bhnrc/fsrg, published 2012.
3. Position of the American Dietetic Association and Dietitians of Canada: Vegetarian diets, *Journal of the American Dietetic Association* 109 (2009): 1266–1282.
4. Committee on Dietary Reference Intakes, *Dietary Reference Intakes: Energy, Carbohydrate, Fiber, Fat, Fatty Acids, Cholesterol, Protein, and Amino Acids* (Washington, D.C.: National Academies Press, 2005), p. 694.
5. S. R. Preis and coauthors, Dietary protein and risk of ischemic heart disease in middle-aged men, *American Journal of Clinical Nutrition* 92 (2010): 1265–1272.
6. P. M. Clifton, Protein and coronary heart disease: The role of different protein sources, *Current Atherosclerosis Reports* 13 (2011): 493–498; D. G. Hackam and coauthors, The 2010 Canadian Hypertension Education Program recommendations for the management of hypertension: Part 2—Therapy, *Canadian Journal of Cardiology* 26 (2010): 249–258.
7. J. B. J. vanMeurs and coauthors, Common genetic loci influencing plasma homocysteine concentrations and their effect on risk of coronary artery disease, *American Journal of Clinical Nutrition* 98 (2013): 668–676; Q. Yang and coauthors, Prospective study of methylenetetrahydrofolate reductase (*MTHFR*) variant C677T and risk of all-cause and cardiovascular disease mortality among US adults, *American Journal of Clinical Nutrition* 95 (2012): 1245–1253.
8. R. J. Glynn, Complex relations of genetic polymorphisms with nutritionally influenced biomarkers, *American Journal of Clinical Nutrition* 95 (2012): 1001–1002; R. Clarke and coauthors, Homocysteine and vascular disease: Review of published results of the homocysteine-lowering trials, *Journal of Inherited Metabolic Disease* 34 (2011): 83–91.
9. M. Hoffman, Hypothesis: Hyperhomocysteinemia is an indicator of oxidant stress, *Medical Hypotheses* 77 (2011): 1088–1093.
10. P. Tighe and coauthors, A dose-finding trial of the effect of long-term folic acid intervention: Implications for food fortification policy, *American Journal of Clinical Nutrition* 93 (2011): 11–18.
11. J. D. Spence and M. J. Stampfer, Understanding the complexity of homocysteine lowering with vitamins: The potential role of subgroup analyses, *Journal of the American Medical Association* 306 (2011): 2610–2611; S. Eilat-Adar and U. Goldbourt, Nutritional recommendations for preventing coronary heart disease in women: Evidence concerning whole foods and supplements, *Nutrition, Metabolism, and Cardiovascular Disease* 20 (2010): 459–466.
12. L. Chao-Qiang, *MAT1A* variants are associated with hypertension, stroke, and markers of DNA damage and are modulated by plasma vitamin B-6 and folate, *American Journal of Clinical Nutrition* 91 (2010): 1377–1386; J. M. Armitage and coauthors, Effects of homocysteine-lowering with folic acid plus vitamin B_{12} vs placebo on mortality and major morbidity in myocardial infarction survivors: A randomized trial, *Journal of the American Medical Association* 303 (2010): 2486–2494.
13. U. N. Das and coauthors, L-arginine, NO and asymmetrical dimethylarginine in hypertension and type 2 diabetes, *Frontiers in Bioscience* 16 (2011): 13–20; D. Tousoulis and coauthors, Novel therapeutic strategies targeting vascular endothelium in essential hypertension, *Expert Opinion on Investigational Drugs* 19 (2010): 1395–1412.

14. B. Magalhães, B. Peleteiro, and N. Lunet, Dietary patterns and colorectal cancer: Systematic review and meta-analysis, *European Journal of Cancer Prevention* 21 (2012): 15–23; S. C. Larsson and A. Wolk, Red and processed meat consumption and risk of pancreatic cancer: Meta-analysis of prospective studies, *British Journal of Cancer* 106 (2012): 603–607; R. Takachi and coauthors, Red meat intake may increase the risk of colon cancer in Japanese, a population with relatively low red meat consumption, *Asia Pacific Journal of Clinical Nutrition* 20 (2011): 603–612; A. T. Chan and E. L. Giovannucci, Primary prevention of colorectal cancer, *Gastroenterology* 138 (2010): 2029–2043.
15. Committee on Dietary Reference Intakes, 2005, p. 841; Committee on Dietary Reference Intakes, *Dietary Reference Intakes for Calcium and Vitamin D* (Washington, D.C.: National Academies Press, 2011).
16. J. Calvez and coauthors, Protein intake, calcium balance and health consequences, *European Journal of Clinical Nutrition* 66 (2012): 281–295; M. P. Thorpe and E. M. Evans, Dietry protein and bone health: Harmonizing conflicting theories, *Nutrition Reviews* 9 (2011): 215–230; J. J. Cao, L. K. Johnson, and J. R. Hunt, A diet high in meat protein and potential renal acid load increases fractional calcium absorption and urinary calcium excretion without affecting markers of bone resorption or formation in postmenopausal women, *Journal of Nutrition* 141 (2011): 391–397; J. M. Beasley and coauthors, Is protein intake associated with bone mineral density in young women? *American Journal of Clinical Nutrition* 91 (2010): 1311–1316.
17. J. J. Cao and F. H. Nielsen, Acid diet (high-meat protein) effects on calcium metabolism and bone health, *Current Opinion in Clinical Nutrition and Metabolic Care* 13 (2010): 698–702.
18. D. Bujnowski and coauthors, Longitudinal association between animal and vegetable protein intake and obesity among men in the United States: The Chicago Western Electric Study, *Journal of the American Dietetic Association* 111 (2011): 1150–1155.
19. G. A. Bray and coauthors, Effect of dietary protein content on weight gain, energy expenditure, and body composition during overeating: A randomized controlled trial, *Journal of the American Medical Association* 307 (2012): 47–55.
20. Z. Li and D. Heber, Overeating and overweight: Extra calories increase fat mass while protein increases lean mass, *Journal of the American Medical Association* 307 (2012): 86–87.
21. A. Belza and coauthors, Contribution of gastroenteropancreatic appetite hormones to protein-induced satiety, *American Journal of Clinical Nutrition* 97 (2013): 980–989.
22. Committee on Dietary Reference Intakes, *Dietary Reference Intakes: The Essential Guide to Nutrient Requirements* (Washington, D.C.: National Academies Press, 2006), p. 152.
23. J. D. Fernstrom, Effects and side effects associated with the non-nutritional use of tryptophan by humans, *Journal of Nutrition* 142 (2012): 2236S–2244S.

HIGHLIGHT > 6
Nutritional Genomics

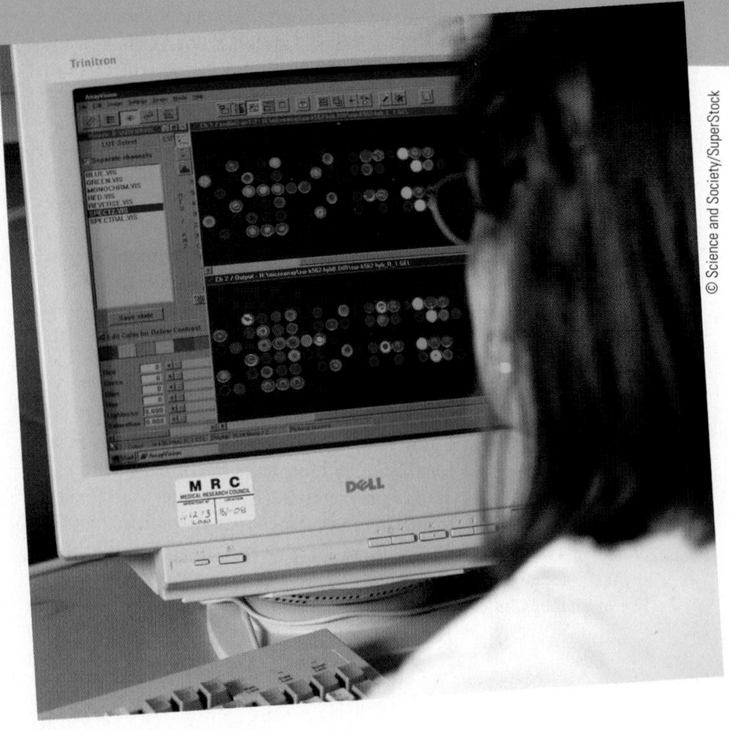

> LEARN IT Explain how nutrients influence gene activity (nutrigenomics) and how genes influence the activities of nutrients (nutrigenetics).

Imagine this scenario: A physician scrapes a sample of cells from inside your cheek and submits it to a **genomics** lab. The lab returns a report based on your genetic profile that reveals which diseases you are most likely to develop, and your physician recommends specific lifestyle changes and medical treatments that can help you maintain good health. You may also be given a prescription for an individualized diet and dietary supplements that will best meet your personal nutrient requirements. This scenario may one day become a common reality as scientists uncover the relationships among **genetics,** diet, and disease.[1] Such genetic testing holds great promise, but consumers need to know that current genetic test kits commonly available to the public are unproven and may create more problems than they resolve; the American Academy of Pediatrics strongly discourages direct-to-consumer testing and advises against testing children for diseases that typically develop in adulthood.[2]

Figure H6-1 introduces **nutritional genomics,** a new field of study that examines how nutrients influence gene activity (nutrigenomics) and how **genes** influence the activities of nutrients (nutrigenetics). The accompanying glossary defines related terms.

The recent surge in genomics research grew from the Human Genome Project, an international effort by industry and government scientists to identify and describe all of the genes in the **human genome**—that is, all the genetic information contained within a person's cells. Completed in 2003, this project developed many of the research technologies needed to study genes and genetic variation. Scientists are now working on the human **proteome** and hope to identify each of the proteins made by the genes, the genes associated with aging and diseases, and the dietary and lifestyle choices that most influence the expression of those genes. Such information will have major implications for society in general, and for health care in particular.[3]

A Genomics Primer

Figure H6-2 (p. 196) shows the relationships among the materials that comprise the genome. As Chapter 6's discussion of protein synthesis points out, genetic information is encoded in DNA molecules within the nucleus of cells. The **DNA (deoxyribonucleic acid)** molecules and associated proteins are packed within 46 **chromosomes.** The genes are segments of a DNA strand that can eventually be translated into one or more proteins. The sequence of **nucleotide bases** within each gene determines the amino acid sequence of a particular protein. Scientists currently estimate that there are between 20,000 and 25,000 protein-coding genes in the human genome.

GLOSSARY

chromosomes: structures within the nucleus of a cell made of DNA and associated proteins. Human beings have 46 chromosomes in 23 pairs. Each chromosome has many genes.

DNA (deoxyribonucleic acid): the double helix molecules of which genes are made.

epigenetics: the study of heritable changes in gene function that occur without a change in the DNA sequence.

gene expression: the process by which a cell converts the genetic code into RNA and protein.

genes: sections of chromosomes that contain the instructions needed to make one or more proteins.

genetics: the study of genes and inheritance.

genomics: the study of all the genes in an organism and their interactions with environmental factors.

human genome (GEE-nome): the complete set of genetic material (DNA) in a human being.

methylation: the addition of a methyl group (CH_3).

microarray technology: research tools that analyze the expression of thousands of genes simultaneously and search for particular gene changes associated with a disease. DNA microarrays are also called *DNA chips.*

mutations: permanent changes in the DNA that can be inherited.

nucleotide bases: the nitrogen-containing building blocks of DNA and RNA—cytosine (C), thymine (T), uracil (U), guanine (G), and adenine (A). In DNA, the base pairs are A–T and C–G and in RNA, the base pairs are A–U and C–G.

nucleotides: the subunits of DNA and RNA molecules, composed of a phosphate group, a 5-carbon sugar (deoxyribose for DNA and ribose for RNA), and a nitrogen-containing base.

nutritional genomics: the science of how nutrients affect the activities of genes *(nutrigenomics)* and how genes affect the activities of nutrients *(nutrigenetics).*

phenylketonuria (FEN-il-KEY-toe-NEW-ree-ah) or **PKU:** an inherited disorder characterized by failure to metabolize the amino acid phenylalanine to tyrosine.

proteome: all proteins in a cell. The study of all proteins produced by a species is called *proteomics.*

RNA (ribonucleic acid): a compound similar to DNA, but RNA is a single strand with a ribose sugar instead of a deoxyribose sugar and uracil instead of thymine as one of its bases.

> **FIGURE H6-1 Nutritional Genomics**

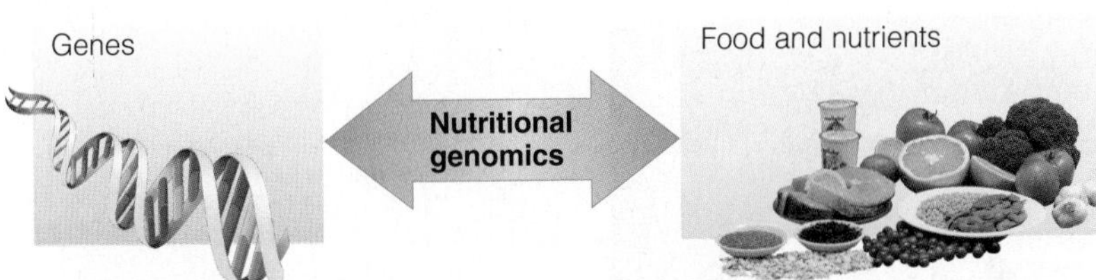

Nutritional genomics examines the interactions of genes and nutrients. These interactions include both nutrigenetics and nutrigenomics.

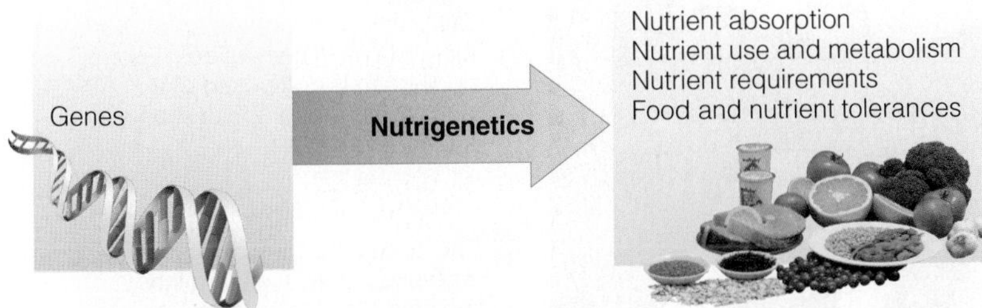

Nutrigenetics (or nutritional genetics) examines how genes influence the activities of nutrients.

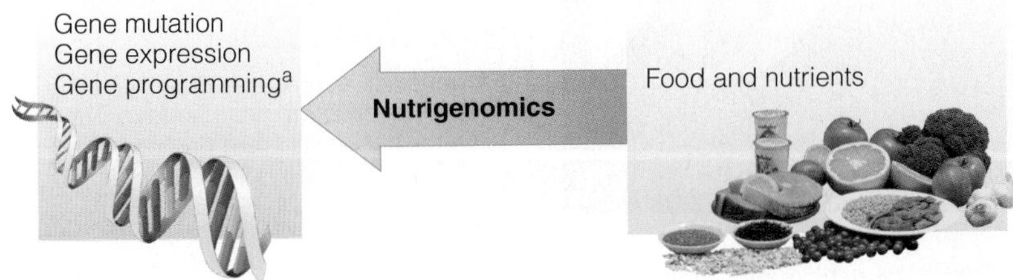

Nutrigenomics, which includes epigenetics, examines how nutrients influence the activities of genes.

[a]Chapter 15 introduces fetal programming and describes how a mother's nutrition can permanently change gene expression in the fetus with consequences for future generations.

As Figure 6-7 (p. 178) explains, when cells make proteins, a DNA sequence is used to make messenger **RNA (ribonucleic acid).** The **nucleotide** sequence in messenger RNA then determines the amino acid sequence to make a protein. This process—from genetic information to protein synthesis—is known as **gene expression.** Gene expression can be determined by measuring the amounts of messenger RNA in a tissue sample. **Microarray technology** (see photo on the previous page) allows researchers to detect messenger RNA and analyze the expression of thousands of genes simultaneously. These patterns of gene expression help to explain the development of diseases and relationships between diet and diseases.[4]

Simply having a certain gene does not determine that its associated trait will be expressed; the gene has to be activated. (Similarly, owning lamps does not ensure you will have light in your home unless you turn them on.) Nutrients are among many environmental factors that play key roles in either activating or silencing genes. Switching genes on and off does not change the DNA itself, but it can have dramatic consequences for a person's health.

The area of study that examines how environmental factors influence gene expression without changing the DNA is known as **epigenetics.**[5] To turn genes on, enzymes attach proteins near the beginning of a gene. If enzymes attach a methyl group (CH_3) instead, the protein is blocked from binding to the gene and the gene remains switched off. Other factors influence gene expression as well, but methyl groups are currently the most well understood.[6] They also are known to have dietary connections.[7]

The accompanying photo of two mice illustrates epigenetics and how diet can influence genetic traits such as hair color and body weight. Both mice have a gene that tends to produce fat, yellow pups, but their mothers were given different diets during pregnancy. The mother of the mouse on the right was given a dietary supplement containing the B vitamins folate and vitamin B_{12}. These nutrients silenced the gene for "yellow and fat," resulting in brown pups with normal appetites. As Chapter 10 explains, one of the main roles of these B vitamins is to transfer methyl groups. In the case of the supplemented mice, methyl groups migrated onto DNA and silenced several genes, thus producing brown coats and protecting against the development of obesity (and consequently, some related diseases). Keep in mind that these changes occurred epigenetically. In other words, the DNA sequence within the genes of the mice remained the same. Nutrition and other environmental factors can influence genes in a way that creates inheritable changes in the body's metabolism and susceptibility to disease.In this way, the dietary habits of parents, and even grandparents, can influence future generations.

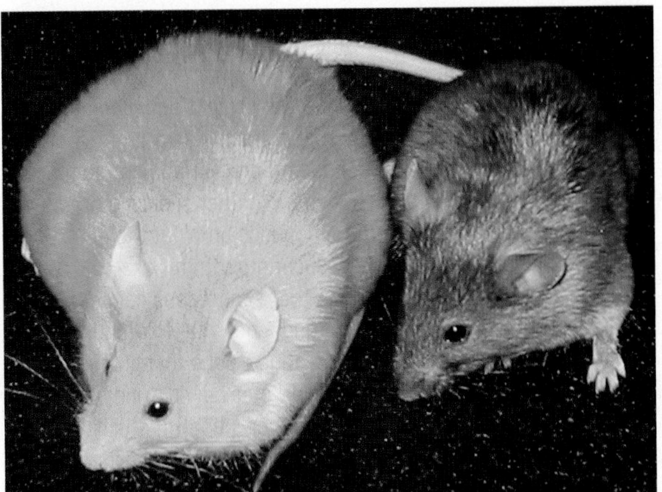

Both of these mice have the gene that tends to produce fat, yellow pups, but their mothers had different diets. The mother of the mouse on the right received a dietary supplement, which silenced the gene, resulting in brown pups with normal appetites.

> FIGURE H6-2 The Human Genome

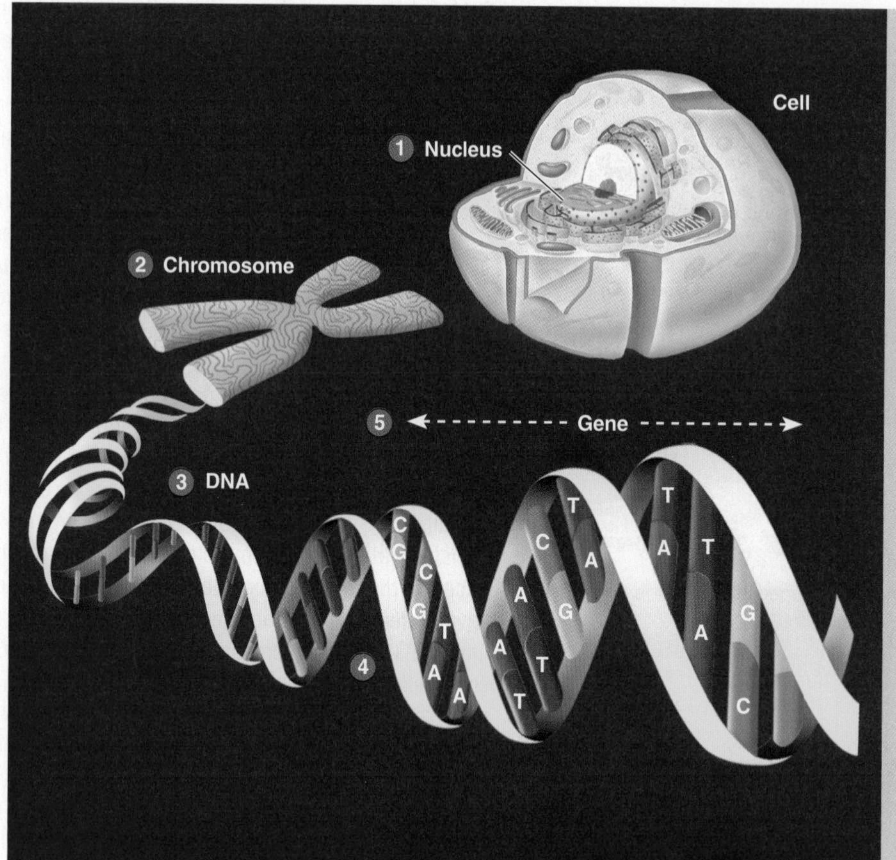

Cell
1 Nucleus
2 Chromosome
5 Gene
3 DNA
4
1 The human genome is a complete set of genetic material organized into 46 chromosomes, located within the nucleus of a cell.
2 A chromosome is made of DNA and associated proteins.
3 The double helical structure of a DNA molecule is made up of two long chains of nucleotides. Each nucleotide is composed of a phosphate group, a 5-carbon sugar, and a base.
4 The sequence of nucleotide bases (C, G, A, T) determines the amino acid sequence of proteins. These bases are connected by hydrogen bonding to form base pairs—adenine (A) with thymine (T) and guanine (G) with cytosine (C).
5 A gene is a segment of DNA that includes the information needed to synthesize one or more proteins.

SOURCE: Adapted from "A Primer: From DNA to Life," Human Genome Project, US Department of Energy Office of Science, accessed at www.orn.gov/sci/techresources/human_genome/primer-pic.shtml.

Many nutrients and phytochemicals regulate gene expression and influence health through their involvement in DNA **methylation.** Some, such as folate, silence genes and protect against some cancers by increasing methylation.[8] Others, such as a phytochemical found in green tea, activate genes and protect against some cancers by inhibiting methylation activity. Whether silencing or activating a gene is beneficial or harmful depends on what the gene does. Silencing a gene that stimulates cancer growth, for example, would be beneficial, but silencing a gene that suppresses cancer growth would be harmful. Similarly, activating a gene that defends against obesity would be beneficial, but activating a gene that promotes obesity would be harmful. Figure H6-3 illustrates how nutrient regulation of gene expression can influence a person's health. Much research is under way to determine which nutrients activate or silence which genes. Such knowledge is expected to help researchers reverse the epigenetic changes that lead to cancer.[9] Similarly, researchers exploring how kcalorie-restricted diets influence DNA methylation are gaining new insights on the regulation of appetite and the metabolism of weight loss.[10]

Genetic Variation and Disease

Except for identical twins, no two persons are genetically identical. Even then, a particular gene may become active in one twin and silenced in the other because of epigenetic changes.

The variation in the genomes of any two persons is only about 0.1 percent, a difference of only one nucleotide base in every 1000. Yet it is this incredibly small difference that makes each of us unique and explains why, given the same environmental influences, some of us develop certain diseases and others do not. Similarly, genetic variation explains why some of us respond to interventions such as diet and others do not. For example, following a diet low in saturated fats will significantly lower LDL cholesterol for most people, but the degree of change varies dramatically among individuals, with some people having only a small decrease or even a slight increase. In other words, dietary factors may be more helpful or more harmful depending on a person's particular genetic variations. Such findings help to explain some of the conflicting results from research studies. One of the goals of nutritional genomics is to custom design *specific* recommendations

> FIGURE H6-3 **Nutrient Regulation of Gene Expression**

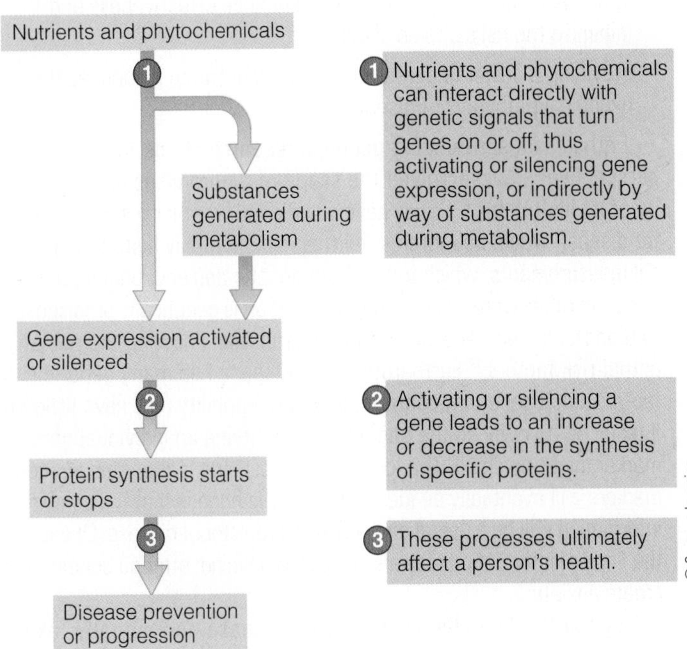

Nutrients and phytochemicals
1
Substances generated during metabolism
1 Nutrients and phytochemicals can interact directly with genetic signals that turn genes on or off, thus activating or silencing gene expression, or indirectly by way of substances generated during metabolism.
Gene expression activated or silenced
2
2 Activating or silencing a gene leads to an increase or decrease in the synthesis of specific proteins.
Protein synthesis starts or stops
3
3 These processes ultimately affect a person's health.
Disease prevention or progression
© Cengage Learning

that fit the needs of *each* individual. Such personalized recommendations are expected to provide more effective disease prevention and treatment solutions.

Diseases characterized by a single-gene disorder are genetically predetermined, usually exert their effects early in life, and greatly affect those touched by them; such diseases are relatively rare. The cause and effect of single-gene disorders is clear—those with the genetic defect get the disease and those without it don't. In contrast, the more common diseases, such as heart disease and cancer, are influenced by many genes and typically develop over several decades. These chronic diseases have multiple genetic components that *predispose* the prevention or development of a disease, depending on a variety of environmental factors (such as smoking, diet, and physical activity). Both types of diseases are of interest to researchers studying nutritional genomics.

Single-Gene Disorders

Some disorders are caused by **mutations** in single genes that are inherited at birth. The consequences of a missing or malfunctioning protein can seriously disrupt metabolism and may require significant dietary or medical intervention. A classic example of a diet-related, single-gene disorder is **phenylketonuria,** or **PKU.**

Approximately one in every 15,000 infants in the United States is born with PKU. PKU arises from mutations in the gene that codes for the enzyme that converts the essential amino acid phenylalanine to the amino acid tyrosine. Without this enzyme, phenylalanine and its metabolites accumulate and damage the nervous system, resulting in mental retardation, seizures, and behavior abnormalities. At the same time, the body cannot make tyrosine or compounds made from it (such as the neurotransmitter epinephrine). Consequently, tyrosine becomes a conditionally essential amino acid: because the body cannot make it, the diet must supply it.

Although the most debilitating effect is on brain development, other symptoms of PKU become evident if the condition is left untreated. Infants with PKU may have poor appetites and grow slowly. They may be irritable or have tremors or seizures. Their bodies and urine may have a musty odor. Their skin coloring may be unusually pale, and they may develop skin rashes.

The effect of nutrition intervention in PKU is remarkable. In fact, the only current treatment for PKU is a diet that restricts phenylalanine and supplies tyrosine to maintain blood levels of these amino acids within safe ranges. Because all foods containing protein provide phenylalanine, the diet must depend on a special formula to supply a phenylalanine-free source of energy, amino acids, vitamins, and minerals. If the restricted diet is conscientiously followed, the symptoms can be prevented. Because phenylalanine is an essential amino acid, the diet cannot exclude it completely. Children with PKU need phenylalanine to grow, but they cannot handle excesses without detrimental effects. Therefore, their diets must provide enough phenylalanine to support normal growth and health but not enough to cause harm. The diet must also provide tyrosine. To ensure that blood concentrations of phenylalanine and tyrosine are close to normal, children and adults who have PKU must have blood tests periodically and adjust their diets as necessary.

Multigene Disorders

In multigene disorders, several genes can influence the progression of a disease, but no single gene causes the disease on its own. For this reason, genomics researchers must study the expression and interactions of *multiple* genes. Because multigene disorders are often sensitive to interactions with environmental influences, they are not as straightforward as single-gene disorders.[11]

Heart disease provides an example of a chronic disease with multiple gene and environmental influences.[12] Consider that major risk factors for heart disease include elevated blood cholesterol levels, obesity, diabetes, and hypertension. Each of these risk factors has multiple underlying genetic and environmental causes, many of which are not completely understood. Research in nutritional genomics involves coordinating multiple findings on each of these risk factors and explaining the interactions among several genes, biological pathways, and nutrients in relatively little time. Studies have been quite successful in examining the genome and identifying multiple pathways in the development of complex diseases.[13] This information could then guide physicians and dietitians to prescribe the most appropriate medical and dietary interventions from among many possible solutions. Finding the best option for each person is a challenge given the many possible interactions between genes and environmental factors and the millions of possible gene variations in the human genome that make each individual unique.

The results of genomic research are helping to explain findings from previous nutrition research. Consider dietary fat and heart disease, for example. As Highlight 5 explains, epidemiological and clinical studies have found that a diet high in omega-3 polyunsaturated fatty acids benefits heart health. Now genetic studies offer an underlying explanation of this relationship: diets rich in omega-3 polyunsaturated fatty acids alter gene expression of immune cells to suppress inflammation and inhibit plaque build-up. Both actions support a healthy heart.

To learn more about how individuals respond to diet, researchers examine the genetic differences among people. The most common genetic differences involve a change in a single nucleotide base located in a particular region of a DNA strand—thymine replacing cytosine, for example. Such variations are called single nucleotide polymorphisms (SNPs), and they commonly occur throughout the genome. Many SNPs (commonly pronounced "snips") have no effect on cell activity. In fact, SNPs are significant only if they affect the amino acid sequence of a protein in a way that alters its function *and* if that function is critical to the body's well-being. In these cases, SNPs may reveal fascinating answers to previously unexplained findings. Consider that research on a gene that plays a key role in lipid metabolism reveals differences in a person's response to diet depending on whether the gene has a common SNP. People with the SNP have lower LDL when eating a diet rich in polyunsaturated fatty acids—and higher LDL with a low intake—than those without the SNP. These findings clearly show how diet (in this case, polyunsaturated fat) interacts with a gene (in this case, a fat metabolism gene with a SNP) to influence the development of a disease (changing blood lipids implicated in heart disease).[14]

Clinical Concerns

Because multigene, chronic diseases are common, an understanding of the human genome will have widespread ramifications for health care.[15] This new understanding of the human genome is expected to change health care by:

- Providing knowledge of an individual's genetic predisposition to specific diseases[16]
- Allowing physicians to develop "designer" therapies—prescribing the most effective schedule of screening, behavior changes (including diet), and medical interventions based on each individual's genetic profile
- Enabling manufacturers to create new medications for each genetic variation so that physicians can prescribe the best medicine in the exact dose and frequency to enhance effectiveness and minimize the risks of side effects
- Providing a better understanding of how nutrition influences the biological pathways of diseases

Enthusiasm surrounding genomic research needs to be put into perspective, however, given the scope of its promises and the reality of its limitations.[17] Critics have questioned whether genetic markers for disease would be more useful than simple family history and clinical measurements, which reflect both genetic *and* environmental influences. In other words, knowing that a person is genetically predisposed to diabetes is not necessarily more useful than knowing the person's actual risk factors.[18] Furthermore, if a disease has many genetic risk factors, each gene that contributes to susceptibility may have little influence on its own, so the benefits of identifying an individual genetic marker might be small. The long-range possibility is that many genetic markers will eventually be identified, and the hope is that the combined information will be a useful and accurate predictor of disease. Of course, the flood of information may also be overwhelming, offer no benefit, and create anxiety.

Having the knowledge to prevent disease and actually taking action do not always coincide. Despite the abundance of current dietary recommendations, many people are unwilling to make behavior changes known to improve their health—especially when they can simply blame their genes.[19] For example, it has been estimated that heart disease and type 2 diabetes are 90 percent preventable when people adopt an appropriate diet, maintain a healthy body weight, and exercise regularly. Yet these two diseases remain among the leading causes of death. Given the difficulty that many people have with current recommendations, it may be unrealistic to expect that they will enthusiastically adopt an even more detailed list of lifestyle modifications. Then again, compliance may be better when it is supported by information based on a person's own genetic profile and the knowledge that the epigenetic profile can be changed.

The debate over nature versus nurture—whether genes or the environment are more influential—has quieted. The focus has shifted. Scientists acknowledge the important roles of each and understand the real answers lie within the myriad interactions. Current research is sorting through how nutrients and other dietary factors interact with genes to confer health benefits or risks. Answers from genomic research may not become apparent for years to come, but the opportunities and rewards may prove well worth the efforts.

CRITICAL THINKING QUESTIONS

A. How might nutritional genomics influence health care in the future?

B. You may have heard about the diet that is based on a person's blood type and claims to restore the body's natural genetic rhythms and improve health. Research may one day reveal exactly which foods might best turn on and off specific genes to defend against specific chronic diseases. No doubt marketers will rush to fill grocery shelves with foods manufactured to match genetic profiles. Why do you think these genetic approaches to diet and health might be more or less appealing than eating patterns that include a variety of fruits, vegetables, whole grains, milk products, and meats?

REFERENCES

1. W. G. Feero, A. E. Guttmacher, and F. S. Collins, Genomic medicine: An updated primer, *New England Journal of Medicine* 362 (2010): 2001–2011.
2. American Academy of Pediatrics, Policy statement: Ethical and policy issues in genetic testing and screening of children, *Pediatrics* 131 (2013): 620–622; Government Accountability Office, *Direct-to-consumer genetic tests: Misleading test results are further complicated by deceptive marketing and other questionable practices*, GAO-10-847T (Washington D.C.: July 22, 2010); J. P. Annes, M. A. Giovanni, and M. F. Murray, Risks of presymptomatic direct-to-consumer genetic testing, *New England Journal of Medicine* 363 (2010): 1100–1101; L. Esserman and V. Kaklamani, Lessons learned from genetic testing, *Journal of the American Medical Association* 304 (2010): 1011–1012; J. P. Evans, D. C. Dale, and C. Fomous, Preparing for a consumer-driven genomic age, *New England Journal of Medicine* 363 (2010): 1099–1103.
3. Position of the Academy of Nutrition and Dietetics: Nutritional genomics, *Journal of the Academy of Nutrition and Dietetics* 114 (2014): 299–312; G. S. Ginsburg, Realizing the opportunities of genomics in health care, *Journal of the American Medical Association* 309 (2013): 1463–1464; K. L. Hudson, Genomics, health care, and society, *New England Journal of Medicine* 365 (2011): 1033–1041; H. Varmus, Ten years on: The human genome and medicine, *New England Journal of Medicine* 362 (2010): 2028–2029.
4. J. C. Jiménez-Chillarón and coauthors, The role of nutrition on epigenetic modifications and their implications on health, *Biochimie* 94 (2012): 2242–2263; M. P. Keller and A. D. Attie, Physiological insights gained from gene expression analysis in obesity and diabetes, *Annual Review of Nutrition* 30 (2010): 341–364; M. I. McCarthy, Genomics, type 2 diabetes, and obesity, *New England Journal of Medicine* 363 (2010): 2339–2350.
5. S. W. Choi and S. Friso, Epigenetics: A new bridge between nutrition and health, *Advances in Nutrition* 1 (2010): 8–16.
6. O. S. Anderson, K. E. Sant, D. C. Dolinoy, Nutrition and epigenetics: An interplay of dietary methyl donors, one-carbon metabolism and DNA methylation, *Journal of Nutritional Biochemistry* 23 (2012): 853–859.
7. L. K. Park, S. Friso, and S. W. Choi, Vitamins, infectious and chronic disease during adulthood and aging: Nutritional influences on epigenetics and age-related disease, *Proceedings of the Nutrition Society* 71 (2012): 75–83.
8. R. A. Stein, Epigenetics—The link between infectious diseases and cancer, *Journal of the American Medical Association* 305 (2011): 1484–1485.
9. M. A. Dawson, T. Kouzarides, and B. J. P. Huntly, Targeting epigenetic readers in cancer, *New England Journal of Medicine* 367 (2012): 647–657; S. Sharma, T. K. Kelly, and P. A. Jones, Epigenetics in cancer, *Carcinogenesis* 31 (2010): 27–36.
10. L. Bouchard and coauthors, Differential epigenomic and transcriptomic responses in subcutaneous adipose tissue between low and high responders to caloric restriction, *American Journal of Clinical Nutrition* 91 (2010): 309–320.
11. H. G. Brunner, The variability of genetic disease, *New England Journal of Medicine* 367 (2012): 1350–1352.
12. W. G. Feero and A. E. Guttmacher, Genomics of cardiovascular disease, *New England Journal of Medicine* 365 (2011): 2098–2109.
13. T. A. Manolio, Genomewide association studies and assessment of the risk of disease, *New England Journal of Medicine* 363 (2010): 166–176.
14. L. A. Afman and M. Müller, Human nutrigenomics of gene regulation by dietary fatty acids, *Progress in Lipid Research* 51 (2012): 63–70; R. Do and coauthors, The effect of chromosome 9p21 variants on cardiovascular disease may be modified by dietary intake: Evidence from a case/control and a prospective study, *PLoS Medicine* 9 (2011): e1001106.
15. W. G. Feero and E. D. Green, Genomics education for health care professionals in the 21st century, *Journal of the American Medical Association* 306 (2011): 989–990.
16. R. P. Lifton, Individual genomes on the horizon, *New England Journal of Medicine* 362 (2010): 1235–1236.
17. C. Klein, K. Lohmann, and A. Ziegler, The promise and limitations of genome-wide association studies, *Journal of the American Medical Association* 308 (2012): 1867–1868.
18. N. P. Paynter and coauthors, Association between a literature-based genetic risk score and cardiovascular events in women, *Journal of the American Medical Association* 303 (2010): 631–637.
19. S. C. O'Neill and coauthors, Preferences for genetic and behavioral health information: The impact of risk factors and disease attributions, *Annals of Behavioral Medicine* 40 (2010): 127–173.

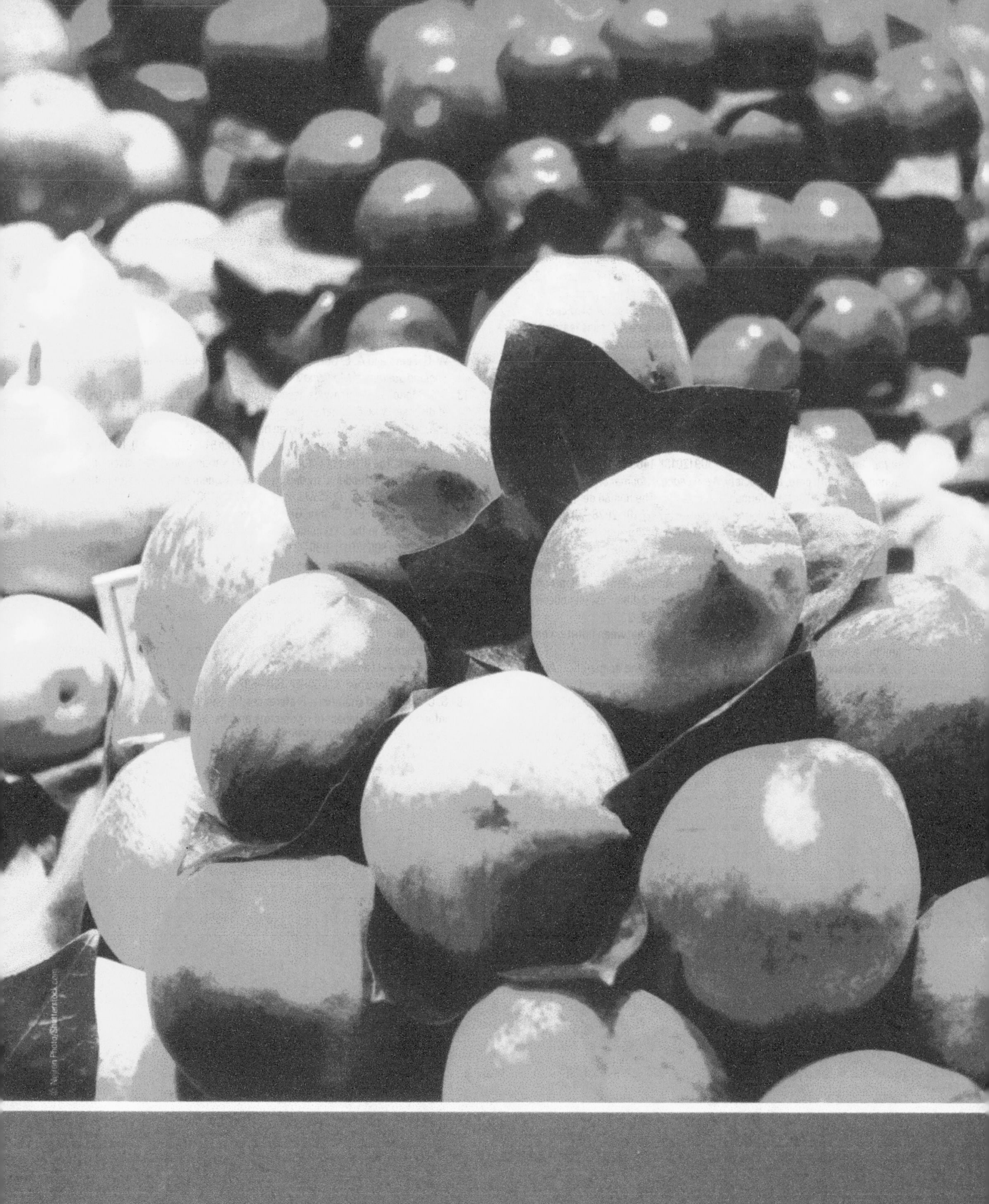

8

Energy Balance and Body Composition

Nutrition in Your Life

It's simple: energy balance occurs when energy in = energy out. The reality, of course, is much more complex. One day you may devour a dozen doughnuts at midnight and sleep through your morning workout—tipping the scales toward weight gain. Another day you may snack on veggies and train for this weekend's 10K race—shifting the balance toward weight loss. Your body weight—especially as it relates to your body fat—and your level of fitness have consequences for your health. So, how are you doing? In the Nutrition Portfolio at the end of this chapter, you can see how your "energy in" and "energy out" balance and whether your body weight and fat measures are consistent with good health.

LEARNING GPS

As Chapter 7 explains, the body's remarkable metabolism can cope with variations in the diet. When the diet delivers too little energy, carbohydrate, or protein, the body uses its fat to meet energy needs and degrades its lean tissue to meet glucose and protein needs. When the diet delivers too much energy—whether from excess carbohydrate, excess protein, or excess fat—the body stores fat.

Both excessive and deficient body fat result from an energy imbalance. The simple picture is as follows. People who consume more food energy than they expend store the surplus as body fat. To reduce body fat, they need to expend more energy than they take in from food. In contrast, people who consume too little food energy to support their bodies' activities must rely on their bodies' fat stores and possibly some of their lean tissues as well. To gain weight, these people need to take in more food energy than they expend. As you will see, though, the details of energy balance and weight regulation are quite complex.[1] This chapter describes energy balance and body composition and examines the health problems associated with having too much or too little body fat. The next chapter presents strategies toward resolving these problems.

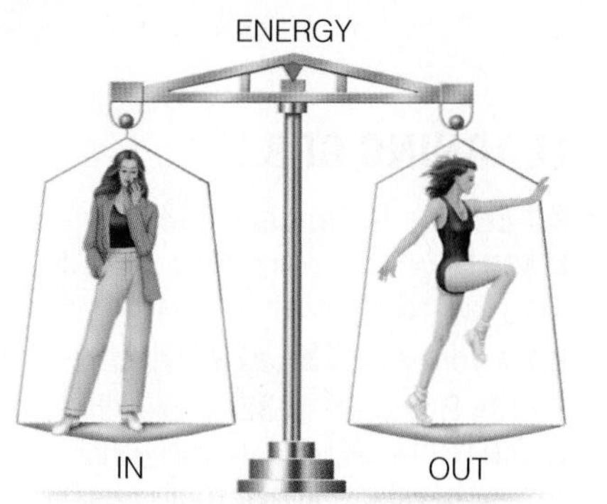

When energy in balances with energy out, a person's body weight is stable.

8.1 Energy Balance

› LEARN IT Describe energy balance and the consequences of not being in balance.

People expend energy continuously and eat periodically to refuel. Ideally, their energy intakes cover their energy expenditures with little, or no, excess. Excess energy is stored as fat, and stored fat is used for energy between meals. The fat stores of even a healthy-weight adult represent an ample reserve of energy—50,000 to 200,000 kcalories.

The amount of body fat a person deposits in, or withdraws from, storage on any given day depends on the **energy balance** for that day—the amount consumed (energy in) versus the amount expended (energy out). When a person is maintaining weight, energy in equals energy out. When the balance shifts, weight changes.

A classic rule states that for each 3500 kcalories eaten in excess, a pound of body fat is stored; similarly, a pound of fat is lost for each 3500 kcalories expended beyond those consumed.* To that end, many diet plans recommend lowering energy intake by 500 kcalories a day to incur a weight loss of 1 pound per week. This "3500 kcalorie rule" has been used for more than 50 years, but it has several limitations.[2] For one, as a person loses weight, the deficit in energy needed to continue losing weight shifts; in general, the kcalorie deficit is relatively low and weight loss is relatively rapid in the early phase but then it is followed by a markedly slower weight loss that plateaus as the kcalorie deficit needed to continue losing weight gradually increases. For another, body composition differs dramatically for men and women and for obese and lean people; in general, the kcalorie deficit needed for weight loss is relatively larger for women than for men and for obese than for lean people. Understanding the dynamic nature of weight loss may help people adopt more realistic expectations than a fixed 3500-kcalorie rule provides.

Quick changes in body weight are not simple changes in fat stores. Weight gained or lost rapidly includes some fat, large amounts of fluid, and some lean tissues such as muscle proteins and bone minerals. Because water constitutes about 60 percent of an adult's body weight, retention or loss of water can greatly influence body weight. Even over the long term, the composition of weight gained or lost is normally about 75 percent fat and 25 percent lean. During starvation, losses of fat and lean are about equal. (Recall from Chapter 7 that without adequate carbohydrate, protein-rich lean tissues break down to provide glucose.) Invariably, though, *fat* gains and losses are gradual. The next two sections examine the two sides of the energy-balance equation—energy in and energy out. As you read, keep in mind that this simple equation falls short of fully explaining the many metabolic changes that cause obesity.[3]

› FIGURE 8-1 Bomb Calorimeter

When food is burned, energy is released in the form of heat. Heat energy is measured in kcalories.

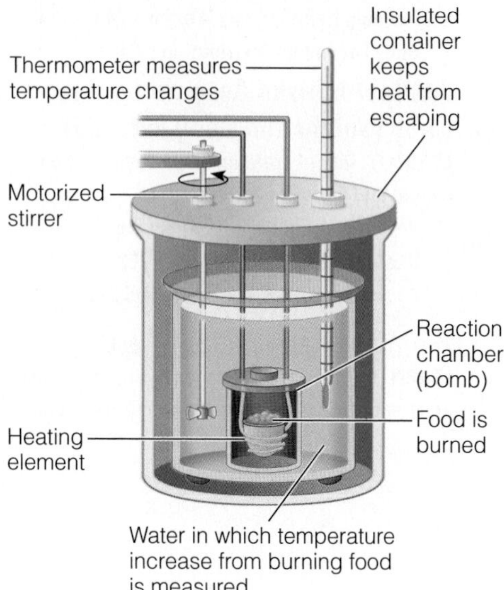

› REVIEW IT Describe energy balance and the consequences of not being in balance.

When energy consumed equals energy expended, a person is in energy balance and body weight is stable. If more energy is taken in than is expended, a person gains weight. If more energy is expended than is taken in, a person loses weight.

8.2 Energy In: The kCalories Foods Provide

› LEARN IT Discuss some of the physical, emotional, and environmental influences on food intake.

Foods and beverages provide the "energy in" part of the energy-balance equation. How much energy a person receives depends on the composition of the foods and beverages and on the amount the person eats and drinks.

Food Composition To find out how many kcalories a food provides, a scientist can burn the food in a **bomb calorimeter** (see Figure 8-1). When the

energy balance: the energy (kcalories) consumed from foods and beverages compared with the energy expended through metabolic processes and physical activities.

bomb calorimeter (KAL-oh-RIM-eh-ter): an instrument that measures the heat energy released when foods are burned, thus providing an estimate of the potential energy of the foods.

- **calor** = heat
- **metron** = measure

*Body fat, or adipose tissue, is composed of a mixture of mostly fat, some protein, and water. A pound of body fat (454 g) is approximately 87 percent fat, or (454 × 0.87) 395 g, and 395 g × 9 kcal/g = 3555 kcal.

food burns, energy is released in the form of heat. The amount of heat given off provides a *direct* measure of the food's energy value (remember that kcalories are units of heat energy).* In addition to releasing heat, these reactions generate carbon dioxide and water—just as the body's cells do when they metabolize the energy-yielding nutrients from foods. Details of the chemical reactions in a calorimeter and in the body differ, but the overall process is similar: when the food burns and the chemical bonds break, the carbons (C) and hydrogens (H) combine with oxygens (O) to form carbon dioxide (CO_2) and water (H_2O). The amount of oxygen consumed gives an *indirect* measure of the amount of energy released.

A bomb calorimeter measures the available energy in foods but overstates the **physiological fuel value**—the amount of energy that the human body derives from foods. The body is less efficient than a calorimeter and cannot metabolize all of the energy-yielding nutrients in a food completely. Researchers can correct for this discrepancy mathematically to create useful tables of the energy values of foods (such as Appendix H). These values provide reasonable estimates, but they do not reflect the *precise* amount of energy a person will derive from the foods consumed.

The energy values of foods can also be computed from the amounts of carbohydrate, fat, and protein (and alcohol, if present) in the foods.** For example, a food containing 12 grams of carbohydrate, 5 grams of fat, and 8 grams of protein will provide 48 carbohydrate kcalories, 45 fat kcalories, and 32 protein kcalories, for a total of 125 kcalories. (To review how to calculate the energy foods provide, turn to the "How To" feature on p. 10.)

Food Intake To achieve energy balance, the body must meet its needs without taking in too much or too little energy. **Appetite** prompts a person to eat—or not to eat. Somehow the body decides how much and how often to eat—when to start eating and when to stop. As you will see, many signals—from both the environment and genetics—initiate or delay eating.[4]

Hunger People eat for a variety of reasons, most obviously (although not necessarily most commonly) because they are hungry. Most people recognize **hunger** as an irritating feeling that prompts thoughts of food and motivates them to start eating. In the body, hunger is the physiological response to a need for food triggered by nerve signals and chemical messengers originating and acting in the brain, primarily in the **hypothalamus**. Hunger can be influenced by the presence or absence of nutrients in the bloodstream, the size and composition of the preceding meal, customary eating patterns, climate (heat reduces food intake; cold increases it), physical activity, hormones, and illnesses. Hunger determines what to eat, when to eat, and how much to eat.

The stomach is ideally designed to handle periodic batches of food, and people typically eat meals at roughly 4-hour intervals. Four hours after a meal, most, if not all, of the food has left the stomach. Most people do not feel like eating again until the stomach is either empty or almost so. Even then, a person may not feel hungry for quite a while.

Satiation During the course of a meal, as food enters the GI tract and hunger diminishes, **satiation** occurs. As receptors in the stomach stretch and hormones such as cholecystokinin become active, the person begins to feel full. The response: satiation, which prompts the person to stop eating.

Satiety After a meal, the feeling of **satiety** continues to suppress hunger and allows a person to not eat again for a while. Whereas *satiation* tells us to "stop eating," *satiety* reminds us to "not start eating again." Figure 8-2 (p. 238) summarizes the relationships among hunger, satiation, and satiety. Of course, people can override these signals, especially when presented with stressful situations or favorite foods.

*As Chapter 1 mentions, many scientists measure food energy in *kilojoules* (a measure of work energy). Conversion factors for these and other measures can be found in Appendix K.

**Some of the food energy values in the table of food composition in Appendix H were derived by bomb calorimetry, and many were calculated from their energy-yielding nutrient contents.

physiological fuel value: the number of kcalories that the body derives from a food, in contrast to the number of kcalories determined by calorimetry.

appetite: the integrated response to the sight, smell, thought, or taste of food that initiates or delays eating.

hunger: the painful sensation caused by a lack of food that initiates food-seeking behavior.

hypothalamus (high-po-THAL-ah-mus): a brain center that controls activities such as maintenance of water balance, regulation of body temperature, and control of appetite.

satiation (say-she-AY-shun): the feeling of satisfaction and fullness that occurs during a meal and halts eating. Satiation determines how much food is consumed during a meal.

satiety (sah-TIE-eh-tee): the feeling of fullness and satisfaction that occurs after a meal and inhibits eating until the next meal. Satiety determines how much time passes between meals.

> FIGURE 8-2 **Hunger, Satiation, and Satiety**

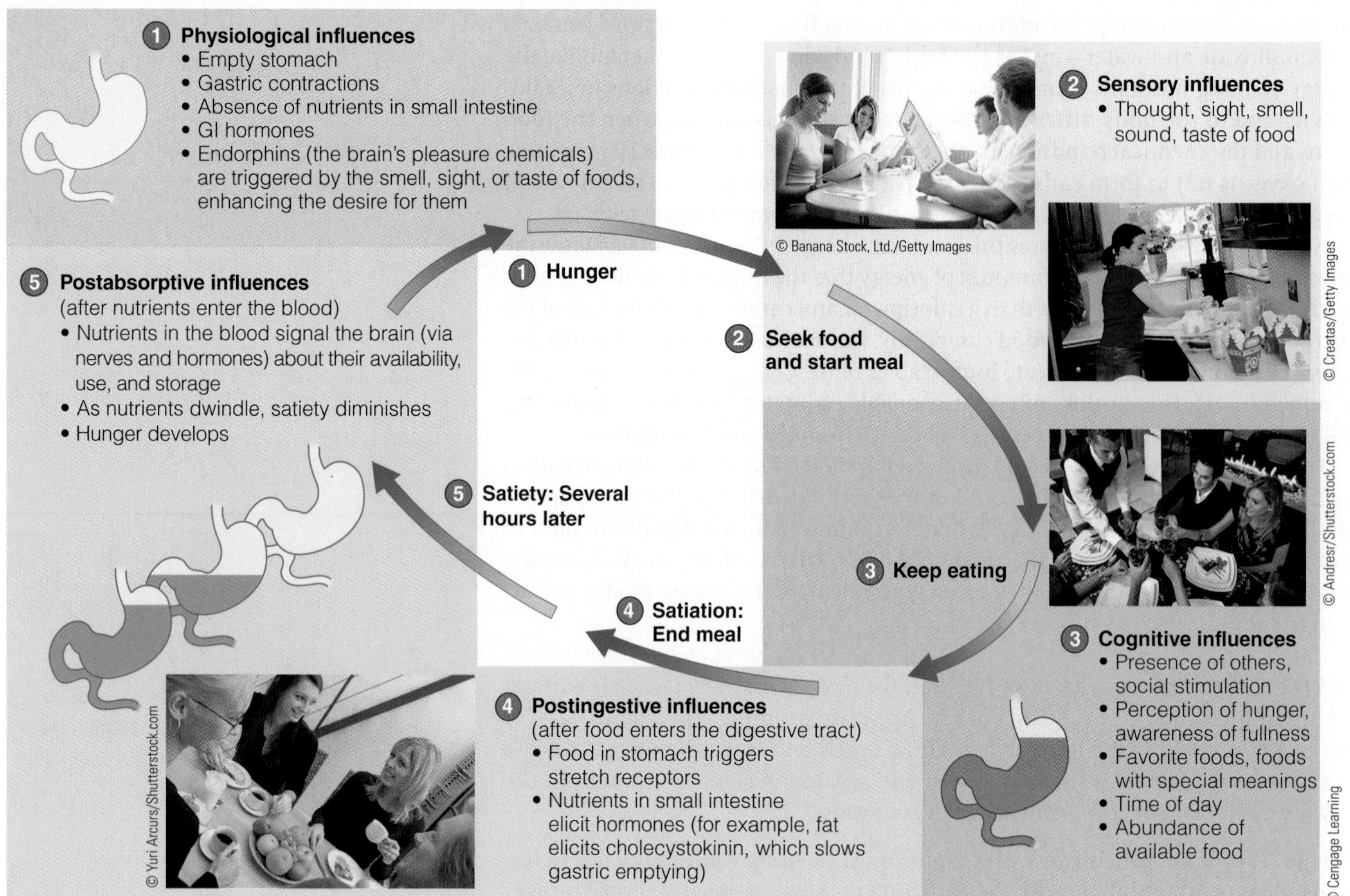

1 Physiological influences
• Empty stomach
• Gastric contractions
• Absence of nutrients in small intestine
• GI hormones
• Endorphins (the brain's pleasure chemicals) are triggered by the smell, sight, or taste of foods, enhancing the desire for them
2 Sensory influences
• Thought, sight, smell, sound, taste of food
© Banana Stock, Ltd./Getty Images
© Creatas/Getty Images
1 Hunger
2 Seek food and start meal
5 Postabsorptive influences
(after nutrients enter the blood)
• Nutrients in the blood signal the brain (via nerves and hormones) about their availability, use, and storage
• As nutrients dwindle, satiety diminishes
• Hunger develops
5 Satiety: Several hours later
3 Keep eating
© Andresr/Shutterstock.com
4 Satiation: End meal
3 Cognitive influences
• Presence of others, social stimulation
• Perception of hunger, awareness of fullness
• Favorite foods, foods with special meanings
• Time of day
• Abundance of available food
4 Postingestive influences
(after food enters the digestive tract)
• Food in stomach triggers stretch receptors
• Nutrients in small intestine elicit hormones (for example, fat elicits cholecystokinin, which slows gastric emptying)
© Yuri Arcurs/Shutterstock.com
© Cengage Learning

Overriding Hunger and Satiety Not surprisingly, eating can be triggered by signals other than hunger, even when the body does not need food. Some people experience food cravings when they are bored or anxious. In fact, they may eat in response to any kind of stress, negative or positive. ("What do I do when I'm grieving? Eat. What do I do when I'm celebrating? Eat!") Not too surprisingly, repeatedly eating to relieve chronic stress can lead to overeating and weight gain.

Many people respond to external cues such as the time of day ("It's time to eat") or the availability, sight, and taste of food ("I'd love a piece of chocolate even though I'm full"). Environmental influences such as large portion sizes, favorite foods, or an abundance or variety of foods stimulate eating and increase energy intake. Cognitive influences—such as perceptions, memories, intellect, and social interactions—can easily lead to weight gain. Those who are overweight or obese may be especially susceptible to external cues that trigger hunger and the desire to eat.[5]

Eating can also be suppressed by signals other than satiety, even when a person is hungry. People with the eating disorder anorexia nervosa, for example, use tremendous discipline to ignore the pangs of hunger. Some people simply cannot eat during times of stress, negative or positive. ("I'm too sad to eat." "I'm too excited to eat!") Why some people overeat in response to stress and others cannot eat at all remains a bit of a mystery, although researchers are beginning to understand the connections between stress hormones, brain activity, and "comfort foods." Factors that appear to be involved include how the person perceives the stress and whether usual eating behaviors are restrained. (Highlight 8 features anorexia nervosa and other eating disorders.)

Sustaining Satiation and Satiety The extent to which foods produce satiation and sustain satiety depends in part on the nutrient composition of a meal. Of the

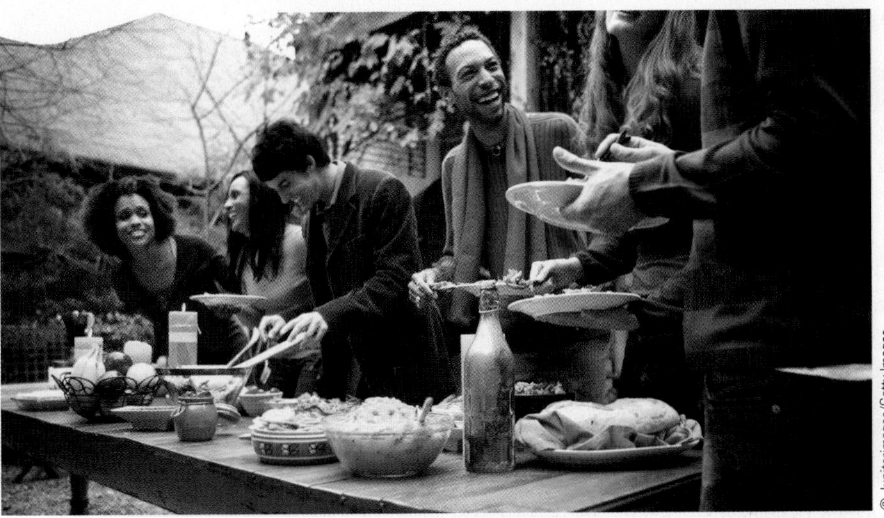

Regardless of hunger, people typically overeat when offered the abundance and variety of a buffet. To limit unhealthy weight gains, listen to hunger and satiety signals.

three energy-yielding nutrients, protein is considered the most **satiating.** In fact, too little protein in the diet can leave a person feeling hungry. Including some protein—such as drinking milk—provides satiety and decreases energy intake at the next meal.[6] In contrast, fructose in a sugary fruit drink seems to stimulate appetite and increase food intake.

Chapter 1 explains that energy density is a measure of the energy a food provides relative to the amount of food (kcalories per gram). Foods with a high energy density provide more kcalories, and those with low energy density provide fewer kcalories, for the same amount of food. Foods low in energy density are also more satiating. High-fiber foods effectively provide satiation by filling the stomach and delaying the absorption of nutrients. For this reason, eating a large salad as a first course helps a person eat less during the meal. In contrast, fat has a weak effect on satiation; consequently, eating high-fat foods may lead to passive overconsumption. High-fat foods are flavorful, which stimulates the appetite and entices people to eat more. High-fat foods are also energy dense; consequently, they deliver more kcalories per bite. (Chapter 9 describes how considering a food's energy density can help with weight management.) Although fat provides little satiation during a meal, it produces strong satiety signals once it enters the intestine. Fat in the intestine triggers the release of cholecystokinin—a hormone that signals satiety and inhibits food intake.

Eating high-fat foods while trying to limit energy intake requires small portion sizes, which can leave a person feeling unsatisfied. Portion size correlates directly with a food's satiety. Instead of eating small portions of high-fat foods and feeling deprived, a person can feel satisfied by eating large portions of low-fat, high-fiber, and low-energy-density foods. Figure 8-3 (p. 240) illustrates how fat influences portion size.

Message Central—The Hypothalamus As you can see, eating is a complex behavior controlled by a variety of genetic, psychological, social, metabolic, and physiological factors.[7] The hypothalamus appears to be the control center, integrating messages about energy intake, expenditure, and storage from other parts of the brain and from the mouth, GI tract, and liver.[8] Some of these messages influence satiation, which helps control the size of a meal; others influence satiety, which helps determine the frequency of meals.*

Dozens of gastrointestinal hormones influence appetite control and energy balance.[9] By understanding the action of these hormones, researchers may one day be able to develop anti-obesity treatments. An added challenge is to sort out

*Gastrointestinal hormones that regulate food intake include amylin, cholecystokinin (CCK), enterostatin, ghrelin, glucagon-like peptide-1 (GLP-1), oxyntomodulin, pancreatic polypeptide (PP), and peptide YY (PYY).

satiating: having the power to suppress hunger and inhibit eating.

> **FIGURE 8-3 How Fat Influences Portion Sizes**

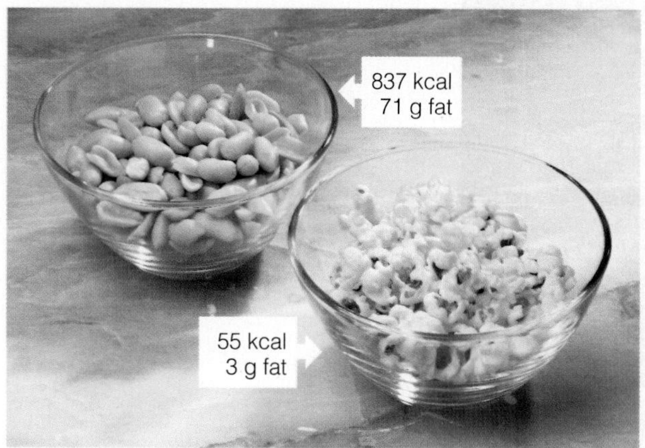

For the same size portion, peanuts deliver more than 15 times the kcalories and 20 times the fat of popcorn.

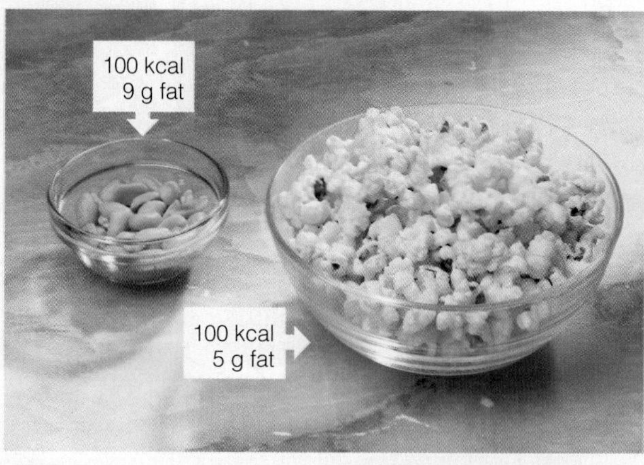

For the same number of kcalories, a person can have a few high-fat peanuts or almost 2 cups of high-fiber popcorn. (This comparison used oil-based popcorn; using air-popped popcorn would double the amount of popcorn in this example.)

the many actions of related brain chemicals. For example, one brain chemical, **neuropeptide Y,** causes carbohydrate cravings, initiates eating, decreases energy expenditure, and increases fat storage—all factors favoring a positive energy balance and weight gain.

neuropeptide Y: a chemical produced in the brain that stimulates appetite, diminishes energy expenditure, and increases fat storage.

thermogenesis: the generation of heat; used in physiology and nutrition studies as an index of how much energy the body is expending.

basal metabolism: the energy needed to maintain life when a body is at complete digestive, physical, and emotional rest.

> **REVIEW IT** Discuss some of the physical, emotional, and environmental influences on food intake.

A mixture of signals governs a person's eating behaviors. Hunger and appetite initiate eating, whereas satiation and satiety stop and delay eating, respectively. Each responds to messages from the nervous and hormonal systems. Superimposed on these signals are complex factors involving emotions, habits, and other aspects of human behavior.

8.3 Energy Out: The kCalories the Body Expends

> **LEARN IT** List the components of energy expenditure and factors that might influence each.

Chapter 7 explains that heat is released whenever the body breaks down carbohydrate, fat, or protein for energy and again when that energy is used to do work. The generation of heat, known as **thermogenesis,** can be measured to determine the amount of energy expended. The total energy a body expends reflects three main categories of thermogenesis:

- Energy expended for basal metabolism
- Energy expended for physical activity
- Energy expended for food consumption

A fourth category is sometimes involved:

- Energy expended for adaptation

> **FIGURE 8-4 Components of Energy Expenditure**

The amount of energy expended in voluntary physical activities has the greatest variability, depending on a person's activity patterns. For a sedentary person, physical activities may account for less than half as much energy as basal metabolism, whereas an extremely active person may expend as much on physical activity as for basal metabolism.

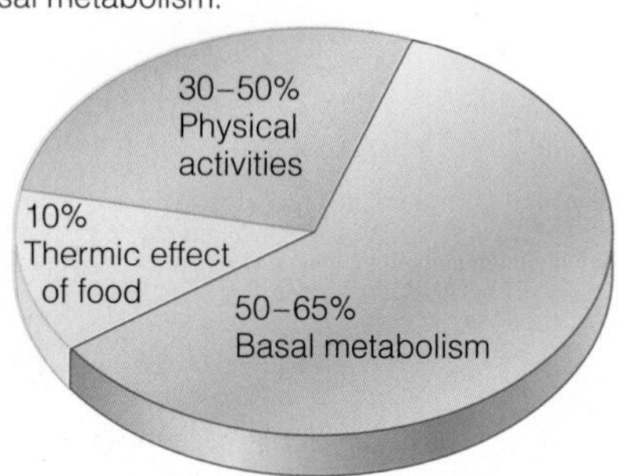

The amount of energy expended in a day differs for each individual, but in general, basal metabolism is the largest component of energy expenditure and thermic effect of food is the smallest.

Components of Energy Expenditure

People expend energy when they are physically active, of course, but they also expend energy when they are resting quietly. In fact, quiet metabolic activities account for the largest share of most people's energy expenditures, as Figure 8-4 shows.

Basal Metabolism About two-thirds of the energy the average person expends in a day supports the body's **basal metabolism.** Metabolic activities include the lungs inhaling and exhaling air, the bone marrow making new red blood cells,

TABLE 8-1 Estimating Energy Expended on Basal Metabolism

	BMR Estimates	BMR Equations
Men	Slightly >1 kcal/min (1.1 to 1.3 kcal/min) or 24 kcal/kg/day	$(10 \times \text{wt}) + (6.25 \times \text{ht}) - (5 \times \text{age}) + 5$
Women	Slightly <1 kcal/min (0.8 to 1.0 kcal/min) or 23 kcal/kg/day	$(10 \times \text{wt}) + (6.25 \times \text{ht}) - (5 \times \text{age}) - 161$
Note	For perspective, a burning candle or a 75-watt light bulb releases about 1 kcal/min	Use actual weight in kilograms, height in centimeters, and age in years

the heart beating 100,000 times a day, and the kidneys filtering wastes—in short, they support all the basic processes of life.

The **basal metabolic rate (BMR)** is the rate at which the body expends energy for these life-sustaining activities. The rate may vary from person to person and may vary for the same individual with a change in circumstance or physical condition. The rate is slowest when a person is sleeping undisturbed, but it is usually measured in a room with a comfortable temperature when the person is awake, but lying still, after a restful sleep and an overnight (12 to 14 hour) fast. A similar measure of energy output—called the **resting metabolic rate (RMR)**—is slightly higher than the BMR because its criteria for recent food intake and physical activity are not as strict. When energy needs cannot be measured, equations can provide reasonably accurate estimates (see Table 8-1).

In general, the more a person weighs, the more *total* energy is expended on basal metabolism, but the amount of energy *per pound* of body weight may be lower. For example, an adult's BMR might be 1500 kcalories per day and an infant's only 500, but compared to body weight, the infant's BMR is more than twice as fast. Similarly, a normal-weight adult may have a metabolic rate one and a half times that of an obese adult when compared to body weight because lean tissue is metabolically more active than body fat.

Table 8-2 (p. 242) summarizes the factors that raise and lower the BMR. For the most part, the BMR is highest in people who are growing (children, adolescents, and pregnant women) and in those with considerable **lean body mass** (physically fit people and males). One way to increase the BMR, then, is to participate in endurance and strength-training activities regularly to maximize lean body mass. The BMR is also high in people with fever or under stress and in people with highly active thyroid glands. The BMR slows down with a loss of lean body mass and during fasting and malnutrition.

Physical Activity The second component of a person's energy output is physical activity: voluntary movement of the skeletal muscles and support systems. Physical activity is the most variable—and the most changeable—component of energy expenditure. Consequently, its influence on both weight gain and weight loss can be significant.

During physical activity, the muscles need extra energy to move, and the heart and lungs need extra energy to deliver nutrients and oxygen and dispose of wastes. The amount of energy needed for any activity, whether playing tennis or studying for an exam, depends on three factors: muscle mass, body weight, and activity. The larger the muscle mass and the heavier the weight of the body part being moved, the more energy is expended. Table 8-3 (p. 242) gives average energy expenditures for various activities. The activity's duration, frequency, and intensity also influence energy expenditure: the longer, the more frequent, and the more intense the activity, the more kcalories expended. (Chapter 14 describes how an activity's duration, frequency, and intensity also influence the body's use of the energy-yielding nutrients.)

basal metabolic rate (BMR): the rate of energy use for metabolism under specified conditions: after a 12-hour fast and restful sleep, without any physical activity or emotional excitement, and in a comfortable setting. It is usually expressed as kcalories per kilogram body weight per hour.

resting metabolic rate (RMR): similar to the basal metabolic rate (BMR), a measure of energy use for a person at rest in a comfortable setting, but with less stringent criteria for recent food intake and physical activity. Consequently, the RMR is slightly higher than the BMR.

lean body mass: the body minus its fat.

TABLE 8-2 Factors that Affect the BMR

Factor	Effect on BMR
Age	Lean body mass diminishes with age, slowing the BMR.[a]
Height	In tall, thin people, the BMR is higher.[b]
Growth	In children, adolescents, and pregnant women, the BMR is higher.
Body composition (gender)	The more lean tissue, the higher the BMR (which is why males usually have a higher BMR than females). The more fat tissue, the lower the BMR.
Fever	Fever raises the BMR.[c]
Stresses	Stresses (including many diseases and certain drugs) raise the BMR.
Environmental temperature	Both heat and cold raise the BMR.
Fasting/starvation	Fasting/starvation lowers the BMR.[d]
Malnutrition	Malnutrition lowers the BMR.
Hormones	The thyroid hormone thyroxine, for example, can speed up or slow down the BMR.[e] Premenstrual hormones slightly raise the BMR.
Smoking	Nicotine increases energy expenditure.
Caffeine	Caffeine increases energy expenditure.
Sleep	BMR is lowest when sleeping.

[a]The BMR begins to decrease in early adulthood (after growth and development cease) at a rate of about 2 percent/decade. A reduction in voluntary activity as well brings the total decline in energy expenditure to about 5 percent/decade.
[b]If two people weigh the same, the taller, thinner person will have the faster metabolic rate, reflecting the greater skin surface, through which heat is lost by radiation, in proportion to the body's volume (see Figure 8-5, p. 244).
[c]Fever raises the BMR by 7 percent for each degree Fahrenheit.
[d]Prolonged starvation reduces the total amount of metabolically active lean tissue in the body, although the decline occurs sooner and to a greater extent than body losses alone can explain. More likely, the neural and hormonal changes that accompany fasting are responsible for changes in the BMR.
[e]The thyroid gland releases hormones that travel to the cells and influence cellular metabolism. Thyroid hormone activity can speed up or slow down the rate of metabolism by as much as 50 percent.

TABLE 8-3 Estimating Energy Expended on Physical Activities

The values listed in this table reflect both the energy expended in physical activity and the amount used for BMR. To calculate kcalories spent per minute of activity for your own body weight, multiply kcal/lb/min (or kcal/kg/min) by your exact weight and then multiply that number by the number of minutes spent in the activity. For example, if you weigh 142 pounds, and you want to know how many kcalories you spent doing 30 minutes of vigorous aerobic dance: 0.062 × 142 = 8.8 kcalories per minute; 8.8 × 30 minutes = 264 total kcalories expended.

Activity	kCal/lb min	kCal/kg min
Aerobic dance (vigorous)	.062	.136
Basketball (vigorous, full court)	.097	.213
Bicycling		
13 mph	.045	.099
15 mph	.049	.108
17 mph	.057	.125
19 mph	.076	.167
21 mph	.090	.198
23 mph	.109	.240
25 mph	.139	.306
Canoeing, flat water, moderate pace	.045	.099
Cross-country skiing 8 mph	.104	.229
Gardening	.045	.099
Golf (carrying clubs)	.045	.099
Handball	.078	.172
Horseback riding (trot)	.052	.114
Rowing (vigorous)	.097	.213
Running		
5 mph	.061	.134
6 mph	.074	.163
7.5 mph	.094	.207
9 mph	.103	.227
10 mph	.114	.251
11 mph	.131	.288
Soccer (vigorous)	.097	.213
Studying	.011	.024
Swimming		
20 yd/min	.032	.070
45 yd/min	.058	.128
50 yd/min	.070	.154
Table tennis (skilled)	.045	.099
Tennis (beginner)	.032	.070
Vacuuming and other household tasks	.030	.066
Walking		
3.5 mph	.035	.077
4.5 mph	.048	.106
Weight lifting		
light-to-moderate	.024	.053
vigorous	.048	.106
Wheelchair basketball	.084	.185
Wheeling self in wheelchair	.030	.066
Wii games		
bowling	.021	.046
boxing	.021	.047
tennis	.022	.048

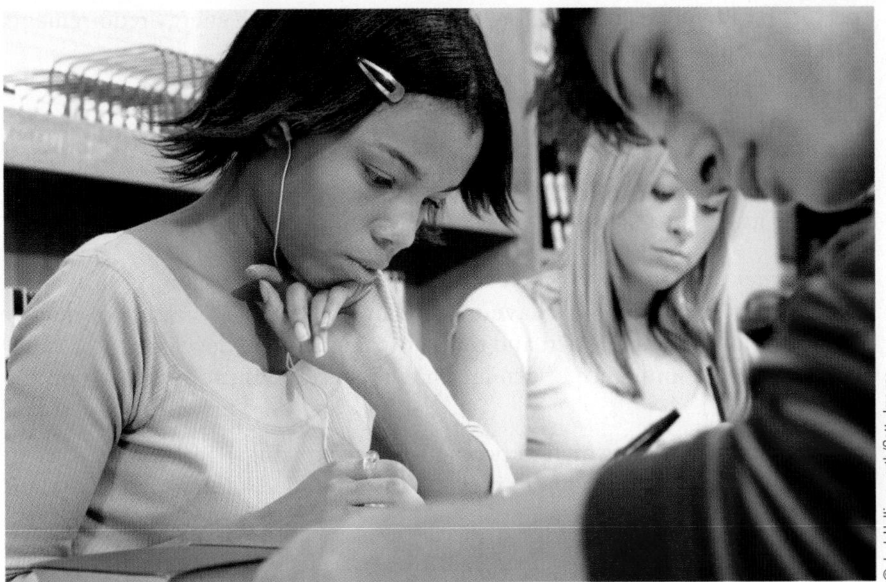

© Jack Hollingsworth/Getty Images

It feels like work and it may make you tired, but studying requires only one or two kcalories per minute.

Thermic Effect of Food When a person eats, the GI tract muscles speed up their rhythmic contractions, the cells that manufacture and secrete digestive juices become active, and some nutrients require energy to be absorbed. This acceleration of activity requires energy and produces heat; it is known as the **thermic effect of food (TEF).**

The thermic effect of food is proportional to the food energy taken in and is usually estimated at 10 percent of energy intake. Thus a person who ingests 2000 kcalories probably expends about 200 kcalories on the thermic effect of food. The proportions vary for different foods, however, and are also influenced by factors such as meal size and frequency. In general, the thermic effect of food is greater for high-protein foods than for high-fat foods (see Table 8-4) and for a meal eaten all at once rather than spread out over a couple of hours. For most purposes, however, the thermic effect of food can be ignored when estimating energy expenditure because its contribution to total energy output is smaller than the probable errors involved in estimating overall energy intake and output.

Adaptive Thermogenesis Additional energy is expended when circumstances in the body are dramatically changed. A body challenged to physical conditioning, extreme cold, overfeeding, starvation, trauma, or other types of stress must adapt; it has extra work to do and uses extra energy to build the tissues and produce the enzymes and hormones necessary to cope with the demand. This energy is known as **adaptive thermogenesis,** and in some circumstances (for example, in burn victims), it makes a considerable difference in the total energy expended. Because this component of energy expenditure is so variable and

TABLE 8-4 Estimating Energy Expended on Thermic Effect of Foods

Food Component	Energy Expended
Carbohydrate	5–10%
Fat	0–5%
Protein	20–30%
Alcohol	15–20%

NOTE: Percentages are calculated by dividing the energy expended during digestion and absorption (above basal) by the energy content of the food.

© Cengage Learning

thermic effect of food (TEF): an estimation of the energy required to process food (digest, absorb, transport, metabolize, and store ingested nutrients); also called the *specific dynamic effect (SDE)* of food or the *specific dynamic activity (SDA)* of food. The sum of the TEF and any increase in the metabolic rate due to overeating is known as *diet-induced thermogenesis (DIT).*

adaptive thermogenesis: adjustments in energy expenditure related to changes in environment such as extreme cold and to physiological events such as overfeeding, trauma, and changes in hormone status.

> FIGURE 8-5 How Body Size Influences BMR

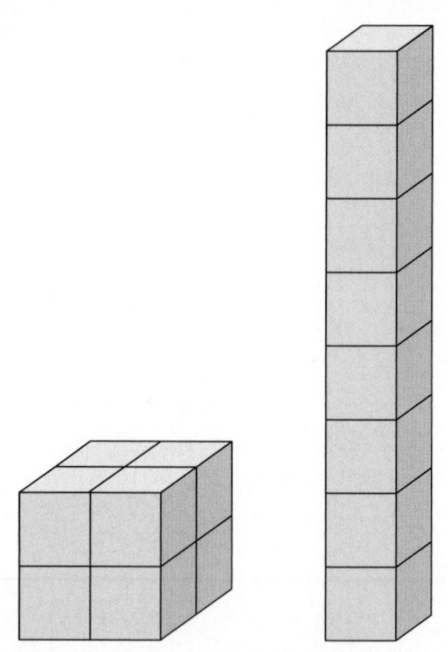

Each of these structures is made of eight blocks. They weigh the same, but they are arranged differently. The short, wide structure has 24 sides exposed and the tall, thin one has 34. Because the tall, thin structure has a greater surface area, it will lose more heat (expend more energy) than the short, wide one. Similarly, two people of different heights might weigh the same, but the taller, thin one will have a higher BMR (expending more energy) because of the greater skin surface.

specific to individuals, it is not included when estimating energy requirements for most healthy people.

Estimating Energy Requirements In estimating energy requirements, the DRI Committee developed equations based on research measuring total daily energy expenditure. These equations consider how the following factors influence BMR and consequently energy expenditure:

- *Gender.* In general, women have a lower BMR than men, in large part because men typically have more lean body mass. Two sets of energy equations—one for men and one for women—were developed to accommodate the influence of gender on energy expenditure (provided on the next page).
- *Growth.* The BMR is high in people who are growing. For this reason, pregnant and lactating women, infants, children, and adolescents have their own sets of energy equations.
- *Age.* The BMR declines during adulthood as lean body mass diminishes. This change in body composition occurs, in part, because some hormones that influence appetite, body weight, and metabolism become more, or less, active with age. Physical activities tend to decline as well, bringing the average reduction in energy expenditure to about 5 percent per decade. The decline in BMR that occurs when a person becomes less active reflects the loss of lean body mass and may be minimized with ongoing physical activity. Because age influences energy expenditure, it is also factored into the energy equations.
- *Physical activity.* Using individual values for various physical activities (as in Table 8-3 on p. 242) is time-consuming and impractical for estimating the energy needs of a population. Instead, various activities are clustered according to the typical intensity of a day's efforts. Energy equations include a physical activity factor for various levels of intensity for each gender.
- *Body composition and body size.* The BMR is high in people who are tall and so have a large surface area, as illustrated in Figure 8-5. Similarly, the more a person weighs, the more energy is expended on basal metabolism. For these reasons, energy equations include a factor for both height and weight.

As just explained, energy needs vary between individuals depending on such factors as gender, growth, age, physical activity, and body size and composition. Even when two people are similarly matched, however, their energy needs still differ because of genetic differences. Perhaps one day genetic research will reveal how to estimate requirements for each individual. For now, the "How To" feature provides instructions on estimating energy requirements using the DRI equations and physical activity factors. Appendix F presents a table that provides a shortcut to estimating daily energy needs by age, gender, and activity level, based on the DRI equations using reference heights and weights.

> REVIEW IT List the components of energy expenditure and factors that might influence each.

A person in energy balance takes in energy from food and expends much of it on basal metabolism, some of it on physical activities, and a little on the thermic effect of food. Energy requirements vary from person to person, depending on such factors as gender, age, weight, and height as well as the intensity and duration of physical activity. All of these factors must be considered when estimating energy requirements.

>How To

Estimate Energy Requirements

To determine your estimated energy requirement (EER), use the appropriate equation, inserting your age in years, weight (wt) in kilograms, height (ht) in meters, and physical activity (PA) factor from the accompanying table. (To convert pounds to kilograms, divide by 2.2; to convert inches to meters, divide by 39.37.)

- For men 19 years and older:
  EER = [662 − (9.53 × age)] + PA × [(15.91 × wt) + (539.6 × ht)]
- For women 19 years and older:
  EER = [354 − (6.91 × age)] + PA × [(9.36 × wt) + (726 × ht)]

For example, consider an active 30-year-old male who is 5 feet 11 inches tall and weighs 178 pounds. First, he converts his weight from pounds to kilograms and his height from inches to meters, if necessary:

$$178 \text{ lb} \div 2.2 = 80.9 \text{ kg}$$

$$71 \text{ in} \div 39.37 = 1.8 \text{ m}$$

Next, he considers his level of daily physical activity and selects the appropriate PA factor from the accompanying table. (In this example, 1.25 for an active male.) Then, he inserts his age, PA factor, weight, and height into the appropriate equation:

$$\text{EER} = [662 - (9.53 \times 30)] + 1.25 \times [(15.91 \times 80.9) + (539.6 \times 1.8)]$$

(A reminder: Do calculations within the parentheses first.) He calculates:

$$\text{EER} = [662 - 286] + 1.25 \times [1287 + 971]$$

(Another reminder: Do calculations within the brackets next.)

$$\text{EER} = 376 + 1.25 \times 2258$$

(One more reminder: Do multiplication before addition.)

$$\text{EER} = 376 + 2823$$

$$\text{EER} = 3199$$

The estimated energy requirement for an active 30-year-old male who is 5 feet 11 inches tall and weighs 178 pounds is about 3200 kcalories/day. His actual requirement probably falls within a range of 200 kcalories above and below this estimate.

NOTE: Appendix F provides estimates of energy needs based on EER equations, using reference heights and weights for each age-gender group.

Physical Activity (PA) Factors for EER Equations

	Men	Women	Physical Activity
Sedentary	1.0	1.0	Typical daily living activities
Low active	1.11	1.12	plus 30–60 min moderate activity
Active	1.25	1.27	plus ≥ 60 min moderate activity
Very active	1.48	1.45	plus ≥ 60 min moderate activity and 60 min vigorous or 120 min moderate activity

NOTE: Moderate activity is equivalent to walking at 3 to 4½ mph.

> TRY IT Estimate your energy requirement based on your current age, weight, height, and activity level.

8.4 Body Weight and Body Composition

> LEARN IT Distinguish between body weight and body composition, including methods to assess each.

A person 5 feet 10 inches tall who weighs 150 pounds may carry only about 30 of those pounds as fat.* The rest is mostly water and lean tissues—muscles, organs such as the heart and liver, and the bones of the skeleton. Direct measures of **body composition** are impossible in living human beings; instead, researchers assess body composition indirectly based on the following assumption:

$$\text{Body weight} = \text{fat} + \text{lean tissue (including water)}$$

Weight gains and losses tell us nothing about how the body's composition may have changed, yet weight is the measure most people use to judge their "fatness." For many people, overweight is overfat, but this is not always the case. Athletes with dense bones and well-developed muscles may be overweight by some standards but have little body fat. Conversely, inactive people may seem to have acceptable weights, when, in fact, they may have too much body fat.

*In metric terms, a person 1.78 meters tall who weighs 68 kilograms may carry only about 14 of those kilograms as fat.

body composition: the proportions of muscle, bone, fat, and other tissue that make up a person's total body weight.

Defining Healthy Body Weight How much should a person weigh? How can a person know if her weight is appropriate for her height? How can a person know if his weight is jeopardizing his health? Such questions seem so simple, yet the answers can be complex—and quite different depending on whom you ask.

The Criterion of Fashion In asking what is ideal, people often mistakenly turn to friends and fashion for the answer and judge body weight by appearances. No doubt our society sets unrealistic ideals for body weight, especially for women. Magazines, movies, and television all convey the message that to be thin is to be beautiful and happy. As a result, the media have a great influence on the weight concerns and dieting patterns of people of all ages, but most tragically on young, impressionable children and adolescents.

Importantly, perceived body image may have little to do with actual body weight or size. People of all shapes, sizes, and ages—including extremely thin fashion models with anorexia nervosa and fitness instructors with ideal body composition—have learned to be unhappy with their "overweight" bodies. Such dissatisfaction can lead to damaging behaviors, such as starvation diets, diet pill abuse, and health-care avoidance. The first step toward making healthy changes may be self-acceptance. Keep in mind that fashion is fickle; the body shapes valued by our society change with time. Furthermore, body shapes valued by one society differ from those of other societies. The standards defining "ideal" are subjective and may have little in common with health. Table 8-5 offers some tips for adopting health as an ideal.

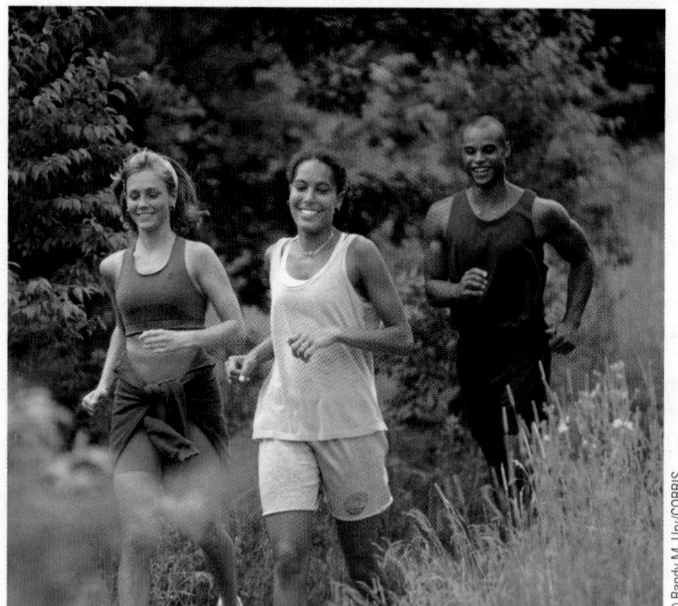

A healthy body contains enough lean tissue to support health and the right amount of fat to meet body needs.

The Criterion of Health Even if our society were to accept fat as beautiful, obesity is still a major risk factor for several life-threatening diseases, including heart disease, type 2 diabetes, and some cancers. For this reason, the most important criterion for determining how much a person should weigh and how much body fat a person needs is not appearance but good health and longevity. Ideally, a person has enough fat to meet basic needs but not so much as to incur health risks. This range of healthy body weights has been identified using a common measure of weight and height—the body mass index.

Body Mass Index The **body mass index (BMI)** describes relative weight for height:

$$\text{BMI} = \frac{\text{weight (kg)}}{\text{height (m)}^2} \text{ or } \frac{\text{weight (lb)}}{\text{height (in)}^2} \times 703$$

Weight classifications based on BMI are presented in Table 8-6. Notice that healthy weight falls between a BMI of 18.5 and 24.9, with **underweight** below 18.5, **overweight** above 25, and **obese** above 30. Figure 8-6 shows examples of body shapes with different BMI. More than two-thirds of adults in the United States have a BMI greater than 25, as Figure 8-7 shows.[10]

body mass index (BMI): a measure of a person's weight relative to height; determined by dividing the weight (in kilograms) by the square of the height (in meters).

underweight: body weight lower than the weight range that is considered healthy; BMI less than 18.5.

overweight: body weight greater than the weight range that is considered healthy; BMI 25 to 29.9.

obese: too much body fat with adverse health effects; BMI 30 or more.

TABLE 8-5 Tips for Accepting a Healthy Body Weight

- Value yourself and others for human attributes other than body weight. Realize that prejudging people by weight is as harmful as prejudging them by race, religion, or gender.
- Use positive, nonjudgmental descriptions of your body.
- Accept positive comments from others.
- Focus on your whole self, including your intelligence, social grace, and professional and scholastic achievements.
- Accept that no magic diet exists.
- Stop dieting to lose weight. Adopt a lifestyle of healthy eating and physical activity permanently.
- Follow the USDA Food Patterns. Never restrict food intake below the minimum levels that meet nutrient needs.
- Become physically active, not because it will help you get thin but because it will make you feel good and improve your health.
- Seek support from loved ones. Tell them of your plan for a healthy life in the body you have been given.
- Seek professional counseling from someone who can help you make gains in self-esteem without weight as the primary focus.
- Appreciate body weight for its influence on health, not appearance.

TABLE 8-6 Body Mass Index (BMI)

	Underweight	Healthy Weight						Overweight					Obese										
	(<18.5)	(18.5–24.9)						(25–29.9)					(≥30)										
	18	19	20	21	22	23	24	25	26	27	28	29	30	31	32	33	34	35	36	37	38	39	40
Height	***Body weight (pounds)***																						
4′10″	86	91	96	100	105	110	115	119	124	129	134	138	143	148	153	158	162	167	172	177	181	186	191
4′11″	89	94	99	104	109	114	119	124	128	133	138	143	148	153	158	163	168	173	178	183	188	193	198
5′0″	92	97	102	107	112	118	123	128	133	138	143	148	153	158	163	168	174	179	184	189	194	199	204
5′1″	95	100	106	111	116	122	127	132	137	143	148	153	158	164	169	174	180	185	190	195	201	206	211
5′2″	98	104	109	115	120	126	131	136	142	147	153	158	164	169	175	180	186	191	196	202	207	213	218
5′3″	102	107	113	118	124	130	135	141	146	152	158	163	169	175	180	186	191	197	203	208	214	220	225
5′4″	105	110	116	122	128	134	140	145	151	157	163	169	174	180	186	192	197	204	209	215	221	227	232
5′5″	108	114	120	126	132	138	144	150	156	162	168	174	180	186	192	198	204	210	216	222	228	234	240
5′6″	112	118	124	130	136	142	148	155	161	167	173	179	186	192	198	204	210	216	223	229	235	241	247
5′7″	115	121	127	134	140	146	153	159	166	172	178	185	191	198	204	211	217	223	230	236	242	249	255
5′8″	118	125	131	138	144	151	158	164	171	177	184	190	197	203	210	216	223	230	236	243	249	256	262
5′9″	122	128	135	142	149	155	162	169	176	182	189	196	203	209	216	223	230	236	243	250	257	263	270
5′10″	126	132	139	146	153	160	167	174	181	188	195	202	209	216	222	229	236	243	250	257	264	271	278
5′11″	129	136	143	150	157	165	172	179	186	193	200	208	215	222	229	236	243	250	257	265	272	279	286
6′0″	132	140	147	154	162	169	177	184	191	199	206	213	221	228	235	242	250	258	265	272	279	287	294
6′1″	136	144	151	159	166	174	182	189	197	204	212	219	227	235	242	250	257	265	272	280	288	295	302
6′2″	141	148	155	163	171	179	186	194	202	210	218	225	233	241	249	256	264	272	280	287	295	303	311
6′3″	144	152	160	168	176	184	192	200	208	216	224	232	240	248	256	264	272	279	287	295	303	311	319
6′4″	148	156	164	172	180	189	197	205	213	221	230	238	246	254	263	271	279	287	295	304	312	320	328
6′5″	151	160	168	176	185	193	202	210	218	227	235	244	252	261	269	277	286	294	303	311	319	328	336
6′6″	155	164	172	181	190	198	207	216	224	233	241	250	259	267	276	284	293	302	310	319	328	336	345

Obesity-related diseases become evident beyond a BMI of 25. For this reason, a BMI of 25 for adults represents a healthy goal for overweight people and an upper limit for others. The lower end of the healthy range may be a reasonable target for severely underweight people. BMI values slightly below the healthy range may

> FIGURE 8-6 BMI and Body Shapes

Standard silhouette figures such as those shown below are commonly used in research studies (without the BMI numbers) to determine how accurately people perceive their body size.

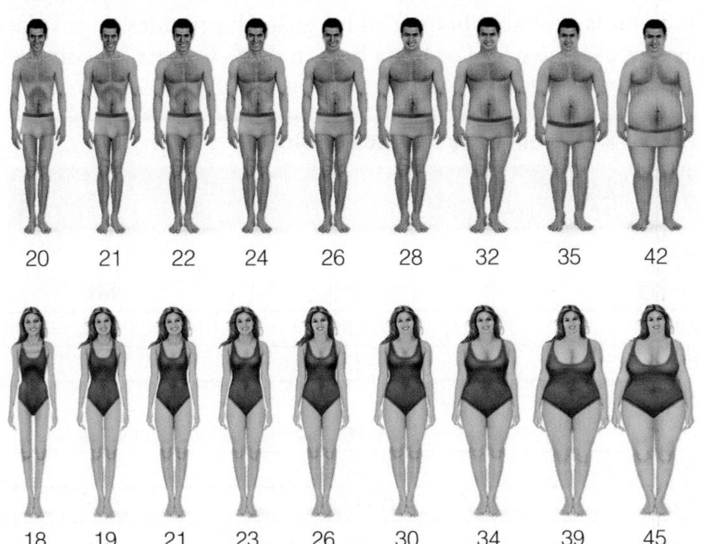

Source: A. J. Stunkard, T. Sorensen, and F. Schulsinger, Use of the Danish Adoption Register for the study of obesity and thinness, Research Publications: Association for Research in Nervous and Mental Disorders 60 (1983): 115–120.

> FIGURE 8-7 Distribution of Body Weights in US Adults

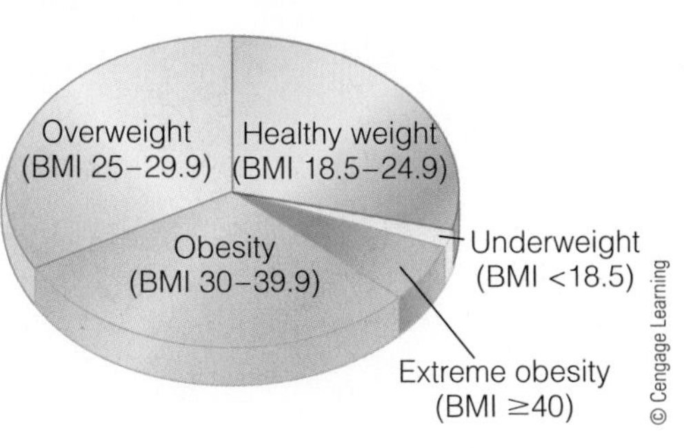

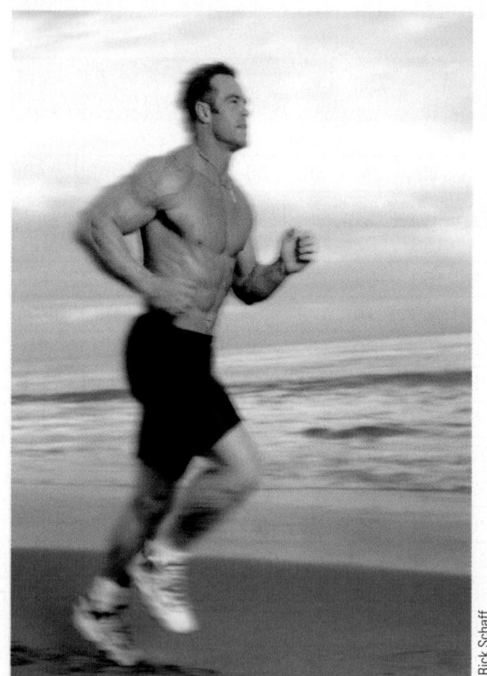
© Rick Schaff

At 6 feet 4 inches tall and 250 pounds (1.93 meters and 113 kilograms), this runner would be considered over*weight* by most standards. Yet he is clearly not over*fat*.

TABLE 8-7 Percent Body Fat at Various BMI

	BMI 18.5	BMI 25	BMI 30	BMI 35	BMI 40
Men	12–19%	23–28%	27–32%	31–35%	34–38%
Women	25–32%	35–40%	40–44%	43–47%	46–49%

NOTE: In general, women have roughly 12% more body fat than men at the same BMI.

SOURCE: Adapted from M. Heo and coauthors, Percentage of body fat cutoffs by sex, age, and race-ethnicity in the US adult population from NHANES 1999–2004, American Journal of Clinical Nutrition 95 (2012): 594–602.

be compatible with good health if food intake is adequate, but signs of illness, reduced work capacity, and poor reproductive function become apparent when BMI is below 17. The "How To" feature describes how to determine your BMI and how to find a goal weight based on a desired BMI.

Keep in mind that BMI reflects height and weight measures and not body composition. Consequently, muscular athletes may be classified as over*weight* by BMI standards and not be over*fat*. At the peak of his bodybuilding career, Arnold Schwarzenegger won the Mr. Olympia competition with a BMI of 31, the same BMI as the man running in the accompanying photo. Yet neither would be considered obese. Striking differences in body composition are also apparent among people of different ages and various ethnic and racial groups, making standard BMI guidelines inappropriate for some populations. For example, blacks tend to have a greater bone density and protein content than whites; consequently, using BMI as the standard may overestimate the prevalence of overweight and obesity among blacks.

Body Fat and Its Distribution Although weight measures are inexpensive, easy to take, and highly accurate, they fail to reveal two valuable pieces of information in assessing disease risk: how much of the weight is fat and where the fat is located.[11] The ideal amount of body fat depends partly on the person. Table 8-7 shows the percent body fat in the US population at various BMI and Table 8-8 compares percent body fat values of healthy weight, average fitness individuals with averages from national surveys.

Some People Need Less Body Fat For many athletes, a lower percentage of body fat may be ideal—just enough fat to provide fuel, insulate and protect the body, assist in nerve impulse transmissions, and support normal hormone activity, but not so much as to burden the body with excess bulk. Percent body fat for athletes, then, might be 7 to 16 percent for young men and 15 to 22 percent for young women. (Review the runner's photo to appreciate what 8 percent body fat looks like—even with a BMI greater than 30.)

Some People Need More Body Fat For an Alaska fisherman, a higher percentage of body fat is probably beneficial because fat provides an insulating blanket to prevent excessive loss of body heat in cold climates. A woman starting a

TABLE 8-8 Percent Body Fat: Ideal vs Actual

Age (yr)	Ideal (Healthy weight, average fitness)	Actual (US average)
Male		
20–39	18–21%	26%
40–59	22–25%	29%
60+	24–27%	31%
Female		
20–39	23–26%	38%
40–59	28–32%	41%
60+	31–34%	42%

SOURCE: L. G. Borrud and coauthors, Body composition data for individuals 8 years of age and older: US population, 1999–2004, *Vital and Health Statistics* 11 (2010): 1–87; *ACSM's Health-Related Physical Fitness Assessment Manual*, 2nd ed. (Baltimore, MD: Lippincott Williams & Wilkins, 2008), p. 59.

>How To

Determine BMI

To calculate your body mass index (BMI), use one of the following equations:

$$\text{BMI} = \frac{\text{weight (lb)}}{\text{height (in)}^2} \times 703$$

or

$$\text{BMI} = \frac{\text{weight (kg)}}{\text{height (m)}^2}$$

Consider, for example, a person who is 5′5″ (1.65 m) tall and weighs 174 lb (79 kg):

$$\text{BMI} = \frac{174 \text{ lb}}{65 \text{ in}^2} \times 703 = 29$$

or

$$\text{BMI} = \frac{79 \text{ kg}}{1.65 \text{ m}^2} = 29$$

This person has a BMI of 29 and is considered overweight.

You could also use Table 8-6 (p. 247) to determine your BMI. Locate your height in the first column (in this example, 5′5″). Then look across the row until you find the number that is closest to your weight (in this example, 174). The number at the top of that column identifies your BMI (in this example, 29).

A reasonable initial target for most overweight people is a BMI 2 units below their current one. To determine a goal weight based on a desired BMI, locate your height in the first column and then look across the row until you reach the column with the desired BMI at the top. In this example, to reach a BMI of 27, this person's goal weight is 162 pounds, which represents a 12-pound weight loss. Such a determination can help a person set realistic weight goals using health risk as a guide.

> TRY IT Calculate your BMI and determine whether you are underweight, healthy weight, overweight, or obese. If your BMI is less than 18.5 or greater than 25, identify a weight that takes your BMI 2 units closer to the healthy weight range.

pregnancy needs sufficient body fat to support conception and fetal growth. Below a certain threshold for body fat, hormone synthesis falters, and individuals may become infertile, develop depression, experience abnormal hunger regulation, or become unable to keep warm. These thresholds differ for each function and for each individual; much remains to be learned about them.

Fat Distribution The location of fat on the body may influence health as much, or more than, total fat alone. **Visceral fat** that is stored around the organs of the abdomen is referred to as **central obesity** or upper-body fat (see Figure 8-8 on p. 250). Much research supports the widely held belief that central obesity—significantly and independently of BMI—contributes to heart disease, cancers, diabetes, and related deaths.[12]

Visceral fat is most common in men and to a lesser extent in women past menopause. Even when total body fat is similar, men have more visceral fat than women. **Subcutaneous fat** around the hips and thighs, sometimes referred to as lower-body fat, is most common in women during their reproductive years, and is associated with lower heart disease risks.[13] Figure 8-9 (p. 250) compares the body shapes of people with upper-body fat and lower-body fat.

Waist Circumference A person's **waist circumference** is a good indicator of central obesity and its associated health risks.[14] In general, women with a waist circumference of greater than 35 inches (88 centimeters) and men with a waist circumference of greater than 40 inches (102 centimeters) have a high risk of central obesity–related health problems. To simplify the message, waist circumference should be less than half of a person's height; the waist-to-height ratio is also a useful measure of disease risks.[15] As waist circumference increases, disease risks increase. Appendix E includes instructions for measuring waist circumference and assessing abdominal fat.

Some researchers use the waist-to-hip ratio as an indicator of disease risks. The ratio requires another step or two (measuring the hips and comparing that

visceral fat: fat stored within the abdominal cavity in association with the internal abdominal organs; also called *intra-abdominal fat.*

central obesity: excess fat around the trunk of the body; also called *abdominal fat* or *upper-body fat.*

subcutaneous fat: fat stored directly under the skin.

- **sub** = beneath
- **cutaneous** = skin

waist circumference: an anthropometric measurement used to assess a person's abdominal fat.

> **FIGURE 8-8 Central Obesity**

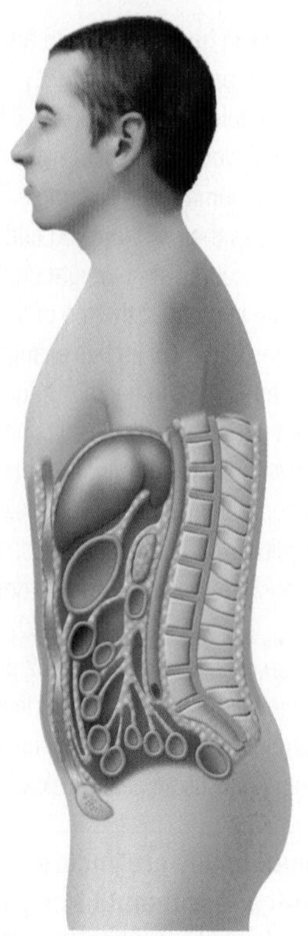

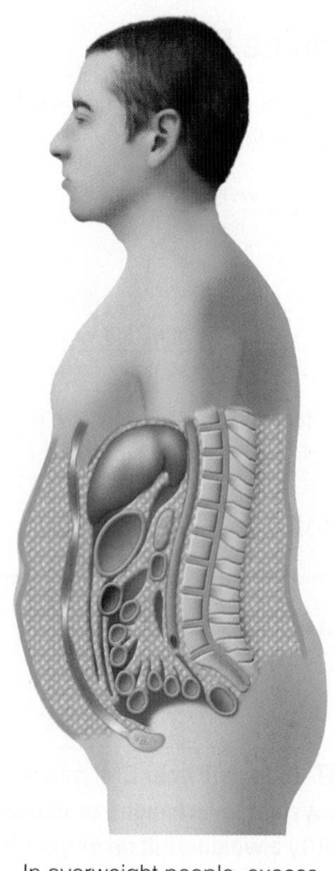

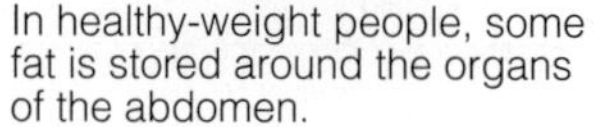

In healthy-weight people, some fat is stored around the organs of the abdomen.

In overweight people, excess abdominal fat increases the risks of diseases.

> **FIGURE 8-9 "Apple" and "Pear" Body Shapes Compared**

Popular articles sometimes call bodies with upper-body fat "apples" and those with lower-body fat, "pears." Researchers sometimes refer to upper-body fat as "android" (manlike) obesity and to lower-body fat as "gynoid" (womanlike) obesity.

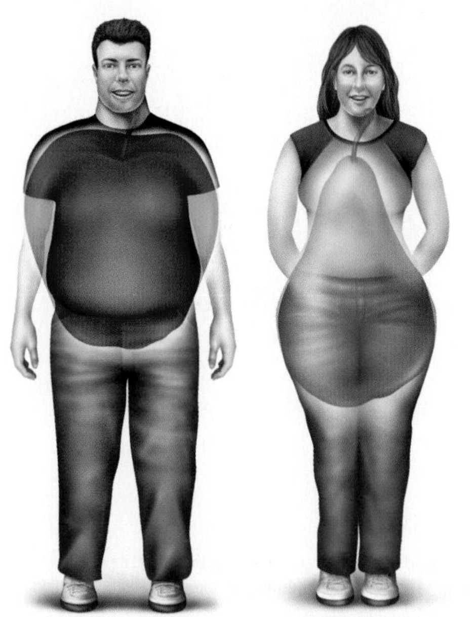

Upper-body fat is more common in men than in women and may be more closely associated with chronic diseases.

Lower-body fat is more common in women than in men and is not usually associated with chronic diseases.

SOURCE: R.E.C. Wildman and D. M. Medeiros, *Advanced Human Nutrition* (Boca Raton, FL: CRC Press, 2000), pp. 321–323.

measurement to the waist measurement), but it does not provide any additional information. Therefore, waist circumference alone is the preferred method for assessing abdominal fat in a clinical setting.

Other Measures of Body Composition Health-care professionals commonly use BMI and waist circumference measurements because they are relatively easy and inexpensive. Together, these two measurements prove most valuable in assessing a person's health risks and monitoring changes over time.[16] Researchers needing more precise measures of body composition may choose any of several other techniques to estimate body fat and its distribution (see Figure 8-10). Mastering these techniques requires proper instruction and practice to ensure reliability. In addition to the methods shown in Figure 8-10, researchers sometimes estimate body composition using these methods: total body water, radioactive potassium count, near-infrared spectrophotometry, ultrasound, computed tomography, and magnetic resonance imaging. Each method has advantages and disadvantages with respect to cost, technical difficulty, and precision of estimating body fat. Appendix E provides additional details and includes many of the tables and charts routinely used in assessment procedures.

> **REVIEW IT** Distinguish between body weight and body composition, including methods to assess each.

The body mass index (BMI) is based on weight relative to height and serves as a reliable indicator of chronic disease risks, but it says little about body composition. The ideal amount of body fat varies from person to person, but researchers have found that body fat in excess of 22 percent for young men and 27 percent for young women (the levels rise slightly with age) poses health risks. Central obesity is measured by waist circumference and indicates excess abdominal fat distributed around the trunk of the body. Central obesity contributes to chronic diseases.

> FIGURE 8-10 **Common Methods Used to Assess Body Fat**

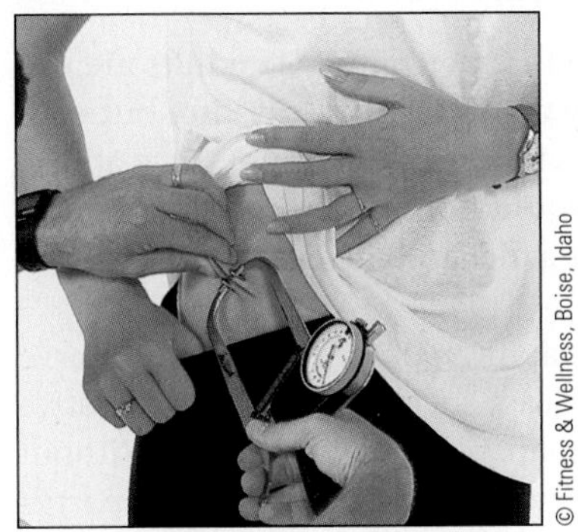

Skinfold measures estimate body fat by using a caliper to gauge the thickness of a fold of skin on the back of the arm (over the triceps), below the shoulder blade (subscapular), and in other places (including lower-body sites), and then comparing these measurements with standards.

© Fitness & Wellness, Boise, Idaho

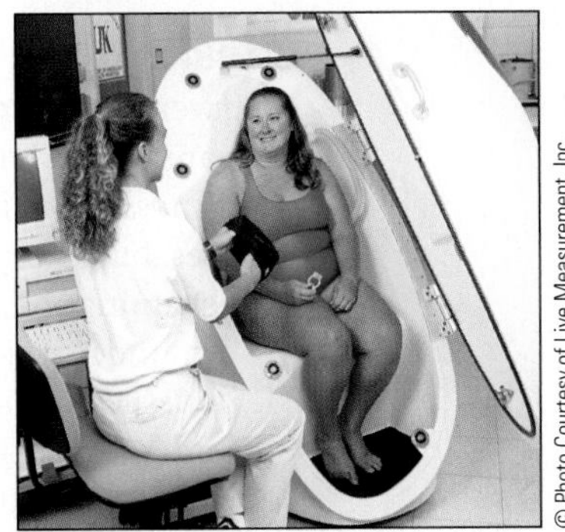

Air displacement plethysmography (commonly called the *bod pod*) estimates body composition by having a person sit inside a chamber while computerized sensors determine the amount of air displaced by the person's body.

© Photo Courtesy of Live Measurement, Inc.

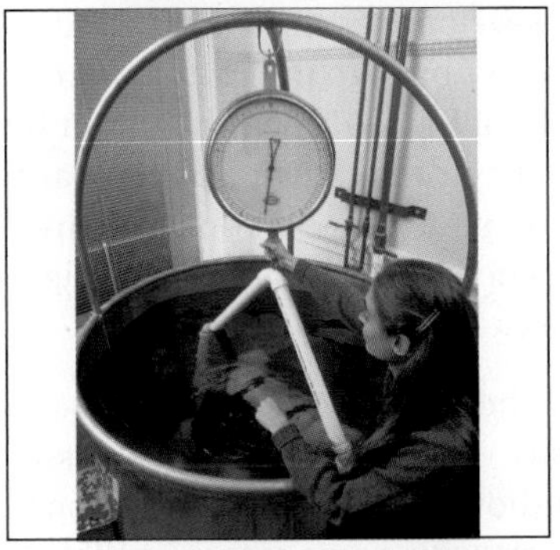

Hydrodensitometry measures body density by weighing the person first on land and then again while submerged in water. The difference between the person's actual weight and underwater weight provides a measure of the body's volume. A mathematical equation using the two measurements (volume and actual weight) determines body density, from which the percentage of body fat can be estimated.

Yoav Levy/Phototake

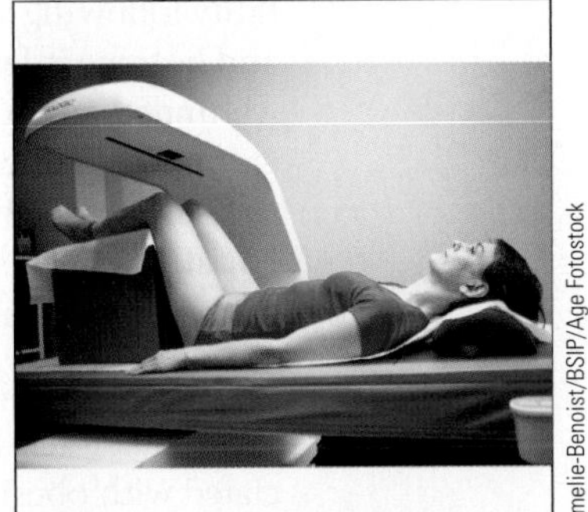

Dual energy X-ray absorptiometry (DEXA) uses two low-dose X-rays that differentiate among fat-free soft tissue (lean body mass), fat tissue, and bone tissue, providing a precise measurement of total fat and its distribution in all but extremely obese subjects.

Amelie-Benoist/BSIP/Age Fotostock

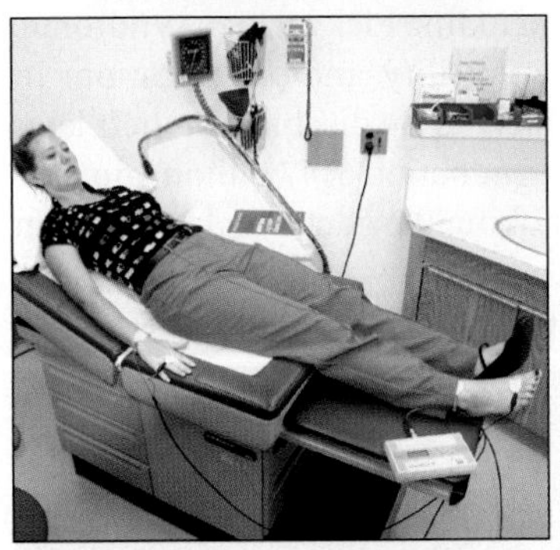

Bioelectrical impedance measures body fat by using a low-intensity electrical current. Because electrolyte-containing fluids, which readily conduct an electrical current, are found primarily in lean body tissues, the leaner the person, the less resistance to the current. The measurement of electrical resistance is then used in a mathematical equation to estimate the percentage of body fat.

© Geri Engberg Photography

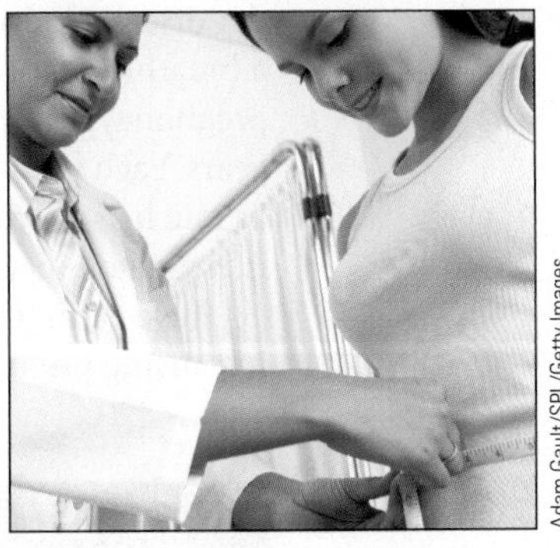

Waist circumference measures central obesity by placing a nonstretchable measuring tape around the waist just above the bony crest of the hip. The tape runs parallel to the floor and is snug, but does not compress the skin.

Adam Gault/SPL/Getty Images

8.5 Health Risks Associated with Body Weight and Body Fat

› LEARN IT Identify relationships between body weight and chronic diseases.

Body weight and body fat correlate with disease risks and life expectancy. The correlation suggests a greater *likelihood* of developing chronic diseases and shortening life expectancy for those with a higher BMI and waist circumference.[17] Not all overweight and underweight people will get sick and die before their time nor will all normal-weight people live long healthy lives. *Correlations* are not *causes.* For the most part though, people with a BMI between 18.5 and 24.9 have relatively few weight-related health risks; risks increase as BMI falls below or rises above this range, indicating that both too little and too much body fat impair health. Epidemiological data show a J- or U-shaped relationship between body weights and mortality (see Figure 8-11).[18] People who are extremely underweight or extremely obese carry higher risks of early deaths than those whose weights fall within the healthy or even the slightly overweight range.[19] These mortality risks decline with age.

Independently of BMI, factors such as smoking habits raise health risks, and physical fitness lowers them. A man with a BMI of 22 who smokes two packs of

> FIGURE 8-11 **BMI and Mortality**

This J-shaped curve describes the relationship between body mass index (BMI) and mortality and shows that both underweight and overweight present risks of a premature death.

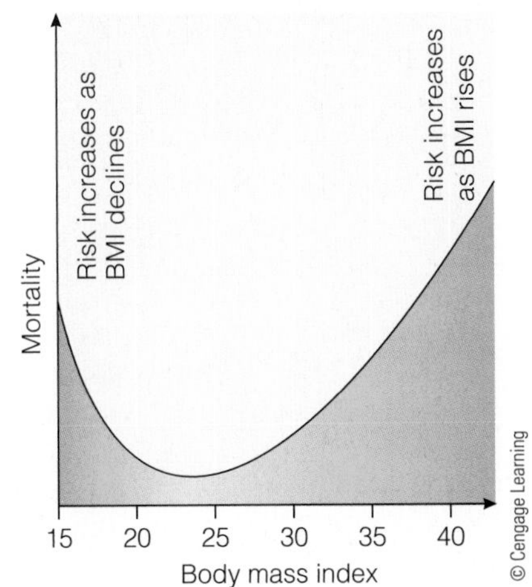

© Cengage Learning

cigarettes a day is jeopardizing his health, whereas a woman with a BMI of 32 who walks briskly for an hour a day is improving her health.

Health Risks of Underweight Fewer than 2 percent of US adults are underweight.[20] Some underweight people enjoy an active, healthy life, but others are underweight because of malnutrition, smoking habits, substance abuse, or illnesses. Weight and fat measures alone would not reveal these underlying causes, but a complete assessment that includes a diet and medical history, physical examination, and laboratory tests would.

An underweight person, especially an older adult, may be unable to preserve lean tissue during the fight against a wasting disease such as cancer or a digestive disorder, especially when the disease is accompanied by malnutrition. Without adequate nutrient and energy reserves, an underweight person will have a particularly tough battle against such medical stresses and face increased risks of mortality following surgeries.[21] Underweight women develop menstrual irregularities and become infertile. Those who do conceive may give birth to unhealthy infants. An underweight woman can improve her chances of having a healthy infant by gaining weight prior to conception, during pregnancy, or both. Underweight and significant weight loss are also associated with osteoporosis and bone fractures. For all these reasons, underweight people may benefit from enough of a weight gain to provide an energy reserve and protective amounts of all the nutrients.

Health Risks of Overweight As for excessive body fat, the health risks are so many that it has been designated a disease—obesity. Among the health risks associated with obesity are diabetes, hypertension, cardiovascular disease, sleep apnea (abnormal ceasing of breathing during sleep), osteoarthritis, some cancers, gallbladder disease, kidney stones, respiratory problems (including Pickwickian syndrome, a breathing blockage linked with sudden death), infertility, and complications in pregnancy and surgery. Obese people are more likely to be disabled in their later years. Each year, these obesity-related illnesses cost our nation $147 billion—in fact, as much as, or more than, the medical costs of smoking. An additional $73 billion is estimated in a loss of productivity at work due to mortality and disability.[22]

The cost in terms of lives is also great. In fact, obesity is second only to tobacco in causing premature deaths.[23]

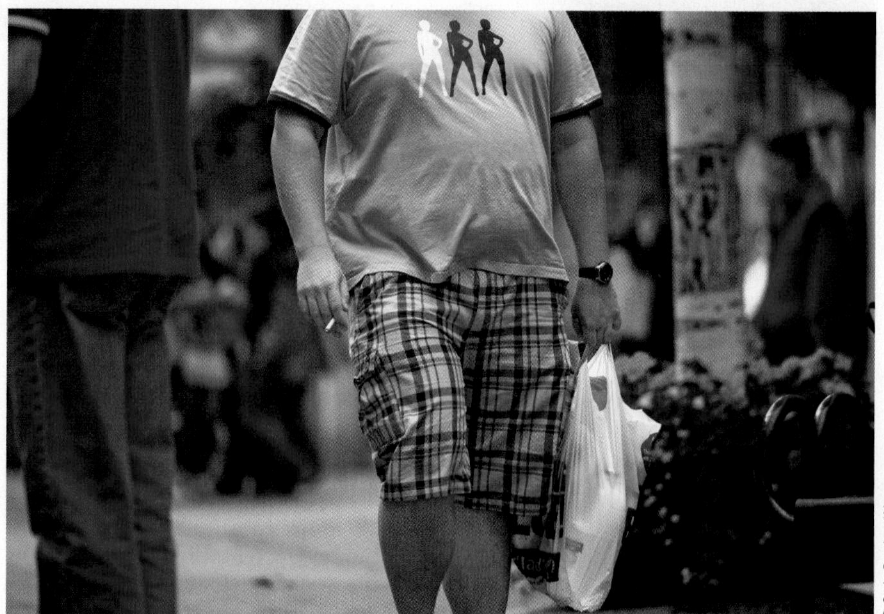

© Craig Stephen/Alamy

Smoking is the leading cause of preventable illnesses and early deaths. Obesity is a close second. A BMI of 40 or greater is equivalent to a lifetime of smoking, representing 10 years' loss of life.

Cardiovascular Disease The relationship between obesity and cardiovascular disease risk is strong, with links to both elevated blood cholesterol and hypertension.[24] Central obesity may raise the risk of heart attack and stroke as much as the three leading risk factors (high LDL cholesterol, hypertension, and smoking) do. In addition to body fat, weight gain also increases the risk of cardiovascular disease. Weight loss, on the other hand, can effectively reverse atherosclerosis and lower both blood cholesterol and blood pressure in overweight and obese people.[25] Of course, lean and normal-weight people may also have high blood cholesterol and blood pressure, and these factors are just as dangerous in lean people as in obese people. Obese people who do not have high blood cholesterol, high blood pressure, or other indicators of heart disease tend to have more a favorable fat distribution and may be described as "metabolically healthy" with lower risks for heart disease.[26]

Type 2 Diabetes The incidence of diabetes has risen dramatically in recent decades, as the nation's population has grown more overweight. Most adults with type 2 diabetes are overweight or obese.[27] Type 2 diabetes is three times more likely to develop in an obese person than in a nonobese person. Furthermore, the person with type 2 diabetes often has central obesity. Central-body fat cells appear to be larger and more insulin-resistant than lower-body fat cells. The association between **insulin resistance** and obesity is strong, and both are major risk factors for the development of type 2 diabetes.

Diabetes appears to be influenced by weight gains as well as by body weight. A weight gain of more than 10 pounds (4.5 kilograms) after the age of 18 doubles the risk of developing diabetes, even in adults of average weight. In contrast, weight loss is effective in improving glucose tolerance and insulin resistance.[28]

Inflammation and the Metabolic Syndrome Chronic **inflammation** accompanies obesity, and inflammation contributes to chronic diseases.[29] As a person grows fatter, lipids first fill the adipose tissue and then migrate into other tissues such as the muscles and liver. Fatty liver is a major contributor to the many diseases associated with obesity.[30] This accumulation of fat, especially in the abdominal region, changes the body's metabolism, resulting in insulin resistance (and high blood glucose), low HDL cholesterol, high triglycerides, and high blood pressure.[31] This cluster of symptoms—collectively known as the metabolic syndrome—increases the risks for diabetes, hypertension, and atherosclerosis. Fat accumulation, especially in the abdominal region, activates genes that code for proteins (adipokines) involved in inflammation.[32] Furthermore, although relatively few immune cells are commonly found in adipose tissue, weight gain significantly increases their number and their role in inflammation. Elevated blood lipids—whether due to obesity or to a high-fat diet—also promote inflammation. Together, these factors help to explain why chronic inflammation accompanies obesity and how obesity contributes to the metabolic syndrome and the progression of chronic diseases.[33] Even in healthy youngsters, body fat correlates positively with chronic inflammation. As might be expected, weight loss improves insulin resistance, reduces the number of immune cells in adipose tissue, and changes gene expression to reduce inflammation.

Cancer The risk of some cancers increases with both body weight and weight gain, but researchers do not fully understand the relationships.[34] One possible explanation may be that obese people have elevated levels of hormones that could influence cancer development. For example, adipose tissue is the major site of estrogen synthesis in women, obese women have elevated levels of estrogen, and estrogen has been implicated in the development of cancers of the female reproductive system—cancers that account for half of all cancers in women. Another possible explanation may be that the chronic inflammation that accompanies obesity is a risk factor for several cancers.[35]

Fit and Fat versus Sedentary and Slim

Importantly, BMI and weight gains and losses do not tell the whole story. Cardiorespiratory and muscular fitness play major roles in health and longevity, independently of body weight. Normal-weight people who are fit have a lower risk of mortality than normal-weight

insulin resistance: the condition in which a normal amount of insulin produces a subnormal effect in muscle, adipose, and liver cells, resulting in an elevated fasting glucose; a metabolic consequence of obesity that precedes type 2 diabetes.

inflammation: an immunological response to cellular injury characterized by an increase in white blood cells.

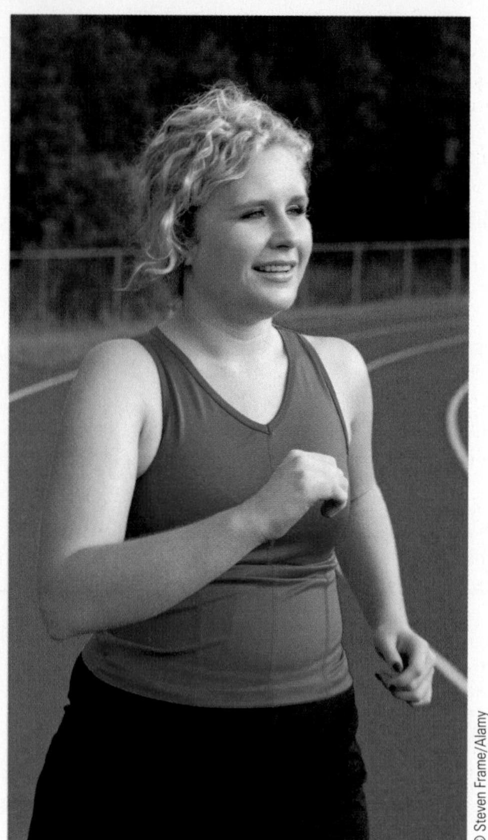

Being active—even if overweight—is healthier than being sedentary.

people who are unfit. Furthermore, overweight but fit people have lower risks than normal-weight, unfit ones.[36] Fit people are also likely to gain less weight over the years. Clearly, a healthy body weight is good, but it may not be good enough. Fitness, in and of itself, offers many health benefits, as Chapter 14 confirms.

› REVIEW IT Identify relationships between body weight and chronic diseases.
The weight appropriate for an individual depends largely on factors specific to that individual, including body fat distribution, family health history, and current health status. At the extremes, both overweight and underweight carry clear risks to health.

This chapter has described energy balance and body composition with a focus on the health problems associated with too much or too little body weight and body fat. Highlight 8 examines the health problems that arise when efforts to control body weight become eating disorders. The next chapter continues the discussion with a look at weight management and the benefits of choosing nutritious foods and exercising regularly.

Nutrition Portfolio

When combined with fitness, a healthy body weight will help you to defend against chronic diseases. Go to Diet & Wellness Plus and choose one of the days on which you have tracked your diet for the entire day. Go to the Energy Balance report; use this report to help you answer the following questions:

- Describe how your daily food intake and physical activity balance with each other.
- What did the diet analysis program estimate as your daily energy requirement? What information was this based on?
- Describe any health risks that may be of concern for a person who continuously has inadequate or excessive energy intakes for many years.

DIET & WELLNESS PLUS To complete this exercise, go to your Diet & Wellness Plus at www.cengagebrain.com.

› STUDY IT To review the key points of this chapter and take a practice quiz, go to the study cards at the end of the book.

REFERENCES

1. M. B. Katan and D. S. Ludwig, Extra calories cause weight gain: But how much? *Journal of the American Medical Association* 303 (2010): 65–66.
2. S. B. Heymsfield and coauthors, Energy content of weight loss: Kinetic features during voluntary caloric restriction, *Metabolism* 61 (2012): 937–943; K. D. Hall and coauthors, Energy balance and its components: Implications for body weight regulation, *American Journal of Clinical Nutrition* 95 (2012): 989–994.
3. K. D. Hall, Modeling metabolic adaptations and energy regulation in humans, *Annual Review of Nutrition* 32 (2012): 35–54; J. C. K. Wells and M. Siervo, Obesity and energy balance: Is the tail wagging the dog? *European Journal of Clinical Nutrition* 65 (2011): 1173–1189.
4. E. R. Grimm and N. I. Steinle, Genetics of eating behavior: Established and emerging concepts, *Nutrition Reviews* 69 (2011): 52–60.
5. D. Ferriday and J. M. Brunstrom, "I just can't help myself": Effects of food-cue exposure in overweight and lean individuals, *International Journal of Obesity* 35 (2011): 142–149; L. B. Shomaker and coauthors, Eating in the absence of hunger in adolescents: Intake after a large-array meal compared with that after a standardized meal, *American Journal of Clinical Nutrition* 92 (2010): 697–703.
6. J. A. Gilbert and coauthors, Milk supplementation facilitates appetite control in obese women during weight loss: A randomized, single-blind, placebo-controlled trial, *British Journal of Nutrition* 105 (2011): 133–143.
7. E. Egecioglu and coauthors, Hedonic and incentive signals for body weight control, *Reviews in Endocrine and Metabolic Disorders* 12 (2011): 141–151.
8. J. A. Parker and S. R. Bloom, Hypothalamic neuropeptides and the regulation of appetite, *Neuropharmacology* 63 (2012): 18–30.
9. H. Schloegl and coauthors, Peptide hormones regulating appetite: Focus on neuroimaging studies in humans, *Diabetes/Metabolism Research and Reviews* 27 (2011): 104–112; K. A. Simpson and S. R. Bloom, Appetite and hedonism: Gut hormones and the brain, *Endocrinology and Metabolism Clinics of North America* 39 (2010): 729–743; S. Zac-Varghese, T. Tan, and S. R. Bloom, Hormonal interactions between gut and brain, *Discovery Medicine* 10 (2010): 543–552.

10. C. D. Fryar, M. D. Carroll, and C. L. Ogden, Prevalence of overweight, obesity, and extreme obesity among adults: United States, trends 1960–1962 through 2009–2010, *NCHS Health E-Stats*, September 2012.
11. A. G. Dulloo and coauthors, Body composition phenotypes in pathways to obesity and the metabolic syndrome, *International Journal of Obesity* 3 (2010): S4–S17.
12. K. A. Britton and coauthors, Body fat distribution, incident cardiovascular disease, cancer, and all-cause mortality, *Journal of the American College of Cardiology* 62 (2013): 921–925; A. M. Sironi and coauthors, Impact of increased visceral and cardiac fat on cardiometabolic risk and disease, *Diabetic Medicine* 29 (2012): 622–627; The InterAct Consortium, Long-term risk of incident type 2 diabetes and measures of overall and regional obesity: The EPIC-InterAct case-cohort study, *PLoS Medicine* 9 (2012): e1001230; T. Coutinho and coauthors, Central obesity and survival in subjects with coronary artery disease: A systematic review of the literature and collaborative analysis with individual subject data, *Journal of the American College of Cardiology* 57 (2011): 1877–1886; D. Sluik and coauthors, Associations between general and abdominal adiposity and mortality in individuals with diabetes mellitus, *American Journal of Epidemiology* 174 (2011): 22–34; B. J. Arsenault and coauthors, Physical inactivity, abdominal obesity and risk of coronary heart disease in apparently healthy men and women, *International Journal of Obesity* 34 (2010): 340–347; E. J. Jacobs and coauthors, Waist circumference and all-cause mortality in a large US cohort, *Archives of Internal Medicine* 170 (2010): 1293–1301.
13. K. Karastergiou and coauthors, Sex differences in human adipose tissues—the biology of pear shape, *Biology of Sex Differences* 3 (2013): 13.
14. P. T. Katzmarzyk, S. B. Heymsfield, and C. Bouchard, Clinical utility of visceral adipose tissue for the identification of cardiometabolic risk in white and African American adults, *American Journal of Clinical Nutrition* 97 (2013): 480–486.
15. M. Ashwell, P. Gunn, and S. Gibson, Waist-to-height ratio is a better screening tool than waist circumference and BMI for adult cardiometabolic risk factors: Systematic review and meta-analysis, *Obesity Reviews* 13 (2012): 275–286.
16. Position of the American Dietetic Association: Weight management, *Journal of the American Dietetic Association* 109 (2009): 330–346.
17. A. E. Staiano and coauthors, Body mass index versus waist circumference as predictors of mortality in Canadian adults, *International Journal of Obesity* 36 (2012): 1450–1454; N. Y. Krakauer and J. C. Krakauer, A new body shape index predicts mortality hazard independently of body mass index, *PLoS One* 7 (2012): e39504.
18. A. Berrington de Gonzalez and coauthors, Body-mass index and mortality among 1.46 million white adults, *New England Journal of Medicine* 363 (2010): 2211–2219.
19. K. M. Flegal and coauthors, Association of all-cause mortality with overweight and obesity using standard body mass index categories: A systematic review and meta-analysis, *Journal of the American Medical Association* 309 (2013): 71–82.
20. C. D. Fryar and C. L. Ogden, Prevalence of underweight among adults aged 20 years and over: United States, 1960–1962 through 2007–2010, *NCHS Health E-Stat*, September 2012.
21. F. E. Turrentine and coauthors, The relationship between body mass index and 30-day mortality risk, by principal surgical procedure, *Archives of Surgery* 147 (2012): 236–242; R. Gupta and coauthors, The effect of low body mass index on outcome in critically ill surgical patients, *Nutrition in Clinical Practice* 26 (2011): 593–597.
22. E. A. Finkelstein and coauthors, The costs of obesity in the workplace, *Journal of Occupational and Environmental Medicine* 52 (2010): 971–976; Society of Actuaries, Obesity and its relation to mortality and morbidity costs, www.soa.org/files/research/projects/research-2011-obesity-relation-mortality.pdf, December 2010.
23. H. Jia and E. I. Lubetkin, Trends in quality-adjusted life-years lost contributed by smoking and obesity, *American Journal of Preventive Medicine* 38 (2010): 138–144.
24. C. W. Mende, Obesity and hypertension: A common coexistence, *Journal of Clinical Hypertension* 14 (2012): 137–138.
25. C. DeCiuceis and coauthors, Effects of weight loss on structural and functional alterations of subcutaneous small arteries in obese patients, *Hypertension* 58 (2011): 29–36; I Shai and coauthors, Dietary intervention to reverse carotid atherosclerosis, *Circulation* 121 (2010): 1200–1208.
26. M. Hamer and E. Stamatakis, Metabolically healthy obesity and risk of all-cause and cardiovascular disease mortality, *Journal of Clinical Endocrinology and Metabolism* 97 (2012): 2482–2488.
27. M. L. Biggs and coauthors, Association between adiposity in midlife and older age and risk of diabetes in older adults, *Journal of the American Medical Association* 303 (2010): 2504–2512.
28. B. Kowall and coauthors, Impact of weight and weight change on normalization of prediabetes and on persistence of normal glucose tolerance in an older population: The KORA S4/F4 Study, *International Journal of Obesity* 36 (2012): 826–833.
29. F. P. deHeredia, S. C. Gómez-Martínezm, and A. Marcos, Chronic and degenerative diseases: Obesity, inflammation, and the immune system, *Proceedings of the Nutrition Society* 71 (2012): 332–338; N. Lumeng and A. R. Saltiel, Inflammatory links between obesity and metabolic disease, *Journal of Clinical Investigation* 121 (2011): 2111–2117; B. B. Aggarwal, Targeting inflammation-induced obesity and metabolic diseases by curcumin and other nutraceuticals, *Annual Review of Nutrition* 30 (2010): 173–199.
30. E. M. McCarthy and M. E. Rinella, The role of diet and nutrient composition in nonalcoholic fatty liver disease, *Journal of the Academy of Nutrition and Dietetics* 112 (2012): 401–409; K. L. Kopec and D. Burns, Nonalcoholic fatty liver disease: A review of the spectrum of disease, diagnosis, and therapy, *Nutrition in Clinical Practice* 26 (2011): 565–576; N. N. Kumashiro and coauthors, Cellular mechanism of insulin resistance in nonalcoholic fatty liver disease, *Proceedings of the National Academy of Sciences* 108 (2011): 16381–16385; J. C. Cohen, J. D. Horton, and H. H. Hobbs, Human fatty liver disease: Old questions and new insights, *Science* 332 (2011): 1519–1523.
31. E. J. Gallagher, D. Leroith, and E. Karnieli, Insulin resistance in obesity as the underlying cause for the metabolic syndrome, *Mt. Sinai Journal of Medicine* 77 (2010): 511–523; E. W. Demerath, Causes and consequences of human variation in visceral adiposity, *American Journal of Clinical Nutrition* 91 (2010): 1–2.
32. J. M. Northcott and coauthors, Adipokines and the cardiovascular system: Mechanisms mediating health and disease, *Canadian Journal of Physiology and Pharmacology* 90 (2012): 1029–1059; R. Stienstra and coauthors, The inflammasome puts obesity in the danger zone, *Cell Metabolism* 15 (2012): 10–18; E. Dalmas and coauthors, Variations in circulating inflammatory factors are related to changes in calorie and carbohydrate intakes early in the course of surgery-induced weight reduction, *American Journal of Clinical Nutrition* 94 (2011): 450–458.
33. S. Sun and coauthors, Mechanisms of inflammatory responses in obese adipose tissue, *Annual Review of Nutrition* 32 (2012): 261–286; R. Lorenzet and coauthors, Thrombosis and obesity: Cellular bases, *Thrombosis Research* 129 (2012): 285–289; A. Das and S. Mukhopadhyay, The evil axis of obesity, inflammation and type-2 diabetes, *Endocrine, Metabolic and Immune Disorders Drug Targets* 11 (2011): 23–31; A. L. Marsland and coauthors, Systemic inflammation and the metabolic syndrome among middle-aged community volunteers, *Metabolism: Clinical and Experimental* 59 (2010): 1801–1808.
34. Institute of Medicine, *The role of obesity in cancer survival and recurrence: Workshop summary*, Washington, DC: National Academies Press, 2012; C. Eheman and coauthors, Annual report to the nation on the status of cancer, 1975–2008, featuring cancers associated with excess weight and lack of sufficient physical activity, *Cancer* 118 (2012): 2338–2366; N. Parekh, U. Chandran, and E. V, Bandera, Obesity in cancer survival, *Annual Review of Nutrition* 32 (2012): 311–342.
35. S. Pendyala and coauthors, Diet-induced weight loss reduces colorectal inflammation: Implications for colorectal carcinogenesis, *American Journal of Clinical Nutrition* 93 (2011): 234–242.
36. D. E. Larson-Meyer and coauthors, Caloric restriction with or without exercise: The fitness versus fatness debate, *Medicine and Science in Sports and Exercise* 42 (2010): 152–159.

HIGHLIGHT > 8
Eating Disorders

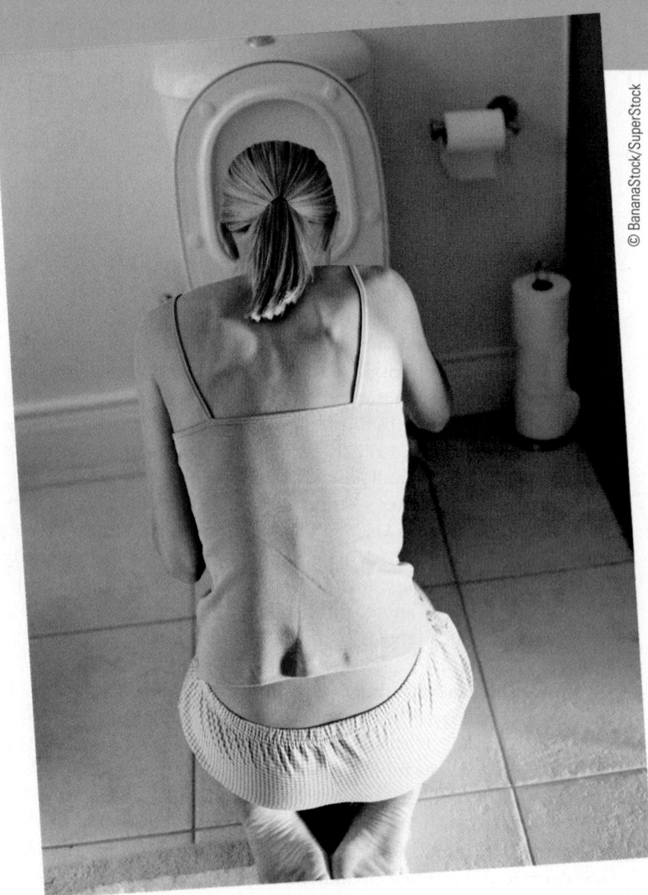
© BananaStock/SuperStock

› LEARN IT Compare the diagnoses, characteristics, and treatments of the different eating disorders.

For some people, the struggle with body weight manifests itself as an **eating disorder**. (The accompanying glossary defines this and related terms.) Three eating disorders—anorexia nervosa, bulimia nervosa, and binge eating disorder—are relatively uncommon, but present real concerns because of their health consequences.[1] Findings from large national surveys suggest that 0.9 percent of women and 0.3 percent of men suffer from anorexia nervosa at some time in their lives. Prevalence of bulimia nervosa is slightly higher, with 1.5 percent of women and 0.5 percent of men. Binge eating disorder is higher still, with 3.5 percent of women and 2 percent of men. Many more suffer from other unspecified eating disorders that do not meet the strict diagnostic criteria but still imperil a person's well-being.[2]

Why do so many people in our society suffer from eating disorders? Most experts agree that the causes include multiple factors: sociocultural, psychological, and perhaps neurochemical. Excessive pressure to be thin is at least partly to blame. Family attitudes concerning body shape and eating habits can have profound effects. Young people may have learned to identify discomforts such as anger, jealousy, or disappointment with "feeling fat." They often have other psychological issues such as depression, anxiety, or substance abuse. As weight issues become more of a focus, psychological problems worsen, and the likelihood of developing eating disorders intensifies. Unfortunately, few seek health care for eating disorders. Athletes and dancers are among those most likely to develop eating disorders.

Disordered Eating in Athletes

At age 14, Suzanne was a top contender for a spot on the state gymnastics team. Each day her coach reminded team members that they must weigh no more than their assigned weights to qualify for competition. The coach chastised gymnasts who gained weight, and Suzanne was terrified of being singled out. Convinced that the less she weighed the better she would perform, Suzanne weighed herself several times a day to confirm that she had not exceeded her 80-pound limit. Driven to excel in her sport, Suzanne kept her weight down by eating very little and training very hard. Unlike many of her friends, Suzanne never began to menstruate. A few months before her fifteenth birthday, Suzanne's coach dropped her back to the second-level team. Suzanne blamed her poor performance on a slow-healing stress fracture. Mentally stressed and physically exhausted, she quit gymnastics and began overeating between periods of self-starvation. Suzanne had developed the dangerous combination of problems originally known as the **female athlete triad,** which focused

GLOSSARY

amenorrhea (ay-MEN-oh-REE-ah): the absence of or cessation of menstruation. *Primary amenorrhea* is menarche delayed beyond 15 years of age. *Secondary amenorrhea* is the absence of three consecutive menstrual cycles.

anorexia (an-oh-RECK-see-ah) **nervosa:** an eating disorder characterized by a refusal to maintain a minimally normal body weight and a distortion in perception of body shape and weight.

- **an** = without
- **orex** = mouth
- **nervos** = of nervous origin

binge-eating disorder: an eating disorder characterized by recurring episodes of eating a significant amount of food in a short period of time with marked feelings of lack of control.

bulimia (byoo-LEEM-ee-ah) **nervosa:** an eating disorder characterized by repeated episodes of binge eating usually followed by self-induced vomiting, misuse of laxatives or diuretics, fasting, or excessive exercise.

cathartic (ka-THAR-tik): a strong laxative.

disordered eating: eating behaviors that are neither normal nor healthy, including restrained eating, fasting, binge eating, and purging.

eating disorder: any of several psychological disorders characterized by serious disturbances in eating behavior that jeopardize a person's physical or psychological health.

emetic (em-ETT-ic): an agent that causes vomiting.

female athlete triad: a potentially fatal combination of three medical problems—disordered eating, amenorrhea, and osteoporosis.

muscle dysmorphia (dis-MORE-fee-ah): a psychiatric disorder characterized by a preoccupation with building body mass.

relative energy deficiency in sport (RED-S): a syndrome of impaired physiological functions caused by relative energy deficiency (too little energy intake for the energy expended).

stress fractures: bone damage or breaks caused by stress on bone surfaces during exercise.

on disordered eating, amenorrhea, and osteoporosis.[3] Because the problems reach beyond these three components and male athletes are also affected, a more comprehensive term is now being used: **Relative Energy Deficiency in Sport (RED-S).**

Relative Energy Deficiency

Central to RED-S is an energy deficiency—the athlete's diet is providing too little energy given the amount of energy expended to support health, activities of daily living, growth, and sports. Sometimes energy deficiencies develop as the result of mismanaged athletic programs to quickly reduce body weight. Consider David, for example. Each week throughout the season, David drastically restricts his food and fluid intake before a wrestling match in an effort to "make weight." He believes that competing in a lower weight class will give him a competitive advantage over smaller opponents. To that end, David intensifies his exercise, skips meals, restricts fluids, practices in plastic suits, and trains in heated rooms to lose 4 to 7 pounds rapidly.[4] He hopes to replenish the lost fluids, glycogen, and lean tissue during the hours between weigh-in and competition, but the body needs days to correct this metabolic mayhem. Reestablishing fluid and electrolyte balances may take 1 to 2 days, replenishing glycogen stores may take 2 to 3 days, and replacing lean tissue may take even longer.

Ironically, the combination of food deprivation and dehydration impairs physical performance by reducing muscle strength, decreasing anaerobic power, and reducing endurance capacity. For optimal performance, athletes need to first achieve their competitive weight during the off-season and then eat well-balanced meals and drink plenty of fluids during the competitive season.

Energy deficiencies sometimes occur when athletes participate in unsupervised weight loss regimens or fail to eat enough during times of extreme exercise. Most often, however, **disordered eating** underlies energy deficiencies in athletes.

Disordered Eating

One reason many athletes engage in disordered eating is that they and their coaches have embraced unsuitable weight standards. An athlete's body must be heavier for a given height than a nonathlete's body because the athlete's body is dense, containing more healthy bone and muscle and less fat. When athletes rely only on the scales, they may mistakenly believe they are too fat because weight standards, such as the BMI, do not provide adequate information about body composition.

Many young athletes severely restrict energy intakes to improve performance, enhance appearance, or meet the weight guidelines of a specific sport. They fail to realize that the loss of lean tissue that accompanies energy restriction actually impairs their physical performance. Risk factors for eating disorders among athletes include:

- Young age (adolescence)
- Pressure to excel at a chosen sport
- Focus on achieving or maintaining an "ideal" body weight or body fat percentage
- Participation in sports or competitions that emphasize a lean appearance or judge performance on aesthetic appeal such as gymnastics, wrestling, figure skating, or dance
- Weight-loss dieting at an early age
- Unsupervised dieting

Disordered eating among athletes usually involves energy deficits and weight loss, but some athletes, usually males, go to extreme measures to bulk up and *gain* weight. People afflicted with **muscle dysmorphia** eat high-protein diets, take dietary supplements, weight train for hours at a time, and often abuse steroids in an attempt to increase muscle mass. Their bodies are large and muscular, yet they see themselves as puny 90-pound weaklings. They are preoccupied with the idea that their bodies are too small or inadequately muscular. Like others with distorted body images, people with muscle dysmorphia weigh themselves frequently and center their lives on diet and exercise. Paying attention to diet and pumping iron for fitness is admirable, but obsessing over it can cause serious social, occupational, and physical problems.

Adverse Consequences

A prolonged, inadequate energy intake has numerous adverse consequences, as outlined in Table H8-1. It leads to nutrient deficiencies (including anemia), chronic fatigue, and increased risk of infections and illnesses. Protein synthesis decreases and blood lipids increase, favoring heart disease. All of these consequences harm health and impair performance.

As mentioned earlier, females commonly develop **amenorrhea.** The prevalence of amenorrhea among premenopausal women in the United States is about 2 to 5 percent overall, but among female athletes, it may be as high as 65 to 70 percent. Body fat stores and hormone levels are too inadequate to support normal menstruation. Amenorrhea is often accompanied by bone mineral losses.

TABLE H8-1 Consequences of Relative Energy Deficiency in Sport (RED-S)

Physiological functions	Psychological problems	Physical performance
Altered hormone activities	Decreased concentration	Decreased coordination
Anemia	Depression	Decreased endurance
Bone loss	Impaired judgment	Decreased muscle strength
Decreased glycogen stores	Irritability	Decreased training response
Decreased protein synthesis		Increased injuries
Impaired metabolism		
Menstrual dysfunction		
Poor growth		

SOURCE: Adapted from M. Mountjoy and coauthors, The IOC statement: Beyond the Female Athlete Triad—Relative Energy Deficiency in Sport (RED-S), *British Journal of Sports Medicine* 48 (2014): 491–497.

In general, weight-bearing physical activity, dietary calcium, and the hormone estrogen protect against the bone loss of osteoporosis, but in women with disordered eating and amenorrhea, strenuous activity can increase bone turnover, impair bone health, and increase the risks of **stress fractures.**[5] To grow strong bones, athletes should be encouraged to consume 1300 milligrams of calcium each day, to eat nutrient-dense foods, and to obtain enough energy to support both a healthy body weight and the energy expended in physical activity. Nutrition is critical to bone recovery.

Preventing Eating Disorders in Athletes

To prevent eating disorders in athletes and dancers, the performers, their coaches, and their parents must learn about inappropriate body weight ideals, improper weight-loss techniques, eating disorder development, proper nutrition, and safe weight-management strategies. Young people naturally search for identity and will often follow the advice of a person in authority without question. Therefore, coaches and dance instructors should never encourage unhealthy weight loss to qualify for competition or to conform to distorted artistic ideals. Athletes who need to lose weight for health's sake should try to do so during the off-season and under the supervision of a health-care professional.

Table H8-2 includes suggestions to help athletes and dancers protect themselves against developing eating disorders. The remaining sections describe eating disorders that anyone, athlete or nonathlete, may experience.

Anorexia Nervosa

Julie, 18 years old, is a superachiever in school. She watches her diet with great care, and she exercises daily, maintaining a rigorous schedule of self-discipline. She is thin, but she is determined to lose more weight.

TABLE H8-2 Tips for Combating Eating Disorders

General Guidelines

- Never restrict food amounts to below those suggested for adequacy by the USDA Food Patterns (see Table 2-3 on p. 43).
- Eat frequently. Include healthy snacks between meals. The person who eats frequently never gets so hungry as to allow hunger to dictate food choices.
- If not at a healthy weight, establish a reasonable weight goal based on a healthy body composition.
- Allow a reasonable time to achieve the goal. A reasonable loss of excess fat can be achieved at the rate of about 10 percent of body weight in 6 months.
- Establish a weight-maintenance support group with people who share interests.

Specific Guidelines for Athletes and Dancers

- Adopt realistic and health-promoting goals related to weight and body composition instead of weight restrictive guidelines.
- Disregard critical comments about weight and body composition.
- Recognize that eating disorders impair health and physical performance. Seek professional treatment if needed.
- Emphasize nutrition as an important key to optimal performance.

She is 5 feet 6 inches tall and weighs 104 pounds (roughly 1.68 meters and 47 kilograms). Her BMI is less than 17. She has **anorexia nervosa.**

Characteristics of Anorexia Nervosa

Julie is unaware that she is undernourished, and she sees no need to obtain treatment. She developed amenorrhea several months ago and has become moody and chronically depressed. She views normal healthy body weight as too fat and insists that she needs to lose weight, although her eyes are sunk in deep hollows in her face. Julie denies that she is ever tired, although she is close to physical exhaustion and no longer sleeps easily. Her family is concerned, and though reluctant to push her, they have finally insisted that she see a psychiatrist. Julie's psychiatrist has diagnosed anorexia nervosa using specific criteria that describe such characteristics as a significantly low body weight caused by persistent restriction of energy intake; an intense fear of gaining weight or becoming fat, or persistent behaviors that interfere with weight gains; and a disturbance in self-perceived weight or shape.[6] She is prescribed group therapy as a start and if she does not begin to gain weight soon, she may need to enter a residential program or be hospitalized.

Central to the diagnosis of anorexia nervosa is a distorted body image that overestimates personal body fatness. When Julie looks at herself in the mirror, she sees a "fat" 104-pound body. The more Julie overestimates her body size, the more resistant she is to treatment, and the more unwilling she is to examine her faulty values and misconceptions. In fact, she finds value in her condition. Malnutrition and weight loss affect brain functioning and judgment in this way, causing lethargy, confusion, and delirium and influencing mood, anxiety, and emotions.

Anorexia nervosa cannot be self-diagnosed. Many people in our society are engaged in the pursuit of thinness, and denial runs high among people with anorexia nervosa. Some women have all the attitudes and behaviors associated with the condition, but without the dramatic weight loss.

How can a person as thin as Julie continue to starve herself? Julie uses tremendous discipline against her hunger to strictly limit her portions of low-fat, high-fiber, low-kcalorie foods. She will deny her hunger, and having adapted to eating so little food, she feels full after nibbling on a few carrot sticks. She knows the kcalorie intake of various foods and the kcalorie expenditure of different physical activities. If she feels that she has gained an ounce of weight, she runs or jumps rope until she is sure she has exercised it off. If she fears that the food she has eaten outweighs her physical activity, she may take laxatives to hasten the passage of food from her system. She drinks water incessantly to fill her stomach, risking dangerous mineral imbalances. She is desperately hungry. In fact, she is starving, but she doesn't eat because her need for self-control dominates.

Many people, on learning of this disorder, say they wish they had "a touch" of it to get thin. They mistakenly think that people with anorexia nervosa feel no hunger. They also fail to recognize the pain of the associated psychological and physical trauma.

The starvation of anorexia nervosa damages the body just as the starvation of war and poverty does. In fact, most people with anorexia

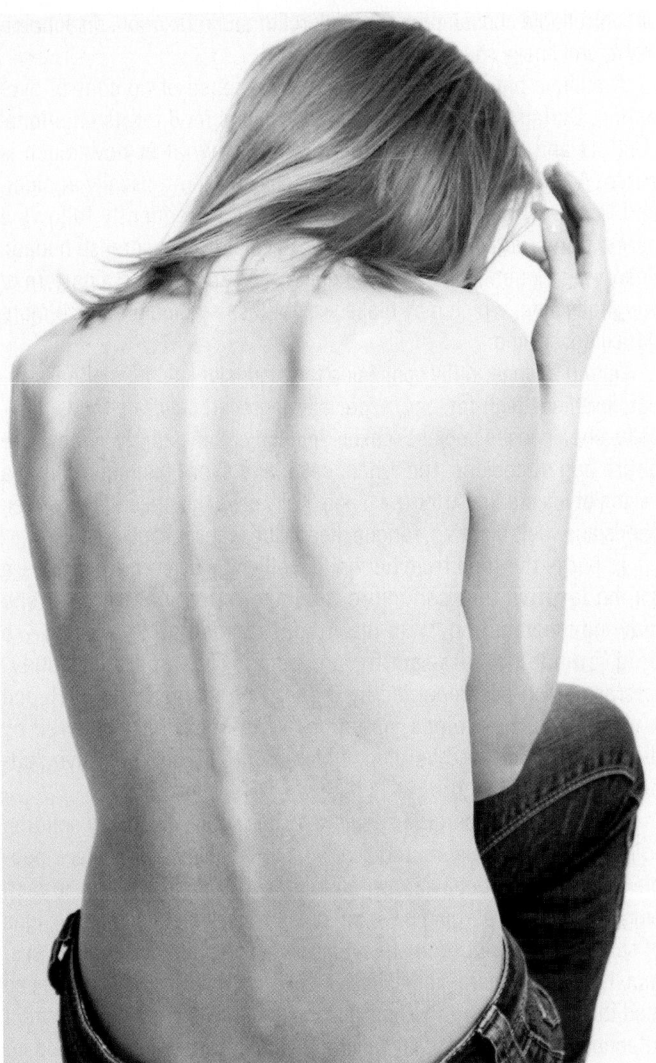

People with anorexia nervosa see themselves as fat, even when they are dangerously underweight.

Sniegirova Mariia/Shutterstock.com

nervosa are malnourished. Their bodies have been depleted of both body fat and protein. Victims are dying to be thin—quite literally. In young people, growth ceases and normal development falters. They lose so much lean tissue that their basal metabolic rate slows. In addition, the heart pumps inefficiently and irregularly, the heart muscle becomes weak and thin, the chambers diminish in size, and the blood pressure falls. Minerals that help to regulate heartbeat become unbalanced. Many deaths occur because of multiple organ system failure when the heart, kidneys, and liver cease to function.

Starvation brings other physical consequences as well, such as loss of brain tissue, impaired immune response, anemia, and a loss of digestive functions that worsen malnutrition. Peristalsis becomes sluggish, the stomach empties slowly, and the lining of the intestinal tract atrophies. The pancreas slows its production of digestive enzymes. The deteriorated GI tract fails to provide sufficient digestive enzymes and absorptive surfaces for handling any food that is eaten. The person may suffer from diarrhea, further worsening malnutrition.

Other effects of starvation include altered blood lipids, high blood vitamin A and vitamin E, low blood proteins, dry thin skin, abnormal nerve functioning, reduced bone density, low body temperature, low blood pressure, and the development of fine body hair (the body's attempt to keep warm). The electrical activity of the brain becomes abnormal, and insomnia is common. Both women and men lose their sex drives. In short, the metabolic mayhem of anorexia nervosa results in numerous physical complications, many of them life-threatening.[7]

Women with anorexia nervosa commonly develop amenorrhea. In young girls, the onset of menstruation is delayed. Menstrual periods typically resume with recovery, although some women never restart even after they have gained weight. Should an underweight woman with anorexia nervosa become pregnant, she is likely to give birth to an underweight baby—and low-birthweight babies face many health problems (as Chapter 15 explains). Mothers with anorexia nervosa may underfeed their children, who then fail to grow and may also suffer the other consequences of starvation.

Treatment of Anorexia Nervosa

Treatment of eating disorders requires a multidisciplinary approach.[8] Teams of physicians, nurses, psychiatrists, family therapists, and dietitians work together to resolve two sets of issues and behaviors: those relating to food and weight and those involving relationships with oneself and others.

The first dietary objective is to stop weight loss while establishing regular eating patterns. Appropriate diet is crucial to recovery and must be tailored to each individual's needs. Because body weight is low and fear of weight gain is high, initial food intake may be small—perhaps only 1200 kcalories per day. A variety of foods and foods with a higher energy density help to ensure greater success.[9] As eating becomes more comfortable, clients should gradually increase energy intake. Initially, clients may be unwilling to eat for themselves. Those who do eat will have a good chance of recovering without additional interventions. Even after recovery, however, energy intakes and eating behaviors may not fully return to normal. Furthermore, weight gains may be slow because energy needs may be slightly elevated due to anxiety, abdominal pain, and cigarette smoking.

Because anorexia nervosa is like starvation physically, health-care professionals classify clients based on indicators of malnutrition. Low-risk clients need dietary counseling. Intermediate-risk clients may need supplements such as high-kcalorie, high-protein formulas in addition to regular meals. High-risk clients may require hospitalization and may need to be fed by tube at first to prevent death. Residential programs that provide intensive behavioral treatment may be most appropriate for those who do not respond to less intensive approaches.

Denial runs high among those with anorexia nervosa. Few seek treatment on their own. About half of the women who are treated can maintain their body weight at 85 percent or more of a healthy weight, and at that weight, many of them may begin menstruating again. The other half have poor to fair treatment outcomes, relapse into abnormal eating behaviors, or die. Anorexia nervosa has one of the highest mortality rates among psychiatric disorders—most commonly from cardiac complications or by suicide.[10] Much like treatment for drug addictions, treatment for eating disorders engages family members. Therapists help family members to understand how their past interactions have enabled the client to continue destructive behaviors and how new ways of interacting can support change.

Before drawing conclusions about someone who is extremely thin or who eats very little, remember that diagnosis requires professional assessment. Several national organizations offer information for people who are seeking help with anorexia nervosa, either for themselves or for others.

Bulimia Nervosa

Kelly is a charming, intelligent, 30-year-old flight attendant of normal weight who thinks constantly about food. She alternates between starving herself and secretly bingeing, and when she has eaten too much, she makes herself vomit. Most readers recognize these symptoms as those of **bulimia nervosa.**

Characteristics of Bulimia Nervosa

Bulimia nervosa is distinct from anorexia nervosa and is more prevalent, although the true incidence is difficult to establish because bulimia nervosa is not as physically apparent. More men suffer from bulimia nervosa than from anorexia nervosa, but bulimia nervosa is still more common in women than in men. The secretive nature of bulimic behaviors makes recognition of the problem difficult, but once it is recognized, diagnosis is based on such criteria as number and frequency of binge eating episodes, inappropriate compensatory behaviors to prevent weight gain (such as self-induced vomiting or misuse of laxatives), and self-evaluation unduly influenced by body shape and weight.[11]

Like the typical person with bulimia nervosa, Kelly is single, female, and white. She is well educated and close to her ideal body weight, although her weight fluctuates over a range of 10 pounds or so every few weeks. She prefers to weigh less than the weight that her body maintains naturally.

Kelly seldom lets her eating disorder interfere with work or other activities, although a third of all bulimics do. From early childhood, she has been a high achiever and emotionally dependent on her parents. As a young teen, Kelly frequently followed severely restricted diets but could never maintain the weight loss. Kelly feels anxious at social events and cannot easily establish close personal relationships. She is usually depressed, is often impulsive, and has low self-esteem. When crisis hits, Kelly responds by replaying events, worrying excessively, and blaming herself but never asking for help—behaviors that interfere with effective coping.

Like the person with anorexia nervosa, the person with bulimia nervosa spends much time thinking about body image and food. The preoccupation with food manifests itself in secret binge-eating episodes, which usually progress through several emotional stages: anticipation and planning, anxiety, urgency to begin, rapid and uncontrollable consumption of food, relief and relaxation, disappointment, and finally shame or disgust.

A bulimic binge is characterized by a sense of no control over eating. During a binge, the person consumes food for its emotional comfort and cannot stop eating or control what or how much is eaten. A typical binge occurs periodically, in secret, usually at night, and lasts an hour or more. Because a binge frequently follows a period of restrictive dieting, eating is accelerated by intense hunger. Energy restriction followed by bingeing can set in motion a pattern of weight cycling, which may make weight loss and maintenance more difficult over time.

During a binge, Kelly consumes thousands of kcalories of easy-to-eat, low-fiber, high-fat, and, especially, high-carbohydrate foods. Typically, she chooses cookies, cakes, and ice cream—and she eats the entire bag of cookies, the whole cake, and every last spoonful in a carton of ice cream. After the binge, Kelly pays the price with swollen hands and feet, bloating, fatigue, headache, nausea, and pain.

To purge the food from her body, Kelly may use a **cathartic**—a strong laxative that can injure the lower intestinal tract. Or she may induce vomiting, with or without the use of an **emetic**—a drug intended as first aid for poisoning. These purging behaviors are often accompanied by feelings of shame or guilt. Hence a vicious cycle develops: negative self-perceptions followed by dieting, bingeing, and purging, which in turn lead to negative self-perceptions (see Figure H8-1).

On first glance, purging seems to offer a quick and easy solution to the problems of unwanted kcalories and body weight. Many people perceive such behavior as neutral or even positive, when, in fact, binge eating and purging have serious physical consequences. Signs of subclinical malnutrition are evident in a compromised immune system. Fluid and mineral imbalances caused by vomiting or diarrhea can lead to abnormal heart rhythms and injury to the kidneys. Urinary tract infections can lead to kidney failure. Vomiting causes irritation and infection of the pharynx, esophagus, and salivary glands; painful sores in the mouth; erosion of the teeth; and dental caries. The esophagus

> FIGURE H8-1 **The Vicious Cycle of Restrictive Dieting and Binge Eating**

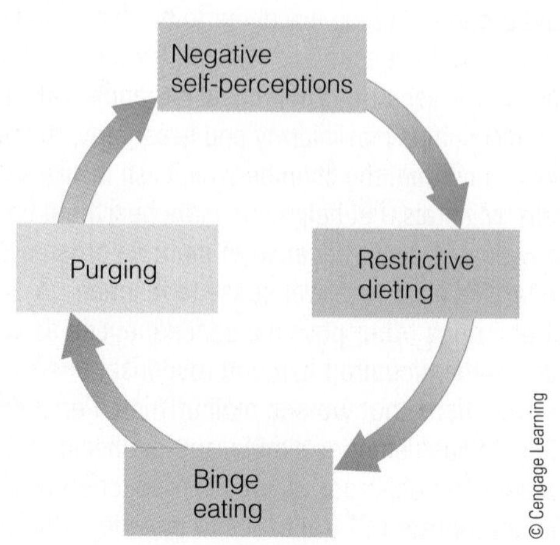

may rupture or tear, as may the stomach. Sometimes the eyes become red from pressure during vomiting. The hands may be calloused or cut by the teeth while inducing vomiting. Overuse of emetics depletes potassium concentrations and can lead to death by heart failure.

Unlike Julie, Kelly is aware that her behavior is abnormal, and she is deeply ashamed of it. She wants to recover, and this makes recovery more likely for her than for Julie, who clings to denial. Feeling inadequate ("I can't even control my eating"), Kelly tends to be passive and to look to others for confirmation of her sense of worth. When she experiences rejection, either in reality or in her imagination, her bulimia nervosa becomes worse. If Kelly's depression deepens, she may seek solace in drug or alcohol abuse or in other addictive behaviors. Clinical depression is common in people with bulimia nervosa, and the rates of substance abuse are high.

Treatment of Bulimia Nervosa

Kelly needs to establish regular eating patterns. She may also benefit from a regular exercise program. Weight maintenance, rather than cyclic weight gains and losses, is the treatment goal. Major steps toward recovery include discontinuing purging and restrictive dieting habits and learning to eat three meals a day plus snacks. Initially, energy intake should provide enough food to satisfy hunger and maintain body weight. Table H8-3 offers diet strategies to correct the eating problems of bulimia nervosa. Most women diagnosed with bulimia nervosa recover within 5 to 10 years, with or without treatment, but treatment probably speeds the recovery process. Cognitive behavioral therapy may be more effective than other types of treatment.[12] A mental health professional should be on the treatment team to help clients with their depression and addictive behaviors.

Anorexia nervosa and bulimia nervosa are distinct eating disorders, yet they sometimes overlap in important ways. Anorexia victims may purge, and victims of both disorders are overly concerned with body image and have a tendency to drastically undereat. Many perceive foods as "forbidden" and "give in" to an eating binge. The two disorders can also appear in the same person, or one can lead to the other. Treatment is challenging and relapses are common. Another common eating disorder is **binge-eating disorder.**

TABLE H8-3 Diet Strategies for Combating Bulimia Nervosa

Planning Principles

- Plan meals and snacks; record plans in a food diary prior to eating.
- Plan meals and snacks that require eating at the table and using utensils.
- Refrain from finger foods.
- Refrain from "dieting" or skipping meals.

Nutrition Principles

- Eat a well-balanced diet and regularly timed meals consisting of a variety of foods.
- Include raw vegetables, salad, or raw fruit at meals to prolong eating times.
- Choose whole-grain, high-fiber breads, pasta, rice, and cereals to increase bulk.
- Consume adequate fluid, particularly water.

Other Tips

- Choose foods that provide protein and fat for satiety and bulky, fiber-rich carbohydrates for immediate feelings of fullness.
- Try including soups and other water-rich foods for satiety.
- Choose portions that meet the definition of "a serving" according to the USDA Food Patterns (pp. 42–43).
- For convenience (and to reduce temptation) select foods that naturally divide into portions. Select one potato, rather than rice or pasta that can be overloaded onto the plate; purchase yogurt and cottage cheese in individual containers; look for small packages of precut steak or chicken; choose frozen dinners with measured portions.
- Include 30 minutes of physical activity every day—exercise may be an important tool in defeating bulimia.

Binge-Eating Disorder

Charlie is a 40-year-old schoolteacher who has been overweight all his life. His friends and family are forever encouraging him to lose weight, and he has come to believe that if he only had more willpower, dieting would work. He periodically gives dieting his best shot—restricting energy intake for a day or two only to succumb to uncontrollable cravings, especially for high-fat foods. Like Charlie, up to half of the obese people who try to lose weight periodically binge; unlike people with bulimia nervosa, however, they typically do not purge. Binge-eating disorder has its own specific diagnostic criteria based on recurring episodes of binge eating, with a marked sense of lack of control. It can occur in people of normal weight as well as those who are severely overweight. Obesity alone is not an eating disorder.

Clinicians note differences between people with bulimia nervosa and those with binge-eating disorder. People with binge-eating disorder typically consume less during a binge, rarely purge, and exert less restraint during times of dieting. Similarities also exist, including feeling out of control, disgusted, depressed, embarrassed, guilty, or distressed because of their self-perceived gluttony.

There are also differences between obese binge eaters and obese people who do not binge. Those with binge-eating disorder report higher rates of self-loathing, disgust about body size, depression, and anxiety. Their eating habits differ as well. Obese binge eaters tend to consume more kcalories and more dessert and snack-type foods during regular meals and binges than obese people who do not binge. Binge eating may incur health risks greater than those of obesity alone.[13]

Some of the characteristics seen in people with binge-eating disorder are similar to those seen in people with substance-use disorders: strong cravings, poor self-control, a diminished sensitivity to pleasure, and patterns of compulsive use.[14] These resemblances have given rise to the concept of *food addictions* and may reflect the same biological and psychological systems that are involved in rewards and self-control.[15] When the reward of delicious foods tempts a person, the ability to resist depends on self-control.[16] Neural images show that certain foods (especially those with added sugars and solid fats) have effects on the brain similar to those seen with addictive drugs. Dopamine activity—which helps to regulate emotional and motivational behavior—is also similarly altered in both drug addicts and those with compulsive eating behaviors.[17]

Binge eating can be resolved with treatment. Reducing binge eating makes participation in weight-control programs easier. It also improves physical health, mental health, and the chances of success in breaking the cycle of rapid weight losses and gains.

Eating Disorders in Society

Society plays a central role in eating disorders. Consider that the average US woman is 5 feet 4 inches tall and weighs 140 pounds, whereas the average US model is 7 inches taller and weighs 23 pounds less. Adolescent girls and women of all ages who obsess over weight loss and envy beautiful models are likely to engage in unhealthy eating habits. Further proof of society's influence is found in the demographic distribution of eating disorders—they are known only in developed nations, and they become more prevalent as wealth increases and food becomes plentiful. Some people point to the vomitoriums of ancient times and claim that bulimia nervosa is not new, but the two are actually distinct. Ancient people were eating for pleasure, without guilt, and in the company of others; they vomited so that they could rejoin the feast. Bulimia nervosa is a disorder of isolation and is often accompanied by low self-esteem.

Chapter 8 describes how our society sets unrealistic ideals for body weight, especially in women, and devalues those who do not conform to them. Anorexia nervosa and bulimia nervosa are not a form of rebellion against these unreasonable expectations, but rather an exaggerated acceptance of them. In fact, some people fail to recognize the health dangers and endorse eating disorders as a lifestyle choice. Some 200 websites encourage, support, and motivate users to continue their lives with anorexia and bulimia.[18]

The incidence and prevalence of eating disorders in young people has increased steadily since the 1950s.[19] Most alarming is the rising prevalence at progressively younger ages. Restrained eating, fasting, binge eating, purging, fear of fatness, and distortion of body image are extraordinarily common among children and adolescents. Most are "on diets," and many are poorly nourished. Some eat too little food to support normal growth, thus they miss out on their adolescent growth spurts and may never catch up. Many eat so little that hunger propels them into binge-purge cycles. Disordered eating behaviors set a pattern that likely continues into young adulthood.[20]

Perhaps a person's best defense against these disorders is to learn to appreciate his or her own uniqueness. When people discover and honor their body's real physical needs, they become unwilling to sacrifice health for conformity. To respect and value oneself may be lifesaving.

CRITICAL THINKING QUESTIONS

A. How do eating disorders affect health?

B. You overheard someone saying that eating disorders aren't really diseases and that if people who have anorexia or bulimia would just eat normally, they'd be cured. What is your opinion of this position? How can you make a distinction between someone with an eating disorder and others who are concerned with managing their body weight?

REFERENCES

1. F. R. E. Smink, D. vanHocken, and H. W. Hock, Epidemiology of eating disorders: Incidence, prevalence and mortality rates, *Current Psychiatry Reports* 14 (2012): 406–414.
2. R. D. Grave, Eating disorders: Progress and challenges, *European Journal of Internal Medicine* 22 (2011): 153–160.
3. J. C. Gibbs, N. I. Williams, and M. J. deSouza, Prevalence of individual and combined components of the female athlete triad, *Medicine and Science in Sports and Exercise* 45 (2013): 985–996; T. G. Nazem and K. E. Ackerman, The female athlete triad, *Sports Health* 4 (2012): 302–311.
4. G. G. Artioli and coauthors, Prevalence, magnitude, and methods of rapid weight loss among judo competitors, *Medicine and Science in Sports and Exercise* 42 (2010): 436–442.
5. C. A. Hincapié and J. D. Cassidy, Disordered eating, menstrual disturbances, and low bone mineral density in dancers: A systematic review, *Archives of Physical Medicine and Rehabilitation* 91 (2010): 1777–1789; E. Waugh and coauthors, Effects of exercise on bone mass in young women with anorexia nervosa, *Medicine and Science in Sports and Exercise* 43 (2011): 755–763; M. T. Barrack and coauthors, Physiologic and behavioral indicators of energy deficiency in female adolescent runners with elevated bone turnover, *American Journal of Clinical Nutrition* 92 (2010): 652–659.
6. American Psychiatric Association, *Diagnostic and Statistical Manual of Mental Disorders,* (Washington, D.C.: American Psychiatric Publishing, 2013).
7. A. P. Winston, The clinical biochemistry of anorexia nervosa, *Annals of Clinical Biochemistry* 49 (2012): 132–143.
8. Position of the American Dietetic Association: Nutrition intervention in the treatment of eating disorders, *Journal of the American Dietetic Association* 111 (2011): 1236–1241.
9. J. E. Schebendach and coauthors, Food choice and diet variety in weight-restored patients with anorexia nervosa, *Journal of the American Dietetic Association* 111 (2011): 732–736.
10. M. J. Krantz and coauthors, Factors influencing QT prolongation in patients hospitalized with severe anorexia nervosa, *General Hospital Psychiatry* 34 (2012): 173–177.
11. American Psychiatric Association, *Diagnostic and Statistical Manual of Mental Disorders* (Washington, D.C.: American Psychiatric Publishing, 2013).
12. ECRI Institute, *Bulimia Nervosa: Comparative Efficacy of Available Psychological and Pharmacological Treatments*, as cited in M. Mitka, Reports weighs options for bulimia nervosa treatment, *Journal of the American Medical Association* 305 (2011): 875.
13. J. I. Hudson and coauthors, Longitudinal study of the diagnosis of components of the metabolic syndrome in individuals with binge-eating disorder, *American Journal of Clinical Nutrition* 91 (2010): 1568–1573.
14. American Psychiatric Association, *Diagnostic and Statistical Manual of Mental Disorders* (Washington, D.C.: American Psychiatric Publishing), 2013.

15. D. G. Smith and T. W. Robbins, The neurobiological underpinnings of obesity and binge eating: A rationale for adopting the food addiction model, *Biological Psychiatry* 73 (2013): 804–810; N. D. Volkow and coauthors, Obesity and addiction: Neurobiological overlaps, *Obesity Reviews* 14 (2013): 2–18; J. L. Fortuna, The obesity epidemic and food addiction: Clinical similarities to drug dependence, *Journal of Psychoactive Drugs* 44 (2012): 56–63; C. Moreno and R. Randon, Should overeating and obesity be classified as an addictive disorder in DSM-5? *Current Pharmaceutical Design* 17 (2011): 1128–1131.
16. N. D. Volkow and coauthors, The addictive dimensionality of obesity, *Biological Psychiatry* 73 (2013): 811–818.
17. J. H. Baik, Dopamine signaling in food addiction: Role of Dopamine D2 receptors, *BMB Reports* (2013): pii: 2509.
18. D. L. G. Borzekowski and coauthors, e-Ana and e-Mia: A content analysis of pro-eating disorder web sites, *American Journal of Public Health* 100 (2010): 1526–1534.
19. D. S. Rosen and the Committee on Adolescence, Clinical report: Identification and management of eating disorders in children and adolescents, *Pediatrics* 126 (2010): 1240–1253.
20. D. Neumark-Sztainer and coauthors, Dieting and disordered eating behaviors from adolescence to young adulthood: Findings from a 10-year longitudinal study, *Journal of the American Dietetic Association* 111 (2011): 1004–1011.

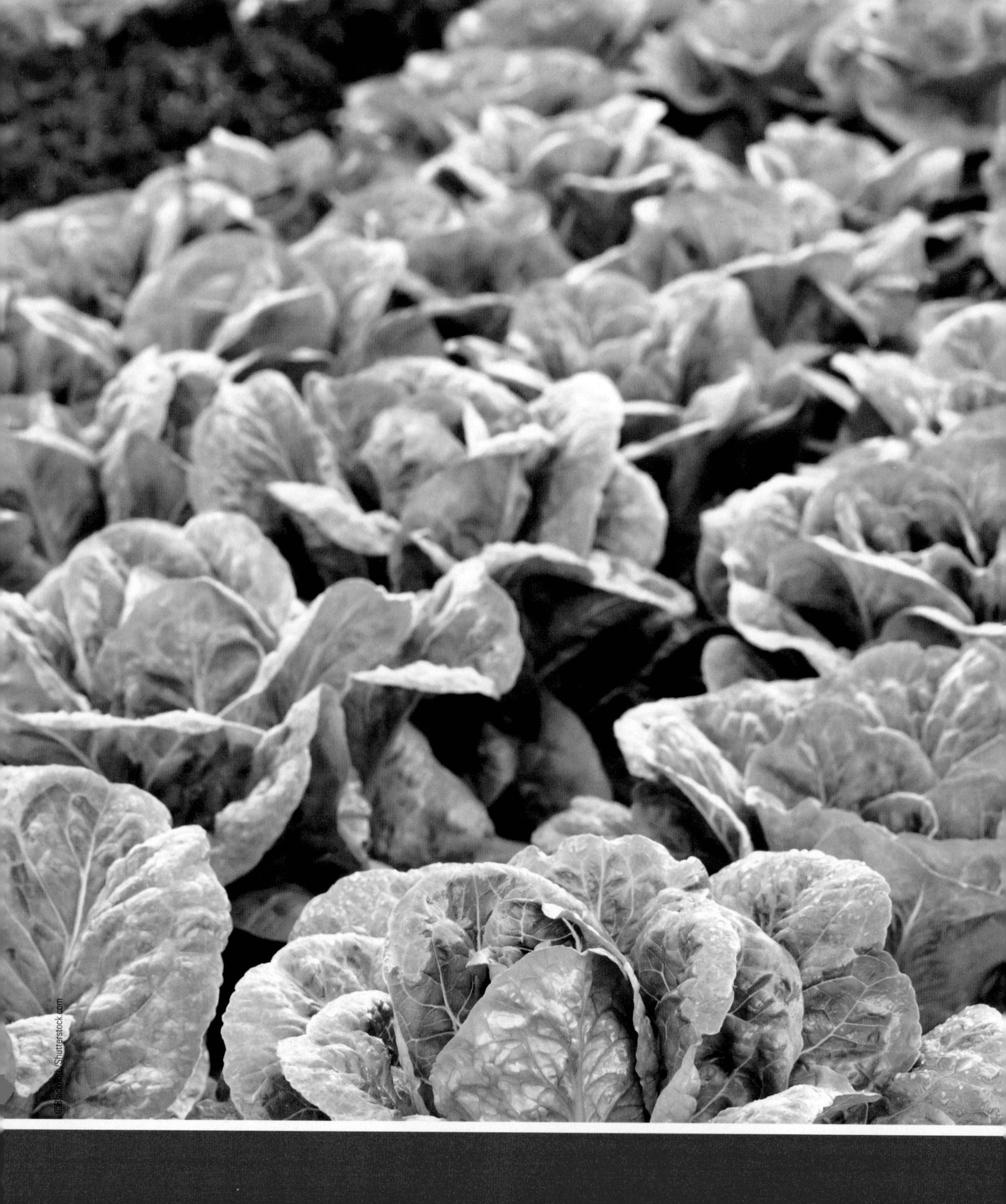

9

Weight Management: Overweight, Obesity, and Underweight

Nutrition in Your Life

Are you pleased with your body weight? If so, you are a rare individual. Most people in our society think they should weigh more or less (mostly less) than they do. Usually, their primary concern is appearance, but they often understand that physical health is also somehow related to body weight. One does not necessarily cause the other—that is, an ideal body weight does not ensure good health. Instead, both depend on diet and physical activity. A well-balanced diet and active lifestyle support good health—and help maintain body weight within a reasonable range. In the Nutrition Portfolio at the end of this chapter, you can consider whether your eating habits and physical activities are supporting good health and a reasonable body weight.

The previous chapter described how body weight is stable when energy in equals energy out. Weight gains occur when energy intake exceeds energy expended, and conversely, weight losses occur when energy expended exceeds energy intake. At the extremes, both overweight and underweight present health risks. **Weight management** is a key component of good health. To that end, this chapter offers strategies to help achieve and maintain a healthy body weight. It also explores overweight and obesity by examining some of the causes, consequences, and treatments.

This chapter emphasizes overweight (BMI 25 to 29.9) and obesity (BMI ≥30), partly because they have been more intensively studied and partly because they represent a major health problem in the United States and a growing concern worldwide. Underweight (BMI <18.5) is a far less prevalent problem. Information on underweight is presented at the end of the chapter. The highlight that follows this chapter examines fad diets.

LEARNING GPS

weight management: maintaining body weight in a healthy range by preventing gradual weight gains over time and losing weight if overweight, and by preventing weight losses and gaining weight if underweight.

> **FIGURE 9-1 Increasing Prevalence of Obesity (BMI ≥30) among US Adults**

1995

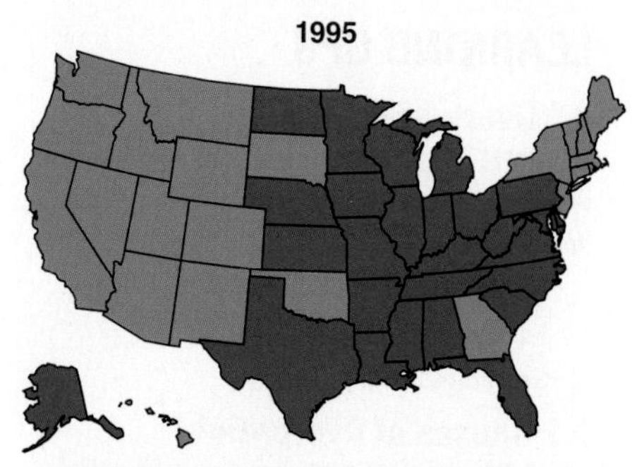

10%–14%	15%–19%	20%–24%	25%–29%	≥30%
23 states	27 states	0 states	0 states	0 states

2000

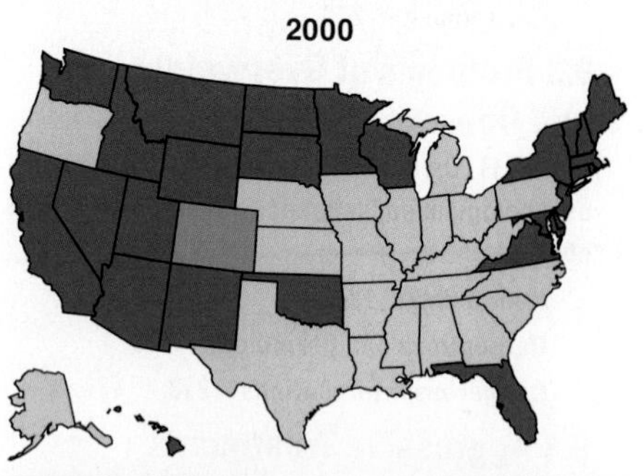

10%–14%	15%–19%	20%–24%	25%–29%	≥30%
1 state	27 states	22 states	0 states	0 states

2005

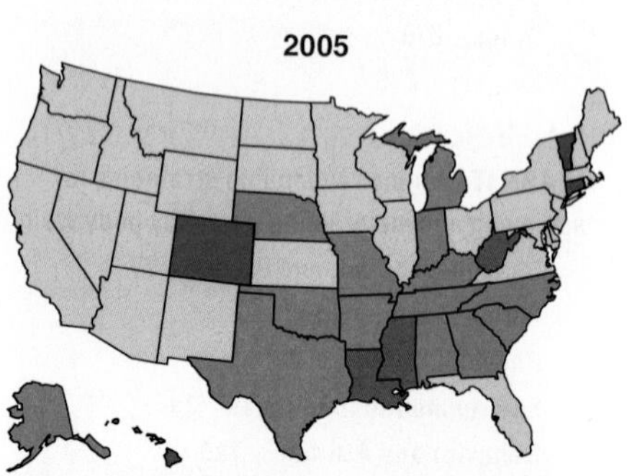

10%–14%	15%–19%	20%–24%	25%–29%	≥30%
0 states	4 states	29 states	14 states	3 states

2010

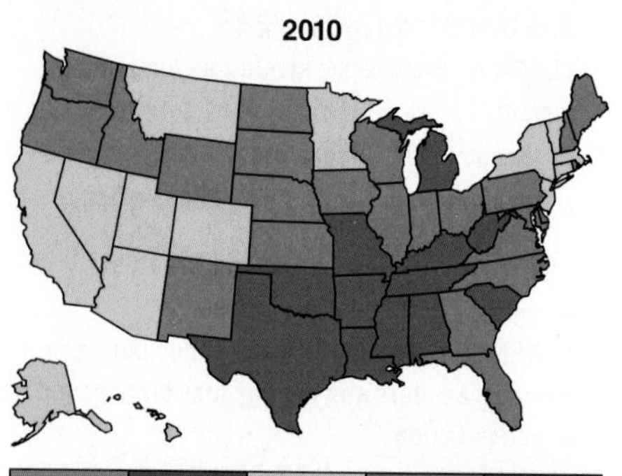

10%–14%	15%–19%	20%–24%	25%–29%	≥30%
0 states	0 states	14 states	24 states	12 states

SOURCE: www.cdc.gov/obesity/data/adult.html

9.1 Overweight and Obesity

> **LEARN IT** Describe how body fat develops and why it can be difficult to maintain weight gains and losses.

Despite our preoccupation with body image and weight loss, the prevalence of overweight and obesity in the United States continues to be high.[1] In the past four decades, obesity increased in every state, in both genders, and across all ages, races, and educational levels (see Figure 9-1).* An estimated 69 percent of the adults in the United States are now considered overweight or obese, as defined by a BMI of 25 to 29.9, or 30 and greater, respectively.[2] The prevalence of overweight is especially high among women, the poor, blacks, and Mexican Americans.

The prevalence of overweight among children in the United States has also risen at an alarming rate. An estimated 32 percent of children and adolescents aged 2 to 19 years are either overweight or obese.[3] Chapter and Highlight 16 present information on overweight during childhood and adolescence.

Obesity in the United States is widespread. Prevalence increased rapidly over the past four decades, but seems to have leveled out in recent years.[4] This **epidemic** of obesity has spread worldwide, affecting 1.4 billion adults and 40 million children younger than age 5.[5] Increasing rates of obesity in countries around the world reflects a global food system that delivers an abundance of energy-dense, processed, affordable, and effectively marketed products.[6] Before examining the suspected causes of obesity and the various strategies used to treat it, it is helpful to understand the development and metabolism of body fat.

Fat Cell Development When "energy in" exceeds "energy out," much of the excess energy is stored in the fat cells of adipose tissue. The amount of fat in adipose tissue reflects both the number and the size of the fat cells.** The number of fat cells increases most rapidly during the growing years of late childhood and early puberty. After growth ceases, fat cell numbers may continue to increase whenever energy balance is positive.[7] Obese people have more fat cells than healthy-weight people; their fat cells are also larger.

As fat cells accumulate triglycerides, they expand in size (review Figure 5-18 on p. 148). When the cells enlarge, they stimulate cell proliferation so that their numbers increase again. Thus obesity develops when a person's fat cells increase in number, in size, or quite often both. Figure 9-2 illustrates fat cell development.

When "energy out" exceeds "energy in," the size of fat cells dwindles, but not their number. People with extra fat cells tend to regain lost weight rapidly; with weight gain, their many fat cells readily fill. In contrast, people with an average number of enlarged fat cells may be more successful in maintaining weight losses; when their cells shrink, both cell size and number are normal. Prevention of obesity is most critical, then, during the growing years of childhood and adolescence when fat cells increase in number. Researchers are exploring ways to induce fat cell death—which would decrease the number.[8]***

As mentioned, excess fat first fills the body's natural storage site—adipose tissue. If fat is still abundant, the excess is deposited in organs such as the heart and liver and plays a key role in the development of diseases such as heart failure and fatty liver, respectively.[9]**** As adipose tissue produces adipokines, metabolic changes that indicate disease risk—such as insulin resistance—become apparent and chronic inflammation develops.[10] The adipokine profile begins to improve with as little as a 5 percent weight loss and a decrease in fat cell size, suggesting that other metabolic changes might also occur at that time to improve disease risks.

*Figure 9.1 maps offer a glimpse at the dramatic changes in obesity prevalence over the past several decades. Because of changes in methodology, however, estimates of obesity prevalence from 2011 forward cannot be compared to estimates from previous years.

**Obesity due to an increase in the *number* of fat cells is *hyperplastic obesity*. Obesity due to an increase in the *size* of fat cells is *hypertrophic obesity*.

***Cell death is known as as *apoptosis*.

****The adverse effect of fat in nonadipose tissue is known as *lipotoxicity*.

> FIGURE 9-2 **Fat Cell Development**

Fat cells are capable of increasing their size by 20-fold and their number by several thousandfold.

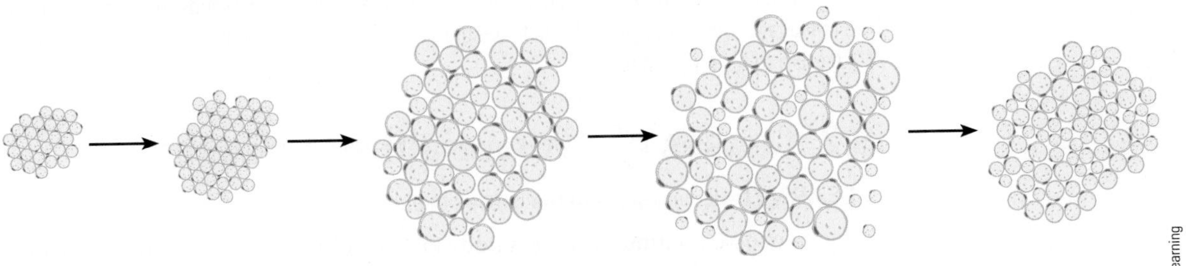

During growth, fat cells increase in number.

When energy intake exceeds expenditure, fat cells increase in size.

When fat cells have enlarged and energy intake continues to exceed energy expenditure, fat cells may increase in number again.

With fat loss, the size of the fat cells shrinks but not the number.

Fat Cell Metabolism The enzyme **lipoprotein lipase (LPL)** plays a major role in the metabolism and transport of lipids, and consequently is a participant in the development of obesity.[11] One of its roles is to remove triglycerides from the blood for storage in both adipose tissue and muscle cells. Obese people generally have much more LPL activity in their adipose cells than lean people do (their muscle cell LPL activity is similar, though). This high LPL activity makes fat storage especially efficient. Consequently, even modest excesses in energy intake have a more dramatic impact on obese people than on lean people. When obese people eat less in an effort to lose weight, their LPL activity diminishes.

The activity of LPL in different regions of the body is partially influenced by gender. In women, fat cells in the breasts, hips, and thighs produce abundant LPL, storing fat in those body sites; in men, fat cells in the abdomen produce abundant LPL. This enzyme activity explains why men tend to develop central obesity around the abdomen (apple-shaped) whereas women more readily develop lower-body fat around the hips and thighs (pear-shaped).

Gender differences are also apparent in the activity of the lipase enzymes controlling the release and breakdown of fat in various parts of the body. The release of lower-body fat is less active in women than in men, whereas the release of upper-body fat is similar. Furthermore, the rate of fat breakdown is lower in women than in men. Consequently, women may have a more difficult time losing fat in general, and from the hips and thighs in particular.

Enzyme activity may also explain why some people who lose weight regain it so easily. After weight loss and weight stabilization, adipose tissue LPL is increased and its response to meals is heightened. It's as if the LPL enzyme gene is saying "Make more fat-storing enzymes." People easily regain weight after having lost it because they are battling against enzymes that want to store fat. Fat storage is efficient, and fat oxidation is not. Dietary fat oxidation correlates negatively with body fatness: obese people have the least activity. The activities of these and other proteins provide an explanation for the observation that some biological mechanism seems to set a person's body weight or composition at a fixed point; the body will make adjustments to restore that **set point** if the person tries to change it.

Set-Point Theory Many physiological variables, such as blood glucose, blood pH, and body temperature, remain fairly stable under a variety of conditions. The hypothalamus and other regulatory centers constantly monitor and delicately adjust conditions to maintain homeostasis. The stability of such complex systems may depend on set-point regulators that maintain variables within specified limits.

Researchers have confirmed that after weight losses, the body adjusts its metabolism. The decrease in the metabolic rate after weight loss is greater than would be expected based on body composition alone.[12] This adaptation helps to explain why it can be difficult for an overweight person to maintain weight losses. While set point answers some questions regarding the biology of energy balance, it fails to explain the many other influences contributing to the population's obesity epidemic.[13]

epidemic (ep-ih-DEM-ick): the appearance of a disease (usually infectious) or condition that attacks many people at the same time in the same region.

- **epi** = upon
- **demos** = people

lipoprotein lipase (LPL): an enzyme that hydrolyzes triglycerides passing by in the bloodstream and directs their parts into the cells, where they can be metabolized or reassembled for storage.

set point: the point at which controls are set (for example, on a thermostat). The set-point theory that relates to body weight proposes that the body tends to maintain a certain weight by means of its own internal controls.

> **REVIEW IT** Describe how body fat develops and why it can be difficult to maintain weight gains and losses.
>
> Fat cells develop by increasing in number and size. Obesity prevention depends on maintaining a reasonable number of fat cells. With weight gains or losses, the body adjusts in an attempt to return to its set-point weight.

9.2 Causes of Overweight and Obesity

› LEARN IT Review some of the causes of obesity.

Why do people accumulate excess body fat? The obvious answer is that they take in more energy from foods and beverages than they expend in physical activity and metabolic processes. But that answer falls short of explaining why they do this. Is it genetic? Environmental? Cultural? Behavioral? Socioeconomic? Psychological? Metabolic? All of these? Most likely the latter. Many factors contribute to the development of obesity and most are interrelated. This section reviews the two major contributing and interacting factors—genetics and the environment.[14]

Genetics and Epigenetics Genetics plays a true causative role in relatively few cases of obesity, for example, in Prader-Willi syndrome—a genetic disorder characterized by excessive appetite, massive obesity, short stature, and often mental retardation. Most cases of obesity, however, do not stem from a single gene, yet multiple genetic influences do seem to be involved. Highlight 6 describes epigenetics—the influence of environmental factors, such as diet and physical activity, on gene expression. Obesity provides a classic example of epigenetic regulation.[15]

Researchers have found that adopted children tend to be more similar in weight to their biological parents than to their adoptive parents.[16] Studies of twins yield similar findings: compared with fraternal twins, identical twins are far more likely to weigh the same.[17] These findings suggest an important role for genetics in determining a person's *susceptibility* to obesity.[18] In other words, genes interact with the diet and activity patterns that lead to obesity and the metabolic pathways that influence satiety and energy balance. Even identical twins with identical genes become different over the years as epigenetic changes accumulate. This raises an important point: you cannot change the genome you inherit, but you can influence the epigenome. Physical activity, for example, can minimize the genetic influences on BMI.[19] Likewise, high-fat diets, sugar-sweetened beverages, and low physical activity can accentuate the genetic influences on obesity.[20]

Clearly, something genetic makes a person more or less likely to gain or lose weight when overeating or undereating. Some people gain more weight than others on comparable energy intakes. Given an extra 1000 kcalories a day for 100 days, some pairs of identical twins gain less than 10 pounds while others gain up to 30 pounds. Within each pair, the amounts of weight gained, percentages of body fat, and locations of fat deposits are similar. Similarly, some people lose more weight than others following comparable exercise routines.

Researchers have been examining the human genome in search of genetic and epigenetic answers to obesity questions. As the section on protein synthesis in Chapter 6 describes, each cell expresses only the genes for the proteins it needs, and each protein performs a unique function. The following paragraphs describe only a couple of the proteins that help explain appetite control, energy regulation, and obesity development.

Leptin Researchers have identified an obesity gene, called *ob,* that is expressed primarily in the adipose tissue and codes for the protein **leptin**. Leptin acts as a hormone, primarily in the hypothalamus. Leptin maintains homeostasis by regulating food intake and energy expenditure in response to adipose tissue. When body fat increases, leptin increases—which suppresses appetite. When body fat decreases, leptin decreases—which stimulates appetite and suppresses energy expenditure.

Mice with a defective *ob* gene do not produce leptin and can weigh up to three times as much as normal mice and have five times as much body fat (see Figure 9-3).

leptin: a protein produced by fat cells under direction of the *ob* gene that decreases appetite and increases energy expenditure.

- **leptos** = thin

When injected with a synthetic form of leptin, the mice rapidly lose body fat. (Because leptin is a protein, it would be destroyed during digestion if given orally; consequently, it must be given by injection.) The fat cells not only lose fat, but they self-destruct (reducing cell number), which may explain why weight gains are delayed when the mice are fed again.

Although extremely rare, a genetic deficiency of leptin or genetic mutation of its receptor has been identified in human beings as well. Extremely obese children with barely detectable blood levels of leptin have little appetite control; they are constantly hungry and eat considerably more than their siblings or peers. Given daily injections of leptin, these children lose a substantial amount of weight, confirming leptin's role in regulating appetite and body weight.

Very few obese people have a leptin deficiency, however. In fact, leptin levels increase as BMI increases. Leptin rises but fails to suppress appetite or enhance energy expenditure—a condition researchers describe as leptin resistance.[21] With weight loss, leptin levels decline, which reduces satiation and challenges weight loss maintenance; leptin injections effectively increase satiation after weight loss.[22]

> FIGURE 9-3 Mice with and without Leptin Compared

Both of these mice have a defective *ob* gene. Consequently, they do not produce leptin. They both became obese, but the one on the right received daily injections of leptin, which suppressed food intake and increased energy expenditure, resulting in weight loss.

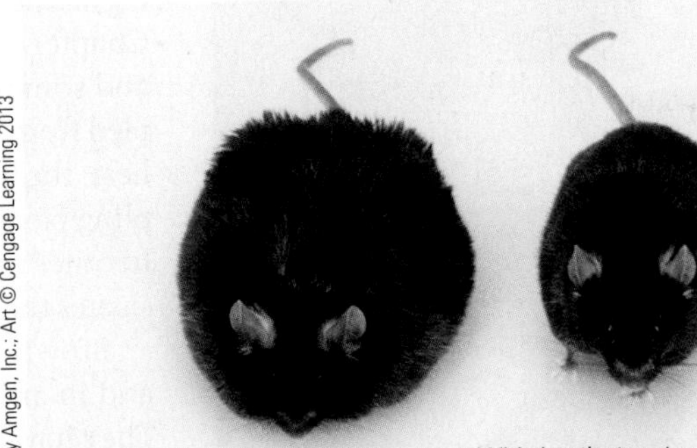

Without leptin, this mouse weighs almost three times as much as a normal mouse.
With leptin treatment, this mouse lost a significant amount of weight but still weighs almost one and a half times as much as a normal mouse.

Ghrelin Another protein, known as **ghrelin**, also acts as a hormone primarily in the hypothalamus. In contrast to leptin, ghrelin is secreted primarily by the stomach cells and promotes eating and weight gain by increasing smell sensitivity, stimulating appetite, and promoting efficient energy storage.[23]

Ghrelin triggers the desire to eat. Blood levels of ghrelin typically rise before and fall after a meal—reflecting the hunger and satiety that precede and follow eating. On average, ghrelin levels are high whenever the body is in negative energy balance, as occurs during low-kcalorie diets, for example. This response may help explain why weight loss is so difficult to maintain. Weight loss is more successful with exercise and after gastric bypass surgery, in part because ghrelin levels are relatively low. Ghrelin levels decline again whenever the body is in positive energy balance, as occurs with weight gains.

Findings from an interesting research study suggest that a person's mindset also influences ghrelin's response to a meal.[24] Young adults were given beverages on two separate occasions—either a beverage labeled as a high-fat, 620-kcalorie "indulgent" milkshake or one labeled as a low-fat, 140-kcalorie "sensible" milkshake. Ghrelin's rise in anticipation of drinking the indulgent milkshake and its decline afterward was much steeper than for the sensible milkshake. In reality, though, the two milkshakes were identical (380 kcalories). Not only was the ghrelin response different, but the participants' satiety differed, reflecting their perceptions of the products. Drinking the sensible milkshake was not as satisfying, despite having the exact same nutrient contents as the indulgent milkshake. The sensible mindset with its relatively flat ghrelin response leaves a person with an increased appetite. These researchers suggest there may be a physiological benefit to adopting a psychological mindset of indulgence when eating low-energy-density, healthy foods.

Some research indicates that ghrelin also promotes sleep. Interestingly, a lack of sleep increases the hunger hormone ghrelin and decreases the satiety hormone leptin—which may help to explain the association between inadequate sleep and overweight.[25]

These two proteins—leptin and ghrelin—illustrate some of the complex factors involved in the regulation of food intake and energy homeostasis. Scientists have identified numerous proteins expressed by dozens of genes linked to obesity and several others associated with fat distribution in the body. Each of these genes has slight variations that differ among individuals.[26] Furthermore, these genes interact with one another and with the environment. The complexity of it all creates a multitude of possible genetic explanations.[27]

ghrelin (GRELL-in): a protein produced by the stomach cells that enhances appetite and decreases energy expenditure.
- **ghre** = growth

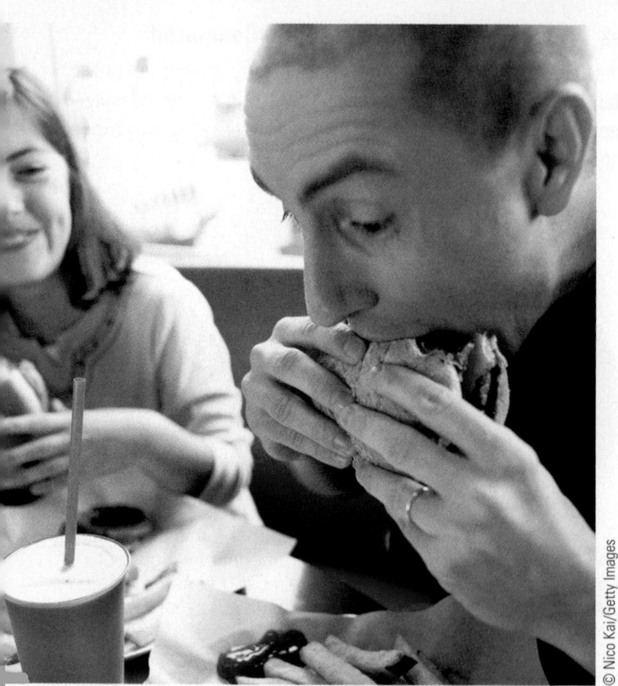

The food industry spends billions of dollars a year on advertising. The message? "Eat more."

Uncoupling Proteins Genes also code for proteins involved in energy metabolism. These proteins may influence the storing or expending of energy with different efficiencies or in different types of fat. The body has two main types of fat: white and **brown adipose tissue.** White adipose tissue stores fat for other cells to use for energy; brown adipose tissue releases stored energy as heat, thus defending against cold and preventing obesity. Recall from Chapter 7 that when fat is oxidized, some of the energy is released in heat and some is captured in ATP. In brown adipose tissue, oxidation is uncoupled from ATP formation, producing heat only.* By radiating energy away as heat, the body expends, rather than stores, energy. In contrast, efficient coupling facilitates synthesis reactions, including the making of fat for storage. In other words, weight gains or losses may depend on whether the body dissipates the energy from an ice cream sundae as heat or stores it in body fat.

Brown fat and heat production is particularly important in newborns and in animals exposed to cold weather, especially those that hibernate. They have plenty of brown adipose tissue. In contrast, human adults have little brown fat, stored primarily around the neck and clavicles.[28] Brown fat is most metabolically active during exposure to cold.[29] Importantly, brown fat activity declines with age and with obesity; overweight and obese individuals have less brown fat activity than others.[30] The role of brown fat in body weight regulation is not yet fully understood, but such an understanding may prove most useful in developing obesity treatments.[31]

Recent research has revealed that some white fat cells can undergo a process known as browning as they take on characteristics of brown fat, most notably the activity of uncoupled proteins; these fat cells have been named **brite adipocytes.**[32] Brite fat cells are far more abundant than brown fat cells in adults.[33] By learning how browning is regulated, researchers hope to tilt energy balance from storage to expenditure in the effort to fight obesity. Interestingly, among the factors that trigger browning is physical activity. During exercise, muscle cells release a protein (the myokine irisin) that triggers the transformation of white fat cells into brite fat cells.[34] Such findings help to explain one of the many ways physical activity expends energy and supports weight management.

Environment With obesity rates rising and the **gene pool** remaining relatively unchanged, environment must also play a role in obesity. Obesity reflects the interactions between genes and the environment. An **obesogenic environment** includes all of the circumstances that we encounter daily that push us toward fatness. Over the past 4 decades, the demand for physical activity has decreased as the abundance of food has increased.

Keep in mind that genetic and environmental factors are not mutually exclusive; in fact, their *interactions* create the epigenetics that provide a greater understanding of obesity and related diseases. Genes can influence eating behaviors, for example, and food and activity behaviors influence the genes that regulate body weight. Interestingly, even social relationships can influence the development of obesity.[35] The likelihood that a person will become obese increases when a friend, sibling, or spouse becomes obese.

Overeating One explanation for obesity is that overweight people overeat, although diet histories may not always reflect high intakes. Diet histories are not always accurate records of actual intakes; both normal-weight and obese people commonly misreport their dietary intakes. Most importantly, current dietary intakes may not reflect the eating habits that led to obesity. Obese people who had a positive energy balance for years and accumulated excess body fat may not currently have a positive energy balance. This reality highlights an important point: the energy-balance equation must consider time. Both present *and* past eating and activity patterns influence current body weight.

*In *coupled reactions,* the energy released from the breakdown of one compound is used to create a bond in the formation of another compound. In *uncoupled reactions,* the energy is released as heat.

brown adipose tissue: masses of specialized fat cells packed with pigmented mitochondria that produce heat instead of ATP.

brite adipocytes: white fat cells with brown fat cell characteristics; also called *beige adipocytes.*

gene pool: all the genetic information of a population at a given time.

obesogenic (oh-BES-oh-JEN-ick) **environment:** all the factors surrounding a person that promote weight gain, such as increased food intake, especially of unhealthy choices, and decreased physical activity.

We live in an environment that exposes us to an abundance of high-kcalorie, high-fat foods that are readily available, relatively inexpensive, heavily advertised, and reasonably tasty. Food is available everywhere, all the time—thanks largely to fast food. Our highways are lined with fast-food restaurants. Convenience stores and service stations offer fast food and snacks as well. Fast food is available in our schools, malls, and airports. The mere proximity of fast food increases the risk of obesity. It's convenient and it's available morning, noon, and night—and all times in between. Consequently, we are eating more meals more frequently than in decades past—and energy intake has risen accordingly.[36]

Most alarming are the extraordinarily large portions and ready-to-go combo-meals. Eating large portion sizes multiple times a day accounts for much of the weight increase seen over the decades.[37] People buy the large portions and combinations, perceiving them to be a good value, but then they eat more than they need—a bad deal. In fact, one research study calculated that for the 67 cents extra to upsize a meal, consumers receive an extra 400 kcalories, an extra 36 grams of body fat, and an extra $1 to $7 in health-care costs.[38]

Simply put, large portion sizes deliver more kcalories. And portion sizes of virtually all foods and beverages have increased markedly in the past several decades, most notably at fast-food restaurants. Not only have portion sizes increased over time, but they are now two to eight times larger than standard serving sizes. The trend toward large portion sizes parallels the increasing prevalence of overweight and obesity in the United States, beginning in the 1970s, increasing sharply in the 1980s, and continuing today.

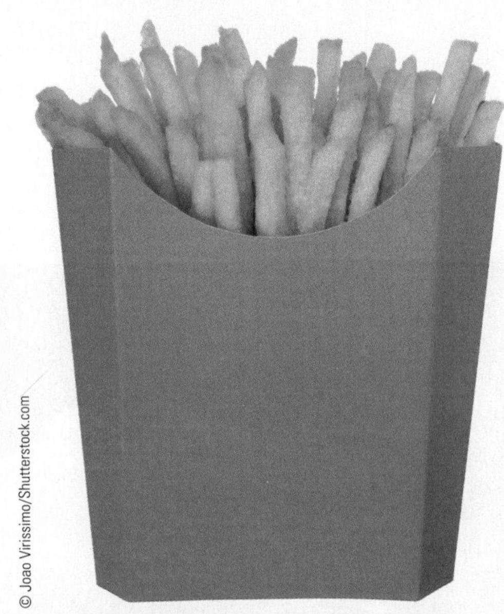

"Want fries with that?" A supersize portion delivers more than 600 kcalories.

Restaurant food, especially fast food, contributes significantly to the development of obesity.[39] Fast food is often energy-dense food, which increases energy intake, BMI, and body fatness. The combination of large portions and energy-dense foods is a double whammy. Reducing portion sizes is somewhat helpful, but the real kcalorie savings come from lowering the energy density. Low-energy-density foods such as fruits and vegetables can help with weight loss.

Physical Inactivity Our environment fosters physical inactivity as well.[40] Life requires little exertion—escalators carry us up stairs, automobiles take us across town, and remote controls change television channels from a distance. Modern technology has replaced physical activity at home, at work, and in transportation.[41] Inactivity contributes to weight gain and poor health. Most physical inactivity occurs when watching television, playing video games, and using the computer. The more time people spend in these sedentary activities, the more likely they are to be overweight—and to incur the metabolic risk factors of heart disease (high blood lipids, high blood pressure, and high blood glucose).[42]

Sedentary activities contribute to weight gain in several ways. First, they require little energy beyond the resting metabolic rate. Second, they replace time spent in more vigorous activities. Third, watching television influences food purchases and correlates with between-meal snacking on the high-kcalorie, solid fat and added sugars foods and beverages most heavily advertised.

Some obese people are so extraordinarily inactive that even when they eat less than lean people, they still have an energy surplus. Reducing their food intake further would incur nutrient deficiencies and jeopardize health. Physical activity is a necessary component of nutritional health. People must be physically active if they are to eat enough food to deliver all the nutrients they need without unhealthy weight gain. In fact, *to prevent weight gain,* the DRI suggests an accumulation of 60 minutes of moderately intense physical activities every day in addition to the less intense activities of daily living. Recommendations *to lose weight* encourage even greater duration, intensity, or frequency of physical activity (as a later section of the chapter discusses).

People may be obese, therefore, not because they eat too much, but because they move too little—both in purposeful exercise and in the activities of daily life. Studies report that the differences in the time obese and lean people spend lying, sitting, standing, and moving accounts for about 350 kcalories a day. In general, lean people tend to be more spontaneously active in their occupations and their leisure time. The energy expended in these everyday spontaneous activities—called *nonexercise activity thermogenesis (NEAT)*—plays a pivotal role in energy balance and weight management.

› REVIEW IT Review some of the causes of obesity.
Obesity has many causes and most interact, creating a complex scenario. Environmental factors, such as overeating and physical inactivity, may influence a person's genetic susceptibility to obesity.

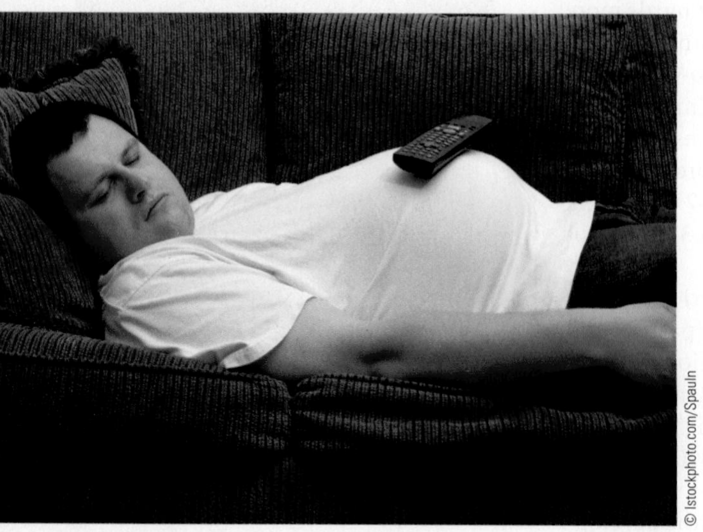
© Istockphoto.com/Spauln

Lack of physical activity fosters obesity.

9.3 Problems of Overweight and Obesity

› LEARN IT Discuss the physical, social, and psychological consequences of overweight and obesity.

Millions of US adults are trying to lose weight on any given day. Some of these people may not even need to lose weight. Others may benefit from weight loss, but they will not be successful. Relatively few people succeed in losing weight, and even fewer succeed permanently. For many, improving diet and activity habits to simply prevent further weight gains may be sufficient. Whether a person will benefit from weight loss is a question of health.

Health Risks Chapter 8 describes some of the health problems that commonly accompany obesity. In evaluating the risks to health from obesity, health-care professionals use three indicators:

- Body mass index (25 to 29.9 for overweight and ≥30 for obese)
- Waist circumference (>40 inches for men and >35 inches for women)
- Disease risk profile

Importantly, the disease risk profile takes into account family history, life-threatening diseases, and common risk factors for chronic diseases (such as blood lipid profile). The higher the BMI, the greater the waist circumference, and the more risk factors—the greater the urgency to treat obesity.

People can best decide whether weight loss might be beneficial by considering their health status. People who are overweight by BMI standards, but otherwise in good health, might not benefit from losing weight; they might focus on preventing further weight gains instead. In contrast, those who are obese and suffering from a life-threatening disease such as diabetes might improve their health substantially by adopting a diet and activity plan that supports weight loss.

Overweight in Good Health Often a person's motivations for weight loss have nothing to do with health. A healthy young woman with a BMI of 26 might want to lose a few pounds for spring break, but doing so might not improve her health. In fact, if she opts for a starvation diet or diet pills, she would be healthier *not* trying to lose weight. In any case, she should try to avoid additional weight gains.

Obese or Overweight with Risk Factors Weight loss is recommended for people who are obese and those who are overweight with one or more of the following risk factors for chronic diseases:

- Hypertension
- Cigarette smoking
- Abnormal blood lipids
- Diabetes or prediabetes
- Family history of heart disease
- Men 45 or older and women 55 or older

A 50-year-old man with a BMI of 28 who has high blood pressure and a family history of heart disease can improve his health by adjusting his diet and engaging in a regular exercise plan.

Obese or Overweight with Life-Threatening Condition Weight loss is also recommended for a person who is either obese or overweight and suffering from a life-threatening condition such as heart disease, type 2 diabetes, or sleep apnea. The health benefits of weight loss are clear. For example, a 30-year-old man with a BMI of 40 might be able to prevent or control diabetes by losing 75 pounds. Although the effort required to do so may be great, it may be no greater than the effort and consequences of living with diabetes.

> FIGURE 9-4 **The Psychology of Weight Cycling**

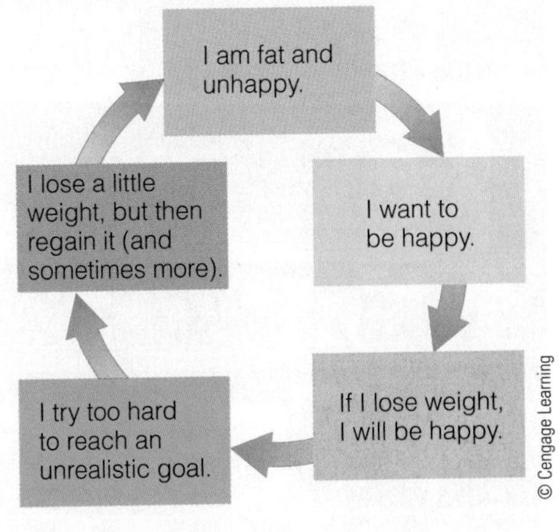

I am fat and unhappy.
I want to be happy.
If I lose weight, I will be happy.
I try too hard to reach an unrealistic goal.
I lose a little weight, but then regain it (and sometimes more).
© Cengage Learning

Perceptions and Prejudices

Many people assume that every obese person can achieve slenderness and should pursue that goal. First consider that most obese people do not—for whatever reason—successfully lose weight and maintain their losses. Then consider the prejudice involved in that assumption. People come with varying weight tendencies, just as they come with varying potentials for height and physical talents, yet we do not expect tall people to shrink or fast runners to slow down in an effort to become "normal."

Social Consequences Large segments of our society place such enormous value on thinness that obese people face prejudice and discrimination on the job, at school, and in social situations: they are judged on their appearance more than on their character. Socially, obese people are negatively stereotyped as lazy and lacking in self-control. Such a critical view of overweight is not prevalent in many other cultures, including segments of our own society. Instead, overweight is simply accepted or even embraced as a sign of robust health and beauty. To free society of its obsession with body weight and prejudice against obesity, people must first learn to judge others—and themselves—for who they are and not for what they weigh.

Psychological Problems Psychologically, obese people may suffer embarrassment when others treat them with hostility and contempt, and many have come to view their own bodies as flawed. Feelings of rejection, shame, and depression are common among obese people. Anxiety and depression, in turn, may contribute to the development of obesity, which perpetuates the problem.[43]

Most weight-loss programs assume that the problem can be solved simply by applying willpower and hard work. If determination were the only factor involved, though, the success rate would be far greater than it is. Overweight people may readily assume blame for failure to lose weight and maintain the losses when, in fact, it is the programs that have failed. Ineffective treatment and its associated sense of failure add to a person's psychological burden. Figure 9-4 illustrates how the devastating psychological effects of obesity and dieting perpetuate themselves.

Dangerous Interventions

Some people attach so many dreams of happiness to weight loss that they willingly risk huge sums of money for the slightest chance of success. As a result, weight-loss schemes flourish. Of the tens of thousands of claims, treatments, and theories for losing weight, few are effective—and many are downright dangerous. The negative consequences must be carefully considered before embarking on any weight-loss program. Some interventions entail greater dangers than the risk of being overweight. Physical, metabolic, and psychosocial problems may arise from fad diets and "yo-yo" dieting.[44] Wise consumers scrutinize fad diets, magic potions, and wonder gizmos with a healthy dose of skepticism.

Some of the nation's most popular diet books and weight-loss programs have misled consumers with unsubstantiated claims and deceptive testimonials. Furthermore, they fail to provide an assessment of the short- and long-term results of their treatment plans, even though such evaluations are possible and would permit consumers to make informed decisions. Of course, some weight-loss programs are better than others in terms of cost, approach, and customer satisfaction. Reputable weight-loss programs will explain the risks associated with their plans and provide honest predictions of success.

Fad Diets **Fad diets** often sound good, but they typically fall short of delivering on their promises. They espouse exaggerated or false theories of weight loss and advise consumers to follow inadequate diets. Some fad diets are hazardous to

fad diets: popular eating plans that promise quick weight loss. Most fad diets severely limit certain foods or overemphasize others (for example, never eat potatoes or pasta, or eat cabbage soup daily).

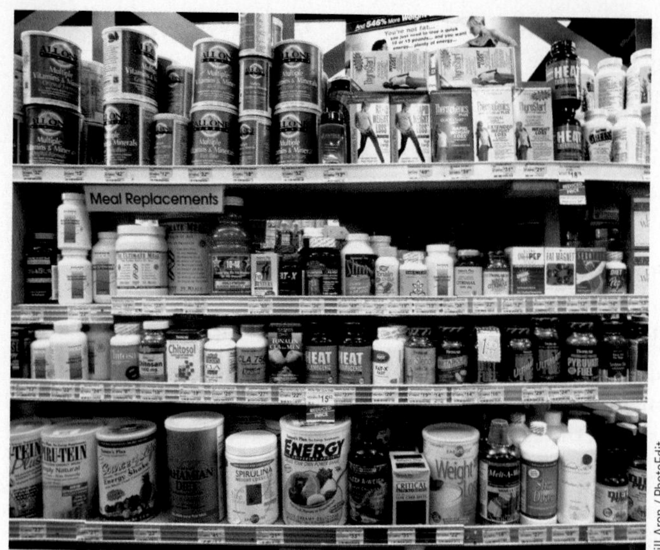

Bill Aron / PhotoEdit

So many promises, so little success.

health as Highlight 9 explains. Adverse reactions can be as minor as headaches, nausea, and dizziness or as serious as death. The "How To" on p. 299 offers guidelines for identifying unsound weight-loss schemes and fad diets.

Weight-Loss Products Millions of people in the United States use over-the-counter weight-loss products. Most users are women, especially young overweight women, but almost 10 percent are of normal weight.

In their search for weight-loss magic, some consumers turn to "natural" herbal products and dietary supplements, even though few have proved to be effective and many have proved to be harmful.[45] For example, in addition to the many cautions that accompany the use of all herbal remedies, consumers should be aware that St. John's wort is often prepared in combination with the herbal stimulant ephedrine. Ephedrine-containing supplements promote modest short-term weight loss (about 2 pounds a month), but with great risks. These supplements have been implicated in numerous heart attacks and seizures, resulting in about 100 deaths. For this reason, the FDA has banned the sale of ephedrine-containing supplements, but they are still readily available on the Internet.* Similarly, the FDA has issued warnings for another herbal weight loss supplement called Que She, which contains not only ephedrine but two weight-loss drugs that have been withdrawn from the market and another drug used to treat heart conditions.

Highlight 18 explores the possible benefits and potential dangers of herbal products and other alternative therapies. As it explains, dietary supplements do not need to be approved by the FDA, and manufacturers do not need to test the safety or effectiveness of any product. In other words, consumers cannot assume that an herbal product or dietary supplement is safe or effective just because it is available on the market. In fact, the FDA has identified more than 75 products that contain undeclared, active pharmaceutical ingredients that can have serious consequences such as seizures and heart attacks.[46] These ingredients are not listed on the labels, and consumers have no way of knowing what the products actually contain. Anyone considering whether to use dietary supplements for weight loss should consult with a physician and research the product with the FDA (www.fda.gov).

Other Gimmicks Other gimmicks don't help with weight loss either. Hot baths do not speed up metabolism so that pounds can be lost in hours. Steam and sauna baths do not melt the fat off the body, although they may dehydrate people so that they lose water weight. Brushes, sponges, wraps, creams, and massages intended to move, burn, or break up fat do nothing of the kind.

> **› REVIEW IT** Discuss the physical, social, and psychological consequences of overweight and obesity.
>
> The question of whether a person should lose weight depends on many factors: among them are the extent of overweight, age, health, and genetic makeup. Not all obesity will cause disease or shorten life expectancy. Just as there are unhealthy, normal-weight people, there are healthy, overweight people. Some people may risk more in the process of losing weight than in remaining overweight. Fad diets and weight-loss supplements can be as physically and psychologically damaging as excess body weight.

9.4 Aggressive Treatments for Obesity

› LEARN IT Explain the risks and benefits, if any, of aggressive ways to treat obesity.

The appropriate strategies for weight loss depend on the degree of obesity and the risk of disease. An overweight person in good health may need only to improve eating habits and increase physical activity, but someone with **clinically severe obesity** may need more aggressive treatment options—drugs or surgery. Drugs appear

clinically severe obesity: a BMI of 40 or greater or a BMI of 35 or greater with additional medical problems. A less preferred term used to describe the same condition is *morbid obesity.*

*Ephedrine is an amphetamine-like substance extracted from the Chinese ephedra herb *ma huang.* The FDA has banned the sale of *ma huang* in the United States.

to be modestly effective and safe, at least in the short term; surgery appears to be dramatically effective but can have severe complications, at least for some people.

Drugs Based on new understandings of obesity's genetic basis and its classification as a chronic disease, much research effort has focused on drug treatments for obesity. Experts reason that if obesity is a chronic disease, it should be treated as such—and the treatment of most chronic diseases includes drugs. The challenge, then, is to develop an effective drug—or more likely, a combination of drugs—that can be used over time without adverse side effects or the potential for abuse. Weight-loss drugs should be prescribed only to those with medical risks—not for cosmetic reasons—and in tandem with a healthy diet and activity program.

Several drugs for weight loss have been tried over the years, with varying degrees of effectiveness and safety.[47] When used as part of a long-term, comprehensive weight-loss program, drugs can help with modest weight loss. Because weight regain commonly occurs with the discontinuation of drug therapy, treatment must be long term. Yet the long-term use of drugs poses risks. We don't yet know whether a person would be harmed more from maintaining a 100-pound excess or from taking a drug for a decade to keep the 100 pounds off. Physicians must prescribe drugs appropriately, inform consumers of the potential risks, and monitor side effects carefully. Table 9-1 presents the drugs to treat obesity that meet the FDA mandate that "benefits must exceed risks."[48]

Some physicians prescribe drugs that have not been approved for weight loss, a practice known as "off-label" use. These drugs have been approved for other conditions (such as seizures) and incidentally cause modest weight loss. Physicians using off-label drugs must be well-informed of the drugs' use and effects and monitor their patients' responses closely.

Surgery The US prevalence of clinically severe obesity (BMI >40) is estimated at 6 percent.[49] At this level of obesity, lifestyle changes and modest weight losses can improve disease risks a little, but the most effective treatment is surgery.[50] Surgery may be an option for people with all of the following conditions:

- Unable to achieve adequate weight loss with diet and exercise
- BMI ≥40 or BMI ≥35 with weight-related health problems (such as diabetes or hypertension)
- No medical or psychological contraindications
- Understanding of risks and strong motivation to comply with post-surgery treatment plan

More than 100,000 such surgeries are performed in the United States annually.[51] As Figure 9-5 (p. 276) shows, the two most common surgical procedures effectively

TABLE 9-1 FDA-Approved Drugs for Weight Loss

Drug	Action	Side Effects
Orlistat (OR-leh-stat), trade names: Alli, Xenical	Inhibits pancreatic lipase activity in the GI tract, thus blocking digestion and absorption of dietary fat and limiting energy intake	GI cramping, diarrhea, gas, frequent bowel movements, reduced absorption of fat-soluble vitamins; rare cases of liver injury
Phentermine (FEN-ter-mean),diethylpropion (DYE-eth-ill-PRO-pee-on), phendimetrazine (FEN-dye-MEH-tra-zeen)	Enhances the release of the neurotransmitter norepinephrine, which suppresses appetite	Increased blood pressure and heart rate, insomnia, nervousness, dizziness, headache
Lorcaserin hydrochloride, trade name: Belviq (BELL-veek)	Interacts with brain serotonin receptors to increase satiety and reduce food intake	Headache, dizziness, fatigue, nausea, dry mouth, and constipation; low blood glucose in people with diabetes; serotonin syndrome, including agitation, confusion, fever, loss of coordination, rapid or irregular heart rate, shivering, seizures, and unconsciousness; cannot be safely used by pregnant or lactating women or people with heart-valve problems; high doses cause hallucinations
Phentermine (an appetite suppressant) and topiramate (a seizure/migraine medication) combination, trade name: Qsymia (kyoo-sim-EE-uh)	Enhances the release of the neurotransmitter norepinephrine, which suppresses appetite, and increases the feeling of being full, making foods taste less appealing	Increased heart rate; can cause birth defects if taken in the first weeks or months of pregnancy; increased heart rate; suicidal thoughts; may worsen glaucoma and other eye problems

NOTE: Weight-loss drugs are most effective when taken as directed and used in combination with reduced-kcalorie diet and increased physical activity.

> **FIGURE 9-5 Gastric Surgery Used in the Treatment of Clinically Severe Obesity**

Both of these surgical procedures limit the amount of food that can be comfortably eaten.

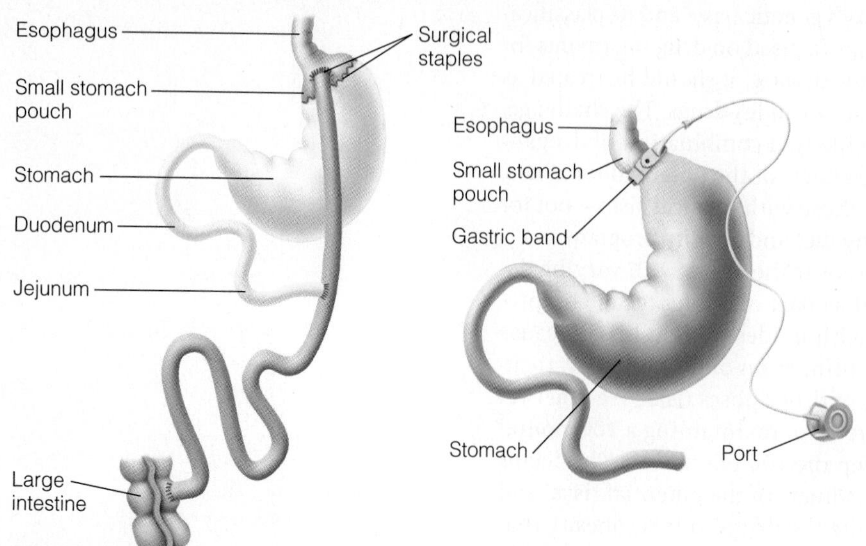

In gastric bypass, the surgeon constructs a small stomach pouch and creates an outlet directly to the small intestine, bypassing most of the stomach, the entire duodenum, and some of the jejunum. (Dark areas highlight the flow of food through the GI tract; pale areas indicate bypassed sections.)

Advantages:
- No foreign object in abdomen or need for adjustments
- More durable, reliable, and effective

In gastric banding, the surgeon uses a gastric band to create a small stomach pouch. The size of the opening can be adjusted by inflating or deflating the band by way of a port placed in the abdomen just beneath the skin.

Advantages:
- No malabsorption
- More flexible, less invasive, safer

limit food intake by reducing the capacity of the stomach. In addition, gastric bypass suppresses hunger by changing production of gastrointestinal hormones.[52] Changes in food preferences and GI microbes may also influence weight losses.[53] The results are significant: depending on the type of surgery, nearly 50 percent of the excess weight remains lost after 15 years.[54] Importantly, most people experience dramatic and lasting improvements in their diabetes, blood lipids, and blood pressure—even before significant weight loss.[55] Improvements in depression and anxiety are not as likely. Whether surgery is a reasonable option for obese teens is the subject of much debate among pediatricians and **bariatric** surgeons (see Chapter 16).[56]

Because the long-term safety and effectiveness of surgery depend, in large part, on compliance with dietary instructions, nutrition care plays an important role in follow-up treatment.[57] Vitamin and mineral deficiencies are common, and dietary supplements are routinely prescribed.[58] Weight regain may occur and psychological problems—such as disordered eating behaviors—may also develop.[59] Lifelong medical supervision is necessary, but the possible health benefits of weight loss—improved blood lipid profile, blood pressure, and insulin sensitivity—may outweigh the risks. Overall risk of death and heart disease is lower for obese people after successful surgery than for obese people who do not undergo surgery.[60]

Another surgical procedure removes some fat deposits by liposuction. This cosmetic procedure has little effect on body weight (less than 10 pounds), but can alter body shape slightly in specific areas. Liposuction is a popular procedure in part because of its perceived safety, but immediate and delayed complications can arise.[61] Furthermore, removing adipose tissue by way of liposuction does not provide the health benefits that typically accompany weight loss. In other words, liposuction does not improve blood pressure, inflammation, blood lipid profile, or insulin sensitivity. Perhaps most surprisingly, a year after liposuction, body fat returns and redistributes itself from the thighs to the abdomen.[62]

> **REVIEW IT** Explain the risks and benefits, if any, of aggressive ways to treat obesity.

Overweight and obese people may benefit most from improving eating and activity habits. Those with clinically severe obesity and high risks of medical problems may need more aggressive treatment, including drugs or surgery. Such treatments may offer benefits, but also incur some risks.

9.5 Weight-Loss Strategies

> **LEARN IT** Outline reasonable strategies for achieving and maintaining a healthy body weight.

From the bustling activity of a cell making fat to the inactivity of a person watching television, the factors contributing to obesity are numerous and complex. Each

bariatric: pertaining to the field of medicine that specializes in treating obesity.

interacts with many others. Efforts to combat obesity must integrate healthy eating patterns, physical activities, supportive environments, and psychosocial support.[63]

Changes, Losses, and Goals Successful weight-loss strategies embrace changes, celebrate losses, and set goals. A comprehensive lifestyle approach that includes low-kcalorie, nutrient-dense foods and regular physical activity supports both weight loss and health benefits. In keeping with this philosophy, the *Dietary Guidelines for Americans* advise those who need to lose weight to "consume fewer kcalories from foods and beverages, increase physical activity, and reduce time in sedentary behaviors."

> **DIETARY GUIDELINES FOR AMERICANS**
> Strive to achieve and maintain a healthy body weight through improved eating and physical activity behaviors.

Even modest weight loss brings health benefits. Modest weight loss, even when a person is still overweight, can improve blood glucose and reduce the risks of heart disease by lowering blood pressure and blood cholesterol, especially for those with central obesity. Improvements in physical capabilities and quality of life become evident with even a 5 percent weight loss.[64] For these reasons, parameters such as blood pressure, blood cholesterol, or even vitality are more useful than body weight in marking success. People less concerned with disease risks may prefer to set goals for personal fitness, such as being able to play with children or climb stairs without becoming short of breath. Importantly, they can focus on healthy eating and activity habits instead of weight loss.

Depending on initial body weight, a reasonable rate of loss for overweight adults is ½ to 2 pounds a week, or 5 to 10 percent of body weight over 6 months. For a person weighing 250 pounds, a 10 percent loss is 25 pounds, or about 1 pound a week for 6 months. Such gradual weight losses are more likely to be maintained than rapid losses. Keep in mind that pursuing good health is a lifelong journey. Most adults are keenly aware of their body weights and shapes and realize that what they eat and what they do can make a difference to some extent. Those who are most successful at weight management seem to have fully incorporated healthful eating and physical activity into their daily lives.

Eating Patterns Contrary to the claims of fad diets, no single food plan is magical, and no specific food must be included or avoided in a weight-management program. In designing an eating pattern, people need only consider foods that they like or can learn to like, that are available, and that are within their means. Creating a healthful eating pattern is the first step. The important next step is following it for the rest of one's life. Achieving and maintaining a healthy weight requires permanent lifestyle changes.

Be Realistic about Energy Intake The main characteristic of a weight-loss diet is that it provides less energy than the person needs to maintain present body weight. If food energy is restricted too severely, dieters may not receive sufficient nutrients. Rapid weight loss usually means excessive loss of lean tissue, a lower BMR, and rapid weight regains to follow. The composition of regained weight is more fat and less lean than the composition of the originally lost weight.[65] In addition, restrictive eating may create stress or foster unhealthy behaviors of eating disorders as described in Highlight 8.[66]

Energy intake should provide nutritional adequacy without excess—that is, somewhere between deprivation and complete freedom to eat whatever, whenever. A reasonable suggestion for overweight and obese adults is to increase activity and reduce food intake enough to create a deficit of 500 to 750 kcalories per day. Such a deficit produces a weight loss of 1 to 2 pounds per week—a rate that supports the loss of fat efficiently while retaining lean tissue.[67] In general, weight-loss diets need to provide about 1200 to 1500 kcalories per day for women and 1500 to 1800 kcalories a day for men.

Some people skip meals, typically breakfast, in an effort to reduce energy intake and lose weight. Research does not support such a causal relationship between breakfast and body weight, but it does suggest some interesting associations.[68] Breakfast frequency is inversely associated with obesity and its associated risk factors—that is, people who frequently eat breakfast have a lower BMI, blood pressure, and blood cholesterol than those who tend to skip breakfast.[69] Furthermore, eating breakfast, especially a protein-rich breakfast, improves satiety and diet quality—two factors that support healthy body weight.[70] One study found that even when total kcalories were the same on two weight-loss diets, the "breakfast diet" (big breakfast, medium lunch, and small dinner) had better results than the "dinner diet" (small breakfast, medium lunch, and big dinner).[71] After three months, the women on the breakfast diet lost 10 more pounds than the others; had better triglycerides, HDL, blood glucose, and waist circumference measures; and were less hungry.

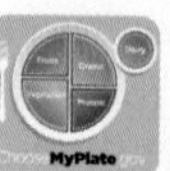

> DIETARY GUIDELINES FOR AMERICANS

Control total kcalorie intake to manage body weight. For people who are overweight or obese, this will mean consuming fewer kcalories from foods and beverages.

Emphasize Nutritional Adequacy Healthy diet plans make nutritional adequacy a priority. Nutritional adequacy is difficult to achieve on fewer than 1200 kcalories a day, and most healthy adults need never consume any less. A plan that provides an adequate intake supports a healthier and more successful weight loss than a restrictive plan that creates feelings of starvation and deprivation, which can lead to an irresistible urge to binge.

Table 9-2 specifies the amounts of foods from each food group for diets providing 1200 to 1800 kcalories. Such an intake would allow most people to lose weight and still meet their nutrient needs with careful, low-kcalorie, nutrient-dense food selections. Keep in mind, too, that well-balanced diets that emphasize fruits, vegetables, whole grains, lean protein foods, and low-fat milk products offer many health rewards even when they don't result in weight loss. A dietary supplement providing vitamins and minerals—especially iron and calcium for women—at or below 100 percent of the Daily Values can help people following low-kcalorie diets to achieve nutrient adequacy.

Eat Small Portions As mentioned earlier, portion sizes at markets, at restaurants, and even at home have increased dramatically over the years, contributing significantly to energy intake and weight gains.[72] We have come to expect large portions, and we have learned to clean our plates. Many of us pay more attention to these external cues defining how much to eat than to our internal cues of hunger and satiety. For health's sake, we may need to learn to eat less food at each meal—one piece of chicken for dinner instead of two, a teaspoon of butter on vegetables instead of a tablespoon, and one cookie for dessert instead of six. The goal is to eat enough food for adequate energy, abundant vitamins and minerals, and some pleasure, but not more. This amount should leave a person feeling satisfied—not stuffed. A saying credited to Confucius captures this concept—hara hachi bu—which translates to "eat until you are 80 percent full."

TABLE 9-2 Daily Amounts from Each Food Group for 1200- to 1800-kCalorie Diets

Food Group	1200 kCalories	1400 kCalories	1600 kCalories	1800 kCalories
Fruit	1 c	1½ c	1½ c	1½ c
Vegetables	1½ c	1½ c	2 c	2½ c
Grains	4 oz	5 oz	5 oz	6 oz
Protein foods	3 oz	4 oz	5 oz	5 oz
Milk and milk products	2½ c	2½ c	3 c	3 c
Oils	4 tsp	4 tsp	5 tsp	5 tsp

Keep in mind that even fat-free and low-fat foods can deliver a lot of kcalories when a person eats large quantities. A low-fat cookie or two can be a sweet treat even on a weight-loss diet, but larger portions defeat the savings.

People who have difficulty making low-kcalorie selections or controlling portion sizes may find it easier to use prepared meal plans. Prepared meals that provide low-kcalorie, nutritious meals or snacks can support weight loss while easing the task of diet planning.[73] Ideally, those using a prepared meal plan will also receive counsel from a registered dietitian nutritionist to learn how to select appropriately from conventional food choices as well.

Slow Down Eating can be a pleasurable experience, and taking the time to savor the flavors can help with weight management. Eating slowly, taking small bites, and chewing thoroughly all help to decrease food intake.[74] A person who slows down and savors each bite eats less before hormones signal satiety and the end of a meal.[75] Consequently, energy intake is lower when meals are eaten slowly. Savoring each bite also activates the pleasure centers of the brain. Some research suggests that people may overeat when the brain doesn't sense enough gratification from food. Faster eating correlates with higher BMI.[76]

Lower Energy Density Most people take their cues about how much to eat based on portion sizes, and the larger the portion size, the more they eat. To lower energy intake, a person can either reduce the portion size or reduce the energy density. Reducing energy density while maintaining or even increasing food quantity, especially by reducing fat and including fruits and vegetables, seems to be a successful strategy to control hunger and manage weight.[77] This concept of using large quantities of low-energy-density foods is sometimes referred to as *volumetrics*. Figure 9-6 illustrates how water, fiber, and fat influence energy density, and the accompanying "How To" feature (p. 280) compares foods based on their energy density. Foods containing water, those rich in fiber, and those low in fat help to lower energy density, providing more satiety for fewer kcalories. Because a low-energy-density diet is a low-fat, high-fiber diet rich in many vitamins and minerals, it supports good health in addition to weight loss.

Remember Water In addition to lowering the energy density of foods, water seems to help those who are trying to lose or maintain weight.[78] For one, foods with high water content (such as broth-based soups) increase fullness, reduce hunger, and consequently reduce energy intake. For another, drinking a large glass of water before a meal eases hunger, fills the stomach, and consequently reduces energy intake.[79] Importantly, water adds no kcalories. The average US diet delivers an estimated 75 to 150 kcalories a day from sweetened beverages. Simply replacing nutrient-poor, energy-dense beverages with water can help a person achieve a 5 percent weight loss at 6 months.[80] Water also helps the GI tract adapt to a high-fiber diet.

> FIGURE 9-6 Energy Density

Decreasing the energy density (kcal/g) of foods allows a person to eat satisfying portions while still reducing energy intake. To lower energy density, select foods high in water or fiber and low in fat.

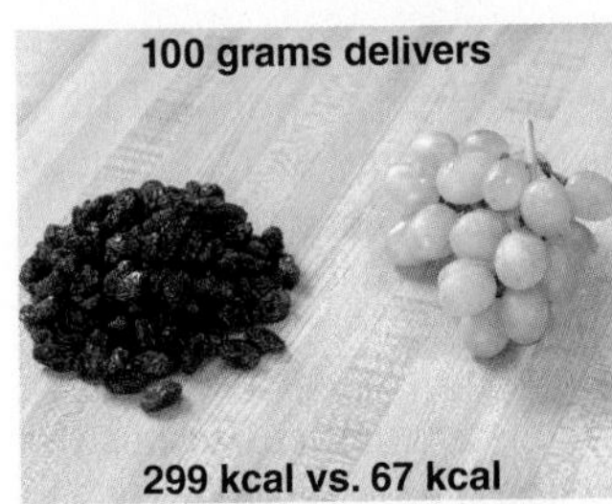

Selecting grapes with their high water content instead of raisins increases the volume and cuts the energy intake.

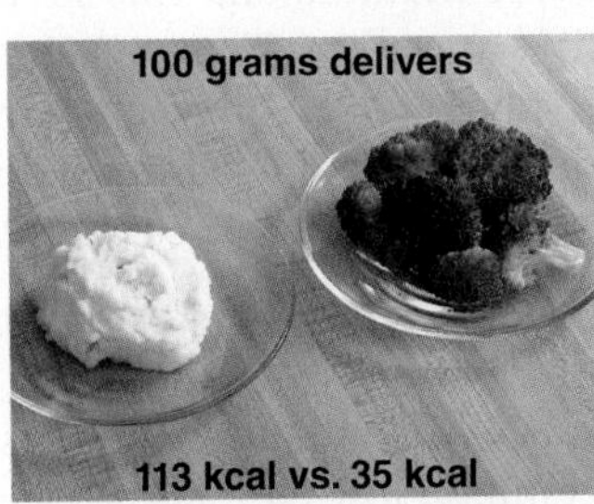

Even at the same weight and similar serving sizes, the fiber-rich broccoli delivers twice the fiber for about one-third the energy.

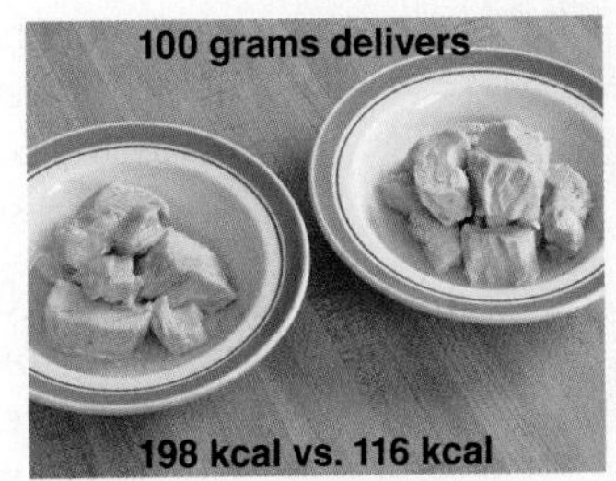

By selecting the water-packed tuna (on the right) instead of the oil-packed tuna (on the left), a person can enjoy the same amount for fewer kcalories.

>How To

Compare Foods Based on Energy Density

Chapter 2 describes how to evaluate foods based on their nutrient density—their nutrient contribution per kcalorie. Another way to evaluate foods is to consider their energy density—their energy contribution per gram. This example compares carrot sticks with french fries. The conclusion is no surprise, but understanding the mathematics may offer valuable insight into the concept of energy density. A carrot weighing 72 grams delivers 31 kcalories. To calculate the energy density, divide kcalories by grams:

$$\frac{31 \text{ kcal}}{72 \text{ g}} = 0.43 \text{ kcal/g}$$

Do the same for french fries weighing 50 grams and contributing 167 kcalories:

$$\frac{167 \text{ kcal}}{50 \text{ g}} = 3.34 \text{ kcal/g}$$

The more kcalories per gram, the greater the energy density. French fries are more energy dense than carrots. They provide more energy per gram—and per bite. Considering a food's energy density is especially useful in planning diets for weight management. Foods with a high energy density help with weight gain, whereas foods with a low energy density help with weight loss.

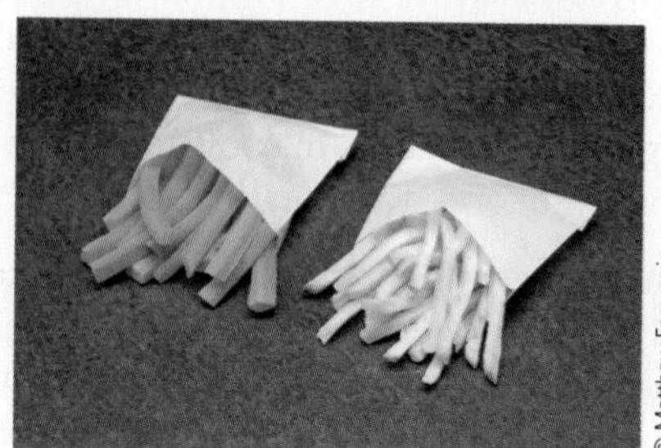
© Matthew Farruggio

> TRY IT Compare the energy density of a hard-boiled egg (50 grams and 78 kcalories) with light tuna canned in water (57 grams and 66 kcalories).

Focus on Fiber High-fiber foods such as fresh fruits, vegetables, legumes, and whole grains may help with weight management. By offering abundant vitamins, minerals, and fiber but little fat, these foods tend to be relatively low in energy and high in nutrients. Eating high-fiber foods also takes time, which eases hunger and promotes satiety.

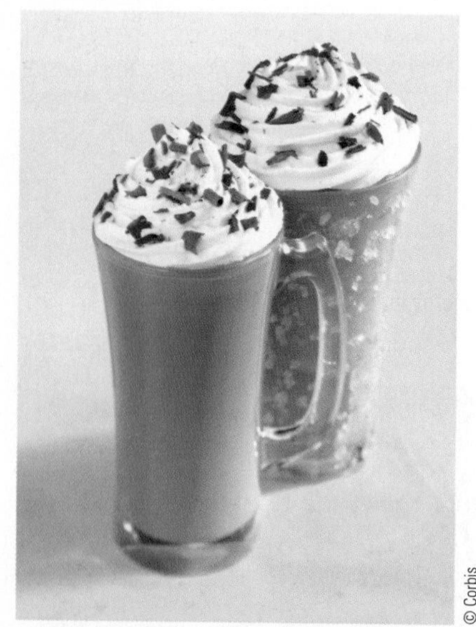
© Corbis

If you want to lose weight, steer clear of the empty kcalories in fancy coffee drinks. A 16-ounce caffè mocha delivers 400 kcalories—half of them from fat and the other half from sugar.

Choose Fats Sensibly One way to lower energy intake is to lower fat intake. Lowering the fat content of a food lowers its energy density—for example, selecting fat-free milk instead of whole milk. That way, a person can consume the usual amount (say, a cup of milk) at a lower energy intake (85 instead of 150 kcalories).

Fat has a weak satiating effect, and satiation plays a key role in determining food intake during a meal. Consequently, a person eating a high-fat meal increases energy intake in two ways—more food and more fat kcalories. For these reasons, measure fat with extra caution. (Review p. 157 for strategies to lower fat in the diet.) Be careful not to take this advice to extremes, however; too little fat incurs health risks as well, as Chapter 5 explains.

Lowering the amount of fat in the diet can lead to weight loss, but an important point to notice in any discussion on weight-loss diets is total energy intake.[81] A low-fat diet supports weight loss only when energy intake is less than energy expenditure.

Select Carbohydrates Carefully Another popular way to lower energy intake is to lower carbohydrate intake. Highlight 4's discussion of carbohydrate-restricted and carbohydrate-modified diets reaches the same conclusion as the previous paragraph on low-fat diets: they work only when energy intake is less than energy expenditure.

Chapter 4 describes how foods with added sugars increase energy intake and contribute to weight gain. Limiting consumption of foods with added sugars can help with weight management. One way people try to control weight is to use foods and beverages sweetened with artificial sweeteners. Using artificial sweeteners instead of sugars can lower energy intake and may support modest weight loss, or at least prevent weight gain, although evidence is inconsistent; in fact, some research indicates that artificial sweeteners may stimulate appetite and lead to weight gain.[82] One study offers a possible explanation. People who regularly drink diet sodas have decreased activity in the brain center that signals reward and controls food intake.[83] Such an alteration makes it more likely that these people would eat more later in the day.

To what extent artificial sweeteners can help someone lose weight depends in part on the person's motivations and actions. For example, one person might drink an artificially sweetened beverage now so as to be able to eat a high-kcalorie food later. This person's energy intake might stay the same or increase. A person trying to control energy intake might drink an artificially sweetened beverage now and choose a low-kcalorie food later. This plan would help reduce the person's total energy intake. Using artificial sweeteners will not automatically lower energy intake. To control energy intake successfully, a person needs to make informed diet and activity decisions throughout the day.

Watch for Other Empty kCalories A person trying to achieve or maintain a healthy weight needs to pay attention not only to fat and sugar, but to alcohol too. Not only does alcohol add kcalories, but accompanying mixers can also add both kcalories and fat, especially in creamy drinks such as piña coladas (review Table H7-3 on p. 229). Furthermore, drinking alcohol reduces a person's inhibitions, which can lead to excessive eating.[84]

A person who adopts a lifelong "eating plan for good health" rather than a "diet for weight loss" will be more likely to keep the lost weight off. Table 9-3 provides several tips for successful weight management.

Physical Activity

Whether trying to minimize weight gains or support weight losses, the best approach includes physical activity.[85] To prevent weight gains and support weight losses, current recommendations advise 200 to 300 minutes of moderately intense physical activity a week in addition to activities of daily life.[86] People who combine diet and exercise typically lose more fat, retain more muscle, and regain less weight than those who only follow a weight-loss diet. Even when they do not lose more weight, they seem to follow their diet plans more closely and maintain their losses better than those who do not exercise. Consequently, they benefit from taking in a little less energy from the diet

TABLE 9-3 Weight-Loss Strategies

Food	Activities
• To maintain weight, consume foods and drinks to meet, not exceed, kcalorie needs. To lose weight, energy out should exceed energy in by about 500 kcalories/day. • Emphasize foods with a low energy density and a high nutrient density; make legumes, whole grains, vegetables, and fruits central to your diet plan. • Eat slowly. • Drink water before you eat and while you eat; drink plenty of water throughout the day. • Track food and kcalorie intake. • Plan ahead to make better food choices. • Limit kcalorie intake from solid fats and added sugars. • Reduce portions, especially of high-kcalorie foods. • Cook and eat more meals at home, instead of eating out. When eating out, think about choosing healthy options.	• Limit screen time. • Choose moderate- or vigorous-intensity physical activities. • Avoid inactivity. Some physical activity is better than none. • Gradually increase the frequency, intensity, and duration of physical activities.

as well as from expending a little more energy in physical activity. Importantly, those who exercise reap important health benefits—reduced abdominal obesity and improved blood pressure, insulin resistance, and cardiorespiratory fitness—regardless of weight loss.[87] Fitness benefits—such as strength and balance—also improve when exercise is part of a weight-loss program.[88] Chapter 14 presents the many benefits of physical activity; the focus here is on its role in weight management.

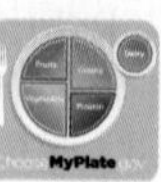

> **DIETARY GUIDELINES FOR AMERICANS**
> Increase physical activity and reduce time spent in sedentary behaviors.

Activity and Energy Expenditure Table 8-3 (p. 242) shows how much energy each of several activities uses. The number of kcalories spent in an activity depends on body weight, intensity, and duration. For example, a person who weighs 150 pounds and walks 3½ miles in 60 minutes expends about 315 kcalories. That same person running 3 miles in 30 minutes uses a similar amount. By comparison, a 200-pound person running 3 miles in 30 minutes expends an additional 100 kcalories or so. The goal is to expend as much energy as your time allows. The greater the energy deficit created by exercise, the greater the fat loss. And be careful not to compensate for the energy expended in exercise by eating more food.[89] Otherwise, energy balance won't shift, and fat loss will be less significant.

Activity and Discretionary kCalories Chapter 2 introduced the concept of discretionary kcalories as the difference between the kcalories needed to supply nutrients and those needed to maintain energy balance. Because exercise expends energy, the energy allowance to maintain weight increases with increased physical activity—yet the energy needed to deliver needed nutrients remains about the same. In this way, physical activity increases discretionary kcalories (see Figure 9-7). Having more discretionary kcalories puts a little wiggle room in a weight-loss diet for such options as second helpings, sweet treats, or alcoholic beverages on occasion. Of course, selecting nutrient-dense foods and *not* using discretionary kcalories will maximize weight loss.

Activity and Metabolism Activity also contributes to energy expenditure in an indirect way—by speeding up metabolism. It does this both immediately and over the long term. On any given day, metabolism remains elevated for several hours after vigorous and prolonged exercise.[90] This postexercise effect may raise the energy expenditure of exercise up to 15 percent. Over the long term, a person who engages in daily vigorous activity gradually develops more lean tissue. Metabolic rate rises accordingly, and this supports continued weight loss or maintenance.

> FIGURE 9-7 **Influence of Physical Activity on Discretionary kCalories**

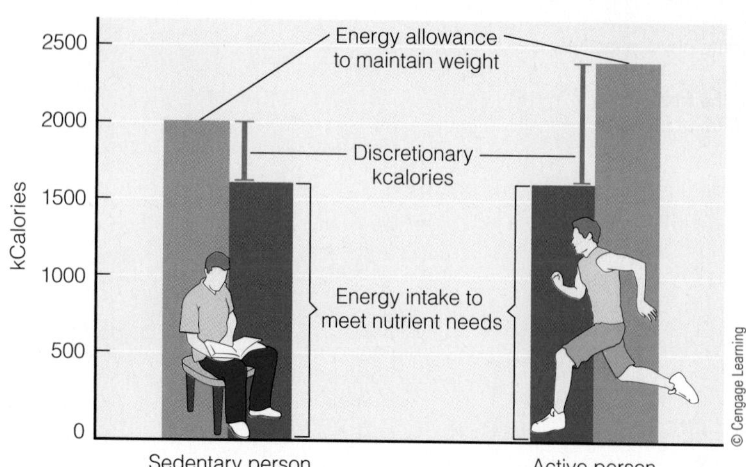

Activity and Body Composition Physically active people have less body fat than sedentary people do—even if they have the same BMI. Physical activity, even without weight loss, changes body composition: body fat decreases and lean body mass increases; high-intensity intermittent exercises may be even more effective at reducing body fat than other types of exercise.[91] Furthermore, physical activity reduces abdominal fat even without weight loss.[92]

Activity and Appetite Control Some people think that being active will increase hunger, but research does not show that exercise causes overeating; in fact, when sedentary people participate in an ongoing activity program, they reduce their energy intake.[93] Active people do have healthy appetites, but appetite is suppressed after an aerobic workout.[94] The body has released fuels from storage to support the exercise, so glucose and fatty acids are abundant in the blood. At the same time, the body has suppressed its digestive functions. Hard physical work and eating are not compatible. A person must calm down, put energy fuels back in storage, and relax before eating. At that time, a physically active person may eat more than a sedentary person, but not so much as to fully compensate for the energy expended in exercise.

Exercise may also help curb the inappropriate appetite that accompanies boredom, anxiety, or depression. Weight-management programs encourage people who feel the urge to eat when not particularly hungry to exercise instead. The activity passes time, relieves anxiety, and prevents inappropriate eating.

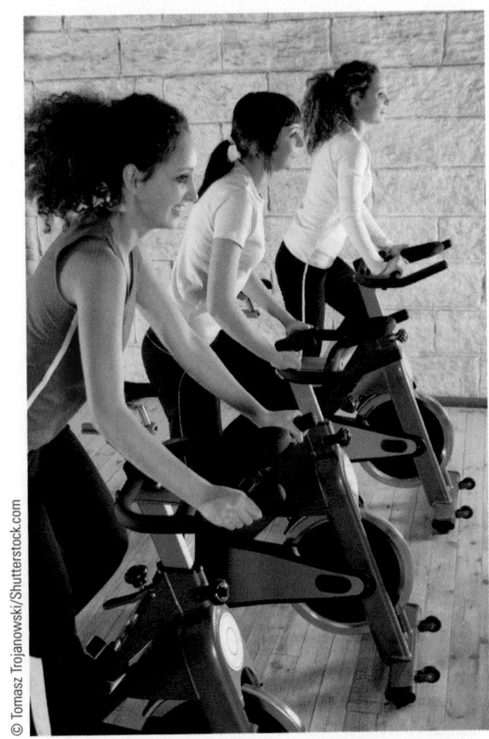
© Tomasz Trojanowski/Shutterstock.com

The key to good health is to combine sensible eating with regular exercise.

Activity and Psychological Benefits Activity also helps reduce stress, which is especially helpful for people who respond to stress with inappropriate eating. In addition, physical activity helps to improve body image and separate the connections between body weight and self-worth.[95] A physically active person begins to look and feel healthy and, as a result, gains self-esteem. High self-esteem motivates a person to continue seeking good health and fitness, which keeps the beneficial cycle going. The benefits of physical activity in a weight-management program include:

- Short-term increase in energy expenditure (from exercise and from a slight rise in metabolism)
- Long-term increase in BMR (from an increase in lean tissue)
- Improved body composition
- Appetite control
- Stress reduction and control of stress eating
- Physical, and therefore psychological, well-being
- Improved self-esteem

Chapter 14 presents additional benefits of physical activity.

Choosing Activities Clearly, physical activity is a plus in a weight-management program. What kind of physical activity is best? People should choose activities that they enjoy and are willing to do regularly. What schedule of physical activity is best? It doesn't matter; a person can benefit from either several short bouts of exercise or one continuous workout. Any activity is better than being sedentary. For an active life, limit sedentary activities, engage in strength and flexibility activities, enjoy leisure activities often, engage in vigorous activities regularly, and be as active as possible every day.

Health-care professionals frequently advise people to engage in activities of low-to-moderate intensity for a long duration, such as an hour-long, fast-paced walk. The reasoning behind such advice is that walking offers the health benefits of aerobic physical activity with low risk of injury. It can be done almost anywhere at any time. A person who stays with an activity routine long enough to enjoy the rewards will be less inclined to give it up and will, over the long term, reap many health benefits. A regular walking program can prevent or slow the weight gain that commonly occurs in most adults. An average of 60 minutes a day of moderate-intensity activity or an expenditure of at least 2000 kcalories per week is especially helpful for weight management.[96] Higher levels of duration, frequency, or intensity produce greater losses.

In addition to exercise, a person can incorporate hundreds of energy-expending activities into daily routines: take the stairs instead of the elevator, walk to the neighbor's apartment instead of making a phone call, and rake the leaves instead of using a blower. Remember that sitting uses more kcalories than lying down, standing uses more kcalories than sitting, and moving uses more kcalories than standing. A 175-pound person who replaces a 30-minute television program with a 2-mile walk a day can expend enough energy to lose (or at least not gain) 18 pounds in a year. Even walking in place during the commercials of a one-hour program can increase activity time by 25 minutes, steps taken by 2100, and kcalories expended by 150.[97] Meeting an activity goal of 10,000 steps a day is an excellent way to support a healthy BMI. By wearing a pedometer, a person can easily increase physical activity, lose weight, and lower blood pressure without measuring miles or watching the clock. The point is to be active. Walk. Run. Swim. Dance. Cycle. Climb. Skip. Do whatever you enjoy doing—and do it often.

Spot Reducing People sometimes ask about "spot reducing." Unfortunately, muscles do not "own" the fat that surrounds them. Fat cells all over the body release fat in response to the demand of physical activity for use by whatever muscles are active. Specific exercises—whether moderate or intense—do not influence the site of adipose tissue loss.

Exercise can help with trouble spots in another way, though. The "trouble spot" for most men is the abdomen, their primary site of fat storage. During aerobic exercise, abdominal fat readily releases its stores, providing fuel to the physically active body. With regular exercise and weight loss, men will deplete these abdominal fat stores before those in the lower body. Women may also deplete abdominal fat with exercise, but their "trouble spots" are more likely to be their hips and thighs.

In addition to aerobic activity, strength training can help to improve the tone of muscles in a trouble area, and stretching to gain flexibility can help with associated posture problems. A combination of aerobic, strength, and flexibility workouts best improves fitness and physical appearance.

Environmental Influences Chapter 8 describes how hormones regulate hunger, satiety, and satiation, but people don't always pay close attention to such internal signals. Instead, their eating behaviors are often dictated by environmental factors—those surrounding the eating experience as well as those pertaining to the food itself. Changing any of these factors can influence how much a person eats.

Atmosphere The environment surrounding a meal or snack influences its duration. When the lighting, décor, aromas, and sounds of an environment are pleasant and comfortable, people tend to spend more time eating and thus eat more. A person needn't eat under neon lights with offensive music to eat less, of course. Instead, after completing a meal, remove food from the table and enjoy the ambience—without the presence of visual cues to stimulate additional eating.

Accessibility Among the strongest influences on how much we eat are the accessibility, ease, and convenience of obtaining food. In general, the less effort needed to obtain food, the more likely food will be eaten. Think about it. Are you more likely to eat if half a leftover pizza is in your refrigerator or if you have to drive to the grocery store, buy a frozen pizza, and bake it for 45 minutes? Similarly you are more likely to reach for a second helping of potatoes or another piece of chicken if they are on the dining table in front of you than if the leftovers have already been wrapped and refrigerated. Having food nearby and visible encourages eating—regardless of hunger. The message is clear. For people wanting to eat fewer empty-kcalorie or high-kcalorie foods, keep them out of sight in an inconvenient place, or better yet, don't even bring them home. In contrast, a bowl of fruit on the counter and vegetables in the refrigerator promote healthy eating options.

Socializing People tend to eat more when socializing with others. Pleasant conversations extend the duration of a meal, allowing a person more time to eat more, and the longer the meal, the greater the consumption. In addition, by taking a visual cue from companions, a person might eat more when others at the table eat large portions or go to the buffet line for seconds.[98] One way to eat less is to pace yourself with the person who seems to be eating the least and slowest.

Social interactions also distract a person from paying attention to how much has been eaten. In some cases, socializing with friends during a meal may provide comfort and lower a person's motivation to limit consumption. In other cases, socializing with unfamiliar people during a meal—during a job interview or blind date, for example—may create stress and reduce food consumption. To eat less while socializing, pay attention to portion size.

Distractions Distractions influence food intake by initiating eating, interfering with internal controls to stop eating, and extending the duration of eating. Some people start eating dinner when a favorite television program comes on, regardless of hunger. Other people continue eating breakfast until they finish reading the newspaper. Such mindless eating can easily become overeating. Distractions interfere with a person's ability to perceive and regulate how much is consumed. Not only do people tend to eat more and feel less full after eating a meal while distracted, they tend to eat more at the next meal.[99] If distractions are a part of the eating experience, extra care is needed to control portion sizes.

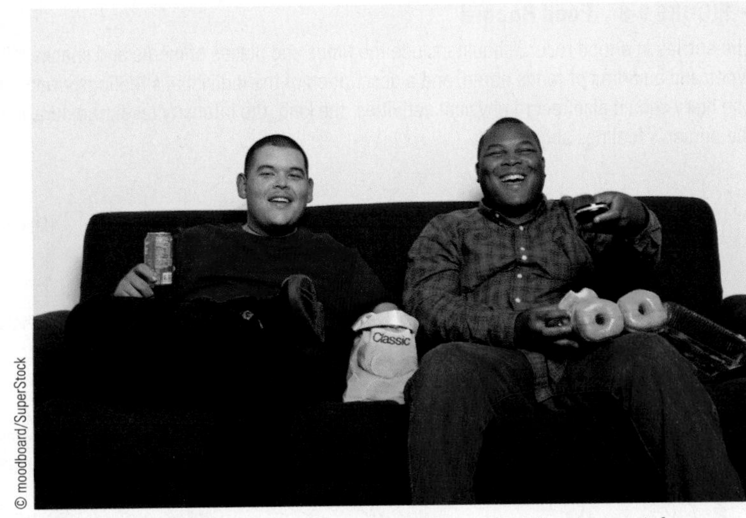

Eating from the package while distracted by television is a weight-gaining combination.

Multiple Choices When offered a large assortment of foods, or several flavors of the same food, people tend to eat more. To limit intake, then, focus on a limited number of foods per meal; eating the same meal everyday tends to lower energy intake.[100] Be careful not to misunderstand and abandon variety in diet planning. Eating a variety of nutrient-dense foods from each of the food groups is still a healthy plan.

Package and Portion Sizes As noted earlier, the sizes of packages in grocery stores as well as portion sizes at restaurants and at home have increased dramatically in recent decades, contributing to the increase in obesity in the United States. Put simply, we tend to clean our plates and finish the package. The larger the bag of potato chips, the greater the intake. To keep from overeating, repackage snacks into smaller containers or eat a measured portion from a plate, not directly from the package.

Serving Containers We often use plates, utensils, and glasses as visual cues to guide our decisions on how much to eat and drink. If you plan to eat a bowl of ice cream, it matters whether the bowl you select holds 8 ounces or 24 ounces. Large dinner plates and wide glasses create illusions and misperceptions about quantities consumed. A scoop of mashed potatoes on a small plate looks larger than the same-size scoop on a large plate, leading a person to underestimate the amount of food eaten. To control portion sizes, use small bowls and plates, small serving spoons, and tall, narrow glasses. Of course, using a small plate will not result in less food eaten if multiple servings are taken.

Behavior and Attitude

Changes in behavior and attitude can be very effective in supporting efforts to achieve and maintain appropriate body weight and composition. **Behavior modification** focuses on how to change behaviors to increase energy expenditure and decrease energy intake. A person must commit to taking action. Adopting a positive, matter-of-fact attitude helps to ensure success. Healthy eating and activity choices are an essential part of healthy living and should simply be incorporated into the day—much like brushing one's teeth or wearing a safety belt.

Become Aware of Behaviors To solve a problem, a person must first identify all the behaviors that created the problem. Keeping a record will help to identify eating and exercise behaviors that may need changing (see Figure 9-8, p. 286). Such self-monitoring raises awareness, establishes a baseline against which to measure future progress, and improves compliance.[101]

In this era of technology, many companies have developed weight-loss applications for smartphones to help users manage their daily food and physical activity behaviors.* Applications include diet analysis tools that can track eating habits, scanning devices that can quickly enter food data, customized activity and meal

behavior modification: the changing of behavior by the manipulation of antecedents (cues or environmental factors that trigger behavior), the behavior itself, and consequences (the penalties or rewards attached to behavior).

*Reliable reviews of food and nutrition apps are available at www.eatright.org/appreviews.

> FIGURE 9-8 Food Record

The entries in a food record should include the times and places of meals and snacks, the types and amounts of foods eaten, and a description of the individual's feelings when eating. The diary should also record physical activities: the kind, the intensity level, the duration, and the person's feelings about them.

Time	Place	Activity or food eaten	People present	Mood
10:30–10:40	School vending machine	6 peanut butter crackers and 12 oz. cola	by myself	starved
12:15–12:30	Restaurant	Sub sandwich and 12 oz. cola	friends	relaxed & friendly
3:00–3:45	Gym	Weight training	work out partner	tired
4:00–4:10	Snack bar	Small frozen yogurt	by myself	OK

plans that can be sent to users, and support programs that deliver encouraging messages and helpful tips. Social media sites allow users to upload progress reports and receive texts. Using these applications can help a person become more aware of behaviors that lead to weight gains and losses.[102]

Change Behaviors Behavior modification strategies focus on learning desired eating and activity behaviors and eliminating unwanted behaviors. Examples include not grocery shopping when hungry and exercising when watching television. With so many possible behavior changes, a person can feel overwhelmed. Start with small time-specific goals for each behavior—for example, "I'm going to take a 30-minute walk after dinner every evening" instead of "I'm going to run in a marathon someday." Practice desired behaviors until they become routine. Addressing multiple behaviors that focus on a common goal simultaneously may better support changes than taking on one at a time. Using a reward system also seems to effectively support weight-loss efforts.

Cognitive Skills Successful behavior changes depend in part on two cognitive skills—problem solving and cognitive restructuring. Problem-solving skills enable a person to identify the problem, generate potential solutions, list the pros and cons of each, implement the most feasible solution, and evaluate whether behaviors should be continued or abandoned. Cognitive restructuring requires a person to replace negative thoughts that derail success with positive thoughts that support behavior change. In general, people who believe they can complete tasks and reach goals are more likely to follow a diet plan and achieve success than those lacking that confidence.[103] Cognitive behavioral treatment for weight loss can be most effective in helping families work together to reduce energy intake and increase physical activity.[104]

The effectiveness of cognitive behavioral treatment in weight-loss extends to other health behaviors as well. Overweight smokers who participate in a cognitive program for weight management lose weight, make healthy food choices, increase their confidence in managing their eating and smoking habits, decrease the number of cigarettes smoked, and increase their readiness to quit smoking. Such findings highlight the need to include dietary strategies in smoking cessation programs. Smoking a cigarette overrides feelings of hunger. When smokers receive a hunger signal, they can quiet it with cigarettes instead of food. Such behavior ignores body signals and postpones energy and nutrient intake. Indeed, smokers tend to weigh less than nonsmokers and to gain weight when they stop smoking. People contemplating giving up cigarettes should know that the average weight gain is about 10 pounds in the first year. Smokers wanting to quit should prepare for the possibility of weight gain and adjust their diet and activity habits so as to maintain weight during and after quitting.

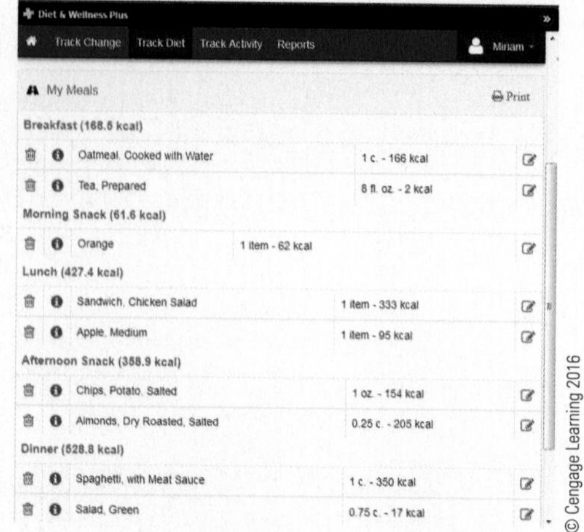

Diet analysis programs help people identify high-kcalorie foods and monitor their eating habits.

Personal Attitude For many people, overeating and being overweight have become an integral part of their identity. Those who fully understand their personal relationships with food are best prepared to make healthful changes in eating and activity behaviors.

Sometimes habitual behaviors that are hazardous to health, such as smoking or drinking alcohol, contribute positively by helping people adapt to stressful situations. Similarly, many people overeat to cope with the stresses of life. Weight gains, in turn, contribute to psychosocial stress, thus creating an unhealthy cycle.

To break out of that pattern, they must first identify the particular stressors that trigger the urge to overeat. Then, when faced with these situations, they must learn and practice problem-solving skills that will help them to respond appropriately. Learning to reduce episodes of emotional eating can help lead to weight loss.

All this is not to imply that psychotherapy holds the magic answer to a weight problem. Still, efforts to improve one's general well-being may result in healthy eating and activity habits even when weight loss is not the primary goal. When the problems that trigger the urge to overeat are resolved in alternative ways, people may find they eat less. They may begin to respond appropriately to internal cues of hunger rather than inappropriately to external cues of stress. Sound emotional health supports a person's ability to take care of physical health in all ways—including nutrition, weight management, and fitness.

Support Groups Group support can prove helpful when making life changes. Some people find it useful to join a group such as Take Off Pounds Sensibly (TOPS), Weight Watchers (WW), Overeaters Anonymous (OA), or others. Some dieters prefer to form their own self-help groups or find support online. The Internet offers numerous opportunities for weight-loss education and counseling that may be effective alternatives to face-to-face or telephone counseling programs.[105] As always, consumers need to choose wisely and avoid rip-offs.

Weight Maintenance The prevalence of **successful weight-loss maintenance** is difficult to determine, in part because researchers have used different criteria. Some look at success after 1 year and others after 5 years; some quantify success as 10 or more pounds lost and others as 5 or 10 percent of initial body weight lost. Furthermore, most research studies examine the success of one episode of weight loss in a structured program, but this scenario does not necessarily reflect the experiences of the general population. In reality, most people have lost weight several times in their lifetimes and did so on their own, not in a formal program. An estimated one out of every six overweight adults in the United States has successfully maintained at least a 10 percent loss for at least a year.[106]

Those who are successful in maintaining their weight loss have established regular exercise regimens and careful eating patterns, taking in less energy than the national average. Because formerly overweight people are more efficient at

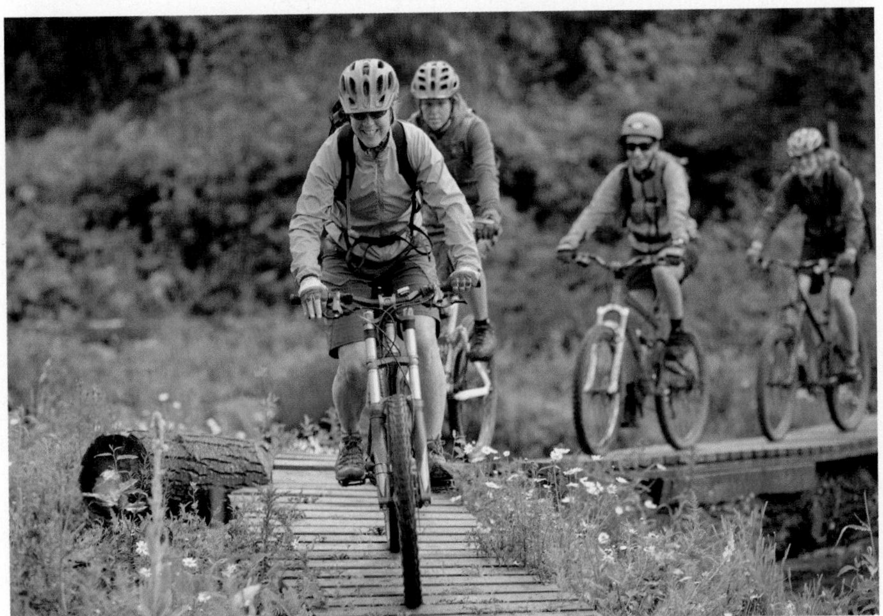

Maintaining a healthy body weight requires maintaining the vigorous physical activities and careful eating habits that supported weight loss.

successful weight-loss maintenance: achieving a weight loss of at least 5 to 10 percent of initial body weight and maintaining the loss for at least 1 year.

storing fat, they do not have the same flexibility in their food and activity habits as their friends who have never been overweight. With weight loss, hormones involved in appetite regulation shift in a way that encourages weight gain, and metabolism shifts downward so that formerly overweight people require less energy than might be expected given their current body weight and body composition.[107] These hormonal and metabolic changes persist over time.[108] Consequently, to keep weight off, they must either eat less or exercise more than people the same size who have never been obese. Put simply, it takes more effort to prevent weight regain than to prevent weight gain.

Physical activity plays a key role in preventing weight gains and maintaining weight losses.[109] Those who consistently exercise are far more successful than those who are inactive. Weight maintenance may require a person to expend at least 2500 kcalories in physical activity per week. To accomplish this, a person might exercise either moderately (such as brisk walking at 4 miles per hour) for 60 minutes a day or vigorously (such as fast bicycling at 18 miles per hour) for 30 minutes a day, for example. Being active during both work hours and leisure time also helps a person expend more energy and maintain weight loss.[110]

In addition to limiting energy intake and exercising regularly, one other strategy helps with weight maintenance: frequent self-monitoring. People who weigh themselves periodically and monitor their eating and exercise habits regularly can detect weight gains in the early stages and promptly initiate changes to prevent relapse.

Losing weight and maintaining the loss may not be easy, but it is possible. The National Weight Control Registry tracks over 10,000 individuals who have maintained a significant weight loss over time. Strategies of those who have been successful may differ in the details, but in general, most do the following:[111]

- Eat a low-kcalorie diet (usually small portions four to five times a day).
- Follow a diet that is high in nutrient density and low in energy density.
- Eat breakfast (curbs hunger).
- Engage in physical activity regularly (at least 60 minutes of moderate activity daily).
- Monitor weight frequently (at least weekly) and take prompt action with small gains.
- Use productive problem-solving skills and positive self-talk.
- Limit television time (less than 10 hours a week).
- Consult a registered dietitian nutritionist, physician, or other support person (or group).

Importantly, people who are successful losing weight find that it gets easier with time—the changes in diet and activity patterns become permanent.

Prevention Given the information presented up to this point in the chapter, the adage "An ounce of prevention is worth a pound of cure" seems particularly apropos. Obesity is a major risk factor for numerous diseases, and losing weight is challenging and often temporary. Many of the strategies for preventing weight gain are very similar to those for losing weight, with one exception: they begin early. Over the years, these strategies become an integral part of a person's life:

- Eat regular meals and limit snacking
- Drink water instead of high-kcalorie beverages
- Select sensible portion sizes and limit daily energy intake to no more than energy expended
- Become physically active and limit sedentary activities

It is much easier for a person to resist doughnuts for breakfast if he rarely eats them. Similarly, a person will have little trouble walking each morning if she has always been active.

TABLE 9-4 National Strategies to Prevent Obesity

- Provide a variety of opportunities to help make physical activity an integral and routine part of life.
- Create environments that ensure healthy foods and beverages are visible, attractive, and easy-to-obtain.
- Encourage media messages that promote physically active lifestyles and nutritionally healthy diets.
- Support health care providers in offering information on weight management and employers in offering wellness programs.
- Make schools centers for health and wellness.

SOURCE: *Accelerating Progress in Obesity Prevention: Solving the Weight of the Nation,* (Washington, DC: Institute of Medicine of the National Academies), 2012.

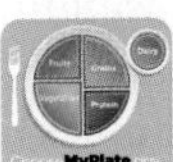

> DIETARY GUIDELINES FOR AMERICANS

Maintain appropriate kcalorie balance during each stage of life—childhood, adolescence, adulthood, pregnancy and lactation, and older age.

Community Programs Reversing the US obesity epidemic is a challenge in an environment of abundant food and physical inactivity. Success may depend on community actions to promote healthy lifestyle choices. Table 9-4 lists health strategies to speed the progress in obesity prevention in the United States.[112] Whether changes in public policy—such as providing pedestrian-friendly streets or taxing sugar-sweetened beverages and high-fat snacks—will influence activity or diet habits remains to be seen.[113] Clearly, effective strategies will need to reach beyond individuals to address social networks, community institutions, and government policies.

> REVIEW IT Outline reasonable strategies for achieving and maintaining a healthy body weight.

A surefire remedy for obesity has yet to be found, although many people find a combination of approaches to be most effective. Diet and exercise shift energy balance so that more energy is expended than is taken in. Behavior modification and cognitive restructuring retrain habits to support a healthy eating and activity plan. Such a plan requires time, individualization, and sometimes the assistance of a registered dietitian nutritionist or support group.

9.6 Underweight

> LEARN IT Summarize strategies for gaining weight.

Underweight is a far less prevalent problem than overweight, affecting no more than 2 percent of US adults (review Figure 8-7 on p. 247). Whether an underweight person needs to gain weight is a question of health and, like weight loss, a highly individual matter. There are no compelling reasons for people who are healthy at their present weight to try to gain weight. Those who are thin because of malnourishment or illness, however, might benefit from a diet that supports weight gain. Medical advice can help make the distinction.

Thin people may find gaining weight difficult. Unlike the genes expressed in obesity, the genes in lean people protect against energy excesses. Those who wish to gain weight for appearance's sake or to improve their athletic performance need to be aware that healthful weight gains can be achieved only by physical conditioning combined with high energy intakes. On a high-kcalorie diet alone, a person may gain weight, but it will be mostly fat. Even if the gain improves appearance, it can be detrimental to health and might impair athletic performance. Therefore, in weight gain, as in weight loss, physical activity and energy intake are essential components of a sound plan.

Problems of Underweight The causes of underweight may be as diverse as those of overweight—genetic tendencies; hunger, appetite, and satiety

underweight: body weight lower than the weight range that is considered healthy; BMI less than 18.5.

irregularities; psychological traits; and metabolic factors. Habits learned early in childhood, especially food aversions, may perpetuate themselves.

The high demand for energy to support physical activity and growth may contribute to underweight. An active, growing boy may need more than 4000 kcalories a day to maintain his weight and may be too busy to take time to eat adequately. In addition, underweight people may find it hard to gain weight because they are expending energy in adaptive thermogenesis. So much energy may be expended adapting to a higher food intake that at first as many as 750 to 800 extra kcalories a day may be needed to gain a pound a week. Like those who want to lose weight, people who want to gain must learn new habits and learn to like new foods. They are also similarly vulnerable to potentially harmful schemes.

As described in Highlight 8, the underweight condition anorexia nervosa sometimes develops in people who employ self-denial to control their weight. They go to such extremes that they become severely undernourished, achieving final body weights of 70 pounds or even less. One difference between a person with anorexia nervosa and other underweight people is that starvation is intentional. (See Highlight 8 for a review of anorexia nervosa and other eating disorders.)

Weight-Gain Strategies Adequacy and balance are the key diet-planning strategies for weight gain. Meals focus on energy-dense foods to provide many kcalories in a small volume and exercise to build muscle. By using the USDA Food Pattern recommendations for the higher kcalorie levels (see Table 2-3 on p. 43), a person can gain weight while meeting nutrient needs.

Energy-Dense Foods Energy-dense foods (the very ones eliminated from a successful weight-loss diet) hold the key to weight gain. Pick the highest-kcalorie items from each food group—that is, milk shakes instead of fat-free milk, salmon instead of snapper, avocados instead of cucumbers, a cup of grape juice instead of a small apple, and whole-wheat muffins instead of whole-wheat bread. Because fat provides more than twice as many kcalories per teaspoon as sugar does, fat adds kcalories without adding much bulk.

Although eating high-kcalorie, high-fat foods is not healthy for most people, it may be essential for an underweight individual who needs to gain weight. An underweight person who is physically active and eating a nutritionally adequate diet can afford a few extra kcalories from fat. For health's sake, it is wise to select foods with monounsaturated and polyunsaturated fats instead of those with saturated or *trans* fats: for example, sautéing vegetables in olive oil instead of butter or hydrogenated margarine.

Regular Meals Daily People who are underweight need to make meals a priority and take the time to plan, prepare, and eat each meal. They should eat at least three healthy meals every day. Another suggestion is to eat meaty appetizers or the main course first and leave the soup or salad until later.

Large Portions Underweight people need to learn to eat more food at each meal. For example, they can add extra slices of ham and cheese on a sandwich for lunch, drink milk from a larger glass, and eat cereal from a larger bowl.

The person should expect to feel full. Most underweight individuals are accustomed to small quantities of food. When they begin eating significantly more, they feel uncomfortable. This is normal and passes over time.

Extra Snacks Because a substantially higher energy intake is needed each day, in addition to eating more food at each meal, it is necessary to eat more frequently. Between-meal snacks can readily lead to weight gains. For example, a student might make three sandwiches in the morning and eat them between classes in addition to the day's three regular meals. Snacking on dried fruit, nuts, and seeds is also an easy way to add kcalories.

Juice and Milk Beverages provide an easy way to increase energy intake. Consider that 6 cups of cranberry juice add almost 1000 kcalories to the day's intake.

TABLE 9-5 Weight-Gain Strategies

- Energy in should exceed energy out by at least 500 kcalories/day. Eat enough to store more energy than you expend in exercise. Exercise and eat to build muscles.
- Expect weight gain to take time (1 pound per month would be reasonable).
- Emphasize energy-dense foods.
- Eat at least three meals a day.
- Eat large portions of foods and expect to feel full.
- Eat snacks between meals.
- Drink plenty of juice and milk.

kCalories can be added to milk by mixing in powdered milk or packets of instant breakfast.

For people who are underweight because of illness, liquid dietary supplements are often recommended because a weak person can swallow them easily. Used in addition to regular meals, these high-protein, high-kcalorie formulas can help an underweight person maintain or gain weight easily.

Exercising to Build Muscles To gain weight, use strength training primarily, and increase energy intake to support that exercise. Eating extra food to provide an additional 500 to 1000 kcalories a day above normal energy needs can support the exercise as well as build muscle.

› REVIEW IT Summarize strategies for gaining weight.

Both the incidence of underweight and the health problems associated with it are less prevalent than overweight and its associated problems. To gain weight, a person must train physically and increase energy intake by selecting energy-dense foods, eating regular meals, taking larger portions, and consuming extra snacks and beverages. Table 9-5 includes a summary of weight-gain strategies.

Achieving and maintaining a healthy weight requires vigilant attention to diet and physical activity. Taking care of oneself is a lifelong responsibility.

Nutrition Portfolio

To enjoy good health and maintain a reasonable body weight, combine sensible eating habits and regular physical activity. Go to Diet & Wellness Plus and choose one of the days on which you have tracked your diet for the entire day. Go to the Energy Balance and Intake vs. Goals reports.

- Calculate your BMI and consider whether you need to maintain, lose, or gain weight for the sake of good health. If you do need to gain or lose weight, do the Diet Analysis reports give you insight into why you may be overweight or underweight?
- Reflect on your weight over the past year or so and explain any weight gains or losses. Using the Intake vs. Goals report, can you identify areas in which you need to adjust your food intake, perhaps eating more or less?
- Describe the potential risks and possible benefits of fad diets and over-the-counter weight-loss drugs or herbal supplements.

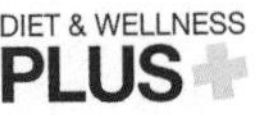

To complete this exercise, go to your Diet & Wellness Plus at **www.cengagebrain.com.**

› STUDY IT To review the key points of this chapter and take a practice quiz, go to the study cards at the end of the book.

REFERENCES

1. K. M. Flegal and coauthors, Prevalence of obesity and trends in the distribution of body mass index among US adults, 1999–2010, *Journal of the American Medical Association* 307 (2012): 491–497.
2. Centers for Disease Control and Prevention, Obesity and overweight, www.cdc.gov/nchs/fastats/overwt.htm, accessed November 2013.
3. C. L. Ogden and coauthors, Prevalence of obesity and trends in body mass index among US children and adolescents, 1999–2010, *Journal of the American Medical Association* 307 (2012): 483–490.
4. C. L. Ogden and coauthors, Prevalence of obesity in the United States, 2009–2010, NCHS data brief, no 82 (Hyattsville, MD: National Center for Health Statistics), 2012.
5. World Health Organization, www.who.int/features/factfiles/obesity, accessed November 2013.
6. B. M. Popkin, L. S. Adair, and S. W. Ng, Global nutrition transition and the pandemic of obesity in developing countries, *Nutrition Reviews* 70 (2012): 3–21; B. A. Swinburn and coauthors, The global obesity pandemic: Shaped by global drivers and local environments, *Lancet* 378 (2011): 804–814; R. W. Kimokoti and B. E. Millen, Diet, the global obesity epidemic, and prevention, *Journal of the American Dietetic Association* 111 (2011): 1137–1140.
7. Y. D. Tchoukalova and coauthors, Regional differences in cellular mechanisms of adipose tissue gain with overfeeding, *Proceedings of the National Academic of Sciences of the United States of America* 107 (2010): 18226–18231.
8. C. A. Baile and coauthors, Effect of resveratrol on fat mobilization, *Annals of the New York Academy of Sciences* 1215 (2011): 40–47.
9. M. Krawczyk, L. Bonfrate, and P. Portincasa, Nonalcoholic fatty liver disease, *Best Practice and Research, Clinical Gastroenterology* 24 (2010): 695–708; D. M. Muoio, Metabolism and vascular fatty acid transport, *New England Journal of Medicine* 363 (2010): 291–293; G. Tarantino, S. Savastano, and A. Colao, Hepatic steatosis, low-grade chronic inflammation and hormone/growth factor/adipokine imbalance, *World Journal of Gastroenterology* 16 (2010): 4773–4783.
10. P. Trayhurn, C. A. Drevon, and J. Eckel, Secreted proteins from adipose tissue and skeletal muscle: Adipokines, myokines and adipose/muscle cross-talk, *Archives of Physiology and Biochemistry* 117 (2011): 47–56; N. Ouchi and coauthors, Adipokines in inflammation and metabolic disease, *Nature Reviews Immunology* 11 (2011): 85–97; C. Stryjecki and D. M. Mutch, Fatty acid-gene interactions, adipokines and obesity, *European Journal of Clinical Nutrition* 65 (2011): 285–297.
11. H. Wong and R. H. Eckel, Lipoprotein lipase in the brain and nervous system, *Annual Review of Nutrition* 32 (2012): 147–160.
12. S. Camps, S. Verhoef, and K. R. Westerterp, Weight loss, weight maintenance, and adaptive thermogenesis, *American Journal of Clinical Nutrition* 97 (2013): 990–994.
13. J. R. Speakman and coauthors, Set points, settling points and some alternative models: Theoretical options to understand how genes and environments combine to regulate body adiposity, *Disease Models and Mechanisms* 4 (2011): 733–745.
14. J. R. Speakman, Evolutionary perspectives on the obesity epidemic: Adaptive, maladaptive, and neutral viewpoints, *Annual Review of Nutrition* 33 (2013): 289–317; L. Dubois and coauthors, Genetic and environmental contributions to weight, height, and BMI from birth to 19 years of age: An international study of over 12,000 twin pairs, *PLoS One* 7 (2012): e30153; B. Levin, Developmental gene x environment interactions affecting systems regulating energy homeostasis and obesity, *Frontiers in Neuroendocinology* 31 (2010): 270–283.
15. C. Lavebratt, M. Almgren, and T. J. Ekström, Epigenetic regulation in obesity, *International Journal of Obesity* 36 (2012): 757–765.
16. K. Silventoinen and coauthors, The genetic and environmental influences on childhood obesity: A systematic review of twin and adoption studies, *International Journal of Obesity* 34 (2010): 29–40.
17. J. Naukkarinen and coauthors, Causes and consequences of obesity: The contribution of recent twin studies, *International Journal of Obesity* 36 (2012): 1017–1024.
18. J. Cecil and coauthors, Obesity and eating behaviour in children and adolescents: Contribution of common gene polymorphisms, *International Review of Psychiatry* 24 (2012): 200–210; M. Manco and B. Dallapiccola, Genetics of pediatric obesity, *Pediatrics* 130 (2012): 123–133.
19. P. T. Williams, Attenuated inheritance of body weight by running in monozygotic twins, *Medicine and Science in Sports and Exercise* 44 (2012): 98–103; S. Li and coauthors, Physical activity attenuates the genetic predisposition to obesity in 20,000 men and women from EPIC-Norfolk prospective population study, *PLoS Medicine* 7 (2010): e1000331.
20. J. Mattei and coauthors, *TCF7L2* genetic variants modulate the effect of dietary fat intake on changes in body composition during a weight-loss intervention, *American Journal of Clinical Nutrition* 96 (2012): 1129–1136; Q. Qibin and coauthors, Sugar-sweetened beverages and genetic risk of obesity, *New England Journal of Medicine* 367 (2012): 1387–1396.
21. Y. Xu and Q. Tong, Expanding neurotransmitters in the hypothalamic neurocircuitry for energy balance, *Protein Cell* 2 (2011): 800–813; L. Gautron and J. K. Elmquist, Sixteen years and counting: An update on leptin in energy balance, *Journal of Clinical Investigation* 121 (2011): 2087–2093.
22. H. R. Kissileff and coauthors, Leptin reverses declines in satiation in weight-reduced obese humans, *American Journal of Clinical Nutrition* 95 (2012): 309–317.
23. J. Tong and coauthors, Ghrelin enhances olfactory sensitivity and exploratory sniffing in rodents and humans, *Journal of Neuroscience* 31 (2011): 5841–5846; T. R. Castañeda and coauthors, Ghrelin in the regulation of body weight and metabolism, *Frontiers in Neuroendocrinology* 31 (2010): 44–60.
24. A. J. Crum and coauthors, Mind over milkshakes: Mindsets, not just nutrients, determine ghrelin response, *Health Psychology* 30 (2011): 424–429.
25. M. St. Onge and coauthors, Sleep restriction leads to increased activation of brain regions sensitive to food stimuli, *American Journal of Clinical Nutrition* 95 (2012): 818–824; H. K. J. Gonnissen and coauthors, Effect of a phase advance and phase delay of the 24-h cycle on energy metabolism, appetite, and related hormones, *American Journal of Clinical Nutrition* 96 (2012): 689–697; C. Benedict and coauthors, Acute sleep deprivation reduces energy expenditure in healthy men, *American Journal of Clinical Nutrition* 93 (2011): 1229–1236; R. Hursel and coauthors, Effects of sleep fragmentation in healthy men on energy expenditure, substrate oxidation, physical activity, and exhaustion measured over 48 h in a respiratory chamber, *American Journal of Clinical Nutrition* 94 (2011): 804–808; P. Lyytikäinen and coauthors, Sleep problems and major weight gain: A follow-up study, *International Journal of Obesity* 35 (2011): 109–114; L. Brondel and coauthors, Acute partial sleep deprivation increases food intake in healthy men, *American Journal of Clinical Nutrition* 91 (2010): 1550–1559.
26. S. Li and coauthors, Cumulative effects and predictive value of common obesity-susceptibility variants identified by genome-wide association studies, *American Journal of Clinical Nutrition* 91 (2010): 184–190.
27. M. M. Hetherington and J. E. Cecil, Gene-environment interactions in obesity, *Forum of Nutrition* 63 (2010): 195–203; C. Bouchard, Defining the genetic architecture of the predisposition to obesity: A challenging but not insurmountable task, *American Journal of Clinical Nutrition* 91 (2010): 5–6.
28. M. E. Lidell and coauthors, Evidence for two types of brown adipose tissue in humans, *Nature Medicine* 19 (2013): 631–634; B. Cannon and J. Nedergaard, Yes, even human brown fat is on fire! *Journal of Clinical Investigation* 122 (2012): 486–489.
29. K. A. Virtanen and P. N. Muutila, Brown adipose tissue in humans, *Current Opinion in Lipidology* 22 (2011): 49–54.
30. A. Bartelt and J. Heeren, The holy grail of metabolic disease: Brown adipose tissue, *Current Opinion in Lipidology* 23 (2012): 190–195.

31. T. J. Schulz and Y. H. Tseng, Brown adipose tissue: Development, metabolism and beyond, *Biochemical Journal* 453 (2013): 167–178; E. Ravussin and J. E. Galgani, The implication of brown adipose tissue for humans, *Annual Review of Nutrition* 31 (2011): 33–47.
32. K. A. Lo and L. Sun, Turning WAT into BAT: A review on regulators controlling the browning of white adipocytes, *Bioscience Reports* 33 (2013): 711–719; G. E. Beranger, In vitro brown and "brite"/"beige" adipogenesis: Human cellular models and molecular aspects, *Biochimica et Biophysica Acta* 1831 (2013): 905–914; M. L. Bonet, P. Oliver, and A. Palou, Pharmacological and nutritional agents promoting browning of white adipose tissue, *Biochimica et Biophysica Acta* 1831 (2013): 969–985; J. Wu and coauthors, Beige adipocytes are a distinct type of thermogenic fat cell in mouse and human, *Cell* 150 (2012): 366–376.
33. L. Z. Sharp and coauthors, Human BAT possesses molecular signatures that resemble beige/brite cells, *PLoS One* 7 (2012): doi 10.1371.
34. B. K. Pedersen, A muscular twist on the fate of fat, *New England Journal of Medicine* 366 (2012): 1544–1545.
35. J. M. McCaffery and coauthors, Effects of social contact and zygosity on 21-y weight change in male twins, *American Journal of Clinical Nutrition* 94 (2011): 404–409.
36. B. M. Popkin and K. J. Duffey, Does hunger and satiety drive eating anymore? Increasing eating occasions and decreasing time between eating occasions in the United States, *American Journal of Clinical Nutrition* 91 (2010): 1342–1347.
37. K. J. Duffey and B. M. Popkin, Energy density, portion size, and eating occasions: Contributions to increased energy intake in the United States, 1977–2006, *PLoS Medicine* 8 (2011): e1001050.
38. R. N. Close and D. A. Schoeller, The financial reality of overeating, *Journal of the American College of Nutrition* 25 (2006): 203–209.
39. I. N. Bezerra, C. Curioni, and R. Sichieri, Association between eating out of home and body weight, *Nutrition Reviews* 70 (2012): 65–79.
40. J. F. Sallis and coauthors, Role of built environments in physical activity, obesity, and cardiovascular disease, *Circulation* 125 (2012): 729–737.
41. T. S. Church and coauthors, Trends over 5 decades in US occupation-related physical activity and their association with obesity, *PLoS ONE* 6 (2011): e19657.
42. K. Wijndaele and coauthors, Increased cardiometabolic risk is associated with increased TV viewing time, *Medicine and Science in Sports and Exercise* 42 (2010): 1511–1518.
43. H. Konttinen and coauthors, Emotional eating and physical activity self-efficacy as pathways in the association between depressive symptoms and adiposity indicators, *American Journal of Clinical Nutrition* 92 (2010): 1031–1039.
44. D. P. Beavers and coauthors, Cardiometabolic risk after weight loss and subsequent weight regain in overweight and obese postmenopausal women, *Journals of Gerontology Series A: Biological Sciences and medical Sciences* 68 (2013): 691–698; K. Stohacker and B. K. McFarlin, Influence of obesity, physical inactivity, and weight cycling on chronic inflammation, *Frontiers in Bioscience (Elite Edition)* 2 (2010): 98–104.
45. K. Poddar and coauthors, Nutraceutical supplements for weight loss: A systematic review, *Nutrition in Clinical Practice* 26 (2011): 539–552.
46. FDA, Tainted weight loss products, http://www.fda.gov/drugs/resourcesforyou/consumers/buyingusingmedicinesafely/medicationhealthfraud/ucm234592.htm, accessed November 2013; M. H. Tang and coauthors, Case series on a diversity of illicit weight-reducing agents: From the well known to the unexpected, *British Journal of Clinical Pharmacology* 71 (2011): 250–253.
47. A. Astrup, Drug management of obesity: Efficacy versus safety, *New England Journal of Medicine* 363 (2010): 288–290.
48. E. H. Morrato and D. B. Allison, FDA approval of obesity drugs: A difference in risk-benefit perceptions, *Journal of the American Medical Association* 308 (2012): 1097–1098; E. Colman and coauthors, The FDA's assessment of two drugs for chronic weight management, *New England Journal of Medicine* 367 (2012): 1577–1579.
49. C. D. Fryar, M. D. Carroll, and C. L. Ogden, Prevalence of overweight, obesity, and extreme obesity among adults: United States, trends 1960–1962 through 2009–2010, *NCHS Health E-Stats*, September 2012.
50. R. Padwal and coauthors, Bariatric surgery: A systematic review of the clinical and economic evidence, *Journal of Internal Medicine* 26 (2011): 1183–1194; A. Nagle, Bariatric surgery: A surgeon's perspective, *Journal of the American Dietetic Association* 110 (2010): 520–523; G. L. Blackburn, S. Wollner, and S. B. Heymsfield, Lifestyle interventions for the treatment of class III obesity: A primary target for nutrition medicine in the obesity epidemic, *American Journal of Clinical Nutrition* 91 (2010): 289S–292S.
51. E. H. Livingston, The incidence of bariatric surgery has plateaued in the U.S., *American Journal of Surgery* 200 (2010): 378–385.
52. B. Laferrère, Diabetes remission after bariatric surgery: Is it just the incretins? *International Journal of Obesity* 35 (2011): S22–S25; L. M. Beckman, T. R. Beckman, and C. P. Earthman, Changes in gastrointestinal hormones and leptin after Roux-en-Y gastric bypass procedure: A review, *Journal of the American Dietetic Association* 110 (2010): 571–584.
53. L. Kong and coauthors, Gut microbiota after gastric bypass in human obesity: Increased richness and associations of bacterial genera with adipose tissue genes, *American Journal of Clinical Nutrition* 98 (2013): 16–24; A. D. Miras and coauthors, Gastric bypass surgery for obesity decreases the reward value of a sweet-fat stimulus as assessed in a progressive ratio task, *American Journal of Clinical Nutrition* 96 (2012): 467–473.
54. P. E. O'Brien and coauthors, Long-term outcomes after bariatric surgery: Fifteen-year follow-up of adjustable gastric banding and a systematic review of the bariatric surgical literature, *Annals of Surgery* 257 (2013): 87–94.
55. T. D. Adams, Health benefits of gastric bypass surgery after 6 years, *Journal of the American Medical Association* 308 (2012): 1122–1131; G. Mingrone and coauthors, Bariatric surgery versus conventional medical therapy for type 2 diabetes, *New England Journal of Medicine* 366 (2012): 1577–1585; D. Sandoval, Bariatric surgeries: Beyond restriction and malabsorption, *International Journal of Obesity* 35 (2011): S45–S49.
56. E. H. Livingston, Surgical treatment of obesity in adolescence, *Journal of the American Medical Association* 303 (2010): 559–560.
57. L. Beckman and C. Earthman, Nutritional implications of bariatric surgery and the role of registered dietitians, *Journal of the Academy of Nutrition and Dietetics* 113 (2013): 398–399; Y. Chen, Acute bariatric surgery complications: Managing parenteral nutrition in the morbidly obese, *Journal of the American Dietetic Association* 110 (2010): 1734–1737; D. Kulick, L. Hark, and D. Deen, The bariatric surgery patient: A growing role for registered dietitians, *Journal of the American Dietetic Association* 110 (2010): 593–599; G. Snyder-Marlow, D. Taylor, and J. Lenhard, Nutrition care for patients undergoing laparoscopic sleeve gastrectomy for weight loss, *Journal of the American Dietetic Association* 110 (2010): 600–607.
58. E. Saltzman and J. P. Karl, Nutrient deficiencies after gastric bypass surgery, *Annual Review of Nutrition* 33 (2013): 183–203; S. P. Donadelli and coauthors, Daily vitamin supplementation and hypovitaminosis after obesity surgery, *Nutrition* 28 (2012): 391–396; R. Welbourn and D. Pournaras, Bariatric surgery: A cost-effective intervention for morbid obesity; functional and nutritional outcomes, *Proceedings of the Nutrition Society* 69 (2010): 528–535.
59. M. Kruseman and coauthors, Dietary, weight, and psychological changes among patients with obesity, 8 years after gastric bypass, *Journal of the American Dietetic Association* 110 (2010): 527–534.
60. L. Sjöström and coauthors, Bariatric surgery and long-term cardiovascular events, *Journal of the American Medical Association* 301 (2012): 56–65.
61. P. J. Stephan and J. M. Kenkel, Updates and advances in liposuction, *Aesthetic Surgery Journal* 30 (2010) 83–97.
62. T. L. Hernandez and coauthors, Fat redistribution following suction lipectomy: Defense of body fat and patterns of restoration, *Obesity* 19 (2011): 1388–1395.
63. D. Laddu and coauthors, A review of evidence-based strategies to treat obesity in adults, *Nutrition in Clinical Practice* 26 (2011): 512–525; D. Heber, An integrative view of obesity, *American Journal of Clinical Nutrition* 91 (2010): 280S–283S.
64. M. D. Jensen and coauthors, *2013 AHA/ACC/TOS Guideline for the Management of Overweight and Obesity in Adults*, 2013.

65. K. M. Beavers and coauthors, Is lost lean mass from intentional weight loss recovered during weight regain in postmenopausal women? *American Journal of Clinical Nutrition* 94 (2011): 767–774.
66. A. J. Tomiyama and coauthors, Low calorie dieting increases cortisol, *Psychosomatic Medicine* 72 (2010): 357–364.
67. H. M. Seagle and coauthors, Position of the American Dietetic Association: Weight management, *Journal of the American Dietetic Association* 109 (2009): 330–346.
68. A. W. Brown, M. M. B. Brown, and D. B. Allison, Belief beyond the evidence: Using the proposed effect of breakfast on obesity to show 2 practices that distort scientific evidence, *American Journal of Clinical Nutrition* 98 (2013): 1298–1308.
69. P. Deshmukh-Taskar and coauthors, The relationship of breakfast skipping and type of breakfast consumed with overweight/obesity, abdominal obesity, other cardiometabolic risk factors and the metabolic syndrome in young adults. The National Health and Nutrition Examination Survey (NHANES): 1999–2006, *Public Health Nutrition* 16 (2013): 2073–2082; S. P. P. Tin and coauthors, Breakfast skipping and change in body mass index in young children, *International Journal of Obesity* 35 (2011): 899–906; K. J. Smith and coauthors, Skipping breakfast: Longitudinal associations with cardiometabolic risk factors in the Childhood Determinants of Adult Health Study, *American Journal of Clinical Nutrition* 92 (2010): 1316–1325.
70. H. J. Leidy and coauthors, Beneficial effects of a higher-protein breakfast on the appetitive, hormonal, and neural signals controlling energy intake regulation in overweight/obese, "breakfast skipping," late-adolescent girls, *American Journal of Clinical Nutrition* 97 (2013): 677–688; P. R. Deshmukh-Taskar and coauthors, The relationship of breakfast skipping and type of breakfast consumption with nutrient intake and weight status in children and adolescents: The National Health and Nutrition Examination Survey 1999–2006, *Journal of the American Dietetic Association* 110 (2010): 869–878.
71. D. Jakubowicz and coauthors, High caloric intake at breakfast vs. dinner differentially influences weight loss of overweight and obese women, *Obesity* (2013): doi:10.1002/oby.20460.
72. K. J. Duffey and B. M. Popkin, Energy density, portion size, and eating occasions: Contributions to increased energy intake in the United States, 1977–2006, *PLoS Medicine* 8 (2011): e1001050.
73. C. L. Rock and coauthors, Effect of a free prepared meal and incentivized weight loss program on weight loss and weight loss maintenance in obese and overweight women: A randomized controlled trial, *Journal of the American Medical Association* 304 (2010): 1803–1810; Position of the American Dietetic Association: Weight management, *Journal of the American Dietetic Association* 109 (2009): 330–346.
74. J. Li and coauthors, Improvement in chewing activity reduces energy intake in one meal and modulates plasma gut hormone concentrations in obese and lean young Chinese men, *American Journal of Clinical Nutrition* 94 (2011): 709–716.
75. A. Kokkinos and coauthors, Eating slowly increases the postprandial response of the anorexigenic gut hormones, peptide YY and glucagon-like peptide-1, *Journal of Clinical Endocrinology and Metabolism* 95 (2010): 333–337.
76. S. L. Leong and coauthors, Faster self-reported speed of eating is related to higher body mass index in a nationwide survey of middle-aged women, *Journal of the American Dietetic Association* 111 (2011): 1192–1197.
77. R. A. Williams, L. S. Roe, and B. J. Rolls, comparison of three methods to reduce energy density: Effects on daily energy intake, *Appetite* 66 (2013): 75–83; R. Pérez-Escamilla and coauthors, Dietary energy density and body weight in adults and children: A systematic review, *Journal of the Academy of Nutrition and Dietetics* 112 (2012): 671–684; H. A. Raynor and coauthors, The effects of an energy density prescription on diet quality and weight loss: A pilot randomized controlled trial, *Journal of the Academy of Nutrition and Dietetics* 112 (2012): 1397–1402.
78. R. Muckelbauer and coauthors, Association between water consumption and body weight outcomes: A systematic review, *American Journal of Clinical Nutrition* 98 (2013): 282–299.
79. M. C. Daniels and B. M. Popkin, Impact of water intake on energy intake and weight status: A systematic review, *Nutrition Reviews* 68 (2010): 505–521.
80. D. F. Tate and coauthors, Replacing caloric beverages with water or diet beverages for weight loss in adults: Main results of the Choose Healthy Options Consciously Everyday (CHOICE) randomized clinical trial, *American Journal of Clinical Nutrition* 95 (2012): 555–563.
81. L. Hooper and coauthors, Effect of reducing total fat intake on body weight: Systematic review and meta-analysis of randomised controlled trials and cohort studies, *British Medical Journal* 345 (2012): e766.
82. M. A. Pereira, Diet beverages and the risk of obesity, diabetes, and cardiovascular disease: A review of the evidence, *Nutrition Reviews* 71 (2013): 433–440.
83. E. Green and C. Murphy, Altered processing of sweet taste in the brain of diet soda drinkers, *Physiology and Behavior* 107 (2012): 560–567.
84. C. D. Chapman and coauthors, Lifestyle determinants of the drive to eat: A meta-analysis, *American Journal of Clinical Nutrition* 96 (2012): 492–497.
85. B. H. Goodpaster and coauthors, Effects of diet and physical activity interventions on weight loss and cardiometabolic risk factors in severely obese adults: A randomized study, *Journal of the American Medical Association* 304 (2010): 1795–1802; A. L. Hankinson and coauthors, Maintaining a high physical activity level over 20 years and weight gain, *Journal of the American Medical Association* 304 (2010): 2603–2610.
86. J. E. Donnelly and coauthors, American College of Sports Medicine Position Stand: Appropriate physical activity intervention strategies for weight loss and prevention of weight regain for adults, *Medicine and Science in Sports and Exercise* 41 (2009): 459–471; Committee on Dietary Reference Intakes, *Dietary Reference Intakes for Energy, Carbohydrate, Fiber, Fat, Fatty Acids, Cholesterol, Protein, and Amino Acids* (Washington, D.C.: National Academies Press, 2005).
87. Goodpaster and coauthors, 2010; M. Hamer and G. O'Donovan, Cardiorespiratory fitness and metabolic risk factors in obesity, *Current Opinion in Lipidology* 21 (2010): 1–7; D. E. Larson-Meyer and coauthors, Caloric restriction with or without exercise: The fitness versus fatness debate, *Medicine and Science in Sports and Exercise* 42 (2010): 152–159.
88. D. T. Villareal and coauthors, Weight loss, exercise, or both and physical function in obese older adults, *New England Journal of Medicine* 364 (2011): 1218–1229.
89. J. E. Turner and coauthors, Nonprescribed physical activity energy expenditure is maintained with structured exercise and implicates a compensatory increase in energy intake, *American Journal of Clinical Nutrition* 92 (2010): 1009–1016.
90. A. M. Knab and coauthors, A 45-minute vigorous exercise bout increases metabolic rate for 14 hours, *Medicine and Science in Sports and Exercise* 43 (2011): 1643–1648.
91. S. H. Boutcher, High-intensity intermittent exercise and fat loss, *Journal of Obesity* 2011 (2011): doi 10.1155.2011.868305.
92. U. Ekelund and coauthors, Physical activity and gain in abdominal adiposity and body weight: Prospective cohort study in 288,498 men and women, *American Journal of Clinical Nutrition* 93 (2011): 826–835; C. A. Slentz and coauthors, The effects of aerobic versus resistance training on visceral and liver fat stores, liver enzymes and HOMA from STRRIDE AT/RT: A randomized trial, *American Journal of Physiology: Endocrinology and Metaolism* 301 (2011): E1033-E1039; J. W. Bea and coauthors, Resistance training predicts 6-yr body composition change in postmenopausal women, *Medicine and Science in Sports and Exercise* 42 (2010): 1286–1295.
93. C. W. Bales and coauthors, Aerobic and resistance training effects on energy intake: The STRRIDE-AT/RT Study, *Medicine and Science in Sports and Exercise* 44 (2012): 2033–2039; D. Stensel, Exercise, Appetite and appetite-regulating hormones: Implications for food intake and weight control, *Annals of Nutrition and Metabolism* 57 (2010): 36–42; J. A. King and coauthors, Influence of brisk walking on appetite, energy intake, and plasma acylated ghrelin, *Medicine and Science in Sports and Exercise* 42 (2010): 485–492.

94. K. J. Guelfi, C. E. Conges, R. Duffield, Beneficial effects of 12 weeks of aerobic compared with resistance exercise training on perceived appetite in previously sedentary overweight and obese men, *Metabolism: Clinical and Experimental* 62 (2013): 235–243; K. Deighton, J. C. Zahra, and D. J. Stensel, Appetite, energy intake and resting metabolic responses to 60 min treadmill running performed in a fasted versus a postprandial state, *Appetite* 58 (2012): 946–954.
95. E. V. Carraca and coauthors, Physical activity predicts changes in body image during obesity treatment in women, *Medicine and Science in Sports and Exercise* 44 (2012): 1604–1612.
96. I. M. Lee and coauthors, Physical activity and weight gain prevention, *Journal of the American Medical Association* 303 (2010): 1173–1179.
97. J. A. Steeves, D. L. Thompson, and D. R. Bassett Jr., Energy cost of stepping in place while watching television commercials, *Medicine and Science in Sports and Exercise* 44 (2012): 330–335.
98. B. McFerran and coauthors, I'll have what she's having: Effects of social influence and body type on the food choices of others, *Journal of Consumer Research* 36 (2010): 915–929.
99. E. Robinson and coauthors, Eating attentively: A systematic review and meta-analysis of the effect of food intake memory and awareness on eating, *American Journal of Clinical Nutrition* 97 (2013): 728–742; R. E. Oldham-Cooper and coauthors, Playing a computer game during lunch affects fullness, memory for lunch, and later snack intake, *American Journal of Clinical Nutrition* 93 (2011): 308–313.
100. L. H. Epstein and coauthors, Long-term habituation to food in obese and nonobese women, *American Journal of Clinical Nutrition* 94 (2011): 371–376.
101. A. Kong and coauthors, Self-monitoring and eating-related behaviors are associated with 12-month weight loss in postmenopausal overweight-to-obese women, *Journal of the Academy of Nutrition and Dietetics* 112 (2012): 1428–1435; M. B. Conroy and coauthors, Physical activity self-monitoring and weight loss: 6-month results of the SMART Trial, *Medicine and Science in Sports and Exercise* 43 (2011): 1568–1574; L. E. Burke, J. Wang, and M. A. Sevick, Self-monitoring in weight loss: A systematic review of the literature, *Journal of the American Dietetic Association* 111 (2011): 92–102.
102. S. D. Acharya and coauthors, Using a personal digital assistant for self-monitoring influences diet quality in comparison to a standard paper record among overweight/obese adults, *Journal of the American Dietetic Association* 111 (2011): 583–588.
103. H. Shin and coauthors, Self-efficacy improves weight loss in overweight/obese postmenopausal women during a 6-month weight loss intervention, *Nutrition Research* 31 (2011): 822–828.
104. R. Rossini and coauthors, Effects of cognitive-behavioral treatment for weight loss in family members, *Journal of the American Dietetic Association* 111 (2011): 1712–1719.
105. S. Kodama and coauthors, Effect of web-based lifestyle modification on weight control: A meta-analysis, *International Journal of Obesity* 36 (2012): 675–685; L. J. Appel and coauthors, Comparative effectiveness of weight-loss interventions in clinical practice, *New England Journal of Medicine* 365 (2011): 1959–1968.
106. J. L. Kraschnewski and coauthors, Long-term weight loss maintenance in the United States, *International Journal of Obesity* 34 (2010): 1644–1654.
107. C. B. Ebbeling and coauthors, Effects of dietary composition on energy expenditure during weight-loss maintenance, *Journal of the American Medical Association* 307 (2012): 2627–2634.
108. P. Sumithran and coauthors, Long-term persistence of hormonal adaptations to weight loss, *New England Journal of Medicine* 365 (2011): 1597–1604.
109. J. L. Unick, J. M. Jakicic, and B. H. Marcus, Contribution of behavior intervention components to 24-month weight loss, *Medicine and Science in Sports and Exercise* 42 (2010): 745–753.
110. E. Manthou and coauthors, Behavioral compensatory adjustments to exercise training in overweight women, *Medicine and Science in Sports and Medicine* 42 (2010): 1221–1228.
111. National Weight Loss Registry, www.nwlr.ws, accessed November 2013; S. F. L. Kirk and coauthors, Effective weight management practice: A review of the lifestyle intervention evidence, *International Journal of Obesity* 36 (2012): 178–185; N. R. Reyes and coauthors, Similarities and differences between weight loss maintainers and regainers: A qualitative analysis, *Journal of the Academy of Nutrition and Dietetics* 112 (2012): 499–505; J. P. Moreno and C. A. Johnston, Successful habits of weight loss, *American Journal of Lifestyle Medicine* 6 (2012): 113–115; J. L. Bachman and coauthors, Eating frequency is higher in weight loss maintainers and normal-weight individuals than in overweight individuals, *Journal of the American Dietetic Association* 111 (2011): 1730–1734; S. N. Grief and R. L. Miranda, Weight loss maintenance, *American Family Physician* 82 (2010): 630–634.
112. *Accelerating Progress in Obesity Prevention: Solving the Weight of the Nation*, (Washington, DC: Institute of Medicine of the National Academies), 2012.
113. J. C. Giesen and coauthors, Exploring how calorie information and taxes on high-calorie foods influence lunch decisions, *American Journal of Clinical Nutrition* 93 (2011): 689–694; E. A. Finkelstein and coauthors, Impact of targeted beverage taxes on higher- and lower-income households, *Archives of Internal Medicine* 170 (2010): 2028–2034.

HIGHLIGHT > 9

The Latest and Greatest Weight-Loss Diet—Again

> LEARN IT Contrast the differences between popular fad diets and weight-loss diets based on sound nutrition.

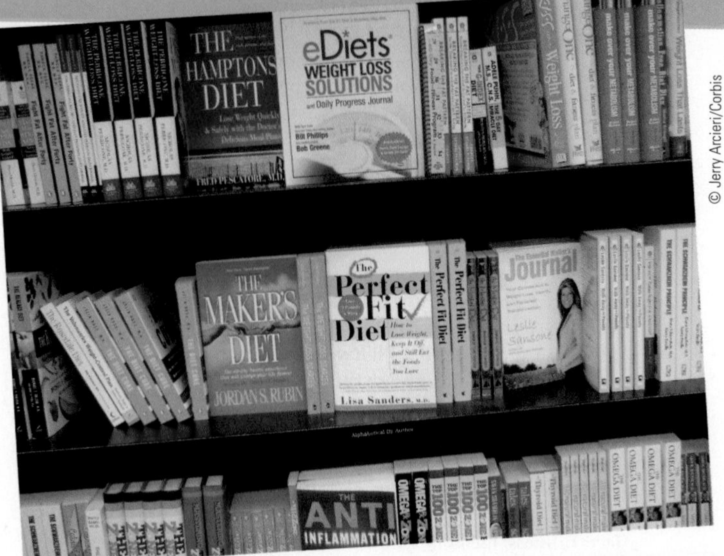

To paraphrase William Shakespeare, "A fad diet by any other name would still be a fad diet." Year after year, "new and improved" diets appear on bookstore shelves and circulate among friends.* People of all sizes eagerly try the best diet ever on the market, hoping that this one will really work. Sometimes these diets seem to work for a while, but more often than not, their success is short-lived. Then another diet takes the spotlight. Here's how Dr. K. Brownell, an obesity researcher and dean at Duke University's Sanford School of Public Policy, describes this phenomenon: "When I get calls about the latest diet fad, I imagine a trick birthday cake candle that keeps lighting up and we have to keep blowing it out."

Realizing that fad diets do not offer a safe and effective long-term plan for weight loss, health professionals speak out, but they never get the candle blown out permanently. New fad diets can keep making outrageous claims because no one requires their advocates to prove what they say. Fad diet gurus do not have to conduct credible research on the benefits or dangers of their diets. They can simply make recommendations and then later, if questioned, search for bits and pieces of research that support the conclusions they have already reached. That's backward. Diet and health recommendations should *follow* years of sound scientific research *before* being offered to the public.

Because anyone can publish anything—in books or on the Internet—peddlers of fad diets can make unsubstantiated statements that fall far short of the truth but sound impressive to the uninformed. They often offer distorted bits of legitimate research. They may start with one or more actual facts but then leap from one erroneous conclusion to the next. Anyone who wants to believe these claims has to wonder how the thousands of scientists working on obesity research over the past century could possibly have missed such obvious connections.

Fad diets come in almost as many shapes and sizes as the people who search them out. Some restrict fats or carbohydrates, some limit portion sizes, some focus on food combinations, and some claim that a person's genetic type or blood type determines the foods best suited to manage weight and prevent disease. A lack of scientific evidence just doesn't seem to stop diets from making claims.[1] Table H9-1 compares some of today's popular diets.

Fad Diets' Appeal

With more than half of our nation's adults overweight and many more concerned about their weight, the market for a weight-loss book, product, or program is huge (no pun intended). Americans spend an estimated $33 billion a year on weight-loss books and products. Even a plan that offers only minimal weight-loss success easily attracts a following.

Perhaps the greatest appeal of fad diets is that they tend to ignore dietary recommendations. Foods such as meats and milk products that need to be selected carefully to limit saturated fat can be eaten with abandon. Whole grains, legumes, vegetables, and fruits that should be eaten in abundance can now be bypassed. For some people, this is a dream come true: steaks without the potatoes, ribs without the coleslaw, and meatballs without the pasta. Who can resist the promise of weight loss while eating freely from a list of favorite foods?

Dieters are also lured into fad diets by sophisticated—yet often erroneous—explanations of the metabolic consequences of eating certain foods. Terms such as *eicosanoids* and *de novo lipogenesis* are scattered about, often intimidating readers into believing that the authors must be right given their brilliance in understanding the body.

If fad diets were as successful as some people claim, then consumers who tried them would lose weight, and their obesity problems would be solved. But this is not the case. Similarly, if fad diets were as worthless as others claim, then consumers would eventually stop pursuing them. Clearly, this is not happening either. Most fad diets have enough going for them that they work for some people at least for a short time, but they fail to produce long-lasting results for most people.

Don't Count kCalories

Who wants to count kcalories? Even experienced dieters find counting kcalories burdensome, not to mention timeworn. They want a new, easy way to lose weight, and fad diet plans seem to offer this boon. But, though fad diets often claim to disregard kcalories, their design typically ensures a low energy intake. Most of the sample menu plans,

*The Academy of Nutrition and Dietetics offers evaluations of popular diets for your review. Look for reviews of popular diets at their website, **www.eatright.org/dietreviews.**

TABLE H9-1 **Popular Diets Compared**

Diet	Claim(s)	Strong Point(s)	Weak Point(s)
The 4-Hour Body	• Small, simple changes produce big, long-lasting results. • The Slow-Carb diet supports a 20-pound weight loss in 30 days without exercise.	• Encourages lean proteins, legumes, and vegetables. • Organized format provides simple plan.	• Excludes fruit, whole grains, and milk (except cottage cheese), which may lead to nutrient deficiencies. • Lacks variety.
The 17 Day Diet	• Changing the way you eat every few days creates "body confusion," which prevents metabolism from settling into homeostasis. • You can boost metabolism by "eating clean," which means no sugar, no processed food, and no fried foods.	• Prevents boredom by alternating between cycles. • Fairly well-balanced diet promotes healthy eating.	• Lacks scientific evidence that changing the diet creates "body confusion." • Does not provide individualized kcalorie goals. • Promotes its own processed foods.
The 100	• Restricting sugar consumption to 100 kcalories a day will reduce insulin levels (the weight-gaining hormone), speed weight loss, improve health, and boost metabolism. • The real problem causing weight gains is hidden sugars in healthy foods such as yogurt and fruit.	• Limits processed foods. • Encourages consumption of vegetables and fiber-rich foods.	• Focuses on very basic food choices and lacks variety. • Limits important food groups such as low-fat dairy, legumes, and fruits, which may lead to nutrient deficiencies.
Biggest Loser Diet	• Lose weight, gain health, feel young, and take control of your life using portion control, progressively lowering energy intake, and a following a customized food pyramid.	• Provides motivation and promotes selecting low-fat foods and drinking water. • Stresses the importance of exercise.	• Recommends energy intakes below the recommended minimum of 1200 kcalories a day, which may lead to nutrient deficiencies.
Cinch!	• A nutrient-dense diet composed mainly of plant-based foods will help you lose weight and lower the risk of disease.	• Recommends a plant-based, nutrient-dense diet. • Stresses the importance of exercise.	• A little confusing and dense with facts.
The Dukan Diet	• A high-protein, low-kcalorie diet promotes rapid and permanent weight loss.	• Encourages daily exercise, moderate salt intake, and lifelong weight management. • Provides a highly structured plan.	• Restricts carbohydrates to induce ketosis, which can cause nausea, light-headedness, and fatigue and can worsen medical problems such as kidney disease. • Not suited for vegetarians and others who prefer not to emphasize animal proteins.
The Fast Diet	• Lose weight by eating "normally" for five days while choosing two nonconsecutive days to "fast"—limiting kcalories to 500 for women and 600 for men.	• Focuses only on two days of the week. • Promotes lean protein and low glycemic foods on "fast" days.	• Little research supporting the health benefits of intermittent fasting diets. • Fasting can cause irritability, sleeplessness or sleepiness, and dehydration.
New Sonoma Diet	• Enjoying portion-controlled Coastal California style foods supports weight loss and promotes good health.	• Emphasizes nutrient-dense foods. • Limits processed foods.	• No individualized kcalorie plan.
Wheat Belly	• Lose weight and reverse health problems by eliminating all forms of wheat.	• Creates a low-kcalorie diet.	• Restrictive diet would likely be low in B vitamins, calcium, and vitamin D.
The Zen Diet Revolution	• Combine spiritual wisdom and dietary adjustments to reduce fat cells without counting kcalories. • Visualization, meditation, and mindfulness can change mental, dietary, lifestyle, and activity habits.	• Offers a basic nutrition approach that does no harm. • Reminds you to make food meaningful and treat your body with respect.	• Recommendations to use fat-burning herbs, supplements, and green tea to decrease fat cells are unsubstantiated and expensive.

SOURCE: Adapted from Academy of Nutrition and Dietetics, *Consumer Diet and Lifestyle Book Reviews*, www.eatright.org/dietreviews, accessed November 2013.

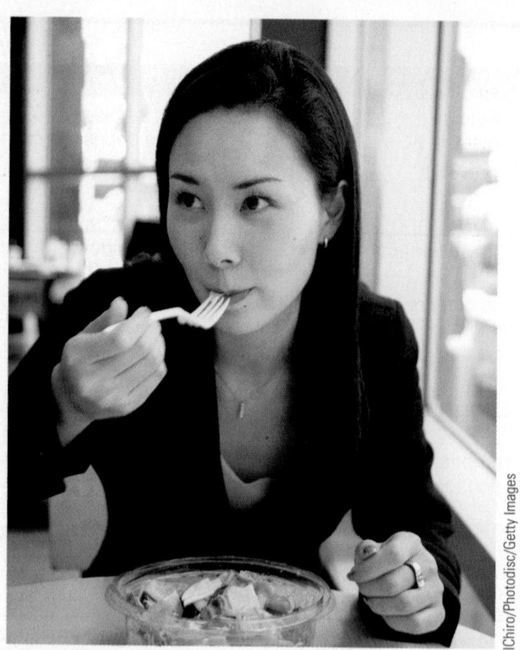
IChiro/Photodisc/Getty Images

The wise consumer seeks a diet that supports not only weight loss, but also health gains.

especially in the early stages, are designed to deliver an average of 1200 kcalories a day.

Even when counting kcalories is truly not necessary, total kcalories tend to be low simply because food intake is so limited. Diets that omit hundreds of foods and several food groups limit a person's options and lack variety. Chapter 2 praises variety as a valuable way to ensure an adequate intake of nutrients, but variety also entices people to eat more food and gain more weight. Without variety, some people lose interest in eating, which further reduces energy intake. Even if the allowed foods are favorites, eating the same foods week after week can become monotonous.

Without its refried beans, tortilla wrapping, and chopped vegetables, a burrito is reduced to a pile of ground beef. Without the baked potato, there's no need for butter and sour cream. Weight loss occurs because of the low energy intake. This is an important point. Any diet can produce weight loss, at least temporarily, if intake is restricted. The real value of a diet is determined by its ability to maintain weight loss and support good health over the long term. The goal is not simply weight loss, but health gains—and most fad diets cannot support optimal health over time. In fact, some weight-loss diets can create or exacerbate health problems.[2]

When food choices are limited, nutrient intakes may be inadequate. To help shore up some of these inadequacies, fad diets often recommend a dietary supplement. Conveniently, many of the companies selling fad diets also peddle these supplements. But as Highlights 10 and 11 explain, foods offer many more health benefits than any supplement can provide. Quite simply, if the diet is inadequate, it needs to be improved.

Follow a Plan

Most people need specific instructions and examples to make dietary changes. Popular diets offer dieters a plan. The user doesn't have to decide what foods to eat, how to prepare them, or how much to eat. Unfortunately, these instructions serve only short-term weight-loss needs. They do not provide for long-term changes in lifestyle that will support weight maintenance or health goals.

The success of any weight-loss diet depends on the person adopting the plan and sticking with it. People who prefer a high-protein, low-carbohydrate diet over a high-carbohydrate, low-fat diet, for example, may have more success at sticking with it, perhaps because of protein's role in providing satiety.[3] Keep in mind, though, that weight loss occurs because of the duration of a low-kcalorie plan—not the proportion of energy nutrients.[4]

The Real Deal

Fad diets attribute magical powers to their weight-loss plans, but in reality, the magic is in tipping the energy balance so that metabolic and physical activities expend more kcalories than foods bring in. Because new diets emerge in the market regularly, it can be challenging to sort the fad diets from the healthy options. Furthermore, it can be difficult determining how a diet's overall quality rates and how it compares with others.

Keep in mind that healthy weight loss requires long-term lifestyle changes in eating and activity habits—not quick, short-term fixes. A healthy plan may not be quick, but it allows for flexibility and a variety of foods, including some favorite treats on occasion.

Some currently popular diet plans offer a sensible approach to weight loss and healthy eating. The challenge is sorting through "the good, the bad, and the ugly." The accompanying "How To" feature offers tips for identifying fad diets and other weight-loss scams. Fad diets may not harm healthy people if used for only a little while, but they cannot support optimal health for long. Chapter 9 includes reasonable approaches to weight management and concludes that the ideal diet is one you can live with for the rest of your life. Keep that criterion in mind when you evaluate the next "latest and greatest weight-loss diet" that comes along.

>How To

Identify a Fad Diet or Weight-Loss Scam

It may be a fad diet or weight-loss scam if it:

- Sounds too good to be true.
- Recommends using a single food consistently as the key to the program's success.
- Promises quick and easy weight loss with no effort. "Lose weight while you sleep!"
- Eliminates an entire food group such as grains or milk and milk products.
- Guarantees an unrealistic outcome in an unreasonable time period. "Lose 10 pounds in 2 days!"
- Bases evidence for its effectiveness solely on anecdotal stories.
- Requires you to buy special products that are not readily available in the marketplace at affordable prices.
- Specifies a proportion for the energy nutrients that falls outside the recommended ranges—carbohydrate (45 to 65 percent), fat (20 to 35 percent), and protein (10 to 35 percent).
- Claims to alter your genetic code or reset your metabolism.
- Fails to mention potential risks or additional costs.
- Promotes products or procedures that have not been proven safe and effective.
- Neglects plans for weight maintenance following weight loss.

› TRY IT Review an advertisement for a popular weight-loss plan and explain why you think it might—or might not—be a fad diet.

CRITICAL THINKING QUESTIONS

A. What patterns are evident in fad weight-loss diets?

B. A fad diet website says it all: 30 ways to lose 5 pounds in a week. Millions of people have tried hundreds of crash diets in search of short-term fixes to their weight problems. It's amazing to think about what people are willing to do to avoid eating a well-balanced diet and exercising regularly—wire their jaws closed, swallow a parasite, drink nothing but salt water for a week. Why do you think consumers continue to pursue fad diets? How would you design a weight loss plan that would be appealing to most people *and* produce long-lasting results?

REFERENCES

1. L. Cusack and coauthors, Blood type diets lack supporting evidence: A systematic review, *American Journal of Clinical Nutrition* 98 (2013): 99–104.
2. P. Sjögren and coauthors, Mediterranean and carbohydrate-restricted diets and mortality among elderly men: A cohort study in Sweden, *American Journal of Clinical Nutrition* 92 (2010): 967–974.
3. M. S. Westerterp-Plantenga, S. G. Lemmens, and K. R. Westerterp, Dietary protein: Its role in satiety, energetics, weight loss and health, *British Journal of Nutrition* 108 (2012): S105–S112; T. M. Larsen and coauthors, Diets with high or low protein content and glycemic index for weight-loss maintenance, *New England Journal of Medicine* 363 (2010): 2102–2113.
4. W. S. Yancy and coauthors, A randomized trial of a low-carbohydrate diet vs orlistat plus a low-fat diet for weight loss, *Archives of Internal Medicine* 170 (2010): 121–123.

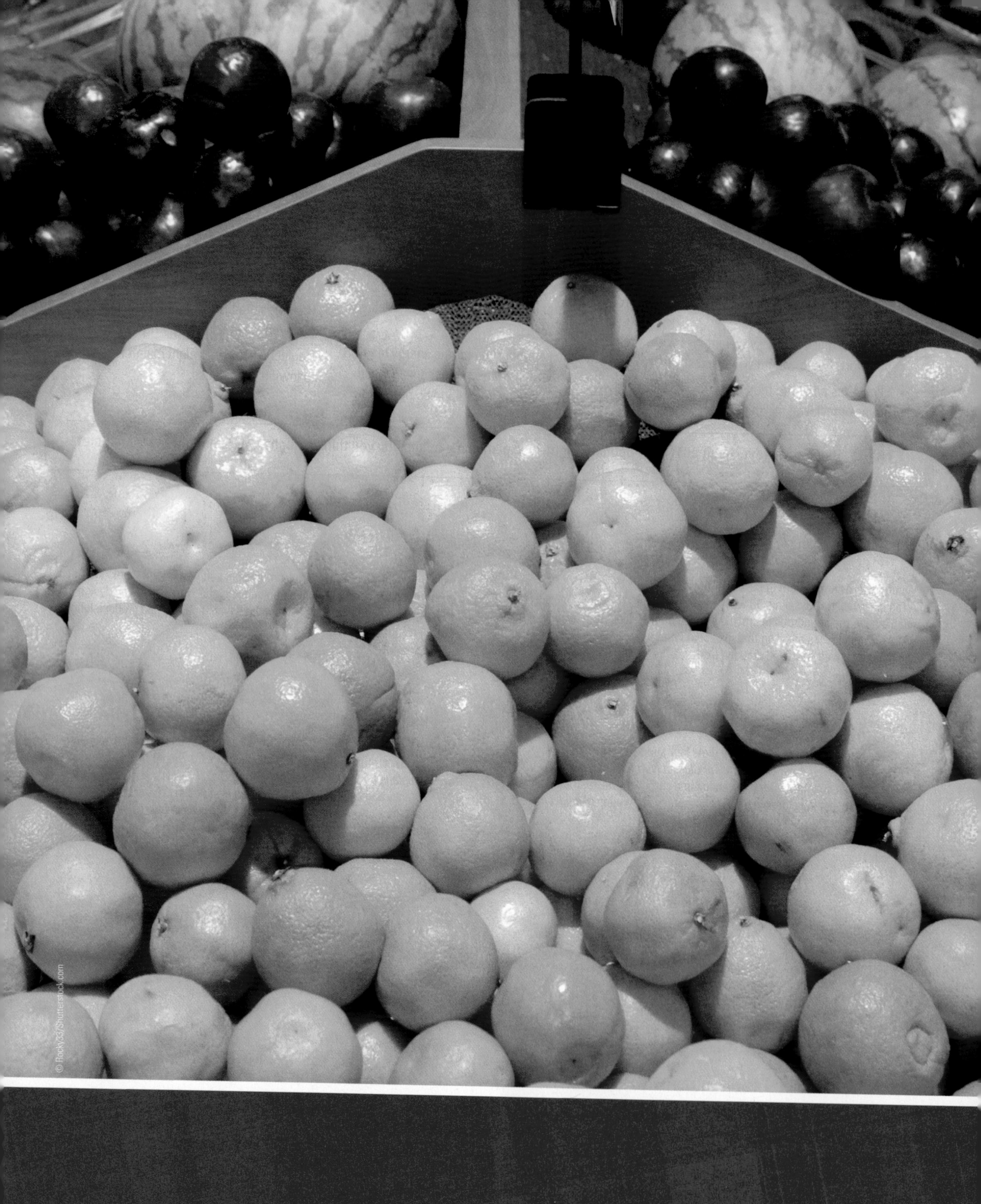

10

The Water-Soluble Vitamins: B Vitamins and Vitamin C

Nutrition in Your Life

If you were playing a word game and your partner said "vitamins," how would you respond? If "pills" and "supplements" immediately come to mind, you may be missing the main message of the vitamin story—that hundreds of foods deliver more than a dozen vitamins that participate in thousands of activities throughout your body. Quite simply, foods supply vitamins to support all that you are and all that you do—and supplements of any one of them, or even a combination of them, can't compete with foods in keeping you healthy. In the Nutrition Portfolio at the end of this chapter, you can determine whether the foods you are eating are meeting your water-soluble vitamin needs.

LEARNING GPS

Earlier chapters focused on the energy-yielding nutrients—carbohydrates, fats, and proteins. This chapter begins with an overview of the **vitamins** and then examines each of the water-soluble vitamins; the next chapter features the fat-soluble vitamins. Researchers first recognized in the early 1900s that foods contain substances that are "vital to life."[1] Since then, the world of vitamins has opened up dramatically.

Vitamins are powerful, as their *absence* attests. Vitamin A deficiency can cause blindness; a lack of the B vitamin niacin can cause dementia; and without vitamin D, bones fail to grow. The *presence* of vitamins also attests to their power. The B vitamin folate helps to prevent birth defects, and vitamin K creates blood clots. Every year, people spend billions of dollars on supplements, hoping to cure their ailments (see Highlight 10). Vitamins do support good health, but they do not cure all ills nor do supplements provide all of the many disease-preventing benefits of vitamin-rich foods such as vegetables, fruits, and whole grains (as Highlight 11 explains).

vitamins: organic, essential nutrients required in small amounts by the body for health. Vitamins regulate body processes that support growth and maintain life.
- **vita** = life
- **amine** = containing nitrogen (the first vitamins discovered contained nitrogen)

10.1 The Vitamins—An Overview

› LEARN IT Describe how vitamins differ from the energy nutrients and how fat-soluble vitamins differ from water-soluble vitamins.

The vitamins differ from carbohydrates, fats, and proteins in the following ways:

- *Structure.* Vitamins are individual units; they are not linked together (as are molecules of glucose or amino acids). Appendix C presents the chemical structure for each of the vitamins.
- *Function.* Vitamins do not yield energy when metabolized; many of them do, however, assist the enzymes that participate in the release of energy from carbohydrates, fats, and proteins.
- *Food contents.* The amounts of vitamins people ingest from foods and the amounts they require daily are measured in *micrograms* (μg) or *milligrams* (mg), rather than grams (g).*

The vitamins are similar to the energy-yielding nutrients, though, in that they are essential, organic, and available from foods.

Bioavailability Some water-soluble vitamins are synthesized by GI tract bacteria and absorbed by the large intestine, but not in quantities great enough to meet the body's needs; foods must supply these essential nutrients.[2] The amount of vitamins available from foods depends not only on the quantity provided by a food but also on the amount absorbed and used by the body—referred to as the vitamins' **bioavailability.** The quantity of vitamins in a food can be determined relatively easily. Researchers analyze foods to determine the vitamin contents and publish the results in tables of food composition such as Appendix H. Determining the bioavailability of a vitamin is a more complex task because it depends on many factors, including:

- Efficiency of digestion and time of transit through the GI tract
- Previous nutrient intake and nutrition status
- Method of food preparation (raw, cooked, or processed)
- Source of the nutrient (synthetic, fortified, or naturally occurring)
- Other foods consumed at the same time

Chapters 10 through 13 describe factors that inhibit or enhance the absorption of individual vitamins and minerals. Experts consider these factors when estimating recommended intakes.

Precursors Some of the vitamins are available from foods in inactive forms known as **precursors,** or provitamins. Once inside the body, the precursor is converted to an active form of the vitamin. For example, beta-carotene, a red-orange pigment found in fruits and vegetables, is a precursor to vitamin A. Thus, in measuring a person's vitamin intake, it is important to count both the amount of the active vitamin and the potential amount available from its precursors. The discussions and summary tables throughout this chapter and the next indicate which vitamins have precursors.

Organic Nature Fresh foods naturally contain vitamins, but because these vitamins are organic, they can be readily destroyed during processing. Therefore, processed foods should be used sparingly, and fresh foods should be handled with care during storage and in cooking. Prolonged heating may destroy much of the thiamin in food. Because riboflavin can be destroyed by the ultraviolet rays of the sun or by fluorescent light, foods stored in transparent glass containers are most likely to lose riboflavin. Oxygen destroys vitamin C, so losses occur when foods are cut, processed, and stored; these losses may be enough to reduce its action in the body. Table 10-1 summarizes ways to minimize nutrient losses in the kitchen, and Chapter 19 provides more details.

Solubility As you may recall, carbohydrates and proteins are hydrophilic and lipids are hydrophobic. The vitamins divide along the same lines—the hydrophilic,

*For perspective, a dollar bill weighs about 1 g; 1 g = 1000 mg, and 1 mg = 1000 μg. Appendix K explains how to convert a measurement from one unit of measure to another.

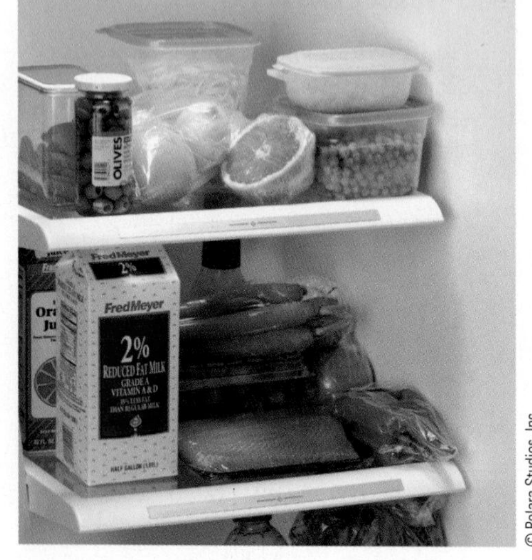

To minimize vitamin losses, wrap cut fruits and vegetables or store them in airtight containers.

bioavailability: the rate at and the extent to which a nutrient is absorbed and used.

precursors: substances that precede others; with regard to vitamins, compounds that can be converted into active vitamins; also known as *provitamins.*

TABLE 10-1 Minimizing Nutrient Losses

- To slow the degradation of vitamins, refrigerate (most) fruits and vegetables.
- To minimize the oxidation of vitamins, store fruits and vegetables that have been cut in airtight wrappers, and store juices that have been opened in closed containers (and refrigerate them).
- To prevent vitamin losses during washing, rinse fruits and vegetables before cutting (not after).
- To minimize vitamin losses during cooking, use a microwave oven or steam vegetables in a small amount of water. Add vegetables after water has come to a boil. Use the cooking water in mixed dishes such as casseroles and soups. Avoid high temperatures and long cooking times.

water-soluble ones are the B vitamins (thiamin, riboflavin, niacin, biotin, pantothenic acid, vitamin B_6, folate, and vitamin B_{12}) and vitamin C; the hydrophobic, fat-soluble ones are vitamins A, D, E, and K. As each vitamin was discovered, it was given a name and sometimes a letter and number as well. Many of the vitamins have multiple names, which has led to some confusion. The summary tables throughout this chapter and the next provide both the standard and the common alternative names.

Solubility is apparent in the food sources of the different vitamins, and it affects their absorption, transport, storage, and excretion by the body. The water-soluble vitamins are found in the watery compartments of foods; the fat-soluble vitamins usually occur together in the fats and oils of foods. On being absorbed, the water-soluble vitamins move directly into the blood. Like fats, the fat-soluble vitamins must first enter the lymph, then the blood. Once in the blood, many of the water-soluble vitamins travel freely, whereas many of the fat-soluble vitamins require transport proteins. Upon reaching the cells, water-soluble vitamins freely circulate in the water-filled compartments whereas fat-soluble vitamins are held in fatty tissues and the liver until needed. The kidneys, monitoring the blood that flows through them, detect and remove small excesses of water-soluble vitamins; large excesses, however, may overwhelm the system, creating adverse effects. Fat-soluble vitamins tend to remain in fat-storage sites in the body rather than being excreted, and so are more likely to reach toxic levels when consumed in excess.

Because the body stores fat-soluble vitamins, they can be eaten in large amounts once in a while and still meet the body's needs over time. Water-soluble vitamins are retained for varying lengths of time in the body. The water-soluble vitamins must be eaten more regularly than the fat-soluble vitamins, although a single day's omission from the diet does not create a deficiency.

Toxicity Knowledge about some of the amazing roles of vitamins has prompted many people to take vitamin supplements, assuming that "more is better." Just as an inadequate intake can cause harm, so can an excessive intake. Even some of the water-soluble vitamins have adverse effects when taken in large doses.

That a vitamin can be both essential and harmful may seem surprising, but the same is true of most nutrients. The effects of every substance depend on its dose, and this is one reason consumers should not self-prescribe supplements. Figure 10-1 (p. 304) shows three possible relationships between dose levels and effects. The third diagram in Figure 10-1 represents the situation with nutrients—more is better up to a point, but beyond that point, still more can be harmful.

The Committee on Dietary Reference Intakes (DRI) addresses the possibility of adverse effects from high doses of nutrients by establishing Tolerable Upper Intake Levels (UL). The UL defines the highest amount of a nutrient that is likely not to cause harm for most healthy people when consumed daily. The risk of harm increases as intakes rise above the UL. Of the nutrients discussed in this chapter, niacin, vitamin B_6, folate, choline, and vitamin C have UL, and these values are presented in their respective summary tables. Data are lacking to establish UL for the remaining B vitamins, but this does not mean that excessively high intakes would be without risk. (The inside front cover pages present UL for the vitamins and minerals.)

> FIGURE 10-1 **Dose Levels and Effects**

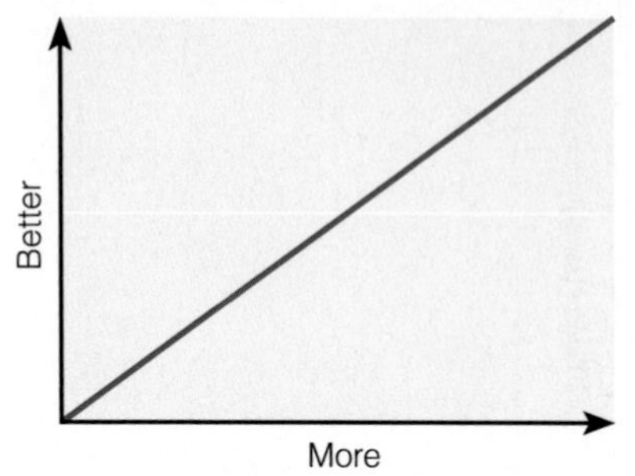

As you progress in the direction of more, the effect gets better and better, with no end in sight (real life is seldom, if ever, like this).

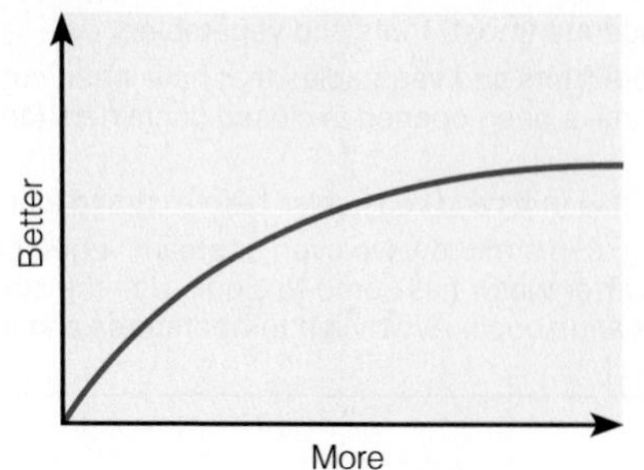

As you progress in the direction of more, the effect reaches a maximum and then a plateau, becoming no better with higher doses.

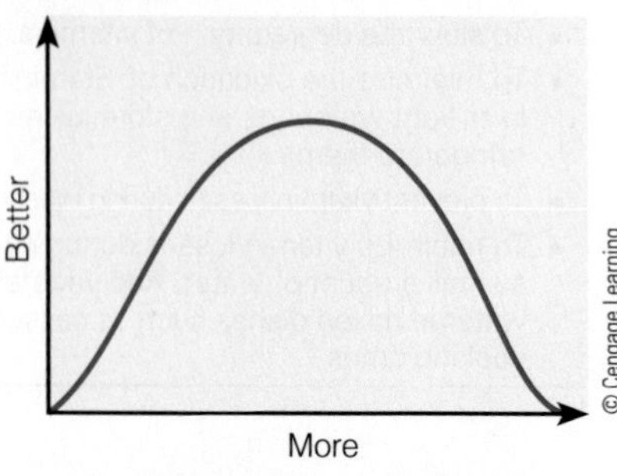

As you progress in the direction of more, the effect reaches an optimum at some intermediate dose and then declines, showing that more is better up to a point and then harmful. That too much can be as harmful as too little represents the situation with most nutrients.

TABLE 10-2 **Water-Soluble and Fat-Soluble Vitamins Compared**

	Water-Soluble Vitamins: B Vitamins and Vitamin C	Fat-Soluble Vitamins: Vitamins A, D, E, and K
Absorption	Directly into the blood	First into the lymph, then the blood
Transport	Travel freely	Many require transport proteins
Storage	Circulate freely in water-filled parts of the body	Stored in the cells associated with fat
Excretion	Kidneys detect and remove excess in urine	Less readily excreted; tend to remain in fat-storage sites
Toxicity	Possible to reach toxic levels when consumed from supplements	Likely to reach toxic levels when consumed from supplements
Requirements	Needed in frequent doses (perhaps 1 to 3 days)	Needed in periodic doses (perhaps weeks or even months)

NOTE: Exceptions occur, but these differences between the water-soluble and fat-solule vitamins are valid generalizations.

> **REVIEW IT** Describe how vitamins differ from the energy nutrients and how fat-soluble vitamins differ from water-soluble vitamins.

The vitamins are essential nutrients needed in tiny amounts in the diet both to prevent deficiency diseases and to support optimal health. The water-soluble vitamins are the B vitamins and vitamin C; the fat-soluble vitamins are vitamins A, D, E, and K. Table 10-2 summarizes the differences between the water-soluble and fat-soluble vitamins.

The discussion of B vitamins that follows begins with a brief description of each of them, then offers a look at the ways they work together. Thus, a preview of the individual vitamins is followed by a discussion of their interactions.

10.2 The B Vitamins

> **LEARN IT** Identify the main roles, deficiency symptoms, and food sources for each of the B vitamins.

Despite supplement advertisements that claim otherwise, the vitamins do not provide the body with fuel for energy. It is true, though, that without B vitamins the body would lack energy. The energy-yielding nutrients—carbohydrate, fat, and protein—are used for fuel; the B vitamins help the body to use that fuel. Several of the B vitamins—thiamin, riboflavin, niacin, pantothenic acid, and biotin—form part of the **coenzymes** that assist enzymes in the release of energy from carbohydrate, fat, and protein. Other B vitamins play other indispensable

coenzymes: complex organic molecules that work with enzymes to facilitate the enzymes' activity. Many coenzymes have B vitamins as part of their structures.

> **FIGURE 10-2 Coenzyme Action**

Some vitamins form part of the coenzymes that enable enzymes either to synthesize compounds (as illustrated by the lower enzymes in this figure) or to dismantle compounds (as illustrated by the upper enzymes).

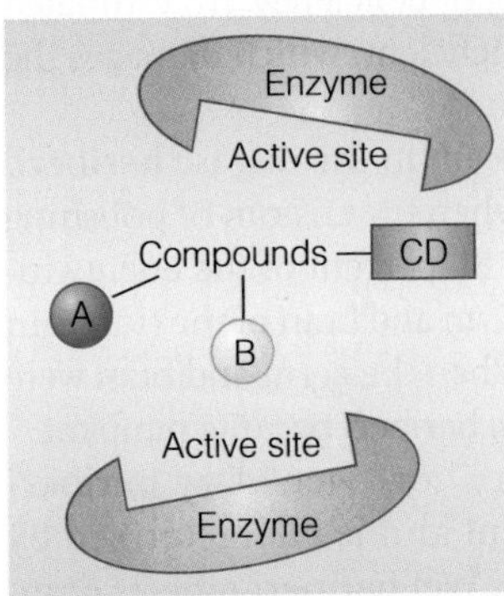

Without coenzymes, compounds A, B, and CD don't respond to their enzymes.

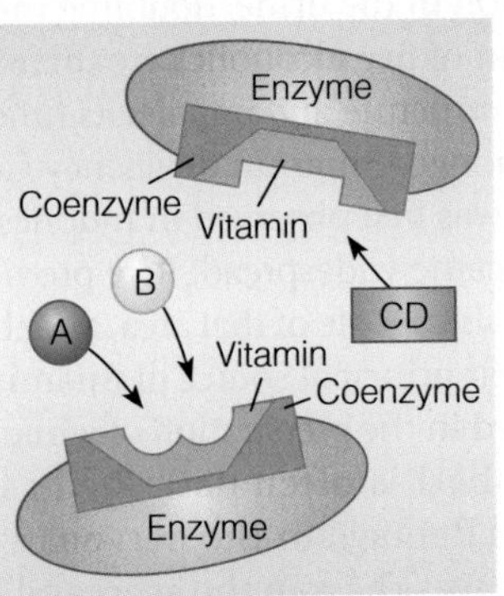

With the coenzymes in place, compounds are attracted to their sites on the enzymes . . .

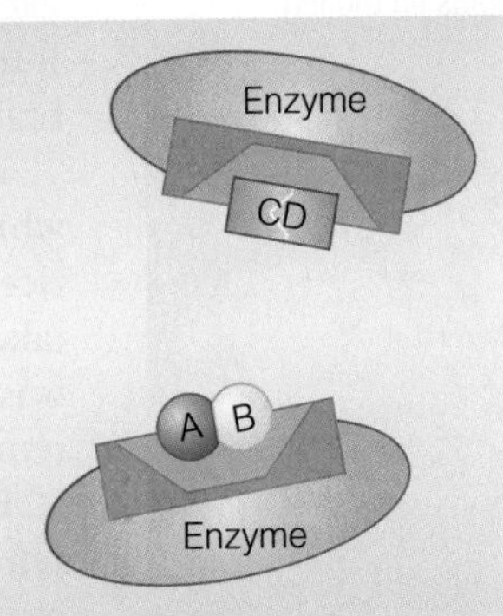

. . . and the reactions proceed instantaneously. The coenzymes often donate or accept electrons, atoms, or groups of atoms.

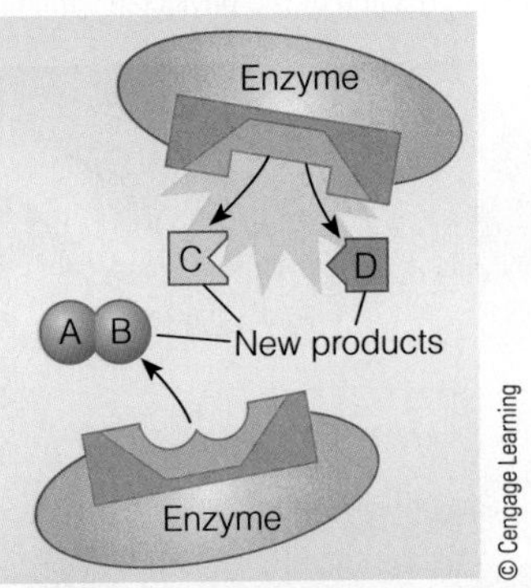

The reactions are completed with either the formation of a new product, AB, or the breaking apart of a compound into two new products, C and D, and the release of energy.

roles in metabolism. Vitamin B_6 assists enzymes that metabolize amino acids. Folate and vitamin B_{12} help cells to multiply. Among these cells are the red blood cells and the cells lining the GI tract—cells that deliver energy to all the others.

The vitamin portion of a coenzyme allows a chemical reaction to occur; the remaining portion of the coenzyme binds to the enzyme. Without its coenzyme, an enzyme cannot function. Thus symptoms of B vitamin deficiencies directly reflect the disturbances of metabolism caused by a lack of coenzymes. Figure 10-2 illustrates coenzyme action.

The following sections describe the roles of individual B vitamins and note many coenzymes and metabolic pathways. Keep in mind that a later discussion assembles these pieces of information into a whole picture. The following sections also present the recommendations, deficiency and toxicity symptoms, and food sources for each vitamin. For thiamin, riboflavin, niacin, vitamin B_6, folate, vitamin B_{12}, and vitamin C, sufficient data were available to establish an RDA; for biotin, pantothenic acid, and choline, an Adequate Intake (AI) was set; only niacin, vitamin B_6, folate, choline, and vitamin C have UL. These values appear in the summary tables and figures that follow and on the pages of the inside front cover.

Thiamin

Thiamin is the vitamin part of the coenzyme TPP (thiamin pyrophosphate) that assists in energy metabolism. The TPP coenzyme participates in the conversion of pyruvate to acetyl CoA (described in Chapter 7). Recall how important this step is in allowing carbohydrate fuel to enter the TCA cycle and produce much more ATP than during glycolysis. The reaction removes 1 carbon from the 3-carbon pyruvate to make the 2-carbon acetyl CoA and carbon dioxide (CO_2). In a similar step in the TCA cycle, TPP helps convert a 5-carbon compound to a 4-carbon compound. Besides playing these pivotal roles in energy metabolism, thiamin occupies a special site on the membranes of nerve cells. Consequently, nerve activity and muscle activity in response to nerves depend heavily on thiamin.

Thiamin Recommendations

Dietary recommendations are based primarily on thiamin's role in enzyme activity. Generally, thiamin needs will be met if a person eats enough food to meet energy needs—if that energy comes from nutritious foods. The average thiamin intake in the United States meets or exceeds recommendations.

Thiamin Deficiency and Toxicity

People who fail to eat enough food to meet energy needs risk nutrient deficiencies, including thiamin deficiency. Inadequate thiamin intakes have been reported among the nation's malnourished and homeless people. Similarly, people who derive most of their energy from empty-kcalorie foods and beverages risk thiamin deficiency. Alcohol provides a good example of how empty

thiamin (THIGH-ah-min): a B vitamin. The coenzyme form is *TPP* (*thiamin pyrophosphate*).

> **FIGURE 10-3 Thiamin-Deficiency Symptom—The Edema of Beriberi**

Physical examination confirms that this person has wet beriberi. Notice how the impression of the physician's thumb remains on the leg.

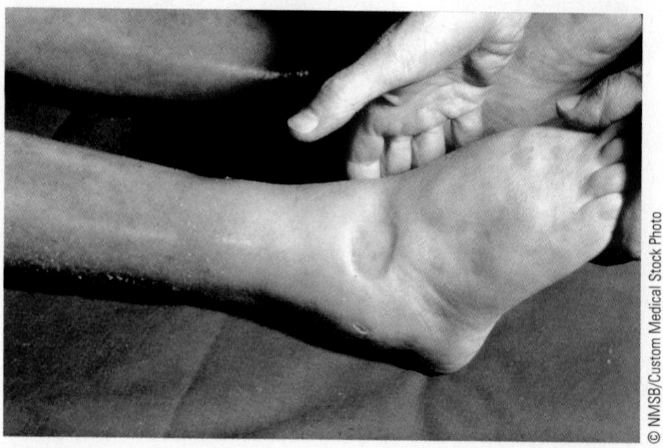

kcalories can lead to thiamin deficiency. Alcohol contributes energy but provides few, if any, nutrients and often displaces food. In addition, alcohol impairs thiamin absorption and enhances thiamin excretion in the urine, doubling the risk of deficiency. An estimated four out of five alcoholics are thiamin deficient, which damages the brain's structure and impairs its function.[3]*

Prolonged thiamin deficiency can result in the disease **beriberi,** which was first observed in Indonesia when the custom of polishing rice became widespread. Rice provided 80 percent of the energy intake of the people of that area, and the germ and bran of the rice grain was their principal source of thiamin. When the germ and bran were removed in the preparation of white rice, beriberi became rampant.

Beriberi is often described as "dry" or "wet." Dry beriberi reflects damage to the nervous system and is characterized by muscle weakness in the arms and legs. Wet beriberi reflects damage to the cardiovascular system and is characterized by dilated blood vessels, which cause the heart to work harder and the kidneys to retain salt and water, resulting in edema. Typically, both types of beriberi appear together, with one set of symptoms predominating. Figure 10-3 presents the edema of beriberi. No adverse effects have been associated with excesses of thiamin, and no UL has been determined.

Thiamin Food Sources Before examining Figure 10-4, you may want to read the accompanying "How To" feature, which describes the content in this and similar figures found in this chapter and the next three chapters. When you look at Figure 10-4, notice that thiamin occurs in small quantities in many nutritious foods. The long red bar near the bottom of the graph shows that meats in the

beriberi: the thiamin-deficiency disease characterized by muscle weakness, edema, or both.

- **beri** = weakness
- **beriberi** = "I can't, I can't"

*Severe thiamin deficiency in alcohol abusers is called the *Wernicke-Korsakoff* (VER-nee-key KORE-sah-kof) *syndrome.* Symptoms include disorientation, loss of short-term memory, jerky eye movements, and staggering gait.

>How To

Evaluate Foods for Their Nutrient Contributions

Figure 10-4 is the first of a series of figures in this and the next three chapters that present the vitamins and minerals in foods. Each figure presents the same 24 foods, which were selected to ensure a variety of choices representative of each of the food groups as suggested by the USDA Food Patterns. For example, a bread, a cereal, and a pasta were chosen from the grain group. The suggestion to include a variety of vegetables was also considered: dark green vegetables (broccoli); orange and red vegetables (carrots); starchy vegetables (potatoes); legumes (pinto beans) and other vegetables (tomato juice). The selection of fruits followed suggestions to use whole fruits (bananas); citrus fruits (oranges); melons (watermelon); and berries (strawberries). Items were selected from the milk group and protein foods in a similar way. In addition to the 24 foods that appear in all of the figures, three different foods were selected for each of the nutrients to add variety and often reflect excellent, and sometimes unusual, sources.

Notice that the figures list the food, the serving size, and the food energy (kcalories) on the left. The amount of the nutrient per serving is presented in the graph on the right along with the RDA (or AI) for adults, so you can see how many servings would be needed to meet recommendations.

The colored bars show at a glance which food groups best provide a nutrient: yellow for grains; green for vegetables; purple for fruits; white for milk and milk products; brown for legumes; and red for protein foods. Because the USDA Food Patterns include legumes with both the protein foods group and the vegetable group and because legumes are especially rich in many vitamins and minerals, they have been given their own color to highlight their nutrient contributions.

Notice how the bar graphs shift in the various figures. Careful study of all of the figures taken together will confirm that variety is the key to nutrient adequacy.

Another way to evaluate foods for their nutrient contributions is to consider their nutrient density (their thiamin *per 100 kcalories*, for example). Quite often, vegetables rank higher on a nutrient-per-kcalorie list than they do on a nutrient-per-serving list (see p. 39 to review how to evaluate foods based on nutrient density). The left column in the figure highlights about five foods that offer the best nutrient density. Notice how many of them are vegetables.

Realistically, people cannot eat for single nutrients. Fortunately, most foods deliver more than one nutrient, allowing people to combine foods into nourishing meals.

> **TRY IT** Calculate which food provides more riboflavin per 1-ounce serving—a pork chop (3 oz, 291 kcal, 0.25 mg riboflavin) or cheddar cheese (1½ oz, 165 kcal, 0.11 mg riboflavin). Which food is more nutrient dense with respect to riboflavin?

> FIGURE 10-4 Thiamin in Selected Foods

Food	Serving size (kcalories)
Bread, whole wheat	1-oz slice (70 kcal)
Cornflakes, fortified	1 oz (110 kcal)
Spaghetti pasta	½ c cooked (99 kcal)
Tortilla, flour	1 10" round (234 kcal)
Broccoli	½ c cooked (22 kcal)
Carrots	½ c shredded raw (24 kcal)
Potato	1 medium baked w/skin (133 kcal)
Tomato juice	¾ c (31 kcal)
Banana	1 medium raw (109 kcal)
Orange	1 medium raw (62 kcal)
Strawberries	½ c fresh (22 kcal)
Watermelon	1 slice (92 kcal)
Milk	1 c reduced-fat 2% (121 kcal)
Yogurt, plain	1 c low-fat (155 kcal)
Cheddar cheese	1½ oz (171 kcal)
Cottage cheese	½ c low-fat 2% (101 kcal)
Pinto beans	½ c cooked (117 kcal)
Peanut butter	2 tbs (188 kcal)
Sunflower seeds	1 oz dry (165 kcal)
Tofu (soybean curd)	½ c (76 kcal)
Ground beef, lean	3 oz broiled (244 kcal)
Chicken breast	3 oz roasted (140 kcal)
Tuna, canned in water	3 oz (99 kcal)
Egg	1 hard cooked (78 kcal)
Excellent, and sometimes unusual, sources:	
Pork chop, lean	3 oz broiled (169 kcal)
Soy milk	1 c (81 kcal)
Squash, acorn	½ c baked (69 kcal)

Milligrams
0
0.25
0.50
0.75
1.00
1.25
RDA for men
RDA for women
THIAMIN
Many different foods contribute some thiamin, but few are rich sources. Together, several servings of a variety of nutritious foods will help meet thiamin needs. Grain selections should be either whole grain or enriched.
Key:
Grains
Vegetables
Fruits
Milk and milk products
Legumes, nuts, seeds
Meats, poultry, seafood
Best sources per kcalorie

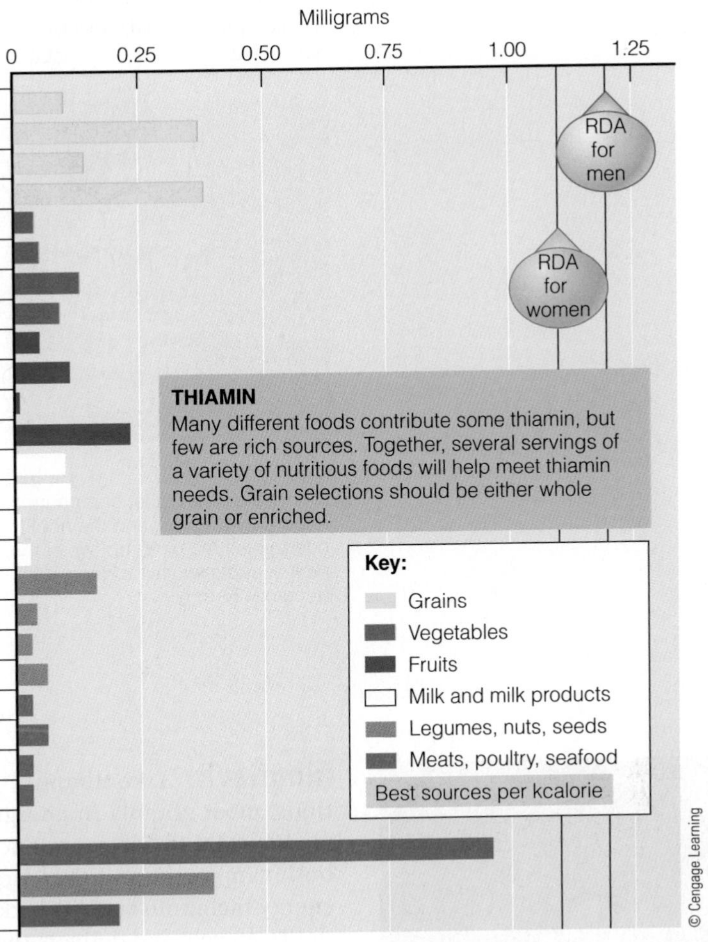

pork family are exceptionally rich in thiamin. Yellow bars confirm that grains—whole grains or enriched—are a reliable source of thiamin.

As mentioned earlier, prolonged cooking can destroy thiamin. Also, like other water-soluble vitamins, thiamin leaches into water when foods are boiled or blanched. Cooking methods that require little or no water such as steaming and microwave heating conserve thiamin and other water-soluble vitamins. The accompanying table provides a summary of thiamin.

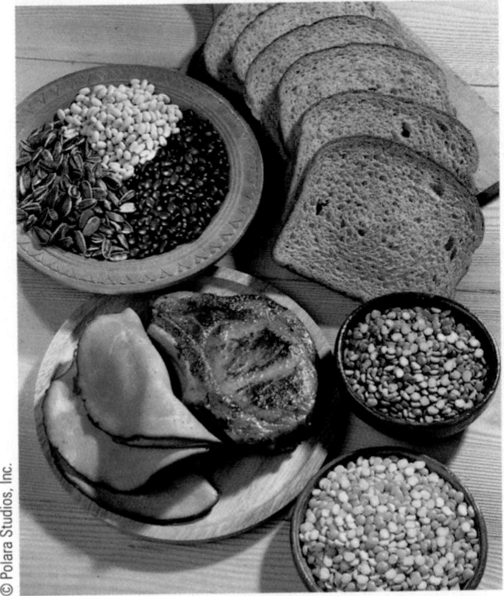

Pork is the richest source of thiamin, but enriched or whole-grain products typically make the greatest contribution to a day's intake because of the quantities eaten. Legumes such as split peas are also valuable sources of thiamin.

> REVIEW IT Thiamin

Other Names

Vitamin B_1

RDA

Men: 1.2 mg/day

Women: 1.1 mg/day

Chief Functions in the Body

Part of coenzyme TPP (thiamin pyrophosphate) used in energy metabolism

Significant Sources

Whole-grain, fortified, or enriched grain products; moderate amounts in all nutritious food; pork

Easily destroyed by heat

Deficiency Disease

Beriberi (wet, with edema; dry, with muscle wasting)

Deficiency Symptoms[a]

Enlarged heart, cardiac failure; muscular weakness; apathy, poor short-term memory, confusion, irritability; anorexia, weight loss

Toxicity Symptoms

None reported

[a]Severe thiamin deficiency is often related to heavy alcohol consumption with limited food consumption (Wernicke-Korsakoff syndrome).

> **FIGURE 10-5 Riboflavin Coenzyme, Accepting and Donating Hydrogens**

This figure shows the chemical structure of the riboflavin portion of the coenzyme only; the remainder of the coenzyme structure is represented by dotted lines (see Appendix C for the complete chemical structures of FAD and FMN). The reactive sites that accept and donate hydrogens are highlighted in white.

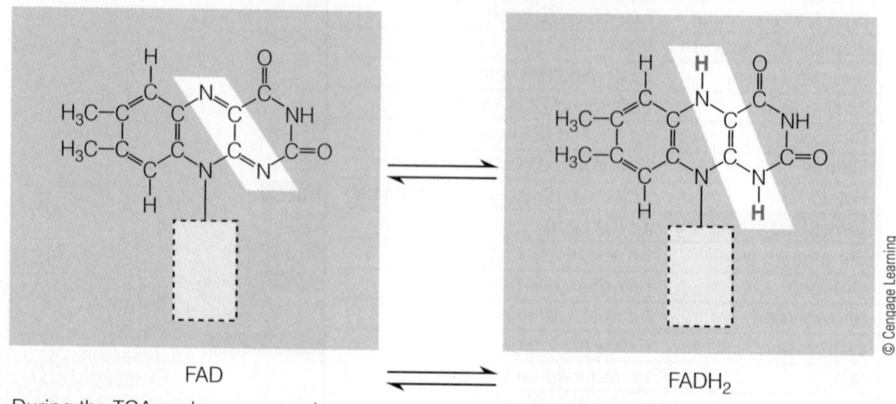

FAD

During the TCA cycle, compounds release hydrogens, and the riboflavin coenzyme FAD picks up two of them. As it accepts two hydrogens, FAD becomes $FADH_2$.

$FADH_2$

$FADH_2$ carries the hydrogens to the electron transport chain. At the end of the electron transport chain, the hydrogens are accepted by oxygen, creating water, and $FADH_2$ becomes FAD again. For every $FADH_2$ that passes through the electron transport chain, two ATP are generated.

Riboflavin

Like thiamin, **riboflavin** serves as a coenzyme in many reactions, most notably in energy metabolism. The coenzyme forms of riboflavin are FMN (flavin mononucleotide) and FAD (flavin adenine dinucleotide); both can accept and then donate two hydrogens (see Figure 10-5). During energy metabolism, FAD picks up two hydrogens (with their electrons) from the TCA cycle and delivers them to the electron transport chain (described in Chapter 7).

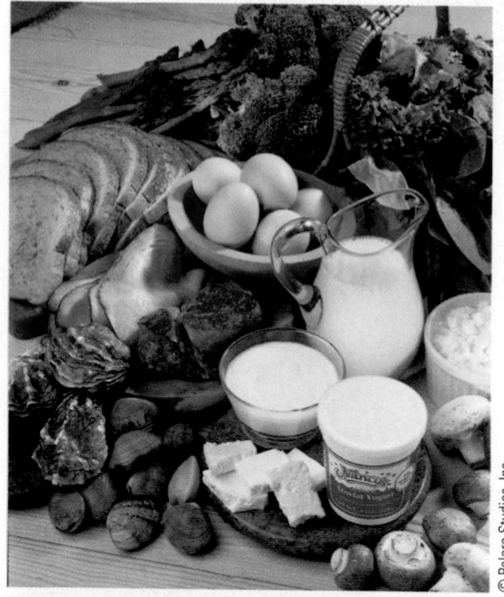

© Polara Studios, Inc.

All of these foods are rich in riboflavin, but milk and milk products provide much of the riboflavin in the diets of most people.

Riboflavin Recommendations Like thiamin's RDA, riboflavin's RDA is based primarily on its role in enzyme activity. Most people in the United States meet or exceed riboflavin recommendations.

Riboflavin Deficiency and Toxicity Riboflavin deficiency most often accompanies other nutrient deficiencies.* Lack of the vitamin causes inflammation of the membranes of the mouth, skin, eyes, and GI tract. Excesses of riboflavin appear to cause no harm, and no UL has been established.

Riboflavin Food Sources The greatest contributions of riboflavin come from milk and milk products (see Figure 10-6). Whole-grain or enriched grains are also valuable sources because of the quantities people typically consume. When riboflavin sources are ranked by nutrient density (per kcalorie), many dark green, leafy vegetables (such as broccoli, turnip greens, asparagus, and spinach) appear high on the list. Vegans and others who don't use milk must rely on ample servings of dark greens and enriched grains for riboflavin. Nutritional yeast is another good source.

Ultraviolet light and irradiation destroy riboflavin. For these reasons, milk is sold in cardboard or opaque plastic containers, instead of clear glass bottles. In contrast, riboflavin is stable to heat, so cooking does not destroy it. The accompanying table provides a summary of riboflavin.

riboflavin (RYE-boh-flay-vin): a B vitamin. The coenzyme forms are *FMN (flavin mononucleotide)* and *FAD (flavin adenine dinucleotide)*.

*Riboflavin deficiency is called *ariboflavinosis* (ay-RYE-boh-FLAY-vin-oh-sis).

> **FIGURE 10-6 Riboflavin in Selected Foods**

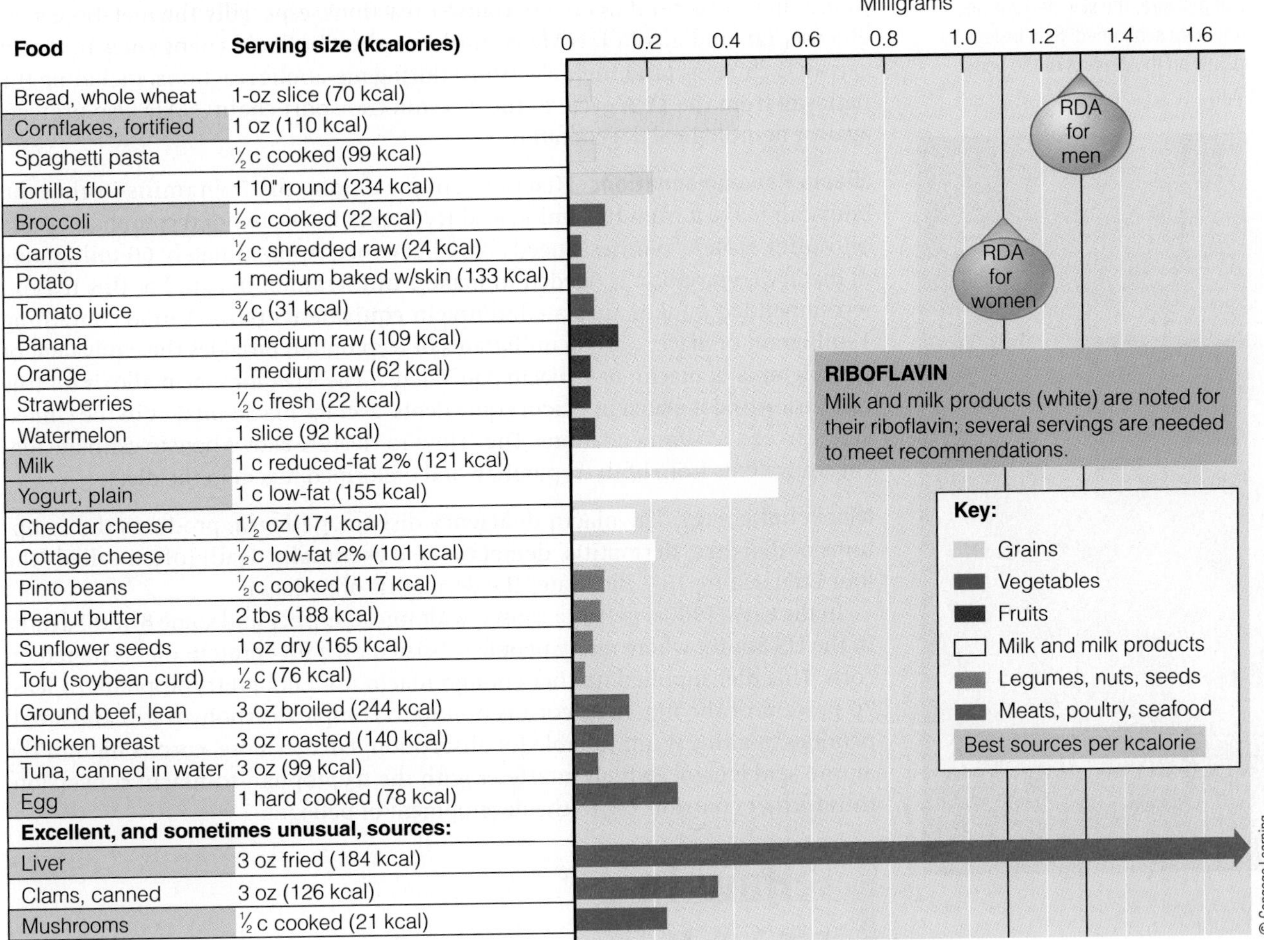

Milligrams
0
0.2
0.4
0.6
0.8
1.0
1.2
1.4
1.6
Food
Serving size (kcalories)
Bread, whole wheat 1-oz slice (70 kcal)
Cornflakes, fortified 1 oz (110 kcal)
Spaghetti pasta ½ c cooked (99 kcal)
Tortilla, flour 1 10" round (234 kcal)
Broccoli ½ c cooked (22 kcal)
Carrots ½ c shredded raw (24 kcal)
Potato 1 medium baked w/skin (133 kcal)
Tomato juice ¾ c (31 kcal)
Banana 1 medium raw (109 kcal)
Orange 1 medium raw (62 kcal)
Strawberries ½ c fresh (22 kcal)
Watermelon 1 slice (92 kcal)
Milk 1 c reduced-fat 2% (121 kcal)
Yogurt, plain 1 c low-fat (155 kcal)
Cheddar cheese 1½ oz (171 kcal)
Cottage cheese ½ c low-fat 2% (101 kcal)
Pinto beans ½ c cooked (117 kcal)
Peanut butter 2 tbs (188 kcal)
Sunflower seeds 1 oz dry (165 kcal)
Tofu (soybean curd) ½ c (76 kcal)
Ground beef, lean 3 oz broiled (244 kcal)
Chicken breast 3 oz roasted (140 kcal)
Tuna, canned in water 3 oz (99 kcal)
Egg 1 hard cooked (78 kcal)
Excellent, and sometimes unusual, sources:
Liver 3 oz fried (184 kcal)
Clams, canned 3 oz (126 kcal)
Mushrooms ½ c cooked (21 kcal)
RDA for men
RDA for women
RIBOFLAVIN
Milk and milk products (white) are noted for their riboflavin; several servings are needed to meet recommendations.
Key:
Grains
Vegetables
Fruits
Milk and milk products
Legumes, nuts, seeds
Meats, poultry, seafood
Best sources per kcalorie

> **REVIEW IT** Riboflavin

Other Names

Vitamin B_2

RDA

Men: 1.3 mg/day

Women: 1.1 mg/day

Chief Functions in the Body

Part of coenzymes FMN (flavin mononucleotide) and FAD (flavin adenine dinucleotide) used in energy metabolism

Significant Sources

Milk products (yogurt, cheese); whole-grain, fortified, or enriched grain products; liver

Easily destroyed by ultraviolet light and irradiation

Deficiency Disease

Ariboflavinosis (ay-RYE-boh-FLAY-vin-oh-sis)

Deficiency Symptoms

Sore throat; cracks and redness at corners of mouth;[a] painful, smooth, purplish red tongue;[b] inflammation characterized by skin lesions covered with greasy scales

Toxicity Symptoms

None reported

[a]Cracks at the corners of the mouth are called *angular stomatitis* or *cheilosis* (kye-LOH-sis or kee-LOH-sis).

[b]Smoothness of the tongue is caused by loss of its surface structures and is termed *glossitis* (gloss-EYE-tis).

Niacin Niacin refers to two chemical structures: nicotinic acid and nicotinamide (also known as niacinamide). The body can easily convert nicotinic acid to nicotinamide, which is the major form of niacin in the blood.

niacin (NIGH-a-sin): a B vitamin. The coenzyme forms are NAD (*nicotinamide adenine dinucleotide*) and NADP (*the phosphate form of NAD*). Niacin can be eaten preformed or made in the body from its precursor, tryptophan, an essential amino acid.

> FIGURE 10-7 **Niacin-Deficiency Symptom—The Dermatitis of Pellagra**

In the dermatitis of pellagra, the skin darkens and flakes away as if it were sunburned. Skin lesions typically develop only on those parts of the body exposed to the sun.

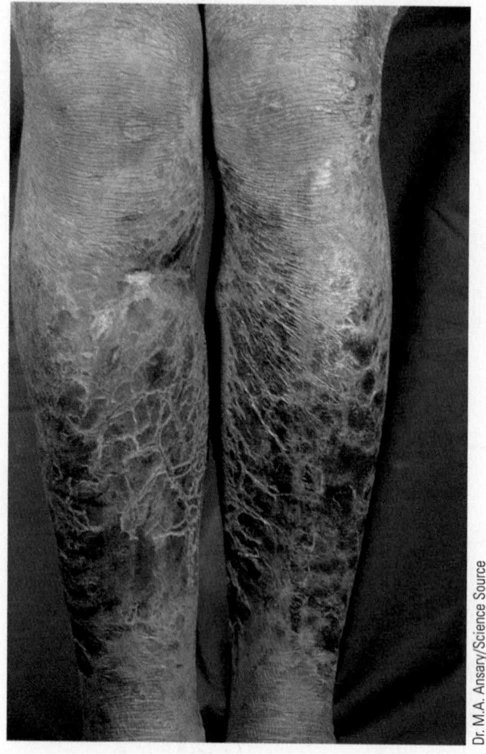

Dr. M.A. Ansary/Science Source

The two coenzyme forms of niacin, NAD (nicotinamide adenine dinucleotide) and NADP (the phosphate form), participate in numerous metabolic reactions. They are central in energy-transfer reactions, especially the metabolism of glucose, fat, and alcohol. NAD is similar to the riboflavin coenzymes in that it carries hydrogens (and their electrons) during metabolic reactions, including the pathway from the TCA cycle to the electron transport chain. NAD also protects against neurological degeneration.

Niacin Recommendations Niacin is unique among the B vitamins in that the body can make it from the amino acid tryptophan. This use of tryptophan occurs only after protein synthesis needs have been met. Approximately 60 milligrams of dietary tryptophan is needed to make 1 milligram of niacin. For this reason, recommended intakes are stated in **niacin equivalents (NE).** A food containing 1 milligram of niacin and 60 milligrams of tryptophan provides the equivalent of 2 milligrams of niacin, or 2 niacin equivalents. The RDA for niacin allows for this conversion and is stated in niacin equivalents; average niacin intakes in the United States exceed recommendations. The "How To" feature shows how to estimate niacin equivalents from both tryptophan and preformed niacin in the diet.

Niacin Deficiency The niacin-deficiency disease, **pellagra,** produces the symptoms of diarrhea, dermatitis, dementia, and eventually death (often called "the four Ds"). Figure 10-7 illustrates the dermatitis of pellagra.

In the early 1900s, pellagra caused widespread misery and some 87,000 deaths in the US South, where many people subsisted on a low-protein diet centered on corn. This diet supplied neither enough niacin nor enough tryptophan. At least 70 percent of the niacin in corn is bound to complex carbohydrates and small peptides, making it unavailable for absorption. Furthermore, corn is high in the amino acid leucine, which interferes with the tryptophan-to-niacin conversion, thus further contributing to the development of pellagra.

>How To

Estimate Niacin Equivalents

Niacin recommendations are expressed as niacin equivalents (NE), but diet analysis programs and food composition tables report only preformed niacin. To estimate niacin equivalents from the tryptophan in dietary protein:

- Assume that most dietary proteins contain about 1 percent tryptophan. To determine the amount of tryptophan in protein, divide grams of protein by 100.
- Multiply by 1000 to convert grams of tryptophan to milligrams.
- Because it takes 60 milligrams of tryptophan to make 1 milligram of niacin, divide milligrams of tryptophan by 60 to get niacin equivalents.
- Add the amount of preformed niacin obtained in the diet.

Consider, for example, a person who consumes 80 grams of protein and 5 milligrams of preformed niacin.

- Estimate the amount of tryptophan in 80 grams of protein and convert to milligrams:

  80 g protein ÷ 100 = 0.8 g tryptophan

  0.8 g tryptophan × 1000 = 800 mg tryptophan

- Convert milligrams of tryptophan to niacin equivalents:

  800 mg tryptophan ÷ 60 = 13 mg NE

To determine the total amount of niacin available from the diet, add the amount available from tryptophan to the amount preformed in the diet.

13 mg NE + 5 mg preformed niacin = 18 mg NE

> TRY IT Calculate how many niacin equivalents a person receives from a diet that delivers 60 grams of protein and 6 milligrams of niacin.

niacin equivalents (NE): the amount of niacin present in food, including the niacin that can theoretically be made from its precursor, tryptophan, present in the food.

- 1 NE = 1 mg niacin or 60 mg tryptophan

pellagra (pell-AY-gra): the niacin-deficiency disease, characterized by diarrhea, dermatitis, dementia, and eventually death.

- **pellis** = skin
- **agra** = rough

Pellagra was originally believed to be caused by an infection. Medical researchers spent many years and much effort searching for infectious microbes until they realized that the problem was not what was *present* in the food but what was *absent* from it. That a disease such as pellagra could be caused by diet inadequacies—and not by pathogens—was a groundbreaking discovery. It contradicted commonly held medical opinions that diseases were caused only by infectious agents. By carefully following the scientific method (as described in Chapter 1), researchers advanced the science of nutrition dramatically.

Niacin Toxicity When a normal dose of a nutrient (levels commonly found in foods) provides a normal blood concentration, the nutrient is having a *physiological* effect. When a large dose (levels commonly available only from supplements) overwhelms the body and raises blood concentrations to abnormally high levels, the nutrient is acting like a drug and having a *pharmacological* effect. Naturally occurring niacin from foods has a physiological effect that causes no harm. Large doses of nicotinic acid from supplements or drugs, however, produce a variety of pharmacological effects, most notably **"niacin flush."** Niacin flush occurs when nicotinic acid is taken in doses only three to four times the RDA. It dilates the capillaries and causes a tingling sensation that can be painful. The nicotinamide form does not produce this effect.

Large doses of nicotinic acid can effectively lower LDL cholesterol and triglycerides and raise HDL cholesterol—all factors that help to protect against heart disease.[4] As effective as niacin therapy is in improving blood lipids, however, it may not benefit patients with heart disease whose blood lipids are already being controlled with statin drugs.[5] The use of niacin as a drug may benefit other patients, but its use must be closely monitored. People with the following conditions may be particularly susceptible to the toxic effects of niacin: liver disease, diabetes, peptic ulcers, gout, irregular heartbeats, inflammatory bowel disease, migraine headaches, and alcoholism. The nicotinamide form does not improve blood cholesterol levels.[6]

Niacin Food Sources Tables of food composition typically list preformed niacin only, but as mentioned, niacin can also be made in the body from the amino acid tryptophan. Dietary tryptophan could meet about half the daily niacin need for most people, but the average diet easily supplies enough preformed niacin.

Figure 10-8 (p. 312) presents niacin in selected foods. Meat, poultry, fish, legumes, and enriched and whole grains contribute about half the niacin people consume. Mushrooms, potatoes, and tomatoes are among the richest vegetable sources, and they can provide abundant niacin when eaten in generous amounts.

Niacin is less vulnerable to losses during food preparation and storage than other water-soluble vitamins. Being fairly heat resistant, niacin can withstand reasonable cooking times, but like other water-soluble vitamins, it will leach into cooking water. The accompanying table provides a summary of niacin.

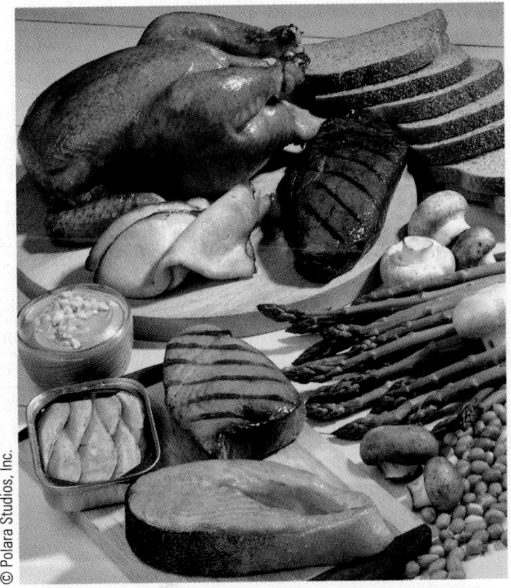

Protein-rich foods such as meat, fish, poultry, and peanut butter contribute much of the niacin in people's diets. Enriched breads and cereals and a few vegetables are also rich in niacin.

› REVIEW IT Niacin

Other Names
Nicotinic acid, nicotinamide, niacinamide, vitamin B_3; precursor is dietary tryptophan (an amino acid)

RDA
Men: 16 mg NE/day
Women: 14 mg NE/day

UL[a]
Adults: 35 mg/day

Chief Functions in the Body
Part of coenzymes NAD (nicotinamide adenine dinucleotide) and NADP (its phosphate form) used in energy metabolism

Significant Sources
Milk, eggs, meat, poultry, fish; whole-grain, fortified, and enriched grain products; nuts and all protein-containing foods

Deficiency Disease
Pellagra

Deficiency Symptoms
Diarrhea, abdominal pain, vomiting; inflamed, swollen, smooth, bright red tongue;[b] depression, apathy, fatigue, loss of memory, headache; bilateral symmetrical rash on areas exposed to sunlight

Toxicity Symptoms
Painful flush, hives, and rash ("niacin flush"); nausea and vomiting; liver damage; impaired glucose tolerance

[a]The UL applies to synthetic forms obtained from supplements, fortified foods, or a combination.
[b]Smoothness of the tongue is caused by loss of its surface structures and is termed *glossitis* (gloss-EYE-tis).

niacin flush: a temporary burning, tingling, and itching sensation that occurs when a person takes a large dose of nicotinic acid; often accompanied by a headache and reddened face, arms, and chest.

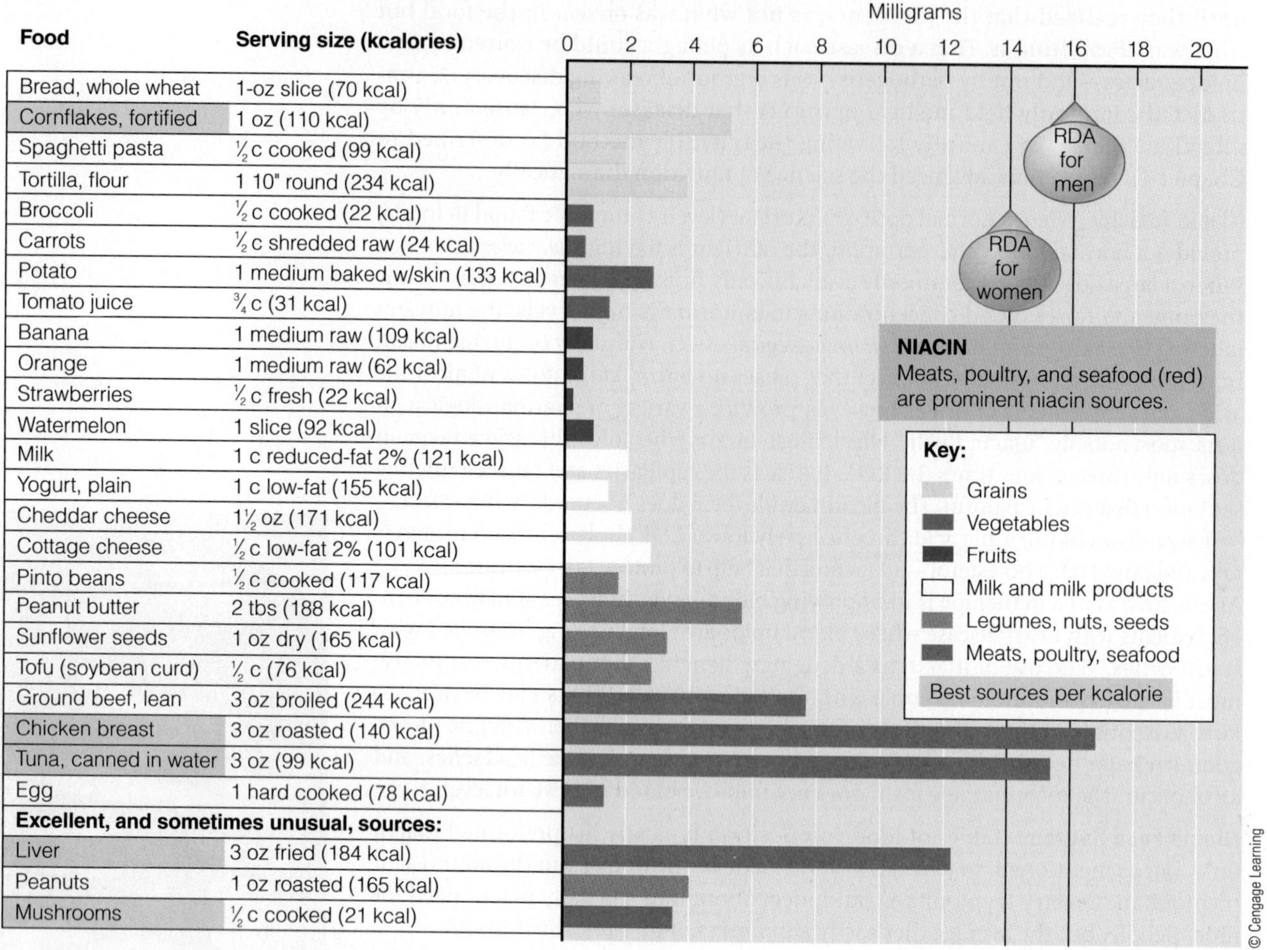

Food
Serving size (kcalories)
Milligrams
0 2 4 6 8 10 12 14 16 18 20
Bread, whole wheat | 1-oz slice (70 kcal)
Cornflakes, fortified | 1 oz (110 kcal)
Spaghetti pasta | ½ c cooked (99 kcal)
Tortilla, flour | 1 10" round (234 kcal)
Broccoli | ½ c cooked (22 kcal)
Carrots | ½ c shredded raw (24 kcal)
Potato | 1 medium baked w/skin (133 kcal)
Tomato juice | ¾ c (31 kcal)
Banana | 1 medium raw (109 kcal)
Orange | 1 medium raw (62 kcal)
Strawberries | ½ c fresh (22 kcal)
Watermelon | 1 slice (92 kcal)
Milk | 1 c reduced-fat 2% (121 kcal)
Yogurt, plain | 1 c low-fat (155 kcal)
Cheddar cheese | 1½ oz (171 kcal)
Cottage cheese | ½ c low-fat 2% (101 kcal)
Pinto beans | ½ c cooked (117 kcal)
Peanut butter | 2 tbs (188 kcal)
Sunflower seeds | 1 oz dry (165 kcal)
Tofu (soybean curd) | ½ c (76 kcal)
Ground beef, lean | 3 oz broiled (244 kcal)
Chicken breast | 3 oz roasted (140 kcal)
Tuna, canned in water | 3 oz (99 kcal)
Egg | 1 hard cooked (78 kcal)
Excellent, and sometimes unusual, sources:
Liver | 3 oz fried (184 kcal)
Peanuts | 1 oz roasted (165 kcal)
Mushrooms | ½ c cooked (21 kcal)
RDA for men
RDA for women
NIACIN
Meats, poultry, and seafood (red) are prominent niacin sources.
Key:
Grains
Vegetables
Fruits
Milk and milk products
Legumes, nuts, seeds
Meats, poultry, seafood
Best sources per kcalorie

> **FIGURE 10-8** **Niacin in Selected Foods**

Biotin Biotin plays an important role in metabolism as a coenzyme that carries activated carbon dioxide. This role is critical in the TCA cycle: biotin delivers a carbon to 3-carbon pyruvate, thus replenishing oxaloacetate, the 4-carbon compound needed to combine with acetyl CoA to keep the TCA cycle turning (review Figure 7-15 on p. 214). The biotin coenzyme also participates in gluconeogenesis, fatty acid synthesis, and the breakdown of certain fatty acids and amino acids.

Biotin Recommendations Biotin is needed in very small amounts. Because there is insufficient research on biotin requirements, an Adequate Intake (AI) has been determined, instead of an RDA.

Biotin Deficiency and Toxicity Biotin deficiencies rarely occur. Researchers can induce a biotin deficiency in animals or human beings by feeding them raw egg whites, which contain a protein that binds biotin and thus prevents its absorption.* Biotin-deficiency symptoms include skin rash, hair loss, and neurological impairment. More than two dozen raw egg whites must be consumed daily for several months to produce these effects; cooking eggs denatures the binding protein. Because no adverse effects have been reported from high biotin intakes, a UL has not been set.

Biotin Food Sources Biotin is widespread in foods (including egg yolks), so eating a variety of foods protects against deficiencies. Some biotin is also synthesized by GI tract bacteria, but this amount does not contribute much to the biotin absorbed. The accompanying table provides a summary of biotin.

biotin (BY-oh-tin): a B vitamin that functions as a coenzyme in metabolism.

*The protein *avidin* (AV-eh-din) in egg whites binds biotin.

› REVIEW IT Biotin

AI	**Deficiency Symptoms**
Adults: 30 μg/day	Depression, lethargy, hallucinations, numb or tingling sensation in the arms and legs; red, scaly rash around the eyes, nose, and mouth; hair loss
Chief Functions in the Body	**Toxicity Symptoms**
Part of a coenzyme used in energy metabolism, fat synthesis, amino acid metabolism, and glycogen synthesis	None reported
Significant Sources	
Widespread in foods; liver, egg yolks, soybeans, fish, whole grains; also produced by GI bacteria	

Pantothenic Acid

Pantothenic acid is part of the chemical structure of coenzyme A—the same CoA that forms acetyl CoA, a key compound in several metabolic pathways featured in Chapter 7, including the TCA cycle. (Appendix C presents the chemical structures of these two molecules and shows that coenzyme A is made up in part of pantothenic acid.) As such, it is involved in more than 100 different steps in the synthesis of lipids, neurotransmitters, steroid hormones, and hemoglobin.

Pantothenic Acid Recommendations An Adequate Intake (AI) for pantothenic acid has been set. It reflects the amount needed to replace daily losses.

Pantothenic Acid Deficiency and Toxicity Pantothenic acid deficiency is rare. Its symptoms involve a general failure of all the body's systems and include fatigue, GI distress, and neurological disturbances. The "burning feet" syndrome that affected prisoners of war in Asia during World War II is thought to have been caused by pantothenic acid deficiency. No toxic effects have been reported, and no UL has been established.

Pantothenic Acid Food Sources Pantothenic acid is widespread in foods, and typical diets seem to provide adequate intakes. Beef, poultry, whole grains, potatoes, tomatoes, and broccoli are particularly good sources. Losses of pantothenic acid during food production can be substantial because it is readily destroyed by the freezing, canning, and refining processes. The accompanying table provides a summary of pantothenic acid.

› REVIEW IT Pantothenic Acid

AI	**Deficiency Symptoms**
Adults: 5 mg/day	Vomiting, nausea, stomach cramps; insomnia, fatigue, depression, irritability, restlessness, apathy; hypoglycemia, increased sensitivity to insulin; numbness, muscle cramps, inability to walk
Chief Functions in the Body	**Toxicity Symptoms**
Part of coenzyme A, used in energy metabolism	None reported
Significant Sources	
Widespread in foods; chicken, beef, potatoes, oats, tomatoes, liver, egg yolk, broccoli, whole grains	
Easily destroyed by food processing	

Vitamin B_6

Vitamin B_6 occurs in three forms—pyridoxal, pyridoxine, and pyridoxamine. All three can be converted to the coenzyme PLP (pyridoxal phosphate), which is active in more than 100 reactions, including carbohydrate, fatty acid, and amino acid metabolism.[7] Because PLP can transfer amino groups (NH_2) from an amino acid to a keto acid, the body can make nonessential amino acids (review Figure 6-12 on p. 183). The ability to add and remove amino groups makes PLP valuable in protein and urea metabolism as well. The conversions of the amino acid tryptophan to niacin or to the neurotransmitter serotonin also depend on PLP.

pantothenic (PAN-toe-THEN-ick) **acid:** a B vitamin. The principal active form is part of coenzyme A, called "CoA" throughout Chapter 7.

- **pantos** = everywhere

vitamin B_6: a family of compounds—pyridoxal, pyridoxine, and pyridoxamine. The primary active coenzyme form is *PLP* (*pyridoxal phosphate*).

In addition, PLP participates in the synthesis of heme (the nonprotein portion of hemoglobin), nucleic acids (such as DNA and RNA), and lecithin (a phospholipid).

Vitamin B_6 Recommendations The RDA for vitamin B_6 is based on the amounts needed to maintain adequate levels of its coenzymes. Unlike other water-soluble vitamins, vitamin B_6 is stored extensively in muscle tissue. Research does not support claims, however, that large doses of vitamin B_6 enhance muscle strength or physical endurance.

Vitamin B_6 Deficiency Without adequate vitamin B_6, synthesis of key neurotransmitters diminishes, and abnormal compounds produced during tryptophan metabolism accumulate in the brain. Early symptoms of vitamin B_6 deficiency include depression and confusion; advanced symptoms include abnormal brain wave patterns and convulsions. Low levels of vitamin B_6 are associated with increased risks of some cancers and cardiovascular disease.[8]

Alcohol contributes to the destruction and loss of vitamin B_6 from the body. As Highlight 7 describes, when the body breaks down alcohol, it produces acetaldehyde. If allowed to accumulate, acetaldehyde dislodges the PLP coenzyme from its enzymes; once loose, PLP breaks down and is excreted.

Another drug that acts as a vitamin B_6 **antagonist** is isoniazid, a medication that inhibits the growth of the tuberculosis bacterium.* This drug has saved countless lives, but because isoniazid binds and inactivates vitamin B_6, it can induce a deficiency. Whenever isoniazid is used to treat tuberculosis, vitamin B_6 supplements must be given to protect against deficiency. Oral contraceptives also seem to decrease the body's vitamin B_6 reserves.[9]

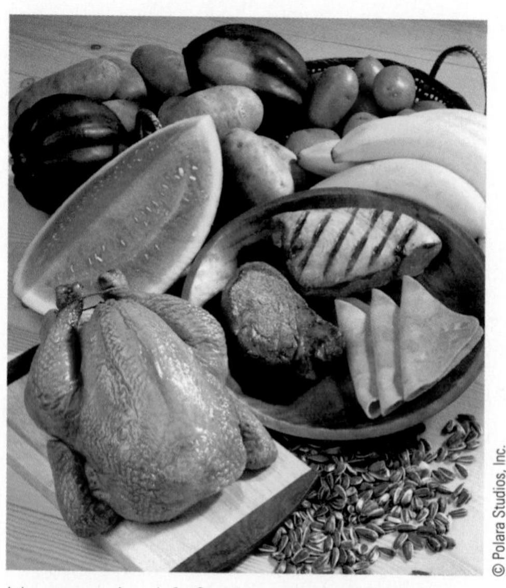

Most protein-rich foods such as meat, fish, and poultry provide ample vitamin B_6; some vegetables and fruits are good sources too.

Vitamin B_6 Toxicity The first major report of vitamin B_6 toxicity appeared in the early 1980s. Until that time, most researchers and dietitians believed that, like the other water-soluble vitamins, vitamin B_6 could not reach toxic concentrations in the body. The report described neurological damage in people who had been taking more than 2 *grams* of vitamin B_6 daily (20 times the current UL of 100 *milligrams* per day) for 2 months or more.

Vitamin B_6 Food Sources As you can see from the colors in Figure 10-9, meats, fish, and poultry (red bars), potatoes and a few other vegetables (green bars), and fruits (purple bars) offer vitamin B_6. As is true of most of the other vitamins, fruits and vegetables rank considerably higher when foods are judged by nutrient density (vitamin B_6 per kcalorie). Several servings of vitamin B_6–rich foods are needed to meet recommended intakes.

Foods lose vitamin B_6 when heated. Information is limited, but vitamin B_6 bioavailability from plant-derived foods seems to be lower than from animal-derived foods. Fiber does not appear to interfere with vitamin B_6 absorption. The accompanying table provides a summary of vitamin B_6.

› REVIEW IT Vitamin B_6

Other Names

Pyridoxine, pyridoxal, pyridoxamine

RDA

Adults (19–50 yr): 1.3 mg/day

UL

Adults: 100 mg/day

Chief Functions in the Body

Part of coenzymes PLP (pyridoxal phosphate) and PMP (pyridoxamine phosphate) used in amino acid and fatty acid metabolism; helps to convert tryptophan to niacin and to serotonin; helps to make red blood cells

Significant Sources

Meats, fish, poultry, potatoes and other starchy vegetables, legumes, noncitrus fruits, fortified cereals, liver, soy products

Easily destroyed by heat

Deficiency Symptoms

Scaly dermatitis; anemia (small-cell type);[a] depression, confusion, convulsions

Toxicity Symptoms

Depression, fatigue, irritability, headaches, nerve damage causing numbness and muscle weakness leading to an inability to walk and convulsions; skin lesions

[a]Small-cell-type anemia is called *microcytic anemia.*

antagonist: a competing factor that counteracts the action of another factor. When a drug displaces a vitamin from its site of action, the drug renders the vitamin ineffective and thus acts as a vitamin antagonist.

*Isoniazid (eye-so-NYE-uh-zid) is also known as INH (isonicotinic acid hydrazide).

> FIGURE 10-9 **Vitamin B_6 in Selected Foods**

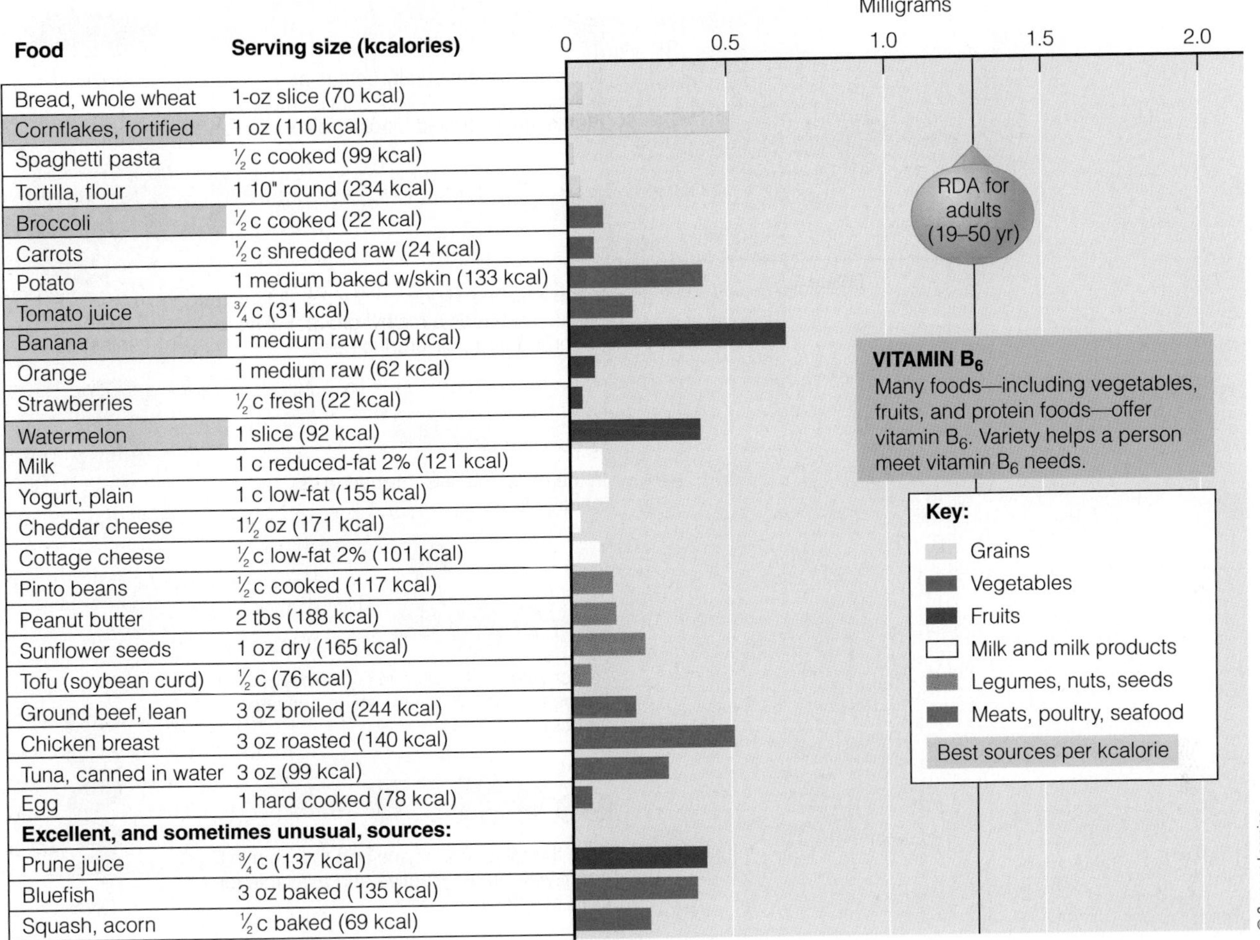

Folate Folate, also known as folacin or folic acid, has a chemical name that would fit a flying dinosaur: pteroylglutamic acid (PGA for short). Its primary coenzyme form, THF (tetrahydrofolate), serves as part of an enzyme complex that transfers 1-carbon compounds that arise during metabolism.[10] This action converts vitamin B_{12} to one of its coenzyme forms, synthesizes the DNA required for all rapidly growing cells, and regenerates the amino acid methionine from homocysteine.

Figure 10-10 (p. 316) summarizes folate's absorption, activation, and relationship with vitamin B_{12}. It explains that foods deliver folate mostly in the "bound" form—that is, combined with a string of amino acids (all glutamate), known as polyglutamate. (See Appendix C for the chemical structure.) Enzymes on the intestinal cell surfaces hydrolyze the polyglutamate to monoglutamate—folate with only one glutamate attached—and several single glutamates. The monoglutamate is then attached to a methyl group (CH_3) and delivered to the liver and other body cells. To activate folate, the methyl group must be removed by an enzyme that requires the help of vitamin B_{12}. Without that help, folate becomes trapped inside cells in its methyl form, unavailable to support DNA synthesis and cell growth.

The liver incorporates excess folate into bile that is then sent to the gallbladder and GI tract. Thus folate travels in the same enterohepatic circulation as bile (review Figure 5-14 on p. 144).

This complicated system for handling folate is vulnerable to GI tract injuries. Because folate is actively secreted back into the GI tract with bile, it can be

folate (FOLE-ate): a B vitamin; also known as folic acid, folacin, or pteroylglutamic (tare-o-EEL-glue-TAM-ick) acid (PGA). The coenzyme forms are *DHF (dihydrofolate)* and *THF (tetrahydrofolate)*.

> FIGURE 10-10 Folate's Absorption and Activation

COOH – CH₂ – CH₂ – CH – COOH, with O=C–NH– linking to ring structure

Ring structure + Glutamate

Folate

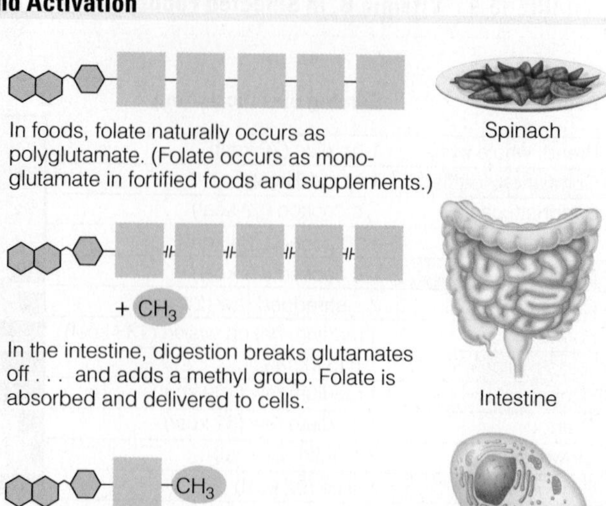

In foods, folate naturally occurs as polyglutamate. (Folate occurs as monoglutamate in fortified foods and supplements.)

In the intestine, digestion breaks glutamates off . . . and adds a methyl group. Folate is absorbed and delivered to cells.

$-CH_3$

In the cells, folate is trapped in its inactive form.

Cell

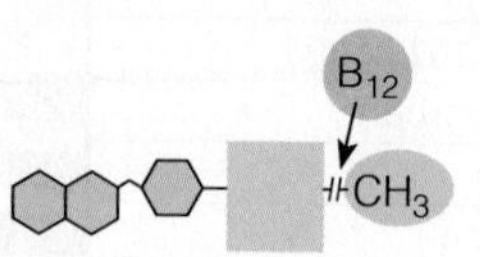

To activate folate, vitamin B_{12} removes and keeps the methyl group, which activates vitamin B_{12}.

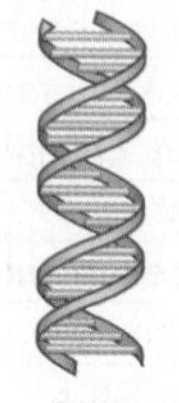

Both the folate coenzyme and the vitamin B_{12} coenzyme are now active and available for DNA synthesis.

reabsorbed repeatedly. If the GI tract cells are damaged, then folate is lost. Such is the case in alcohol abuse; folate deficiency rapidly develops and, ironically, further damages the GI tract. Remember, folate is active in cell multiplication—and the cells lining the GI tract are among the most rapidly replaced cells in the body. When unable to make new cells, the GI tract deteriorates and not only loses folate, but fails to absorb other nutrients as well.

Folate Recommendations The bioavailability of folate ranges from 50 percent for foods to 100 percent for supplements taken on an empty stomach. These differences in bioavailability must be considered when establishing folate recommendations.[11] The DRI committee gives naturally occurring folate from foods full credit. Synthetic folate from fortified foods and supplements is given extra credit because, on average, it is 1.7 times more available than naturally occurring food folate. Thus a person consuming 100 micrograms of folate from foods and 100 micrograms from a supplement (multiplied by 1.7) receives 270 **dietary folate equivalents (DFE).** The "How To" feature (p. 317) describes how to estimate dietary folate equivalents. The need for folate rises considerably during pregnancy and whenever cells are multiplying, so the recommendations for pregnant women are considerably higher than for other adults.

Folate and Neural Tube Defects The brain and spinal cord develop from the **neural tube,** and defects in its orderly formation during the early weeks of pregnancy may result in various central nervous system disorders and death. (Figure 15-5 in Chapter 15 includes an illustration of spina bifida, a neural tube defect.)

dietary folate equivalents (DFE): the amount of folate available to the body from naturally occurring sources, fortified foods, and supplements, accounting for differences in the bioavailability from each source.

- DFE = µg food folate + (1.7 × µg synthetic folate)

neural tube: the embryonic tissue that forms the brain and spinal cord.

>How To

Estimate Dietary Folate Equivalents

Folate is expressed in terms of DFE (dietary folate equivalents) because synthetic folate from supplements and fortified foods is absorbed at almost twice (1.7 times) the rate of naturally occurring folate from other foods. Use the following equation to calculate:

$$\text{DFE} = \mu\text{g food folate} + (1.7 \times \mu\text{g synthetic folate})$$

Consider, for example, a pregnant woman who takes a supplement and eats a bowl of fortified cornflakes, 2 slices of fortified bread, and a cup of fortified pasta. From the supplement and fortified foods, she obtains synthetic folate:

Supplement	100 µg folate
Fortified cornflakes	100 µg folate
Fortified bread	40 µg folate
Fortified pasta	60 µg folate
	300 µg folate

To calculate the DFE, multiply the amount of synthetic folate by 1.7:

$$300\ \mu\text{g} \times 1.7 = 510\ \mu\text{g DFE}$$

Now add the naturally occurring folate from the other foods in her diet—in this example, another 90 µg of folate.

$$510\ \mu\text{g DFE} + 90\ \mu\text{g} = 600\ \mu\text{g DFE}$$

Notice that if we had not converted synthetic folate from supplements and fortified foods to DFE, then this woman's intake would appear to fall short of the 600 µg recommendation for pregnancy (300 µg + 90 µg = 390 µg). But as our example shows, her intake does meet the recommendation. Recent revisions to food labels now list folate in µg DFE, making such calculations unnecessary.

› TRY IT Calculate how many dietary folate equivalents a person receives from 200 µg of folate from a supplement, 75 µg of folate from fortified cereal, and 120 µg of folate from other foods.

Folate supplements taken 1 month before conception and continued throughout the first trimester of pregnancy can help prevent **neural tube defects.** For this reason, all women of childbearing age who are capable of becoming pregnant should consume 0.4 milligram (400 micrograms) of folate daily—easily accomplished by eating folate-rich foods, folate-fortified foods, or a multivitamin supplement daily. Because half of the pregnancies each year are unplanned and because neural tube defects occur early in development before most women realize they are pregnant, the Food and Drug Administration (FDA) has mandated that grain products be fortified to deliver folate to the US population.* Labels on fortified products may claim that "adequate intake of folate has been shown to reduce the risk of neural tube defects." Fortification has improved folate status in women of childbearing age and lowered the prevalence rate of neural tube defects, as Figure 10-11 (p. 318) shows.

© Wellcome Trust Library/Custom Medical Stock Photo

Folate helps to protect against spina bifida, a neural tube defect characterized by the incomplete closure of the spinal cord and its bony encasement.

Some research suggests that folate taken before and during pregnancy may also prevent congenital birth defects, such as cleft lip and cleft palate, and neurodevelopmental disorders, such as autism.[12] Such findings strengthen recommendations for women to pay attention to their folate needs.

Folate fortification raises safety concerns as well. Because high intakes of folate can mask a vitamin B_{12} deficiency, folate consumption should not exceed 1 milligram daily without close medical supervision. The risks and benefits of folate fortification continue to be a topic of current debate, especially given that 5 percent of the US population exceed the UL for folate.[13]

neural tube defects: malformations of the brain, spinal cord, or both during embryonic development that often result in lifelong disability or death. The two main types of neural tube defects are *spina bifida* (literally "split spine") and *anencephaly* ("no brain").

*Bread products, flour, corn grits, cornmeal, farina, rice, macaroni, and noodles must be fortified with 140 micrograms of folate per 100 grams of grain. For perspective, 100 grams is roughly 3 slices of bread; 1 cup of flour; ½ cup of corn grits, cornmeal, farina, or rice; or ¾ cup of macaroni or noodles.

> **FIGURE 10-11 Decreasing Prevalence of Neural Tube Defects since Folate Fortification**

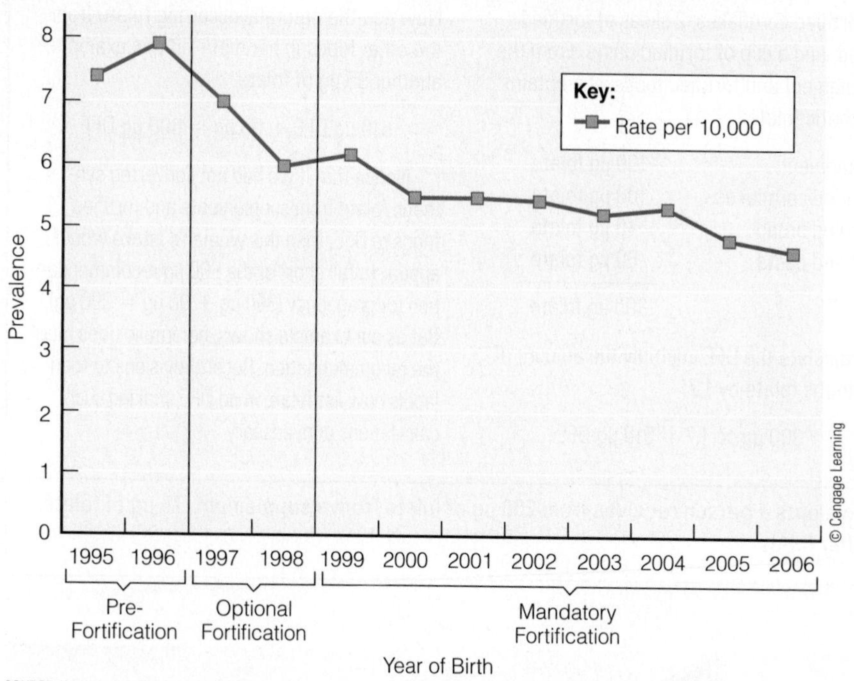

SOURCE: National Center for Health Statistics, Centers for Disease Control and Prevention, www.cdc.gov, updated January 2010.

Folate and Heart Disease The FDA's decision to fortify grain products with folate was strengthened by research suggesting a role for folate in protecting against heart disease.[14] One of folate's key roles in the body is to break down the amino acid homocysteine. Without folate, homocysteine accumulates, which seems to enhance formation of blood clots and atherosclerotic lesions. Fortified foods and folate supplements raise blood folate and reduce blood homocysteine, but do not seem to reduce the risk of heart attacks, strokes, or death from cardiovascular causes.[15]

Folate and Cancer Because the synthesis of DNA and the transfer of methyl groups depend on folate, its relationships with cancer are complex, depending on the type of cancer and the timing of folate supplementation. Some research suggests that sufficient folate may protect against the initiation of cancer, whereas other studies report that high intakes may enhance progression once cancer has begun.[16] In general, foods containing folate probably reduce the risk of pancreatic cancer.[17] Limited evidence suggests that folate may also reduce the risk of esophageal and colorectal cancer.[18]

Folate Deficiency Folate deficiency impairs cell division and protein synthesis—processes critical to growing tissues. In a folate deficiency, the replacement of red blood cells and GI tract cells falters. Not surprisingly, then, two of the first symptoms of a folate deficiency are **anemia** and GI tract deterioration.

The anemia of folate deficiency is known as *macrocytic* or *megaloblastic anemia* and is characterized by large, immature red blood cells (see Figure 10-12). Without folate, DNA damage destroys many of the red blood cells as they attempt to divide and mature. The result is fewer, but larger, red blood cells that cannot carry oxygen or travel through the capillaries as efficiently as normal red blood cells. Since the implementation of folate fortification in the United States, the prevalence of macrocytic anemia has decreased dramatically.[19]

Primary folate deficiencies may develop from inadequate intake and have been reported in infants who were fed goat's milk, which is notoriously low in folate. Secondary folate deficiencies may result from impaired absorption or an unusual metabolic need for the vitamin. Metabolic needs increase in situations where cell multiplication must speed up, such as pregnancies involving twins and triplets; cancer; skin-destroying diseases such as chicken pox and measles; and burns, blood loss, GI tract damage, and the like.

Of all the vitamins, folate appears to be most vulnerable to interactions with drugs, which can also lead to a secondary deficiency. Some medications, notably anticancer drugs, have a chemical structure similar to folate's structure and can displace the vitamin from enzymes and interfere with normal metabolism. Like all cells, cancer cells need the real vitamin to multiply—without it, they die. Unfortunately, anticancer drugs affect both cancerous cells and healthy cells, creating a folate deficiency for all cells. (Highlight 17 discusses nutrient-drug interactions, and Figure H17-1 illustrates the similarities between the vitamin folate and the anticancer drug methotrexate.)

anemia (ah-NEE-me-ah): literally, "too little blood." Anemia is any condition in which too few red blood cells are present, or the red blood cells are immature (and therefore large) or too small or contain too little hemoglobin to carry the normal amount of oxygen to the tissues. Anemia is not a disease itself but can be a consequence of many different disease conditions, including many nutrient deficiencies, bleeding, excessive red blood cell destruction, and defective red blood cell formation.

- **an** = without
- **emia** = blood

> **FIGURE 10-12 Normal Blood Cells and Blood Cells in Macrocytic Anemia Compared**

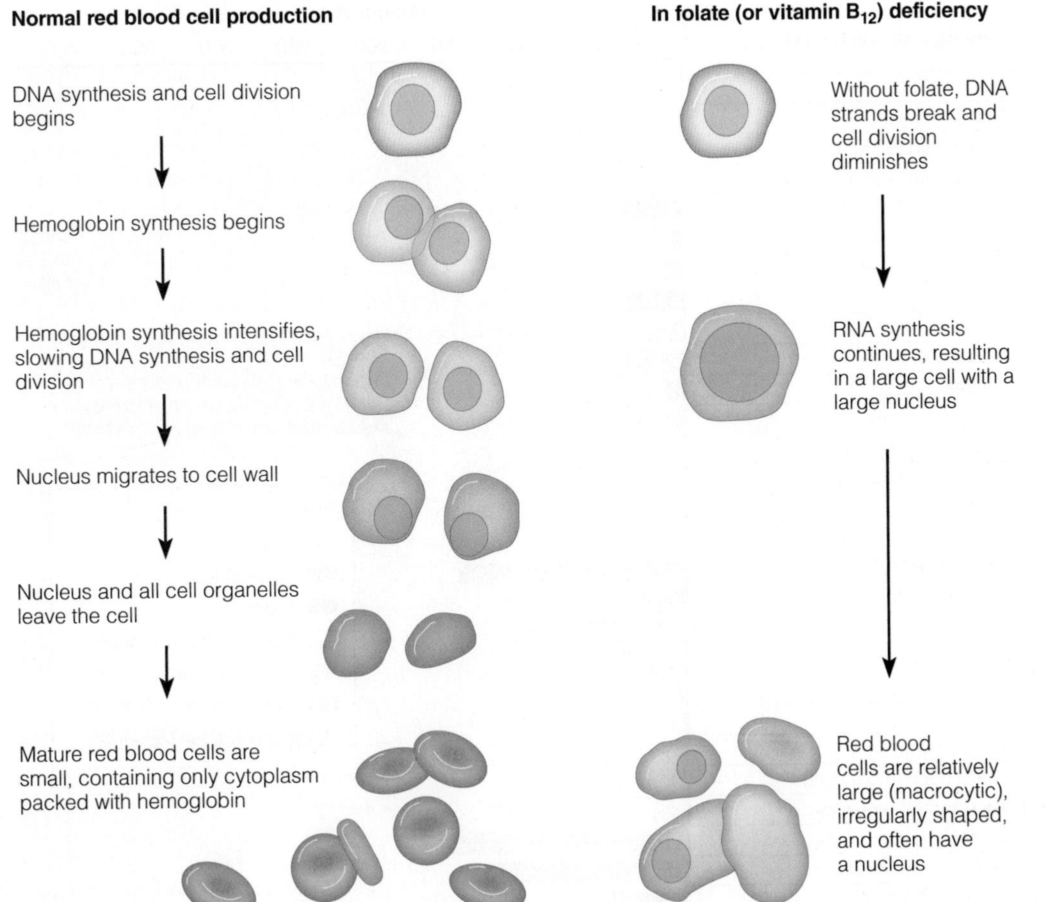

Normal red blood cell production
DNA synthesis and cell division begins
Hemoglobin synthesis begins
Hemoglobin synthesis intensifies, slowing DNA synthesis and cell division
Nucleus migrates to cell wall
Nucleus and all cell organelles leave the cell
Mature red blood cells are small, containing only cytoplasm packed with hemoglobin
In folate (or vitamin B_{12}) deficiency
Without folate, DNA strands break and cell division diminishes
RNA synthesis continues, resulting in a large cell with a large nucleus
Red blood cells are relatively large (macrocytic), irregularly shaped, and often have a nucleus

Aspirin and antacids also interfere with the body's folate status: aspirin inhibits the action of folate-requiring enzymes, and antacids limit the absorption of folate. Healthy adults who use these drugs to relieve an occasional headache or upset stomach need not be concerned, but people who rely heavily on aspirin or antacids should be aware of the nutrition consequences.

Folate Toxicity A UL has been established for folate from fortified foods or supplements (see the inside front cover). Commonly consumed amounts of folate from both natural sources and fortified foods appear to cause no harm. The small percentage of adults who also take high-dose folate supplements, however, can reach levels that are high enough to obscure a vitamin B_{12} deficiency and delay diagnosis of neurological damage.[20]

Folate Food Sources Figure 10-13 (p. 320) shows that folate is especially abundant in legumes, fruits, and vegetables. The vitamin's name suggests the word *foliage,* and indeed, dark green, leafy vegetables are outstanding sources. With fortification, grain products also contribute folate. The small red and white bars in Figure 10-13 indicate that meats and milk products are poor folate sources. Heat and oxidation during cooking and storage can destroy as much as half of the folate in foods. The table on p. 320 provides a summary of folate.

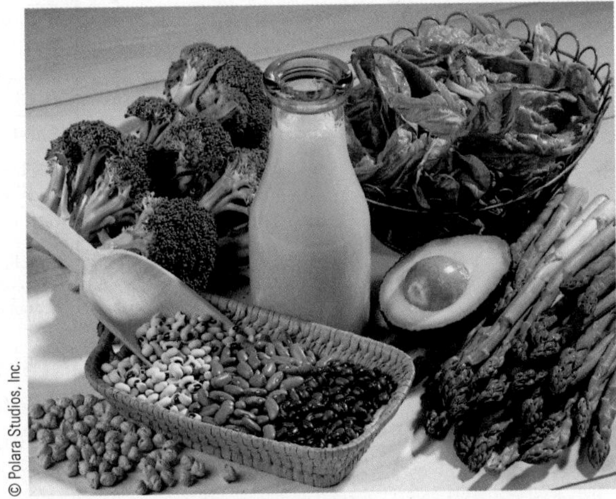

Dark green and leafy vegetables (such as spinach and broccoli), legumes (such as black beans, kidney beans, and black-eyed peas), liver, and some fruits (notably citrus fruits and juices) are naturally rich in folate.

> **FIGURE 10-13 Folate in Selected Foods**

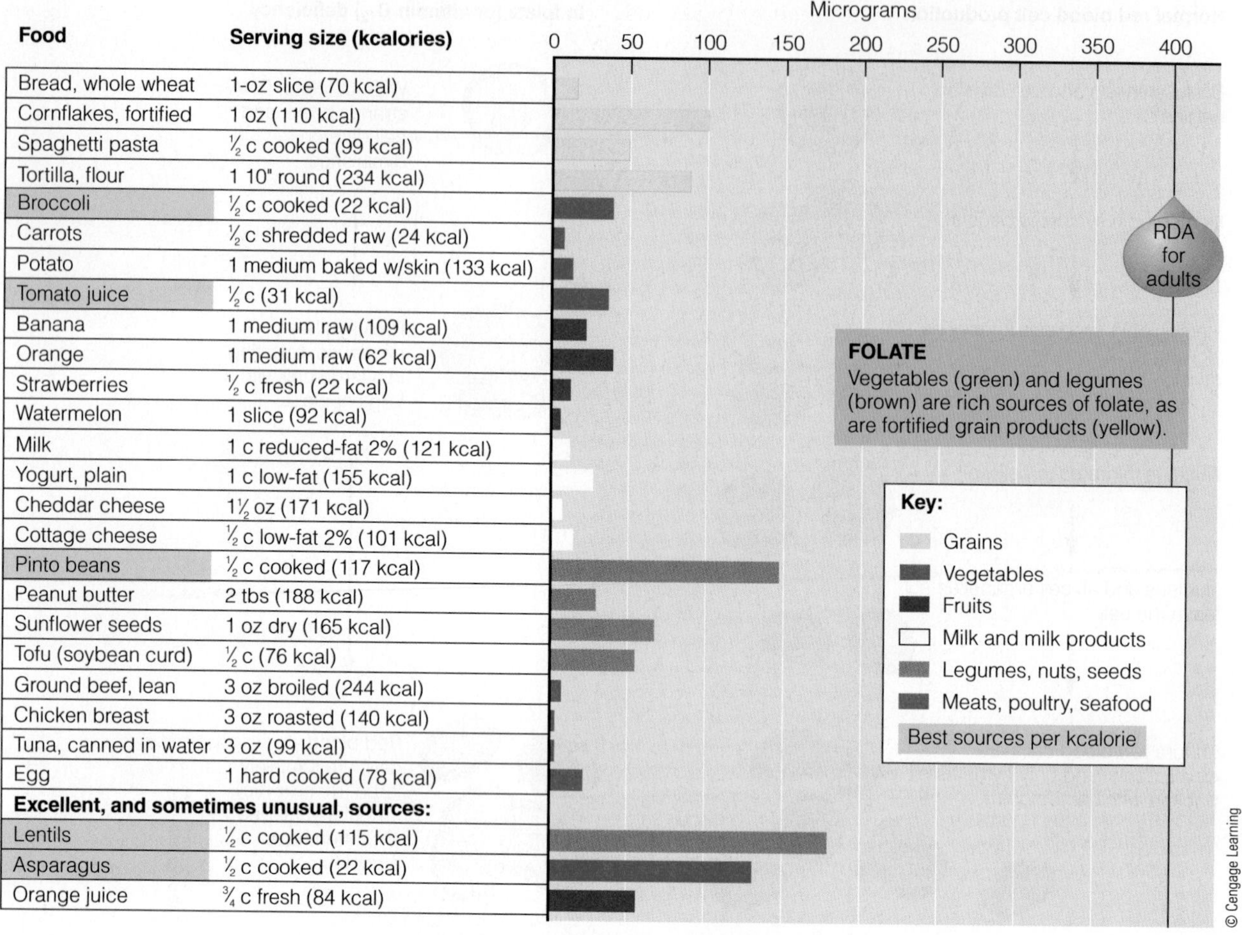

Food	Serving size (kcalories)
Bread, whole wheat	1-oz slice (70 kcal)
Cornflakes, fortified	1 oz (110 kcal)
Spaghetti pasta	½ c cooked (99 kcal)
Tortilla, flour	1 10" round (234 kcal)
Broccoli	½ c cooked (22 kcal)
Carrots	½ c shredded raw (24 kcal)
Potato	1 medium baked w/skin (133 kcal)
Tomato juice	½ c (31 kcal)
Banana	1 medium raw (109 kcal)
Orange	1 medium raw (62 kcal)
Strawberries	½ c fresh (22 kcal)
Watermelon	1 slice (92 kcal)
Milk	1 c reduced-fat 2% (121 kcal)
Yogurt, plain	1 c low-fat (155 kcal)
Cheddar cheese	1½ oz (171 kcal)
Cottage cheese	½ c low-fat 2% (101 kcal)
Pinto beans	½ c cooked (117 kcal)
Peanut butter	2 tbs (188 kcal)
Sunflower seeds	1 oz dry (165 kcal)
Tofu (soybean curd)	½ c (76 kcal)
Ground beef, lean	3 oz broiled (244 kcal)
Chicken breast	3 oz roasted (140 kcal)
Tuna, canned in water	3 oz (99 kcal)
Egg	1 hard cooked (78 kcal)
Excellent, and sometimes unusual, sources:	
Lentils	½ c cooked (115 kcal)
Asparagus	½ c cooked (22 kcal)
Orange juice	¾ c fresh (84 kcal)

› REVIEW IT Folate

Other Names

Folic acid, folacin, pteroylglutamic acid (PGA)

RDA

Adults: 400 µg/day

UL[a]

Adults: 1000 µg/day

Chief Functions in the Body

Part of coenzymes THF (tetrahydrofolate) and DHF (dihydrofolate) used in DNA synthesis and therefore important in new cell formation

Significant Sources

Fortified grains, leafy green vegetables, legumes, seeds, liver

Easily destroyed by heat and oxygen

Deficiency Symptoms

Anemia (large-cell type);[b] smooth, red tongue;[c] mental confusion, weakness, fatigue, irritability, headache; shortness of breath; elevated homocysteine

Toxicity Symptoms

Masks vitamin B_{12}–deficiency symptoms

[a]The UL applies to synthetic forms obtained from supplements, fortified foods, or a combination.
[b]Large-cell-type anemia is known as either *macrocytic* or *megaloblastic anemia*.
[c]Smoothness of the tongue is caused by loss of its surface structures and is termed *glossitis* (gloss-EYE-tis).

Vitamin B_{12}

Vitamin B_{12} and folate are closely related: each depends on the other for activation. Recall that vitamin B_{12} removes a methyl group to activate the folate coenzyme. When folate gives up its methyl group, the vitamin B_{12} coenzyme becomes activated (review Figure 10-10 on p. 316).

The regeneration of the amino acid methionine and the synthesis of DNA and RNA depend on both folate and vitamin B_{12}.* In addition, without any help from folate, vitamin B_{12} maintains the sheath that surrounds and protects nerve fibers

vitamin B_{12}: a B vitamin characterized by the presence of cobalt (see Figure 13-2). The active forms of coenzyme B_{12} are *methylcobalamin* and *deoxyadenosylcobalamin*.

*In the body, methionine serves as a methyl (CH_3) donor. In doing so, methionine can be converted to other amino acids. Some of these amino acids can regenerate methionine, but methionine is still considered an essential amino acid that is needed in the diet.

and promotes their normal growth. Bone cell activity and metabolism also depend on vitamin B_{12}.

The digestion and absorption of vitamin B_{12} depends on several steps. In the stomach, hydrochloric acid and the digestive enzyme pepsin release vitamin B_{12} from the proteins to which it is attached in foods. Then as vitamin B_{12} passes from the stomach to the small intestine, it binds with a stomach secretion called **intrinsic factor.** Bound together, intrinsic factor and vitamin B_{12} travel to the end of the small intestine, where receptors recognize the complex. Importantly, the receptors do not recognize vitamin B_{12} without intrinsic factor. The vitamin is gradually absorbed into the bloodstream as the intrinsic factor is degraded. Transport of vitamin B_{12} in the blood depends on specific binding proteins.

Like folate, vitamin B_{12} enters the enterohepatic circulation—continuously being secreted into bile and delivered to the intestine, where it is reabsorbed. Because most vitamin B_{12} is reabsorbed, healthy people rarely develop a deficiency even when their intake is minimal.

Vitamin B_{12} Recommendations The RDA for adults is only 2.4 micrograms of vitamin B_{12} a day—just over two-millionths of a gram. The ink in the period at the end of this sentence may weigh about that much. As tiny as this amount appears to the human eye, it contains billions of molecules of vitamin B_{12}, enough to provide coenzymes for all the enzymes that need its help.

Vitamin B_{12} Deficiency and Toxicity Most vitamin B_{12} deficiencies reflect inadequate absorption, not poor intake. Inadequate absorption typically occurs for one of two reasons: a lack of hydrochloric acid or a lack of intrinsic factor. Without hydrochloric acid, the vitamin is not released from the dietary proteins and so is not available for binding with the intrinsic factor. Without the intrinsic factor, the vitamin cannot be absorbed.

Vitamin B_{12} deficiency is common among the elderly. Many older adults develop **atrophic gastritis,** a condition that damages the cells of the stomach. Atrophic gastritis may also develop in response to iron deficiency or infection with *Helicobacter pylori,* the bacterium implicated in ulcer formation. Without healthy stomach cells, production of hydrochloric acid and intrinsic factor diminishes. Even with an adequate intake from foods, vitamin B_{12} status suffers. The vitamin B_{12} deficiency caused by atrophic gastritis and a lack of intrinsic factor is known as **pernicious anemia.**

Some people inherit a defective gene for the intrinsic factor. In such cases, or when the stomach has been injured and cannot produce enough of the intrinsic factor, vitamin B_{12} must be given by injection to bypass the need for intestinal absorption. Alternatively, the vitamin may be delivered by nasal spray; absorption is rapid, high, and well tolerated.

Because vitamin B_{12} is found primarily in foods derived from animals, people who follow a vegetarian diet may develop a vitamin B_{12} deficiency.[21] It may take several years for people who stop eating animal-derived foods to develop deficiency symptoms because the body recycles much of its vitamin B_{12}, reabsorbing it over and over again. Even when the body fails to absorb vitamin B_{12}, deficiency may take up to 3 years to develop because the body conserves its supply. Neurological degeneration, a sign of vitamin B_{12} deficiency, appears more rapidly in infants born to mothers with unsupplemented vegan diets or untreated pernicious anemia.

Because vitamin B_{12} is required to convert folate to its active form, one of the most obvious vitamin B_{12}–deficiency symptoms is the anemia commonly seen in folate deficiency. This anemia is characterized by large, immature red blood cells, which indicate slow DNA synthesis and an inability to divide (see Figure 10-12, p. 319). When folate is trapped in its inactive (methyl folate) form because of vitamin B_{12} deficiency or is unavailable because of folate deficiency itself, DNA synthesis slows.

First to be affected in a vitamin B_{12} or folate deficiency are the rapidly growing blood cells. Either vitamin B_{12} or folate will clear up the anemia, but if folate is given when vitamin B_{12} is needed, the result is disastrous: devastating neurological symptoms. Remember that vitamin B_{12}, but not folate, maintains the sheath that

intrinsic factor: a glycoprotein (a protein with short polysaccharide chains attached) secreted by the stomach cells that binds with vitamin B_{12} in the small intestine to aid in the absorption of vitamin B_{12}.

- **intrinsic** = on the inside

atrophic (a-TRO-fik) **gastritis** (gas-TRY-tis): chronic inflammation of the stomach accompanied by a diminished size and functioning of the mucous membranes and glands. This condition is also characterized by inadequate hydrochloric acid and intrinsic factor—two substances needed for vitamin B_{12} absorption.

- **atrophy** = wasting
- **gastro** = stomach
- **itis** = inflammation

pernicious (per-NISH-us) **anemia:** a blood disorder that reflects a vitamin B_{12} deficiency caused by lack of intrinsic factor and characterized by abnormally large and immature red blood cells. Other symptoms include muscle weakness and irreversible neurological damage.

- **pernicious** = destructive

surrounds and protects nerve fibers and promotes their normal growth. Folate "cures" the *blood* symptoms of a vitamin B_{12} deficiency, but cannot stop the *nerve* symptoms from progressing. By doing so, folate "masks" a vitamin B_{12} deficiency.

Marginal vitamin B_{12} deficiency impairs cognition.[22] Advanced neurological symptoms include a creeping paralysis that begins at the extremities and works inward and up the spine. Early detection and correction are necessary to prevent permanent nerve damage and paralysis. With sufficient folate in the diet, the neurological symptoms of vitamin B_{12} deficiency can develop without evidence of anemia and the cognitive decline is especially rapid. Such interactions between folate and vitamin B_{12} highlight some of the safety issues surrounding the use of supplements and the fortification of foods. No adverse effects have been reported for excess vitamin B_{12}, and no UL has been set.

Vitamin B_{12} Food Sources Vitamin B_{12} is unique among the vitamins in being found almost exclusively in foods derived from animals. Its bioavailability is greatest from milk and fish. Anyone who eats reasonable amounts of animal-derived foods is most likely to have an adequate intake, including vegetarians who use milk products or eggs. Vegans, who restrict all foods derived from animals, need a reliable source, such as vitamin B_{12}–fortified soy milk or vitamin B_{12} supplements. Yeast grown on a vitamin B_{12}–enriched medium and mixed with that medium provides some vitamin B_{12}, but yeast itself does not contain active vitamin B_{12}. Similarly, neither fermented soy products such as miso (a soybean paste) nor sea algae such as spirulina provide active vitamin B_{12}. Extensive research shows that the amounts listed on the labels of these plant products are inaccurate and misleading because the vitamin B_{12} is in an inactive, unavailable form.

As mentioned earlier, the water-soluble vitamins are particularly vulnerable to losses in cooking. For most of these nutrients, microwave heating minimizes losses as well as, or better than, traditional cooking methods. Such is not the case for vitamin B_{12}, however. Microwave heating inactivates vitamin B_{12}. To preserve this vitamin, use the oven or stovetop instead of a microwave to cook meats and milk products (major sources of vitamin B_{12}). The accompanying table provides a summary of vitamin B_{12}.

› REVIEW IT Vitamin B_{12}

Other Names

Cobalamin (and related forms)

RDA

Adults: 2.4 μg/day

Chief Functions in the Body

Part of coenzymes methylcobalamin and deoxyadenosylcobalamin used in new cell synthesis; helps to maintain nerve cells; reforms folate coenzyme; helps to break down some fatty acids and amino acids

Significant Sources

Foods of animal origin (meat, fish, poultry, shellfish, milk, cheese, eggs), fortified cereals

Easily destroyed by microwave cooking

Deficiency Disease

Pernicious anemia[a]

Deficiency Symptoms

Anemia (large-cell type);[b] fatigue, degeneration of peripheral nerves progressing to paralysis; sore tongue, loss of appetite, constipation

Toxicity Symptoms

None reported

[a]The name *pernicious anemia* refers to the vitamin B_{12} deficiency caused by atrophic gastritis and a lack of intrinsic factor, but not to that caused by inadequate dietary intake.

[b]Large-cell-type anemia is known as either *macrocytic* or *megaloblastic anemia*.

Choline Although not defined as a vitamin, choline is an essential nutrient that is commonly grouped with the B vitamins. The body uses choline to make the neurotransmitter acetylcholine and the phospholipid lecithin. During fetal development, choline supports the structure and function of the brain and spinal cord, by supporting neural tube closure and enhancing learning performance.

Choline Recommendations The body can make choline from the amino acid methionine, but without dietary choline, synthesis alone appears to be insufficient to meet the body's needs. For this reason, the DRI Committee established an Adequate Intake (AI) for choline.

Choline Deficiency and Toxicity Average choline intakes fall below the AI, but the impact of deficiencies are not fully understood. The UL for choline is based on its life-threatening effect in lowering blood pressure.

Choline Food Sources Choline is found in a variety of common foods such as milk, eggs, and peanuts and as part of lecithin, a food additive commonly used as an emulsifying agent (review Figure 5-8 on p. 140). The accompanying table provides a summary of choline.

› REVIEW IT Choline

AI

Men: 550 mg/day

Women: 425 mg/day

UL

Adults: 3500 mg/day

Chief Functions in the Body

Needed for the synthesis of the neurotransmitter acetylcholine and the phospholipid lecithin

Deficiency Symptoms

Liver damage

Toxicity Symptoms

Body odor, sweating, salivation, reduced growth rate, low blood pressure, liver damage

Significant Sources

Milk, liver, eggs, peanuts

Nonvitamins

Some substances have been mistaken for vitamins, but they are not essential nutrients. Among them are the compounds **inositol** and **carnitine,** which can be made by the body. Inositol is a part of cell membrane structures, and carnitine transports long-chain fatty acids from the cytosol to the mitochondria for oxidation. Other nonvitamins include PABA (para-aminobenzoic acid, a component of folate's chemical structure), the bioflavonoids (vitamin P or hesperidin), pyrroloquinoline quinone (methoxatin), orotic acid, lipoic acid, and ubiquinone (coenzyme Q_{10}). Other names erroneously associated with vitamins are "vitamin O" (oxygenated saltwater), "vitamin B_5" (another name for pantothenic acid), "vitamin B_{15}" (also called "pangamic acid," a hoax), and "vitamin B_{17}" (laetrile, an alleged "cancer cure" and not a vitamin or a cure by any stretch of the imagination—in fact, laetrile is a potentially dangerous substance).

Interactions among the B Vitamins

This chapter has described some of the impressive ways that vitamins work individually, as if their many actions in the body could easily be disentangled. In fact, it is often difficult to tell which vitamin is truly responsible for a given effect because the nutrients are interdependent; the presence or absence of one affects another's absorption, metabolism, and excretion. You have already seen this interdependence with folate and vitamin B_{12}.

Riboflavin and vitamin B_6 provide another example. One of the riboflavin coenzymes, FMN, assists the enzyme that converts vitamin B_6 to its coenzyme form PLP. Consequently, a severe riboflavin deficiency can impair vitamin B_6 activity. Thus a deficiency of one nutrient may alter the action of another. Furthermore, a deficiency of one nutrient may create a deficiency of another. For example, both riboflavin and vitamin B_6 (as well as iron) are required for the conversion of tryptophan to niacin. Consequently, an inadequate intake of either riboflavin or vitamin B_6 can diminish the body's niacin supply. These interdependent relationships are evident in many of the roles B vitamins play in the body.

B Vitamin Roles Figure 10-14 (p. 324) summarizes the metabolic pathways introduced in Chapter 7 and conveys an *impression* of the many ways B vitamins assist in

inositol (in-OSS-ih-tall): a nonessential nutrient that can be made in the body from glucose. Inositol is a part of cell membrane structures.

carnitine (CAR-neh-teen): a nonessential, nonprotein amino acid made in the body from lysine that helps transport fatty acids across the mitochondrial membrane.

> **FIGURE 10-14 Metabolic Pathways Involving B Vitamins**

These metabolic pathways are introduced in Chapter 7 and are presented here to highlight the many coenzymes that facilitate the reactions. These coenzymes depend on the following vitamins:

- NAD and NADP: niacin
- TPP: thiamin
- CoA: pantothenic acid
- B_{12}: vitamin B_{12}
- FMN and FAD: riboflavin
- THF: folate
- PLP: vitamin B_6
- Biotin

Pathways leading toward acetyl CoA and the TCA cycle are catabolic, and those leading toward amino acids, glycogen, and fat are anabolic. For further details, see Appendix C.

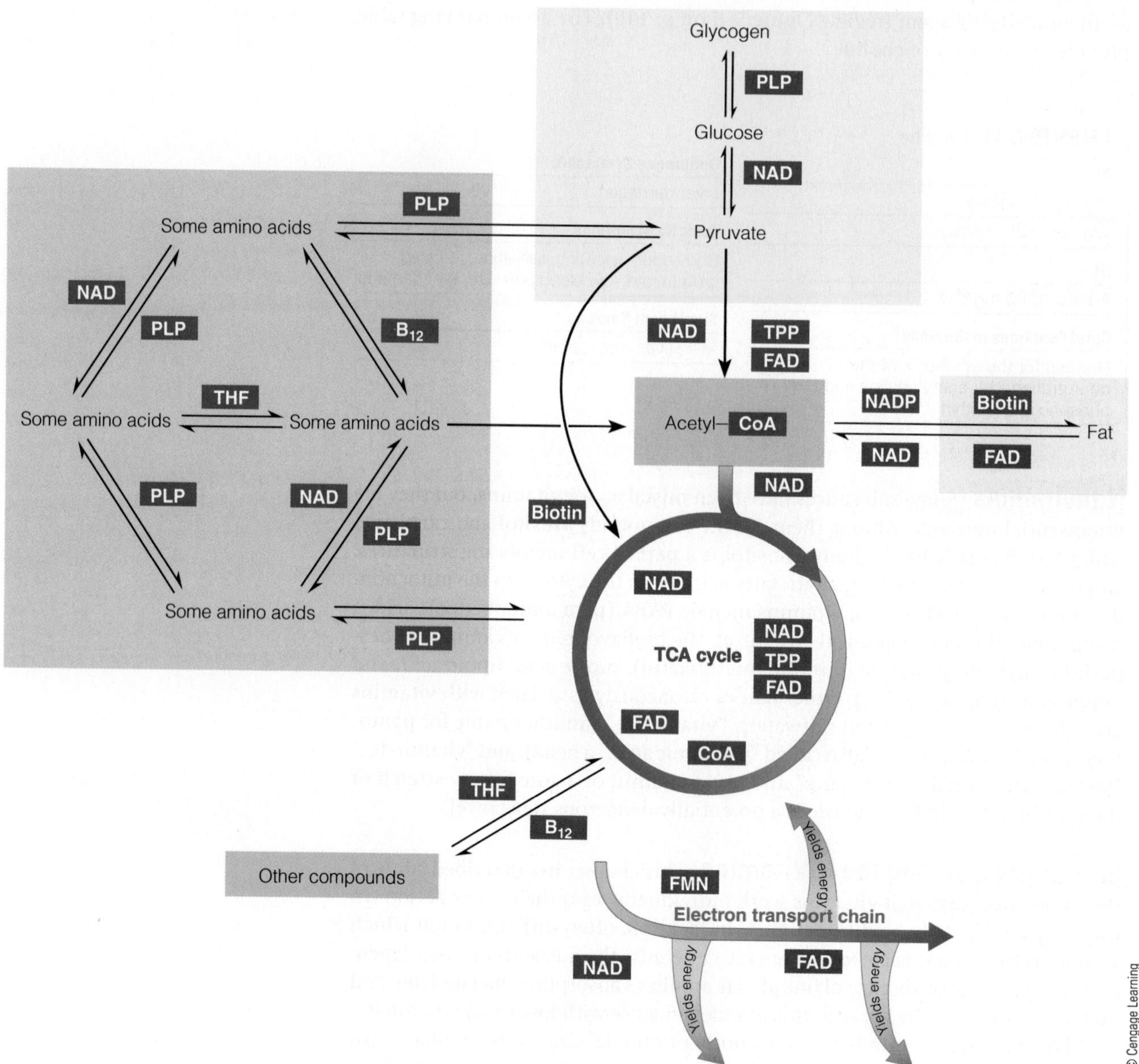

metabolic pathways. Metabolism is the body's work, and the B vitamin coenzymes are indispensable to every step. In scanning the pathways of metabolism depicted in the figure, note the many abbreviations for the coenzymes that keep the processes going.

Look at the now-familiar pathway of glucose breakdown. To break down glucose to pyruvate, the cells must have certain enzymes. For the enzymes to work, they must have the niacin coenzyme NAD. Cells can make NAD, but only if they have enough niacin (or enough of the amino acid tryptophan to make niacin).

The next step is the breakdown of pyruvate to acetyl CoA. The enzymes involved in this step require both NAD and the thiamin and riboflavin coenzymes

TPP and FAD, respectively. The cells can manufacture the enzymes they need from the vitamins, if the vitamins are in the diet.

Another coenzyme needed for this step is CoA. Predictably, the cells can make CoA except for an essential part that must be obtained in the diet—pantothenic acid. Another coenzyme requiring biotin serves the enzyme complex involved in converting pyruvate to oxaloacetate, the compound that combines with acetyl CoA to start the TCA cycle.

These and other coenzymes participate throughout all the metabolic pathways. Vitamin B_6 is an indispensable part of PLP—a coenzyme required for many amino acid conversions, for a crucial step in the making of the iron-containing portion of hemoglobin for red blood cells, and for many other reactions. Folate becomes THF—the coenzyme required for the synthesis of new genetic material and therefore new cells. The vitamin B_{12} coenzyme, in turn, regenerates THF to its active form; thus vitamin B_{12} is also necessary for the formation of new cells.

Thus each of the B vitamin coenzymes is involved, directly or indirectly, in energy metabolism. Some facilitate the energy-releasing reactions themselves; others help build new cells to deliver the oxygen and nutrients that allow the energy reactions to occur.

B Vitamin Deficiencies Now suppose the body's cells lack one of these B vitamins—niacin, for example. Without niacin, the cells cannot make NAD. Without NAD, the enzymes involved in every step of the glucose-to-energy pathway cannot function. Then, because all the body's activities require energy, literally everything begins to grind to a halt. This is no exaggeration. The deadly disease pellagra, caused by niacin deficiency, produces the "devastating four Ds": dermatitis, which reflects a failure of the skin; dementia, a failure of the nervous system; diarrhea, a failure of digestion and absorption; and eventually, as would be the case for any severe nutrient deficiency, death. These symptoms are the obvious ones, but a niacin deficiency affects all other organs, too, because all are dependent on the energy pathways.

All the vitamins are as essential as niacin. With any B vitamin deficiency, many body systems become deranged, and similar symptoms may appear. A lack of any of them can have disastrous and far-reaching effects.

Deficiencies of single B vitamins seldom show up in isolation, however. After all, people do not eat nutrients singly; they eat foods, which contain mixtures of nutrients. Only in two cases described earlier—beriberi and pellagra—have dietary deficiencies associated with single B vitamins been observed on a large scale in human populations. Even in these cases, several vitamins were lacking even though one vitamin stood out above the rest. When foods containing the vitamin known to be needed were provided, the other vitamins that were in short supply came as part of the package.

Major deficiency diseases of epidemic proportions such as pellagra and beriberi are no longer seen in the United States, but lesser deficiencies of nutrients, including the B vitamins, sometimes occur in people whose food choices are poor because of poverty, ignorance, illness, or poor health habits like alcohol abuse. (Review Highlight 7 to fully appreciate how alcohol induces vitamin deficiencies and interferes with energy metabolism.) Remember from Chapter 1 that deficiencies can arise not only from deficient intakes (primary causes), but also for other (secondary) reasons.

In identifying nutrient deficiencies, it is important to realize that a particular sign or symptom may not always have the same cause. The skin and the tongue (shown in Figure 10-15 on p. 326) appear to be especially sensitive to B vitamin deficiencies, but focusing on these body parts gives them undue emphasis. Both the skin and the tongue are readily visible in a physical examination.* The physician sees and reports the deficiency's outward signs, but the full impact of a vitamin deficiency occurs inside the cells of the body. If the skin develops a rash or lesions, other tissues beneath it may be degenerating too. Similarly, the mouth

*The two common signs of B vitamin deficiencies are *glossitis* (gloss-EYE-tis), an inflammation of the tongue, and *cheilosis* (kye-LOH-sis or kee-LOH-sis), a condition of reddened lips with cracks at the corners of the mouth.

> FIGURE 10-15 **B Vitamin–Deficiency Symptoms—The Smooth Tongue of Glossitis and the Skin Lesions of Cheilosis**

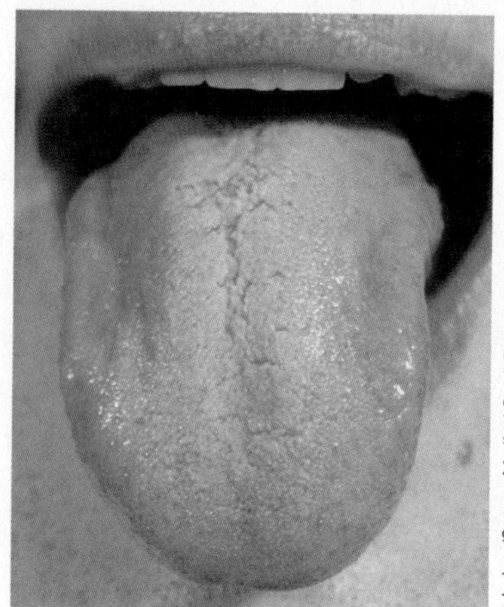

A healthy tongue has a rough and somewhat bumpy surface.

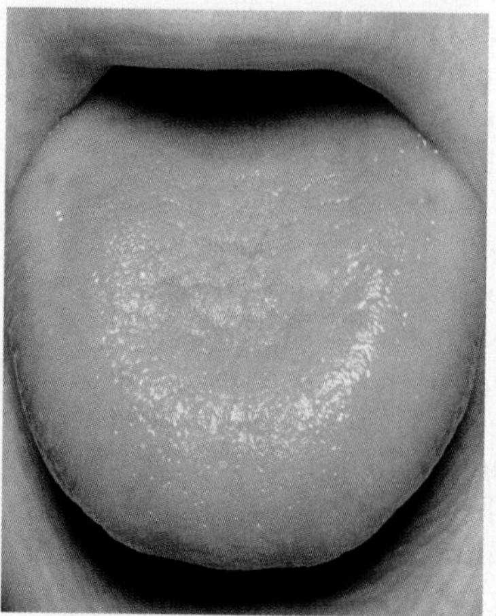

Pulschen/Custom Medical Stock Photo

In a B vitamin deficiency, the tongue becomes smooth and swollen due to atrophy of the tissue (glossitis).

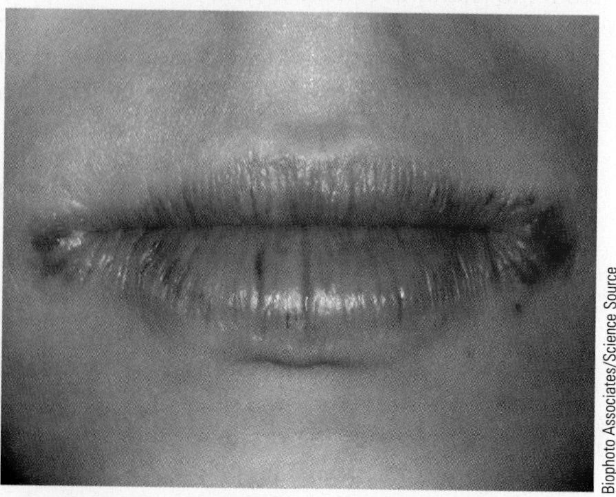

Science Photo Library/Science Source

Biophoto Associates/Science Source

In a B vitamin deficiency, the corners of the mouth become irritated and inflamed (cheilosis).

and tongue are the visible part of the digestive system; if they are abnormal, most likely the rest of the GI tract is as well.

Keep in mind that the cause of a sign or symptom is not always apparent. The summary tables in this chapter show that deficiencies of riboflavin, niacin, biotin, and vitamin B_6 can all cause skin rashes. So can a deficiency of protein, linoleic acid, or vitamin A. Because skin is on the outside and easy to see, it is a useful indicator of "things going wrong inside cells." By itself, a skin condition says nothing about its possible cause.

The same is true of anemia. Anemia is often caused by iron deficiency, but it can also be caused by a folate or vitamin B_{12} deficiency; by digestive tract failure to absorb any of these nutrients; or by such nonnutritional causes as infections, parasites, cancer, or loss of blood. No single nutrient will always cure a given symptom.

A person who feels chronically tired may be tempted to self-diagnose iron-deficiency anemia and self-prescribe an iron supplement. But this will relieve tiredness only if the cause is indeed iron-deficiency anemia. If the cause is a folate deficiency, taking iron will only prolong the fatigue. A person who is better informed may decide to take a vitamin supplement with iron, covering the possibility of a vitamin deficiency. But the symptom may have a nonnutritional cause. If the cause of the tiredness is actually hidden blood loss due to cancer, the postponement of a diagnosis may be life-threatening. When fatigue is caused by a lack of sleep, of course, no nutrient or combination of nutrients can replace a good night's rest. A person who is chronically tired should see a physician rather than self-prescribe. If the condition is nutrition-related, a registered dietitian nutritionist should be consulted as well.

B Vitamin Toxicities Toxicities of the B vitamins from foods alone are unknown, but they can occur when people overuse dietary supplements. With supplements, the quantities can quickly overwhelm the cells. Consider that one small capsule can easily deliver 2 milligrams of vitamin B_6, but it would take more than 3000 bananas, 6600 cups of rice, or 3600 chicken breasts to supply an equivalent amount. When the cells become oversaturated with a vitamin, they must work to eliminate the excess. The cells dispatch water-soluble vitamins to the urine for excretion, but sometimes they cannot keep pace with the onslaught. Homeostasis becomes disturbed and symptoms of toxicity develop.

B Vitamin Food Sources Significantly, deficiency diseases, such as beriberi and pellagra, were eliminated by providing foods. Dietary supplements advertise that vitamins are indispensable to life, but human beings obtained their nourishment from foods for centuries before supplements existed. If the diet lacks a vitamin, the first solution is to adjust food intake to obtain that vitamin.

The bar graphs of selected foods in this chapter, taken together, sing the praises of a balanced diet. The grains deliver thiamin, riboflavin, niacin, and folate. The fruit and vegetable groups excel in folate. Protein foods serve thiamin, niacin, vitamin B_6, and vitamin B_{12} well. The milk group stands out for riboflavin and vitamin B_{12}. A diet that offers a variety of foods from each group, prepared with reasonable care, serves up ample B vitamins.

› REVIEW IT Identify the main roles, deficiency symptoms, and food sources for each of the B vitamins.

The B vitamins serve as coenzymes that facilitate the work of every cell. They are active in carbohydrate, fat, and protein metabolism and in the making of DNA and thus new cells. Historically famous B vitamin–deficiency diseases are beriberi (thiamin), pellagra (niacin), and pernicious anemia (vitamin B_{12}). Pellagra can be prevented by an adequate protein intake because the amino acid tryptophan can be converted to niacin in the body. A high intake of folate can mask the blood symptoms of a vitamin B_{12} deficiency, but it will not prevent the associated nerve damage. Vitamin B_6 participates in amino acid metabolism and can be harmful in excess. Biotin and pantothenic acid serve important roles in energy metabolism and are common in a variety of foods. Many substances that people claim as B vitamins are not. Fortunately, a variety of foods from each of the food groups provides an adequate supply of all of the B vitamins.

10.3 Vitamin C

› LEARN IT Identify the main roles, deficiency symptoms, and food sources for vitamin C.

For many centuries, any man who joined the crew of a seagoing ship knew he had at best a 50–50 chance of returning alive—not because he might be slain by pirates or die in a storm, but because he might contract **scurvy.** As many as two-thirds of a ship's crew could die of scurvy during a long voyage. Only men on short voyages, especially around the Mediterranean Sea, were free of scurvy. No one knew the reason: that on long ocean voyages, the ship's cook used up the fresh fruits and vegetables early and then served only cereals and meats until the return to port.

In the mid-1700s, James Lind, a British physician serving in the navy, devised an experiment to find a cure for scurvy. He divided 12 sailors with scurvy into 6 pairs. Each pair received a different supplemental ration: cider, vinegar, sulfuric acid, seawater, oranges and lemons, or a strong laxative. Those receiving the citrus fruits quickly recovered, but sadly, it was almost 50 years before the British navy required all vessels to provide every sailor with lemon or lime juice daily. The tradition of providing British sailors with citrus juice daily to prevent scurvy gave them the nickname "limeys."

The antiscurvy "something" in citrus and other foods was dubbed the **antiscorbutic factor.** Centuries later, the factor was isolated and found to be a 6-carbon compound similar to glucose; it was named **ascorbic acid.**

Vitamin C Roles

Vitamin C parts company with the B vitamins in its mode of action. In some settings, vitamin C serves as a **cofactor** helping a specific enzyme perform its job, but in others, it acts as an antioxidant participating in more general ways.

As an Antioxidant Vitamin C loses electrons easily, a characteristic that allows it to perform as an antioxidant. In the body, **antioxidants** defend against free radicals. Free radicals are discussed fully in Highlight 11, but for now, a simple definition will suffice. A **free radical** is a molecule with one or more unpaired electrons, which makes it unstable and highly reactive. Antioxidants can neutralize free radicals by donating an electron or two. In doing so, antioxidants protect other substances from free radical damage. Figure 10-16 (p. 328) illustrates how vitamin C can give up electrons and then accept them again to become reactivated. This recycling of vitamin C

scurvy: the vitamin C–deficiency disease.

antiscorbutic (AN-tee-skor-BUE-tik) **factor:** the original name for vitamin C.
- **anti** = against
- **scorbutic** = causing scurvy

ascorbic acid: one of the two active forms of vitamin C (see Figure 10-16). Many people refer to vitamin C by this name.
- **a** = without
- **scorbic** = having scurvy

cofactor: a small, inorganic or organic substance that facilitates the action of an enzyme.

antioxidants: in the body, substances that significantly decrease the adverse effects of free radicals on normal physiological functions.

free radical: an unstable molecule with one or more unpaired electrons.

> FIGURE 10-16 **Active Forms of Vitamin C**

The two hydrogens highlighted in yellow give vitamin C its acidity and its ability to act as an antioxidant.

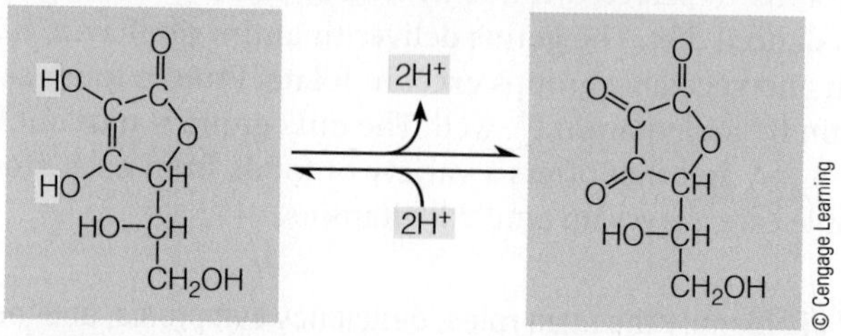

Ascorbic acid protects against oxidative damage by donating its two hydrogens with their electrons to free radicals (molecules with unpaired electrons). In doing so, ascorbic acid becomes dehydroascorbic acid.

Dehydroascorbic acid can readily accept hydrogens to become ascorbic acid. The reversibility of this reaction is key to vitamin C's role as an antioxidant.

is key to limiting losses and maintaining a reserve of antioxidants in the body. Other key antioxidant nutrients include vitamin E, beta-carotene, and selenium.

Vitamin C is like a bodyguard for water-soluble substances; it stands ready to sacrifice its own life to save theirs. In the cells and body fluids, vitamin C protects tissues from the **oxidative stress** of free radicals and thus may play an important role in preventing diseases.[23] In the intestines, vitamin C enhances iron absorption by protecting iron from oxidation. (Chapter 13 provides more details about the relationship between vitamin C and iron.)

As a Cofactor in Collagen Formation Vitamin C helps to form the fibrous structural protein of connective tissues known as **collagen.** Collagen serves as the matrix on which bones and teeth are formed. When a person is wounded, collagen glues the separated tissues together, forming scars. Cells are held together largely by collagen; this is especially important in the walls of the blood vessels, which must withstand the pressure of blood surging with each beat of the heart.

Chapter 6 describes how the body makes proteins by stringing together chains of amino acids. During the synthesis of collagen, each time a proline or lysine is added to the growing protein chain, an enzyme hydroxylates it (adds an OH group), making the amino acid hydroxyproline or hydroxylysine, respectively. These two special amino acids facilitate the binding together of collagen fibers to make strong, ropelike structures. The conversion of proline to hydroxyproline requires both vitamin C and iron. Iron works as a cofactor in the reaction, and vitamin C protects iron from oxidation, thereby allowing iron to perform its duty. Without vitamin C and iron, the hydroxylation step does not occur.

As a Cofactor in Other Reactions Vitamin C also serves as a cofactor in the synthesis of several other compounds. As in collagen formation, vitamin C helps in the hydroxylation of carnitine, a compound that transports fatty acids, especially long-chain fatty acids, across the inner membrane of mitochondria in cells. It also participates in the conversions of the amino acids tryptophan and tyrosine to the neurotransmitters serotonin and norepinephrine, respectively. Vitamin C also assists in the making of hormones, including thyroxine, which regulates the metabolic rate; when metabolism speeds up in times of extreme physical stress, the body's use of vitamin C increases.

In Stress Among the stresses known to increase vitamin C needs are infections; burns; extremely high or low temperatures; intakes of toxic heavy metals such as lead, mercury, and cadmium; the chronic use of certain medications, including aspirin, barbiturates, and oral contraceptives; and cigarette smoking. During stress, the adrenal glands—which contain more vitamin C than any other organ in the body—release vitamin C and hormones into the blood.*

*High amounts of vitamin C are also found in the pituitary glands; medium amounts in the liver, spleen, heart, kidneys, lungs, pancreas, and white blood cells; and small amounts in the muscles and red blood cells.

oxidative stress: a condition in which the production of oxidants and free radicals exceeds the body's ability to handle them and prevent damage.

collagen: the structural protein from which connective tissues such as scars, tendons, ligaments, and the foundations of bones and teeth are made.

When immune system cells are called into action, they use a great deal of oxygen and produce free radicals. In this case, free radicals are helpful. They act as ammunition in an "oxidative burst" that demolishes the offending viruses and bacteria and destroys the damaged cells. Vitamin C steps in as an antioxidant to control this oxidative activity.

In the Prevention and Treatment of the Common Cold Vitamin C has been a popular option for the prevention and treatment of the common cold for decades, but research supporting such claims has been conflicting and controversial. Some studies find no relationship between vitamin C and the occurrence of the common cold, whereas others report modest benefits—fewer colds, fewer days, and shorter duration of severe symptoms, especially for those exposed to physical and environmental stresses. A review of the research on vitamin C in the treatment and prevention of the common cold reveals a slight, but consistent reduction in the duration of the common cold in favor of those taking a daily dose of at least 200 milligrams of vitamin C. The question for consumers to consider is, "Is this enough to warrant routine daily supplementation?"

Discoveries about how vitamin C works in the body provide possible links between the vitamin and the common cold. Anyone who has ever had a cold knows the discomfort of a runny or stuffed-up nose. Nasal congestion develops in response to elevated blood **histamine,** and people commonly take antihistamines for relief. Like an antihistamine, vitamin C comes to the rescue and deactivates histamine.

In Disease Prevention Whether vitamin C may help in preventing or treating cancer, heart disease, cataract, and other diseases is still being studied, and findings are presented in Highlight 11's discussion on antioxidants. Conducting research in the United States can be difficult, however, because diets typically contribute enough vitamin C to provide optimal health benefits.

Vitamin C Recommendations

For decades, vitamin C ranked at the top of dietary supplement sales. How much vitamin C does a person need? As is true of all the vitamins, recommendations are set generously above the minimum requirement to prevent deficiency disease and well below the toxicity level (see Figure 10-17).

The requirement—the amount needed to prevent the overt symptoms of scurvy—is only 10 milligrams daily. Consuming 10 milligrams a day does not saturate all the body tissues, however; higher intakes will increase the body's total vitamin C. At about 100 milligrams per day, 95 percent of the population reaches tissue saturation. (For perspective, 1 cup of orange juice provides more than 100 milligrams of vitamin C.) Recommendations are slightly lower, based on the amounts needed to provide antioxidant protection. At about 200 milligrams, absorption reaches a maximum, and there is little, if any, increase in blood concentrations at higher doses. Excess vitamin C is readily excreted.

As mentioned earlier, cigarette smoking increases the need for vitamin C. Cigarette smoke contains oxidants, which greedily deplete this potent antioxidant. Exposure to cigarette smoke, especially when accompanied by low dietary intakes of vitamin C, depletes the body's vitamin C in both active and passive smokers. People who chew tobacco also have low levels of vitamin C. Because people who smoke cigarettes regularly suffer significant oxidative stress, their requirement for vitamin C is increased an additional 35 milligrams; nonsmokers regularly exposed to cigarette smoke should also be sure to meet their RDA for vitamin C. Smokers are among those most likely to suffer vitamin C deficiency.

Vitamin C Deficiency

Early signs of nutrient deficiencies can be difficult to recognize. Two of the most notable signs of a vitamin C deficiency reflect its role in maintaining the integrity of blood vessels. The gums bleed easily around the teeth, and capillaries under the skin break spontaneously, producing pinpoint hemorrhages (see Figure 10-18 on p. 330).

> FIGURE 10-17 **Vitamin C Intake (mg/day)**

Recommendations for vitamin C are set generously above the minimum requirement and well below the toxicity level.

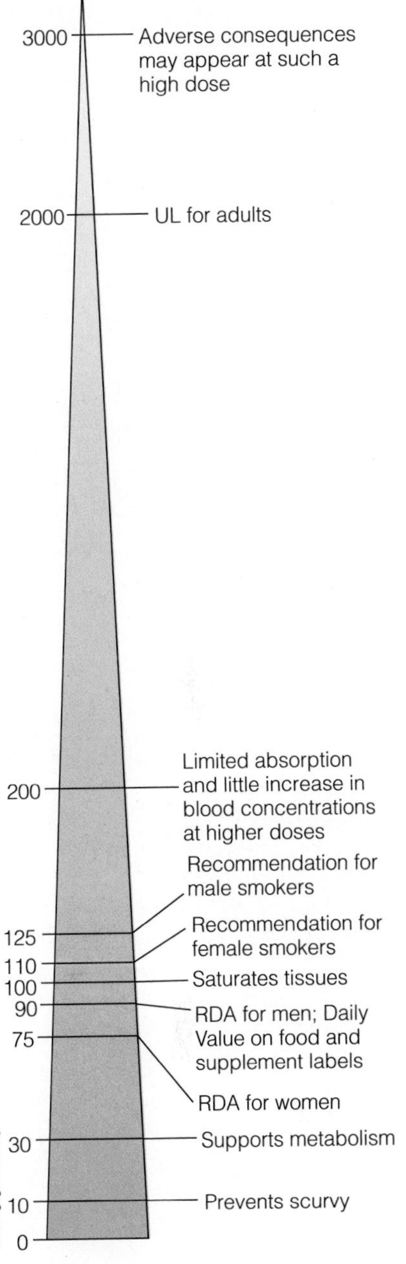

histamine (HISS-tah-mean or HISS-tah-men): a substance produced by cells of the immune system as part of a local immune reaction to an antigen.

> FIGURE 10-18 **Vitamin C–Deficiency Symptoms—Scorbutic Gums and Pinpoint Hemorrhages**

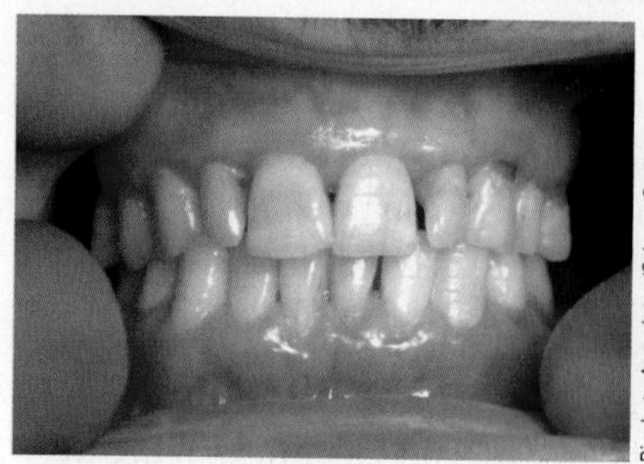

Biophoto Associates/Science Source

Scorbutic gums. Unlike other lesions of the mouth, scurvy presents a symmetrical appearance without infection.

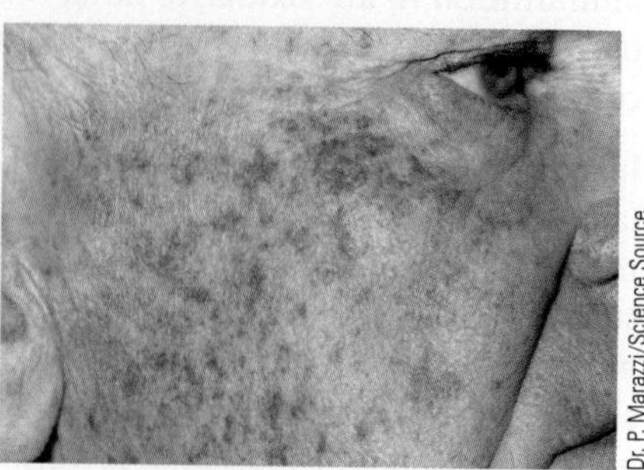

Dr. P. Marazzi/Science Source

Pinpoint hemorrhages. Small red spots appear in the skin, indicating spontaneous bleeding internally.

When vitamin C concentrations fall to about a fifth of optimal levels (this may take more than a month on a diet lacking vitamin C), scurvy symptoms begin to appear. Inadequate collagen synthesis causes further hemorrhaging. Muscles, including the heart muscle, degenerate. The skin becomes rough, brown, scaly, and dry. Wounds fail to heal because scar tissue will not form. Bone rebuilding falters; the ends of the long bones become softened, malformed, and painful, and fractures develop. The teeth become loose as the cartilage around them weakens. Anemia and infections are common. There are also characteristic psychological signs, including hysteria and depression. Sudden death is likely, caused by massive internal bleeding.

Once diagnosed, scurvy is readily resolved by increasing vitamin C intake. Moderate doses in the neighborhood of 100 milligrams per day are sufficient, curing the scurvy within about 5 days. Such an intake is easily achieved by including vitamin C–rich foods in the diet.

Vitamin C Toxicity

The availability of vitamin C supplements and the publication of books recommending vitamin C to prevent colds and cancer have led many people to take large doses of vitamin C. Not surprisingly, side effects of vitamin C supplementation such as gastrointestinal distress and diarrhea have been reported. The UL for vitamin C was established based on these symptoms.

Several instances of interference with medical regimens are also known. Large amounts of vitamin C excreted in the urine obscure the results of tests used to detect glucose or ketones in the diagnosis of diabetes. In some instances, excess vitamin C gives a **false positive** result; in others, a **false negative.** People taking anticlotting medications may unwittingly counteract the effect if they also take massive doses of vitamin C. Those with kidney disease, a tendency toward gout, or a genetic abnormality that alters vitamin C's breakdown to its excretion products are prone to forming kidney stones if they take large doses of vitamin C.* Vitamin C supplements may adversely affect people with iron overload. As Chapter 13 explains, vitamin C enhances iron absorption and releases iron from body stores; too much free iron causes the kind of cellular damage typical of free radicals. These adverse consequences illustrate how vitamin C can act as a *pro*oxidant when quantities exceed the body's needs.

Vitamin C Food Sources

Fruits and vegetables can easily provide a generous amount of vitamin C. A cup of orange juice at breakfast, a salad for lunch, and a stalk of broccoli and a potato for dinner alone provide more than 300 milligrams. (For perspective, review Figure 10-17, p. 329.) Clearly, a person making such food choices does not need vitamin C supplements.

Figure 10-19 shows the amounts of vitamin C in various common foods. The overwhelming abundance of purple and green bars reveals not only that the

*Vitamin C is inactivated and degraded by several routes, and sometimes oxalate, which can form kidney stones, is produced along the way. People may also develop oxalate crystals in their kidneys regardless of vitamin C status.

false positive: a test result indicating that a condition is present (positive) when in fact it is not present (therefore false).

false negative: a test result indicating that a condition is not present (negative) when in fact it is present (therefore false).

> FIGURE 10-19 Vitamin C in Selected Foods

Food	Serving size (kcalories)
Bread, whole wheat	1-oz slice (70 kcal)
Cornflakes, fortified	1 oz (110 kcal)
Spaghetti pasta	½ c cooked (99 kcal)
Tortilla, flour	1 10" round (234 kcal)
Broccoli	½ c cooked (22 kcal)
Carrots	½ c shredded raw (24 kcal)
Potato	1 medium baked w/skin (133 kcal)
Tomato juice	¾ c (31 kcal)
Banana	1 medium raw (109 kcal)
Orange	1 medium raw (62 kcal)
Strawberries	½ c fresh (22 kcal)
Watermelon	1 slice (92 kcal)
Milk	1 c reduced-fat 2% (121 kcal)
Yogurt, plain	1 c low-fat (155 kcal)
Cheddar cheese	1½ oz (171 kcal)
Cottage cheese	½ c low-fat 2% (101 kcal)
Pinto beans	½ c cooked (117 kcal)
Peanut butter	2 tbs (188 kcal)
Sunflower seeds	1 oz dry (165 kcal)
Tofu (soybean curd)	½ c (76 kcal)
Ground beef, lean	3 oz broiled (244 kcal)
Chicken breast	3 oz roasted (140 kcal)
Tuna, canned in water	3 oz (99 kcal)
Egg	1 hard cooked (78 kcal)
Excellent, and sometimes unusual, sources:	
Red bell pepper	½ c raw chopped (20 kcal)
Kiwi	1 (46 kcal)
Brussels sprouts	½ c cooked (30 kcal)

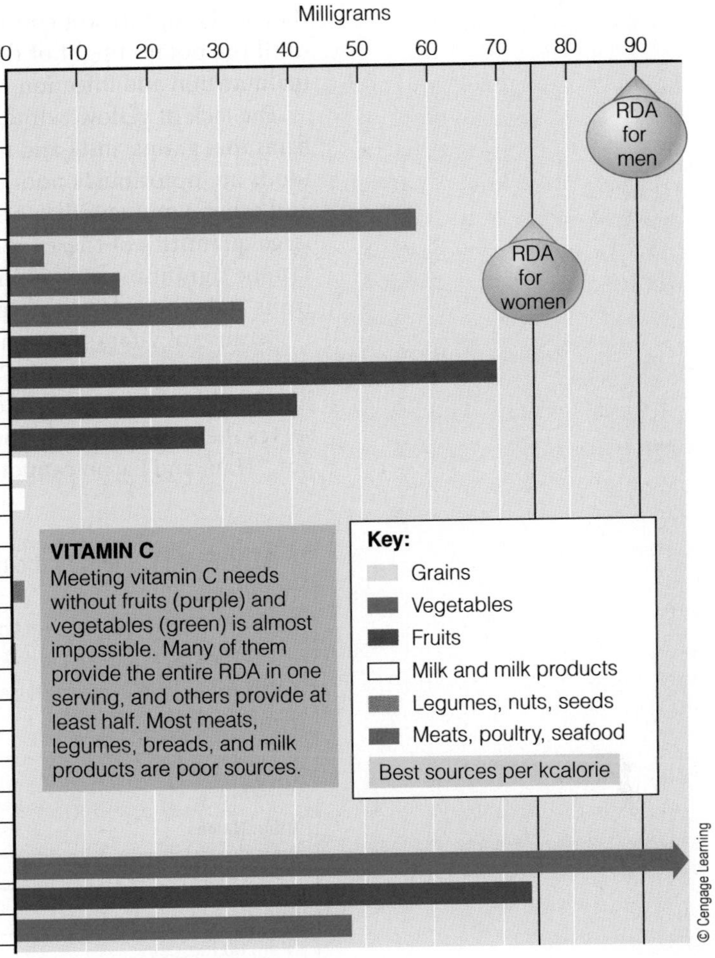

citrus fruits are justly famous for being rich in vitamin C, but that other fruits and vegetables are in the same league. A half cup of broccoli, bell pepper, or strawberries provides more than 50 milligrams of the vitamin (and an array of other nutrients). Because vitamin C is vulnerable to heat, raw fruits and vegetables usually have a higher nutrient density than their cooked counterparts. Similarly, because vitamin C is readily destroyed by oxygen, foods and juices should be stored properly and consumed within a week of opening.

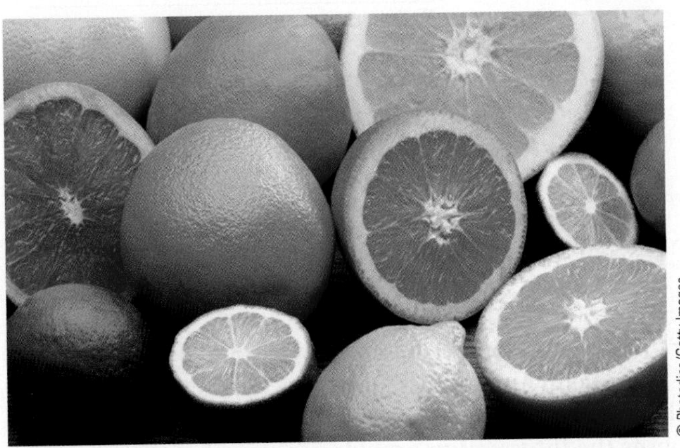

When dietitians say "vitamin C," people think "citrus fruits" . . .

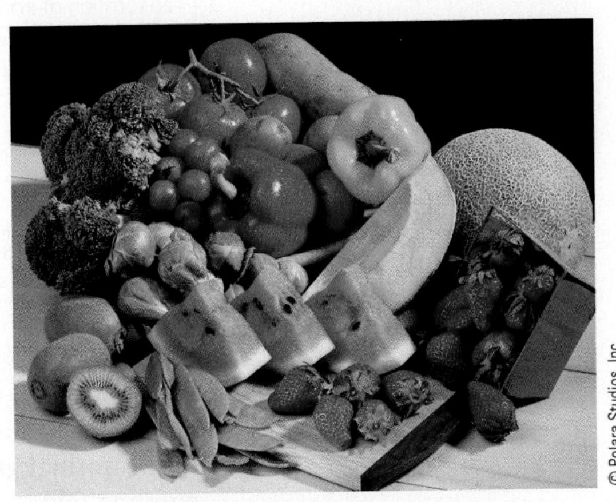

. . . but these foods are also rich in vitamin C.

The potato is an important source of vitamin C, not because one potato by itself meets the daily need, but because potatoes are such a common staple that they make significant contributions. In fact, scurvy was unknown in Ireland until the potato blight of the mid-1840s, when some 2 million people died of malnutrition and infection.

The lack of yellow, white, brown, and red bars in Figure 10-19 (p. 331) confirms that grains, milk and milk products (except breast milk), and most protein foods are notoriously poor sources of vitamin C. Organ meats (liver, kidneys, and others) and raw meats contain some vitamin C, but most people don't eat large quantities of these foods. Raw meats and fish contribute enough vitamin C to be significant sources in parts of Alaska, Canada, and Japan, but elsewhere fruits and vegetables are necessary to supply sufficient vitamin C.

Because of vitamin C's antioxidant property, food manufacturers sometimes add a variation of vitamin C to some beverages and most cured meats, such as luncheon meats, to prevent oxidation and spoilage. This compound safely preserves these foods, but it does not have vitamin C activity in the body. Simply put, "Ham and bacon cannot replace fruits and vegetables."

› REVIEW IT Identify the main roles, deficiency symptoms, and food sources for vitamin C.

Vitamin C acts primarily as an antioxidant and a cofactor. Recommendations are set well above the amount needed to prevent the deficiency disease scurvy. A variety of fruits and vegetables—most notably citrus fruits—provide generous amounts of vitamin C. The accompanying table provides a summary of vitamin C.

Vitamin C

Other Names	Ascorbic acid
RDA	Men: 90 mg/day Women: 75 mg/day Smokers: +35 mg/day
UL	Adults: 2000 mg/day
Chief Functions in the Body	Collagen synthesis (strengthens blood vessel walls, forms scar tissue, provides matrix for bone growth), antioxidant, thyroxine synthesis, amino acid metabolism, strengthens resistance to infection, helps in absorption of iron
Significant Sources	Citrus fruits, cabbage-type vegetables (such as brussels sprouts and cauliflower), dark green vegetables (such as bell peppers and broccoli), cantaloupe, strawberries, lettuce, tomatoes, potatoes, papayas, mangoes Easily destroyed by heat and oxygen
Deficiency Disease	Scurvy
Deficiency Symptoms	Anemia (small-cell type),[a] atherosclerotic plaques, pinpoint hemorrhages; bone fragility, joint pain; poor wound healing, frequent infections; bleeding gums, loosened teeth; muscle degeneration, pain, hysteria, depression; rough skin, blotchy bruises
Toxicity Symptoms	Nausea, abdominal cramps, diarrhea; headache, fatigue, insomnia; hot flashes; rashes; interference with medical tests, aggravation of gout symptoms, urinary tract problems, kidney stones[b]

[a]Small-cell-type anemia is *microcytic anemia*.

[b]People with kidney disease, a tendency toward gout, or a genetic abnormality that alters the breakdown of vitamin C are prone to forming kidney stones. Vitamin C is inactivated and degraded by several routes, sometimes producing oxalate, which can form stones in the kidneys.

Vita means life. After this discourse on the vitamins, who could dispute that they deserve their name? Their regulation of metabolic processes makes them vital to the normal growth, development, and maintenance of the body. The accompanying table condenses the information provided in this chapter for a quick review. The remarkable roles of the vitamins continue in the next chapter.

› REVIEW IT The Water-Soluble Vitamins

Vitamin and Chief Functions	Deficiency Symptoms	Toxicity Symptoms	Food Sources
Thiamin Part of coenzyme TPP in energy metabolism	Beriberi (edema or muscle wasting), anorexia, weight loss, neurological disturbances, muscular weakness, heart enlargement and failure	None reported	Enriched, fortified, or whole-grain products; pork
Riboflavin Part of coenzymes FAD and FMN in energy metabolism	Inflammation of the mouth, skin, and eyelids	None reported	Milk products; enriched, fortified, or whole-grain products; liver
Niacin Part of coenzymes NAD and NADP in energy metabolism	Pellagra (diarrhea, dermatitis, and dementia)	Niacin flush, liver damage, impaired glucose tolerance	Protein-rich foods
Biotin Part of coenzyme in energy metabolism	Skin rash, hair loss, neurological disturbances	None reported	Widespread in foods; GI bacteria synthesis
Pantothenic acid Part of coenzyme A in energy metabolism	Digestive and neurological disturbances	None reported	Widespread in foods
Vitamin B_6 Part of coenzymes used in amino acid and fatty acid metabolism	Scaly dermatitis, depression, confusion, convulsions, anemia	Nerve degeneration, skin lesions	Protein-rich foods
Folate Activates vitamin B_{12}; helps synthesize DNA for new cell growth	Anemia, glossitis, neurological disturbances, elevated homocysteine	Masks vitamin B_{12} deficiency	Legumes, vegetables, fortified grain products
Vitamin B_{12} Activates folate; helps synthesize DNA for new cell growth; protects nerve cells	Anemia; nerve damage and paralysis	None reported	Foods derived from animals
Vitamin C Synthesis of collagen, carnitine, hormones, neurotransmitters; antioxidant	Scurvy (bleeding gums, pinpoint hemorrhages, abnormal bone growth, and joint pain)	Diarrhea, GI distress	Fruits and vegetables

Nutrition Portfolio

To obtain all the vitamins you need each day, be sure to select from a variety of foods from all the food groups. Go to Diet & Wellness Plus and choose one of the days on which you have tracked your diet for the entire day. Go to the Intake vs. Goals report. Near the bottom of this report, you will see all of the vitamins grouped together; using this section of the report for reference, answer the following questions:

- How was your vitamin intake overall?
- Did you consume too much or too little of any vitamin?
- Which vitamins concerned you most?

Next go to the Intake Spreadsheet report, and looking at each of the vitamins, answer the following questions:

- Which of your foods provided high intakes of vitamins?
- Which of your foods provided few or no vitamins?
- How do your daily choices of whole or enriched grains, dark green vegetables, citrus fruits, and legumes contribute to your vitamin intakes?

- If you are a woman of childbearing age, how many dietary folate equivalents did you receive from folate-rich foods, fortified foods, and supplements? How does this compare to your RDA?
- How do your vitamin intakes from supplements compare with their UL?

DIET & WELLNESS PLUS To complete this exercise, go to your Diet & Wellness Plus at **www.cengagebrain.com.**

› STUDY IT To review the key points of this chapter and take a practice quiz, go to the study cards at the end of the book.

REFERENCES

1. A. Piro and coauthors, Casimir Funk: His discovery of the vitamins and their deficiency disorders, *Annals of Nutrition and Metabolism* 57 (2010): 85–88.
2. H. M. Said, Intestinal absorption of water-soluble vitamins in health and disease, *Biochemical Journal* 437 (2011): 357–372.
3. S. S. Jhala and A. S. Hazell, Modeling neurodegenerative disease pathophysiology in thiamine deficiency: Consequences of impaired oxidative metabolism, *Neurochemistry International* 58 (2011): 248–260.
4. J. E. Digby, N. Ruparelia, and R. P. Choudhury, Niacin in cardiovascular disease: Recent preclinical and clinical developments, *Arteriosclerosis, Thrombosis, and Vascular Biology* 32 (2012): 582–588; J. C. Creider, R. A. Hegele, and T. R. Joy, Niacin: Another look at an underutilized lipid-lowering medication, *Nature Reviews: Endocrinology* 8 (2012): 517–528; J. M. Backes, R. J. Padley, and P. M. Moriarty, Important considerations for treatment with dietary supplement versus prescription niacin products, *Postgraduate Medicine* 123 (2011): 70–83.
5. K. M. Ali and coauthors, Cardiovascular risk and HDL cholesterol, *British Journal of Pharmacology* 167 (2012): 1177–1194; M. R. Kolber, N. Ivers, and G. M. Allan, Niacin added to statins for cardiovascular disease, *Canadian Family Physician* 58 (2012): 842; The AIM-HIGH Investigators, Niacin in patients with low HDL cholesterol levels receiving intensive statin therapy, *New England Journal of Medicine* 365 (2011): 2255–2267.
6. D. MacKay, J. Hathcock, and E. Guarneri, Niacin: Chemical forms, bioavailability, and health effects, *Nutrition Reviews* 70 (2012): 357–366.
7. F. G. Bowling, Pyridoxine supply in human development, *Seminars in Cell and Developmental Biology* 22 (2011): 611–618.
8. S. C. Larsson, N. Orsini, and A. Wolk, Vitamin B_6 and risk of colorectal cancer: A meta-analysis of prospective studies, *Journal of the American Medical Association* 303 (2010): 1077–1083; J. Shen and coauthors, Association of vitamin B-6 status with inflammation, oxidative stress, and chronic inflammatory conditions: The Boston Puerto Rican Health Study, *American Journal of Clinical Nutrition* 91 (2010): 337–342.
9. S. M. C. Wilson and coauthors, Oral contraceptive use: Impact on folate, vitamin B_6, and vitamin B_{12} status, *Nutrition Reviews* 69 (2011): 572–583.
10. A. S. Tibbetts and D. R. Appling, Compartmentalization of mammalian folate-mediated one-carbon metabolism, *Annual Review of Nutrition* 30 (2010): 57–81.
11. M. A. Caudill, Folate bioavailability: Implications for establishing dietary recommendations and optimizing status, *American Journal of Clinical Nutrition* 91 (2010): 1455S–1460S.
12. P. Surén and coauthors, Association between maternal use of folic acid supplements and risk of autism spectrum disorders in children, *Journal of the American Medical Association* 309 (2013): 570–577; R. J. Berry, K. S. Crider, and M. Yeargin-Allsopp, Periconceptional folic acid and risk of autism spectrum disorders, *Journal of American Medical Association* 309 (2013): 611–612; R. J. Schmidt and coauthors, Maternal periconceptional folic acid intake and risk of autism spectrum disorders and developmental delay in the CHARGE (CHildhood Autism Risks from Genetics and Environment) case-control study, *American Journal of Clinical Nutrition* 96 (2012): 80–89; S. H. Blanton and coauthors, Folate pathway and nonsyndromic cleft lip and palate, *Birth Defects Research, Part A, Clinical and Molecular Teratology* 91 (2011): 50–60.
13. P. Verhoef, New insights on the lowest dose for mandatory folic acid fortification? *American Journal of Clinical Nutrition* 93 (2011): 1–2; R. L. Bailey and coauthors, Total folate and folic acid intake from foods and dietary supplements in the United States: 2003–2006, *American Journal of Clinical Nutrition* 91 (2010): 231–237.
14. R. Cui and coauthors, Dietary folate and vitamin B6 and B12 intake in relation to mortality from cardiovascular diseases: Japan collaborative cohort study, *Stroke* 41 (2010): 1285–1289; A. Imamura and coauthors, Low folate levels may be an atherogenic factor regardless of homocysteine levels in young healthy nonsmokers, *Metabolism* 59 (2010): 728–733.
15. J. M. Artmitage and the Study of Effectiveness of Additional Reductions in Cholesterol and Homocysteine (SEARCH) Collaborative Group, Effects of homocysteine-lowering with folic acid plus vitamin B_{12} vs placebo on mortality and major morbidity in myocardial infarction survivors: A randomized trial, *Journal of the American Medical Association* 303 (2010): 2486–2494; P. Tighe and coauthors, A dose-finding trial of the effect of the long-term folic acid intervention: Implications for food fortification policy, *American Journal of Clinical Nutrition* 93 (2011): 11–18.
16. J. B. Mason, Folate consumption and cancer risk: A confirmation and some reassurance, but we're not out of the woods yet, *American Journal of Clinical Nutrition* 94 (2011): 965–966; V. L. Stevens and coauthors, Folate and other one-carbon metabolism-related nutrients and risk of postmenopausal breast cancer in the Cancer Prevention Study II Nutrition Cohort, *American Journal of Clinical Nutrition* 91 (2010): 1708–1715.
17. B. M. Oaks and coauthors, Folate intake, post-folic acid grain fortification, and pancreatic cancer risk in the Prostate, Lung, Colorectal, and Ovarian Cancer Screening Trial, *American Journal of Clinical Nutrition* 91 (2010): 449–455.
18. T. M. Gibson and coauthors, Pre- and postfortification intake of folate and risk of colorectal cancer in a large prospective cohort study in the United States, *American Journal of Clinical Nutrition* 94 (2011): 1053–1062; J. E. Lee and coauthors, Folate intake and risk of colorectal cancer and adenoma: Modification by time, *American Journal of Clinical Nutrition* 93 (2011): 817–825.
19. O. A. Odewole and coauthors, Near-elimination of folate-deficiency anemia by mandatory folic acid fortification in older US adults: Reasons for Geographic and Racial Differences in Stroke study 2003–2007, *American Journal of Clinical Nutrition* 98 (2013): 1042–1047; Centers for Disease Control and Prevention, *Second National Report on Biochemical Indicators of Diet and Nutrition in the U.S. Population, 2012: Executive Summary*, www.cdc.gov/nutritionreport.
20. R. L. Bailey and coauthors, Total folate and folic acid intake from foods and dietary supplements in the United States: 2003–2006, *American Journal of Clinical Nutrition* 91 (2010): 231–237; Q. Yang and coauthors, Folic acid source, usual intake, and folate and vitamin B-12 status in US adults: National Health and Nutrition Examination Survey (NHANES) 2003–2006, *American Journal of Clinical Nutrition* 91 (2010): 64–72.
21. R. Pawlak and coauthors, How prevalent is vitamin B_{12} deficiency among vegetarians? *Nutrition Reviews* 71 (2013): 110–117.
22. M. S. Morris, J. Selhub, and P. F. Jacques, Vitamin B-12 and folate status in relation to decline in scores on the Mini-Mental State Examination in the Framingham Heart Study, *Journal of the American Geriatrics Society* 60 (2012): 1457–1464.
23. M. G. Traber and J. F. Stevens, Vitamins C and E: Beneficial effects from a mechanistic perspective, *Free Radical Biology and Medicine* 51 (2011): 1000–1013.

HIGHLIGHT > 10
Vitamin and Mineral Supplements

› LEARN IT Present arguments for and against the use of dietary supplements.

An estimated 75,000 supplements are currently on the US market. More than half of the adults in the United States take a **dietary supplement** regularly, spending almost $24 billion each year.[1] Many people take supplements as dietary insurance—in case they are not meeting their nutrient needs from foods alone. Others take supplements as health insurance—to protect against certain diseases.

An estimated 40 percent of US adults take multivitamin-mineral supplements regularly. Others take large doses of single nutrients, most commonly, vitamin D and calcium. In many cases, taking supplements is a costly but harmless practice; sometimes, it is both costly and harmful to health.[2]

For the most part, people self-prescribe supplements, taking them on the advice of friends, advertisements, websites, or books that may or may not be reliable. Sometimes, they take supplements on the recommendation of a physician. When such advice follows a valid nutrition assessment, supplementation may be warranted, but even then the preferred course of action is to improve food choices and eating habits.[3] Without an assessment, the advice to take supplements may be inappropriate. A registered dietitian nutritionist can help with the decision.

When people think of dietary supplements, they often think of vitamins, but a diet that lacks vitamins probably lacks several minerals as well. This highlight asks several questions related to vitamin-mineral supplements. (The accompanying glossary defines dietary supplements and related terms.) What are the arguments *for* taking supplements? What are the arguments *against* taking them? Finally, if people do take supplements, how can they choose the appropriate ones? (Amino acid supplements and herbal supplements are discussed in Chapter 6 and Highlight 18, respectively.)

Arguments for Supplements

Vitamin-mineral supplements may be appropriate in some circumstances. In some cases, they can prevent or correct deficiencies; in others, they can reduce the risk of diseases. Consumers should discuss supplement use with their health-care providers, who can help monitor for adverse effects or nutrient-drug interactions.

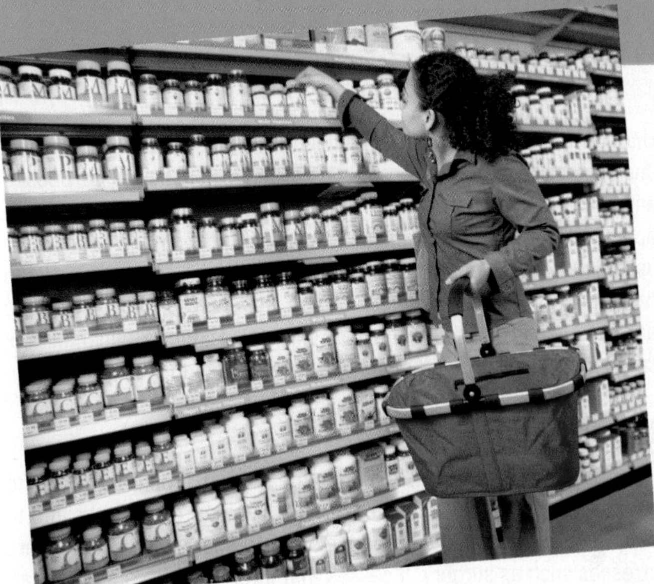
Tanya Constantine/Brand X Pictures/Getty Images

Correct Overt Deficiencies

In the United States, adults rarely suffer nutrient deficiency diseases such as scurvy, pellagra, and beriberi, but nutrient deficiencies do still occur. To correct an overt deficiency disease, a physician may prescribe therapeutic doses two to ten times the RDA (or AI) of a nutrient. At such high doses, the supplement is having a pharmacological effect and acting as a drug.

Support Increased Nutrient Needs

As Chapters 15 through 17 explain, nutrient needs increase during certain stages of life, making it difficult to meet some of those needs without supplementation. For example, women who lose a lot of blood and therefore a lot of iron during menstruation each month may need an iron supplement. Women of childbearing age need folate supplements to reduce the risks of neural tube defects. Similarly, pregnant women and women who are breastfeeding their infants have exceptionally high nutrient needs and so usually need special supplements. Newborns routinely receive a single dose of vitamin K at birth to prevent abnormal bleeding. Infants may need other supplements as well, depending on whether they are breastfed or receiving formula, and on whether the water they drink contains fluoride.

Improve Nutrition Status

In contrast to the classical deficiencies, which present a multitude of symptoms and are relatively easy to recognize, subclinical deficiencies are subtle and easy to overlook—and they are also more likely to occur. Without fortification or supplementation, many adults in the

GLOSSARY

dietary supplement: any pill, capsule, tablet, liquid, or powder that contains vitamins, minerals, herbs, or amino acids intended to increase dietary intake of these substances.

FDA (Food and Drug Administration): a part of the Department of Health and Human Services' Public Health Service that is responsible for ensuring the safety and wholesomeness of all dietary supplements and food processed and sold in interstate commerce except meat, poultry, and eggs (which are under the jurisdiction of the USDA); inspecting food plants and imported foods; and setting standards for food composition and product labeling.

high potency: 100% or more of the Daily Value for the nutrient in a single supplement and for at least two-thirds of the nutrients in a multinutrient supplement.

nanotechnology: a manufacturing technology that manipulates atoms to change the structure of matter.

nanoceuticals: substances with extremely small particles that have been manufactured by nanotechnology.

United States fall short of recommended intakes for several vitamins and minerals.[4] People who do not eat enough food to deliver the needed amounts of nutrients, such as habitual dieters and the elderly, risk developing subclinical deficiencies. Similarly, vegetarians who restrict their use of entire food groups without appropriate substitutions may fail to fully meet their nutrient needs. If there is no way for these people to eat enough nutritious foods to meet their needs, then vitamin-mineral supplements may be appropriate to help prevent nutrient deficiencies.

Improve the Body's Defenses

Health-care professionals may provide special supplementation to people being treated for addictions to alcohol or other drugs and to people with prolonged illnesses, extensive injuries, or other severe stresses such as surgery. Illnesses that interfere with appetite, eating, or nutrient absorption impair nutrition status. For example, the stomach condition atrophic gastritis often creates a vitamin B_{12} deficiency. In addition, nutrient needs are often heightened by diseases or medications. In all these cases, supplements are appropriate.

Reduce Disease Risks

Few people consume the optimal amounts of all the vitamins and minerals by diet alone. Inadequate intakes have been linked to chronic diseases such as heart disease, some cancers, and osteoporosis. For this reason, some physicians recommend that all adults take vitamin-mineral supplements. Such regular supplementation would provide an optimum intake to enhance metabolic harmony and prevent disease at relatively little cost. Others recognize the lack of conclusive evidence and the potential harm of supplementation and advise against such a recommendation.[5] A statement from the National Institutes of Health acknowledges that evidence is insufficient to recommend either for or against the use of supplements to prevent chronic diseases.

Highlight 11 reviews the relationships between supplement use and disease prevention. It describes some of the accumulating evidence suggesting that intakes of certain nutrients at levels much higher than can be attained from foods alone may be beneficial in reducing some disease risks. It also presents research confirming the associated risks. Clearly, consumers must be cautious in taking supplements to prevent disease.

Who Needs Supplements?

In summary, the following list acknowledges that in these specific conditions, these people may need to take supplements:

- People with specific nutrient deficiencies may need specific nutrient supplements.
- People whose energy intakes are particularly low (fewer than 1600 kcalories per day) may need multivitamin-mineral supplements.
- Vegetarians who eat all-plant diets (vegans) and older adults with atrophic gastritis may need vitamin B_{12}.
- People who have lactose intolerance or milk allergies or who otherwise do not consume enough milk products to forestall extensive bone loss may need calcium.
- People in certain stages of the life cycle who have increased nutrient requirements may need specific nutrient supplements. For example, infants may need vitamin D, iron, and fluoride; women of childbearing age and pregnant women may need folate and iron; and the elderly may need vitamin B_{12} and vitamin D.
- People who have inadequate intakes of milk or milk products, limited sun exposure, or heavily pigmented skin may need vitamin D.
- People who have diseases, infections, or injuries or who have undergone surgery that interferes with the intake, absorption, metabolism, or excretion of nutrients may need specific nutrient supplements.
- People taking medications that interfere with the body's use of specific nutrients may need specific nutrient supplements.

Except for people in these circumstances, most adults can get all the nutrients they need by eating a variety of nutrient-dense foods. Even athletes can meet their nutrient needs without the help of supplements, as Chapter 14 explains.

Arguments against Supplements

Foods rarely cause nutrient imbalances or toxicities, but supplements can. The higher the dose, the greater the risk of harm. People's tolerances for high doses of nutrients vary, just as their risks of deficiencies do. Amounts that some can tolerate may be harmful for others, and no one knows who falls where along the spectrum. It is difficult to determine just how much of a nutrient is enough—or too much. The Tolerable Upper Intake Levels (UL) of the DRI answer the question "How much is too much?" by defining the highest amount that appears safe for most healthy people. Table H10-1 presents UL and Daily Values for selected vitamins and minerals.

Who Should Not Take Supplements?

The following list recognizes that in certain circumstances, these people may need to avoid specific supplements:

- Men and postmenopausal women should not take iron supplements given that excess iron is harmful and generally more likely than inadequacies.
- Smokers should not take beta-carotene supplements given that high doses have been associated with increased lung cancer and mortality.
- Postmenopausal women should not take vitamin A supplements given that excess retinol has been associated with increased risk of hip fractures and reduced bone density.
- Surgery patients should not take vitamin E supplements during the week before surgery because vitamin E acts as a blood thinner.

Toxicity

Supplement users are more likely to have excessive intakes of certain nutrients—notably folate, vitamin A, vitamin B_6, vitamin C, calcium, magnesium, iron, and zinc.[6] The extent and severity of supplement toxicity remain unclear. Only a few alert health-care professionals can

TABLE H10-1 Vitamin and Mineral Intakes for Adults

Nutrient	Tolerable Upper Intake Levels[a]	Daily Values
Vitamins		
Vitamin A	3000 μg[b]	900 μg
Vitamin D (as cholecalciferol)	100 μg	20 μg
Vitamin E (as alpha-tocopherol)	1000 mg[b]	15 mg
Vitamin K	—[c]	120 μg
Thiamin	—[c]	1.2 mg
Riboflavin	—[c]	1.3 mg
Niacin (as niacinamide)	35 mg[b]	16 mg
Vitamin B_6 (as pyridoxine)	100 mg	1.7 mg
Folate	1000 μg[b]	400 μg
Vitamin B_{12} (as cyanocobalamin)	—[c]	2.4 μg
Pantothenic acid	—[c]	5 mg
Biotin	—[c]	30 μg
Vitamin C (as ascorbic acid)	2000 mg	90 mg
Choline	3500 mg	550 mg
Minerals		
Chloride	3600 mg	2300 mg
Potasssium	—[c]	4700 mg
Calcium	2500 mg	1300 mg
Phosphorus	4000 mg	1250 mg
Magnesium	350 mg[b]	420 mg
Iron	45 mg	18 mg
Zinc	40 mg	11 mg
Iodine	1100 μg	150 μg
Selenium	400 μg	55 μg
Fluoride	10 mg	—
Copper	10 mg	0.9 mg
Manganese	11 mg	2.3 mg
Chromium	—[c]	35 μg
Molybdenum	2000 μg	45 μg

[a]Unless otherwise noted, Upper Levels represent total intakes from food, water, and supplements.
[b]Upper Levels for vitamin A are for preformed vitamin A only; for vitamin E, niacin, and folate, the UL represent intakes from supplements, fortified foods, or both; for magnesium, the UL represent intakes from supplements only and do not include intakes from food and water.
[c]These nutrients have been evaluated by the DRI Committee for Tolerable Upper Intake Levels, but none were established because of insufficient data. No adverse effects have been reported with intakes of these nutrients at levels typical of supplements, but caution is still advised, given the potential for harm that accompanies excessive intakes.

recognize toxicity, even when it is acute. When it is chronic, with the effects developing subtly and progressing slowly, it often goes unrecognized and unreported.[7] In view of the potential hazards, some authorities believe supplements should bear warning labels, advising consumers that large doses may be toxic.

At a minimum, manufacturers should be held to the same standards required of the drug industry, which may help to prevent toxicities. Consider that more than 200 people reported symptoms of diarrhea, fatigue, hair loss, and joint pain when the selenium supplement they had taken delivered 200 times the selenium concentration listed on the label.[8]

Toxic overdoses of vitamins and minerals in children are more readily recognized and, unfortunately, fairly common. Fruit-flavored, chewable vitamins shaped like cartoon characters entice young children to eat them like candy in amounts that can cause poisoning. Iron supplements (30 milligrams of iron or more per tablet) are especially toxic and are the leading cause of accidental ingestion fatalities among children. Even mild overdoses cause GI distress, nausea, and black diarrhea, which reflects gastric bleeding. Severe overdoses result in bloody diarrhea, shock, liver damage, coma, and death.

Life-Threatening Misinformation

Another problem arises when people who are ill come to believe that high doses of vitamins or minerals can be therapeutic. Not only can high doses be toxic, but the person may take them instead of seeking medical help. Furthermore, there are no guarantees that the supplements will be effective. Taking vitamin supplements instead of medication may sound appealing, but they do not protect against the progression of heart disease or cancers.[9] In some cases, supplements may even be harmful.[10] Supplements of beta-carotene and vitamin A increase the risk of lung cancer and mortality, especially among smokers. Similarly, supplements of vitamin E increase the risk of prostate cancer among healthy men.[11]

Marketing materials for supplements often make health statements that are required to be "truthful and not misleading," but they often fall far short of both. Highlight 18 revisits this topic and includes a discussion of herbal preparations and other alternative therapies.

Unknown Needs

Another argument against the use of supplements is that there are no standards and no one knows exactly how to formulate the "ideal" supplement. What nutrients should be included? Which, if any, of the phytochemicals should be included? How much of each? On whose needs should the choices be based? Surveys have repeatedly shown little relationship between the supplements people take and the nutrients they actually need.

False Sense of Security

Another argument against supplement use is that it may lull people into a false sense of security. A person might eat irresponsibly, thinking, "My supplement will ensure my needs are met." Or, experiencing a warning symptom of a disease, a person might postpone seeking a diagnosis, thinking, "I probably just need a supplement to make this go away." Such self-diagnosis is potentially dangerous.

Other Invalid Reasons

Other invalid reasons people might use for taking supplements include:

- The belief that the food supply or soil contains inadequate nutrients
- The belief that supplements can provide energy

- The belief that supplements can enhance athletic performance or build lean body tissues without physical work or faster than work alone (see Highlight 14)
- The belief that supplements will help a person cope with stress
- The belief that supplements can prevent, treat, or cure conditions ranging from the common cold to cancer

Ironically, people with health problems are more likely to take supplements than other people, yet today's health problems are more likely to be due to overnutrition and poor lifestyle choices than to nutrient deficiencies. The truth—that most people would benefit from improving their eating and activity patterns—is harder to swallow than a supplement pill.

Bioavailability and Antagonistic Actions

In general, the body absorbs nutrients best from foods in which the nutrients are diluted and dispersed among other substances that may facilitate their absorption. Taken in pure, concentrated form, nutrients are likely to interfere with one another's absorption or with the absorption of nutrients in foods eaten at the same time. Documentation of these effects is particularly extensive for minerals: zinc hinders copper and calcium absorption, iron hinders zinc absorption, calcium hinders magnesium and iron absorption, and magnesium hinders the absorption of calcium and iron. Similarly, binding agents in supplements limit mineral absorption.

Although minerals provide the most-familiar and best-documented examples, interference among vitamins is now being seen as supplement use increases. The vitamin A precursor beta-carotene, long thought to be nontoxic, interferes with vitamin E metabolism when taken over the long term as a dietary supplement. Vitamin E, on the other hand, antagonizes vitamin K activity and so should not be used by people being treated for blood-clotting disorders. Consumers who want the benefits of optimal absorption of nutrients should eat foods selected for nutrient density and variety.

Whenever the diet is inadequate, the person should first attempt to improve it so as to obtain the needed nutrients from foods. If that is truly impossible, then the person needs a multivitamin-mineral supplement that supplies between 50 and 150 percent of the Daily Value for each of the nutrients. These amounts reflect the ranges commonly found in foods and therefore are compatible with the body's normal handling of nutrients (its physiologic tolerance). The next section provides some pointers to assist in the selection of an appropriate supplement.

Selection of Supplements

Whenever a physician or registered dietitian nutritionist recommends a supplement, follow the directions carefully. When selecting a supplement yourself, look for a single, balanced vitamin-mineral supplement. Supplements with a USP verification logo have been tested by the US Pharmacopeia (USP) to ensure that the supplement:

- Contains the declared ingredients and amounts listed on the label
- Does not contain harmful levels of contaminants
- Will disintegrate and release ingredients in the body
- Was made under safe and sanitary conditions

If you decide to take a vitamin-mineral supplement, ignore the eye-catching art and meaningless claims. Pay attention to the form the supplements are in, the list of ingredients, and the price. Here's where the truth lies, and from it you can make a rational decision based on facts. You have two basic questions to answer.

Form

The first question: What form do you want—chewable, liquid, or pills? If you'd rather drink your supplements than chew them, fine. If you choose a chewable form, though, be aware that chewable vitamin C can dissolve tooth enamel. If you choose pills, look for statements about the disintegration time. The USP suggests that supplements should completely disintegrate within 30 to 45 minutes. Obviously, supplements that don't dissolve have little chance of entering the bloodstream, so look for a brand that claims to meet USP disintegration standards.

Contents

The second question: What vitamins and minerals do you need? Generally, an appropriate supplement provides vitamins and minerals in amounts that do not exceed recommended intakes. Avoid supplements that, in a daily dose, provide more than the UL for *any* nutrient. Avoid preparations with more than 10 milligrams of iron per dose, except as prescribed by a physician. Iron is hard to get rid of once it's in the body, and an excess of iron can cause problems, just as a deficiency can (see Chapter 13).

Misleading Claims

Manufacturers of *organic* or natural vitamins boast that their pills are purified from real foods rather than synthesized in a laboratory. These supplements are no more effective than others and often cost more. The word *synthetic* may sound like "fake," but to synthesize just means to put together. Think back on the course of human evolution; it is not natural to take any kind of pill. In reality, the finest, most natural vitamin "supplements" available are whole grains, vegetables, fruits, meat, fish, poultry, eggs, legumes, nuts, and milk and milk products.

Avoid products that make **"high potency"** claims. More is not better (review Figure 10-1 on p. 304). Remember that foods are also providing these nutrients. Nutrients can build up and cause unexpected problems. For example, a man who takes vitamins and begins to lose his hair may think his hair loss means he needs more vitamins, when in fact it may be the early sign of a vitamin A overdose. (Of course, it may be completely unrelated to nutrition as well.)

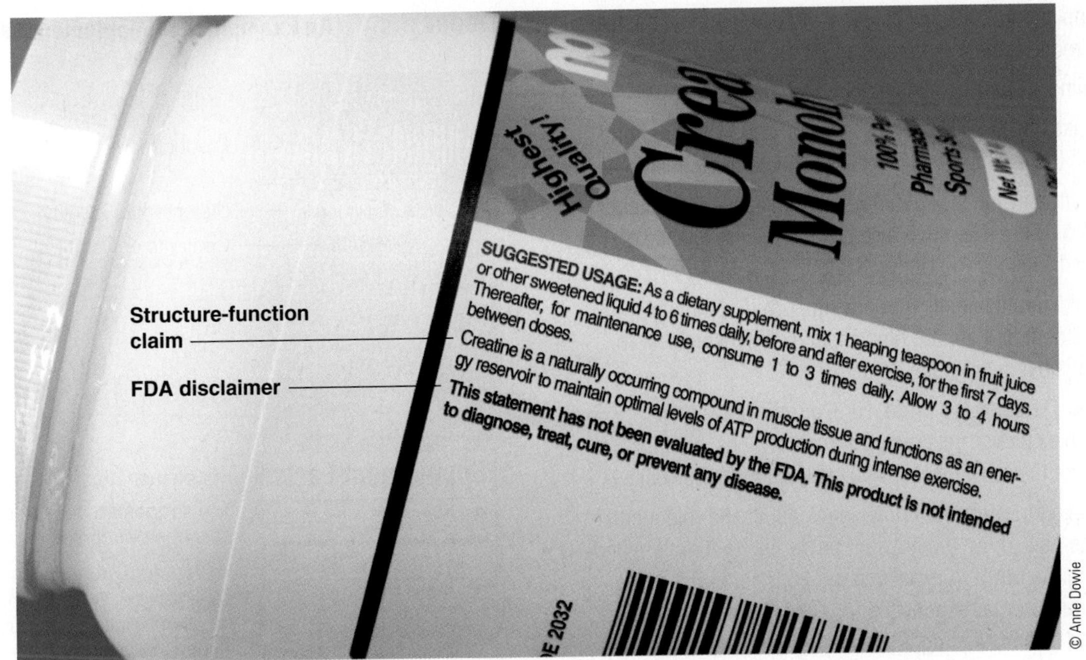

Structure-function claim
FDA disclaimer
Highest Quality!
SUGGESTED USAGE: As a dietary supplement, mix 1 heaping teaspoon in fruit juice or other sweetened liquid 4 to 6 times daily, before and after exercise, for the first 7 days. Thereafter, for maintenance use, consume 1 to 3 times daily. Allow 3 to 4 hours between doses.
Creatine is a naturally occuring compound in muscle tissue and functions as an energy reservoir to maintain optimal levels of ATP production during intense exercise.
This statement has not been evaluated by the FDA. This product is not intended to diagnose, treat, cure, or prevent any disease.
© Anne Dowie

Structure-function claims do not need FDA authorization, but they must be accompanied by a disclaimer.

Be aware that fake vitamins and preparations that contain items not needed in human nutrition, such as carnitine and inositol, reflect a marketing strategy aimed at your pocket, not at your health. The manufacturer wants you to believe that its pills contain the latest "new" nutrient that other brands omit, but in reality, these substances are not known to be needed by human beings.

Realize that the claim that supplements "relieve stress" is another marketing ploy. If you give even passing thought to what people mean by "stress," you'll realize manufacturers could never design a supplement to meet everyone's needs. Is it stressful to take an exam? Well, yes. Is it stressful to survive a major car wreck with third-degree burns and multiple bone fractures? Definitely, yes. The body's responses to these stresses are different. The body does use vitamins and minerals in mounting a stress response, but a body fed a well-balanced diet can meet the needs of most minor stresses. For the major ones, medical intervention is needed. In any case, taking a dietary supplement won't make life any less stressful.

Other marketing tricks to sidestep are "green" pills that contain dehydrated, crushed parsley, alfalfa, and other fruit and vegetable extracts. The nutrients and phytochemicals advertised can be obtained from a serving of vegetables more easily and for less money. Such pills may also provide enzymes, but enzymes are inactivated in the stomach during protein digestion.

Recognize the latest nutrition buzzwords. Manufacturers were marketing "antioxidant" supplements before the print had time to dry on the first scientific reports of antioxidant vitamins' action in the body. Remember, too, that high doses can alter a nutrient's action in the body. An antioxidant in physiological quantities may be beneficial, but in pharmacological quantities, it may act as a prooxidant and cause harm. Highlight 11 explores antioxidants and supplement use in more detail.

Similarly, manufacturers began making dietary supplements using **nanotechnology** before the FDA had created guidelines defining their use in consumer products. These **nanoceuticals** promise enhanced nutrient absorption and activity. Such claims may sound good, but again, more does not always mean better.

Finally, be aware that advertising on the Internet is cheap and not closely regulated. Promotional e-mails can be sent to millions of people in an instant. Internet messages can easily cite references and provide links to other sites, implying an endorsement when in fact none has been given. Be cautious when examining unsolicited information and search for a balanced perspective.

Cost

When shopping for supplements, remember that local or store brands may be just as good as nationally advertised brands. If they are less expensive, it may be because the price does not have to cover the cost of national advertising.

Regulation of Supplements

Dietary supplements are regulated by the **FDA (Food and Drug Administration)** as foods. Details of supplement regulation are defined in the Dietary Supplement Health and Education Act of 1994, which was intended to enable consumers to make informed choices about dietary supplements. The act subjects supplements to the same general labeling requirements that apply to foods. Specifically:

- Nutrition labeling for dietary supplements is required.
- Labels may make nutrient claims (as "high" or "low") according to specific criteria (for example, "an excellent source of vitamin C").
- Labels may claim that the lack of a nutrient can cause a deficiency disease, but if they do, they must also include the prevalence of that deficiency disease in the United States.
- Labels may make health claims that are supported by significant scientific agreement and are not brand specific (for example, "folate protects against neural tube defects").
- Labels may claim to diagnose, treat, cure, or relieve common complaints such as menstrual cramps or memory loss, but may *not* make claims about specific diseases (except as noted previously).
- Labels may make structure-function claims about the role a nutrient plays in the body, how the nutrient performs its function, and how consuming the nutrient is associated with general well-being. The manufacturer is responsible for ensuring that the claims are truthful and not misleading. Claims must be accompanied by an FDA disclaimer statement: "This statement has not been evaluated by the Food and Drug Administration. This product is not intended to diagnose, treat, cure, or prevent any disease." Figure H10-1 provides an example of a supplement label that complies with the requirements.

The multibillion-dollar-a-year supplement industry spends much money and effort influencing these regulations. The net effect of the Dietary Supplement Health and Education Act was a deregulation of the supplement industry. Unlike food additives or drugs, supplements do not need to be proved safe and effective, nor do they need the FDA's approval before being marketed. Furthermore, there are no standards for potency or dosage and no requirements for providing warnings of potential side effects. The FDA can only require good manufacturing practices: that dietary supplements be produced and packaged in a quality manner, do not contain contaminants or impurities, and are accurately labeled to reflect the actual contents.

Should a problem arise, the burden falls to the FDA to prove that the supplement poses a "significant or unreasonable risk of illness or injury." Only then would it be removed from the market. When asked, most Americans express support for greater regulation of dietary supplements. Health professionals agree.[12] To learn more about dietary supplements currently on the US market as well as those that have been recalled, consumers can visit the National Institutes of Health website (www.dsld.nlm.nih.gov/dsld/index.jsp).

> FIGURE H10-1 **An Example of a Supplement Label**

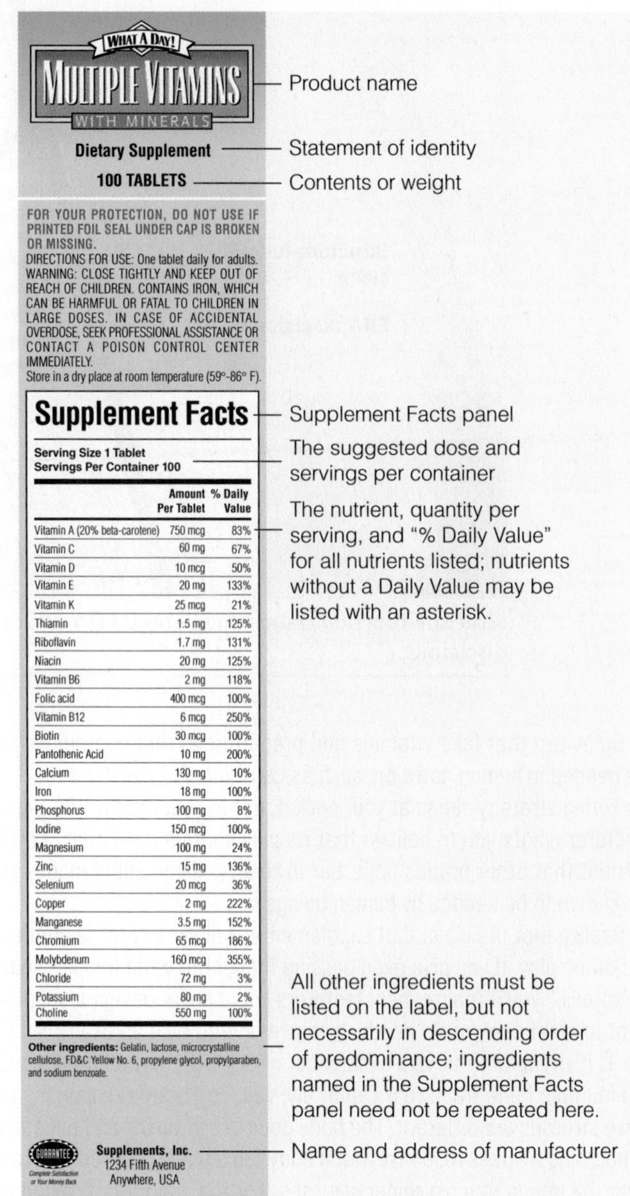

WHAT A DAY!
MULTIPLE VITAMINS
WITH MINERALS
Product name
Dietary Supplement
Statement of identity
100 TABLETS
Contents or weight
FOR YOUR PROTECTION, DO NOT USE IF PRINTED FOIL SEAL UNDER CAP IS BROKEN OR MISSING.
DIRECTIONS FOR USE: One tablet daily for adults.
WARNING: CLOSE TIGHTLY AND KEEP OUT OF REACH OF CHILDREN. CONTAINS IRON, WHICH CAN BE HARMFUL OR FATAL TO CHILDREN IN LARGE DOSES. IN CASE OF ACCIDENTAL OVERDOSE, SEEK PROFESSIONAL ASSISTANCE OR CONTACT A POISON CONTROL CENTER IMMEDIATELY.
Store in a dry place at room temperature (59°-86° F).
Supplement Facts
Supplement Facts panel
Serving Size 1 Tablet
Servings Per Container 100
The suggested dose and servings per container
Amount Per Tablet | % Daily Value
Vitamin A (20% beta-carotene) 750 mcg 83%
Vitamin C 60 mg 67%
Vitamin D 10 mcg 50%
Vitamin E 20 mg 133%
Vitamin K 25 mcg 21%
Thiamin 1.5 mg 125%
Riboflavin 1.7 mg 131%
Niacin 20 mg 125%
Vitamin B6 2 mg 118%
Folic acid 400 mcg 100%
Vitamin B12 6 mcg 250%
Biotin 30 mcg 100%
Pantothenic Acid 10 mg 200%
Calcium 130 mg 10%
Iron 18 mg 100%
Phosphorus 100 mg 8%
Iodine 150 mcg 100%
Magnesium 100 mg 24%
Zinc 15 mg 136%
Selenium 20 mcg 36%
Copper 2 mg 222%
Manganese 3.5 mg 152%
Chromium 65 mcg 186%
Molybdenum 160 mcg 355%
Chloride 72 mg 3%
Potassium 80 mg 2%
Choline 550 mg 100%
The nutrient, quantity per serving, and "% Daily Value" for all nutrients listed; nutrients without a Daily Value may be listed with an asterisk.
Other ingredients: Gelatin, lactose, microcrystalline cellulose, FD&C Yellow No. 6, propylene glycol, propylparaben, and sodium benzoate.
All other ingredients must be listed on the label, but not necessarily in descending order of predominance; ingredients named in the Supplement Facts panel need not be repeated here.
GUARANTEE
Complete Satisfaction or Your Money Back
Supplements, Inc.
1234 Fifth Avenue
Anywhere, USA
Name and address of manufacturer

If all the nutrients we need can come from food, why not just eat food? Foods have so much more to offer than supplements do. Nutrients in foods come in an infinite variety of combinations with a multitude of different carriers and absorption enhancers. They come with water, fiber, and an array of beneficial phytochemicals. Foods stimulate the GI tract to keep it healthy. They provide energy, and as long as you need energy each day, why not have nutritious foods deliver it? Foods offer pleasure, satiety, and opportunities for socializing while eating. Quite simply, foods meet human health needs far better than dietary supplements. For further proof, read Highlight 11.

CRITICAL THINKING QUESTIONS

A. What are the arguments for and against the use of dietary supplements?

B. According to the Health and Education Act of 1994, dietary supplements with familiar ingredients may be marketed without any evidence of effectiveness or safety. Supplements with new ingredients are supposed to provide the FDA with evidence of safety, but this part of the law is rarely enforced. Both the industry and the FDA acknowledge that most supplements are currently on the market without any assessment of safety. What is your position on this situation and what changes to the law, if any, would you propose to support your position?

REFERENCES

1. J. Gahche and coauthors, Dietary supplement use among US adults has increased since NHANES III (1988–1994), *National Center for Health Statistics: Data Brief* 61 (2011): 1–8.
2. D. B. McCormick, Vitamin/mineral supplements: Of questionable benefit for the general population, *Nutrition Reviews* 68 (2010): 207–213.
3. Position of the American Dietetic Association: Nutrient supplementation, *Journal of the American Dietetic Association* 109 (2009): 2073–2085.
4. V. L. Fulgoni III and coauthors, Foods, fortificants, and supplements: Where do Americans get their nutrients? *Journal of Nutrition* 141 (2011): 1847–1854.
5. M. E. Martinez and coauthors, Dietary supplements and cancer prevention: Balancing potential benefits against proven harms, *Journal of the National Cancer Institute* 104 (2012): 732–739.
6. R. L. Bailey and coauthors, Examination of vitamin intakes among US adults by dietary supplement use, *Journal of the Academy of Nutrition and Dietetics* 112 (2012): 657–663; R. L. Bailey and coauthors, Dietary supplement use is associated with higher intakes of minerals from food sources, *American Journal of Clinical Nutrition* 94 (2011): 1376–1381.
7. M. Cellini and coauthors, Dietary supplements: Physician knowledge and adverse event reporting, *Medicine and Science in Sports and Exercise* 45 (2013): 23–28.
8. J. K. MacFarquhar and coauthors, Acute selenium toxicity associated with a dietary supplement, *Archives of Internal Medicine* 170 (2010): 256–261.
9. M. G. O'Doherty and coauthors, Effect of supplementation with B vitamins and antioxidants on levels of asymmetric dimethylarginine (ADMA) and C-reactive protein (CRP): A double-blind, randomized, factorial design, placebo-controlled trial, *European Journal of Nutrition* 49 (2010): 483–492; G. J. Hankey and VITATOPS Trial Study Group, B vitamins in patients with recent transient ischaemic attack or stroke in the VITAmins TO Prevent Stroke (VITATOPS) trial: A randomized, double-blind, parallel, placebo-controlled trial, *The Lancet Neurology* 9 (2010): 855–865.
10. G. Bjelakovic and C. Gluud, Vitamin and mineral supplement use in relation to all-cause mortality in the Iowa Women's Health Study, *Archives of Internal Medicine* 171 (2011): 1633–1634.
11. E. A. Klein and coauthors, Vitamin E and the risk of prostate cancer: The Selenium and Vitamin E Cancer Prevention Trial (SELECT), *Journal of the American Medical Association* 306 (2011): 1549–1556.
12. P. A. Cohen, Hazards of hindsight—Monitoring the safety of nutritional supplements, *New England Journal of Medicine* 370 (2014): 1277–1280.

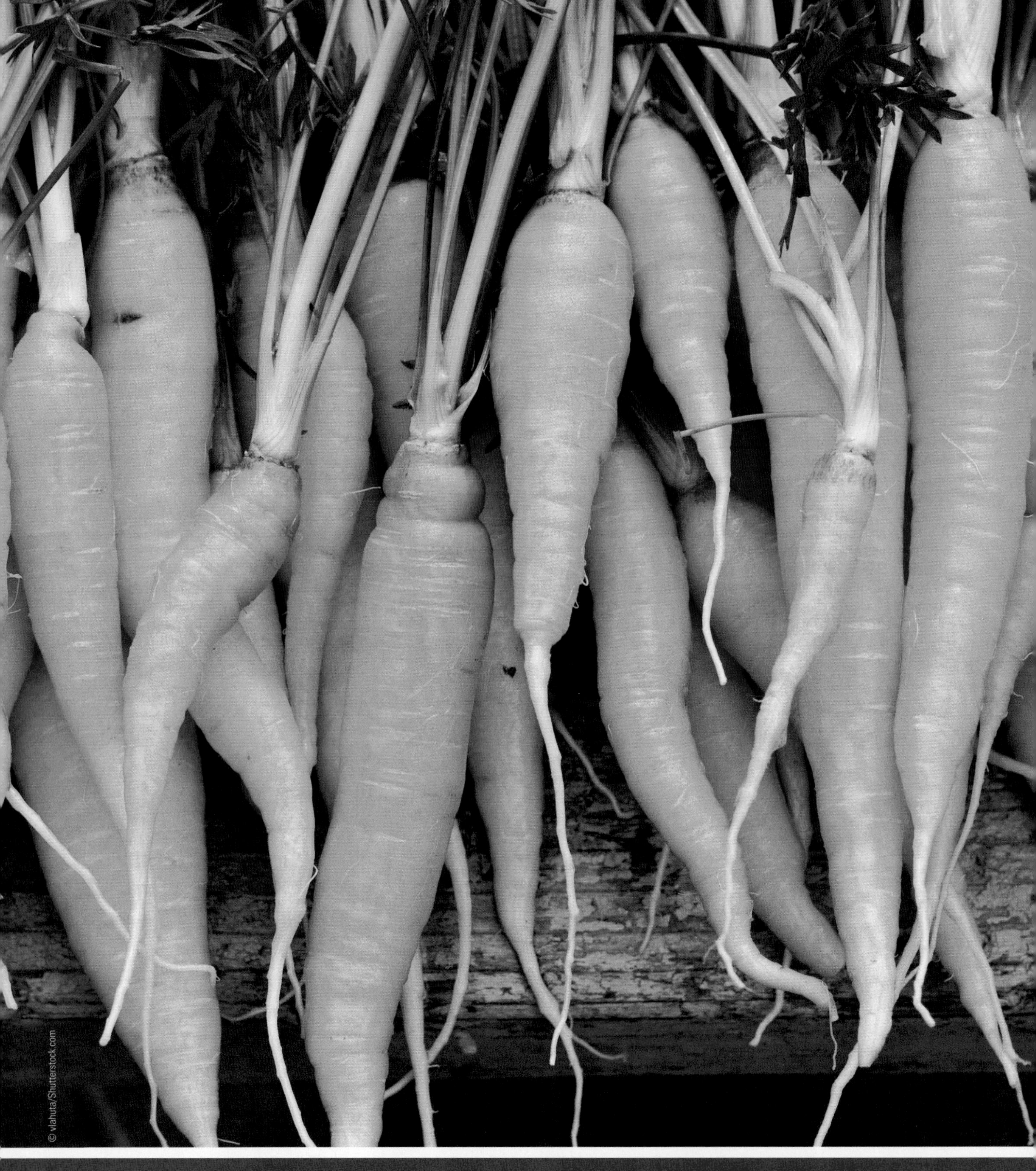

11

The Fat-Soluble Vitamins: A, D, E, and K

Nutrition in Your Life

Realizing that vitamin A from vegetables participates in vision, a mom encourages her children to "eat your carrots" because "they're good for your eyes." A dad takes his children outside to "enjoy the fresh air and sunshine" because they need the vitamin D that is made with the help of the sun. A physician recommends that a patient use vitamin E to slow the progression of heart disease. Another physician gives a newborn a dose of vitamin K to protect against life-threatening blood loss. These common daily occurrences highlight some of the heroic work of the fat-soluble vitamins. In the Nutrition Portfolio at the end of this chapter, you can determine whether the foods you are eating are meeting your fat-soluble vitamin needs.

LEARNING GPS

The fat-soluble vitamins A, D, E, and K differ from the water-soluble vitamins in several significant ways (review Table 10-2 on p. 304). Being insoluble in the watery juices of the GI tract, the fat-soluble vitamins require bile for their digestion and absorption. Upon absorption, fat-soluble vitamins travel through the lymphatic system within chylomicrons before entering the bloodstream, where many of them require protein carriers for transport. The fat-soluble vitamins participate in numerous activities throughout the body, but excesses are stored primarily in the liver and adipose tissue. The body maintains blood concentrations by retrieving these vitamins from storage as needed; thus people can eat less than their daily need for days, weeks, or even months or years without ill effects. They need only ensure that, over time, *average* daily intakes approximate recommendations. By the same token, because fat-soluble vitamins are not readily excreted, the risk of toxicity is greater than it is for the water-soluble vitamins.

11.1 Vitamin A and Beta-Carotene

› LEARN IT Identify the main roles, deficiency symptoms, and food sources for vitamin A.

Vitamin A was the first fat-soluble vitamin to be recognized. More than a century later, vitamin A and its precursor, **beta-carotene,** continue to intrigue researchers with their diverse roles and profound effects on health.

Three different forms of vitamin A are active in the body: **retinol, retinal,** and **retinoic acid.** Collectively known as **retinoids,** these compounds are commonly found in foods derived from animals. Foods derived from plants provide **carotenoids,** some of which can be converted to vitamin A.[1] * The most studied of the carotenoids with **vitamin A activity** is beta-carotene, which can be split to form retinol in the intestine and liver.[2] Figure 11-1 illustrates the structural similarities and differences of these vitamin A compounds and the cleavage of beta-carotene.

The cells can convert retinol and retinal to the other active forms of vitamin A as needed. The conversion of retinol to retinal is reversible, but the further conversion of retinal to retinoic acid is irreversible (see Figure 11-2). This irreversibility is significant because each form of vitamin A performs a specific function that the others cannot.

Several proteins participate in the digestion and absorption of vitamin A. After absorption via the lymph system, vitamin A eventually arrives at the liver, where it is stored. There, a special transport protein, **retinol-binding protein (RBP),** picks up vitamin A from the liver and carries it in the blood. Cells that use vitamin A have special protein receptors for it, and its action within each cell may differ depending on the receptor. For example, retinoic acid can *stimulate* cell growth in the skin and *inhibit* cell growth in tumors.

vitamin A: all naturally occurring compounds with the biological activity of *retinol*, the alcohol form of vitamin A.

beta-carotene (BAY-tah KARE-oh-teen): one of the carotenoids; an orange pigment and vitamin A precursor found in plants.

retinol (RET-ih-nol): the alcohol form of vitamin A.

retinal (RET-ih-nal): the aldehyde form of vitamin A.

retinoic (RET-ih-NO-ick) **acid:** the acid form of vitamin A.

retinoids (RET-ih-noyds): chemically related compounds with biological activity similar to that of retinol; metabolites of retinol.

carotenoids (kah-ROT-eh-noyds): pigments commonly found in plants and animals, some of which have vitamin A activity. The carotenoid with the greatest vitamin A activity is beta-carotene.

vitamin A activity: a term referring to both the active forms of vitamin A and the precursor forms in foods without distinguishing between them.

retinol-binding protein (RBP): the specific protein responsible for transporting retinol.

Roles in the Body

Vitamin A is a versatile vitamin, known to regulate the expression of several hundred genes. Its major roles include:

- Promoting vision
- Participating in protein synthesis and cell differentiation, thereby maintaining the health of epithelial tissues and skin
- Supporting reproduction and regulating growth

As mentioned, each form of vitamin A performs specific tasks. Retinol supports reproduction and is the major transport and storage form of the vitamin.

*Carotenoids with vitamin A activity include alpha-carotene, beta-carotene, and beta-cryptoxanthin; carotenoids with no vitamin A activity include the phytochemicals lycopene, lutein, and zeaxanthin.

› FIGURE 11-1 Forms of Vitamin A

In this diagram, corners represent carbon atoms, as in all previous diagrams in this book. A further simplification here is that methyl groups (CH_3) are understood to be at the ends of the lines extending from corners. (See Appendix C for complete structures.)

Retinol, the alcohol form

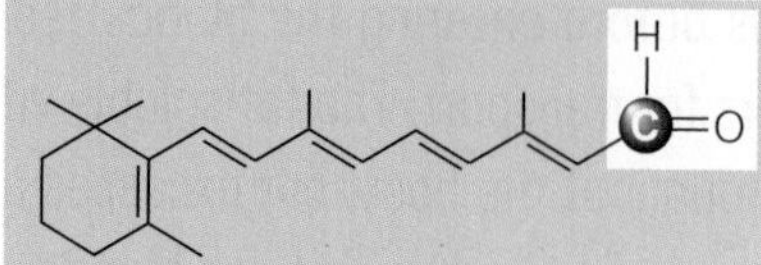

Retinal, the aldehyde form

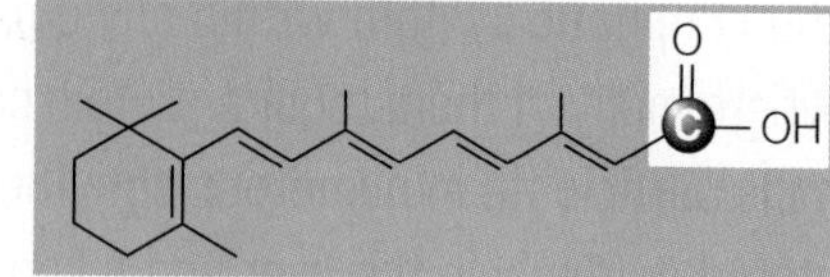

Retinoic acid, the acid form

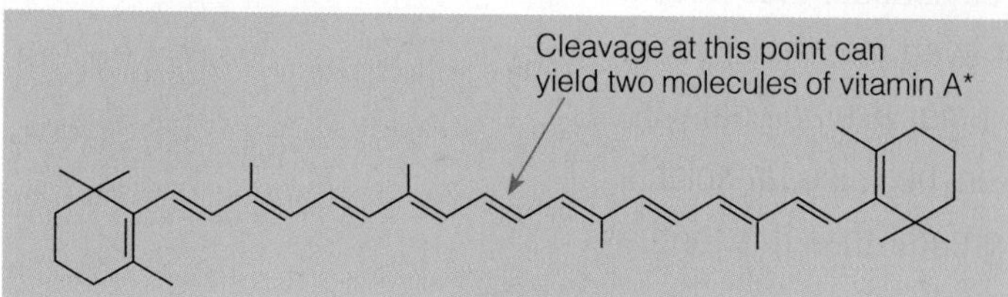

Beta-carotene, a precursor

*Sometimes cleavage occurs at other points as well, so that one molecule of beta-carotene may yield only one molecule of vitamin A. Furthermore, not all beta-carotene is converted to vitamin A, and absorption of beta-carotene is not as efficient as that of vitamin A. For these reasons, 12 μg of beta-carotene are equivalent to 1 μg of vitamin A. Conversion of other carotenoids to vitamin A is even less efficient.

> FIGURE 11-2 Conversion of Vitamin A Compounds

Notice that the conversion from retinol to retinal is reversible, whereas the pathway from retinal to retinoic acid is not.

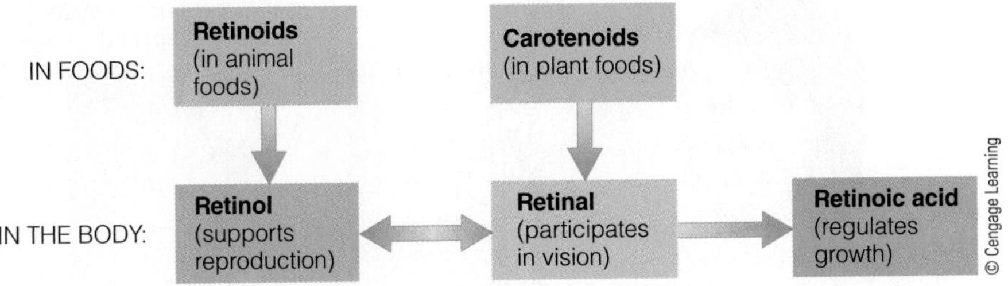

Retinal is active in vision and is also an intermediate in the conversion of retinol to retinoic acid (review Figure 11-2). Retinoic acid acts like a hormone, regulating cell differentiation, growth, and embryonic development. Animals raised on retinoic acid as their only source of vitamin A can grow normally, but they become blind because retinoic acid cannot be converted to retinal (review Figure 11-2).

Vitamin A in Vision Vitamin A plays two indispensable roles in the eye: it helps maintain a crystal-clear outer window, the **cornea,** and it participates in the conversion of light energy into nerve impulses at the **retina** (see Figure 11-3 for details). Some of the photosensitive cells of the retina contain **pigment** molecules called **rhodopsin.** Each rhodopsin molecule is composed of a protein called **opsin** bonded to a molecule of retinal, which plays a central role in vision.[3] When light passes through the cornea of the eye and strikes the retina, rhodopsin responds. As it does, opsin is released and retinal shifts from a *cis* to a *trans* configuration, just as fatty acids do during hydrogenation (see p. 139). These changes generate an electrical impulse that conveys the message to the brain. Much of the retinal is then converted back to its active *cis* form and combined with the opsin protein to regenerate rhodopsin. Some retinal, however, may be oxidized to retinoic acid, a biochemical dead end for the visual process. Visual activity leads to repeated small losses of retinal, necessitating its constant replenishment either directly from foods or indirectly from retinol stores.

Vitamin A in Protein Synthesis and Cell Differentiation Despite its important role in vision, only one-thousandth of the body's vitamin A is in the retina. Much more is in the cells lining the body's surfaces. There, the vitamin participates in protein synthesis and **cell differentiation,** a process by which each type of cell develops to perform a specific function.

cornea (KOR-nee-uh): the transparent membrane covering the outside of the eye.

retina (RET-in-uh): the innermost membrane of the eye, composed of several layers, including one that contains the rods and cones.

pigment: a molecule capable of absorbing certain wavelengths of light so that it reflects only those that we perceive as a certain color.

rhodopsin (ro-DOP-sin): a light-sensitive pigment of the retina that contains the retinal form of vitamin A and the protein opsin.

- **rhod** = red (pigment)
- **opsin** = visual protein

opsin (OP-sin): the protein portion of visual pigment molecules.

cell differentiation (DIF-er-EN-she-AY-shun): the process by which immature cells develop specific functions different from those of the original that are characteristic of their mature cell type.

> FIGURE 11-3 Vitamin A's Role in Vision

More than 100 million photosensitive cells reside in the retina, and each contains about 30 million molecules of vitamin A–containing visual pigments. The rods contain the rhodopsin pigment and respond to faint light; the cones contain the iodopsin pigment and function in color vision.

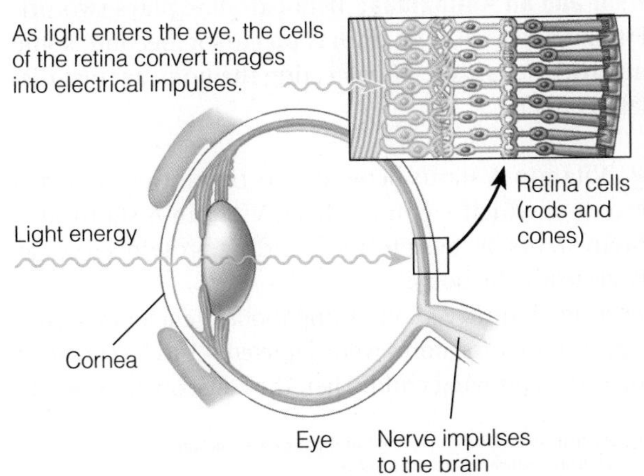

The cells of the retina contain rhodopsin, a molecule composed of opsin (a protein) and *cis*-retinal (vitamin A).

cis-Retinal → *trans*-Retinal

As rhodopsin absorbs light, retinal changes from *cis* to *trans*, which triggers an electrical impulse that carries visual information to the brain through the optic nerve.

© Cengage Learning

> FIGURE 11-4 **Mucous Membrane Integrity**

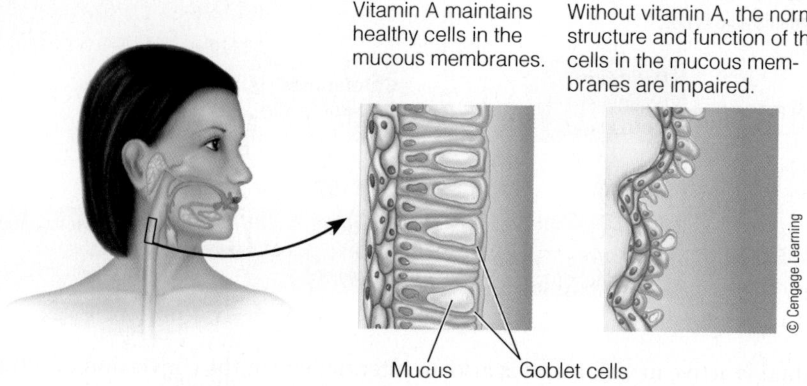

Vitamin A maintains healthy cells in the mucous membranes.
Without vitamin A, the normal structure and function of the cells in the mucous membranes are impaired.
Mucus
Goblet cells
© Cengage Learning

All body surfaces, both inside and out, are covered by layers of cells known as **epithelial cells.** The **epithelial tissue** on the outside of the body is, of course, the skin—and vitamin A and beta-carotene help to protect against skin damage from sunlight.[4] The epithelial tissues that line the inside of the body are the **mucous membranes:** the linings of the mouth, stomach, and intestines; the linings of the lungs and the passages leading to them; the linings of the urinary bladder and urethra; the linings of the uterus and vagina; and the linings of the eyelids and sinus passageways. Within the body, the mucous membranes of the GI tract alone line an area larger than a quarter of a football field, and vitamin A helps to maintain their integrity (see Figure 11-4).

Vitamin A promotes differentiation of epithelial cells and goblet cells, one-celled glands that synthesize and secrete mucus. Mucus coats and protects the epithelial cells from invasive microorganisms and other potentially damaging substances, such as gastric juices.

Vitamin A in Reproduction and Growth As mentioned, vitamin A also supports reproduction and regulates growth.[5] In men, retinol participates in sperm development, and in women, vitamin A supports normal fetal development during pregnancy. Children lacking vitamin A fail to grow; given vitamin A supplements, these children gain weight and grow taller.

The growth of bones illustrates that growth is a complex phenomenon of **remodeling.** To convert a small bone into a large bone, some bone cells must "undo" parts of the bone before other cells can build new bone, and vitamin A participates in the dismantling.* The cells that break down bone contain acid and enzymes that dissolve the minerals and digest the matrix.** With the help of vitamin A, these bone-dismantling cells destroy selected sites in the bone, removing the parts that are not needed. After completing their work, the bone-dismantling cells die, leaving their excavation site to be rebuilt by the bone-building cells.

Beta-Carotene as a Precursor and an Antioxidant Beta-carotene plays two primary roles in the body.[6] First, it serves as a vitamin A precursor. Second, some beta-carotene acts as an antioxidant capable of protecting the body against disease. (Highlight 11 provides details.)

Vitamin A Deficiency

Vitamin A status depends mostly on the adequacy of vitamin A stores, 90 percent of which are in the liver. Vitamin A status also depends on a person's protein status because retinol-binding protein serves as the vitamin's transport carrier inside the body.

If a person were to stop eating vitamin A–containing foods, deficiency symptoms would not begin to appear until after stores were depleted—1 to 2 years for a healthy adult but much sooner for a growing child. Then the consequences would

epithelial (ep-i-THEE-lee-ul) **cells:** cells on the surface of the skin and mucous membranes.

epithelial tissue: the layer of the body that serves as a selective barrier between the body's interior and the environment. Examples are the cornea of the eyes, the skin, the respiratory lining of the lungs, and the lining of the digestive tract.

mucous (MYOO-kus) **membranes:** the membranes, composed of mucus-secreting cells, that line the surfaces of body tissues.

remodeling: the dismantling and re-formation of a structure.

*The cells that dismantle bone during growth are *osteoclasts;* those that build bone are *osteoblasts.*

**The degradative enzymes are contained within *lysosomes* (LYE-so-zomes).

be profound and severe. Vitamin A deficiency is uncommon in the United States, but it is a major nutrition problem in many developing countries, responsible for a million or more unnecessary deaths and cases of blindness each year.[7] Routine vitamin A supplementation and food fortification can be a life-saving intervention.[8]

Infectious Diseases Vitamin A supports immune function and inhibits replication of the measles virus.[9] In developing countries around the world, measles is a devastating infectious disease, killing 430 children each day.[10] The severity of the illness often correlates with the degree of vitamin A deficiency; deaths are usually due to related infections such as pneumonia and severe diarrhea. Providing measles vaccinations and large doses of vitamin A reduces the risk of dying from these infections by more than half.[11]

The World Health Organization (WHO) and UNICEF (the United Nations International Children's Emergency Fund) have made the control of vitamin A deficiency a major goal in their quest to improve child health and survival throughout the developing world. They recommend two doses of vitamin A supplements, given 24 hours apart, for all children with measles. In the United States, the American Academy of Pediatrics recommends vitamin A supplements for certain groups of measles-infected infants and children. Vitamin A supplements also protect against blindness and the complications of other life-threatening infections, including malaria, lung diseases, and HIV (human immunodeficiency virus, the virus that causes AIDS).

Night Blindness **Night blindness** is one of the first detectable signs of vitamin A deficiency and permits early diagnosis. In night blindness, the person loses the ability to recover promptly from the temporary blinding that follows a flash of bright light at night or to see after dark. In many parts of the world, after the sun goes down, vitamin A–deficient people become night-blind. They often cling to others or sit still, afraid that they may trip and fall or lose their way if they try to walk alone.

Blindness (Xerophthalmia) Beyond night blindness is total blindness—failure to see at all. Night blindness is caused by a lack of vitamin A at the back of the eye, the retina; total blindness is caused by a lack of vitamin A at the front of the eye, the cornea. Severe vitamin A deficiency is the leading cause of preventable blindness in the world, causing as many as half a million preschool children to lose their sight each year.

Blindness due to vitamin A deficiency, known as **xerophthalmia,** develops in stages. At first, the cornea becomes dry and hard because of inadequate mucous production—a condition known as **xerosis.** Then xerosis quickly progresses to **keratomalacia,** the softening of the cornea that leads to irreversible blindness.

Keratinization Elsewhere in the body, vitamin A deficiency affects other surfaces. On the body's outer surface, the epithelial cells change shape and begin to secrete the protein **keratin**—the hard, inflexible protein of hair and nails. As Figure 11-5 shows, the skin becomes dry, rough, and scaly as lumps of keratin accumulate (**keratinization**). Without vitamin A, the goblet cells in the GI tract diminish in number and activity, limiting the secretion of mucus. With less mucus, normal digestion and absorption of nutrients falter, and this, in turn, worsens malnutrition by limiting the absorption of whatever nutrients the diet may deliver. Similar changes in the cells of other epithelial tissues weaken defenses, making infections of the respiratory tract, the GI tract, the urinary tract, the vagina, and inner ear likely.

Vitamin A Toxicity

Just as a deficiency of vitamin A affects all body systems, so does a toxicity. Symptoms of toxicity begin to develop when all the binding proteins are loaded, and vitamin A is free to damage cells. Such effects are unlikely when a person depends on a balanced diet for nutrients, but toxicity is a real possibility when concentrated amounts of **preformed vitamin A** in foods derived from animals, fortified foods, or supplements are consumed. Children

> **FIGURE 11-5 Vitamin A–Deficiency Symptom—The Rough Skin of Keratinization**

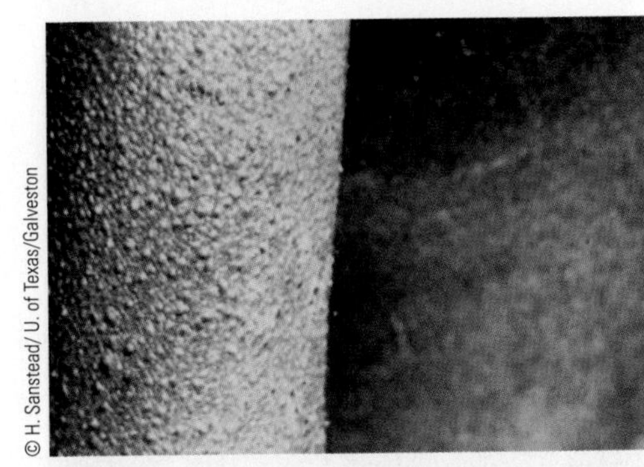

In vitamin A deficiency, the epithelial cells secrete the protein keratin in a process known as *keratinization.* (Keratinization doesn't occur in the GI tract, but mucus-producing cells dwindle and mucus production declines.) The extreme of this condition is *hyperkeratinization* or *hyperkeratosis.* When keratin accumulates around hair follicles, the condition is known as *follicular hyperkeratosis.*

night blindness: slow recovery of vision after flashes of bright light at night or an inability to see in dim light; an early symptom of vitamin A deficiency.

xerophthalmia (zer-off-THAL-mee-uh): progressive blindness caused by inadequate mucus production due to severe vitamin A deficiency.

- **xero** = dry
- **ophthalm** = eye

xerosis (zee-ROW-sis): abnormal drying of the skin and mucous membranes; a sign of vitamin A deficiency.

keratomalacia (KARE-ah-toe-ma-LAY-shuh): softening of the cornea that leads to irreversible blindness; a sign of severe vitamin A deficiency.

keratin (KARE-uh-tin): a water-insoluble protein; the normal protein of hair and nails.

keratinization: accumulation of keratin in a tissue; a sign of vitamin A deficiency.

preformed vitamin A: dietary vitamin A in its active form.

> FIGURE 11-6 Symptom of Beta-Carotene Excess—Discoloration of the Skin

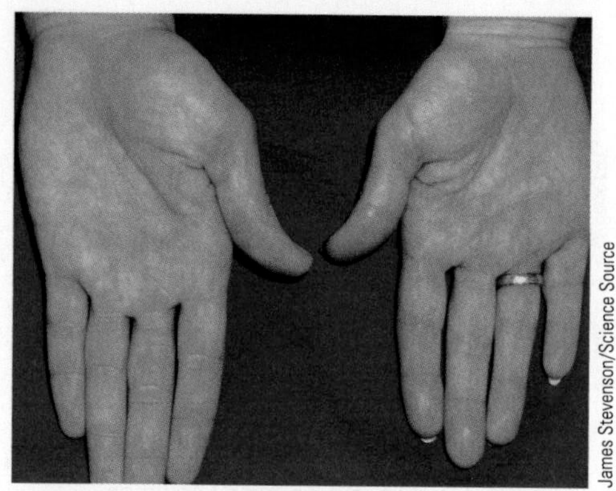

James Stevenson/Science Source

The hand on the right shows the skin yellowing that occurs when blood levels of beta-carotene rise in response to a diet that features carrots, pumpkins, and orange juice. (The hand on the left belongs to someone else and is shown here for comparison.)

are most vulnerable to toxicity because they need less vitamin A and are more sensitive to overdoses. An Upper Level (UL) has been set for preformed vitamin A (see inside front cover). Even multivitamin supplements typically provide 1500 micrograms—much more vitamin A than most people need. (For perspective, the RDA for vitamin A is 700 micrograms for women and 900 micrograms for men.)

Beta-carotene, which is found in a wide variety of fruits and vegetables, is not converted efficiently enough in the body to cause vitamin A toxicity; instead, it is stored in the fat just under the skin. Although overconsumption of beta-carotene from foods may turn the skin yellow, this is not harmful (see Figure 11-6). In contrast, overconsumption of beta-carotene from supplements may be quite harmful. In excess, this antioxidant may act as a prooxidant (as Highlight 11 explains). Adverse effects of beta-carotene supplements are most evident in people who drink alcohol and smoke cigarettes.

Bone Defects Excessive intakes of vitamin A over the years may weaken the bones and contribute to fractures and osteoporosis.[12] Vitamin A suppresses bone-building activity, stimulates bone-dismantling activity, and interferes with vitamin D's ability to maintain normal blood calcium.

Birth Defects Excessive vitamin A during pregnancy leads to abnormal cell death in the spinal cord, which increases the risk of birth defects such as spina bifida and cleft palate.[13] In such cases, vitamin A is considered a **teratogen.** High intakes (daily supplemental intakes of vitamin A equivalent to roughly four times the RDA for women) before the seventh week of pregnancy appear to be the most damaging. For this reason, vitamin A is not given as a supplement in the first trimester of pregnancy without specific evidence of deficiency, which is rare.

Not for Acne Adolescents need to know that massive doses of vitamin A have no beneficial effect on **acne.** The prescription medicine Accutane is made from vitamin A but is chemically different.* Taken orally, Accutane is effective against the deep lesions of cystic acne. It is highly toxic, however, especially during growth, and has caused birth defects in infants when women have taken it during their pregnancies. For this reason, women taking Accutane must agree to pregnancy testing and to using two forms of contraception from at least 1 month before taking the drug through at least 1 month after discontinuing its use. Should they become pregnant, they need to stop taking Accutane immediately and notify their physician.

Another vitamin A relative, Retin-A, fights acne, the wrinkles of aging, and other skin disorders.** Applied topically, this ointment smooths and softens skin; it also lightens skin that has become darkly pigmented after inflammation. During treatment, the skin becomes red and tender and peels.

Vitamin A Recommendations Because the body can derive vitamin A from both retinoids and carotenoids, its content in foods and its recommendations are expressed as **retinol activity equivalents (RAE).** One microgram of retinol counts as 1 RAE, as does 12 micrograms of dietary beta-carotene.*** This difference recognizes that beta-carotene's absorption and conversion are significantly less efficient than those of the retinoids. Until recently, food and supplement labels reported vitamin A contents using International Units (IU), a measure of vitamin activity used before direct chemical analysis was possible. The glossary on the inside back page provides factors that can be used to convert IU to a weight measurement.

*The generic name for Accutane is *isotretinoin*.

**The generic name for Retin-A is *tretinoin topical*.

***For beta-carotene from supplements, 2 micrograms equal 1 µg RAE and for other vitamin A precursor carotenoids, 24 micrograms equal 1 µg RAE.

teratogen (ter-AT-oh-jen): a substance that causes abnormal fetal development and birth defects.

acne: a chronic inflammation of the skin's follicles and oil-producing glands, which leads to an accumulation of oils inside the ducts that surround hairs; usually associated with the maturation of young adults.

retinol activity equivalents (RAE): a measure of vitamin A activity; the amount of retinol that the body will derive from a food containing preformed retinol or its precursor, beta-carotene.

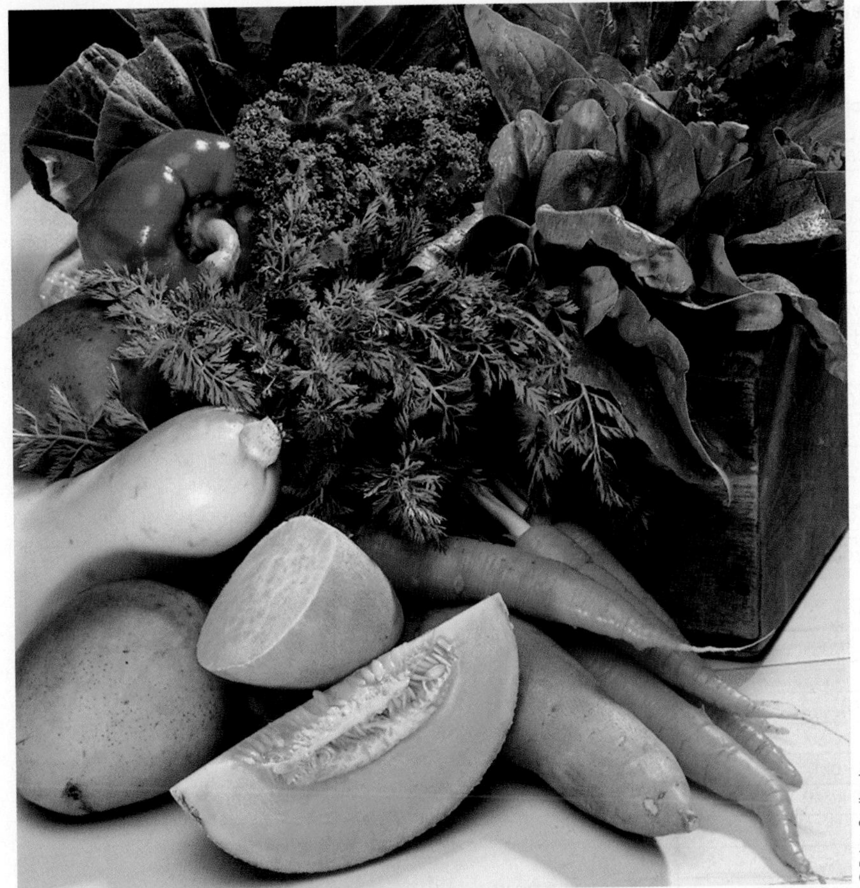

The carotenoids in foods bring colors to meals; the retinoids in our eyes allow us to see them.

Vitamin A in Foods The richest sources of the retinoids are foods derived from animals—liver, fish liver oils, milk and milk products, butter, and eggs. Because vitamin A is fat soluble, it is lost when milk is skimmed. To compensate, reduced-fat, low-fat, and fat-free milks are fortified so as to provide the amount found in whole milk. Margarine is usually fortified to provide the same amount of vitamin A as butter.

Plants contain no retinoids, but many vegetables and some fruits contain vitamin A precursors—the carotenoids. Only a few carotenoids have vitamin A activity; the carotenoid with the greatest vitamin A activity is beta-carotene. Beta-carotene is a rich, deep yellow, almost orange, compound. The beta-carotene in dark green, leafy vegetables is abundant, but masked by large amounts of the green pigment **chlorophyll.** Attractive meals that include colorful fruits and vegetables rich in beta-carotene are likely to provide vitamin A.[14]

The Colors of Vitamin A Foods Dark leafy greens (like broccoli and spinach—not celery or cabbage) and rich yellow or deep orange vegetables and fruits (such as cantaloupe, carrots, and sweet potatoes—not corn or bananas) help people meet their vitamin A needs (see Figure 11-7 on p. 350). A diet including several servings of such carotene-rich sources helps to ensure a sufficient intake.

Bright color is not always a sign of vitamin A activity, however. Beets and corn, for example, derive their colors from the red and yellow **xanthophylls,** which have no vitamin A activity. As for white plant foods such as potatoes, cauliflower, pasta, and rice, they also offer little or no vitamin A. Similarly, fast foods often lack vitamin A. Anyone who dines frequently on hamburgers, french fries, and colas is wise to emphasize colorful vegetables and fruits at other meals.

chlorophyll (KLO-row-fil): the green pigment of plants, which absorbs light and transfers the energy to other molecules, thereby initiating photosynthesis.

xanthophylls (ZAN-tho-fills): pigments found in plants responsible for the color changes seen in autumn leaves.

> **FIGURE 11-7 Vitamin A in Selected Foods**

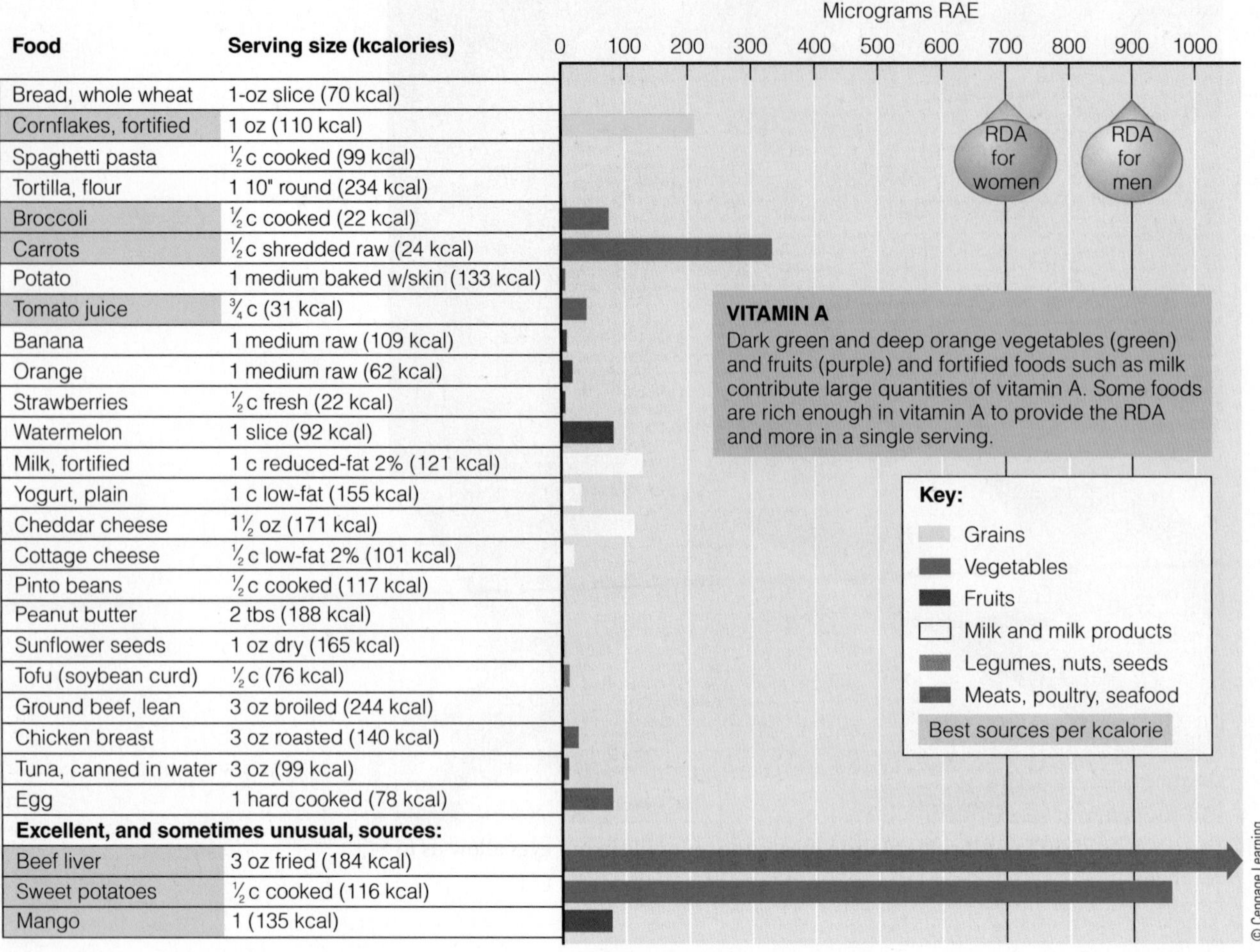

Vitamin A–Rich Liver People sometimes wonder if eating liver too frequently can cause vitamin A toxicity. Liver is a rich source because vitamin A is stored in the livers of animals, just as in humans.* Arctic explorers who have eaten large quantities of polar bear liver have become ill with symptoms suggesting vitamin A toxicity. Liver offers many nutrients, and eating it periodically may improve a person's nutrition status, but caution is warranted not to eat too much too often, especially for pregnant women. With 1 ounce of beef liver providing more than three times the RDA for vitamin A, intakes can rise quickly.

Golden Rice As mentioned earlier, vitamin A deficiency is a major problem in developing countries, impairing growth, causing blindness, and suppressing the immune system. In these developing regions of the world, fruits and vegetables are a scarcity, and rice, which contains no beta-carotene or vitamin A, is the staple food. Through biotechnology, scientists have been able to genetically modify rice to be a significant source of beta-carotene. Commonly called *golden rice* because of its yellowish tinge, this rice offers a promising solution to world malnutrition, but it also raises questions about the potential risks to the environment. More details are provided in Highlight 19's review of food biotechnology and Chapter 20's presentation of world hunger and possible solutions.

*The liver is not the only organ that stores vitamin A. The kidneys, adrenal glands, and other organs do, too, but the liver stores the most and is the most commonly eaten organ meat.

› REVIEW IT Identify the main roles, deficiency symptoms, and food sources for vitamin A.

Vitamin A is found in the body in three forms: retinol, retinal, and retinoic acid. Together, they are essential to vision, healthy epithelial tissues, and growth. Vitamin A deficiency is a major health problem worldwide, leading to infections, blindness, and keratinization. Toxicity can also cause problems and is most often associated with supplement abuse. Animal-derived foods such as liver and whole or fortified milk provide retinoids, whereas brightly colored plant-derived foods such as spinach, carrots, and pumpkins provide beta-carotene and other carotenoids. In addition to serving as a precursor for vitamin A, beta-carotene acts as an antioxidant in the body. The accompanying table provides a summary of vitamin A.

Vitamin A

Other Names	**Deficiency Disease**
Retinol, retinal, retinoic acid; precursors are carotenoids such as beta-carotene	Hypovitaminosis A
RDA	**Deficiency Symptoms**
Men: 900 µg RAE/day Women: 700 µg RAE/day	Night blindness, corneal drying (xerosis), triangular gray spots on eye (Bitot's spots), softening of the cornea (keratomalacia), and corneal degeneration and blindness (xerophthalmia); impaired immunity (infectious diseases); plugging of hair follicles with keratin, forming white lumps (hyperkeratosis)
UL	**Toxicity Disease**
Adults: 3000 µg/day	Hypervitaminosis A[a]
Chief Functions in the Body	**Chronic Toxicity Symptoms**
Vision; maintenance of cornea, epithelial cells, mucous membranes, skin; bone and tooth growth; reproduction; immunity	Increased activity of osteoclasts[b] causing reduced bone density; liver abnormalities; birth defects
Significant Sources	**Acute Toxicity Symptoms**
Retinol: fortified milk, cheese, cream, butter, fortified margarine, eggs, liver Beta-carotene: spinach and other dark green, leafy vegetables, broccoli, deep orange fruits (apricots, cantaloupe) and vegetables (squash, carrots, sweet potatoes, pumpkin)	Blurred vision, nausea, vomiting, vertigo; increase of pressure inside skull, mimicking brain tumor; headaches; muscle incoordination

[a]A related condition, *hypercarotenemia*, is caused by the accumulation of too much of the vitamin A precursor beta-carotene in the blood, which turns the skin noticeably yellow. Hypercarotenemia is not, strictly speaking, a toxicity symptom.
[b]*Osteoclasts* are the cells that destroy bone during its growth. Those that build bone are *osteoblasts*.

11.2 Vitamin D

› LEARN IT Identify the main roles, deficiency symptoms, and sources for vitamin D.

Vitamin D differs from the other nutrients in that the body can synthesize it, with the help of sunlight, from a precursor that the body makes from cholesterol. Therefore, vitamin D is not an essential nutrient; given enough time in the sun, people need no vitamin D from foods.

Also known as **calciferol,** vitamin D comes in two major forms.[15] **Vitamin D_2** derives primarily from plant foods in the diet. **Vitamin D_3** derives from animal foods in the diet and from synthesis in the skin. These two forms of vitamin D are similar and both must be activated before they can fully function.

Figure 11-8 (p. 352) diagrams the pathway for making and activating vitamin D in the body. To make vitamin D, ultraviolet rays from the sun hit a precursor in the skin and convert it to previtamin D_3, which is converted to vitamin D_3 with the help of the body's heat. To activate vitamin D—whether made in the body or consumed from the diet—two hydroxylation reactions must occur. First, the liver adds an OH group, and then the kidneys add another OH group to produce the active vitamin. As you might expect, diseases affecting either the liver or the kidneys can interfere with the activation of vitamin D and produce symptoms of deficiency.

Roles in the Body Though called a vitamin, the active form of vitamin D is actually a hormone—a compound manufactured by one part of the body that

calciferol (kal-SIF-er-ol): vitamin D.

vitamin D_2: vitamin D derived from plants in the diet; also called *ergocalciferol* (ER-go-kal-SIF-er-ol).

vitamin D_3: vitamin D derived from animals in the diet or made in the skin from 7-dehydrocholesterol, a precursor of cholesterol, with the help of sunlight; also called *cholecalciferol* (KO-lee-kal-SIF-er-ol) or *calciol.* After hydroxylation in the liver, calciol becomes *calcidiol* and after hydroxylation in the kidneys, calcidiol becomes *calcitriol.*

> FIGURE 11-8 **Vitamin D Synthesis and Activation**

The final activation step in the kidneys is tightly regulated by hormones.

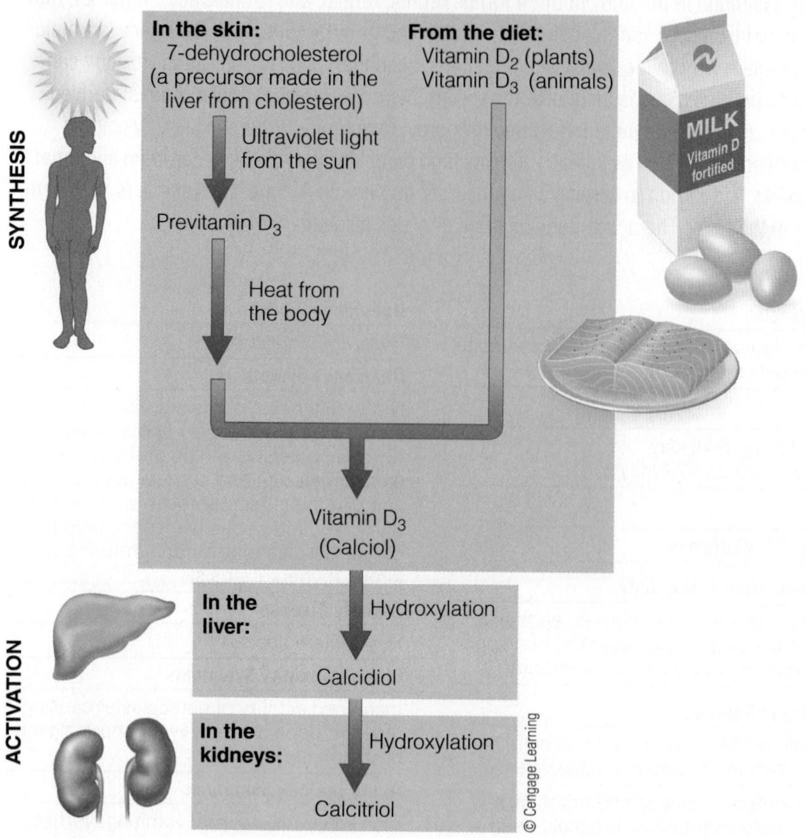

travels through the blood and causes another body part to respond. Like vitamin A, vitamin D has a binding protein that carries it to the target organs—most notably, the intestines, the kidneys, and the bones. All respond to vitamin D by making the minerals needed for bone growth and maintenance available.

Vitamin D in Bone Growth Vitamin D is a member of a large and cooperative bone-making and maintenance team composed of nutrients and other compounds, including vitamins A and K; the hormones parathyroid hormone and calcitonin; the protein collagen; and the minerals calcium, phosphorus, magnesium, and fluoride. Vitamin D's special role in bone health is to assist in the absorption of calcium and phosphorus, thus helping to maintain blood concentrations of these minerals. The bones grow denser and stronger as they absorb and deposit these minerals. Details of calcium balance and mineral deposition appear in Chapter 12, but here's a sneak preview: adequate nutrition and regular exercise are essential to achieving peak bone mass before age 30.

Vitamin D raises blood concentrations of bone minerals in three ways. When the diet is sufficient, vitamin D enhances mineral absorption from the GI tract. When the diet is insufficient, vitamin D provides the needed minerals from other sources: reabsorption by the kidneys and mobilization from the bones into the blood. The vitamin may work alone, as it does in the GI tract, or in combination with parathyroid hormone, as it does in the bones and kidneys.

Vitamin D in Other Roles Scientists have discovered many other tissues that respond to vitamin D, as the following examples describe. In the brain and nerve cells, vitamin D protects against cognitive decline and slows the progression of Parkinson disease.[16] Vitamin D in muscle cells encourages growth in children and preserves strength in adults.[17] Vitamin D signals cells of the immune system to defend against infectious diseases.[18] Vitamin D may also regulate the cells of the adipose tissue in ways that might influence the development of obesity.[19]

In many cases, vitamin D enhances or suppresses the activity of genes that regulate cell growth. As such, it may be valuable in treating a number of diseases. Recent research suggests that vitamin D may protect against metabolic syndrome, type 2 diabetes, tuberculosis, inflammation, multiple sclerosis, macular degeneration, hypertension, and some cancers.[20] Even so, evidence does not support vitamin D supplementation to improve health beyond correcting deficiencies.[21] In fact, some evidence suggests certain cancers are associated with both too little and too much vitamin D, making routine supplementation potentially harmful.[22]

Vitamin D Deficiency Overt signs of vitamin D deficiency are relatively rare, but vitamin D insufficiency is remarkably common.[23] Almost 10 percent of the US population is deficient and another 25 percent are marginal.[24] Factors that contribute to vitamin D deficiency include dark skin, breastfeeding without supplementation, lack of sunlight, and not using fortified milk. In vitamin D deficiency, production of **calbindin,** a protein that binds calcium in the intestinal cells, slows. Thus, even when calcium in the diet is adequate, it passes through the GI tract unabsorbed, leaving the bones undersupplied. Consequently, a vitamin D deficiency creates a calcium deficiency and increases the risks of several chronic diseases and osteoporosis. Vitamin D–deficient adolescents do not reach their peak bone mass.

Rickets Worldwide, the prevalence of the vitamin D–deficiency disease **rickets** is extremely high, affecting more than half of the children in countries such as China and Mongolia, and regions such as sub-Saharan Africa, the Middle East, and Latin America.[25] In the United States, rickets is not common, but when it occurs, black children and adolescents—especially females and overweight teens—are the ones most likely to be affected. To prevent rickets, the American Academy of Pediatrics recommends a supplement for all infants, children, and adolescents who do not receive enough vitamin D.

In rickets, the bones fail to calcify normally, causing growth retardation and skeletal abnormalities. The bones become so weak that they bend when they have to support the body's weight (see Figure 11-9). A child with rickets who is

> FIGURE 11-9 Vitamin D–Deficiency Symptoms—Bowed Legs and Beaded Ribs of Rickets

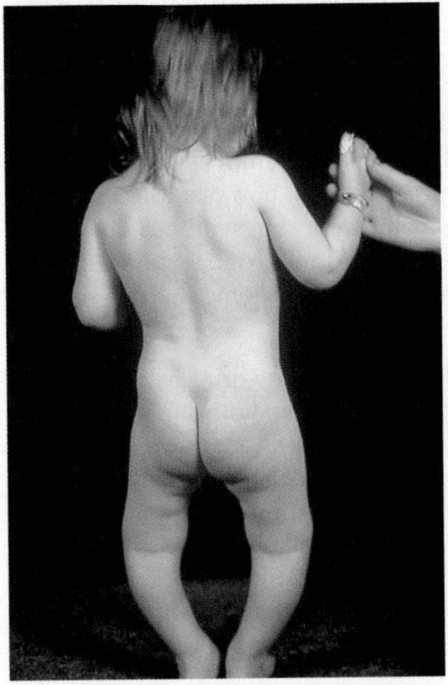

Biophoto Associates/Science Source

Bowed legs. In rickets, the poorly formed long bones of the legs bend outward as weight-bearing activities such as walking begin.

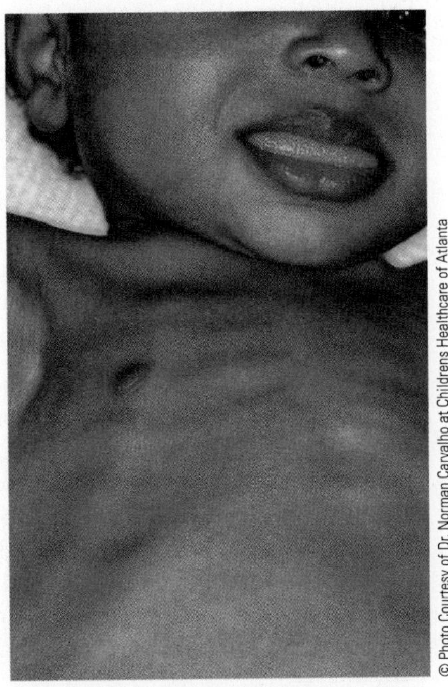

© Photo Courtesy of Dr. Norman Carvalho at Childrens Healthcare of Atlanta

Beaded ribs. In rickets, a series of "beads" develop where the cartilages and bones attach.

calbindin: a calcium-binding transport protein that requires vitamin D for its synthesis.

rickets: the vitamin D–deficiency disease in children characterized by inadequate mineralization of bone (manifested in bowed legs or knock-knees, outward-bowed chest, and "beads" on ribs). A rare type of rickets, not caused by vitamin D deficiency, is known as *vitamin D–refractory rickets.*

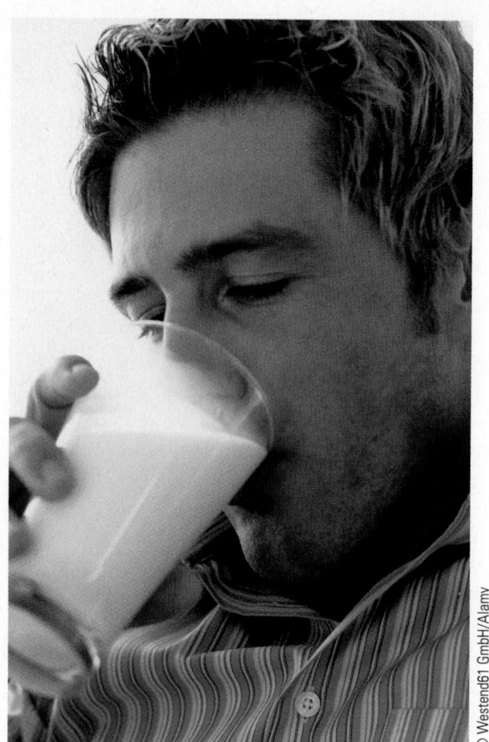
© Westend61 GmbH/Alamy

A cold glass of milk refreshes as it replenishes vitamin D and other bone-building nutrients.

old enough to walk characteristically develops bowed legs, often the most obvious sign of the disease. Another sign is the beaded ribs that result from the poorly formed attachments of the bones to the cartilage.*

Osteomalacia In adults, the poor mineralization of bone results in the painful bone disease **osteomalacia.** The bones become increasingly soft, flexible, brittle, and deformed.

Osteoporosis Any failure to synthesize adequate vitamin D or obtain enough from foods sets the stage for a loss of calcium from the bones, which can result in fractures. Highlight 12 describes the many factors that lead to osteoporosis, a condition of reduced bone density.

The Elderly Vitamin D deficiency is especially likely in older adults for several reasons. For one, the skin, liver, and kidneys lose their capacity to make and activate vitamin D with advancing age. For another, older adults typically drink little or no milk—the main dietary source of vitamin D. And finally, older adults typically spend much of the day indoors, and when they do venture outside, many of them cautiously wear protective clothing or apply sunscreen to all sun-exposed areas of their skin. Dark-skinned adults living in northern regions are particularly vulnerable. All of these factors increase the likelihood of vitamin D deficiency and its consequences: bone losses, osteoporotic fractures, and muscle weakness.[26] Vitamin D supplementation helps to raise blood levels, reduce bone loss, improve muscle performance, and lower the risks of falls and fractures in elderly persons.[27]

Vitamin D Toxicity

Vitamin D clearly illustrates how nutrients in optimal amounts support health, but both inadequacies and excesses create harm. Vitamin D is among the most likely of the vitamins to have toxic effects when consumed in excessive amounts. The amounts of vitamin D made by the skin and found in foods are well within the safe limits set by the UL, but supplements containing the vitamin in concentrated form should be kept out of the reach of children and used cautiously by adults.

Excess vitamin D raises the concentration of blood calcium.** Excess blood calcium tends to precipitate in the soft tissue, forming stones, especially in the kidneys where calcium is concentrated in an effort to excrete it. Calcification may also harden the blood vessels and is especially dangerous in the major arteries of the brain, heart, and lungs, where it can cause death.

Vitamin D Recommendations and Sources

Only a few foods contain vitamin D naturally. Fortunately, the body can make vitamin D with the help of a little sunshine. In setting dietary recommendations, however, the DRI Committee assumed that no vitamin D was available from skin synthesis. In order to reach sufficient levels of vitamin D in the blood without contributions from the sun, dietary recommendations were recently increased.[28] Some research suggests that vitamin D recommendations should be higher still.[29]

Vitamin D in Foods The *Dietary Guidelines* advise consumers to drink at least 2 cups of vitamin D–fortified milk a day. The fortification of milk and other foods with vitamin D is the best guarantee that people will meet their needs.[30]*** Consumers using alternatives such as soy milk or almond milk need to read labels carefully to ensure they are getting vitamin D-fortified products. Despite vitamin D fortification, the average intake in the United States falls short of recommendations. Egg yolks and oily fish such as salmon, mackerel, and sardines are the best natural sources of vitamin D.

Meeting vitamin D needs is difficult without adequate sunshine, fortification, or supplementation. Importantly, feeding infants and young children

osteomalacia (OS-tee-oh-ma-LAY-shuh): a bone disease characterized by softening of the bones. Symptoms include bending of the spine and bowing of the legs. The disease occurs most in adult women.

- **osteo** = bone
- **malacia** = softening

*Because the poorly formed rib attachments resemble rosary beads, this symptom is commonly known as *rachitic* (ra-KIT-ik) *rosary* ("the rosary of rickets").

**High blood calcium is known as *hypercalcemia* and may develop from a variety of disorders, including vitamin D toxicity. It does *not* develop from too much calcium in the diet.

***Vitamin D fortification of milk in the United States is 10 micrograms per quart.

> FIGURE 11-10 Vitamin D Synthesis and Latitude

Above 40° north latitude (and below 40° south latitude in the southern hemisphere), vitamin D synthesis essentially ceases for the 4 months of winter. Synthesis increases as spring approaches, peaks in summer, and declines again in the fall. People living in regions of extreme northern (or extreme southern) latitudes may miss as much as 6 months of vitamin D production.

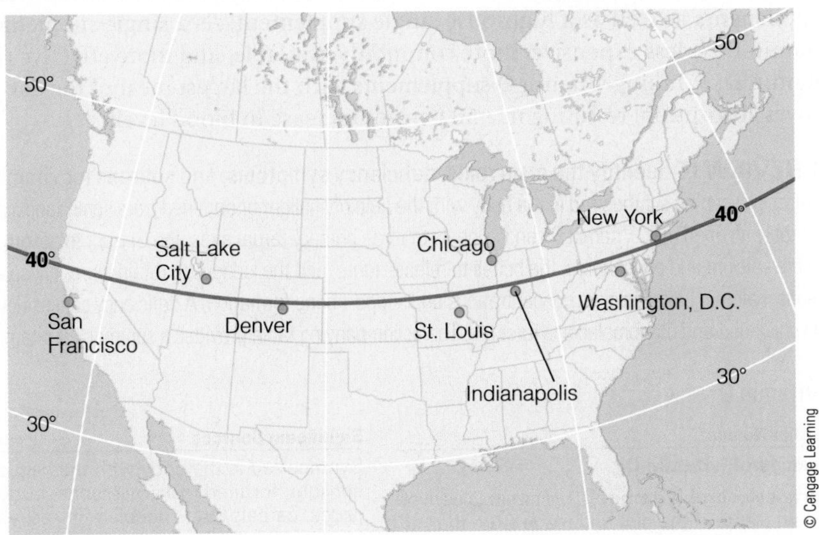

nonfortified "health beverages" instead of milk or infant formula can create severe nutrient deficiencies, including rickets.

Vitamin D from the Sun Most of the world's population relies on natural exposure to sunlight to maintain adequate vitamin D nutrition. The sun imposes no risk of vitamin D toxicity; prolonged exposure to sunlight degrades the vitamin D precursor in the skin, preventing its conversion to the active vitamin.

Prolonged exposure to sunlight can, however, prematurely wrinkle the skin and cause skin cancer. Sunscreens help reduce these risks, but sunscreens with a sun protection factor (SPF) of 8 and higher can also reduce vitamin D synthesis. Still, even with an SPF 15 to 30 sunscreen, sufficient vitamin D synthesis can be obtained in 10 to 20 minutes of sun exposure. Alternatively, a person could apply sunscreen after enough time has elapsed to provide sufficient vitamin D synthesis. For most people, exposing hands, face, and arms on a clear summer day for 5 to 10 minutes two or three times a week should be sufficient to maintain vitamin D nutrition.

The pigments of dark skin provide some protection from the sun's damage, but they also reduce vitamin D synthesis. Dark-skinned people require more sunlight exposure than light-skinned people—perhaps as much as 4 to 6 times longer.[31] Latitude, season, and time of day also have dramatic effects on vitamin D synthesis and status (see Figure 11-10). Heavy cloud cover, smoke, or smog block the ultraviolet (UV) rays of the sun that promote vitamin D synthesis. People who stay in the shade and wear long-sleeved clothing are twice as likely to develop vitamin D deficiency as those who rarely do so.[32] Vitamin D deficiency is especially prevalent in the winter and in the Arctic and Antarctic regions of the world.[33] To ensure an adequate vitamin D status, supplements may be needed. The body's vitamin D supplies from summer synthesis alone are insufficient to meet winter needs.[34]

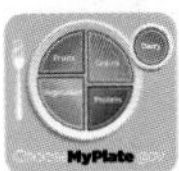

> DIETARY GUIDELINES FOR AMERICANS

Choose foods that provide more vitamin D, a nutrient of concern in American diets. Most dietary vitamin D derives from fortified foods such as milk, yogurt, and breakfast cereals; natural dietary sources of vitamin D include oily fish and egg yolks.

Depending on the radiation used, the UV rays from tanning lamps and tanning beds may also stimulate vitamin D synthesis and increase bone density. The potential

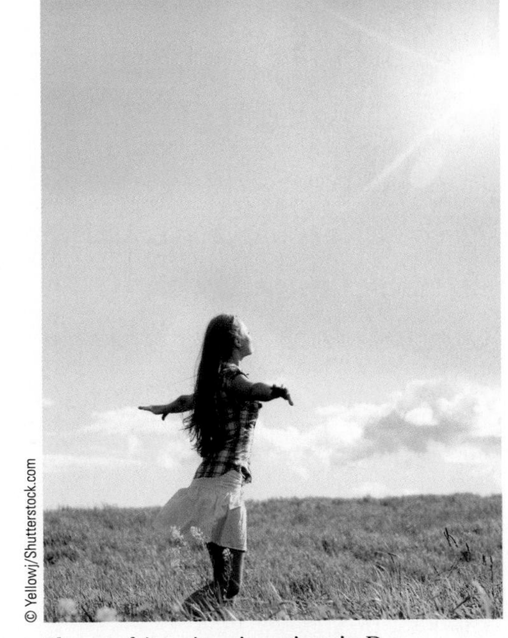

The sunshine vitamin—vitamin D.

hazards of skin damage, however, may outweigh any possible benefits.* The Food and Drug Administration (FDA) warns that if the lamps are not properly filtered, people using tanning booths risk burns, damage to the eyes and blood vessels, and skin cancer.

Vitamin D from Supplements As mentioned, some people may benefit from taking vitamin D supplements. Vitamin D can be found in multivitamin-mineral supplements as well as a high-dose single supplement. As a single supplement, vitamin D_3 is less expensive, more commonly available, and more effective than vitamin D_2.[35] Taking vitamin D supplements with the largest meal of the day improves absorption, resulting in a 50 percent increase in blood levels.[36]

› REVIEW IT Identify the main roles, deficiency symptoms, and sources for vitamin D.

Vitamin D can be synthesized in the body with the help of sunlight or obtained from some foods, most notably fortified milk. Vitamin D sends signals to three primary target sites: the GI tract to absorb more calcium and phosphorus, the bones to release more, and the kidneys to retain more. These actions maintain blood calcium concentrations and support bone formation. A deficiency causes rickets in childhood and osteomalacia in later life. The accompanying table provides a summary of vitamin D.

Vitamin D

Other Names

calciferol (vitamin D)

ergocalciferol (vitamin D_2): vitamin D derived from plants in the diet and made from the yeast and plant sterol ergosterol.

cholecalciferol (vitamin D_3 or **calciol):** vitamin D derived from animals in the diet or made in the skin from 7-dehydrocholesterol, a precursor of cholesterol, with the help of sunlight.

calcidiol (25-hydroxyvitamin D): vitamin D found in the blood that is made from the hydroxylation of calciol in the liver.

calcitriol (1,25-dihydroxyvitamin D): vitamin D that is made from the hydroxylation of calcidiol in the kidneys; the biologically active hormone, sometimes called *active vitamin D.*

RDA

Adults: 15 µg/day or 600 IU/day (19–70 yr)
20 µg/day or 800 IU/day (>70 yr)

UL

Adults: 100 µg/day or 4000 IU/day

Chief Functions in the Body

Mineralization of bones (raises blood calcium and phosphorus by increasing absorption from digestive tract, withdrawing calcium from bones, stimulating retention by kidneys)

Significant Sources

Synthesized in the body with the help of sunlight; fortified milk, margarine, butter, juices, cereals, and chocolate mixes; veal, beef, egg yolks, liver, fatty fish (herring, salmon, sardines) and their oils

Deficiency Diseases

Rickets, osteomalacia

Deficiency Symptoms

Rickets in children:

Inadequate calcification, resulting in misshapen bones (bowing of legs); enlargement of ends of long bones (knees, wrists); deformities of ribs (bowed, with beads or knobs);[a] delayed closing of fontanel, resulting in rapid enlargement of head (see figure below); lax muscles resulting in protrusion of abdomen; muscle spasms

Osteomalacia or osteoporosis in adults:

Loss of calcium, resulting in soft, flexible, brittle, and deformed bones; progressive weakness; pain in pelvis, lower back, and legs

Toxicity Disease

Hypervitaminosis D

Toxicity Symptoms

Elevated blood calcium; calcification of soft tissues (blood vessels, kidneys, heart, lungs, tissues around joints)

Fontanel A fontanel is an open space in the top of a baby's skull before the bones have grown together. In rickets, closing of the fontanel is delayed.

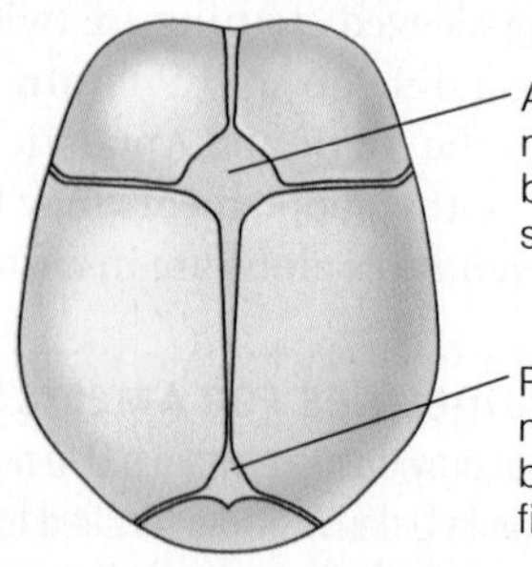

Anterior fontanel normally closes by the end of the second year.
Posterior fontanel normally closes by the end of the first year.
© Cengage Learning

[a]Bowing of the ribs causes the symptoms known as *pigeon breast*. The beads that form on the ribs resemble rosary beads; thus this symptom is known as *rachitic* (ra-KIT-ik) *rosary* ("the rosary of rickets").

*The best wavelengths for vitamin D synthesis are UV-B rays between 290 and 310 nanometers. Some tanning parlors advertise "UV-A rays only, for a tan without the burn," but UV-A rays can damage the skin.

11.3 Vitamin E

› LEARN IT Identify the main roles, deficiency symptoms, and food sources for vitamin E.

The vitamin E family consists of two subgroups—the **tocopherols** and the **tocotrienols**—each containing four members designated by letters of the Greek alphabet (alpha, beta, gamma, and delta). All consist of a complex ring structure with a long saturated (in tocopherols) or unsaturated (in tocotrienols) side chain. The positions of methyl groups (CH_3) on the side chain and their chemical rotations distinguish the four members within each subgroup. (Appendix C provides the chemical structures.)

Of all the members of the vitamin E family, only **alpha-tocopherol** is maintained in the body and can meet the body's needs for the vitamin. The others are not converted to alpha-tocopherol in the body, nor are they recognized by its transport protein. For these reasons, the RDA is based only on alpha-tocopherol.

Most vitamin E research has focused on alpha-tocopherol, but recent studies suggest that the other tocopherols and tocotrienols might also be beneficial. For example, gamma-tocopherol and possibly delta-tocopherol, appear to be most effective in inhibiting inflammation and cancer growth.[37] In addition to preventing cancer, tocotrienols may also protect against osteoporosis, diabetes, heart disease, and neurological disorders.[38]

Vitamin E as an Antioxidant Vitamin E is a fat-soluble antioxidant and one of the body's primary defenders against the adverse effects of free radicals. Its main action is to stop the chain reaction of free radicals from producing more free radicals (see Highlight 11). In doing so, vitamin E protects the vulnerable components of the cells and their membranes from destruction. Most notably, vitamin E prevents the oxidation of the polyunsaturated fatty acids, but it protects other lipids and related compounds (for example, vitamin A) as well.

Accumulating evidence suggests that vitamin E may reduce the risk of heart disease by protecting low-density lipoproteins (LDL) against oxidation and reducing inflammation. The oxidation of LDL and inflammation have been implicated as key factors in the development of heart disease. Highlight 11 explains how vitamin E and other antioxidants might protect against chronic diseases, such as heart disease and cancer, and explores whether foods or supplements might be most helpful—or harmful.

Vitamin E Deficiency A primary deficiency of vitamin E (from poor dietary intake) is rare; deficiency is usually associated with diseases of fat malabsorption such as cystic fibrosis. Without vitamin E, the red blood cells break and spill their contents, probably because of oxidation of the polyunsaturated fatty acids in their membranes. This classic sign of vitamin E deficiency, known as **erythrocyte hemolysis,** is seen in premature infants born before the transfer of vitamin E from the mother to the infant that takes place in the last weeks of pregnancy. Vitamin E treatment corrects **hemolytic anemia.**

Prolonged vitamin E deficiency, as can occur with some genetic disorders, also causes neuromuscular dysfunction.[39] Common symptoms include loss of muscle coordination and reflexes and impaired vision and speech. Vitamin E treatment helps to correct these neurological symptoms of vitamin E deficiency.

Two other conditions seem to respond to vitamin E treatment, although results are inconsistent. One is **fibrocystic breast disease,** a nonmalignant breast disease. The other is **intermittent claudication,** an abnormality of blood flow that causes cramping in the legs.

Vitamin E Toxicity Vitamin E supplement use has risen in recent years as its protective actions against chronic diseases have been recognized. Fortunately, the liver carefully regulates vitamin E concentrations. Toxicity is rare, and vitamin E appears safe across a broad range of intakes. The UL for vitamin E (1000 milligrams)

tocopherols (tuh-KOFF-uh-rawls): members of the vitamin E family having the chemical structure of a complex ring structure with a long saturated side chain. (See Appendix C for chemical structures.)

tocotrienols (TOE-koh-try-EE-nawls): members of the vitamin E family having the chemical structure of a complex ring structure with a long unsaturated side chain. (See Appendix C for chemical structures.)

alpha-tocopherol: the active vitamin E compound.

erythrocyte (eh-RITH-ro-cite) **hemolysis** (he-MOLL-uh-sis): the breaking open of red blood cells (erythrocytes); a symptom of vitamin E–deficiency disease in human beings.

- **erythro** = red
- **cyte** = cell
- **hemo** = blood
- **lysis** = breaking

hemolytic (HE-moh-LIT-ick) **anemia:** the condition of having too few red blood cells as a result of erythrocyte hemolysis.

fibrocystic (FYE-bro-SIS-tik) **breast disease:** a harmless condition in which the breasts develop lumps, sometimes associated with caffeine consumption. In some, it responds to abstinence from caffeine; in others, it can be treated with vitamin E.

- **fibro** = fibrous tissue
- **cyst** = closed sac

intermittent claudication (klaw-dih-KAY-shun): severe calf pain caused by inadequate blood supply. It occurs when walking and subsides during rest.

- **intermittent** = at intervals
- **claudicare** = to limp

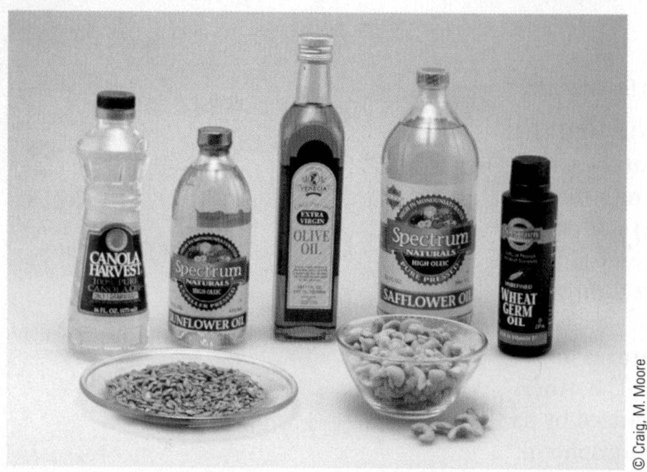

Fat-soluble vitamin E is found predominantly in vegetable oils, seeds, and nuts.

is more than 65 times greater than the recommended intake for adults (15 milligrams). Extremely high doses of vitamin E may interfere with the blood-clotting action of vitamin K and enhance the effects of drugs used to oppose blood clotting, causing hemorrhage.

Vitamin E Recommendations The RDA for vitamin E is based on the alpha-tocopherol form only. As mentioned earlier, the other tocopherols and tocotrienols cannot be converted to alpha-tocopherol, nor do they perform the same metabolic roles in the body. A person who consumes large quantities of polyunsaturated fatty acids needs more vitamin E. Fortunately, vitamin E and polyunsaturated fatty acids tend to occur together in the same foods.

Vitamin E in Foods Vitamin E is widespread in foods. Much of the vitamin E in the diet comes from vegetable oils and products made from them, such as margarine and salad dressings. Wheat germ oil is especially rich in vitamin E.

Because vitamin E is readily destroyed by heat and oxidation, fresh foods are preferable sources. Most processed and convenience foods do not contribute enough vitamin E to ensure an adequate intake.

› REVIEW IT Identify the main roles, deficiency symptoms, and foods sources for vitamin E.

Vitamin E acts as an antioxidant, defending lipids and other components of the cells against oxidative damage. Deficiencies are rare, but they do occur in premature infants, the primary symptom being erythrocyte hemolysis. Vitamin E is found predominantly in vegetable oils and appears to be one of the least toxic of the fat-soluble vitamins. The accompanying table provides a summary of vitamin E.

Vitamin E

Other Names	**Significant Sources**
Alpha-tocopherol	Polyunsaturated plant oils (margarine, salad dressings), dark green, leafy vegetables (spinach, turnip greens, collard greens, broccoli), wheat germ, whole grains, liver, egg yolks, nuts, seeds, fatty meats
RDA	Easily destroyed by heat and oxygen
Adults: 15 mg/day	**Deficiency Symptoms**
UL	Red blood cell breakage,[a] nerve damage
Adults: 1000 mg/day	**Toxicity Symptoms**
Chief Functions in the Body	Augments the effects of anticlotting medication
Antioxidant (stabilization of cell membranes, regulation of oxidation reactions, protection of polyunsaturated fatty acids [PUFA] and vitamin A)	

[a]The breaking of red blood cells is called *erythrocyte hemolysis*.

11.4 Vitamin K

› LEARN IT Identify the main roles, deficiency symptoms, and sources for vitamin K.

Vitamin K appropriately gets its name from the Danish word *koagulation* ("coagulation" or "clotting"). Its primary action is blood clotting, where its presence can make the difference between life and death. Blood has a remarkable ability to remain liquid, but it can clot within seconds when the integrity of that system is disturbed.

Roles in the Body More than a dozen different proteins and the mineral calcium are involved in making a blood clot. Vitamin K is essential for the activation of several of these proteins, among them prothrombin, made by the

> FIGURE 11-11 **Blood-Clotting Process**

Vitamin K is essential for the synthesis of prothrombin and several other clotting factors. Blood clots are formed by a cascade of reactions, with each step creating a compound that activates the next step.

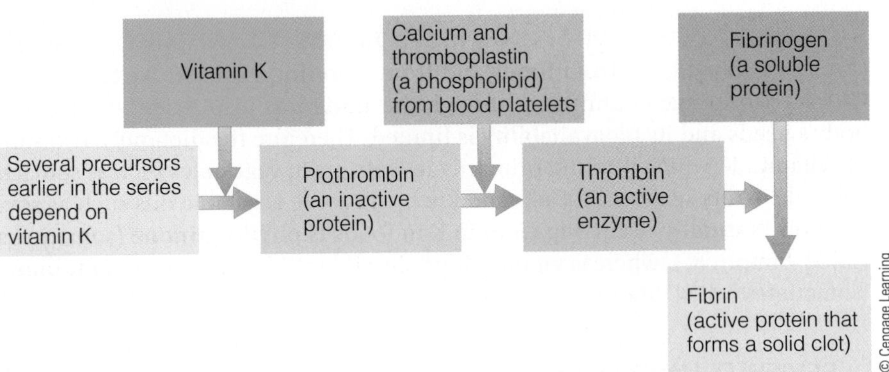

liver as a precursor of the protein thrombin (see Figure 11-11). When any of the blood-clotting factors is lacking, **hemorrhagic disease** results. If an artery or vein is cut or broken, bleeding goes unchecked. Of course, this is not to say that hemorrhaging is always caused by vitamin K deficiency. Another cause is the genetic disorder **hemophilia,** which is neither caused nor cured by vitamin K.

Vitamin K also participates in the metabolism of bone proteins, most notably **osteocalcin.** Without vitamin K, osteocalcin cannot bind to the minerals that normally form bones, resulting in low bone density.* An adequate intake of vitamin K helps to decrease bone turnover and protect against fractures. The effectiveness of vitamin K supplements on bone health is inconclusive.[40]

Vitamin K is historically known for its role in blood clotting, and more recently for its participation in bone building, but researchers continue to discover proteins needing vitamin K's assistance. These proteins have been identified in the plaques of atherosclerosis, the kidneys, and the nervous system.

Vitamin K Deficiency

Chapter 1 explains that a *primary deficiency* develops in response to an inadequate dietary intake whereas a *secondary deficiency* occurs for other reasons. A primary deficiency of vitamin K is rare, but a secondary deficiency may occur in two circumstances. First, whenever fat absorption falters, as occurs when bile production fails, vitamin K absorption diminishes. Second, some drugs disrupt vitamin K's synthesis and action in the body: antibiotics kill the vitamin K–producing bacteria in the intestine, and anticoagulant drugs interfere with vitamin K metabolism and activity. Excessive bleeding due to a vitamin K deficiency can be fatal.

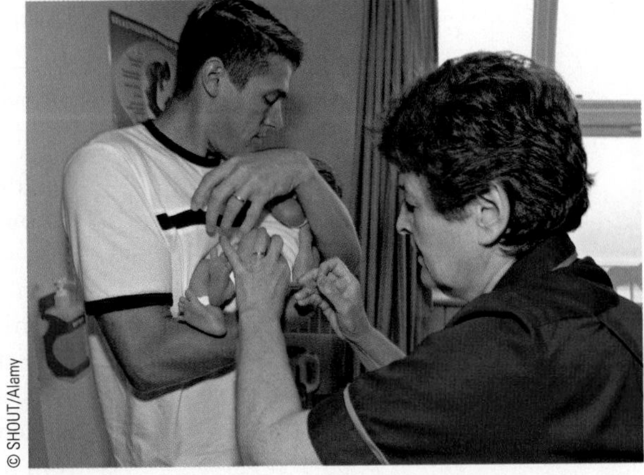

Soon after birth, newborn infants receive a dose of vitamin K to prevent hemorrhagic disease.

Newborn infants present a unique case of vitamin K nutrition because they are born with a **sterile** intestinal tract, and the vitamin K–producing bacteria take weeks to establish themselves. Furthermore, vitamin K is minimally transported across the placenta and its concentration in breast milk is low. At the same time, plasma prothrombin concentrations are low, which reduces the likelihood of fatal blood clotting during the stress of birth. To prevent hemorrhagic disease in the newborn, a single dose of vitamin K is given at birth by intramuscular injection.[41] Concerns that vitamin K given at birth raises the risks of childhood cancer are unfounded.

Vitamin K Toxicity

Toxicity is not common, and no adverse effects have been reported with high intakes of vitamin K. Therefore, a UL has not been established. High doses of vitamin K can, however, reduce the effectiveness of

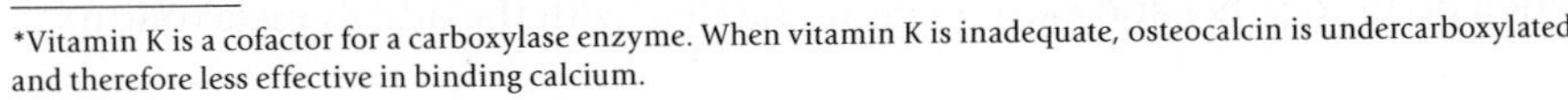
*Vitamin K is a cofactor for a carboxylase enzyme. When vitamin K is inadequate, osteocalcin is undercarboxylated and therefore less effective in binding calcium.

hemorrhagic (hem-oh-RAJ-ik) **disease:** a disease characterized by excessive bleeding.

hemophilia (HE-moh-FEEL-ee-ah): a hereditary disease in which the blood is unable to clot because it lacks the ability to synthesize certain clotting factors.

osteocalcin (os-teo-KAL-sen): a calcium-binding protein in bones, essential for normal mineralization.

sterile: free of microorganisms, such as bacteria.

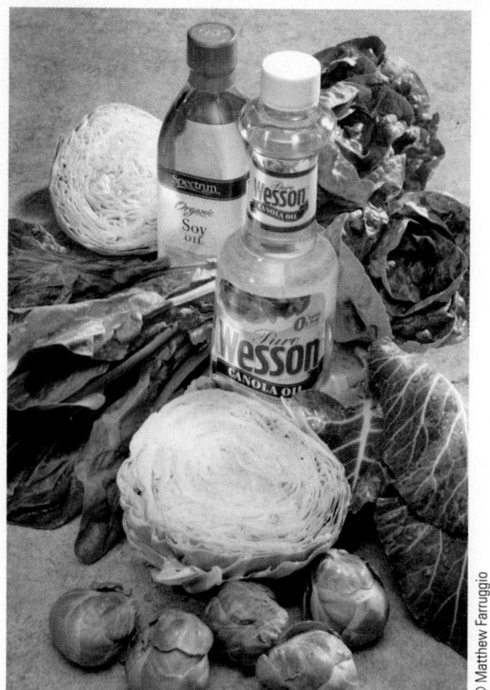

© Matthew Farruggio

Notable food sources of vitamin K include green vegetables such as collards, spinach, bib lettuce, brussels sprouts, and cabbage and vegetable oils such as soybean oil and canola oil.

anticoagulant drugs used to prevent blood clotting. People taking these drugs can continue eating their usual diets. Their blood clotting times should be monitored closely and drug dosages adjusted accordingly.

Vitamin K Recommendations and Sources Like vitamin D, vitamin K can be obtained both from foods and from a nonfood source. Bacteria in the GI tract synthesize vitamin K, although the amount is insufficient to meet the body's needs and its bioavailability is limited. Therefore the diet must also supply vitamin K, which is found primarily in leafy green vegetables such as spinach and kale, fruits such as avocado and kiwi, and some vegetable oils such as soybean oil. Naturally occurring vitamin K in foods is **phylloquinone** (sometimes called vitamin K_1), whereas vitamin K produced by GI bacteria is **menaquinone** (sometimes called vitamin K_2).

› REVIEW IT Identify the main roles, deficiency symptoms, and sources for vitamin K.
Vitamin K helps with blood clotting, and its deficiency causes hemorrhagic disease (uncontrolled bleeding). Bacteria in the GI tract can make the vitamin; people typically receive about half of their requirements from bacterial synthesis and half from foods such as green vegetables and vegetable oils. Because people depend on bacterial synthesis for vitamin K, deficiency is most likely in newborn infants and in people taking antibiotics. The accompanying table provides a summary of vitamin K.

Vitamin K

Other Names	**Significant Sources**
Phylloquinone (vitamin K_1), menaquinone (vitamin K_2), menadione (in supplements)	Bacterial synthesis in the digestive tract;[a] liver; dark green, leafy vegetables, cabbage-type vegetables; milk
AI	**Deficiency Symptoms**
Men: 120 μg/day Women: 90 μg/day	Hemorrhaging
Chief Functions in the Body	**Toxicity Symptoms**
Synthesis of blood-clotting proteins and bone proteins	None known

[a]Vitamin K needs cannot be met from bacterial synthesis alone.

The four fat-soluble vitamins play many specific roles in the growth and maintenance of the body. Their presence affects the health and function of the eyes, skin, GI tract, lungs, bones, teeth, nervous system, and blood; their deficiencies become apparent in these same areas. Toxicities of the fat-soluble vitamins are possible, especially when people use supplements, because the body stores excesses.

As with the water-soluble vitamins, the function of one fat-soluble vitamin often depends on the presence of another. Recall that vitamin E protects vitamin A from oxidation. In vitamin E deficiency, vitamin A absorption and storage are impaired. Three of the four fat-soluble vitamins—A, D, and K—play important roles in bone growth and remodeling. As mentioned, vitamin K helps synthesize a specific bone protein, and vitamin D regulates that synthesis. Vitamin A, in turn, may control which bone-building genes respond to vitamin D. Vitamin E and vitamin K share some metabolic pathways, which can create problems, especially in blood clotting.

Fat-soluble vitamins also interact with minerals. Vitamin D and calcium cooperate in bone formation, and zinc is required for the synthesis of vitamin A's transport protein, retinol-binding protein. Zinc also assists the enzyme that regenerates retinal from retinol in the eye. Vitamin A deficiency and iron deficiency often occur together and each seems to interfere with the other's metabolism.

phylloquinone (fill-oh-KWYN-own): the plant form of vitamin K; also called *vitamin K_1*.

menaquinone (men-ah-KWYN-own): the bacteria-produced form of vitamin K; also called *vitamin K_2*.

The roles of the fat-soluble vitamins differ from those of the water-soluble vitamins, and they appear in different foods—yet they are just as essential to life. The need for them underlines the importance of eating a wide variety of nourishing foods daily. The accompanying table provides a summary of the fat-soluble vitamins.

› REVIEW IT The Fat-Soluble Vitamins

Vitamin and Chief Functions	Deficiency Symptoms	Toxicity Symptoms	Significant Sources
Vitamin A			
Vision; maintenance of cornea, epithelial cells, mucous membranes, skin; bone and tooth growth; reproduction; immunity	Infectious diseases, night blindness, blindness (xerophthalmia), keratinization	Reduced bone mineral density, liver abnormalities, birth defects	Retinol: milk and milk products Beta-carotene: dark green, leafy and deep yellow/orange vegetables
Vitamin D			
Mineralization of bones (raises blood calcium and phosphorus by increasing absorption from digestive tract, withdrawing calcium from bones, stimulating retention by kidneys)	Rickets, osteomalacia	Calcium imbalance (calcification of soft tissues and formation of stones)	Synthesized in the body with the help of sunshine; fortified milk
Vitamin E			
Antioxidant (stabilization of cell membranes, regulation of oxidation reactions, protection of polyunsaturated fatty acids [PUFA] and vitamin A)	Erythrocyte hemolysis, nerve damage	Hemorrhagic effects	Vegetable oils
Vitamin K			
Synthesis of blood-clotting proteins and bone proteins	Hemorrhage	None known	Synthesized in the body by GI bacteria; dark green, leafy vegetables

Nutrition Portfolio

For the fat-soluble vitamins, select colorful fruits and vegetables, fortified milk or soy products, and vegetable oils; use supplements with caution, if at all. Go to Diet & Wellness Plus and choose one of the days on which you tracked your diet for an entire day. Select the MyPlate report and then consider the following questions:

- How was your overall intake in the vegetable group? Do you need improvement in this area? If so, what are some changes you could make?

Now look at the report titled Intake Spreadsheet to answer the following questions:

- Examine your weekly choices of vegetables and evaluate whether you meet the recommendations for dark green or orange and deep yellow vegetables.
- Consider whether you drink enough vitamin D–fortified milk or go outside in the sunshine regularly.
- Describe the vegetable oils you use when you cook and their vitamin contributions.

DIET & WELLNESS PLUS To complete this exercise, go to your Diet & Wellness Plus at www.cengagebrain.com.

› STUDY IT To review the key points of this chapter and take a practice quiz, go to the study cards at the end of the book.

REFERENCES

1. G. Tang, Bioconversion of dietary provitamin A carotenoids to vitamin A in humans, *American Journal of Clinical Nutrition* 91 (2010): 1468S–1473S.
2. J. von Lintig, Colors with functions: Elucidating the biochemical and molecular basis of carotenoid metabolism, *Annual Review of Nutrition* 30 (2010): 35–56.
3. J. C. Saari, Vitamin A metabolism in rod and cone visual cycles, *Annual Review of Nutrition* 32 (2012): 125–145; J. von Lintig, Metabolism of carotenoids and retinoids related to vision, *Journal of Biological Chemistry* 287 (2012): 1627–1634.
4. W. Stahl and H. Sies, β-Carotene and other carotenoids in protection from sunlight, *American Journal of Clinical Nutrition* 96 (2012): 1179S–1184S.
5. M. Clagett-Dame and D. Knutson, Vitamin A in reproduction and development, *Nutrients* 3 (2011): 385–428; N. Noy, Between death and survival: Retinoic acid in regulation of apoptosis, *Annual Review of Nutrition* 30 (2010): 201–217.
6. J. von Lintig, Provitamin A metabolism and functions in mammalian biology, *American Journal of Clinical Nutrition* 96 (2012): 1234S–1244S.
7. A. Sommer and K. S. Vyas, A global clinical view on vitamin A and carotenoids, *American Journal of Clinical Nutrition* 96 (2012): 1204S–1206S.
8. J. C. Sherwin and coauthors, Epidemiology of vitamin A deficiency and xerophthalmia in at-risk populations, *Transactions of the Royal Society of Tropical Medicine and Hygiene* 106 (2012): 205–214; E. Mayo-Wilson and coauthors, Vitamin A supplements for preventing mortality, illness, and blindness in children aged under 5: Systematic review and meta-analysis, *British Medical Journal* 343 (2011): d5094.
9. A. C. Ross, Vitamin A and retinoic acid in T cell-related immunity, *American Journal of Clinical Nutrition* 96 (2012): 1166S–1172S.
10. World Health Organization, Measles fact sheet, February 2013, www.who.int/mediacentre/factsheets/fs286/en/index.html.
11. C. R. Sudfeld, A. M. Navar, and M. A. Halsey, Effectiveness of measles vaccination and vitamin A treatment, *International Journal of Epidemiology* 39 (2010): i48–i55.
12. S. A. Tanumihardjo, Vitamin A and bone health: The balancing act, *Journal of Clinical Densitometry* 16 (2013): 414–419; H. Ahmadieh and A. Arabi, Vitamins and bone health: Beyond calcium and vitamin D, *Nutrition Reviews* 69 (2011): 584–598.
13. M. M. G. Ackermans and coauthors, Vitamin A and clefting: Putative biological mechanisms, *Nutrition Reviews* 69 (2011): 613–624.
14. M. J. Haskell, The challenge to reach nutritional adequacy for vitamin A: β-carotene bioavailability and conversion—evidence in humans, *American Journal of Clinical Nutrition* 96 (2012): 1193S–1203S.
15. G. Jones, Extrarenal vitamin D activation and interactions between vitamin D_2, vitamin D_3, and vitamin D analogs, *Annual Review of Nutrition* 33 (2013): 23–44.
16. X. Cui and coauthors, Low vitamin D concentration exacerbates adult brain dysfunction, *American Journal of Clinical Nutrition* 97 (2013): 907–908; D. J. Llewellyn and coauthors, Vitamin D and risk of cognitive decline in elderly persons, *Archives of Internal Medicine* 170 (2010): 1135–1141.
17. A. S. Grimaldi and coauthors, 25(OH) Vitamin D is associated with greater muscle strength in healthy men and women, *Medicine and Science in Sports and Exercise* 45 (2013): 157–162; T. J. Hazell, J. R. DeGuire, and H. A. Weiler, Vitamin D: An overview of its role in skeletal muscle physiology in children and adolescents, *Nutrition Reviews* 70 (2012): 520–533.
18. I. Laaksi, Vitamins, infectious and chronic disease during adulthood and aging: Vitamin D and respiratory infection in adults, *Proceedings of the Nutrition Society* 71 (2012): 90–97; M. E. Sundaram and L. A. Coleman, Vitamin D and influenza, *Advances in Nutrition: An International Review Journal* 3 (2012): 517–525; M. Hewison, Vitamin D and innate and adaptive immunity, *Vitamins and Hormones* 86 (2011): 23–62; F. Baeke and coauthors, Human T lymphocytes are direct targets of 1,25-dihydroxyvitamin D3 in the immune system, *Journal of Steroid Biochemistry and Molecular Biology* 121 (2010): 221–227.
19. C. P. Earthman and coauthors, The link between obesity and low circulating 25-hydroxyvitamin D concentrations: Considerations and implications, *International Journal of Obesity* 36 (2012): 387–396; C. Ding and coauthors, Vitamin D signalling in adipose tissue, *British Journal of Nutrition* 108 (2012): 1915–1923.
20. S. Lim and coauthors, Association of vitamin D deficiency with incidence of type 2 diabetes in high-risk Asian subjects, *American Journal of Clinical Nutrition* 97 (2013): 524–530; T. D. Cheng and coauthors, Vitamin D intake and lung cancer risk in the Women's Health Initiative, *American Journal of Clinical Nutrition* 98 (2013): 1002–1011; F. M. Yousef and coauthors, Vitamin D status and breast cancer in Saudi Arabian women: Case-control study, *American Journal of Clinical Nutrition* 98 (2013): 105–110; R. E. Stubbins, A. Hakeem, and N. P. Núñez, Using components of the vitamin D pathway to prevent and treat colon cancer, *Nutrition Reviews* 70 (2012): 721–729; G. J. Fung and coauthors, Vitamin D intake is inversely related to risk of developing metabolic syndrome in African American and white men and women over 20 y: The Coronary Artery Risk Development in Young Adults study, *American Journal of Clinical Nutrition* 96 (2012): 24–29; V. Ganji and coauthors, Serum 25-hydroxyvitamin D concentrations are associated with prevalence of metabolic syndrome and various cardiometabolic risk factors in US children and adolescents based on assay-adjusted serum 25-hydroxyvitamin D data from NHANES 2001–2006, *American Journal of Clinical Nutrition* 94 (2011): 225–233; S. A. Chacko and coauthors, Serum 25-hydroxyvitamin D concentrations in relation to cardiometabolic risk factors and metabolic syndrome in postmenopausal women, *American Journal of Clinical Nutrition* 94 (2011): 209–217; J. Mitri, M. D. Muraru, and A. G. Pittas, Vitamin D and type 2 diabetes: A systematic review, *European Journal of Clinical Nutrition* 65 (2011): 1005–1015; E. M. Mowry, Vitamin D: Evidence for its role as a prognostic factor in multiple sclerosis, *Journal of Neurological Science* 311 (2011): 19–22; M. H. Hopkins and coauthors, Effects of supplemental vitamin D and calcium on biomarkers of inflammation in colorectal adenoma patients: A randomized, controlled clinical trial, *Cancer Prevention Research* 4 (2011): 1645–1654; K. Luong and L. T. Nguyen, Impact of vitamin D in the treatment of tuberculosis, *American Journal of Medical Sciences* 341 (2011): 493–498; A. E. Millen and coauthors, Vitamin D status and early age-related macular degeneration in postmenopausal women, *Archives of Ophthalmology* 129 (2011): 481–489; Y. Ma and coauthors, Association between vitamin D and risk of colorectal cancer: A systematic review of prospective studies, *Journal of Clinical Oncology* 29 (2011): 3775–3782; L. N. Anderson and coauthors, Vitamin D and calcium intakes and breast cancer risk in pre- and postmenopausal women, *American Journal of Clinical Nutrition* 91 (2010): 1699–1707; N. Parekh, Protective role of vitamin D against age-related macular degeneration: A hypothesis, *Topics in Clinical Nutrition* 25 (2010): 290–301; A. G. Pittas and coauthors, Systematic review: Vitamin D and cardiometabolic outcomes, *Annals of Internal Medicine* 152 (2010): 307–314; C. D. Toner, C. D. Davis, and J. A. Milner, The vitamin D and cancer conundrum: Aiming at a moving target, *Journal of the American Dietetic Association* 110 (2010): 1492–1500.
21. R. Jorde and G. Grimmes, Vitamin D and metabolic health with special reference to the effect of vitamin D on serum lipids, *Progress in Lipid Research* 50 (2011): 303–312; A. Grey and M. Bolland, Vitamin D: A place in the sun? *Archives of Internal Medicine* 170 (2010): 1099–1100.
22. C. D. Davis and J. A. Milner, Nutrigenomics, vitamin D and cancer prevention, *Journal of Nutrigenetics and Nutrigenomics* 4 (2011): 1–11; K. Michaëlsson and coauthors, Plasma vitamin D and mortality in older men: A community-based prospective cohort study, *American Journal of Clinical Nutrition* 92 (2010): 841–848.
23. C. J. Rosen, Vitamin D insufficiency, *New England Journal of Medicine* 364 (2011): 248–254; A. A. Ginde , M. C. Liu, and C. A. Camargo, Demographic differences and trends of vitamin D insufficiency in the US population, 1988–2004, *Archives of Internal Medicine* 169 (2009): 626–632; S. A. Bowden and coauthors, Prevalence of vitamin D deficiency and insufficiency in children with osteopenia or osteoporosis referred to a pediatric metabolic bone clinic, *Pediatrics* 121 (2008):

e1585–e1590; M. L. Neuhouser and coauthors, Vitamin D insufficiency in a multiethnic cohort of breast cancer survivors, *American Journal of Clinical Nutrition* 88 (2008): 133–139.
24. A. C. Looker and coauthors, Vitamin D status: United States, 2001–2006, *NCHS Data Brief* 59 (2011): 1–8.
25. A. Arabi, R. El Rassi, and G. El-Hajj Fuleihan, Hypovitaminosis D in developing countries–prevalence, risk factors and outcomes, *Nature Reviews: Endocrinology* 6 (2010): 550–561.
26. H. A. Bischoff-Ferrari and coauthors, A pooled analysis of vitamin D dose requirements for fracture prevention, *New England Journal of Medicine* 367 (2012): 40–49; S. R. Mastaglia and coauthors, Effect of vitamin D nutritional status on muscle function and strength in healthy women aged over sixty-five years, *Journal of Nutrition, Health and Aging* 15 (2011): 349–354.
27. P. Lips and coauthors, Once-weekly dose of 8400 IU vitamin D_3 compared with placebo: Effects on neuromuscular function and tolerability in older adults with vitamin D insufficiency, *American Journal of Clinical Nutrition* 91 (2010): 985–991.
28. Committee on Dietary Reference Intakes, *Dietary Reference Intakes for Calcium and Vitamin D*, (Washington, D.C.: National Academies Press, 2011), pp. 75–124.
29. L. M. Hall and coauthors, Vitamin D intake needed to maintain target serum 25-hydroxyvitamin D concentrations in participants with low sun exposure and dark skin pigmentation is substantially higher than current recommendations, *Journal of Nutrition* 140 (2010): 542–550.
30. K. H. Madsern and coauthors, Randomized controlled trial of the effects of vitamin D-fortified milk and bread on serum 25-hydroxyvitamin D concentrations in families in Denmark during winter: The VitmaD study, *American Journal of Clinical Nutrition* 98 (2013): 374–382; R. M. Biancuzzo and coauthors, Fortification of orange juice with vitamin D_2 or vitamin D_3 is as effective as an oral supplement in maintaining vitamin D status in adults, *American Journal of Clinical Nutrition* 91 (2010): 1621–1626.
31. M. D. Farrar and coauthors, Recommended summer sunlight exposure amounts fail to produce sufficient vitamin D status in UK adults of South Asian origin, *American Journal of Clinical Nutrition* 94 (2011): 1219–1224.
32. E. Linos and coauthors, Sun protective behaviors and vitamin D levels in the US population: NHANES 2003–2006, *Cancer Causes and Control* 23 (2012): 133–140.
33. S. Sharma and coauthors, Vitamin D deficiency and disease risk among aboriginal Arctic populations, *Nutrition Reviews* 69 (2011): 468–478.
34. L. A. Houghton and coauthors, Predictors of vitamin D status and its association with parathyroid hormone in young New Zealand children, *American Journal of Clinical Nutrition* 92 (2010): 69–76.
35. U. Lehmann and coauthors, Bioavailability of vitamin D_2 and D_3 in healthy volunteers, a randomised placebo-controlled trial, *Journal of Clinical Endocrinology and Metabolism* 98 (2013): 4339–4345; L. Tripkovic and coauthors, comparison of vitamin D_2 and vitamin D_3 supplementation in raising serum 25-hydroxyvitamin D status: A systematic review and meta-analysis, *American Journal of Clinical Nutrition* 95 (2012): 1357–1364; R. P. Heaney and coauthors, Vitamin D(3) is more potent than vitamin D(2) in humans, *Journal of Clinical Endocrinology and Metabolism* 96 (2011): E447–E452.
36. G. B. Mulligan and A. Licata, Taking vitamin D with the largest meal improves absorption and results in higher serum levels of 25-hydroxyvitamin D, *Journal of Bone and Mineral Research* 25 (2010): 928–930.
37. A. K. Smolarek and N. Suh, chemopreventive activity of vitamin E breast cancer: A focus on γ- and δ-tocopherol, *Nutrients* 3 (2011): 962–986; C. S. Yang and coauthors, Inhibition of inflammation and carcinogenesis in the lung and colon by tocopherols, *Annals of the New York Academy of Sciences* 1203 (2010): 29–34; J. Ju and coauthors, Cancer-preventive activities of tocopherols and tocotrienols, *Carcinogenesis* 31 (2010): 533–542.
38. R. S. Y. Wong and A. K. Radhakrishnan, Tocotrienol research: Past into present, *Nutrition Reviews* 70 (2012): 483–490; P. W. Sylvester and coauthors, The value of tocotriencols in the prevention and treatment of cancer, *Journal of the American College of Nutrition* 29 (2010): 324S–333S; B. B. Aggarwal and coauthors, Tocotrienols, the vitamin E of the 21st century: Its potential against cancer and other chronic disease, *Biochemical Pharmacology* 80 (2010): 1613–1631.
39. R. F. Pfeiffer, Neurologic manifestations of malabsorption syndromes, *Handbook of Clinical Neurology* 120 (2014): 621–632; D. Bromley, P. C. Anderson, and V. Daggett, Sturctural consequences of mutations to the α-tocopherol transfer protein associated with the neurodegenerative disease ataxia with vitamin E deficiency, *Biochemistry* 52 (2013): 4264–4273.
40. M. S. Hamidi, O. Gajic-Velijanoski, and A. M. Cheung, Vitamin K and bone health, *Journal of Clinical Densitometry* 16 (2013): 409–413.
41. M. J. Shearer, X. Fu, and S. L. Booth, Vitamin K nutrition, metabolism, and requirements: Current concepts and future research, *Advances in Nutrition: An International Review Journal* 3 (2012): 182–195; H. J. Ipema, Use of oral vitamin K for prevention of late vitamin K deficiency bleeding in neonates when injectable vitamin K is not available, *Annals of Pharmacotherapy* 46 (2012): 879–883; G. Lippi and M. Franchini, Vitamin K in neonates, Facts and myths, *Blood Transfusion* 9 (2011): 4–9.

HIGHLIGHT > 11

Antioxidant Nutrients in Disease Prevention

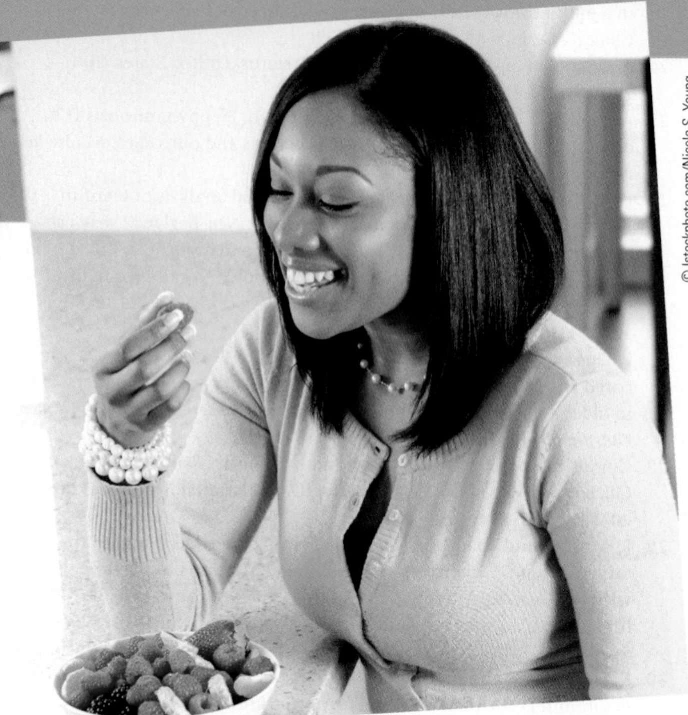

> LEARN IT Describe how antioxidants defend against free radicals that contribute to diseases.

Count on supplement manufacturers to exploit the day's hot topics in nutrition. The moment bits of research news surface, new supplements appear—and terms such as *antioxidants* and *lycopene* become household words. Friendly faces in TV commercials try to persuade us that these supplements hold magic in the fight against aging and disease. New supplements hit the market and sales soar.

In the meantime, scientists and medical experts around the world continue their work to clarify and confirm the roles of antioxidants in preventing chronic diseases. This highlight summarizes some of the accumulating evidence. It also revisits the advantages of foods over supplements. But first it is important to introduce the troublemaker—an unstable molecule known as a **free radical.** (The accompanying glossary defines free radical and related terms.)

Free Radicals and Disease

Chapter 7 describes how the body's cells use oxygen in metabolic reactions. In the process, oxygen reacts with body compounds and produces highly unstable molecules known as free radicals. In addition to normal body processes, environmental factors such as ultraviolet radiation, air pollution, and tobacco smoke generate free radicals.

A free radical is a molecule with one or more unpaired electrons.* An electron without a partner is unstable and highly reactive. To regain its stability, the free radical quickly finds a stable but vulnerable compound from which to steal an electron.

With the loss of an electron, the formerly stable molecule becomes a free radical itself and steals an electron from another nearby molecule. Thus an electron-snatching chain reaction is under way with free radicals producing more free radicals. **Antioxidants** neutralize free radicals by donating one of their own electrons, thus ending the chain reaction. When they lose electrons, antioxidants do not become free radicals because they are stable in either form. (Review Figure 10-16 on p. 328 to see how ascorbic acid can give up two hydrogens with their electrons and become dehydroascorbic acid.)

Free radicals attack. Occasionally, these free-radical attacks are helpful. For example, cells of the immune system use free radicals as ammunition in an "oxidative burst" that demolishes disease-causing viruses and bacteria. Most often, however, free-radical attacks cause widespread damage. They commonly damage the polyunsaturated fatty acids in lipoproteins and in cell membranes, disrupting the transport of substances into and out of cells. Free radicals also alter DNA, RNA, and proteins, creating excesses and deficiencies of specific proteins, impairing cell functions, and eliciting an inflammatory response. All of these actions contribute to cell damage, disease progression, and aging (see Figure H11-1).

The body's natural defenses and repair systems try to control the destruction caused by free radicals, but these systems are not 100 percent effective. In fact, they become less effective with age, and the unrepaired damage accumulates. To some extent, dietary antioxidants defend the body against **oxidative stress,** but if antioxidants are unavailable or if free-radical production becomes excessive, health problems may develop.[1] Oxygen-derived free radicals may cause diseases, not only by indiscriminately destroying the valuable components

*Many free radicals exist, but oxygen-derived free radicals are most common in the human body. Examples of oxygen-derived free radicals include superoxide radical ($O_2^{\cdot -}$), hydroxyl radical ($OH^{\cdot}$), and nitric oxide ($NO^{\cdot}$). (The dots in the symbols represent the unpaired electrons.) Technically, hydrogen peroxide (H_2O_2) and singlet oxygen are not free radicals because they contain paired electrons, but the unstable conformation of their electrons makes radical-producing reactions likely. Scientists sometimes use the term *reactive oxygen species (ROS)* to describe all of these compounds.

GLOSSARY

antioxidants: in the body, substances that significantly decrease the adverse effects of free radicals on normal physiological functions.

free radical: an unstable molecule with one or more unpaired electrons. (See Appendix B for a review of basic chemistry concepts.)

oxidants (OKS-ih-dants): compounds (such as oxygen itself) that oxidize other compounds. Compounds that prevent oxidation are called *antioxidants,* whereas those that promote it are called *prooxidants.*

- **anti** = against
- **pro** = for

oxidative stress: a condition in which the production of oxidants and free radicals exceeds the body's ability to handle them and prevent damage.

phytochemicals: nonnutrient compounds found in plants. Some phytochemicals have biological activity in the body.

prooxidants: substances that significantly induce oxidative stress.

> **FIGURE H11-1 Free-Radical Damage**

Free radicals are highly reactive. They might attack the polyunsaturated fatty acids in a cell membrane, which generates lipid radicals that damage cells and accelerate disease progression. Free radicals might also attack and damage DNA, RNA, and proteins, which interferes with the body's ability to maintain normal cell function, causing disease and premature aging.

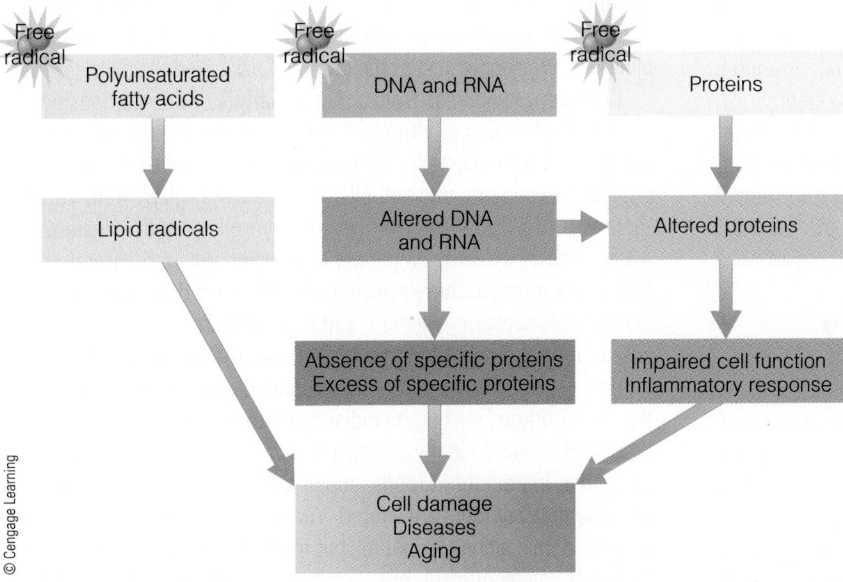

of cells, but also by serving as signals for specific activities within the cells. Scientists have identified oxidative stress as a causative factor and antioxidants as a protective factor in cognitive performance and the aging process as well as in the development of diseases such as cancer, arthritis, cataracts, diabetes, hypertension, and heart disease.[2]

Defending against Free Radicals

The body maintains a couple lines of defense against free-radical damage. A system of enzymes disarms the most harmful **oxidants.*** The action of these enzymes depends on the minerals selenium, copper, manganese, and zinc. If the diet fails to provide adequate supplies of these minerals, this line of defense weakens. The body also uses the antioxidant vitamins—vitamin E, beta-carotene, and vitamin C. Vitamin E defends the body's lipids (cell membranes, nervous tissues, and lipoproteins, for example) by efficiently stopping the free-radical chain reaction.[3] Beta-carotene also acts as an antioxidant in lipid membranes. Vitamin C protects other tissues, such as the skin and fluid of the blood, against free-radical attacks. Vitamin C seems especially adept at neutralizing free radicals from polluted air and cigarette smoke; it also restores oxidized vitamin E to its active state.

Dietary antioxidants also include some of the **phytochemicals** (featured in Highlight 13). Together, nutrients and phytochemicals with antioxidant activity minimize damage and prevent disease in the following ways:[4]

- Limiting free-radical formation
- Destroying free radicals or their precursors
- Stimulating antioxidant enzyme activity
- Repairing oxidative damage
- Stimulating repair enzyme activity
- Supporting a healthy immune system

These actions play key roles in defending the body against chronic diseases such as cancer and heart disease.

*These enzymes include *glutathione peroxidase, thioredoxin reductase, superoxide dismutase,* and *catalase.*

Defending against Cancer

Cancers arise when cellular DNA is damaged—sometimes by free-radical attacks. Antioxidants may reduce cancer risks by protecting DNA from this damage. Many researchers have reported low rates of cancer in people whose diets include abundant vegetables and fruits, rich in antioxidants. Preliminary reports suggest an inverse relationship between DNA damage and vegetable intake and a positive relationship with beef and pork intake.[5]

Foods rich in vitamin C seem to protect against certain types of cancers, especially those of the esophagus. Such a correlation may reflect the benefits of a diet rich in fruits and vegetables and low in fat; evidence that vitamin C supplements reduce the risk of cancer is lacking.

Researchers hypothesize that vitamin E might inhibit cancer formation by attacking free radicals that damage DNA. Evidence that vitamin E supplements help guard against cancer, however, is lacking.

Several studies report a cancer-preventing benefit of vegetables and fruits rich in beta-carotene and the other carotenoids as well. Carotenoids may protect against oxidative damage to DNA. Some research suggests that high concentrations of beta-carotene and the other carotenoids are associated with lower rates of some cancers.[6] Studies do not, however, find a reduction in cancer risk with beta-carotene supplementation. Benefits most likely reflect a healthy diet abundant in fruits and vegetables. In fact, a major review of several large research studies concluded that none produced evidence to justify the use of antioxidant supplements for cancer prevention.[7]

Defending against Heart Disease

Decades of research have contributed to our understanding of how oxidative stress contributes to atherosclerosis and how antioxidants might protect against heart disease, yet questions remain.[8] High blood cholesterol carried in LDL (low-density lipoproteins) is a major risk factor for cardiovascular disease, but how do LDL exert their damage? One scenario is that free radicals within the arterial walls oxidize LDL, changing their structure and function. The oxidized LDL then accelerate the formation of artery-clogging plaques. These free radicals also oxidize the polyunsaturated fatty acids of the cell membranes, sparking additional changes in the arterial walls, which impede the flow of blood. Susceptibility to such oxidative damage within the arterial walls is heightened by a diet high in saturated fat and by cigarette smoke. In contrast, diets that include plenty of fruits and vegetables, especially when saturated fat is low, strengthen antioxidant defenses against LDL oxidation.

Antioxidants, especially vitamin E, may protect against hypertension and cardiovascular disease.[9] Epidemiological studies suggest that people who eat foods rich in vitamin E have relatively few atherosclerotic plaques and low rates of death from heart disease. Among its many protective roles, vitamin E defends against LDL oxidation, inflammation, arterial injuries, and blood clotting. Whether vitamin E supplements slow the progression of heart disease is less clear.

Some studies suggest that vitamin C protects against LDL oxidation, raises HDL, lowers total cholesterol, and improves blood pressure. Vitamin C may also minimize inflammation and the free-radical action within the arterial wall. Like vitamin E, the role of vitamin C supplements in reducing the risk of heart disease remains uncertain.

Foods, Supplements, or Both?

In the process of scavenging and quenching free radicals, antioxidants themselves become oxidized. To some extent, they can be regenerated, but losses still occur and free radicals attack continuously. To maintain defenses, a person must replenish dietary antioxidants regularly. But should antioxidants be replenished from foods or from supplements?

Foods—especially fruits and vegetables—offer not only antioxidants, but an array of other valuable vitamins and minerals as well. Importantly, deficiencies of these nutrients can damage DNA as readily as free radicals can. Eating fruits and vegetables in abundance protects against both deficiencies and diseases—and may protect against inflammation and DNA damage.[10] A major review of the evidence gathered from metabolic studies, epidemiologic studies, and dietary intervention trials identified three dietary strategies most effective in preventing heart disease:

- Use unsaturated fats instead of saturated or *trans* fats (see Highlight 5).
- Select foods rich in omega-3 fatty acids (see Chapter 5).
- Consume a diet high in fruits, vegetables, nuts, and whole grains and low in refined grain products.

Such a diet combined with exercise, weight control, and not smoking serves as the best prescription for health. Notably, taking supplements is not among these disease-prevention recommendations.

Diets that deliver sufficient quantities of antioxidant vitamins may protect against cancer and heart disease—but only a small fraction of the US population consumes recommended amounts. Some research suggests a protective effect from as little as a daily glass of orange juice or carrot juice (rich sources of vitamin C and beta-carotene, respectively). Other intervention studies, however, have used levels of nutrients that far exceed current recommendations and can be achieved only by taking supplements. In making their recommendations for the antioxidant nutrients, members of the DRI Committee considered whether these studies support substantially higher intakes to help protect against chronic diseases. They did raise the recommendations for vitamins C and E, but they do not support taking supplements over eating a healthy diet.

Though fruits and vegetables containing many antioxidant nutrients and phytochemicals have been associated with a diminished risk of many chronic diseases, supplements have not always proved beneficial.[11] In fact, sometimes the benefits are more apparent when the vitamins come from foods rather than from supplements. In other words, the antioxidant actions of fruits and vegetables are greater than their nutrients alone can explain. Without data to confirm the benefits of supplements, we cannot accept the potential risks. And the risks are real.

Consider the findings from a meta-analysis of the relationships between supplements of vitamin A, vitamin E, beta-carotene, or combinations and total mortality. Researchers concluded that supplements provided no benefits and actually *increased* mortality.[12] Beta-carotene *increases* the risk of lung cancer and overall mortality in smokers.[13] A large research study on cancer prevention was prematurely terminated when researchers noted a trend toward developing diabetes in subjects receiving selenium and a slight increased risk of prostate cancer in those receiving vitamin E.[14] Another study concluded that vitamin E supplements increase the risk of some strokes, but reduce the risk of others, making its indiscriminate use unwise.[15]

Even if research clearly proves that a particular nutrient is the ultimate protective ingredient in foods, supplements would not be the answer because their contents are limited. Vitamin E supplements, for example, usually contain alpha-tocopherol, but foods provide an assortment of tocopherols and tocotrienols among other nutrients, many of which provide valuable protection against free-radical damage. In addition to a full array of nutrients, foods provide phytochemicals that also fight against many

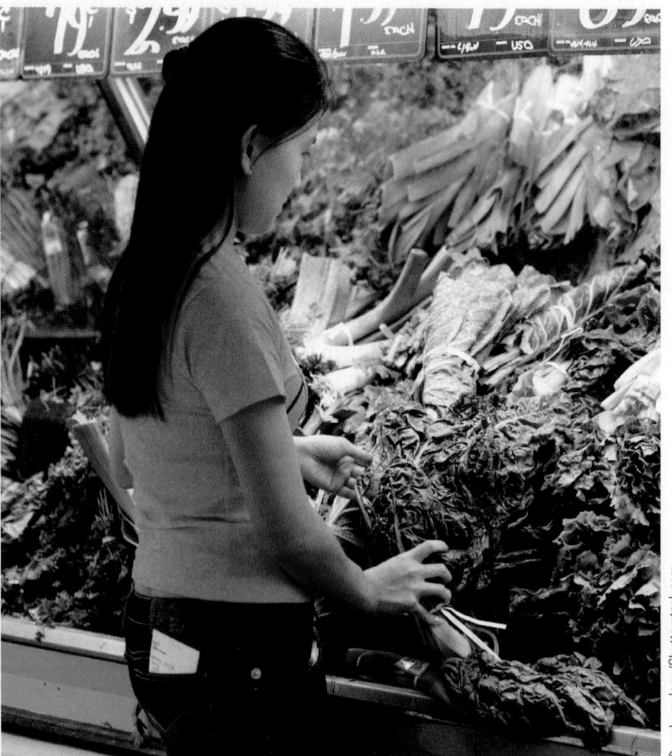

Many cancer-fighting products are available now at your local produce counter.

TABLE H11-1 Antioxidants and Chronic Disease Risk

Antioxidant	Disease	Risk from Foods	Risk from Supplements
Vitamin C	Coronary heart disease	Inconsistent results	Inconsistent results
	Breast cancer	Inconsistent results	—
	Colorectal cancer	Inconsistent results	—
	Gastrointestinal cancer	—	Not known
	Lung cancer	No effect	Not known
Vitamin E	Coronary heart disease	Inconsistent results	No effect or possible increased risk
	Breast cancer	—	No effect
	Colorectal cancer	Inconsistent results	—
	Gastrointestinal cancer	—	No effect
	Lung cancer	No effect	No effect
	Prostate cancer	Decreased risk	Decreased risk in smokers
Beta-carotene	Coronary heart disease	Decreased risk	No effect in nonsmokers, increased risk in smokers
	Lung cancer	Inconsistent results	No effect in nonsmokers, increased risk in smokers
	Colorectal cancer	Decreased risk	—
	Gastrointestinal cancer	—	No effect
	Prostate cancer	No effect	—
Other carotenoids	Lung cancer	Decreased risk for beta-cryptoxanthin	—
	Colorectal cancer	Decreased risk	—
	Prostate cancer	Decreased risk for lycopene	—
Fruits and vegetables	Coronary heart disease	Decreased risk	
	Breast cancer	No effect	
	Colorectal cancer	Inconsistent results	
	Gastric and esophageal cancer	Decreased risk	
	Lung cancer	Decreased risk for fruits, no effect for vegetables	
	Prostate cancer	No effect	
Supplement containing a combination of antioxidants	Coronary heart disease		Possibly increased risk
	Gastrointestinal cancer		Possibly increased risk
	Lung cancer		No effect in nonsmokers, increased risk in smokers

SOURCE: Adapted from H. Verhagen and coauthors, The state of antioxidant affairs, *Nutrition Today* 41 (2006): 244–249.

diseases. Supplements shortchange users. Furthermore, supplements should be used only as an adjunct to other measures such as smoking cessation, weight control, physical activity, and medication as needed.

Clearly, much more research is needed to define optimal and harmful levels of intake. This much we know: antioxidants behave differently under various conditions. At physiological levels typical of a healthy diet, they act as antioxidants, but at pharmacological doses typical of supplements, they may act as **prooxidants,** stimulating the production of free radicals and altering metabolism in a way that may promote disease. A high intake of vitamin C from supplements, for example, may *increase* the risk of heart disease in women with diabetes. Until the optimum intake of antioxidant nutrients can be determined, the risks of supplement use remain unclear. Table H11-1 presents a summary of the relationships between antioxidants and chronic diseases—sorted by foods or supplements. As you can see, many studies report either no effect or inconsistent results. Any decrease in risk is attributed to foods 9 out of 10 times. Any increase in risk is always from supplements, and often in smokers. Clearly, the best way to add antioxidants to the diet is to eat generous servings of fruits and vegetables daily.

It should be clear by now that we cannot know the identity and action of every chemical in every food. Even if we did, why create a supplement to replicate a food? Why not eat foods and enjoy the pleasure, nourishment, and health benefits they provide? The beneficial constituents in foods are widespread among plants. Among the fruits, pomegranates, berries, and citrus rank high in antioxidants; top antioxidant vegetables include kale, spinach, and brussels sprouts; millet and oats contain the most antioxidants among the grains; pinto beans and soybeans are outstanding legumes; and walnuts outshine the other nuts. But don't try to single out one particular food for its "magical" nutrient, antioxidant, or phytochemical. Instead, eat a wide variety of fruits, vegetables, grains, legumes, and nuts every day—and get *all* the benefits these foods have to offer.

CRITICAL THINKING SKILLS

A. What are the arguments for obtaining antioxidants from foods, supplements, or both?
B. The American Heart Association and other health organizations have concluded that consumers should get their antioxidants from foods rather than supplements. They add that taking supplements may even be harmful. Supplement manufacturers claim that such statements are unfair and that their natural botanical extracts provide numerous health benefits. In fact, some suggest that beneficial effects can only be achieved by taking high-dose supplements. Given that there are currently no DRI defining the kinds of antioxidants or the daily quantities needed, how might you ensure a healthy intake of antioxidants? If you decided to take an antioxidant supplement, how might you research the product to determine its safety and effectiveness?

REFERENCES

1. B. Halliwell, Free radicals and antioxidants: Updating a personal view, *Nutrition Reviews* 70 (2012): 257–265.
2. A. Whaley-Connell, P. A. McCullough, and J. R. Sowers, The role of oxidative stress in the metabolic syndrome, *Reviews in Cardiovascular Medicine* 12 (2011): 21–29.
3. M. G. Traber and J. F. Stevens, Vitamins C and E: Beneficial effects from a mechanistic perspective, *Free Radical Biology and Medicine* 51 (2011): 1000–1013.
4. H. Yao and coauthors, Dietary flavonoids as cancer prevention agents, *Environmental Carcinogenesis and Ecotoxicology Reviews* 29 (2011): 1–31.
5. P. Riso and coauthors, DNA damage and repair activity after broccoli intake in young healthy smokers, *Mutagenesis* 25 (2010): 595–602; A. Brevik and coauthors, Polymorphisms in base excision repair genes as colorectal cancer risk factors and modifiers of the effects of diets high in red meat, *Cancer Epidemiology, Biomarkers and Prevention* 19 (2010): 3167–3173.
6. A. H. Eliassen and coauthors, Circulating carotenoids and risk of breast cancer: Pooled analysis of eight prospective studies, *Journal of the National Cancer Institute* 104 (2012): 1905–1916.
7. M. Goodman and coauthors, Clinical trials of antioxidants as cancer prevention agents: Past, present, and future, *Free Radical Biology and Medicine* 51 (2011): 1068–1084.
8. G. Riccioni and coauthors, Carotenoids and vitamins C and E in the prevention of cardiovascular disease, *International Journal for Vitamin and Nutrition Research* 82 (2012): 15–26; D. Farbstein, A. Kozak-Blickstein, and A. P. Levy, Antioxidant vitamins and their use in preventing cardiovascular disease, *Molecules* 15 (2010): 8098–8110.
9. E. L. Schiffrin, Antioxidants in hypertension and cardiovascular disease, *Molecular Interventions* 10 (2010): 354–362.
10. S. N. Bhupathiraju and K. L. Tucker, Greater variety in fruit and vegetable intake is associated with lower inflammation in Puerto Rican adults, *American Journal of Clinical Nutrition* 93 (2011): 37–46; M. K. Shanmugam, R. Kannaiyan, and G. Sethi, Targeting cell signaling and apoptotic pathways by dietary agents: Role in the prevention and treatment of cancer, *Nutrition and Cancer* 63 (2011): 161–173.
11. B. Halliwell, Free radicals and antioxidants: Quo vadis? *Trends in Pharmacological Sciences* 32 (2011): 125–130.
12. G. Bjelakovic, D. Nikolova, and C. Gluud, Antioxidant supplements to prevent mortality, *Journal of the American Medical Association* 310 (2013): 1178–1179.
13. A. M. Mondul and coauthors, Metabolomic profile of response to supplementation with β-carotene in the Alpha-Tocopherol, Beta-Carotene Cancer Prevention Study, *American Journal of Clinical Nutrition* 98 (2013): 488–493.
14. M. C. Ledesma and coauthors, Selenium and vitamin E for prostate cancer: Post-SELECT (Selenium and Vitamin E Cancer Prevention Trial) status, *Molecular Medicine* 17 (2011): 134–143.
15. M. Schürks and coauthors, Effects of vitamin E on stroke subtypes: Meta-analysis of randomised controlled trials, *British Medical Journal* 341 (2010): c5702.

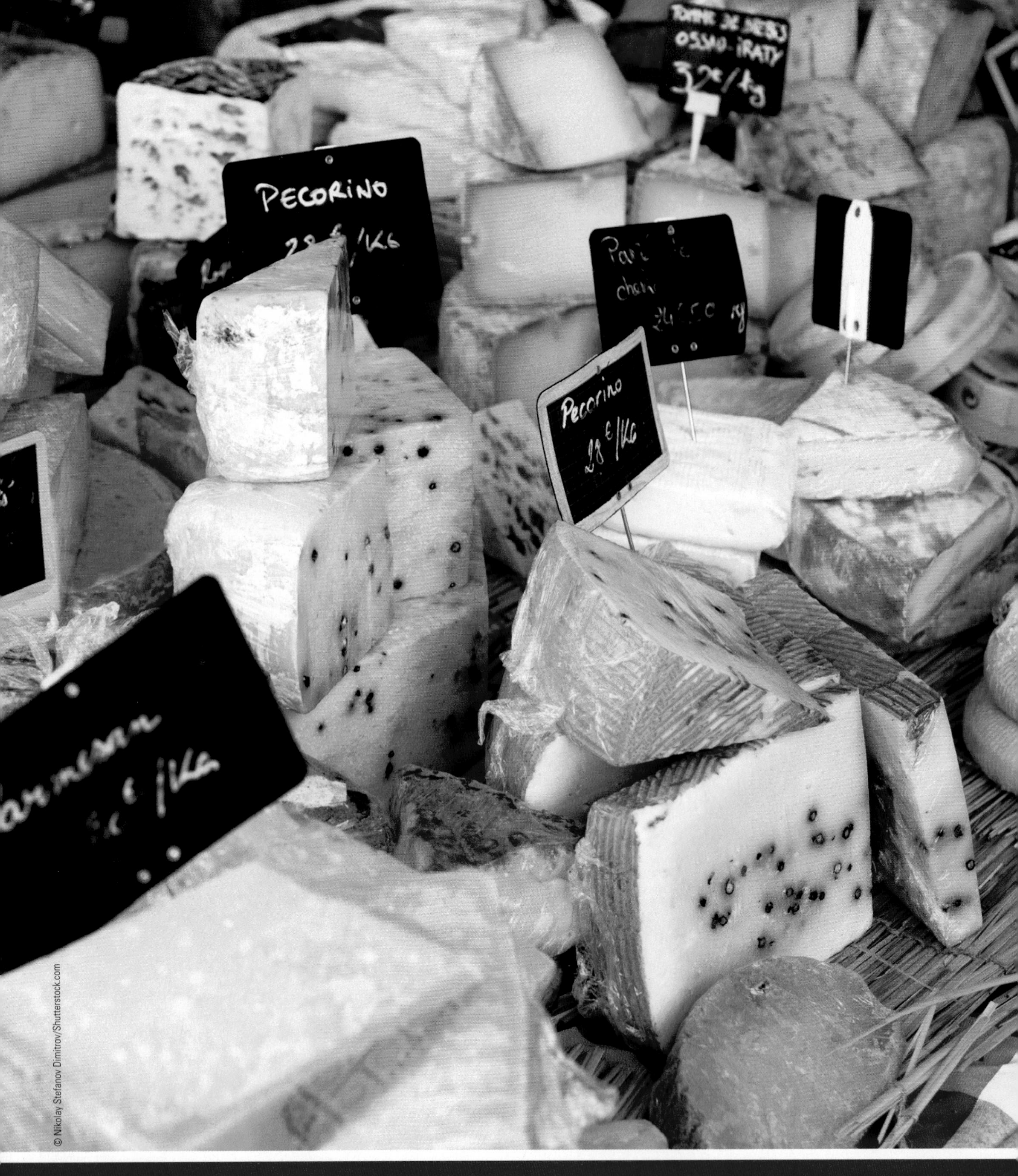
OSSAU-IRATY
PECORINO
Pecorino
28 €/KG

12

Water and the Major Minerals

LEARNING GPS

Nutrition in Your Life

What's your beverage of choice? If you said water, then congratulate yourself for recognizing its importance in maintaining your body's fluid balance. If you answered milk, then pat yourself on the back for taking good care of your bones. Without water, you would realize within days how vital it is to your survival. The consequences of a lack of milk (or other calcium-rich foods) are also dramatic, but may not become apparent for decades. Water, calcium, and all the other major minerals support fluid balance and bone health. Before getting too comfortable reading this chapter, pour yourself a glass of water or milk. Your body will thank you. In the Nutrition Portfolio at the end of this chapter, you can determine whether the foods you are eating are meeting your water and major mineral needs.

Water is an essential nutrient, more important to life than any of the others. The body needs more water each day than any other nutrient. Furthermore, you can survive only a few days without water, whereas a deficiency of the other nutrients may take weeks, months, or even years to develop.

This chapter begins with a look at water and the body's fluids. The body maintains an appropriate balance and distribution of fluids with the help of another class of nutrients—the minerals. In addition to introducing the minerals that help regulate body fluids, this chapter describes many of the other important functions minerals perform in the body. Chapter 19 revisits water as a beverage and addresses consumer concerns about its safety; Chapter 20 looks at water usage in agriculture and food production and examines the impending water shortages we face.

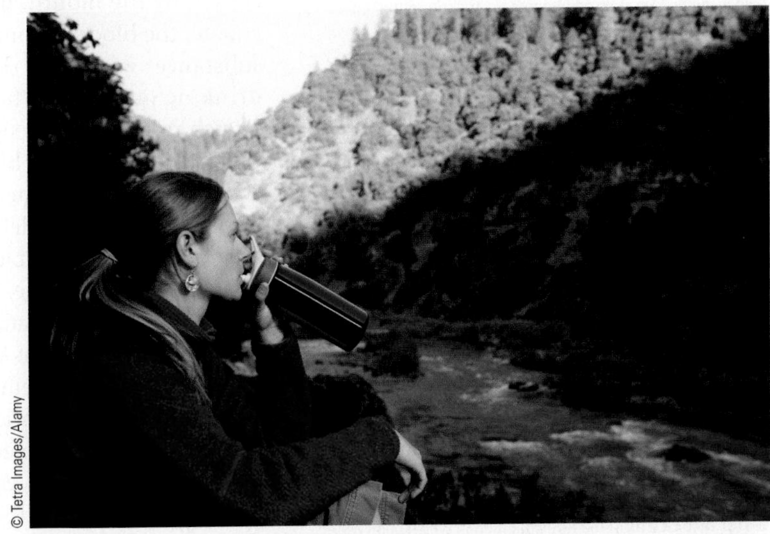

Water is the most indispensable nutrient.

> FIGURE 12-1 One Cell and Its Associated Fluids

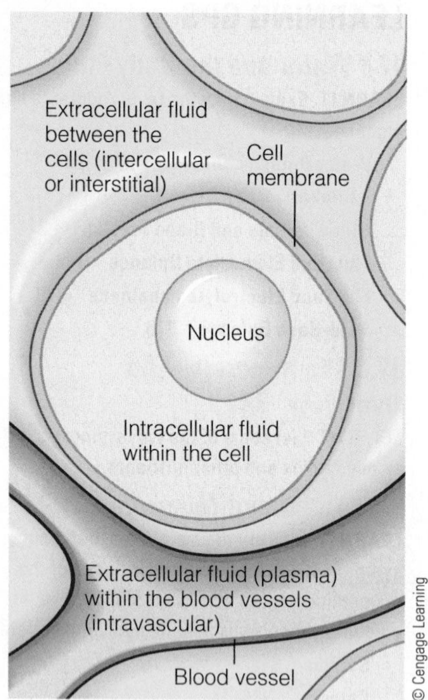

12.1 Water and the Body Fluids

› LEARN IT Explain how the body regulates fluid balance.

Water constitutes about 60 percent of an adult's body weight and a higher percentage of a child's (see Figure 1-1, p. 7). Because water makes up about 75 percent of the weight of lean tissue and less than 25 percent of the weight of fat, a person's body composition influences how much of the body's weight is water. The proportion of water is generally smaller in females, obese people, and the elderly because of their smaller proportion of lean tissue.

In the body, water is the fluid in which all life processes occur. The water in the body fluids:

- Carries nutrients and waste products throughout the body
- Maintains the structure of large molecules such as proteins and glycogen
- Participates in metabolic reactions
- Serves as the solvent for minerals, vitamins, amino acids, glucose, and many other small molecules so that they can participate in metabolic activities
- Acts as a lubricant and cushion around joints and inside the eyes, the spinal cord, and, in pregnancy, the amniotic sac surrounding the fetus in the womb
- Aids in the regulation of normal body temperature, as the evaporation of sweat from the skin removes excess heat from the body
- Maintains blood volume

To support these and other vital functions, the body actively maintains an appropriate **water balance** between intake and output.

Water Balance and Recommended Intakes Every cell contains fluid of the exact composition that is best for that cell. Fluid inside cells is called **intracellular fluid,** whereas fluid outside cells is called **extracellular fluid.** The extracellular fluid that surrounds each cell is called **interstitial fluid,** whereas the extracellular fluid in the blood vessels is called **intravascular fluid**. Figure 12-1 illustrates a cell and its associated fluids. The compositions of intercellular and extracellular fluids differ from each other. They continuously lose and replace their components, yet the composition in each compartment remains remarkably constant under normal conditions. Because imbalances can be devastating, the body quickly responds by adjusting both water intake and excretion as needed. Consequently, the entire system of cells and fluids remains in a delicate, but controlled, state of homeostasis.

Water Intake **Thirst** and satiety influence water intake in response to changes sensed by the mouth, **hypothalamus,** and nerves. When water intake is inadequate, the blood becomes concentrated (having lost water but not the dissolved substances within it), the mouth becomes dry, and the hypothalamus initiates drinking behavior. When water intake is excessive, the stomach expands and stretch receptors send signals to stop drinking. Similar signals are sent from receptors in the heart as blood volume increases.

When too much water is lost from the body and not replaced, **dehydration** develops. A first sign of dehydration is thirst, the signal that the body has lost some fluid. If a person is unable to obtain water or, as in many elderly people, fails to perceive the thirst message, the symptoms of dehydration may progress rapidly from thirst to weakness, exhaustion, and delirium—and end in death if not corrected (see Table 12-1). Notice that an early sign of dehydration is fatigue; keep that in mind when considering caffeinated beverages for an afternoon "pick-me-up" and choose water instead. Dehydration develops with either inadequate water intake or excessive water losses. (Chapter 14 revisits dehydration and the fluid needs of athletes.)

Water intoxication, on the other hand, is rare but can occur with excessive water intake and kidney disorders that reduce urine production. The symptoms may include confusion, convulsions, and even death in extreme cases. Excessive water ingestion (10 to 20 liters) within a few hours dilutes the sodium concentration of the blood and contributes to a dangerous condition known as **hyponatremia.**

water balance: the balance between water intake and output (losses).

intracellular fluid: fluid inside the cells, usually high in potassium and phosphate. Intracellular fluid accounts for approximately two-thirds of the body's water.

- **intra** = within

extracellular fluid: fluid outside the cells. Extracellular fluid includes two main components—the interstitial fluid between cells and the intravascular fluid inside blood vessels. Extracellular fluid accounts for approximately one-third of the body's water.

- **extra** = outside

interstitial (IN-ter-STISH-al) **fluid:** fluid between the cells (intercellular), usually high in sodium and chloride. Interstitial fluid is a large component of extracellular fluid.

- **inter** = in the midst, between

intravascular fluid: fluid within blood vessels.

- **intra** = within

thirst: a conscious desire to drink.

hypothalamus (high-po-THAL-ah-mus): a brain center that controls activities such as maintenance of water balance, regulation of body temperature, and control of appetite.

dehydration: the condition in which body water output exceeds water input. Symptoms include thirst, dry skin and mucous membranes, rapid heartbeat, low blood pressure, and weakness.

water intoxication: the rare condition in which body water contents are too high in all body fluid compartments.

hyponatremia (HIGH-po-na-TREE-me-ah): a decreased concentration of sodium in the blood.

TABLE 12-1 Signs of Dehydration

Body Weight Lost (%)	Symptoms
1–2	Thirst, fatigue, weakness, vague discomfort, loss of appetite
3–4	Impaired physical performance, dry mouth, reduction in urine, flushed skin, impatience, apathy
5–6	Difficulty concentrating, headache, irritability, sleepiness, impaired temperature regulation, increased respiratory rate
7–10	Dizziness, spastic muscles, loss of balance, delirium, exhaustion, collapse

NOTE: The onset and severity of symptoms at various percentages of body weight lost depend on the activity, fitness level, degree of acclimation, temperature, and humidity. If not corrected, dehydration can lead to death.

For this reason, guidelines suggest limiting fluid intake during times of heavy sweating to between 1 and 1.5 liters per hour. (Chapter 14 revisits hyponatremia as sometimes seen in endurance athletes.)

Water Sources The obvious dietary source of water is water itself, which provides about one-third of the total water intake in the United States.[1] In addition, other beverages and nearly all foods also contain water. Most fruits and vegetables contain up to 90 percent water, and many meats and cheeses contain at least 50 percent. See Table 12-2 for selected foods and Appendix H for many more. Also, **metabolic water** is generated as an end product during condensation reactions and the oxidation of energy-yielding nutrients. Recall from Chapter 7 that when the energy-yielding nutrients break down, their carbons and hydrogens combine with oxygen to yield carbon dioxide (CO_2) and water (H_2O). As Table 12-3 shows, the water derived daily from these three sources—beverages, foods, and metabolism—averages about 2500 milliliters (roughly 2.5 quarts or 10.5 cups).

TABLE 12-2 Percentage of Water in Selected Foods

100%	Water
90–99%	Fat-free milk, strawberries, watermelon, lettuce, cabbage, celery, spinach, broccoli
80–89%	Fruit juice, yogurt, apples, grapes, oranges, carrots
70–79%	Shrimp, bananas, corn, potatoes, avocados, cottage cheese, ricotta cheese
60–69%	Pasta, legumes, salmon, ice cream, chicken breast
50–59%	Ground beef, hot dogs, feta cheese
40–49%	Pizza
30–39%	Cheddar cheese, bagels, bread
20–29%	Pepperoni sausage, cake, biscuits
10–19%	Butter, margarine, raisins
1–9%	Crackers, cereals, pretzels, taco shells, peanut butter, nuts
0%	Oils, sugars

Water Losses At the very least, the body must excrete enough water to carry away the waste products generated by a day's metabolic activities. This **obligatory water excretion** is a minimum of about 500 milliliters (about 2 cups) of water each day. Above this amount, excretion adjusts to balance intake. If a person drinks more water, the kidneys excrete more urine, and the urine becomes more dilute. In addition to urine, water is lost from the lungs as vapor and from the skin as sweat; some is also lost in feces.* The amount of fluid lost from each source varies, depending on the environment (such as heat or humidity) and the body's physical condition (such as exercise or fever). On average, daily losses total about 2500 milliliters. Table 12-3 shows how daily water losses and intakes balance; maintaining this balance requires healthy kidneys and an adequate intake of fluids. An adequate intake of fluids, in turn, helps to maintain healthy kidneys and prevent kidney stone formation.[2]

Water Recommendations Because water needs vary depending on diet, activity, environmental temperature, and humidity, a general water requirement is difficult to establish. Recommendations are sometimes expressed in proportion to the amount of energy expended under average environmental conditions; for

TABLE 12-3 Water Balance

Water Sources	Amount (mL)	Water Losses	Amount (mL)
Beverages	550 to 1500	Kidneys (urine)	500 to 1400
Foods	700 to 1000	Skin (sweat)	450 to 900
Metabolism	200 to 300	Lungs (breath)	350
		GI tract (feces)	150
Total	1450 to 2800	Total	1450 to 2800

NOTE: For perspective, 100 milliliters is a little less than ½ cup and 1000 milliliters is a little more than 1 quart (1 mL = 0.03 oz).

*Water lost from the lungs and skin accounts for almost half of the daily losses even when a person is not visibly perspiring; these losses are commonly referred to as *insensible water losses*.

metabolic water: water generated during metabolism.

obligatory (ah-BLIG-ah-TORE-ee) **water excretion:** the minimum amount of water the body has to excrete each day to dispose of its wastes—about 500 milliliters (about 2 cups, or 1 pint).

adults, for example, 1.0 to 1.5 milliliters per kcalorie expended (roughly one-half cup per 100 kcalories). The recommended water intake for a person who expends 2000 kcalories a day, then, is 2 to 3 liters of water (about 8 to 12 cups). This recommendation is in line with the Adequate Intake (AI) for *total* water set by the DRI Committee. Total water includes not only drinking water, but water in other beverages and in foods as well. Only one in five adults in the United States report drinking at least 8 cups of water a day.[3]

Because a wide range of water intakes will prevent dehydration and its harmful consequences, the AI is based on average intakes. People who are physically active or who live in hot environments may need more.

Which beverages are best? Any beverage can readily meet the body's fluid needs, but those with few or no kcalories do so without contributing to weight gain. Given that obesity is a major health problem and that beverages currently represent more than 20 percent of the total energy intake in the United States, water is the best choice for most people. Other choices include tea, coffee, nonfat and low-fat milk and soymilk, artificially sweetened beverages, fruit and vegetable juices, sports drinks, and lastly, sweetened nutrient-poor beverages.

Some research indicates that people who drink caffeinated beverages lose a little more fluid than when drinking water because caffeine acts as a diuretic. The DRI Committee considered such findings in their recommendations for water intake and concluded that caffeinated beverages contribute to the daily total water intake similar to that contributed by non-caffeinated beverages. In other words, it doesn't seem to matter whether people rely on caffeine-containing beverages or other beverages to meet their fluid needs.

As Highlight 7 explains, alcohol acts as a diuretic and can impair a person's health. Alcohol should not be used to meet fluid needs.

Health Effects of Water Water supports good health.[4] Physical and mental performances depend on it, as does the optimal functioning of the GI tract, kidneys, heart, and other body systems.

The kind of water a person drinks may also make a difference to health. Water is usually either hard or soft. **Hard water** has high concentrations of calcium and magnesium; the principal mineral of **soft water** is sodium or potassium. (See the accompanying glossary for other common terms used to describe water.) In practical terms, soft water makes more bubbles with less soap; hard water leaves a ring on the tub, a crust of rocklike crystals in the teakettle, and a gray residue in the laundry.

Soft water may seem more desirable around the house, and some homeowners purchase water softeners that replace magnesium and calcium with sodium. In the body, however, soft water with sodium may aggravate hypertension and heart disease. In contrast, the minerals in hard water may benefit these conditions.

Soft water also more easily dissolves certain contaminant minerals, such as cadmium and lead, from old plumbing pipes. As Chapter 13 explains, these contaminant minerals harm the body by displacing the nutrient minerals from their normal sites of action. People who live in buildings with old plumbing should run the cold water tap a minute or two to flush out harmful minerals whenever the water faucet has been off for more than 6 hours.[5]

Many people select **bottled water,** believing it to be safer than tap water and therefore worth its substantial cost. Chapter 19 offers a discussion of bottled water safety and regulations.

Blood Volume and Blood Pressure

Fluids maintain the blood volume, which in turn influences blood pressure. The kidneys are central to the regulation of blood volume and blood pressure. All day, every day, the kidneys reabsorb needed substances and water and excrete wastes with some water in the urine (see Figure 12-2). The kidneys meticulously adjust the volume and the concentration of the urine to accommodate changes in the body, including variations in the day's food and beverage intakes. Instructions on whether to retain or release substances or water come from ADH, renin, angiotensin, and aldosterone.

hard water: water with a high calcium and magnesium content.

soft water: water with a high sodium or potassium content.

bottled water: drinking water sold in bottles.

> **FIGURE 12-2 A Nephron, One of the Kidney's Many Functioning Units**

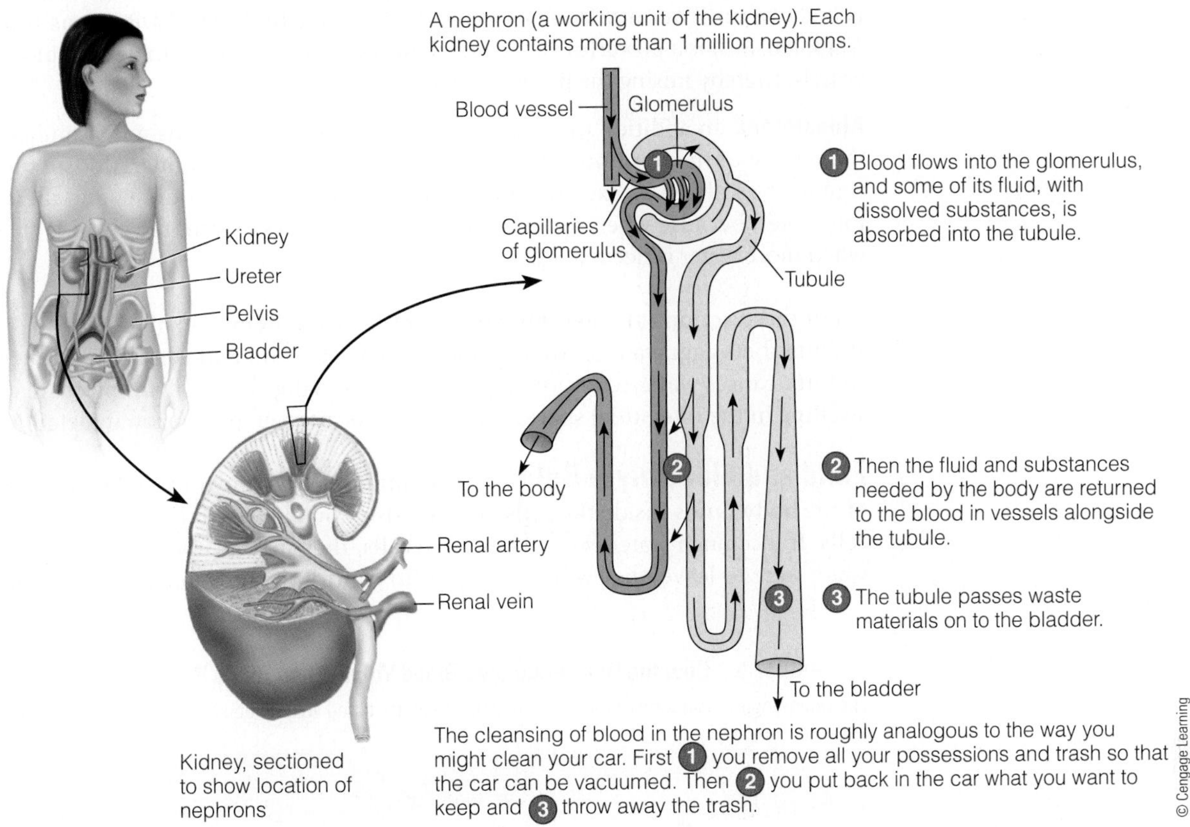
A nephron (a working unit of the kidney). Each kidney contains more than 1 million nephrons.
Blood vessel
Glomerulus
Capillaries of glomerulus
Tubule
1 Blood flows into the glomerulus, and some of its fluid, with dissolved substances, is absorbed into the tubule.
Kidney
Ureter
Pelvis
Bladder
To the body
Renal artery
Renal vein
2 Then the fluid and substances needed by the body are returned to the blood in vessels alongside the tubule.
3 The tubule passes waste materials on to the bladder.
To the bladder
Kidney, sectioned to show location of nephrons

The cleansing of blood in the nephron is roughly analogous to the way you might clean your car. First (1) you remove all your possessions and trash so that the car can be vacuumed. Then (2) you put back in the car what you want to keep and (3) throw away the trash.

ADH Whenever blood volume or blood pressure falls too low, or whenever the extracellular fluid becomes too concentrated, the hypothalamus signals the pituitary gland to release **antidiuretic hormone (ADH).** ADH is a water-conserving hormone that stimulates the kidneys to reabsorb water. Consequently, the more water you need, the less your kidneys excrete. These events also trigger thirst. Drinking water and retaining fluids raise the blood volume and dilute the concentrated fluids, thus helping to restore homeostasis. (Recall from Highlight 7 that alcohol depresses ADH activity, thus promoting fluid losses and dehydration.)

Renin Cells in the kidneys respond to low blood pressure by releasing an enzyme called **renin.** Through a complex series of events, renin causes the kidneys to reabsorb sodium. Sodium reabsorption, in turn, is always accompanied by water retention, which helps to raise blood volume and blood pressure.

antidiuretic hormone (ADH): a hormone produced by the pituitary gland in response to dehydration (or a high sodium concentration in the blood) that stimulates the kidneys to reabsorb more water and therefore to excrete less. In addition to its antidiuretic effect, ADH elevates blood pressure and so is also called *vasopressin* (VAS-oh-PRES-in).

- **vaso** = vessel
- **press** = pressure

renin (REN-in): an enzyme from the kidneys that hydrolyzes the protein angiotensinogen to angiotensin I, which results in the kidneys reabsorbing sodium.

GLOSSARY OF WATER TERMS

artesian water: water drawn from a well that taps a confined aquifer in which the water is under pressure.

carbonated water: water that contains carbon dioxide gas, either naturally occurring or added, that causes bubbles to form in it; also called *bubbling* or *sparkling water.* The FDA defines seltzer, soda, and tonic waters as soft drinks; they are not regulated as water.

distilled water: water that has been vaporized and recondensed, leaving it free of dissolved minerals.

filtered water: water treated by filtration, usually through *activated carbon filters* that reduce the lead in tap water, or by *reverse osmosis* units that force pressurized water across a membrane removing lead, arsenic, and some microorganisms from tap water.

mineral water: water from a spring or well that naturally contains at least 250 parts per million (ppm) of minerals. Minerals give water a distinctive flavor. Many mineral waters are high in sodium.

natural water: water obtained from a spring or well that is certified to be safe and sanitary. The mineral content may not be changed, but the water may be treated in other ways such as with ozone or by filtration.

public water: water from a municipal or county water system that has been treated and disinfected.

purified water: water that has been treated by distillation or other physical or chemical processes that remove dissolved solids. Because purified water contains no minerals or contaminants, it is useful for medical and research purposes.

spring water: water originating from an underground spring or well. It may be bubbly (carbonated), or "flat" or "still," meaning not carbonated. Brand names such as "Spring Pure" do not necessarily mean that the water comes from a spring.

well water: water drawn from groundwater by tapping into an aquifer.

Angiotensin In addition to its role in sodium retention, renin hydrolyzes a protein from the liver called **angiotensinogen** to **angiotensin I.** Angiotensin I is inactive until another enzyme converts it to its active form—**angiotensin II.** Angiotensin II is a powerful **vasoconstrictor** that narrows the diameters of blood vessels, thereby raising the blood pressure.

Aldosterone In addition to acting as a vasoconstrictor, angiotensin II stimulates the release of the hormone **aldosterone** from the **adrenal glands.** Aldosterone signals the kidneys to excrete potassium and to retain more sodium, and therefore water, because when sodium moves, water follows. Again, the effect is that when more water is needed, less is excreted.

All of these actions are presented in Figure 12-3 and help to explain why high-sodium diets aggravate conditions such as hypertension and edema. Too much sodium causes water retention and an accompanying rise in blood pressure or swelling in the interstitial spaces. Chapter 18 discusses hypertension in detail.

Fluid and Electrolyte Balance Maintaining a balance of about two-thirds of the body fluids inside the cells and one-third outside is vital to the life of the cells. If too much water were to enter the cells, they might rupture; if too much water were to leave, they would collapse. To control the movement of water, the

> FIGURE 12-3 **How the Body Regulates Blood Volume and Blood Pressure**

The renin-angiotensin-aldosterone system helps regulate blood volume and therefore blood pressure.

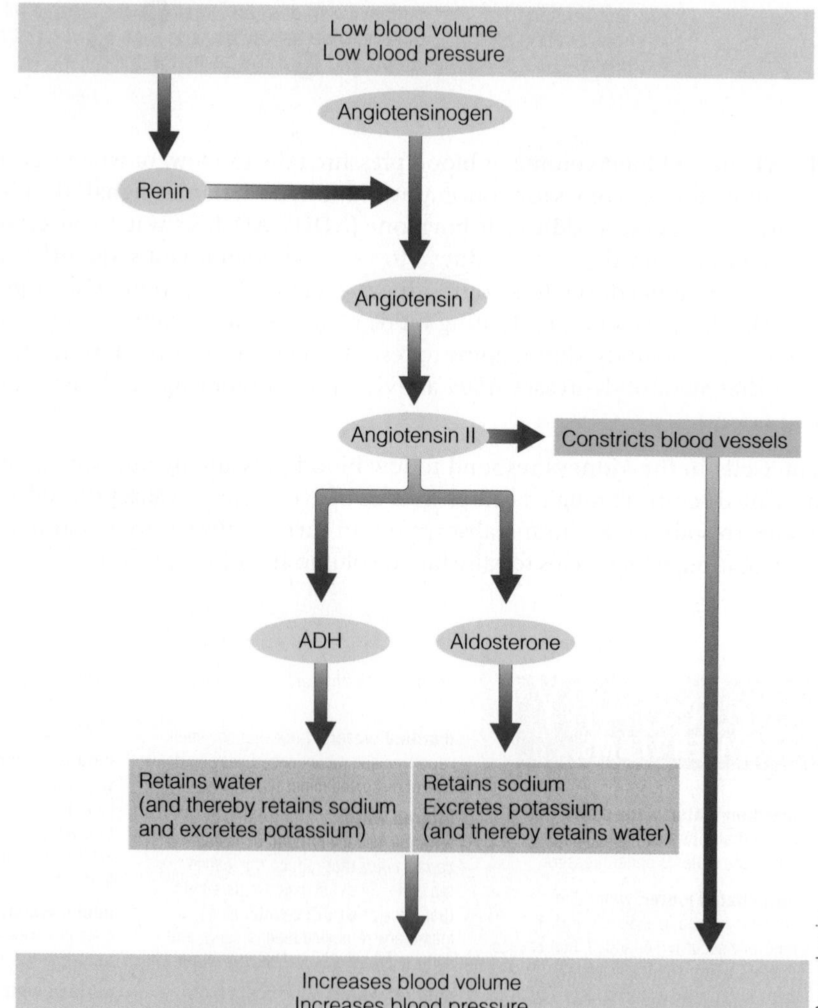

angiotensinogen: a precursor protein that is hydrolyzed to angiotensin I by renin.

angiotensin I (AN-gee-oh-TEN-sin): an inactive precursor that is converted by an enzyme to yield active angiotensin II.

angiotensin II: a hormone involved in blood pressure regulation.

vasoconstrictor (VAS-oh-kon-STRIK-tor): a substance that constricts or narrows the blood vessels.

aldosterone (al-DOS-ter-own): a hormone secreted by the adrenal glands that regulates blood pressure by increasing the reabsorption of sodium by the kidneys. Aldosterone also regulates chloride and potassium concentrations.

adrenal glands: glands adjacent to, and just above, each kidney.

cells direct the movement of the major minerals—sodium, chloride, potassium, calcium, phosphorus, magnesium, and sulfur.

Dissociation of Salt in Water When a mineral **salt** such as sodium chloride (NaCl) dissolves in water, it separates **(dissociates)** into **ions**—positively and negatively charged particles (Na^+ and Cl^-). The positive ions are **cations;** the negative ones are **anions.** (To remember the difference between cations and anions, think of the "t" in cations as a "plus" sign and the "n" in anions as a "negative.") Unlike pure water, which conducts electricity poorly, ions dissolved in water carry electrical current. For this reason, salts that dissociate into ions are called **electrolytes,** and fluids that contain them are **electrolyte solutions.**

In all electrolyte solutions, anion and cation concentrations are balanced (the number of negative and positive charges are equal). If a fluid contains 1000 negative charges, it must contain 1000 positive charges too. If an anion enters the fluid, a cation must accompany it or another anion must leave so that electrical neutrality will be maintained. Thus, whenever sodium (Na^+) ions leave a cell, potassium (K^+) ions enter, for example. In fact, it's a good bet that whenever Na^+ and K^+ ions are moving, they are going in opposite directions.

Table 12-4 shows that, indeed, the positive and negative charges inside and outside cells are perfectly balanced even though the numbers of each kind of ion differ over a wide range. Inside the cells, the positive charges total 202 and the negative charges balance these perfectly. Outside the cells, the amounts and proportions of the ions differ from those inside, but again the positive and negative charges balance. Scientists count these charges in **milliequivalents per liter (mEq/L).**

Electrolytes Attract Water Electrolytes attract water. Each water molecule has a net charge of zero, but the oxygen side of the molecule has a slight negative charge, and the hydrogens have a slight positive charge. Figure 12-4 (p. 378) shows the result in an electrolyte solution: both positive and negative ions attract clusters of water molecules around them. This attraction dissolves salts in water and enables the body to move fluids into appropriate compartments.

Water Follows Electrolytes As Figure 12-5 (p. 378) shows, some electrolytes reside primarily outside the cells (notably, sodium, chloride, and calcium), whereas others reside predominantly inside the cells (notably, potassium, magnesium,

TABLE 12-4 Important Body Electrolytes

Electrolytes	Intracellular (inside cells) Concentration (mEq/L)	Extracellular (outside cells) Concentration (mEq/L)
Cations (positively charged ions)		
Sodium (Na^+)	10	142
Potassium (K^+)	150	5
Calcium (Ca^{++})	2	5
Magnesium (Mg^{++})	40	3
	202	155
Anions (negatively charged ions)		
Chloride (Cl^-)	2	103
Bicarbonate (HCO_3^-)	10	27
Phosphate ($HPO_4^=$)	103	2
Sulfate ($SO_4^=$)	20	1
Organic acids (lactate, pyruvate)	10	6
Proteins	57	16
	202	155

NOTE: The numbers of positive and negative charges in a given fluid are the same. For example, in extracellular fluid, the cations and anions both equal 155 milliequivalents per liter (mEq/L). Of the cations, sodium ions make up 142 mEq/L; and potassium, calcium, and magnesium ions make up the remainder. Of the anions, chloride ions number 103 mEq/L; bicarbonate ions number 27; and the rest are provided by phosphate ions, sulfate ions, organic acids, and protein.

salt: a compound composed of a positive ion other than H^+ and a negative ion other than OH^-. An example is sodium chloride (Na^+Cl^-).
- **Na** = sodium
- **Cl** = chloride

dissociates (dis-SO-see-aites): physically separates.

ions (EYE-uns): atoms or molecules that have gained or lost electrons and therefore have electrical charges. Examples include the positively charged sodium ion (Na^+) and the negatively charged chloride ion (Cl^-). For a closer look at ions, see Appendix B.

cations (CAT-eye-uns): positively charged ions.

anions (AN-eye-uns): negatively charged ions.

electrolytes: salts that dissolve in water and dissociate into charged particles called ions.

electrolyte solutions: solutions that can conduct electricity.

milliequivalents per liter (mEq/L): the concentration of electrolytes in a volume of solution. Milliequivalents reveal characteristics about the solution that are not evident when the concentration is expressed in terms of weight.

> **FIGURE 12-4 Water Dissolves Salts and Follows Electrolytes**

The structural arrangement of the two hydrogen atoms and one oxygen atom enables water to dissolve salts. Water's role as a solvent is one of its most valuable characteristics.

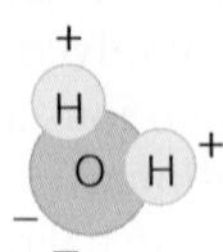

The negatively charged electrons that bond the hydrogens to the oxygen spend most of their time near the oxygen atom. As a result, the oxygen is slightly negative, and the hydrogens are slightly positive (see Appendix B).

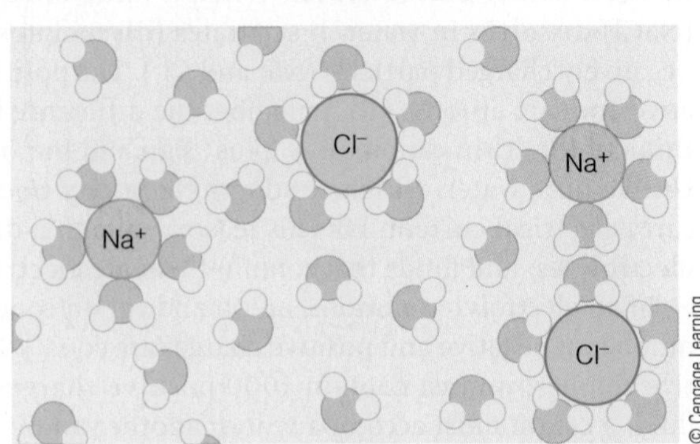

In an electrolyte solution, water molecules are attracted to both anions and cations. Notice that the negative oxygen atoms of the water molecules are drawn to the sodium cation (Na^+), whereas the positive hydrogen atoms of the water molecules are drawn to the chloride ions (Cl^-).

> **FIGURE 12-5 A Cell and Its Electrolytes**

All of these electrolytes are found both inside and outside the cells, but each can be found mostly on one side or the other of the cell membrane.

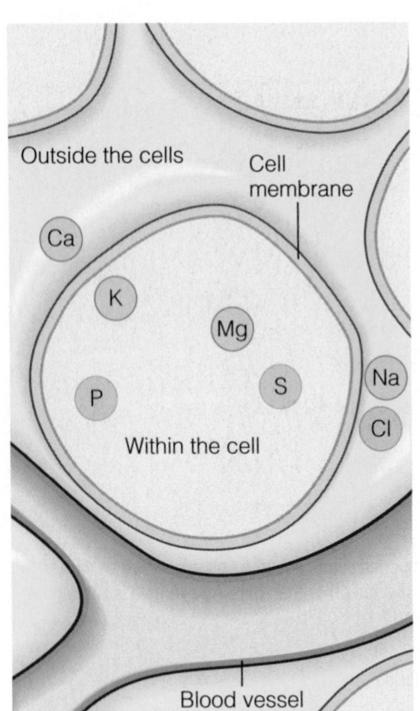

Chemical symbols:
Ca = calcium
Cl = chloride
K = potassium
Mg = magnesium
Na = sodium
P = phosphorus
S = sulfate

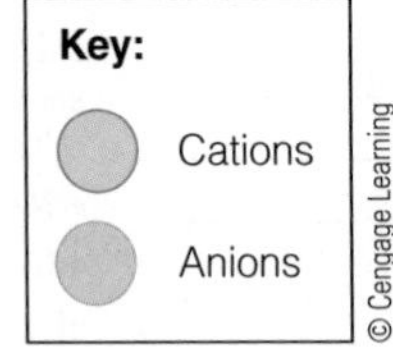

phosphate, and sulfate). Cell membranes are *selectively permeable,* meaning that they allow the passage of some molecules, but not others. Whenever electrolytes move across the membrane, water follows.

The movement of water across a membrane toward the more concentrated **solutes** is called **osmosis.** The amount of pressure needed to prevent the movement of water across a membrane is called the **osmotic pressure.** Figure 12-6 presents osmosis, and the photos of salted eggplant and rehydrated raisins provide familiar examples.

Proteins Regulate Flow of Fluids and Ions Chapter 6 describes how proteins attract water and help to regulate fluid movement. It explains that when proteins leak out of the blood vessels into the spaces between the cells, fluids follow and cause the swelling of edema. In addition, transport proteins in the cell membranes regulate the passage of positive ions and other substances from one side of the membrane to the other. Negative ions follow positive ions, and water flows toward the more concentrated solution.

An example of a protein that regulates the flow of fluids and ions in and out of cells is the sodium-potassium pump. The pump actively exchanges sodium for potassium across the cell membrane, using ATP as an energy source. Figure 6-10 on p. 181 illustrates this action.

Regulation of Fluid and Electrolyte Balance The amounts of various minerals in the body must remain nearly constant. Regulation occurs chiefly at two sites: the GI tract and the kidneys.

Minerals in foods enter the body by way of the GI tract. In addition, the digestive juices of the GI tract contain minerals. These minerals and those from foods are absorbed in the large intestine or excreted as needed. Each day, 8 liters of fluids and associated minerals are recycled this way, providing ample opportunity for the regulation of electrolyte balance.

The kidneys' control of the body's *water* content by way of the hormone ADH has already been described (see p. 375). The kidneys regulate the *electrolyte* contents by responding to the hormone aldosterone (also explained on p. 376). If the body's sodium is low, aldosterone stimulates sodium reabsorption from the

solutes (SOLL-yutes): the substances that are dissolved in a solution. The number of molecules in a given volume of fluid is the *solute concentration.*

osmosis: the movement of water across a membrane *toward* the side where the solutes are more concentrated.

osmotic pressure: the amount of pressure needed to prevent the movement of water across a membrane.

kidneys. As sodium is reabsorbed, potassium (another positive ion) is excreted in accordance with the rule that total positive charges must remain in balance with total negative charges.

Fluid and Electrolyte Imbalance Normally, the body defends itself successfully against fluid and electrolyte imbalances. Certain situations and some medications, however, may overwhelm the body's ability to compensate. Severe, prolonged vomiting and diarrhea as well as heavy sweating, burns, and traumatic wounds may incur such great fluid and electrolyte losses as to precipitate a medical emergency.

Different Solutes Lost by Different Routes Different solutes are lost depending on why fluid is lost. If fluid is lost by vomiting or diarrhea, sodium is lost indiscriminately. If the adrenal glands oversecrete aldosterone, as may occur when they develop a tumor, the kidneys may excrete too much potassium. A person with uncontrolled diabetes may lose glucose, a solute not normally excreted, and large amounts of fluid with it. Each situation results in dehydration, but drinking water alone will not restore electrolyte balance. Medical intervention is required.

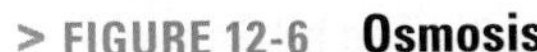

> FIGURE 12-6 **Osmosis**

Water flows in the direction of the more highly concentrated solution.

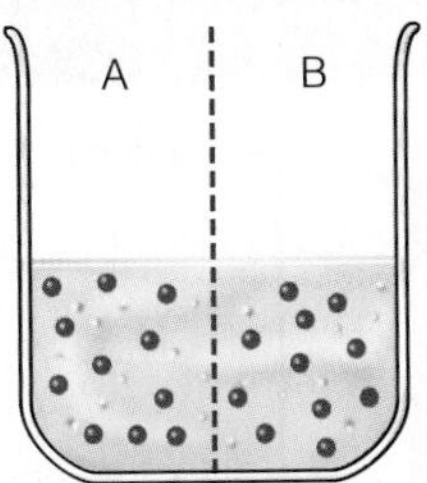

① With equal numbers of solute particles on both sides of the semipermeable membrane, the concentrations are equal, and the tendency of water to move in either direction is about the same.

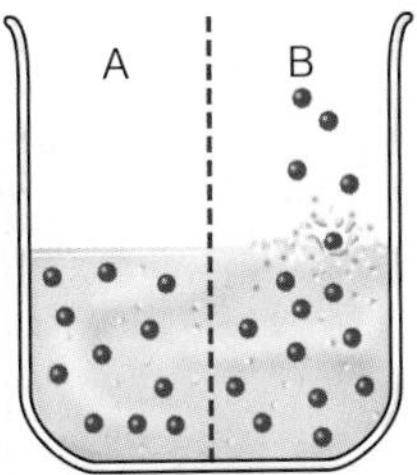

② Now additional solute is added to side B. Solute cannot flow across the divider (in the case of a cell, its membrane).

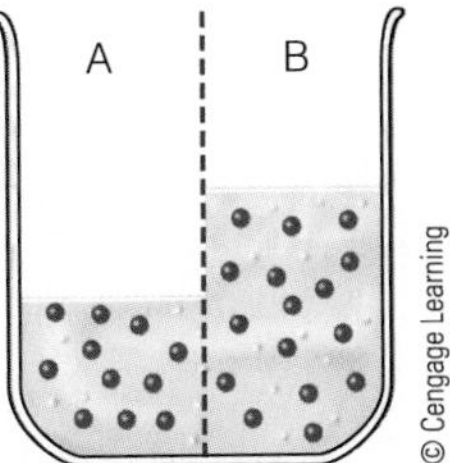

③ Water can flow both ways across the divider, but has a greater tendency to move from side A to side B, where there is a greater concentration of solute. The volume of water becomes greater on side B, and the concentrations on side A and B become equal.

© Cengage Learning

Replacing Lost Fluids and Electrolytes In many cases, people can replace the fluids and minerals lost in sweat or in a temporary bout of diarrhea by drinking plain cool water and eating regular foods. Some cases, however, demand rapid replacement of fluids and electrolytes—for example, when diarrhea threatens the life of a malnourished child. Caregivers around the world have learned to use **oral rehydration therapy (ORT)**—a simple solution of sugar, salt, and water, taken by mouth—to treat dehydration caused by diarrhea. These lifesaving formulas do not require hospitalization and can be prepared from ingredients available locally. Caregivers need only learn to measure ingredients carefully and use sanitary water. Once rehydrated, a person can begin eating foods. (Chapter 14 presents a discussion of sport drinks.)

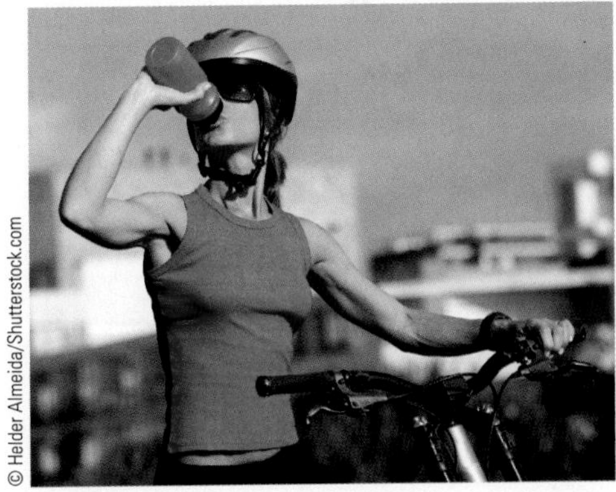

© Helder Almeida/Shutterstock.com

Physically active people must remember to replace their body fluids.

Acid-Base Balance

Acid-Base Balance The body uses its ions not only to help maintain fluid and electrolyte balance, but also to regulate the acidity (pH) of its fluids. The pH scale introduced in Chapter 3 is repeated here, in Figure 12-7 (p. 380), with the

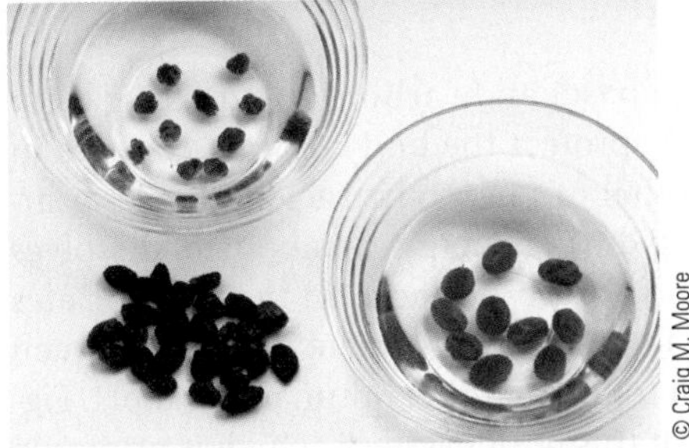

© Craig M. Moore

When immersed in water, raisins become plump because water moves toward the higher concentration of sugar inside the raisins.

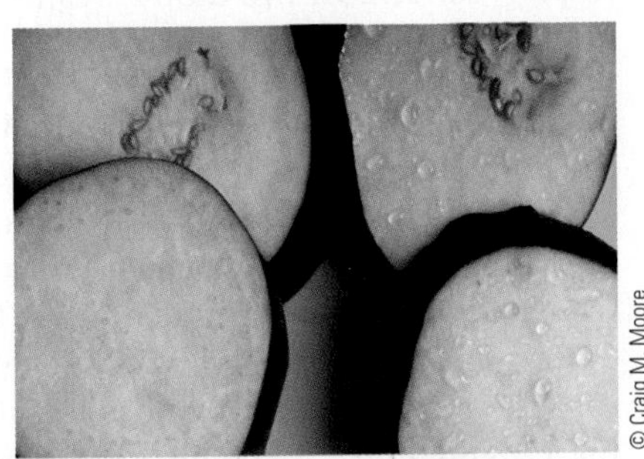

© Craig M. Moore

When sprinkled with salt, eggplant and other vegetables "sweat" because water moves toward the higher concentration of salt outside the vegetable.

oral rehydration therapy (ORT): the administration of a simple solution of sugar, salt, and water, taken by mouth, to treat dehydration caused by diarrhea. A simple ORT recipe (cool before giving):

- ½ L boiling water
- A small handful of sugar (4 tsp)
- 3 pinches of salt (½ tsp)

> **FIGURE 12-7 The pH Scale**

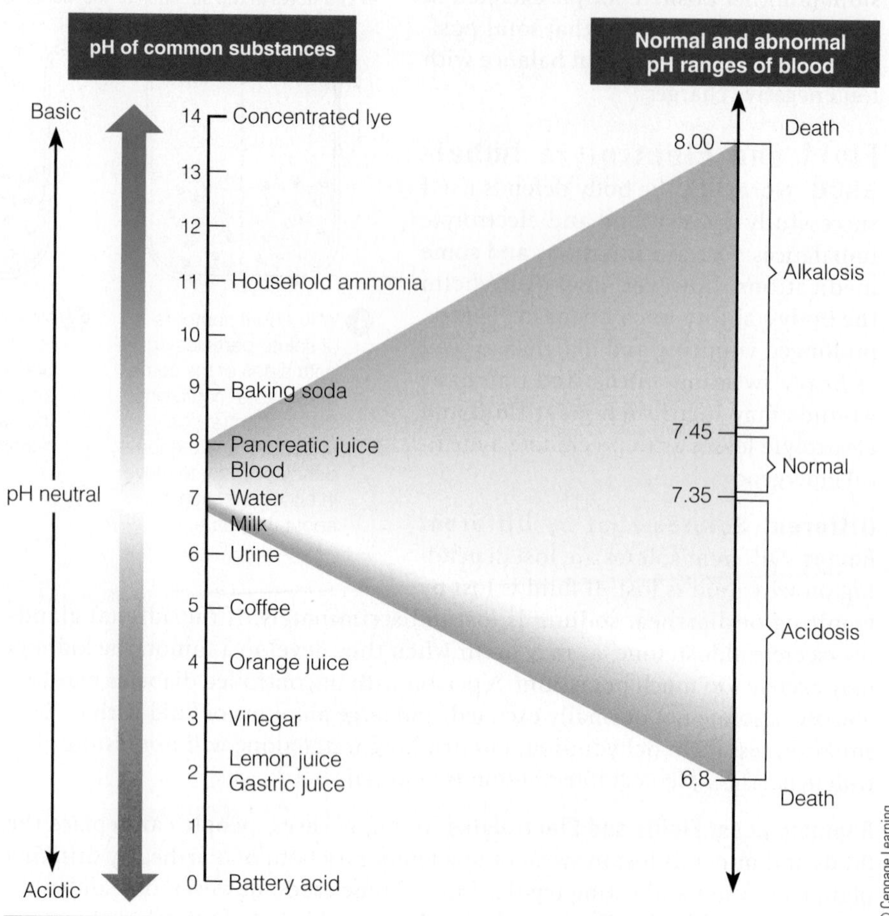

NOTE: Each step is 10 times as concentrated in base (1⁄10 as much as acid, or H^+) as the one below it.

normal and abnormal pH ranges of the blood added. As you can see, the body must maintain the pH within a narrow range to avoid life-threatening consequences. Slight deviations in either direction can denature proteins, rendering them useless. Enzymes couldn't catalyze reactions and hemoglobin couldn't carry oxygen—to name just two examples.

The acidity of the body's fluids is determined by the concentration of hydrogen ions (H^+).* A high concentration of hydrogen ions is acidic. Normal energy metabolism generates hydrogen ions, as well as many other acids, that must be neutralized. Three systems defend the body against fluctuations in pH—buffers in the blood, respiration in the lungs, and excretion in the kidneys.

Regulation by the Buffers **Bicarbonate** (a base) and **carbonic acid** (an acid) in the body fluids, as well as some proteins, protect the body against changes in acidity by acting as **buffers**—substances that can neutralize acids or bases. Carbon dioxide, which is formed all the time during energy metabolism, dissolves in water to form carbonic acid in the blood. Carbonic acid, in turn, dissociates to form hydrogen ions and bicarbonate ions. The appropriate balance between carbonic acid and bicarbonate is essential to maintaining optimal blood pH. Figure 12-8 presents the chemical reactions of this buffer system, which is primarily under the control of the lungs and kidneys.

*The lower the pH, the higher the H^+ ion concentration and the stronger the acid. A pH above 7 is alkaline, or base—a solution in which OH^- ions predominate.

bicarbonate: an alkaline compound with the formula HCO_3 that is produced in all cell fluids from the dissociation of carbonic acid to help maintain the body's acid-base balance. Bicarbonate is also secreted from the pancreas as part of the pancreatic juice.

carbonic acid: a compound with the formula H_2CO_3 that results from the combination of carbon dioxide (CO_2) and water (H_2O); of particular importance in maintaining the body's acid-base balance.

buffers: compounds that keep a solution's pH constant when acids or bases are added.

Respiration in the Lungs The lungs control the concentration of carbonic acid by raising or slowing the respiration rate, depending on whether the pH needs to be increased or decreased. If too much carbonic acid builds up, the respiration rate speeds up; this hyperventilation increases the amount of carbon dioxide exhaled, thereby lowering the carbonic acid concentration and restoring homeostasis. Conversely, if bicarbonate builds up, the respiration rate slows; carbon dioxide is retained and forms more carbonic acid. Again, homeostasis is restored.

Excretion in the Kidneys The kidneys control the concentration of bicarbonate by either reabsorbing or excreting it, depending on whether the pH needs to be increased or decreased, respectively. Their work is complex, but the net effect is easy to sum up. The *body's* total acid burden remains nearly constant; the acidity of the *urine* fluctuates to accommodate that balance.

> FIGURE 12-8 Bicarbonate–Carbonic Acid Buffer System

The reversible reactions of the bicarbonate–carbonic acid buffer system help to regulate the body's pH and maintain homeostasis. Recall from Chapter 7 that carbon dioxide and water are formed during energy metabolism.

Carbon dioxide (CO_2) is a volatile gas that quickly dissolves in water (H_2O), forming carbonic acid (H_2CO_3), which lowers the body's pH:

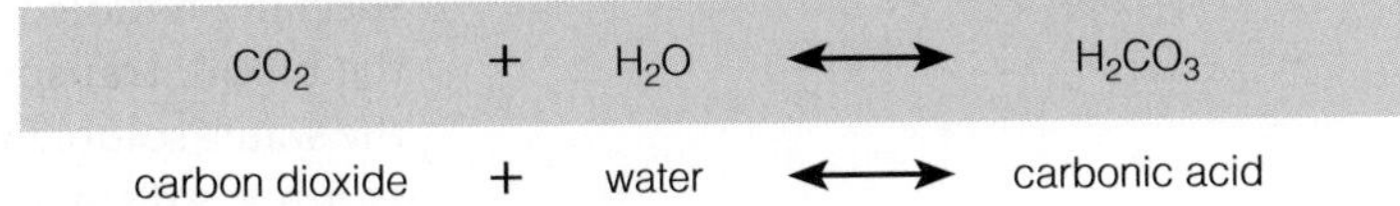

Carbonic acid readily dissociates to a hydrogen ion (H^+) and a bicarbonate ion (HCO_3^-), which raises the body's pH:

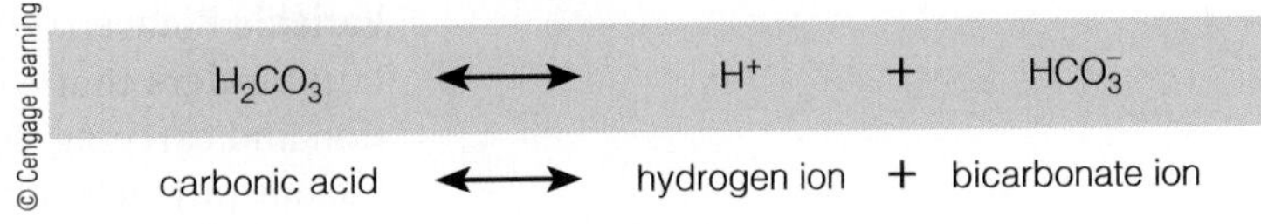

> REVIEW IT Explain how the body regulates fluid balance.

Water makes up about 60 percent of the adult body's weight. It assists with the transport of nutrients and waste products throughout the body, participates in chemical reactions, acts as a solvent, serves as a shock absorber, and regulates body temperature. To maintain water balance, intake from liquids, foods, and metabolism must equal losses from the kidneys, skin, lungs, and GI tract. Whenever the body experiences low blood volume, low blood pressure, or highly concentrated body fluids, the actions of ADH, renin, angiotensin, and aldosterone restore homeostasis. Electrolytes (charged minerals) in the fluids help distribute the fluids inside and outside the cells, thus ensuring the appropriate water balance and acid-base balance to support all life processes. Excessive losses of fluids and electrolytes upset these balances, and the kidneys play a key role in restoring homeostasis.

12.2 The Minerals—An Overview

> LEARN IT List some of the ways minerals differ from vitamins and other nutrients.

Figure 12-9 shows the amounts of the **major minerals** found in the body and, for comparison, some of the **trace minerals.** The distinction between the major and trace minerals does not mean that one group is more important than the other—all minerals are vital. The major minerals are so named because they are present, and needed, in larger amounts in the body. They are shown at the top of the figure and are discussed in this chapter. The trace minerals, shown at the bottom of the figure, are discussed in Chapter 13. A few generalizations pertain to all of the minerals and distinguish them from the vitamins. Especially notable is their chemical nature.

major minerals: essential mineral nutrients the human body requires in relatively large amounts (greater than 100 milligrams per day); sometimes called *macrominerals.*

trace minerals: essential mineral nutrients the human body requires in relatively small amounts (less than 100 milligrams per day); sometimes called *microminerals.*

Inorganic Elements Unlike the organic vitamins, which are easily destroyed, minerals are inorganic elements that always retain their chemical identity. Once minerals enter the body, they remain there until excreted; they cannot be changed into anything else. Iron, for example, may temporarily combine with other charged elements in salts, but it is always iron. Neither can minerals be destroyed by heat, air, acid, or mixing.

> FIGURE 12-9 Minerals in a 60-kilogram (132-pound) Human Body

Not only are the major minerals needed by the body in larger amounts, but they are also present in the body in larger amounts than the trace minerals.

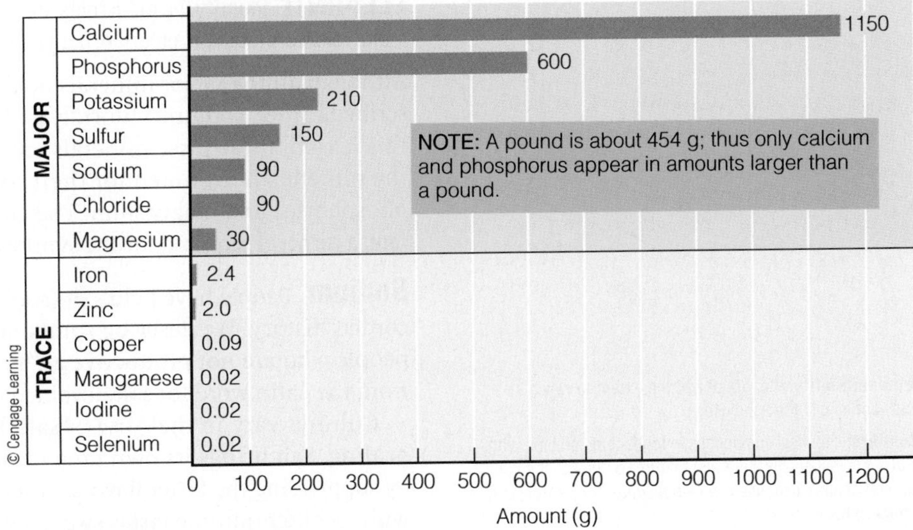

Consequently, little care is needed to preserve minerals during food preparation. In fact, the ash that remains when a food is burned contains all the minerals that were in the food originally. Minerals can be lost from food only when they leach into cooking water that is then poured down the drain.

The Body's Handling of Minerals The minerals also differ from the vitamins in the amounts the body can absorb and in the extent to which they must be specially handled. Some minerals, such as potassium, are easily absorbed into the blood, transported freely, and readily excreted by the kidneys, much like the water-soluble vitamins. Other minerals, such as calcium, are more like fat-soluble vitamins in that they must have carriers to be absorbed and transported. And, like some of the fat-soluble vitamins, minerals consumed in excess can be toxic.

Variable Bioavailability The **bioavailability** of minerals varies. Some foods contain **binders** that combine chemically with minerals, preventing their absorption and carrying them out of the body with other wastes. Examples of binders include phytates, which are found primarily in legumes, seeds, nuts, and grains, and oxalates, which are present in rhubarb, beet greens, sweet potatoes, and spinach, among other vegetables. These foods contain more minerals than the body actually receives for use.

Nutrient Interactions Chapter 10 describes how the presence or absence of one vitamin can affect another's absorption, metabolism, and excretion. The same is true of the minerals. The interactions between sodium and calcium, for example, cause both to be excreted when sodium intakes are high. Phosphorus binds with magnesium in the GI tract, so magnesium absorption is limited when phosphorus intakes are high. These are just two examples of the interactions involving minerals featured in this chapter. Discussions in both this chapter and the next point out additional problems that arise from such interactions. Notice how often they reflect an excess of one mineral creating an inadequacy of another and how supplements—not foods—are most often to blame.

> **› REVIEW IT** List some of the ways minerals differ from vitamins and other nutrients.
> Compared with the trace minerals, major minerals are found, and needed, in larger quantities in the body. Unlike vitamins and the energy-yielding nutrients, minerals are inorganic elements that retain their chemical identities. Minerals usually receive special handling and regulation in the body, and they may bind with other substances or interact with other minerals, thus limiting their absorption.

12.3 The Major Minerals

› LEARN IT Identify the main roles, deficiency symptoms, and food sources for each of the major minerals (sodium, chloride, potassium, calcium, phosphorus, magnesium, and sulfate).

Although all the major minerals help to maintain the body's fluid balance as described earlier, sodium, chloride, and potassium are most noted for that role. For this reason, these three minerals are discussed first here. Later sections describe the minerals most noted for their roles in bone growth and health—calcium, phosphorus, and magnesium. The chapter closes with a brief discussion on sulfate, a mineral required for the synthesis of several sulfur-containing compounds.

Sodium

People have held salt (sodium chloride) in high regard throughout recorded history. We describe someone we admire as "the salt of the earth" and people who are not productive as "not worth their salt." The word *salary* comes from the Latin word for salt, a valued commodity.

Cultures vary in their use of salt, but most people find its taste innately appealing. Salt brings its own tangy taste and enhances other flavors, most likely by suppressing the bitter flavors. You can taste this effect for yourself: tonic water with its bitter quinine tastes sweeter with a little salt added.

bioavailability: the rate at and the extent to which a nutrient is absorbed and used.

binders: chemical compounds in foods that combine with nutrients (especially minerals) to form complexes the body cannot absorb. Examples include *phytates* (FYE-tates) and *oxalates* (OCK-sa-lates).

Sodium Roles in the Body **Sodium** is the principal cation of the extracellular fluid and the primary regulator of its volume. Sodium also helps maintain acid-base balance and is essential to nerve impulse transmission and muscle contraction.*

Sodium is readily absorbed by the intestinal tract and travels freely in the blood until it reaches the kidneys, which filter all the sodium out of the blood. Then, with great precision, the kidneys return to the blood the exact amount of sodium the body needs. Normally, the amount excreted is approximately equal to the amount ingested on a given day. When blood sodium rises, as when a person eats salted foods, thirst signals the person to drink until the appropriate sodium-to-water concentration is restored. Then the kidneys excrete both the excess water and the excess sodium together. Both too much and too little sodium in the diet increase the risk of heart disease.[6] The key to good health, then, is finding the balance that meets the relatively small need for this essential nutrient but does not exceed the amount that leads to hypertension and heart disease.[7]

Sodium Recommendations Diets rarely lack sodium, and even when intakes are low, the body adapts by reducing sodium losses in urine and sweat, thus making deficiencies unlikely. Sodium recommendations are set low enough to protect against high blood pressure, but high enough to allow an adequate intake of other nutrients with a typical diet. Because high sodium intakes correlate with high blood pressure, the Upper Level (UL) for adults is set at 2300 milligrams per day, as is the Daily Value used on food labels. The average sodium intake in the United States is 3400 milligrams, which exceeds recommendations—and most adults will develop hypertension at some point in their lives.[8]

Sodium and Hypertension For years, a high *sodium* intake was considered the primary factor responsible for high blood pressure. Then research pointed to *salt* (sodium chloride) as the dietary culprit. Salt has a greater effect on blood pressure than either sodium or chloride alone or in combination with other ions. The response to a high salt meal may be immediate, reducing blood flow through arteries; this condition is reversible if such meals are not habitual.[9] The elevation of blood pressure in response to a high-salt diet over years is progressive, and the damage caused to blood vessels is irreversible.

Blood pressure increases in response to excesses in salt intake—most notably for those with hypertension, African Americans, and people older than 40 years of age. For them, a high salt intake correlates strongly with heart disease, and salt restriction (to no more than 1500 milligrams of sodium per day) helps to lower blood pressure.

A salt-restricted diet lowers blood pressure and improves heart disease risk in people without hypertension as well.[10] Because reducing salt intake causes no harm and diminishes the risk of hypertension and heart disease, the *Dietary Guidelines for Americans* advise limiting daily *salt* intake to about 1 teaspoon (the equivalent of about 2.3 grams or 2300 milligrams of *sodium*).[11] The American Heart Association goal is to lower blood pressure by reducing sodium intake to less than 1500 milligrams a day.[12] The "How To" feature on p. 384 offers strategies for cutting salt (and therefore sodium) intake.

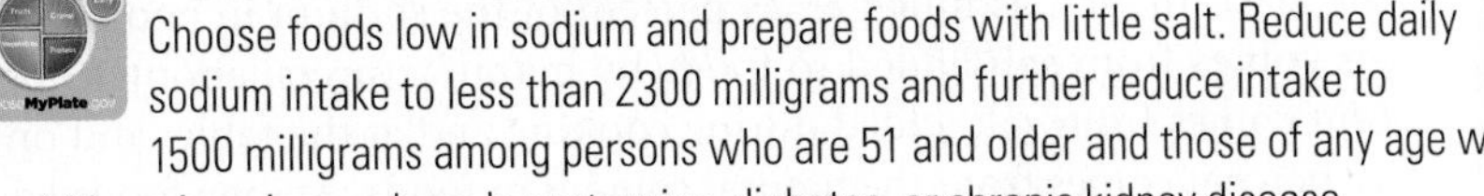

> DIETARY GUIDELINES FOR AMERICANS

Choose foods low in sodium and prepare foods with little salt. Reduce daily sodium intake to less than 2300 milligrams and further reduce intake to 1500 milligrams among persons who are 51 and older and those of any age who are African American or have hypertension, diabetes, or chronic kidney disease.

Given the current US food supply and typical eating habits, creating a nutritionally balanced diet that meets sodium recommendations can be quite a challenge.[13] One eating pattern, known as the DASH (Dietary Approaches to Stop Hypertension) Eating Plan, is especially effective in lowering blood pressure.[14]

*One of the ways the kidneys regulate acid-base balance is by excreting hydrogen ions (H^+) in exchange for sodium ions (Na^+).

sodium: the principal cation in the extracellular fluids of the body; critical to the maintenance of fluid balance, nerve impulse transmissions, and muscle contractions.

>How To

Cut Salt (and Sodium) Intake

Salt (sodium chloride) is about 40% sodium and 60% chloride.

- 1 g salt contributes about 400 mg sodium and 600 mg chloride
- 6 g salt = 1 tsp
- 1 tsp salt contributes about 2300 mg sodium and 3700 mg chloride

Most people eat more salt (and therefore sodium) than they need. Some people can lower their blood pressure by avoiding highly salted foods and removing the salt shaker from the table. Foods eaten without salt may seem less tasty at first, but with repetition, people can learn to enjoy the natural flavors of many unsalted foods. Strategies to cut salt intake include:

- Select fresh or frozen vegetables. If buying canned vegetables, drain and rinse in water to remove some of the sodium or select those labeled low-sodium or no-salt-added.
- Cook with little or no added salt.
- Prepare foods with sodium-free herbs and spices such as basil, bay leaves, curry, garlic, ginger, mint, oregano, pepper, rosemary, and thyme; lemon juice; vinegar; or wine.
- Add little or no salt at the table; taste foods before adding salt.
- Read labels with an eye open for sodium. (See the glossary on p. 61 for terms used to describe the sodium contents of foods on labels.)
- Select low-salt or salt-free products when available.

Use these foods sparingly:

- Foods prepared in brine, such as pickles, olives, and sauerkraut
- Salty or smoked meats, such as bologna, corned or chipped beef, bacon, frankfurters, ham, lunchmeats, salt pork, sausage, and smoked tongue
- Salty or smoked fish, such as anchovies, caviar, salted and dried cod, herring, sardines, and smoked salmon
- Snack items such as potato chips, pretzels, salted popcorn, salted nuts, and crackers
- Condiments such as bouillon cubes; seasoned salts; MSG; soy, teriyaki, Worcestershire, and barbeque sauces; prepared horseradish, ketchup, and mustard
- Cheeses, especially processed types
- Canned and instant soups
- Packaged instant or flavored rice, pasta, and cereal mixes

> TRY IT Compare the sodium contents of 1 ounce of the following foods: a plain bagel, potato chips, and animal crackers.

Like other USDA Food Patterns, the DASH Eating Plan reflects the *Dietary Guidelines* and allows people to stay within their energy allowance, meet nutrient needs, and reduce chronic disease risk. The DASH approach emphasizes potassium-rich fruits, vegetables, and low-fat milk products; includes whole grains, nuts, poultry, and fish; and calls for reduced intakes of sodium, red and processed meats, sweets, and sugar-containing beverages. In combination with a reduced sodium intake, DASH is even more effective at lowering blood pressure than either strategy alone. In addition, DASH lowers the risk of some cancers, heart disease, and stroke.[15] Chapter 18 offers a complete discussion of hypertension and the dietary recommendations for its prevention and treatment.

Sodium and Bone Loss (Osteoporosis) A high salt intake is also associated with increased calcium excretion, but its influence on bone loss is less clear. In addition, potassium may prevent the calcium excretion caused by a high-salt diet. For these reasons, dietary advice to prevent bone loss parallels that suggested for hypertension—a DASH eating pattern that is low in sodium and abundant in potassium-rich fruits and vegetables and calcium-rich low-fat milk.

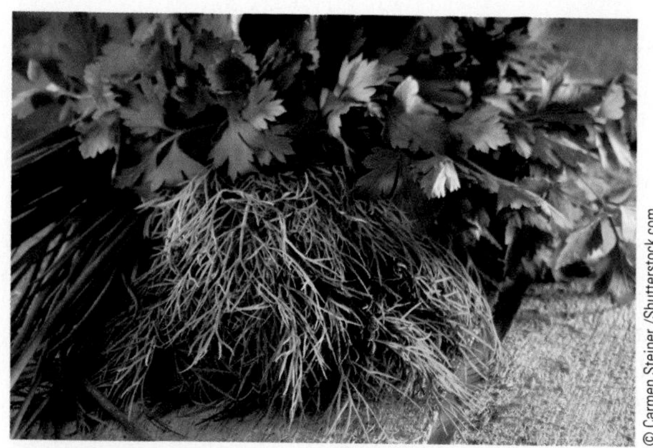

Fresh herbs add flavor to a recipe without adding salt.

Sodium in Foods In general, processed foods have the most sodium, whereas unprocessed foods such as fresh fruits and vegetables have the least. In fact, as much as 75 percent of the sodium in people's diets comes from salt added to foods by manufacturers; about 15 percent comes from salt added during cooking and at the table; and only 10 percent comes from the natural content in foods. Among foods with the highest sodium density (milligrams of sodium per kcalorie) are those from fast food and pizza restaurants.[16] Because sodium intake tends to increase as kcalories increase, making food choices based on low sodium density is a practical and effective way to lower sodium intake.[17]

To help consumers limit their intake, public health organizations and policymakers worldwide are calling for manufacturers and restaurants to reduce sodium in the food supply.[18] In addition to reducing the sodium content of foods, food scientists are designing products to enhance salty perceptions with less salt.[19] Reducing the sodium content in processed foods could prevent an estimated 100,000 deaths and save up to $24 billion in health care costs in the United States annually.[20]

Because processed foods may contain sodium without chloride, as in additives such as sodium bicarbonate or sodium saccharin, they do not always taste salty. Most people are surprised to learn that 1 ounce of some cereals contains more sodium than 1 ounce of salted peanuts—and that ½ cup of instant chocolate pudding contains still more. The peanuts taste saltier because the salt is all on the surface, where the tongue's taste receptors immediately pick it up.

Figure 12-10 shows that processed foods not only contain more sodium than their less-processed counterparts but also have less potassium. Low potassium may be as significant as high sodium when it comes to blood pressure regulation, so processed foods have (at least) two strikes against them.

Sodium Deficiency Sodium deficiency does not develop from an inadequate diet. The body needs so little and diets provide enough. Blood sodium may drop with vomiting, diarrhea, or heavy sweating, and in these cases, both sodium and water must be replenished. Under normal conditions of sweating due to physical activity, salt losses can easily be replaced later in the day with ordinary foods. Salt tablets are not recommended because too much salt, especially if taken with too little water, can induce dehydration. During intense activities, such as ultra-endurance events, athletes can lose so much sodium and drink so much water that they develop hyponatremia—the dangerous condition of having too little sodium in the blood. Symptoms of hyponatremia include headache, confusion, stupor, seizures, and coma. Importantly, hyponatremia is caused by excessive sodium losses, not from inadequate sodium intake. (Chapter 14 offers details about hyponatremia and guidelines for ultra-endurance athletes.)

Sodium Toxicity and Excessive Intakes The immediate symptoms of acute sodium toxicity are edema and high blood pressure. Prolonged excessive sodium intake may contribute to hypertension in some people, as explained earlier.

> FIGURE 12-10 **What Processing Does to the Sodium and Potassium Contents of Foods**

People who eat foods high in salt often happen to be eating fewer potassium-containing foods at the same time. Notice how potassium is lost and sodium is gained as foods become more processed, causing the potassium-to-sodium ratio to fall dramatically. Even when potassium isn't lost, the addition of sodium still lowers the potassium-to-sodium ratio. Selecting fresh, unprocessed foods lowers blood pressure in two ways, then—by lowering sodium intakes and by raising potassium intakes.

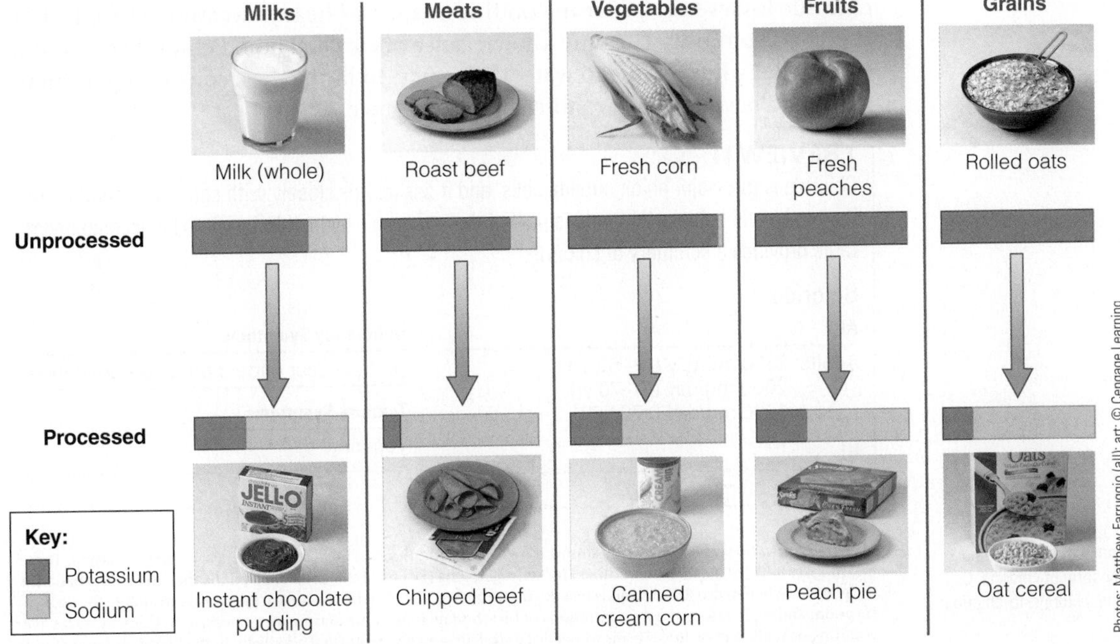

Photos: Matthew Farruggio (all); art: © Cengage Learning

› REVIEW IT

Sodium is the main cation outside cells and one of the primary electrolytes responsible for maintaining fluid balance. Dietary deficiency is unlikely, and excesses raise blood pressure in many people. For this reason, health professionals advise a diet moderate in salt and sodium. The accompanying table provides a summary of sodium.

Sodium

AI	**Deficiency Symptoms**
Adults: 1500 mg/day (19–50 yr) 1300 mg/day (51–70 yr) 1200 mg/day (>70 yr)	Not from inadequate intakes Hyponatremia from excessive losses
UL	**Toxicity Symptoms**
Adults: 2300 mg/day	Edema, acute hypertension
Chief Functions in the Body	**Significant Sources**
Maintains normal fluid and electrolyte balance; assists in nerve impulse transmission and muscle contraction	Table salt, soy sauce; moderate amounts in meats, milks, breads, and vegetables; large amounts in processed foods

Chloride

The element *chlorine* (Cl_2) is a poisonous gas. When chlorine reacts with sodium or hydrogen, however, it forms the negative chloride ion (Cl^-). *Chloride,* an essential nutrient, is required in the diet.

Chloride Roles in the Body **Chloride** is the major anion of the extracellular fluids (outside the cells), where it occurs mostly in association with sodium. Chloride moves passively across membranes through channels and so also associates with potassium inside cells. Like sodium and potassium, chloride maintains fluid and electrolyte balance.

In the stomach, the chloride ion is part of hydrochloric acid, which maintains the strong acidity of gastric juice. One of the most serious consequences of vomiting is the loss of this acid from the stomach, which upsets the acid-base balance.* Such imbalances are commonly seen in bulimia nervosa, as described in Highlight 8.

Chloride Recommendations and Intakes Chloride is abundant in foods (especially processed foods) as part of sodium chloride and other salts. Chloride recommendations are slightly higher than, but still equivalent to, those of sodium. In other words, ¾ teaspoon of salt will deliver some sodium, more chloride, and still meet the AI for both.

Chloride Deficiency and Toxicity Diets rarely lack chloride. Like sodium losses, chloride losses may occur in conditions such as heavy sweating, chronic diarrhea, and vomiting. The only known cause of elevated blood chloride concentrations is dehydration due to water deficiency. In both cases, consuming ordinary foods and beverages can restore chloride balance.

› REVIEW IT

Chloride is the major anion outside cells, and it associates closely with sodium. In addition to its role in fluid balance, chloride is part of the stomach's hydrochloric acid. The accompanying table provides a summary of chloride.

Chloride

AI	**Deficiency Symptoms**
Adults: 2300 mg/day (19–50 yr) 2000 mg/day (51–70 yr) 1800 mg/day (>70 yr)	Do not occur under normal circumstances
	Toxicity Symptoms
	Vomiting
UL	
Adults: 3600 mg/day	

chloride (KLO-ride): the major anion in the extracellular fluids of the body. Chloride is the ionic form of chlorine, Cl^-. See Appendix B for a description of the chlorine-to-chloride conversion.

*Hydrochloric acid secretion into the stomach involves the addition of bicarbonate ions (base) to the plasma. These bicarbonate ions (HCO_3^-) are neutralized by hydrogen ions (H^+) from the gastric secretions that are reabsorbed into the plasma. When hydrochloric acid is lost during vomiting, these hydrogen ions are no longer available for reabsorption, and so, in effect, the concentrations of bicarbonate ions in the plasma are increased. In this way, excessive vomiting of acidic gastric juices leads to *metabolic alkalosis*—an above-normal alkalinity in the blood and body fluids.

› REVIEW IT Chloride *(continued)*

Chief Functions in the Body	Significant Sources
Maintains normal fluid and electrolyte balance; part of hydrochloric acid found in the stomach, necessary for proper digestion	Table salt, soy sauce; moderate amounts in meats, milks, eggs; large amounts in processed foods

Potassium Like sodium, **potassium** is a positively charged ion. In contrast to sodium, potassium is the body's principal intracellular cation, *inside* the body cells.

Potassium Roles in the Body Potassium plays a major role in maintaining fluid and electrolyte balance and cell integrity. During nerve transmissions and muscle contractions, potassium and sodium briefly trade places across the cell membrane. The cell then quickly pumps them back into place. Controlling potassium distribution is a high priority for the body because it affects many aspects of homeostasis, including a steady heartbeat.

Potassium Recommendations and Intakes Potassium is abundant in all living cells. Because cells remain intact unless foods are processed, the richest sources of potassium are *fresh* foods—as Figure 12-11 shows. In contrast, most processed foods such as canned vegetables, ready-to-eat cereals, and luncheon meats contain less potassium—and more sodium (recall Figure 12-10, p. 385). To meet the AI for potassium, most people need to increase their daily intake of fruits and vegetables.

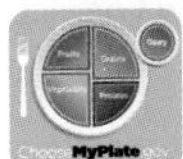

› DIETARY GUIDELINES FOR AMERICANS

Choose foods that provide more potassium, a nutrient of concern in American diets. Potassium is found in all food groups, notably vegetables, fruits, and milk and milk products.

potassium: the principal cation within the body's cells; critical to the maintenance of fluid balance, nerve impulse transmissions, and muscle contractions.

› FIGURE 12-11 Potassium in Selected Foods

Food	Serving size (kcalories)
Bread, whole wheat	1-oz slice (70 kcal)
Cornflakes, fortified	1 oz (110 kcal)
Spaghetti pasta	½ c cooked (99 kcal)
Tortilla, flour	1 10" round (234 kcal)
Broccoli	½ c cooked (22 kcal)
Carrots	½ c shredded raw (24 kcal)
Potato	1 medium baked w/skin (133 kcal)
Tomato juice	¾ c (31 kcal)
Banana	1 medium raw (109 kcal)
Orange	1 medium raw (62 kcal)
Strawberries	½ c fresh (22 kcal)
Watermelon	1 slice (92 kcal)
Milk	1 c reduced-fat 2% (121 kcal)
Yogurt, plain	1 c low-fat (155 kcal)
Cheddar cheese	1½ oz (171 kcal)
Cottage cheese	½ c low-fat 2% (101 kcal)
Pinto beans	½ c cooked (117 kcal)
Peanut butter	2 tbs (188 kcal)
Sunflower seeds	1 oz dry (165 kcal)
Tofu (soybean curd)	½ c (76 kcal)
Ground beef, lean	3 oz broiled (244 kcal)
Chicken breast	3 oz roasted (140 kcal)
Tuna, canned in water	3 oz (99 kcal)
Egg	1 hard cooked (78 kcal)
Excellent, and sometimes unusual, sources:	
Squash, acorn	½ c baked (69 kcal)
Soybeans	½ c cooked (149 kcal)
Artichoke	1 (60 kcal)

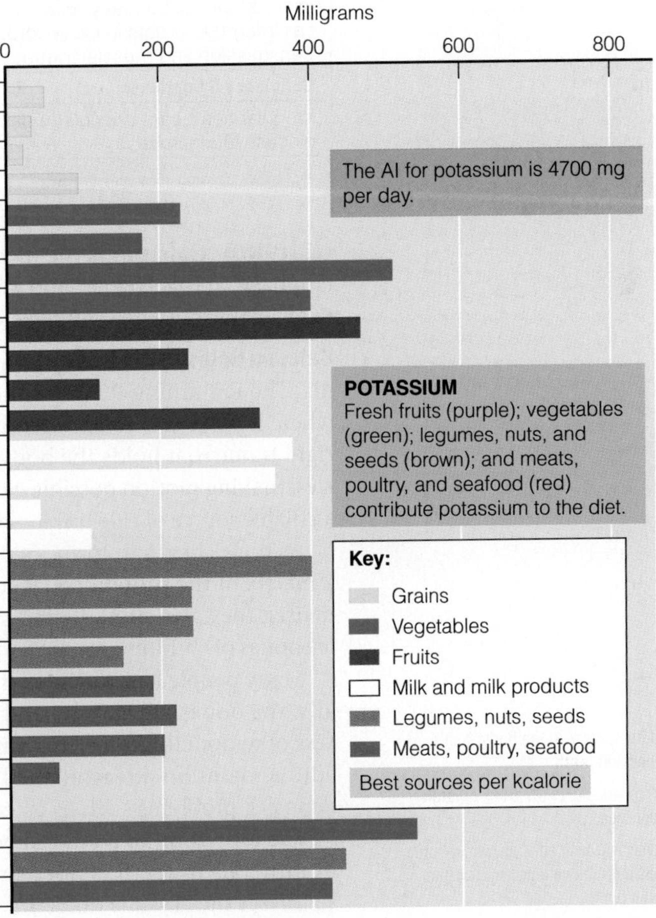

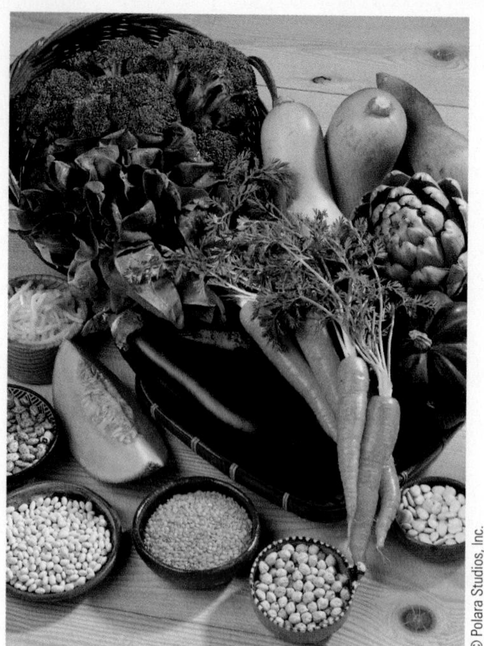

Fresh foods, especially fruits and vegetables, provide potassium in abundance.

Potassium and Hypertension Diets low in potassium, especially when combined with high sodium intakes, raise blood pressure and increase the risk of death from heart disease.[21] In contrast, high potassium intakes, especially when combined with low sodium intakes, appear to both prevent and correct hypertension. Unfortunately, most US adults consume too much sodium and too little potassium.[22] Recall that the DASH eating pattern described earlier is used to lower blood pressure and emphasizes potassium-rich foods such as fruits and vegetables. Potassium-rich fruits and vegetables also appear to reduce the risk of strokes and heart attacks—more so than can be explained by the reduction in blood pressure alone.[23]

Potassium Deficiency Potassium deficiency is characterized by an increase in blood pressure, kidney stones, and bone turnover. As deficiency progresses, symptoms include irregular heartbeats, muscle weakness, and glucose intolerance.

Potassium Toxicity Potassium toxicity does not result from overeating foods high in potassium; therefore a UL has not been set. It can result from overconsumption of potassium salts or supplements (including some "energy fitness shakes") and from certain diseases or treatments. Given more potassium than the body needs, the kidneys accelerate excretion. If potassium is injected directly into a vein, however, it can stop the heart.

› REVIEW IT

Potassium, like sodium and chloride, is an electrolyte that plays an important role in maintaining fluid balance. Potassium is the primary cation inside cells; fresh foods, notably fruits and vegetables, are its best sources. The accompanying table provides a summary of potassium.

Potassium

AI	Toxicity Symptoms
Adults: 4700 mg/day	Muscular weakness; vomiting; if given into a vein, can stop the heart
Chief Functions in the Body	**Significant Sources**
Maintains normal fluid and electrolyte balance; facilitates many reactions; supports cell integrity; assists in nerve impulse transmission and muscle contractions	All whole foods: meats, milks, fruits, vegetables, grains, legumes
Deficiency Symptoms[a]	
Irregular heatbeat, muscular weakness, glucose intolerance	

[a]Deficiency accompanies dehydration.

Calcium

Calcium is the most abundant mineral in the body. It receives much emphasis in this chapter and in the highlight that follows because an adequate intake helps grow a healthy skeleton in early life and minimize bone loss in later life.

Calcium Roles in the Body Only 1 percent of the body's calcium is in the body fluids. The remaining 99 percent of the body's calcium is in the bones (and teeth), where it plays two roles. First, it is an integral part of bone structure, providing a rigid frame that holds the body upright and serves as attachment points for muscles, making motion possible. Second, it serves as a calcium bank, offering a readily available source of calcium to the body fluids should a drop in blood calcium occur.

As bones begin to form, calcium salts form crystals, called **hydroxyapatite,** on a matrix of the protein collagen. During **mineralization,** as the crystals become denser, they give strength and rigidity to the maturing bones. As a result, the long leg bones of children can support their weight by the time they have learned to walk.

Many people have the idea that once a bone is built, it is inert like a rock. Actually, the bones are gaining and losing minerals continuously in an ongoing process of remodeling. Growing children gain more bone than they lose, and healthy adults maintain a reasonable balance. When withdrawals substantially exceed deposits, problems such as osteoporosis develop (as described in Highlight 12).

The formation of teeth follows a pattern similar to that of bones. The turnover of minerals in teeth is not as rapid as in bone, however; fluoride hardens and stabilizes the crystals of teeth, opposing the withdrawal of minerals from them.

calcium: the most abundant mineral in the body; found primarily in the body's bones and teeth.

hydroxyapatite (high-drox-ee-APP-ah-tite): crystals made of calcium and phosphorus.

mineralization: the process in which calcium, phosphorus, and other minerals crystallize on the collagen matrix of a growing bone, hardening the bone.

Although only 1 percent of the body's calcium circulates in the extracellular and intracellular fluids, its presence there is vital to life. Cells throughout the body can detect calcium in the extracellular fluids and respond accordingly. Many of calcium's actions help to maintain normal blood pressure, perhaps by stabilizing the smooth muscle cells of the blood vessels or by releasing relaxing factors from the blood vessel cell walls. Extracellular calcium also participates in blood clotting.

The calcium in intracellular fluids binds to proteins within the cells and activates them. For example, when the protein **calmodulin** binds with calcium, it activates the enzymes involved in breaking down glycogen, which releases energy for muscle contractions. Many such proteins participate in the regulation of muscle contractions, the transmission of nerve impulses, the secretion of hormones, and the activation of some enzyme reactions.

Calcium in Disease Prevention Calcium may protect against some chronic diseases, including hypertension.[24] Considering the success of DASH in lowering blood pressure, restricting sodium to treat hypertension may be narrow advice. The DASH eating pattern is rich in calcium, as well as in magnesium and potassium—all of which help lower blood pressure.

Calcium-rich foods may play a role in reducing body fat, protecting lean tissue, and maintaining a healthy body weight.[25] Some epidemiological studies suggest an inverse relationship between calcium intake and body weight: the higher the calcium intake, the lower the prevalence of overweight. Clinical studies, however, report such small losses (1 to 2 pounds) as to be statistically insignificant.[26] Some would argue that the real-life benefits are significant in that weight gains are diminished and body composition is improved.[27] In addition, calcium-rich foods suppress the inflammation commonly associated with overweight, even without weight loss.[28] Importantly, calcium-rich foods help with weight loss only when used within an energy-restricted diet.[29]

calmodulin (cal-MOD-you-lin): a calcium-binding protein that regulates such cell activities as muscle contractions.

parathyroid hormone: a hormone from the parathyroid glands that regulates blood calcium by raising it when levels fall too low; also known as *parathormone* (PAIR-ah-THOR-moan).

calcitonin (KAL-seh-TOE-nin): a hormone secreted by the thyroid gland that regulates blood calcium by lowering it when levels rise too high.

Calcium Balance Calcium homeostasis involves a system of hormones and vitamin D. Whenever blood calcium falls too low or rises too high, three organ systems respond: the intestines, bones, and kidneys. Figure 12-12 illustrates how vitamin D and two hormones—**parathyroid hormone** and **calcitonin**—return blood calcium to normal.

The calcium in bones provides a nearly inexhaustible bank of calcium for the blood. The blood borrows and returns calcium as needed so that even with an inadequate diet, *blood* calcium remains normal—even as *bone* calcium diminishes (see Figure 12-13 on p. 390). Blood calcium changes only in response to abnormal regulatory control, not to diet. A person can have an inadequate calcium intake for years and have no noticeable symptoms. Only later in life does it become apparent that bone integrity has been compromised.

> FIGURE 12-12 **Calcium Balance**

Low blood calcium Signals the parathyroid glands to secrete parathyroid hormone into the blood		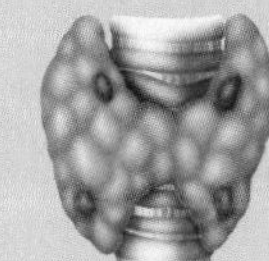 Thyroid gland with parathyroid glands embedded	**High blood calcium** Signals the thyroid gland to secrete calcitonin
Vitamin D	**Parathyroid hormone** Stimulates the activation of vitamin D		**Calcitonin** Inhibits the activation of vitamin D
Stimulates calcium reabsorption from the kidneys into the blood	Stimulates calcium reabsorption from the kidneys into the blood	Kidneys	Prevents calcium reabsorption in the kidneys
Enhances calcium absorption in the intestines		Intestines	Limits calcium absorption in the intestines
Stimulates osteoclast cells to break down bone, releasing calcium into the blood	Stimulates osteoclast cells to break down bone, releasing calcium into the blood	Bones	Inhibits osteoclast cells from breaking down bone, preventing the release of calcium
End results Raised blood calcium	Raised blood calcium Parathyroid hormone secretion inhibited		**End results** Lower blood calcium Calcitonin secretion inhibited

NOTE: Calcitonin plays a major role in defending infants and young children against the dangers of rising blood calcium that can occur when regular feedings of milk deliver large quantities of calcium to a small body. In contrast, calcitonin plays a relatively minor role in adults because their absorption of calcium is less efficient and their bodies are larger, making elevated blood calcium unlikely.

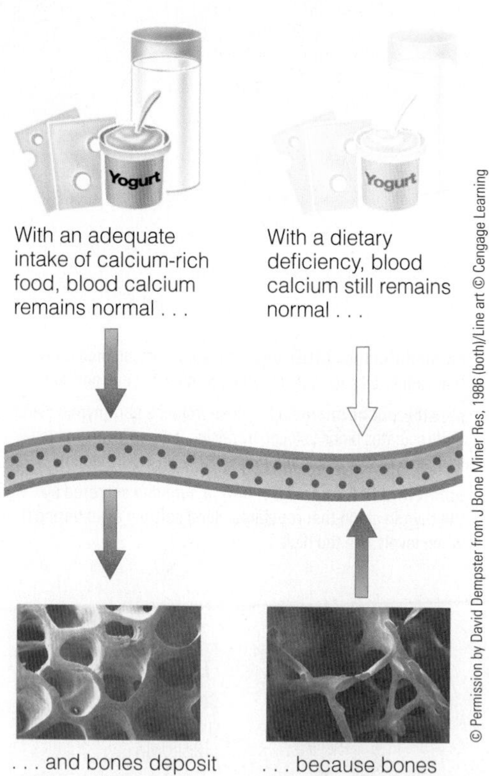

Yogurt
Yogurt
With an adequate intake of calcium-rich food, blood calcium remains normal . . .
With a dietary deficiency, blood calcium still remains normal . . .
. . . and bones deposit calcium. The result is strong, dense bones.
. . . because bones give up calcium to the blood. The result is weak, osteoporotic bones.
© Permission by David Dempster from J Bone Miner Res, 1986 (both)/Line art © Cengage Learning

> **FIGURE 12-13 Maintaining Blood Calcium from the Diet and from the Bones**

Blood calcium above normal results in **calcium rigor:** the muscles contract and cannot relax. Similarly, blood calcium below normal causes **calcium tetany**—also characterized by uncontrolled muscle contraction. These conditions do *not* reflect a *dietary* excess or lack of calcium; they are caused by a lack of vitamin D or by abnormal secretion of the regulatory hormones. A chronic *dietary* deficiency of calcium, or a chronic deficiency due to poor absorption over the years, depletes the bones. Again: the *bones,* not the blood, are robbed by a calcium deficiency.

Calcium Absorption Because many factors affect calcium absorption, the most effective way to ensure adequacy is to increase calcium intake. On average, adults absorb about 30 percent of the calcium they ingest. The stomach's acidity helps to keep calcium soluble, and vitamin D helps to make the **calcium-binding protein** needed for absorption. This relationship explains why calcium-rich milk is a good choice for vitamin D fortification.

Whenever calcium is needed, the body increases its calcium absorption. The result is obvious in the case of a newborn infant, whose calcium absorption is 55 to 60 percent. Similarly, a pregnant woman doubles her absorption of calcium. Growing children and teens absorb up to 50 percent of the calcium they consume. Then, when bone growth slows or stops, absorption falls to the adult level of about 30 percent. In addition, absorption becomes more efficient during times of inadequate intakes.

Many of the conditions that enhance calcium absorption limit its absorption when they are absent. For example, sufficient vitamin D supports absorption, and a deficiency impairs it. In addition, fiber in general, and the binders phytate and oxalate in particular, interfere with calcium absorption, but their effects are relatively minor in typical US diets. Vegetables with oxalates and whole grains with phytates are nutritious foods, of course, but they are not useful calcium sources.

Calcium Recommendations Calcium is unlike most other nutrients in that hormones maintain its *blood* concentration regardless of dietary intake. As Figure 12-13 shows, when calcium intake is high, the *bones* benefit; when intake is low, the *bones* suffer. Calcium recommendations are therefore based on the amount needed to retain the most calcium in bones. By retaining the most calcium possible, the bones can develop to their fullest potential in size and density—their **peak bone mass**—within genetic limits.

Calcium recommendations have been set high enough to accommodate a 30 percent absorption rate. Because obtaining enough calcium during growth helps to ensure that the skeleton will be strong and dense, the recommendation for adolescents to the age of 18 years is 1300 milligrams daily. Between the ages of 19 and 50, recommendations are lowered to 1000 milligrams a day; for women older than 50 and all adults older than 70, recommendations are raised again to 1200 milligrams a day to minimize the bone loss that tends to occur later in life. Some authorities advocate as much as 1500 milligrams a day for women older than 50. Most people in the United States have calcium intakes below current recommendations. Those meeting recommendations for calcium are likely to be using calcium supplements.[30] High intakes of calcium from supplements may have adverse effects such as kidney stone formation. For this reason, a UL has been established.

A high-protein diet increases urinary calcium losses, but does not seem to impair bone health.[31] In fact, protein may even improve calcium absorption and bone strength. The DRI Committee considered these nutrient interactions in establishing the RDA for calcium and did not adjust dietary recommendations based on this information.[32]

Calcium Food Sources Figure 12-14 shows that calcium is found most abundantly in a single food group—milk and milk products. The person who doesn't like to drink milk may prefer to eat cheese or yogurt. Alternatively, milk and milk products can be concealed in foods. Powdered fat-free milk can be added to casseroles, soups, and other mixed dishes during preparation; 5 heaping tablespoons offer the equivalent of 1 cup of milk. This simple step is an excellent way for older women to obtain not only extra calcium, but more protein, vitamins, and minerals as well.

calcium rigor: hardness or stiffness of the muscles caused by high blood calcium concentrations.

calcium tetany (TET-ah-nee): intermittent spasm of the extremities due to nervous and muscular excitability caused by low blood calcium concentrations.

calcium-binding protein: a protein in the intestinal cells, made with the help of vitamin D, that facilitates calcium absorption.

peak bone mass: the highest attainable bone density for an individual, developed during the first three decades of life.

> **FIGURE 12-14 Calcium in Selected Foods**

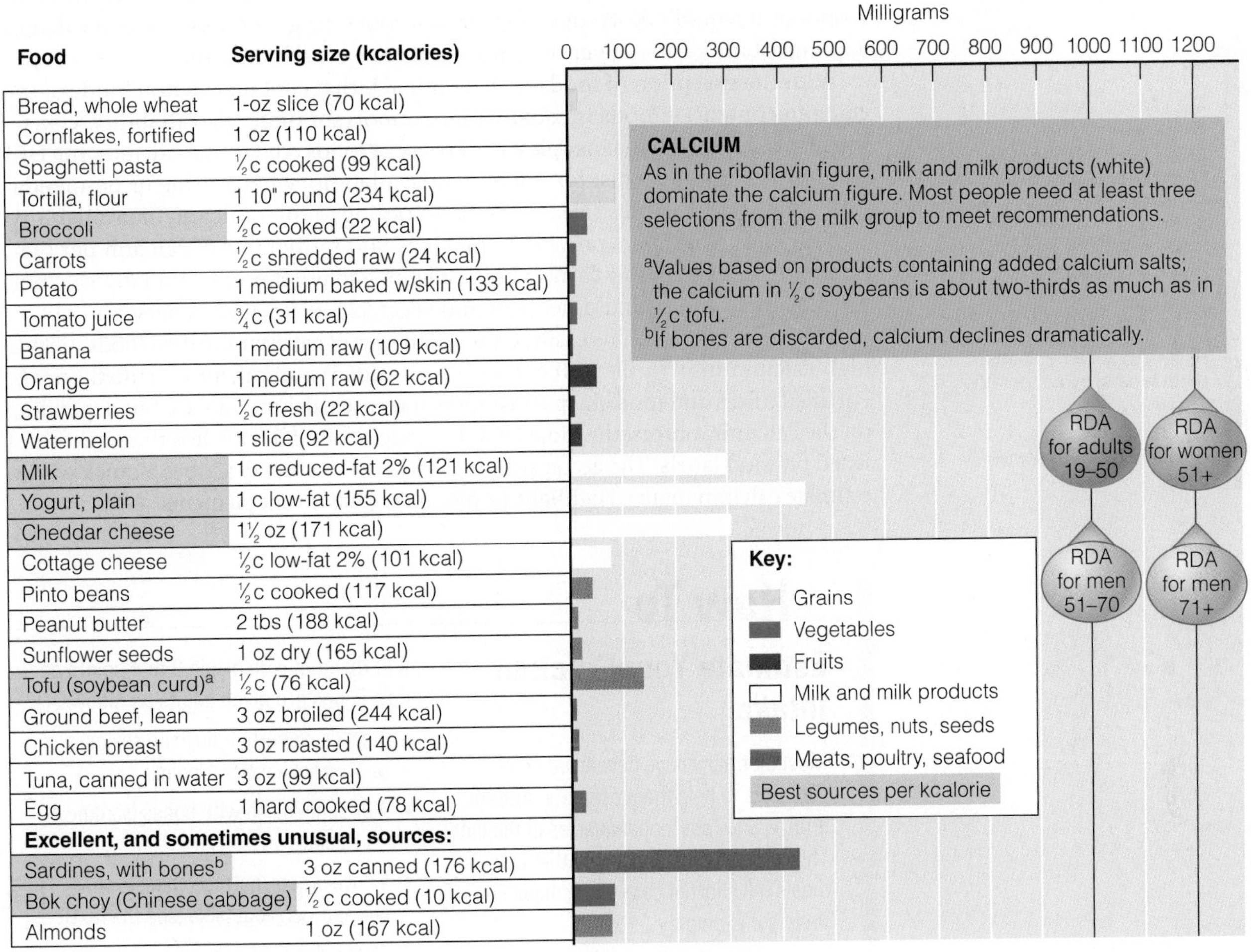

Food	Serving size (kcalories)
Bread, whole wheat	1-oz slice (70 kcal)
Cornflakes, fortified	1 oz (110 kcal)
Spaghetti pasta	½ c cooked (99 kcal)
Tortilla, flour	1 10" round (234 kcal)
Broccoli	½ c cooked (22 kcal)
Carrots	½ c shredded raw (24 kcal)
Potato	1 medium baked w/skin (133 kcal)
Tomato juice	¾ c (31 kcal)
Banana	1 medium raw (109 kcal)
Orange	1 medium raw (62 kcal)
Strawberries	½ c fresh (22 kcal)
Watermelon	1 slice (92 kcal)
Milk	1 c reduced-fat 2% (121 kcal)
Yogurt, plain	1 c low-fat (155 kcal)
Cheddar cheese	1½ oz (171 kcal)
Cottage cheese	½ c low-fat 2% (101 kcal)
Pinto beans	½ c cooked (117 kcal)
Peanut butter	2 tbs (188 kcal)
Sunflower seeds	1 oz dry (165 kcal)
Tofu (soybean curd)[a]	½ c (76 kcal)
Ground beef, lean	3 oz broiled (244 kcal)
Chicken breast	3 oz roasted (140 kcal)
Tuna, canned in water	3 oz (99 kcal)
Egg	1 hard cooked (78 kcal)
Excellent, and sometimes unusual, sources:	
Sardines, with bones[b]	3 oz canned (176 kcal)
Bok choy (Chinese cabbage)	½ c cooked (10 kcal)
Almonds	1 oz (167 kcal)

Milligrams: 0 100 200 300 400 500 600 700 800 900 1000 1100 1200

CALCIUM
As in the riboflavin figure, milk and milk products (white) dominate the calcium figure. Most people need at least three selections from the milk group to meet recommendations.

[a]Values based on products containing added calcium salts; the calcium in ½ c soybeans is about two-thirds as much as in ½ c tofu.
[b]If bones are discarded, calcium declines dramatically.

RDA for adults 19–50; RDA for women 51+; RDA for men 51–70; RDA for men 71+

Key: Grains; Vegetables; Fruits; Milk and milk products; Legumes, nuts, seeds; Meats, poultry, seafood; Best sources per kcalorie

It is especially difficult for children who don't drink milk to meet their calcium needs. The consequences of drinking too little milk during childhood and adolescence persist into adulthood. Women who seldom drank milk as children have lower bone density and greater risk of fractures than those who drank milk regularly. It is possible for people who do not drink milk to obtain adequate calcium, but only if they carefully select other calcium-rich foods.

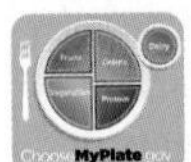

> **DIETARY GUIDELINES FOR AMERICANS**
Choose foods that provide more calcium, a nutrient of concern in American diets. The best sources of calcium are milk and milk products.

Many people, for a variety of reasons, cannot or do not drink milk. Some cultures do not use milk in their cuisines; some vegetarians exclude milk as well as meat; and some people are allergic to milk protein or are lactose intolerant. Others simply do not enjoy the taste of milk. These people need to find other foods to help meet their calcium needs. Some brands of tofu, corn tortillas, some nuts (such as almonds), and some seeds (such as sesame seeds) can supply calcium for the person who doesn't use milk products. A slice of most breads contains only about 5 to 10 percent of the calcium found in milk, but it can be a major source for people who eat many slices because the calcium is well absorbed. Oysters are also a rich source of calcium, as are small fish eaten with their bones, such as canned sardines.

Among the vegetables, mustard and turnip greens, bok choy, kale, parsley, watercress, and broccoli are good sources of available calcium. So are some seaweeds such as the nori popular in Japanese cooking. Some dark green, leafy

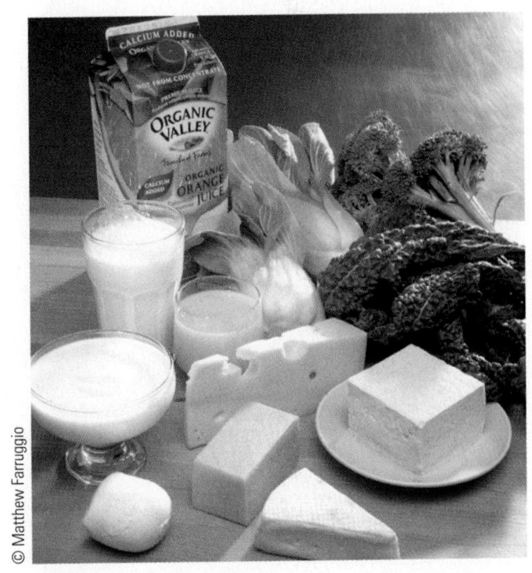

Milk and milk products are well known for their calcium, but calcium-set tofu, bok choy, kale, calcium-fortified orange juice, and broccoli are also rich in calcium.

> FIGURE 12-15 Bioavailability of Calcium from Selected Foods

≥50% absorbed	Cauliflower, watercress, cabbage, brussels sprouts, rutabaga, kale, mustard greens, bok choy, broccoli, turnip greens
≈30% absorbed	Milk, calcium-fortified soy milk, calcium-set tofu, cheese, yogurt, calcium-fortified foods and beverages
≈20% absorbed	Almonds, sesame seeds, pinto beans, sweet potatoes
≤5% absorbed	Spinach, rhubarb, Swiss chard

vegetables—notably spinach and Swiss chard—appear to be calcium-rich but actually provide little, if any, calcium because they contain binders that limit absorption. It would take 8 cups of spinach—containing six times as much calcium as 1 cup of milk—to deliver the equivalent in *absorbable* calcium.

With the exception of foods such as spinach that contain calcium binders, the calcium content of foods is usually more important than bioavailability. Consequently, recognizing that people eat a variety of foods containing calcium, the DRI Committee did not adjust for calcium bioavailability when setting recommendations. Figure 12-15 ranks selected foods according to their calcium bioavailability.

Some mineral waters provide as much as 500 milligrams of calcium per liter, offering a convenient way to meet both calcium and water needs. Similarly, calcium-fortified orange juice and other fruit and vegetable juices allow a person to obtain both calcium and vitamins easily. Other examples of calcium-fortified foods include high-calcium milk (milk with extra calcium added) and calcium-fortified cereals. Fortified juices and foods help consumers increase calcium intakes, but depending on the calcium sources, the bioavailability may be significantly less than quantities listed on food labels. The accompanying "How To" feature describes a quick way to estimate calcium intake. Highlight 12 discusses calcium supplements.

>How To

Estimate Your Calcium Intake

Most dietitians have developed useful shortcuts to help them estimate nutrient intakes and "see" inadequacies in the diet. They can tell at a glance whether a day's meals fall short of calcium recommendations, for example.

To estimate calcium intakes, keep two bits of information in mind:

- A cup of milk provides about 300 milligrams of calcium.
- Adults need between 1000 and 1200 milligrams of calcium per day, which represents 3 to 4 cups of milk—or the equivalent:

$$1000 \text{ mg} \div 300 \text{ mg/c} = 3\tfrac{1}{3} \text{ c}$$
$$1200 \text{ mg} \div 300 \text{ mg/c} = 4 \text{ c}$$

If a person drinks 3 to 4 cups of milk a day, it's easy to see that calcium needs are being met. If not, it takes some detective work to identify the other sources and estimate total calcium intake.

To estimate a person's daily calcium intake, use this shortcut, which compares the calcium in calcium-rich foods to the calcium content of milk. The calcium in a cup of milk is assigned 1 point, and the goal is to attain 3 to 4 points per day. Foods are given points as follows:

- 1 c milk, yogurt, or fortified soy milk or 1½ oz cheese = 1 point
- 4 oz canned fish with bones (sardines) = 1 point
- 1 c ice cream, cottage cheese, or calcium-rich vegetable (see the text) = ½ point

Then, because other foods also contribute small amounts of calcium, together they are given a point.

- Well-balanced diet containing a variety of foods = 1 point

Now consider a day's meals with calcium in mind. Cereal with 1 cup of milk for breakfast (1 point for milk), a ham and cheese sub sandwich for lunch (1 point for cheese), and a cup of broccoli and lasagna for dinner (½ point for calcium-rich vegetable and 1 point for cheese in lasagna)—plus 1 point for all other foods eaten that day—adds up to 4½ points. This shortcut estimate indicates that calcium recommendations have been met, and a diet analysis of these few foods reveals a calcium intake of more than 1000 milligrams. By knowing the best sources of each nutrient, you can learn to scan the day's meals and quickly see if you are meeting your daily goals.

> TRY IT Compare the calcium contents of ½ cup of the following foods: almonds, broccoli, and yogurt.

> FIGURE 12-16 **Phases of Bone Development throughout Life**

The active growth phase occurs from birth to approximately age 20. The phase of peak bone mass development occurs between the ages of 12 and 30. The final phase, when bone resorption exceeds formation, begins between the ages of 30 and 40 and continues through the remainder of life.

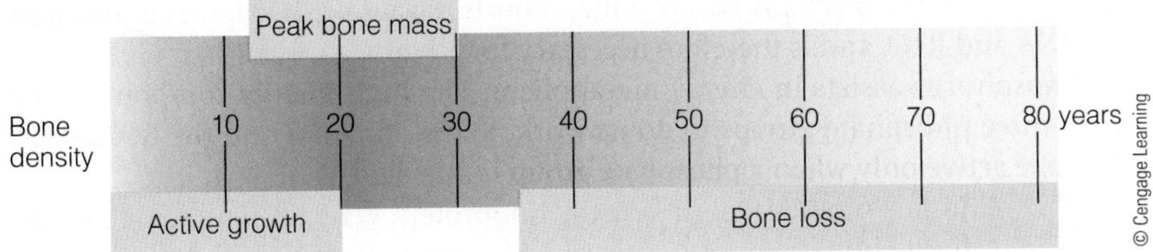

A generalization that has been gaining strength throughout this book is supported by the information given here about calcium. A balanced diet that supplies a variety of foods is the best plan to ensure adequacy for all essential nutrients. All food groups should be included, and none should be overemphasized. In our culture, calcium intake is usually inadequate wherever milk is lacking in the diet. By contrast, iron is usually lacking whenever milk is overemphasized, as Chapter 13 explains.

Calcium Deficiency A low calcium intake during the growing years limits the bones' ability to reach their peak bone mass. Most people achieve a peak bone mass by their late 20s, and dense bones best protect against age-related bone loss and fractures (see Figure 12-16). All adults lose bone as they grow older, beginning between the ages of 30 and 40. When bone losses reach the point of causing fractures under common, everyday stresses, the condition is known as **osteoporosis.** Osteoporosis and low bone mass (osteopenia) affect an estimated 52 million people in the United States, mostly older women.[33]

Unlike many diseases that make themselves known through symptoms such as pain, shortness of breath, skin lesions, tiredness, and the like, osteoporosis is silent. The body sends no signals saying bones are losing their calcium and, as a result, their integrity. Blood samples offer no clues because blood calcium remains normal regardless of bone content, and measures of bone density are not routinely taken until later in life. Highlight 12 suggests strategies to protect against bone loss, of which eating calcium-rich foods is only one.

› REVIEW IT

Most of the body's calcium is in the bones, where it provides a rigid structure and a reservoir of calcium for the blood. Blood calcium participates in muscle contraction, blood clotting, and nerve impulses, and it is closely regulated by a system of hormones and vitamin D. Calcium is found predominantly in milk and milk products. Even when calcium intake is inadequate, blood calcium remains normal, but at the expense of bone loss, which can lead to osteoporosis. The accompanying table provides a summary of calcium.

Calcium

RDA

Adults: 1000 mg/day (adults, 19–50 yr)
1000 mg/day (men, 51–70 yr)
1200 mg/day (men, ≥71 yr)
1200 mg/day (women, ≥51 yr)

UL

Adults: 2500 mg/day (adults, 19–50 yr)
2000 mg/day (adults, ≥51 yr)

Chief Functions in the Body

Mineralization of bones and teeth; also involved in muscle contraction and relaxation, nerve functioning, blood clotting, blood pressure

Deficiency Symptoms

Stunted growth in children; bone loss (osteoporosis) in adults

Toxicity Symptoms

Constipation; increased risk of urinary stone formation and kidney dysfunction; interference with absorption of other minerals

Significant Sources

Milk and milk products, small fish (with bones), calcium-set tofu (bean curd), greens (bok choy, broccoli, chard, kale), legumes

osteoporosis (OS-tee-oh-pore-OH-sis): a disease in which the bones become porous and fragile due to a loss of minerals; also called *adult bone loss.*

- **osteo** = bone
- **porosis** = porous

Phosphorus Phosphorus is the second most abundant mineral in the body. About 85 percent of it is found combined with calcium in the hydroxyapatite crystals of bones and teeth.

Phosphorus Roles in the Body Phosphorus is found not only in bones and teeth, but also in all body cells as part of a major buffer system. Phosphorus is also part of DNA and RNA and is therefore necessary for all growth.

Phosphorus assists in energy metabolism. The high-energy compound ATP uses three phosphate groups to do its work. Many enzymes and the B vitamins become active only when a phosphate group is attached.

Phospholipids provide stability to the lipoprotein vehicles that help to transport lipids in the blood. Phospholipids are also the major structural components of cell membranes, where they control the transport of nutrients into and out of the cells. Some proteins, such as the casein in milk, contain phosphorus as part of their structures (phosphoproteins).

Phosphorus Recommendations and Intakes Because phosphorus is commonly found in almost all foods, dietary deficiencies are unlikely. As Figure 12-17 shows, foods rich in proteins—such as meat, poultry, fish, milk, and cheese—are the best sources of phosphorus. Many processed foods and soft drinks contain phosphate-based additives, and phosphorus intakes in the United States have increased as consumption of these processed foods and beverages has increased.

Phosphate toxicity is rare and usually reflects a significant problem such as kidney failure.[34] Still, phosphorus intakes can be excessive, creating disruptions in normal hormonal functions that contribute to kidney failure, heart disease,

phosphorus: a major mineral found mostly in the body's bones and teeth.

> FIGURE 12-17 **Phosphorus in Selected Foods**

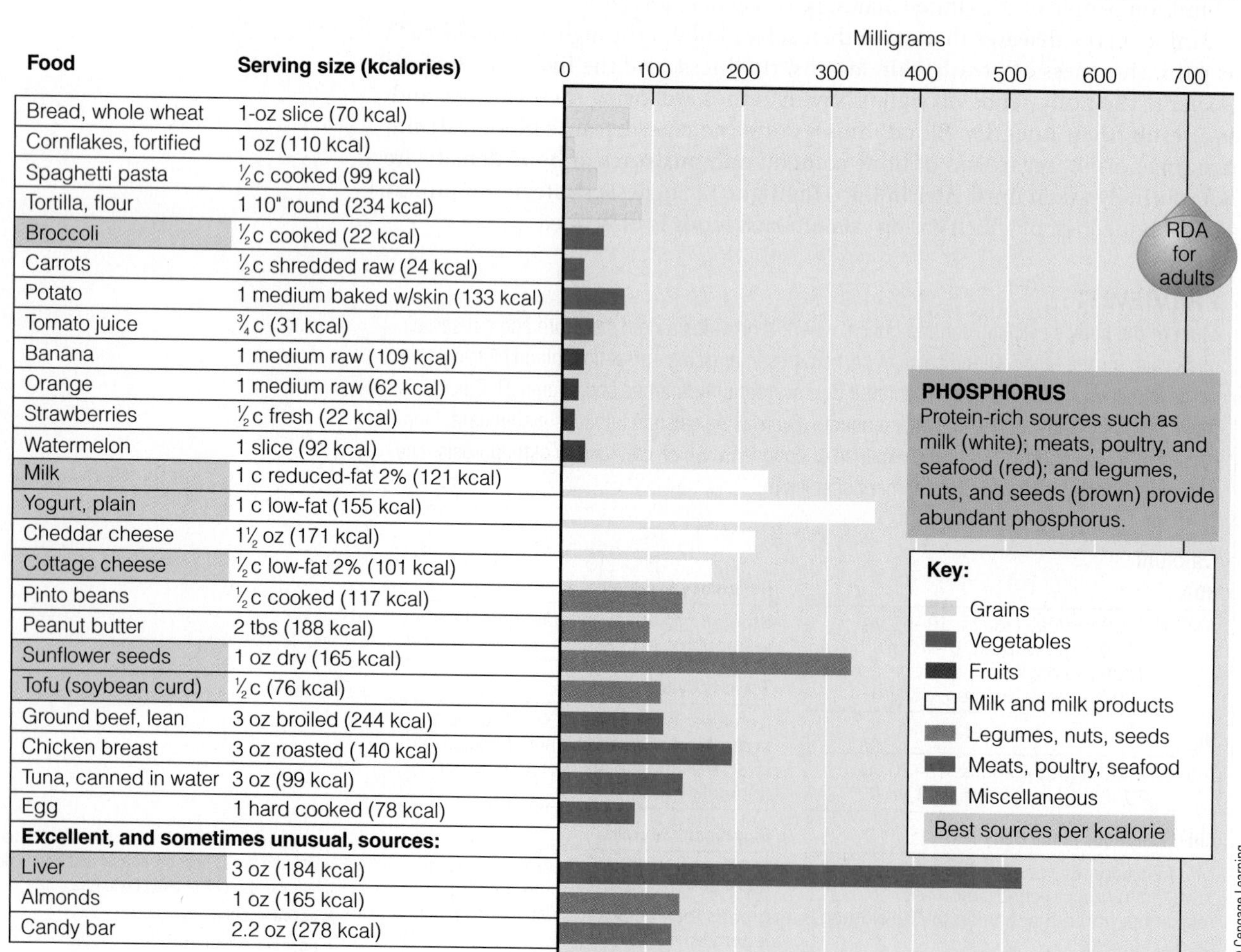

and bone loss.[35] High intakes of phosphorus are not common when diets are based mostly on fresh foods, but can become excessive when processed foods take center stage. A UL of 4000 milligrams has been established.

› REVIEW IT

Phosphorus accompanies calcium both in the crystals of bone and in many foods such as milk. Phosphorus is also important in energy metabolism as part of ATP, in lipid structures as part of phospholipids, and in genetic materials as part of DNA and RNA. The accompanying table provides a summary of phosphorus.

Phosphorus

RDA	Deficiency Symptoms
Adults: 700 mg/day	Muscular weakness, bone pain[a]
UL	**Toxicity Symptoms**
Adults (19–70 yr): 4000 mg/day	Calcification of nonskeletal tissues, particularly the kidneys
Chief Functions in the Body	**Significant Sources**
Mineralization of bones and teeth; part of every cell; important in genetic material, part of phospholipids, used in energy transfer and in buffer systems that maintain acid-base balance	Foods derived from animals (meat, fish, poultry, eggs, milk)

[a]Dietary deficiency rarely occurs, but some drugs can bind with phosphorus making it unavailable and resulting in bone loss that is characterized by weakness and pain.

Magnesium

Only about 1 ounce of **magnesium** is present in the body of a 132-pound person (review Figure 12-9, p. 381). More than half of the body's magnesium is in the bones. Much of the rest is in the muscles and soft tissues, with only 1 percent in the extracellular fluid. As with calcium, bone magnesium may serve as a reservoir to ensure normal blood concentrations.

Magnesium Roles in the Body In addition to maintaining bone health, magnesium acts in all the cells of the soft tissues, where it forms part of the protein-making machinery and is necessary for energy metabolism. It participates in hundreds of enzyme systems. A major role of magnesium is as a catalyst in the reaction that adds the last phosphate to the high-energy compound ATP, making it essential to the body's use of glucose; the synthesis of protein, fat, and nucleic acids; and the cells' membrane transport systems. Together with calcium, magnesium is involved in muscle contraction and blood clotting: calcium promotes the processes, whereas magnesium inhibits them. This dynamic interaction between the two minerals helps regulate blood pressure and lung function. Like many other nutrients, magnesium supports the normal functioning of the immune system.

Magnesium Intakes The brown bars in Figure 12-18 (p. 396) indicate that legumes, nuts, and seeds make significant magnesium contributions. Magnesium is part of the chlorophyll molecule, so dark green, leafy vegetables are also good sources. In areas with hard water, the water contributes both calcium and magnesium to daily intakes. Mineral waters noted earlier for their calcium content may also be magnesium-rich and can be important sources of this mineral for those who drink them. Bioavailability of magnesium from mineral water is about 50 percent, but it improves when the water is consumed with a meal.

Magnesium Deficiency Average magnesium intakes typically fall below recommendations, which may exacerbate inflammation and contribute to chronic diseases such as heart disease, stroke, hypertension, diabetes, and cancer.[36] A severe magnesium deficiency causes a tetany similar to the calcium tetany described earlier. Magnesium deficiencies also impair central nervous system activity and may be responsible for the hallucinations experienced during alcohol withdrawal.

Magnesium and Hypertension Magnesium is critical to heart function and seems to protect against hypertension and heart disease.[37] Interestingly, people living in

magnesium: a cation within the body's cells, active in many enzyme systems.

> **FIGURE 12-18 Magnesium in Selected Foods**

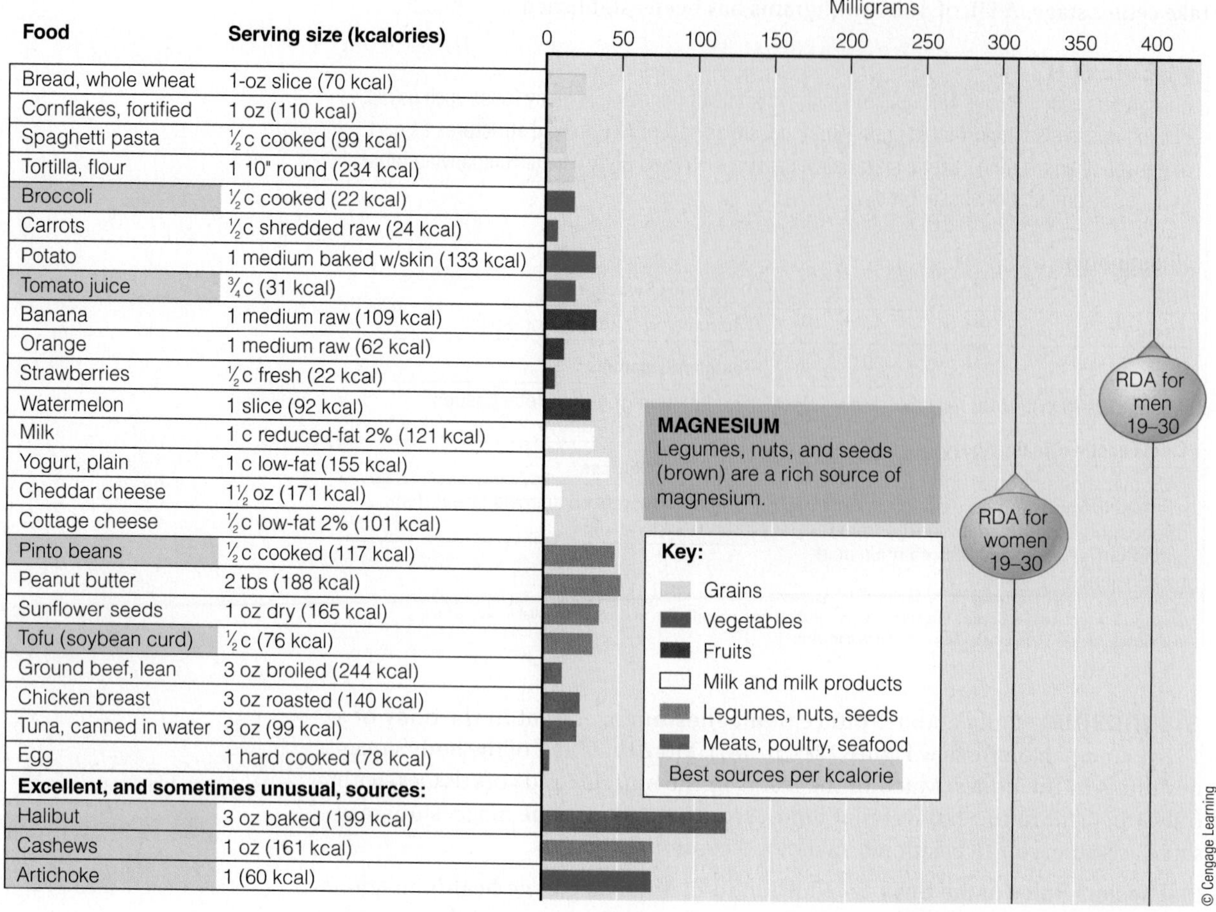

areas of the country with hard water, which contains high concentrations of calcium and magnesium, tend to have low rates of heart disease. With magnesium deficiency, the walls of the arteries and capillaries tend to constrict—a possible explanation for the hypertensive effect.

Magnesium Toxicity Magnesium toxicity is rare, but it can be fatal. The UL for magnesium applies only to nonfood sources such as supplements or magnesium salts.

› REVIEW IT

Like calcium and phosphorus, magnesium supports bone mineralization. Magnesium is also involved in numerous enzyme systems and in heart function. It is found abundantly in legumes and dark green, leafy vegetables and, in some areas, in water. The accompanying table offers a summary of magnesium.

Magnesium

RDA	**Deficiency Symptoms**
Men (19–30 yr): 400 mg/day Women (19–30 yr): 310 mg/day	Weakness; confusion; if extreme, convulsions, bizarre muscle movements (especially of eye and face muscles), hallucinations, and difficulty in swallowing; in children, growth failure[a]
UL	
Adults: 350 mg nonfood magnesium/day	
	Toxicity Symptoms
Chief Functions in the Body	From nonfood sources only; diarrhea, alkalosis, dehydration
Bone mineralization, building of protein, enzyme action, normal muscle contraction, nerve impulse transmission, maintenance of teeth, and functioning of immune system	**Significant Sources** Nuts, legumes, whole grains, dark green vegetables, seafood, chocolate, cocoa

[a]A still more severe deficiency causes tetany, an extreme, prolonged contraction of the muscles similar to that caused by low blood calcium.

Sulfate **Sulfate** is the oxidized form of the mineral **sulfur,** as it exists in foods and water. The body's need for sulfate is easily met by a variety of foods and beverages. In addition, the body receives sulfate from the amino acids methionine and cysteine, which are found in dietary proteins. These sulfur-containing amino acids help determine the contour of protein molecules. The sulfur-containing side chains in cysteine molecules can link to each other via disulfide bridges, which stabilize the protein structure. (See the drawing of insulin with its disulfide bridges in Figure 6-4 on p. 174.) Skin, hair, and nails contain some of the body's more rigid proteins, which have a high sulfur content.

Because the body's sulfate needs are easily met with normal protein intakes, there is no recommended intake for sulfate. Deficiencies do not occur when diets contain protein. Only when people lack protein to the point of severe deficiency will they lack the sulfur-containing amino acids.

sulfate: a salt produced from the oxidation of sulfur.

sulfur: a mineral present in the body as part of some proteins.

› REVIEW IT Identify the main roles, deficiency symptoms, and food sources for each of the major minerals (sodium, chloride, potassium, calcium, phosphorus, magnesium, and sulfate).

Like the other nutrients, minerals' actions are coordinated to get the body's work done. The major minerals, especially sodium, chloride, and potassium, influence the body's fluid balance; whenever an anion moves, a cation moves—always maintaining homeostasis. Sodium, chloride, potassium, calcium, and magnesium are key members of the team of nutrients that direct nerve impulse transmission and muscle contraction. They are also the primary nutrients involved in regulating blood pressure. Phosphorus and magnesium participate in many reactions involving glucose, fatty acids, amino acids, and the vitamins. Calcium, phosphorus, and magnesium combine to form the structure of the bones and teeth. Each major mineral also plays other specific roles in the body. The table provides a summary of the major minerals.

› REVIEW IT The Major Minerals

Chief Functions	Deficiency Symptoms	Toxicity Symptoms	Significant Sources
Sodium Maintains normal fluid and electrolyte balance; assists in nerve impulse transmission and muscle contraction	Muscle cramps, mental apathy, loss of appetite	Edema, acute hypertension	Table salt, soy sauce; moderate amounts in meats, milks, breads, and vegetables; large amounts in processed foods
Chloride Maintains normal fluid and electrolyte balance; part of hydrochloric acid found in the stomach, necessary for proper digestion	Do not occur under normal circumstances	Vomiting	Table salt, soy sauce; moderate amounts in meats, milks, eggs; large amounts in processed foods
Potassium Maintains normal fluid and electrolyte balance; facilitates many reactions; supports cell integrity; assists in nerve impulse transmission and muscle contractions	Irregular heartbeat, muscular weakness, glucose intolerance	Muscular weakness; vomiting; if injected into a vein, can stop the heart	All whole foods; meats, milks, fruits, vegetables, grains, legumes
Calcium Mineralization of bones and teeth; also involved in muscle contraction and relaxation, nerve functioning, blood clotting, and blood pressure	Stunted growth in children; bone loss (osteoporosis) in adults	Constipation; increased risk of urinary stone formation and kidney dysfunction; interference with absorption of other minerals	Milk and milk products, small fish (with bones), tofu, greens (bok choy, broccoli, chard), legumes
Phosphorus Mineralization of bones and teeth; part of every cell; important in genetic material, part of phospholipids, used in energy transfer and in buffer systems that maintain acid-base balance	Muscular weakness, bone pain[a]	Calcification of nonskeletal tissues, particularly the kidneys	All animal tissues (meat, fish, poultry, eggs, milk)
Magnesium Bone mineralization, building of protein, enzyme action, normal muscle contraction, nerve impulse transmission, maintenance of teeth, and functioning of immune system	Weakness; confusion; if extreme, convulsions, bizarre muscle movements (especially of eye and face muscles), hallucinations, and difficulty in swallowing; in children, growth failure[b]	From nonfood sources only; diarrhea, alkalosis, dehydration	Nuts, legumes, whole grains, dark green vegetables, seafood, chocolate, cocoa
Sulfate As part of proteins, stabilizes their shape by forming disulfide bridges; part of the vitamins biotin and thiamin and the hormone insulin	None known; protein deficiency would occur first	Toxicity would occur only if sulfur-containing amino acids were eaten in excess; this (in animals) suppresses growth	All protein-containing foods (meats, fish, poultry, eggs, milk, legumes, nuts)

[a]Dietary deficiency rarely occurs, but some drugs can bind with phosphorus, making it unavailable and resulting in bone loss that is characterized by weakness and pain.

[b]A still more severe deficiency causes tetany, an extreme, prolonged contraction of the muscles similar to that caused by low blood calcium.

With all of the tasks these minerals perform, they are of great importance to life. Consuming enough of each of them every day is easy, given a variety of foods from each of the food groups. Whole-grain breads supply magnesium; fruits, vegetables, and legumes provide magnesium and potassium too; milk products offer calcium and phosphorus; meats, poultry, and seafood offer phosphorus and sulfate as well; all foods provide sodium and chloride, with excesses being more problematic than inadequacies. The message is quite simple and has been repeated throughout this text: for an adequate intake of all the nutrients, including the major minerals, choose a variety of foods from each of the five food groups. And drink plenty of water.

Nutrition Portfolio

Many people may miss the mark when it comes to drinking enough water to keep their bodies well hydrated or obtaining enough calcium to promote strong bones; in contrast, sodium intakes often exceed those recommended for health. Go to Diet & Wellness Plus and choose one of the days on which you tracked your diet for an entire day. Select the Intake vs. Goals report and then consider the following questions.

- Did you exceed, fail to meet, or meet your goal for water intake? Was that a typical day for you? Describe your strategy for ensuring that you drink plenty of water—about eight glasses—every day.
- Take a look at your sodium intake in this report. Most people in the United States exceed the UL. Did you? Explain the importance of selecting and preparing foods with less salt.
- How was your intake of calcium for that day? If you are not getting enough calcium, consult Chapter 12 for ideas to help you get more, then list at least three foods or beverages you would be willing to eat or drink that would improve your intake.

DIET & WELLNESS **PLUS** To complete this exercise, go to your Diet & Wellness Plus at **www.cengagebrain.com.**

› STUDY IT To review the key points of this chapter and take a practice quiz, go to the study cards at the end of the book.

REFERENCES

1. R. S. Sebastian, C. W. Enns, and J. D. Goldman, Drinking water intake in the U.S., *What We Eat in America, NHANES 2005–2008*, September 2011.
2. W. F. Clark and coauthors, "Drink at least 8 glasses of water a day to be healthy???", *Nutrition Today* 48 (2013): S18–S21; G. F. M. Strippoli, Fluids, water, and nutrients and the risk of renal diseases, *Nutrition Today* 47 (2012): S17–S21; M. D. Sorensen and coauthors, Impact of nutritional factors on incident kidney stone formation: A report from the WHI OS, *Journal of Urology* 187 (2012): 1645–1649.
3. A. B. Goodman and coauthors, Behaviors and attitudes associated with low drinking water intake among US adults, food attitudes and behaviors survey, 2007, *Preventing Chronic Disease* 10 (2013): 120248.
4. B. M. Popkin, K. E. D'Anci, and I. H. Rosenberg, Water, hydration, and health, *Nutrition Reviews* 68 (2010): 439–458.
5. Centers for Disease Control and Prevention, http://www.cdc.gov/nceh/lead/tips/water.htm, updated October 15, 2013.
6. M. J. O'Donnell and coauthors, Urinary sodium and potassium excretion and risk of cardiovascular events, *Journal of the American Medical Association* 306 (2011): 2229–2238.
7. T. A. Kotchen, A. W. Cowley, and E. D. Frohlich, Salt in health and disease—A delicate balance, *New England Journal of Medicine* 368 (2013): 1229–1237.
8. A. Carriquiry and coauthors, Trends in the prevalence of excess dietary sodium intake—United States, 2003–2010, *Morbidity and Mortality Weekly Report* 62 (2013): 1021–1025.
9. K. M. Dickinson, P. M. Clifton, and J. B. Keogh, Endothelial function is impaired after a high-salt meal in healthy subjects, *American Journal of Clinical Nutrition* 93 (2011): 500–505.
10. S. C. Eufinger and coauthors, Habitual dietary sodium intake is inversely associated with coronary flow reserve in middle-aged male twins, *American Journal of Clinical Nutrition* 95 (2012): 572–579; J. P. Forman and coauthors, Association between sodium intake and change in uric acid, urine albumin excretion, and the risk of developing hypertension, *Circulation* 125 (2012): 3108–3116.
11. US Department of Agriculture and US Department of Health and Human Services, *Dietary Guidelines for Americans, 2010*, www.dietaryguidelines.gov.

12. P. K. Whelton and coauthors, Sodium, blood pressure, and cardiovascular disease: Further evidence supporting the American Heart Association sodium reduction recommendations, *Circulation* 126 (2012): 2880–2889; L. J. Appel and coauthors, The importance of population-wide sodium reduction as a means to prevent cardiovascular disease and stroke: A call to action from the American Heart Association, *Circulation* 123 (2011): 1138–1143.
13. M. Maillot and A. Drewnowski, A conflict between nutritionally adequate diets and meeting the 2010 Dietary Guidelines for sodium, *American Journal of Preventive Medicine* 42 (2012): 174–179.
14. D. E. Epstein and coauthors, Determinants and consequences of adherence to the Dietary Approaches to Stop Hypertension Diet in African-American and white adults with high blood pressure: Results from the ENCORE Trial, *Journal of the Academy of Nutrition and Dietetics* 112 (2012): 1763–1773.
15. A. Sherzai and coauthors, Stroke, food groups, and dietary patterns: A systematic review, *Nutrition Reviews* 70 (2012): 423–435; T. T. Fung and coauthors, The Mediterranean and Dietary Approaches to Stop Hypertension (DASH) diets and colorectal cancer, *American Journal of Clinical Nutrition* 92 (2010): 1429–1435; S. T. Chen, N. M. Maruthur, and L. J. Appel, The effect of dietary patterns on estimated coronary heart risk: Results from the Dietary Approaches to Stop Hypertension (DASH) Trial, *Circulation: Cardiovascular Quality and Outcomes* 3 (2010): 484–489.
16. A. J. Moshfegh and coauthors, Vital signs: Food categories contributing the most to sodium consumption—United States, 2007–2008, *Morbidity and Mortality Weekly Report* 61 (2012): 92–98.
17. P. M Guenther, J. M. G. Lyon, and L. J. Appel, Modeling dietary patterns to assess sodium recommendations for nutrient adequacy, *American Journal of Clinical Nutrition* 97 (2013): 842–847.
18. J. P. Gunn and coauthors, CDC grand rounds: Dietary sodium reduction—Time for choice, *Morbidity and Mortality Weekly Report* 61 (2012): 89–91; Usual sodium intakes compared with current dietary guidelines—United States, 2005–2008, *Morbidity and Mortality Weekly Report* 60 (2011): 1413–1417; C. N. Mhurchu and coauthors, Sodium content of processed foods in the United Kingdom: Analysis of 44,000 foods purchased by 21,000 households, *American Journal of Clinical Nutrition* 93 (2011): 594–600; C.A.M. Anderson and coauthors, Dietary sources of sodium in China, Japan, the United Kingdom, and the United States, women and men aged 40 to 59 years: The INTERMAP Study, *Journal of the American Dietetic Association* 110 (2010): 736–745; J. L. Webster, E. K. Dunford, and B. C. Neal, *American Journal of Clinical Nutrition* 91 (2010): 413–420.
19. J. L. H. C. Busch, F. Y. S. Yong, and S. J. Goh, Sodium reduction: Optimizing product composition and structure towards increasing saltiness perception, *Trends in Food Science and Technology* 29 (2013): 21–34.
20. K. Bibbins-Domingo and coauthors, Projected effect of dietary salt reductions on future cardiovascular disease, *New England Journal of Medicine* 362 (2010): 590–599; Institute of Medicine (US) Committee on Strategies to Reduce Sodium Intake, *Strategies to Reduce Sodium Intake in the United States* (Washington, D.C.: National Academies Press, 2010).
21. Q. Yang and coauthors, Sodium and potassium intake and mortality among US adults: Prospective data from the third National Health and Nutrition Examination Survey, *Archives of Internal Medicine* 171 (2011): 1183–1191.
22. M. E. Cogswell and coauthors, Sodium and potassium intakes among US adults: NHANES 2003–2008, *American Journal of Clinical Nutrition* 96 (2012): 647–657.
23. M. J. O'Donnell and coauthors, Urinary sodium and potassium excretion and risk of cardiovascular events, *Journal of the American Medical Association* 306 (2011): 2229–2238; M. C. Houston, The importance of potassium in managing hypertension, *Current Hypertension Reports* 13 (2011): 309–317.
24. J. Kaluza and coauthors, Dietary calcium and magnesium intake and mortality: A prospective study of men, *American Journal of Epidemiology* 171 (2010): 801–807; I. R. Reid and coauthors, Effects of calcium supplementation on lipids, blood pressure, and body composition in healthy older men: A randomized controlled trial, *American Journal of Clinical Nutrition* 91 (2010): 131–139.
25. J. L. Rosenblum and coauthors, Calcium and vitamin D supplementation is associated with decreased abdominal visceral adipose tissue in overweight and obese adults, *American Journal of Clinical Nutrition* 95 (2012): 101–108; D. R. Shahar and coauthors, Dairy calcium intake, serum vitamin D, and successful weight loss, *American Journal of Clinical Nutrition* 92 (2010): 1017–1022.
26. I. P. Onakpoya and coauthors, Efficacy of calcium supplementation for management of overweight and obesity: Systematic review of randomized clinical trials, *Nutrition Reviews* 69 (2011): 335–343; M. J. Soares, W. C. S. Ping-Delfos, and M. H. Ghanbari, Calcium and vitamin D for obesity: A review of randomized clinical trials, *European Journal of Clinical Nutrition* 65 (2011): 994–1004.
27. R. P. Heaney, Calcium and obesity: Effect size and clinical relevance, *Nutrition Reviews* 69 (2011): 333–334.
28. M. B. Zemel and coauthors, Effects of dairy compared with soy on oxidative and inflammatory stress in overweight and obese subjects, *American Journal of Clinical Nutrition* 91 (2010): 16–22.
29. M. Chen and coauthors, Effects of dairy intake on body weight and fat: A meta-analysis of randomized controlled trials, *American Journal of Clinical Nutrition* 96 (2012): 735–747.
30. R. L. Bailey and coauthors, Estimation of total usual calcium and vitamin D intakes in the United States, *Journal of Nutrition* 140 (2010): 817–822.
31. J. Calvez and coauthors, Protein intake, calcium balance and health consequences, *European Journal of Clinical Nutrition* 66 (2012): 281–295.
32. S. A. Abrams, Setting Dietary Reference Intakes with the use of bioavailability data: Calcium, *American Journal of Clinical Nutrition* 91 (2010): 1474S–1477S.
33. National Osteoporosis Foundation, www.nof.org, accessed January 2014.
34. M. S. Razzaque, Phosphate toxicity: New insights into an old problem, *Clinical Science* 120 (2011): 91–97.
35. M. S. Calvo and J. Uribarri, Public health impact of dietary phosphorus excess on bone and cardiovascular health in the general population, *American Journal of Clinical Nutrition* 98 (2013): 6–15; E. Takeda and coauthors, Dietary phosphorus in bone health and quality of life, *Nutrition Reviews* 70 (2012): 311–321.
36. M. M. Joosten and coauthors, Urinary and plasma magnesium and risk of ischemic heart disease, *American Journal of Clinical Nutrition* 97 (2013): 1299–1306; L. C. Del Gobbo and coauthors, Circulating and dietary magnesium and risk of cardiovascular disease: A systematic review and meta-analysis of prospective studies, *American Journal of Clinical Nutrition* 98 (2013): 160–173; W. B. Weglicki, Hypomagnesemia and inflammation: Clinical and basic aspects, *Annual Review of Nutrition* 32 (2012) 55–71; J. Sugimoto and coauthors, Magnesium decreases inflammatory cytokine production: A novel innate immunomodulatory mechanism, *Journal of Immunology* 188 (2012): 6338–6346; A. Rosanoff, C. M. Weaver, and R. K. Rude, Suboptimal magnesium status in the United States: Are the health consequences underestimated? *Nutrition Reviews* 70 (2012): 153–164; S. C. Larsson, N. Orsini, and A. Wolk, Dietary magnesium intake and risk of stroke: A meta-analysis of prospective studies, *American Journal of Clinical Nutrition* 95 (2012): 362–366; S. E. Chiuve and coauthors, Plasma and dietary magnesium and risk of sudden cardiac death in women, *American Journal of Clinical Nutrition* 93 (2011): 253–260; M. Shechter, Magnesium and cardiovascular system, *Magnesium Research* 23 (2010): 60–72; F. H. Nielsen, Magnesium, inflammation, and obesity in chronic disease, *Nutrition Reviews* 68 (2010): 333–340.
37. L. Kass, J. Weekes, and L. Carpenter, Effect of magnesium supplementation on blood pressure: A meta-analysis, *European Journal of Clinical Nutrition* 66 (2012): 411–418.

HIGHLIGHT > 12

Osteoporosis and Calcium

› LEARN IT Describe factors that contribute to the development of osteoporosis and strategies to prevent it.

Osteoporosis becomes apparent during the later years, but it develops much earlier—and without warning. Few people are aware that their bones are being robbed of their strength. The problem often first becomes evident when someone's hip suddenly gives way. People say, "She fell and broke her hip," but in fact the hip may have been so fragile that it broke *before* she fell. Even bumping into a table may be enough to shatter a porous bone into fragments so numerous and scattered that they cannot be reassembled. Removing them and replacing them with an artificial joint requires major surgery. An estimated 258,000 people in the United States are hospitalized each year because of hip fractures related to osteoporosis. About one in five die of complications within a year; one in three will never walk or live independently again.[1] Their quality of life slips downward.

This highlight examines low bone density and osteoporosis, one of the most prevalent diseases of aging, affecting an estimated 52 million people in the United States—most of them women older than 50.[2] It reviews the many factors that contribute to the 2 million fractures in the bones of the hips, vertebrae, wrists, arms, and ankles each year. And it presents strategies to reduce the risks, paying special attention to the role of dietary calcium.

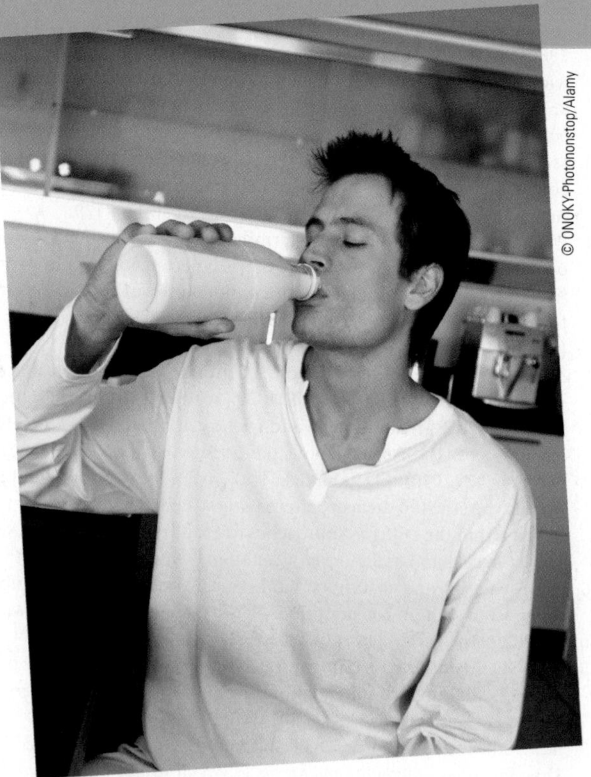
© ONOKY-Photononstop/Alamy

Bone Development and Disintegration

Bone has two compartments: the outer, hard shell of **cortical bone** and the inner, lacy matrix of **trabecular bone.** (The glossary defines these and other bone-related terms.) Both can lose minerals, but in different ways and at different rates. The first photograph in Figure H12-1 shows a human leg bone sliced lengthwise, exposing the lacy, calcium-containing crystals of trabecular bone. These crystals give up calcium to the blood when the diet runs short, and they take up calcium again when the supply is plentiful (review Figure 12-13 on p. 390). For people who have eaten calcium-rich foods throughout the bone-forming years of their youth, these deposits make bones dense and provide a rich reservoir of calcium.

Surrounding and protecting the trabecular bone is a dense, ivorylike exterior shell—the cortical bone. Cortical bone composes the shafts of the long bones, and a thin cortical shell caps the ends of the bones too. Both compartments confer strength on bone: cortical bone provides the sturdy outer wall, and trabecular bone provides support along the lines of stress.

The two types of bone handle calcium in different ways. Supplied with blood vessels and metabolically active, trabecular bone is sensitive to hormones that govern day-to-day deposits and withdrawals of calcium. It readily gives up minerals whenever blood calcium needs replenishing. Losses of trabecular bone start becoming significant for men and women in their 30s, although losses can occur whenever calcium withdrawals exceed deposits. Cortical bone also gives up calcium, but slowly and at a steady pace. Cortical bone losses typically begin at about age 40 and continue slowly but surely thereafter.

As bone loss continues, **bone density** declines, and osteoporosis becomes apparent (see Figure H12-1). Bones become so fragile that even the body's own weight can overburden the spine—vertebrae may suddenly disintegrate and crush down, painfully pinching major nerves. Or the vertebrae may compress into wedge shapes, forming what is

GLOSSARY

antacids: medications used to relieve indigestion by neutralizing acid in the stomach. Calcium-containing preparations (such as Tums) contain available calcium. Antacids with aluminum or magnesium hydroxides (such as Rolaids) can accelerate calcium losses.

bone density: a measure of bone strength. When minerals fill the bone matrix (making it dense), they give it strength.

bone meal or **powdered bone:** crushed or ground bone preparations intended to supply calcium to the diet. Calcium from bone is not well absorbed and is often contaminated with toxic minerals such as arsenic, mercury, lead, and cadmium.

cortical bone: the very dense bone tissue that forms the outer shell surrounding trabecular bone and comprises the shaft of a long bone.

dolomite: a compound of minerals (calcium magnesium carbonate) found in limestone and marble. Dolomite is powdered and is sold as a calcium-magnesium supplement. However, it may be contaminated with toxic minerals, is not well absorbed, and interferes with absorption of other essential minerals.

osteoporosis (OS-tee-oh-pore-OH-sis): a disease in which the bones become porous and fragile due to loss of minerals; also called *adult bone loss.*

oyster shell: a product made from the powdered shells of oysters that is sold as a calcium supplement, but it is not well absorbed by the digestive system.

trabecular (tra-BECK-you-lar) **bone:** the lacy inner structure of calcium crystals that supports the bone's structure and provides a calcium storage bank.

> **FIGURE H12-1 Healthy and Osteoporotic Trabecular Bones**

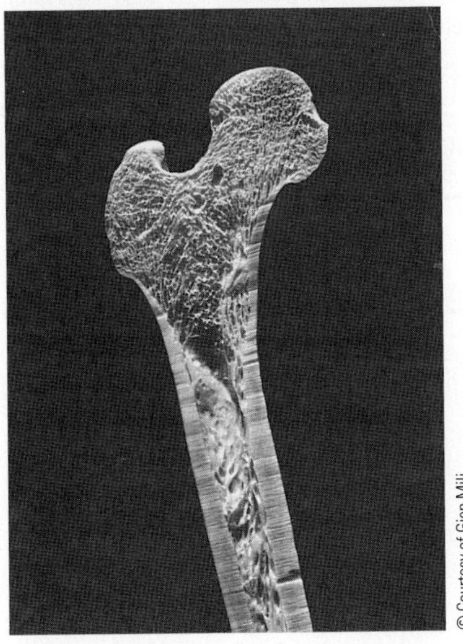

Trabecular bone is the lacy network of calcium-containing crystals that fills the interior. Cortical bone is the dense, ivorylike bone that forms the exterior shell.

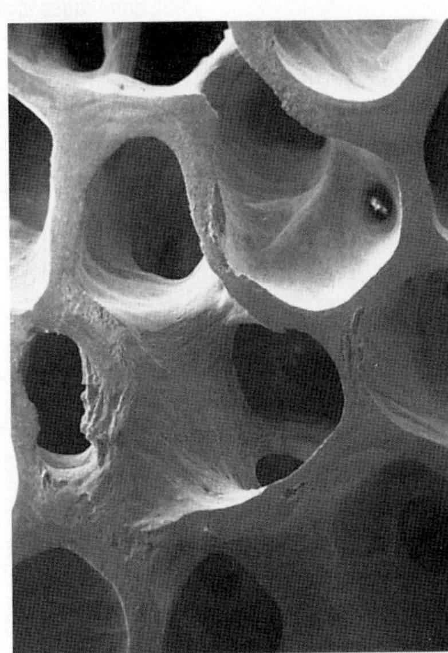

Electron micrograph of healthy trabecular bone.

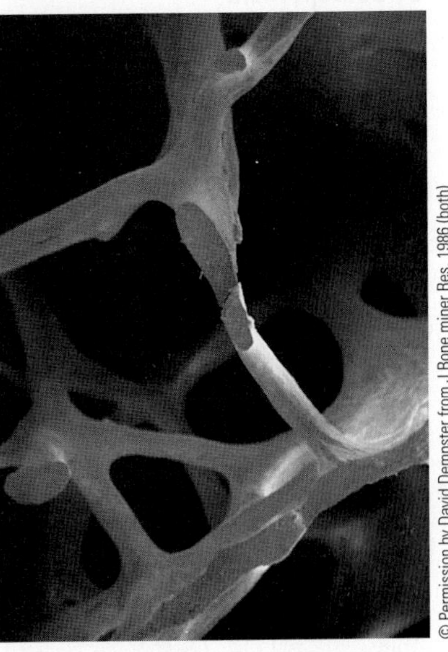

Electron micrograph of trabecular bone affected by osteoporosis.

often called a "dowager's hump," the posture many older people assume as they "grow shorter." Figure H12-2 (p. 402) shows the effect of compressed spinal bone on a woman's height and posture. Because both the cortical shell and the trabecular interior weaken, breaks most often occur in the hip, as mentioned in the introductory paragraph.

Physicians can determine bone loss and diagnose osteoporosis by measuring bone density using dual-energy X-ray absorptiometry (DEXA scan).[3] They also consider risk factors for osteoporosis, including age, personal and family history of fractures, and physical inactivity. Table H12-1 summarizes the major risk factors for osteoporosis. The more risk factors that apply to a person, the greater the chances of bone loss. Notice that several risk factors that are influential in the development of osteoporosis—such as age, gender, and genetics—cannot be changed. Other risk factors—such as diet, physical activity, body weight, smoking, and alcohol use—are personal behaviors that can be changed. By eating a calcium-rich, well-balanced diet; being physically active; abstaining from smoking; and drinking alcohol in moderation (if at all), people can defend themselves against osteoporosis. These decisions are particularly important for those with other risk factors that cannot be changed.

Whether a person develops osteoporosis seems to depend on the interactions of several factors, including nutrition. The strongest predictor of bone density is age.

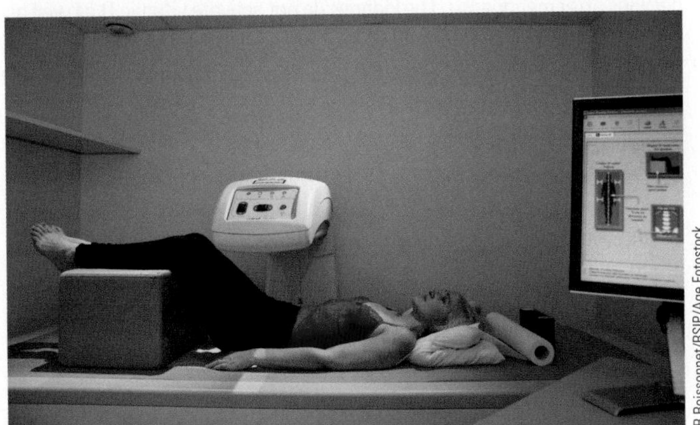

Using a DEXA (dual-energy X-ray absorpiometry) test to measure bone mineral density identifies osteoporosis, determines risks for fractures, and tracks responses to treatment.

TABLE H12-1 Risk Factors for Osteoporosis

Nonmodifiable	Modifiable
• Female gender	• Sedentary lifestyle
• Older age (>50 yr)	• Diet inadequate in calcium and vitamin D
• Small frame	• Diet excessive in protein, sodium, caffeine
• Caucasian, Asian, or Hispanic/Latino	• Cigarette smoking
• Family history of osteoporosis or fractures	• Alcohol abuse
• Personal history of fractures	• Low body weight
• Estrogen deficiency in women (amenorrhea or menopause, especially early or surgically induced); testosterone deficiency in men	• Certain medications, such as glucocorticoids, aluminum-containing antacids, and antiseizure drugs

> **FIGURE H12-2 Loss of Height in a Woman Caused by Osteoporosis**

The woman on the left is about 50 years old. On the right, she is 80 years old. Her legs have not grown shorter. Instead, her back has lost length due to collapse of her spinal bones (vertebrae). Collapsed vertebrae cannot protect the spinal nerves from pressure that causes excruciating pain.

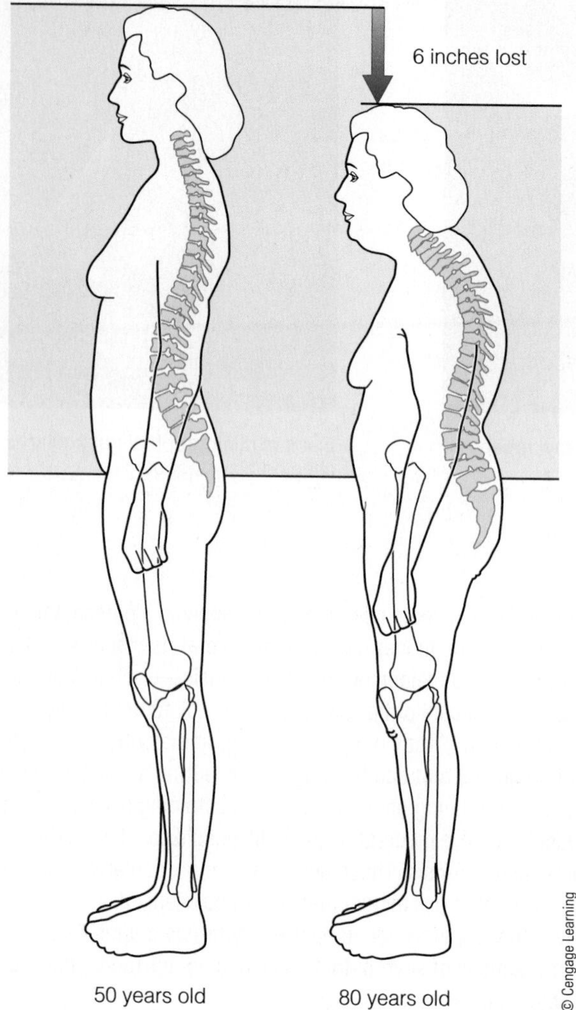

> **FIGURE H12-3 Bone Losses over Time Compared**

Peak bone mass is achieved by age 30. Women gradually lose bone mass until menopause, when losses accelerate dramatically and then gradually taper off.

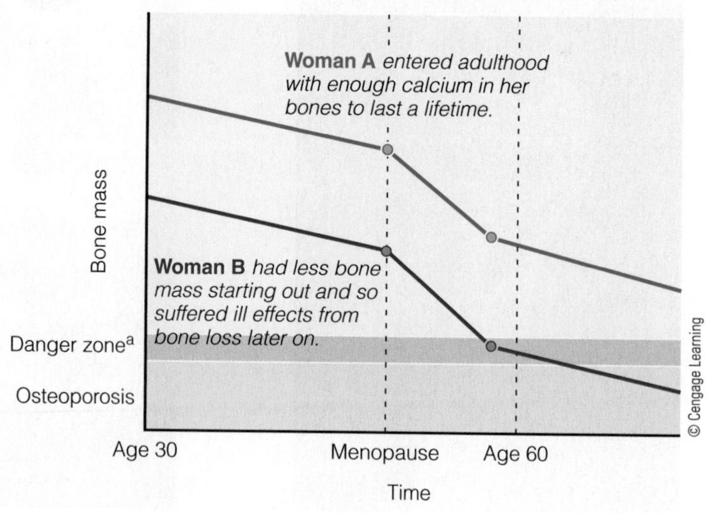

[a]People with a moderate degree of bone mass loss are said to have *osteopenia* and are at increased risk of fractures.

Age and Bone Calcium

Two major stages of life are critical in the development of osteoporosis. The first is the bone-acquiring stage of childhood and adolescence. The second is the bone-losing decades of late adulthood, especially in women after menopause. The bones gain strength and density all through the growing years and into young adulthood. As people age, the cells that build bone gradually become less active, but those that dismantle bone continue working. The result is that bone loss exceeds bone formation. Some bone loss is inevitable, but losses can be curtailed by maximizing bone mass.

Maximizing Bone Mass

To maximize bone mass, the diet must deliver an adequate supply of calcium during the first three decades of life. Children and teens who consume milk products and get enough calcium have denser bones than those with inadequate intakes. With little or no calcium from the diet, the body must depend on bone to supply calcium to the blood—bone mass diminishes, and bones lose their density and strength. When people reach the bone-losing years of middle age, those who formed dense bones during their youth have the advantage. They simply have more bone starting out and can lose more before suffering ill effects. Figure H12-3 demonstrates this effect.

Minimizing Bone Loss

Not only does dietary calcium build strong bones in youth, but it remains important in protecting against losses in the later years. Unfortunately, calcium intakes of older adults are typically low, and calcium absorption declines after menopause. The kidneys do not activate vitamin D as well as they did earlier (recall that vitamin D enhances calcium absorption). Also, sunlight is needed to form vitamin D, and many older people spend little or no time outdoors in the sunshine. For these reasons, and because intakes of vitamin D are typically low anyway, blood levels of vitamin D decline.

Some of the hormones that regulate bone and calcium metabolism—parathyroid hormone, calcitonin, and estrogen—also change with age and accelerate bone loss. Together, these age-related factors contribute to bone loss: inefficient bone remodeling, reduced calcium intakes, impaired calcium absorption, poor vitamin D status, and hormonal changes that favor bone mineral withdrawal.

Gender and Hormones

After age, gender is the next strongest predictor of osteoporosis. The sex hormones play a major role in regulating the rate of bone turnover.[4] Men have greater bone density than women at maturity, and women have greater losses than men in later life. Consequently, men develop bone problems about 10 years later than women, and women account for two out of three cases of osteoporosis.

Menopause imperils women's bones. Bone dwindles rapidly when the hormone estrogen diminishes and menstruation ceases. The lack of estrogen contributes to the release of cytokines that produce inflammation and accelerate bone loss.[5] Women may lose up to 20 percent of their bone mass during the 6 to 8 years following menopause. Eventually, losses taper off so that women again lose bone at the same rate as men their age. Losses of bone minerals continue throughout the remainder of a woman's lifetime, but not at the free-fall pace of the menopause years (review Figure H12-3).

Rapid bone losses also occur when *young* women's ovaries fail to produce enough estrogen, causing menstruation to cease. In some cases, diseased ovaries are to blame and must be removed; in others, the ovaries fail to produce sufficient estrogen because the women suffer from anorexia nervosa and have unreasonably restricted their body weight (see Highlight 8). The amenorrhea and low body weights explain much of the bone loss seen in these young women, even years after diagnosis and treatment.

Estrogen therapy may help some women prevent further bone loss and reduce the incidence of fractures. Because estrogen therapy may increase the risks for breast cancer, women must carefully weigh any potential benefits against the possible dangers. A combination of drugs or of hormone replacement and a drug may be most beneficial.

Several drug therapies have been developed to inhibit bone loss and enhance bone formation.[6] The FDA has approved the following drugs to prevent or treat osteoporosis: biophosphates, calcitonin, estrogens, estrogen antagonists, and parathyroid hormone.[7]

Some women who choose not to use estrogen therapy turn to soy as an alternative treatment. Interestingly, the phytochemicals commonly found in soy mimic the actions of estrogen in the body. Research results have been mixed and controversial, but overall seem to indicate a lack of benefit for soy and its phytochemicals in helping to prevent the rapid bone losses of the menopause years.[8] As is true of all herbal products, there may be risks associated with their use, and in the case of soy, evidence is lacking that the benefits clearly outweigh the potential risks.[9] Because the risks and benefits vary depending on each person's medical history, women should discuss soy options with their physicians.

As in women, sex hormones appear to play a key role in men's bone loss as well.[10] Other common causes of osteoporosis in men include corticosteroid use and alcohol abuse.

Genetics

Risks of osteoporosis appear to run along racial lines and reflect genetic differences in bone development. African Americans, for example, seem to use and retain calcium more efficiently than Caucasians. Consequently, even though their calcium intakes are typically lower, black people have denser bones than white people do. Greater bone density expresses itself in less bone loss, fewer fractures, and a lower rate of osteoporosis among blacks.

The exact role of genetics is unclear.[11] Most likely, genes influence both the peak bone mass achieved during growth and the bone loss incurred during the later years. The extent to which a given genetic potential is realized, however, depends on many outside factors. Diet and physical activity, for example, can maximize peak bone density during growth, whereas alcohol and tobacco abuse can accelerate bone losses later in life. Importantly, these factors are within a person's control.

Physical Activity and Body Weight

Physical activity may be the single most important factor supporting bone growth during adolescence.[12] Muscle strength and bone strength go together. When muscles work, they pull on the bones, stimulating them to grow denser. The hormones that promote new muscle growth also favor the building of bone. As a result, active bones are denser and stronger than sedentary bones.

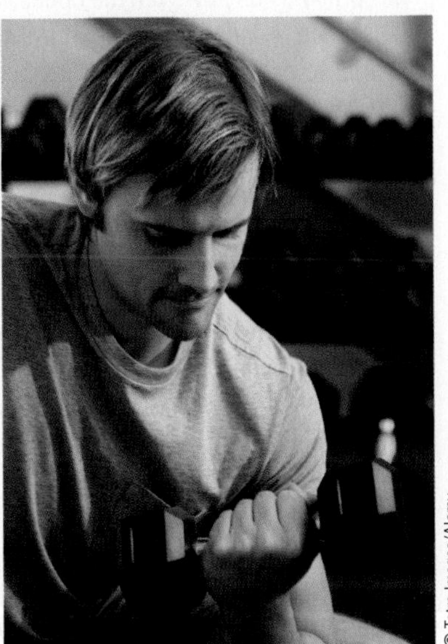
© Tetra Images/Alamy

Strength training helps to build strong bones.

Both the muscle contraction and the gravitational pull of the body's weight create a load that benefits bone metabolism. To keep bones healthy, a person should engage in weight training or weight-bearing endurance activities (such as tennis and jogging or sprint cycling) regularly.[13] Regular physical activity combined with an adequate calcium intake helps to maximize bone density in adolescence. Adults can also maximize and maintain bone density with a regular program of weight training. Even past menopause, when most women are losing bone, weight training improves bone density.

Heavier body weights and weight gains place a similar stress on the bones and promote their density. In contrast, weight losses reduce bone density and increase the risk of fractures—in part because energy restriction diminishes calcium absorption and compromises calcium balance. As mentioned in Highlight 8, the relative energy deficiency that results from a combination of restricted energy intake and extreme daily exercise reliably predicts bone loss.

Smoking and Alcohol

Add bone damage to the list of ill consequences associated with smoking. The bones of smokers are less dense than those of nonsmokers—even after controlling for differences in age, body weight, and physical activity habits. Fortunately, the damaging effects can be reversed with smoking cessation. Blood indicators of beneficial bone activity are apparent 6 weeks after a person stops smoking. In time, bone density is similar for former smokers and nonsmokers.

People who abuse alcohol often suffer from osteoporosis and experience more bone breaks than others. Several factors appear to be involved. Alcohol enhances fluid excretion, leading to excessive calcium losses in the urine; upsets the hormonal balance required for healthy bones; slows bone formation, leading to lower bone density; stimulates bone breakdown; and increases the risk of falling.

Dietary Calcium

Diets that are habitually low in calcium increase the risk of fractures and osteoporosis.[14] For older adults, an adequate calcium intake alone cannot protect against bone fractures. Bone strength later in life depends primarily on how well the bones were built during childhood and adolescence. Adequate calcium nutrition during the growing years is essential to achieving optimal peak bone mass. Simply put, growing children who do not get enough calcium do not develop strong bones. For this reason, the DRI Committee recommends 1300 milligrams of calcium per day for everyone 9 through 18 years of age. Unfortunately, few girls meet the recommendations for calcium during these bone-forming years. (Boys generally obtain intakes close to those recommended because they eat more food.) Consequently, most girls start their adult years with less-than-optimal bone density. As adults, women rarely meet their recommended intakes of 1000 to 1200 milligrams from food. Some authorities suggest 1500 milligrams of calcium for postmenopausal women who are not receiving estrogen.

Other Nutrients

Much research has focused on calcium, but other nutrients support bone health too. Adequate protein protects bones and reduces the likelihood of hip fractures. As mentioned earlier, vitamin D is needed to maintain calcium metabolism and optimal bone health. Vitamin K decreases bone turnover and protects against hip fractures. Vitamin C may slow bone losses. The minerals magnesium and potassium also help to maintain bone mineral density. Vitamin A is needed in the bone-remodeling process, but too much vitamin A may be associated with osteoporosis. Carotenoids may inhibit bone loss. Omega-3 fatty acids may help preserve bone integrity. Additional research points to the bone benefits not of a specific nutrient, but of a diet rich in fruits, vegetables, and whole grains.[15] In contrast, diets containing too much salt are associated with bone losses. Similarly, diets containing too many colas or commercially baked snack and fried foods are associated with low bone mineral density. Clearly, a well-balanced diet that depends on all the food groups to supply a full array of nutrients is central to bone health.

A Perspective on Calcium Supplements

Bone health depends, in part, on calcium. People who do not consume milk products or other calcium-rich foods in amounts that provide even half the recommendation should consider consulting a registered dietitian nutritionist who can assess the diet and suggest food choices to correct any inadequacies. Calcium from foods may support bone health better than calcium from supplements. For those who are unable to consume enough calcium-rich foods, however, taking calcium supplements—especially in combination with vitamin D—may help to enhance bone density and protect against bone loss and fractures.[16] Because some research suggests that calcium supplements may increase the risk of heart attacks and strokes, women should consult their physicians when making this decision.[17]

An estimated 60 percent of women aged 60 and over take calcium supplements.[18] Selecting a calcium supplement requires a little investigative work to sort through the many options. Before examining calcium supplements, recognize that multivitamin-mineral pills contain little or no calcium. The label may list a few milligrams of calcium, but remember that the recommended intake is a gram (1000 milligrams) or more for adults.

Calcium supplements are typically sold as compounds of calcium carbonate (common in **antacids** and fortified chocolate candies), citrate, gluconate, lactate, malate, or phosphate. These supplements often include magnesium, vitamin D, or both. In addition, some calcium supplements are made from **bone meal, oyster shell,** or **dolomite** (limestone). Many calcium supplements, especially those derived from these natural products, contain lead—which impairs health in numerous ways, as Chapter 13 points out. Fortunately, calcium interferes with the absorption and action of lead in the body.

The first question to ask is how much calcium the supplement provides. Most calcium supplements provide between 250 and 1000 milligrams of calcium. To be safe, total calcium intake from both foods and supplements should not exceed the UL. Read the label to find out how much a dose supplies. Unless the label states otherwise, supplements of calcium carbonate are 40 percent calcium; those of calcium citrate are 21 percent; lactate, 13 percent; and gluconate, 9 percent. Select a low-dose supplement and take it several times a day rather than taking a large-dose supplement all at once. Taking supplements in doses of 500 milligrams or less improves absorption. Small doses also help ease the GI distress (constipation, intestinal bloating, and excessive gas) that sometimes accompanies calcium supplement use.

The next question to ask is how well the body absorbs and uses the calcium from various supplements. Most healthy people absorb calcium equally well from milk and any of these supplements: calcium carbonate, citrate, or phosphate. More important than supplement solubility is tablet disintegration. When manufacturers compress large quantities of calcium into small pills, the stomach acid has difficulty penetrating the pill. To test a supplement's ability to dissolve, drop it into a 6-ounce cup of vinegar, and stir occasionally. A high-quality formulation will dissolve within a half-hour.

Finally, people who choose supplements must take them regularly. Furthermore, consideration should be given to the best time to take the supplements. To circumvent adverse nutrient interactions, take calcium supplements between, not with, meals. (Importantly, do not take calcium supplements with iron supplements or iron-rich meals; calcium inhibits iron absorption.) To enhance calcium absorption, take supplements with meals. If such contradictory advice drives you crazy, reconsider the benefits of food sources of calcium. Most experts agree that foods are the best source of most nutrients.

Some Closing Thoughts

Unfortunately, many of the strongest risk factors for osteoporosis are beyond people's control: age, gender, and genetics. But several strategies are effective for prevention. First, ensure an optimal peak bone mass during childhood and adolescence by eating a balanced diet rich in calcium and vitamin D and by engaging in regular physical activity. Then, maintain that bone mass in early adulthood by continuing those healthy diet and activity habits, abstaining from cigarette smoking and using alcohol moderately, if at all. Finally, minimize bone loss in later life by maintaining an adequate nutrition and exercise regimen, and, especially for older women, consult a physician about bone density tests, calcium supplements, or other drug therapies that may be effective both in preventing bone loss and in restoring lost bone.[19] The reward is the best possible chance of preserving bone health throughout life.

CRITICAL THINKING QUESTIONS

A. What behaviors would be most helpful in preventing osteoporosis?

B. Osteoporosis typically develops in old age, yet the time to optimize bone density is during childhood and adolescence—decades away from the realities of hip fractures and spinal collapses. What plan of action might you develop to encourage teens to adopt strategies that will enhance bone development? Be sure to address potential obstacles and reluctances typical of that age.

REFERENCES

1. Centers for Disease Control and Prevention, Hip fractures among older adults, http://www.cdc.gov/homeandrecreationalsafety/falls/adulthipfx.html, September 30, 2013; A. Leboime and coauthors, Osteoporosis and mortality, *Joint Bone Spine* 77 (2010): S107–S112.
2. National Osteoporosis Foundation, www.nof.org, accessed January 2014; R. Nuti and coauthors, Bone fragility in men: Where are we? *Journal of Endocrinological Investigation* 33 (2010): 33–38.
3. R. Lorente-Ramos and coauthors, Dual-energy x-ray absorptiometry in the diagnosis of osteoporosis: A practical guide, *American Journal of Roentgenology* 196 (2011): 897–904.
4. B. Frenkel and coauthors, Regulation of adult bone turnover by sex steroids, *Journal of Cellular Physiology* 224 (2010): 305–310.
5. Y. Imai and coauthors, Minireview: Osteoprotective action of estrogens is mediated by osteoclastic estrogen receptor-alpha, *Molecular Endocrinology* 24 (2010): 877–885.
6. T. D. Rachner, S. Khosla, and L. C. Hofbauer, Osteoporosis: Now and the future, *Lancet* 377 (2011): 1276–1287.
7. National Osteoporosis Foundation, *Clinician's Guide to Prevention and Treatment of Osteoporosis* (Washington, D.C.: National Osteoporosis Foundation, 2010), pp. 21–24.
8. V. S. Lagari and S. Levis, Phytoestrogens in the prevention of postmenopausal bone loss, *Journal of Clinical Densitometry* 16 (2013): 445–449; A. Bitto and coauthors, Genistein aglycone: A dual mode of action anti-osteoporotic soy isoflavone rebalancing bone turnover towards bone formation, *Current Medicinal Chemistry* 17 (2010): 3007–3018.
9. E. Poluzzi and couathors, Phytoestrogens in postmenopause: The state of the art from a chemical pharmacological and regulatory perspective, *Current Medicinal Chemistry* 21 (2014): 417–436; J. Pitkin, Alternative and complementary therapies for the menopause, *Menopause International* 18 (2012): 20–27.
10. E. Gielen and coauthors, Osteoporosis in men, *Best Practice and Research: Clinical Endocrinology and Metabolism* 25 (2011): 321–335; N. Ducharme, Male osteoporosis, *Clinics in Geriatric Medicine* 26 (2010): 301–309; S. Khosla, Update in male osteoporosis, *Journal of Clinical Endocrinology and Metabolism* 95 (2010): 3–10.
11. B. D. Mitchell and L. M. Yerges-Armstrong, The genetics of bone loss: Challenges and prospects, *Journal of Clinical Endocrinology and Metabolism* 96 (2011): 1258–1268.
12. K. F. Janz and coauthors, Early physical activity provides sustained bone health benefits later in childhood, *Medicine and Science in Sports and Exercise* 42 (2010): 1072–1078; A. Guadalupe-Grau and coauthors, Exercise and bone mass in adults, *Sports Medicine* 39 (2009): 439–468.
13. E. A. Marques and coauthors, Response of bone mineral density, inflammatory cytokines, and biochemical bone markers to a 32-week combined loading exercise programme in older men and women, *Archives of Gerontology and Geriatrics* 57 (2013): 226–233; M. T. Korhonen and coauthors, Bone density, structure and strength, and their determinants in aging sprint athletes, *Medicine and Science in Sports and Exercise* 44 (2012): 2340–2349; T. E. Howe and coauthors, Exercise for preventing and treating osteoporosis in postmenopausal women, *Cochrane Database of Systematic Reviews* 7 (2011): CD000333.
14. E. Warensjö and coauthors, Dietary calcium intake and risk of fracture and osteoporosis prospective longitudinal cohort study, *British Medical Journal* 342 (2011): d1473.
15. L. Langsetmo and coauthors, Dietary patterns and incident low-trauma fractures in postmenopausal women and men aged ≥50 y: A population-based cohort study, *American Journal of Clinical Nutrition* 93 (2011): 192–199.
16. R. L. Prentice and coauthors, Health risks and benefits from calcium and vitamin D supplementation Women's Health Initiative clinical trial and cohort study, *Osteoporosis International* 24 (2013): 567–580.
17. D. C. Bauer, Calcium supplements and fracture prevention, *New England Journal of Medicine* 369 (2013): 1537–1543; K. Li and coauthors, Associations of dietary calcium intake and calcium supplementation with myocardial infarction and stroke risk and overall cardiovascular mortality in the Heidelberg cohort of the European Prospective Investigation into Cancer and Nutrition study (EPIC-Heidelberg), *Heart* 98 (2012): 920–925; M. J. Bolland and coauthors, Calcium supplements with or without vitamin D and risk of cardiovascular events: Reanalysis of the Women's Health Initiative limited access dataset and meta-analysis, *British Medical Journal* 342 (2011): d2040.
18. J. Gahche and coauthors, Dietary supplement use among US adults has increased since NHANES III (1988–1994), *NCHS Data Brief* 61 (2011): 1–8.
19. R. C. Hamdy and coauthors, Algorithm for the management of osteoporosis, *Southern Medical Journal* 103 (2010): 1009–1015.

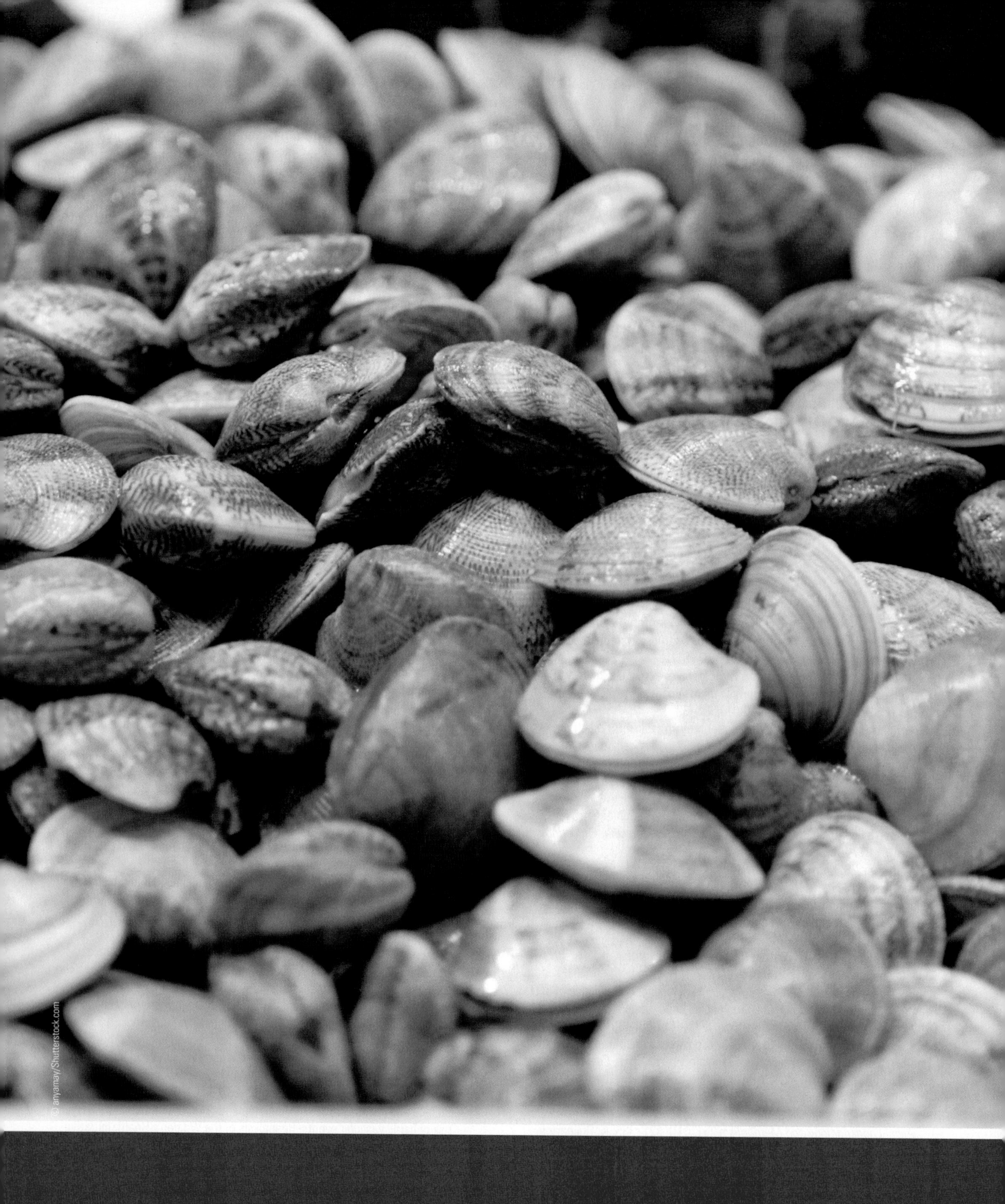

13

The Trace Minerals

Nutrition in Your Life

Trace—barely a perceptible amount. But the trace minerals tackle big jobs. Your blood can't carry oxygen without iron, and insulin can't deliver glucose without chromium. Teeth become decayed without fluoride, and thyroid glands develop goiter without iodine. Together, the trace minerals keep you healthy and strong. Where can you get these amazing minerals? A variety of foods, especially those from the protein foods group, sprinkled with a little iodized salt and complemented by a glass of fluoridated water will do the trick. It's remarkable what your body can do with only a few milligrams—or even micrograms—of the trace minerals. In the Nutrition Portfolio at the end of this chapter, you can determine whether the foods you are eating are meeting your trace mineral needs.

This chapter features the essential **trace minerals**—iron, zinc, iodine, selenium, copper, manganese, fluoride, chromium, and molybdenum. Figure 12-9 in Chapter 12 (p. 381) showed the tiny quantities of trace minerals in the human body. The trace minerals are so named because they are present, and needed, in relatively small amounts in the body. All together, they would hardly fill a teaspoon. Yet they are no less important than the major minerals or any of the other nutrients. Each of the trace minerals performs a vital role. A deficiency of any of them may be fatal, and excesses are equally deadly. Remarkably, a well-balanced diet supplies enough of these minerals to maintain health.

This chapter also mentions other trace minerals—such as arsenic, boron, nickel, bromine, and vanadium—that are not considered nutrients. These minerals may have beneficial roles in the body, but research on them is insufficient to determine essentiality. Also mentioned in this chapter are contaminant minerals that disrupt body processes and impair nutrition status. The highlight that follows examines phytochemicals—compounds that also are not essential nutrients, but that have biological activity in the body. Again, a well-balanced diet—especially one abundant in fruits and vegetables—supplies a full array of phytochemicals to support good health.

LEARNING GPS

trace minerals: essential mineral nutrients the human body requires in relatively small amounts (less than 100 milligrams per day); sometimes called *microminerals*.

13.1 The Trace Minerals—An Overview

› LEARN IT Summarize key factors unique to the trace minerals.

The body requires the trace minerals in minuscule quantities. They participate in diverse tasks all over the body, each having special duties that only it can perform.

Food Sources The trace mineral contents of foods depend on soil and water composition and on how foods are processed. Furthermore, many factors in the diet and within the body affect the minerals' **bioavailability.** Still, outstanding food sources for each of the trace minerals, just like those for the other nutrients, include a wide variety of foods.

Deficiencies Assessing trace mineral status is challenging. Severe deficiencies of the better-known minerals are relatively easy to recognize. Deficiencies of the others may be harder to diagnose, and for all minerals, mild deficiencies are easy to overlook. Because the minerals are active in many body systems—digestive, cardiovascular, circulatory, muscular, skeletal, and nervous—deficiencies can have wide-reaching effects and can affect people of all ages. The most common result of a deficiency in children is failure to grow and thrive.

Toxicities Most of the trace minerals are toxic at intakes only two and a half to eleven times above current recommendations (see Figure 13-1). Thus it is important not to habitually exceed the Upper Level (UL) of recommended

> FIGURE 13-1 **RDA (or AI) and UL Compared for Selected Trace Minerals**

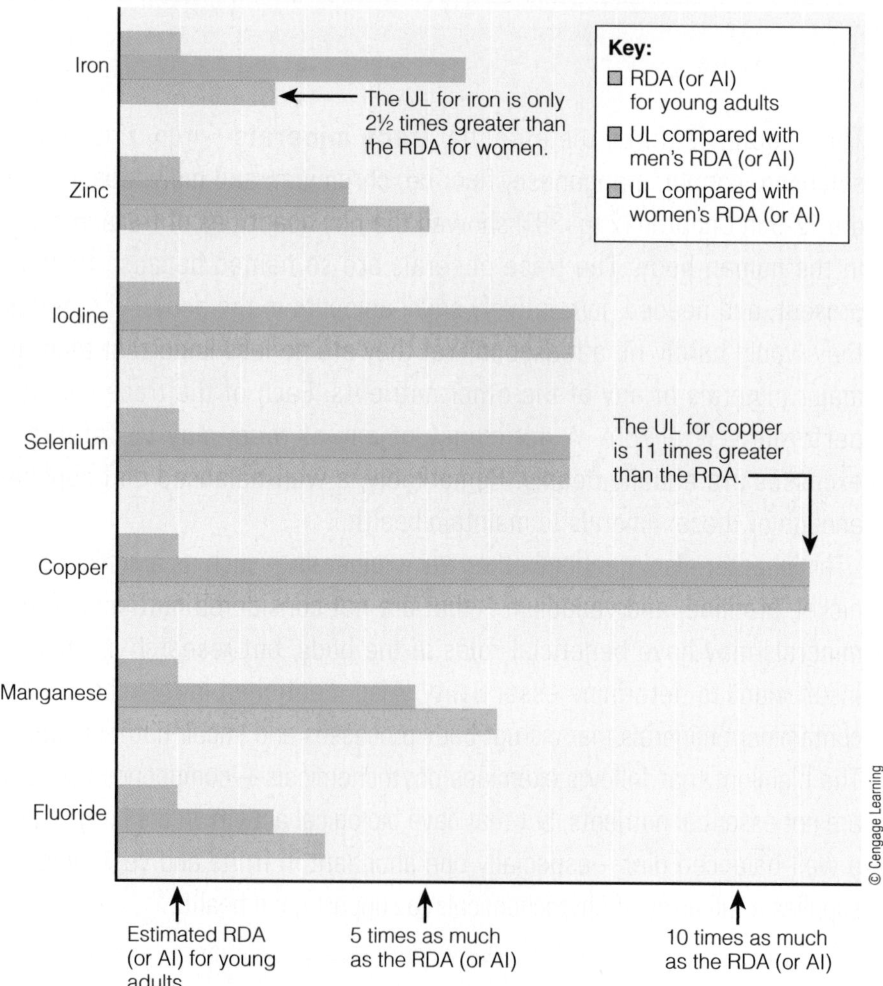

bioavailability: the rate at and the extent to which a nutrient is absorbed and used.

intakes (see inside front pages). Many dietary supplements contain trace minerals, making it easy for users to exceed their needs. Highlight 10 discusses supplement use and some of the regulations included in the Dietary Supplement Health and Education Act. As that discussion notes, consumers have demanded the freedom to choose their own doses of nutrients. By law, the Food and Drug Administration (FDA) has no authority to limit the amounts of trace minerals in supplements. Individuals who take supplements must therefore be aware of the possible dangers and select supplements that contain no more than 100 percent of the Daily Value. It is easier and safer to meet nutrient needs by selecting a variety of foods than by combining an assortment of supplements.

Interactions Interactions among the trace minerals are common and often well coordinated to meet the body's needs. For example, several of the trace minerals support insulin's work, influencing its synthesis, storage, release, and action.

At other times, interactions lead to nutrient imbalances. An excess of one may cause a deficiency of another. (A slight manganese overload, for example, may aggravate an iron deficiency.) A deficiency of one may interfere with the work of another. (A selenium deficiency halts the activation of the iodine-containing thyroid hormones.) A deficiency of a trace mineral may even open the way for a contaminant mineral to cause a toxic reaction. (Iron deficiency, for example, makes the body more vulnerable to lead poisoning.) These examples of nutrient interactions highlight one of the many reasons why people should use supplements conservatively, if at all: supplementation can easily create imbalances.

A good food source of one nutrient may be a poor food source of another, and factors that enhance the action of some trace minerals may interfere with others. Meats, for example, are a good source of iron but a poor source of calcium; vitamin C enhances the absorption of iron but hinders that of copper.

Nonessential Trace Minerals The essential trace minerals featured in this chapter have been well studied; researchers understand the primary roles in the body and the consequences of deficiencies and toxicities. Enough information is available to determine DRI. In contrast, research to determine whether other trace minerals are essential is challenging because quantities in the body are so small and also because human deficiencies are unknown. Identifying their functions in the body can be particularly problematic. Much of the available knowledge comes from research using animals.

Research is currently insufficient to determine the DRI for nickel, bromine, vanadium, cobalt, and boron, even though they may play beneficial roles in the human body. Nickel may serve as a cofactor for certain enzymes. Bromine is involved in the formation of collagen. Vanadium is necessary for growth and bone development and for normal reproduction. Cobalt is a key mineral in the large vitamin B_{12} molecule (see Figure 13-2). Boron may play a key role in bone health, brain activities, and immune response.

In the future, we may discover that these and other trace minerals are essential to growth and health. Even arsenic—famous as a poison used by murderers and known to be a carcinogen—may turn out to be essential for human beings in tiny quantities. It has already proved useful in the treatment of some types of leukemia.[1] Research on all the trace minerals is active, suggesting that we have much more to learn about them.

> REVIEW IT Summarize key factors unique to the trace minerals.

Although the body uses only tiny amounts of the trace minerals, they are vital to health. Because so little is required, the trace minerals can be toxic at levels not far above estimated requirements—a consideration for supplement users. Like the other nutrients, the trace minerals are best obtained by eating a variety of foods.

> FIGURE 13-2 Cobalt in Vitamin B_{12}

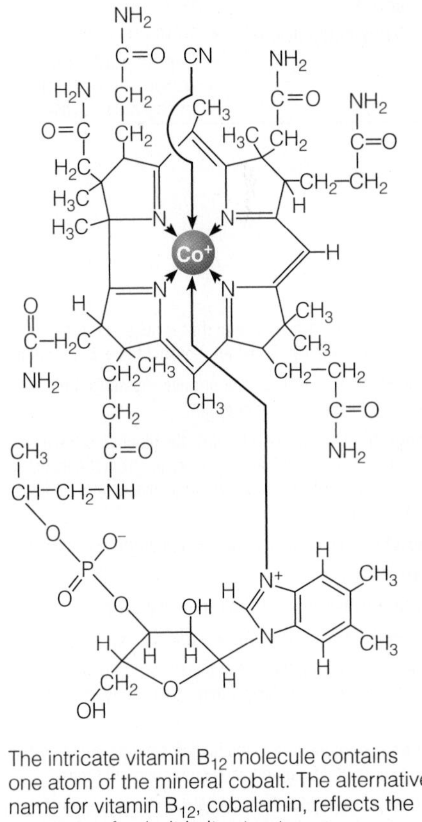

The intricate vitamin B_{12} molecule contains one atom of the mineral cobalt. The alternative name for vitamin B_{12}, cobalamin, reflects the presence of cobalt in its structure.

13.2 The Trace Minerals

› LEARN IT Identify the main roles, deficiency symptoms, and food sources for each of the essential trace minerals (iron, zinc, iodine, selenium, copper, manganese, fluoride, chromium, and molybdenum).

Iron **Iron** is an essential nutrient, vital to many of the cells' activities, but it poses a problem for millions of people. Some people simply don't eat enough iron-containing foods to support their health optimally, whereas others absorb so much iron that it threatens their health. Iron exemplifies the principle that both too little and too much of a nutrient in the body can be harmful. In its wisdom, the body has several ways to maintain iron balance, protecting against both deficiency and toxicity.

Iron Roles in the Body Iron has the knack of switching back and forth between two ionic states. In the reduced state, iron has lost two electrons and therefore has a net positive charge of two; it is known as *ferrous iron* (Fe^{++}). In the oxidized state, iron has lost a third electron, has a net positive charge of three, and is known as *ferric iron* (Fe^{+++}). Ferrous iron can be oxidized to ferric iron, and ferric iron can be reduced to ferrous iron. By doing so, iron can serve as a **cofactor** to enzymes involved in the numerous oxidation-reduction reactions that commonly occur in all cells. Enzymes involved in making amino acids, collagen, hormones, and neurotransmitters all require iron. (For details about ions, oxidation, and reduction, see Appendix B.)

Iron forms a part of the electron carriers that participate in the electron transport chain (discussed in Chapter 7).* These carriers transfer hydrogens and electrons to oxygen, forming water, and in the process, make ATP for the cells' energy use.

Most of the body's iron is found in two proteins: **hemoglobin** in the red blood cells and **myoglobin** in the muscle cells. In both, iron helps accept, carry, and then release oxygen.

TABLE 13-1 Factors That Influence Nonheme Iron Absorption

Enhancing Factors	Inhibiting Factors
• MFP factor • Vitamin C (ascorbic acid) • Acids (citric and lactic) • Sugars (fructose)	• Phytates (legumes, grains, nuts, seeds) • Vegetable proteins (soybeans, legumes, nuts) • Calcium (milk) • Tannic acid (and other polyphenols in tea and coffee)

Iron Absorption The body conserves iron. Because it is difficult to excrete iron once it is in the body, balance is maintained primarily through absorption. More iron is absorbed when stores are empty and less is absorbed when stores are full. Special proteins help the body absorb iron from food (see Figure 13-3).[2] The iron-storage protein **ferritin** captures iron from food and stores it in the cells of the small intestine. When the body needs iron, ferritin releases some iron to an iron transport protein called **transferrin.** If the body does not need iron, it is carried out when the intestinal cells are shed and excreted in the feces; intestinal cells are replaced about every 3 to 5 days. By holding iron temporarily, these cells control iron absorption by either delivering iron when the day's intake falls short or disposing of it when intakes exceed needs.

Iron absorption depends in part on its dietary source. Iron occurs in two forms in foods: as **heme iron,** which is found only in foods derived from the flesh of animals, such as meats, poultry, and fish and as **nonheme iron,** which is found in both plant-derived and animal-derived foods (see Figure 13-4). On average, heme iron represents about 10 percent of the iron a person consumes in a day. Even though heme iron accounts for only a small proportion of the intake, it is so well absorbed that it contributes significant iron. About 25 percent of heme iron and 17 percent of nonheme iron is absorbed, depending on dietary factors and the body's iron stores.[3] In iron deficiency, absorption increases. In iron overload, absorption declines.

Heme iron has a high bioavailability and is not influenced by dietary factors. In contrast, several dietary factors influence nonheme iron absorption (see Table 13-1).[4] Meat, fish, and poultry contain not only the well-absorbed heme iron, but also a peptide (sometimes called the **MFP factor**) that promotes the

iron: an essential trace mineral that is needed for the transport of oxygen and the metabolism of energy nutrients.

cofactor: a small, inorganic or organic substance that facilitates the action of an enzyme.

hemoglobin (HE-moh-GLO-bin): the globular protein of the red blood cells that transports oxygen from the lungs to tissues throughout the body; hemoglobin accounts for 80 percent of the body's iron.

myoglobin: the oxygen-holding protein of the muscle cells.
- **myo** = muscle

ferritin (FAIR-ih-tin): the iron storage protein.

transferrin (trans-FAIR-in): the iron transport protein.

heme (HEEM) **iron:** the iron in foods that is bound to the hemoglobin and myoglobin proteins; found only in meat, fish, and poultry.

nonheme iron: the iron in foods that is not bound to proteins; found in both plant-derived and animal-derived foods.

MFP factor: a peptide released during the digestion of meat, fish, and poultry that enhances nonheme iron absorption.

*The iron-containing electron carriers of the electron transport chain are known as *cytochromes*. See Appendix C for details on the electron transport chain.

> FIGURE 13-3 **Iron Absorption**

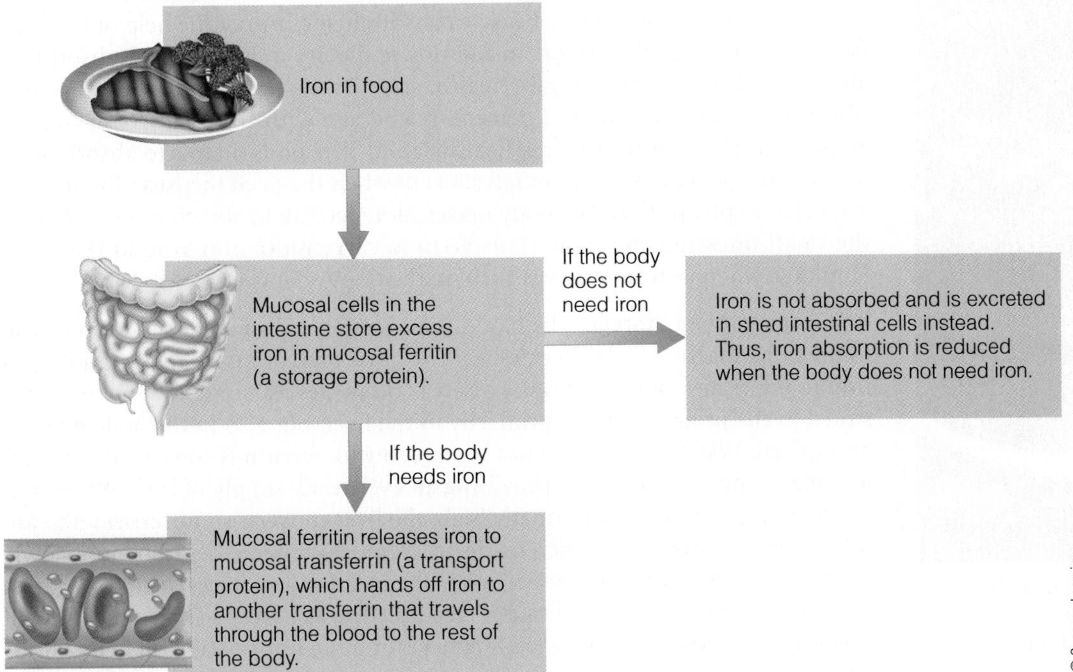

absorption of nonheme iron from other foods eaten at the same meal. Vitamin C (ascorbic acid) also enhances nonheme iron absorption from foods eaten at the same meal by capturing the iron and keeping it in the reduced ferrous form, ready for absorption. Some acids (such as citric acid) and sugars (such as fructose) also enhance nonheme iron absorption.

Iron in food
Mucosal cells in the intestine store excess iron in mucosal ferritin (a storage protein).
If the body does not need iron
Iron is not absorbed and is excreted in shed intestinal cells instead. Thus, iron absorption is reduced when the body does not need iron.
If the body needs iron
Mucosal ferritin releases iron to mucosal transferrin (a transport protein), which hands off iron to another transferrin that travels through the blood to the rest of the body.
© Cengage Learning

Some dietary factors bind with nonheme iron, inhibiting absorption. These factors include the phytates in legumes, whole grains, and rice; the vegetable proteins in soybeans, other legumes, and nuts; the calcium in milk; and the polyphenols (such as tannic acid) in tea, coffee, grain products, oregano, and red wine.

The many dietary enhancers, inhibitors, and their combined effects make it difficult to estimate iron absorption. Most of these factors exert a strong influence individually, but not when combined with the others in a meal. Furthermore, the impact of the combined effects diminishes when a diet is evaluated over several days. When multiple meals are analyzed together, three factors appear to be most relevant: MFP factor and vitamin C as enhancers and phytates as inhibitors.

> FIGURE 13-4 **Heme and Nonheme Iron in Foods**

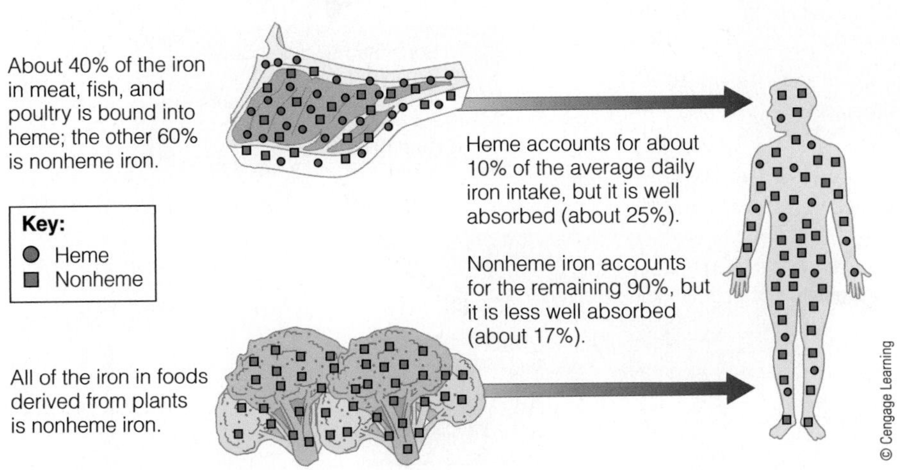

About 40% of the iron in meat, fish, and poultry is bound into heme; the other 60% is nonheme iron.
Key:
Heme
Nonheme
Heme accounts for about 10% of the average daily iron intake, but it is well absorbed (about 25%).
Nonheme iron accounts for the remaining 90%, but it is less well absorbed (about 17%).
All of the iron in foods derived from plants is nonheme iron.
© Cengage Learning

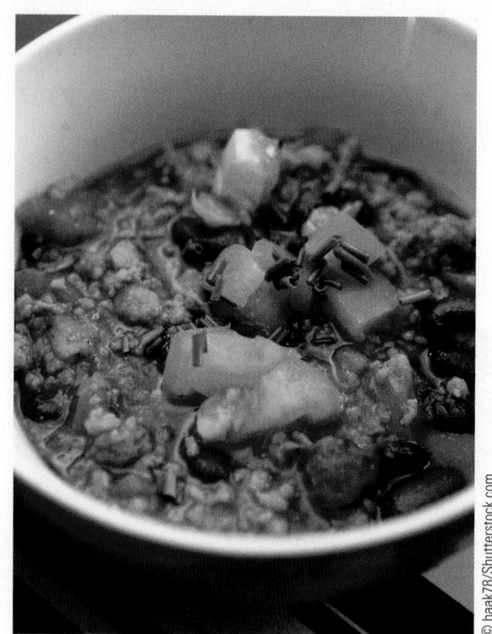

This chili dinner provides several factors that may enhance iron absorption: heme and nonheme iron and the MFP factor from meat, nonheme iron from legumes, and vitamin C from tomatoes.

Overall, about 18 percent of dietary iron is absorbed from mixed diets and only about 10 percent from vegetarian diets. As you might expect, vegetarian diets do not have the benefit of easy-to-absorb heme iron or the help of the MFP factor in enhancing absorption. In addition to dietary influences, iron absorption also depends on an individual's health, stage in the life cycle, and iron status. Absorption can be as low as 2 percent in a person with GI disease or as high as 35 percent in a rapidly growing, healthy child. The body adapts to absorb more iron when a person's iron stores fall short or when the need increases for any reason (such as pregnancy). The body makes more ferritin to absorb more iron from the small intestine and more transferrin to carry more iron around the body. Similarly, when iron stores are sufficient, the body adapts to absorb less iron.

Iron Transport and Storage The blood transport protein transferrin delivers iron to the bone marrow and other tissues. The bone marrow uses large quantities of iron to make new red blood cells, whereas other tissues use less. Surplus iron is stored in the protein ferritin, primarily in the liver, but also in the bone marrow and spleen. When dietary iron has been plentiful, ferritin is constantly and rapidly made and broken down, providing an ever-ready supply of iron. When iron concentrations become abnormally high, the liver converts some ferritin into another storage protein called **hemosiderin.** Hemosiderin releases iron more slowly than ferritin does. Storing excess iron in hemosiderin protects the body against the damage that free iron can cause. Free iron acts as a free radical, attacking cell lipids, DNA, and protein. (See Highlight 11 for more information on free radicals and the damage they can cause.)

The average red blood cell lives about 4 months; then the spleen and liver cells remove it from the blood, take it apart, and prepare the degradation products for excretion or recycling. The iron is salvaged: the liver attaches it to transferrin, which transports it back to the bone marrow to be reused in making new red blood cells. Thus, although red blood cells live for only about 4 months, the iron recycles through each new generation of cells (see Figure 13-5). The body loses some iron daily via the GI tract and, if bleeding occurs, in blood. Only

hemosiderin (heem-oh-SID-er-in): an iron-storage protein primarily made in times of iron overload.

> FIGURE 13-5 Iron Recycled in the Body

Once iron enters the body, most of it is recycled. Some is lost with body tissues and must be replaced by eating iron-containing foods.

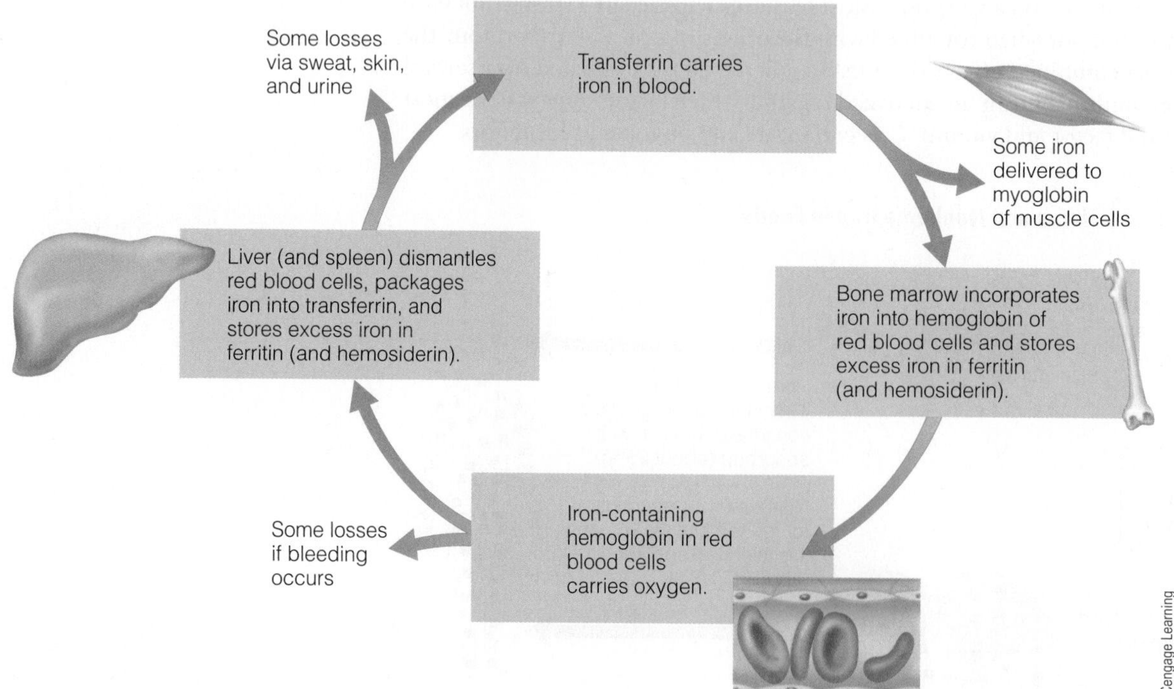

tiny amounts of iron are lost in urine, sweat, and shed skin. Iron excretion differs for men and women. On average, men and women lose about 1.0 milligram of iron per day, with women losing additional iron in menses; menstrual losses vary considerably, but over a month, they average about 0.5 milligram per day.

Maintaining iron balance depends on the careful regulation of iron absorption, transport, storage, recycling, and losses. Central to the regulation of iron balance is the hormone **hepcidin.**[5] Produced by the liver, hepcidin helps to maintain blood iron within the normal range by limiting absorption from the small intestine and controlling release from the liver, spleen, and bone marrow. Hepcidin production increases in iron overload and decreases in iron deficiency.[6]

Iron Deficiency Worldwide, **iron deficiency** is the most common nutrient deficiency, with **iron-deficiency anemia** affecting 1.5 to 2.0 billion people—mostly preschool children and pregnant women.[7] In the United States, iron deficiency is less prevalent, but it still affects about 10 percent of toddlers, adolescent girls, and women of childbearing age. Iron deficiency is also relatively common among those who are overweight. The association between iron deficiency and obesity has yet to be explained, but researchers are currently examining the relationships between the inflammation that develops with excess body fat and reduced iron absorption.[8] The increased production of hepcidin in obesity may also help to explain the relationship between obesity and iron deficiency.[9] Preventing and correcting iron deficiency are high priorities.

Some stages of life demand more iron but provide less, making deficiency likely.[10] Women in their reproductive years are especially prone to iron deficiency because of repeated blood losses during menstruation. Pregnancy demands additional iron to support the added blood volume, growth of the fetus, and blood loss during childbirth. Infants and young children receive little iron from their high-milk diets, yet need extra iron to support their rapid growth and brain development.* Iron deficiency among toddlers in the United States is common. The rapid growth of adolescence, especially for males, and the menstrual losses of females also demand extra iron that a typical teen diet may not provide. An adequate iron intake is especially important during these stages of life.

Bleeding from any site incurs iron losses.** In some cases, such as an active ulcer, the bleeding may not be obvious, but even small chronic blood losses significantly deplete iron reserves. In developing countries, blood loss is often brought on by malaria and parasitic infections of the GI tract. People who donate blood regularly also incur losses and may benefit from iron supplements. As mentioned, menstrual losses can be considerable as they tap women's iron stores regularly.

Assessment of Iron Deficiency Iron deficiency develops in stages. This section provides a brief overview of how to detect these stages, and Appendix E provides more details. In the first stage of iron deficiency, iron stores diminish. Measures of serum ferritin (in the blood) reflect iron stores and are most valuable in assessing iron status at this earliest stage. Unfortunately, serum ferritin increases with infections, which interferes with an accurate diagnosis and estimates of prevalence.[11]

The second stage of iron deficiency is characterized by a decrease in transport iron: serum iron falls, and the iron-carrying protein transferrin *increases* (an adaptation that enhances iron absorption). Together, measurements of serum iron and transferrin can determine the severity of the deficiency—the more transferrin and the less iron in the blood, the more advanced the deficiency is. Transferrin saturation—the percentage of transferrin that is saturated with iron—decreases as iron stores decline.

The third stage of iron deficiency occurs when the lack of iron limits hemoglobin production. Now the hemoglobin precursor, **erythrocyte protoporphyrin,** begins to accumulate as hemoglobin and **hematocrit** values decline.

*The condition of developing iron-deficiency anemia because iron-poor milk displaces iron-rich foods in the diet is sometimes called *milk anemia.*

**The iron content of blood is about 0.5 miligram/100 milliliters of blood. A person donating a pint of blood (approximately 500 milliliters) loses about 2.5 milligrams of iron.

hepcidin: a hormone produced by the liver that regulates iron balance.

iron deficiency: the state of having depleted iron stores.

iron-deficiency anemia: severe depletion of iron stores that results in low hemoglobin and small, pale red blood cells. Iron-deficiency anemia is a *microcytic* (my-cro-SIT-ic) *hypochromic* (high-po-KROME-ic) *anemia.*

- **micro** = small
- **cytic** = cell
- **hypo** = too little
- **chrom** = color

erythrocyte protoporphyrin (PRO-toe-PORE-fe-rin): a precursor to hemoglobin.

hematocrit (hee-MAT-oh-krit): the percentage of total blood volume that consists of red blood cells.

Hemoglobin and hematocrit tests are easy, quick, and inexpensive, so they are the tests most commonly used in evaluating iron status. Their usefulness in detecting iron deficiency is limited, however, because they are late indicators. Furthermore, other nutrient deficiencies and medical conditions can influence their values.

Iron Deficiency and Anemia Notice that iron deficiency and iron-deficiency anemia are not the same: people may be iron deficient without being anemic. The term *iron deficiency* refers to depleted body iron stores without regard to the degree of depletion or to the presence of anemia. The term *iron-deficiency anemia* refers to the severe depletion of iron stores that results in a low hemoglobin concentration. In iron-deficiency anemia, hemoglobin synthesis decreases, resulting in red blood cells that are pale (hypochromic) and small (microcytic), as shown in Figure 13-6. Without adequate iron, these cells can't carry enough oxygen from the lungs to the tissues. Energy metabolism in the cells falters. The result is fatigue, weakness, headaches, apathy, pallor, and poor resistance to cold temperatures. Because hemoglobin is the bright red pigment of the blood, the skin of a fair person who is anemic may become noticeably pale. In a dark-skinned person, the tongue and eye lining, normally pink, is very pale.

The fatigue that accompanies iron-deficiency anemia differs from the tiredness a person experiences from a simple lack of sleep. People with anemia feel fatigue only when they exert themselves. Consequently, their work productivity, voluntary activities, and athletic performance decline.[12] Iron supplementation can relieve the fatigue and improve the body's response to physical activity.[13] (The iron needs of physically active people and the special iron deficiency known as *sports anemia* are discussed in Chapter 14.)

> FIGURE 13-6 **Normal Blood Cells and Blood Cells in Iron Deficiency Anemia Compared**

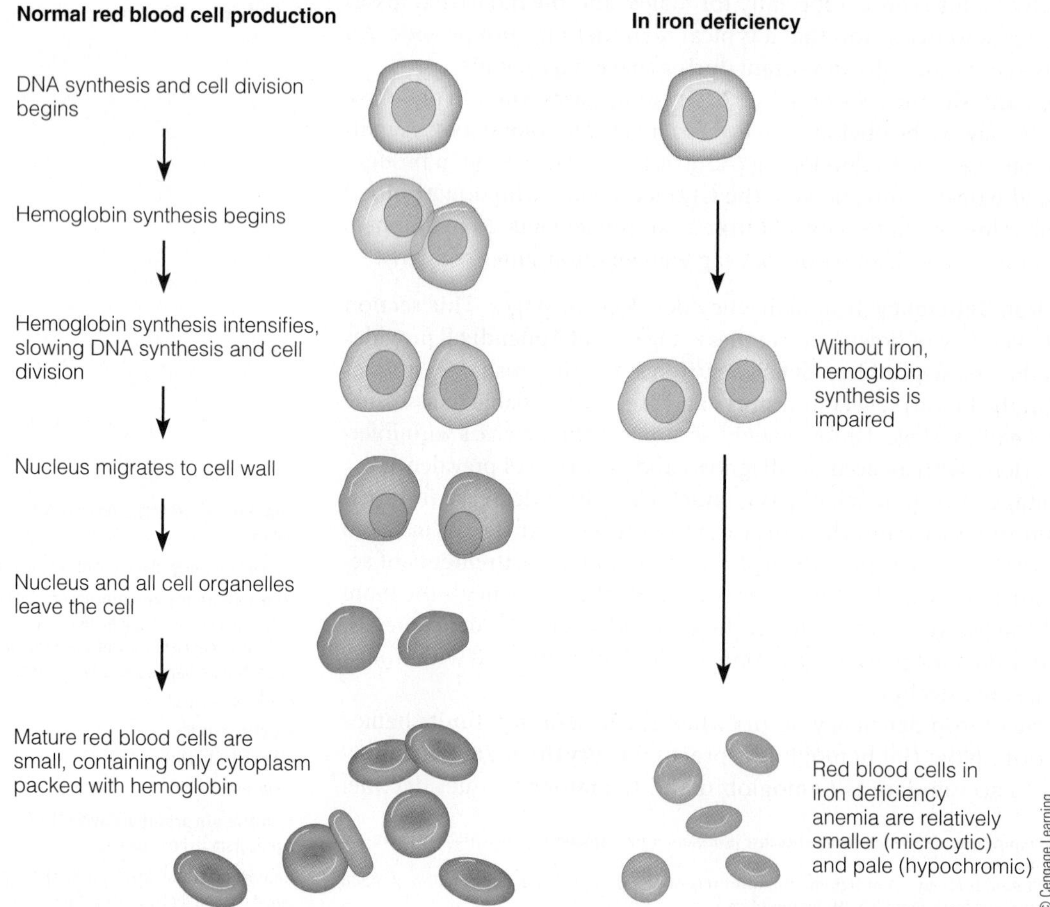

Normal red blood cell production
In iron deficiency
DNA synthesis and cell division begins
Hemoglobin synthesis begins
Hemoglobin synthesis intensifies, slowing DNA synthesis and cell division
Without iron, hemoglobin synthesis is impaired
Nucleus migrates to cell wall
Nucleus and all cell organelles leave the cell
Mature red blood cells are small, containing only cytoplasm packed with hemoglobin
Red blood cells in iron deficiency anemia are relatively smaller (microcytic) and pale (hypochromic)

Iron Deficiency and Behavior Long before the red blood cells are affected and anemia is diagnosed, a developing iron deficiency affects behavior.[14] Even at slightly lowered iron levels, energy metabolism is impaired and neurotransmitter synthesis is altered, reducing physical work capacity and mental productivity.[15] Without the physical energy and mental alertness to work, plan, think, play, sing, or learn, people simply do less. They have no obvious deficiency symptoms; they just appear unmotivated and apathetic.

Many of the symptoms associated with iron deficiency are easily mistaken for behavioral or motivational problems. A restless child who fails to pay attention in class might be thought contrary. An apathetic homemaker who has let housework pile up might be thought lazy. No responsible dietitian would ever claim that all behavioral problems are caused by nutrient deficiencies, but poor nutrition is always a possible contributor to problems like these. When investigating a behavioral problem, check the adequacy of the diet and seek a routine physical examination before undertaking more expensive, and possibly more harmful, treatment options. If iron deficiency is the problem, then treatment with iron supplements may improve mood, cognitive skills, and physical performance. The effects of iron deficiency on children's behavior are discussed further in Chapter 16.

Iron Deficiency and Pica A curious behavior seen in some iron-deficient people, especially in women and children of low-income groups, is **pica**—the craving and consumption of ice, chalk, starch, and other nonfood substances. These substances contain no iron and cannot remedy a deficiency; in fact, clay actually inhibits iron absorption, which may explain the iron deficiency that accompanies such behavior. Pica is poorly understood. Its cause is unknown, but researchers hypothesize that it may be motivated by hunger, nutrient deficiencies, or an attempt to protect against toxins or microbes.[16] The consequence of pica is anemia.

Iron Overload As mentioned earlier, because too much iron can be toxic, its levels in the body are closely regulated and absorption normally decreases when iron stores are full.[17] Even a diet that includes fortified foods usually poses no risk for most people, but some individuals are vulnerable to excess iron. Once considered rare, **iron overload** has emerged as an important disorder of iron metabolism and regulation.

The iron overload disorder known as **hemochromatosis** is caused by a genetic failure to prevent unneeded iron in the diet from being absorbed.[18] Research suggests that just as insulin supports normal glucose homeostasis and its absence or ineffectiveness causes diabetes, the hormone hepcidin supports iron homeostasis and its deficiency or (rarely) resistance causes hemochromatosis.[19] Other causes of iron overload include repeated blood transfusions (which bypass the intestinal defense), massive doses of supplementary iron (which overwhelm the intestinal defense), and other rare metabolic disorders.

Some of the signs and symptoms of iron overload are similar to those of iron deficiency: apathy, lethargy, and fatigue. Therefore, taking iron supplements before assessing iron status is clearly unwise; hemoglobin tests alone would fail to make the distinction because excess iron accumulates in storage. Iron overload assessment tests measure transferrin saturation and serum ferritin.

Iron overload is characterized by a toxic accumulation of iron in the liver, heart, joints, and other tissues. Excess iron in these tissues causes free-radical damage.[20] Infections are likely because viruses and bacteria thrive on iron-rich blood. Symptoms are most severe in alcohol abusers because alcohol damages the small intestine, further impairing its defenses against absorbing excess iron. Untreated iron overload increases the risks of diabetes, liver cancer, heart disease, and arthritis.[21] Currently, treatment involves **phlebotomy,** which removes blood from the body, and chelation therapy, which uses a **chelate** to form a complex with iron and promote its excretion.[22] Research targeting the activity of hepcidin is active and promising.[23]

Iron overload is much more common in men than in women and is twice as prevalent among men as iron deficiency. The widespread fortification of foods with iron makes it difficult for people with hemochromatosis to follow a low-iron

pica (PIE-ka): a craving for and consumption of nonfood substances. Pica is known as *geophagia* (gee-oh-FAY-gee-uh) when referring to eating clay, baby powder, chalk, ash, ceramics, paper, paint chips, or charcoal; *pagophagia* (pag-oh-FAY-gee-uh) when referring to eating large quantities of ice; and *amylophagia* (AM-ee-low-FAY-gee-ah) when referring to eating uncooked starch (flour, laundry starch, or raw rice).

iron overload: toxicity from excess iron.

hemochromatosis (HE-moh-KRO-ma-toe-sis): a genetically determined failure to prevent absorption of unneeded dietary iron that is characterized by iron overload and tissue damage.

phlebotomy: the withdrawal of blood from the body.

chelate (KEY-late): a substance that can grasp the positive ions of a mineral.

- **chele** = claw

diet, and greater dangers lie in the indiscriminate use of iron and vitamin C supplements. Vitamin C not only enhances iron absorption, but also releases iron from ferritin, allowing free iron to wreak the damage typical of free radicals. Thus vitamin C acts as a *pro*oxidant when taken in high doses. (See Highlight 11 for a discussion of free radicals and their effects on disease development.)

Iron and Chronic Diseases Some research suggests a link between heart disease and excess iron.[24] Limited evidence suggests an association between iron and some cancers. Explanations for how iron might be involved in contributing to these chronic diseases focus on its free-radical activity. One of the benefits of a high-fiber diet may be that the accompanying phytates bind iron, making it less available for such reactions.

Iron Poisoning Large doses of iron supplements cause GI distress, including constipation, nausea, vomiting, and diarrhea. These effects may not be as serious as other consequences of iron toxicity, but they are consistent enough to establish a UL of 45 milligrams per day for adults.

Ingestion of iron-containing supplements is a common cause of accidental poisoning in young children.[25] Symptoms of toxicity include nausea, vomiting, diarrhea, a rapid heartbeat, a weak pulse, dizziness, shock, and confusion. As few as five iron tablets containing as little as 200 milligrams of iron have caused death in young children. The exact cause of death is uncertain, but excessive free-radical damage is thought to play a role in heart failure and respiratory distress. Autopsy reports reveal iron deposits and cell death in the stomach, small intestine, liver, and blood vessels (which can cause internal bleeding). As with medicines and other potentially toxic substances, keep iron-containing tablets out of the reach of children. If you suspect iron poisoning, call the nearest poison control center or a physician immediately.

Iron Recommendations The usual diet in the United States provides about 6 to 7 milligrams of iron for every 1000 kcalories. The recommended daily intake for men is 8 milligrams, and because most men eat more than 2000 kcalories a day, they can meet their iron needs with little effort. Women in their reproductive years, however, need 18 milligrams a day. The accompanying "How To" feature explains how the recommended intake was calculated.

>How To

Estimate the Recommended Daily Intake for Iron

To calculate the recommended daily iron intake, the DRI Committee considers a number of factors. For example, for a woman of childbearing age (19 to 50):

- Losses from feces, urine, sweat, and shed skin: 1.0 milligram
- Losses through menstruation: 0.5 milligram (about 14 milligrams total averaged over 28 days)

These losses reflect an average daily need (total) of 1.5 milligrams of *absorbed iron.*

An estimated average requirement is determined based on the daily need and the assumption that an average of 18 percent of ingested iron is absorbed:

1.5 mg iron (needed)
÷ 0.18 (percent iron absorbed)
= 8 mg iron (estimated average requirement)

Then, a margin of safety is added to cover the needs of essentially all women of childbearing age, and the RDA is set at 18 milligrams.

Because the iron bioavailability of typical vegetarian diets is low, the recommendation for iron is 1.8 times higher for vegetarians. To calculate the RDA for vegetarians, multiply by 1.8:

- 8 mg × 1.8 = 14 mg/day (vegetarian men and women >50 yr)
- 18 mg × 1.8 = 32 mg/day (vegetarian women, 19 to 50 yr)

> TRY IT Calculate how many slices of whole-wheat bread, cups of broccoli, ounces of hamburger meat, and cups of milk it takes to provide 18 milligrams of iron.

Because women have higher iron needs and lower energy needs, they sometimes have trouble obtaining enough iron. On average, women receive only 12 to 13 milligrams of iron per day, which is not enough iron for women until after menopause. To meet their iron needs from foods, premenopausal women need to select iron-rich foods at every meal.

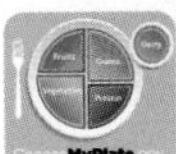

> DIETARY GUIDELINES FOR AMERICANS

Women capable of becoming pregnant should choose foods that supply heme iron, which is more readily absorbed by the body, additional iron sources, and enhancers of iron absorption such as vitamin C. If pregnant, women should take an iron supplement, as recommended by a health-care provider.

Vegetarians need 1.8 times as much iron to make up for the low bioavailability typical of their diets. Good vegetarian sources of iron include soy foods (such as soybeans and tofu), legumes (such as lentils and kidney beans), nuts (such as cashews and almonds), seeds (such as pumpkin seeds and sunflower seeds), cereals (such as cream of wheat and oatmeal), dried fruit (such as apricots and raisins), vegetables (such as mushrooms and potatoes), and blackstrap molasses.

Iron Food Sources To obtain enough iron, people must first select iron-rich foods—both naturally occurring and enriched or fortified—and then take advantage of factors that maximize iron absorption. This discussion begins by identifying iron-rich foods and then reviews the factors affecting absorption. Figure 13-7 (p. 418) shows the amounts of iron in selected foods. Meats, fish, and poultry contribute the most iron per serving; other protein-rich foods such as legumes and eggs are also good sources. Although an indispensable part of the diet, foods in the milk group are notoriously poor in iron. Grain products vary, with whole-grain, enriched, and fortified breads and cereals contributing significantly to iron intakes. Finally, dark greens (such as broccoli) and dried fruits (such as raisins) contribute some iron.

The FDA does not mandate iron enrichment, but most states require manufacturers to enrich flour and grain products with iron.* One serving of enriched bread or cereal provides only a little iron, but because people eat many servings of these foods, the contribution can be significant. Iron added to foods is nonheme iron, which is not absorbed as well as heme iron, but when eaten with absorption-enhancing foods, enrichment iron can increase iron stores and reduce iron deficiency. In cases of iron overload, enrichment may exacerbate the problem.

In general, the bioavailability of iron is high in meats, fish, and poultry, intermediate in grains and legumes, and low in most vegetables, especially those containing oxalates such as spinach. As mentioned earlier, the amount of iron ultimately absorbed from a meal depends on the combined effects of several enhancing and inhibiting factors. For maximum absorption of nonheme iron, eat meat for the MFP factor and fruits or vegetables for vitamin C. The iron of baked beans, for example, will be enhanced by the MFP factor in a piece of pork served with them. The iron of bread will be enhanced by the vitamin C in a slice of tomato on a sandwich.

© Craig M. Moore

When the label on a grain product says "enriched," it means iron and several B vitamins have been added to meet FDA standards.

Iron Contamination In addition to the iron from foods, **contamination iron** from nonfood sources of inorganic iron salts can contribute to the day's intakes. Foods cooked in iron cookware take up iron salts. The more acidic the food and the longer it is cooked in iron cookware, the higher the iron content. The iron content of eggs can triple in the time it takes to scramble them in an iron pan. Admittedly,

contamination iron: iron found in foods as the result of contamination by inorganic iron salts from iron cookware, iron-containing soils, and the like.

*Each pound of enriched flour contains at least 20 milligrams of iron.

> **FIGURE 13-7 Iron in Selected Foods**

Food	Serving size (kcalories)
Bread, whole wheat	1-oz slice (70 kcal)
Cornflakes, fortified	1 oz (110 kcal)
Spaghetti pasta	½ c cooked (99 kcal)
Tortilla, flour	1 10" round (234 kcal)
Broccoli	½ c cooked (22 kcal)
Carrots	½ c shredded raw (24 kcal)
Potato	1 medium baked w/skin (133 kcal)
Tomato juice	½ c (31 kcal)
Banana	1 medium raw (109 kcal)
Orange	1 medium raw (62 kcal)
Strawberries	½ c fresh (22 kcal)
Watermelon	1 slice (92 kcal)
Milk	1 c reduced-fat 2% (121 kcal)
Yogurt, plain	1 c low-fat (155 kcal)
Cheddar cheese	1½ oz (171 kcal)
Cottage cheese	½ c low-fat 2% (101 kcal)
Pinto beans	½ c cooked (117 kcal)
Peanut butter	2 tbs (188 kcal)
Sunflower seeds	1 oz dry (165 kcal)
Tofu (soybean curd)	½ c (76 kcal)
Ground beef, lean	3 oz broiled (244 kcal)
Chicken breast	3 oz roasted (140 kcal)
Tuna, canned in water	3 oz (99 kcal)
Egg	1 hard cooked (78 kcal)
Excellent, and sometimes unusual, sources:	
Clams, canned	3 oz (126 kcal)
Beef liver	3 oz fried (184 kcal)
Parsley	1 c raw (22 kcal)

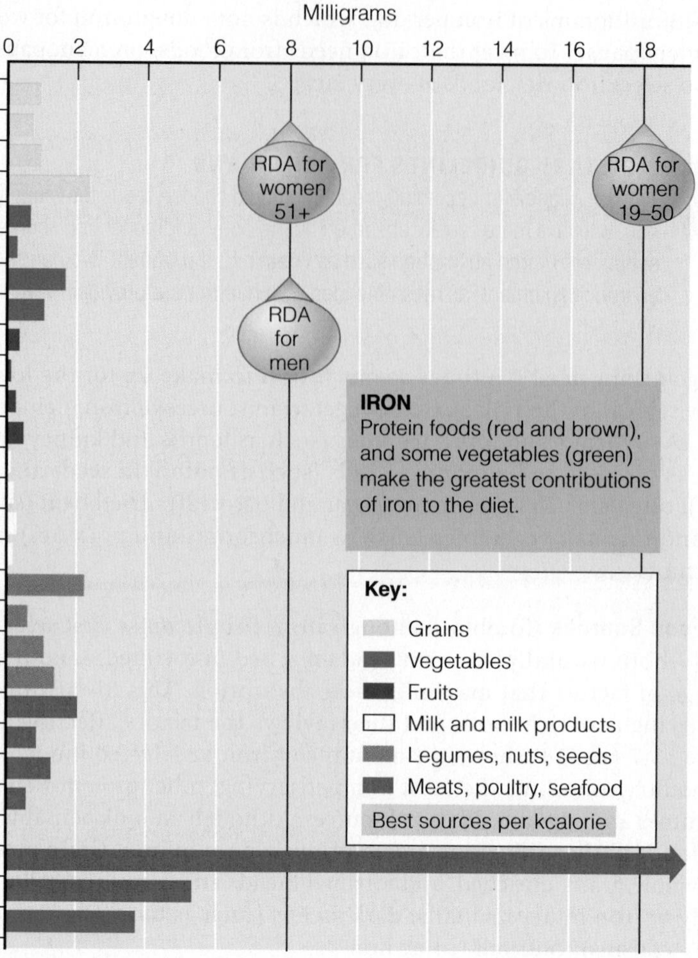

Milligrams: 0 2 4 6 8 10 12 14 16 18

RDA for women 51+ | RDA for men | RDA for women 19–50

IRON
Protein foods (red and brown), and some vegetables (green) make the greatest contributions of iron to the diet.

Key:
Grains
Vegetables
Fruits
Milk and milk products
Legumes, nuts, seeds
Meats, poultry, seafood
Best sources per kcalorie

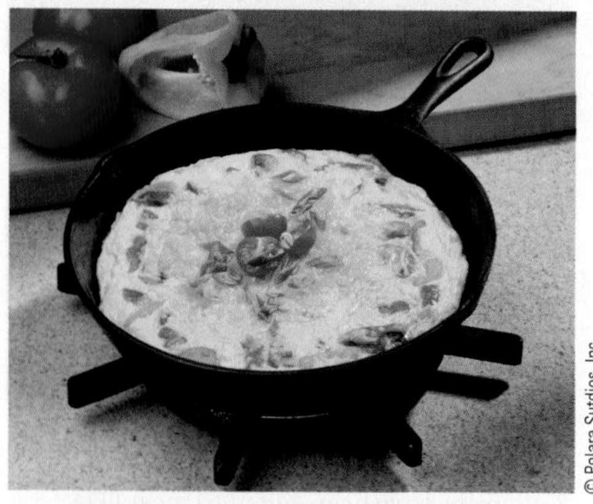

An old-fashioned iron skillet adds iron to foods. Increase in iron content (mg) for selected foods (3 oz) after cooking in iron skillet:

Beef stew	0.66→3.40
Chili	0.96→6.27
Cornbread	0.67→0.86
Hamburger	1.49→2.29
Pancake	0.63→1.31
Rice	0.67→1.97
Scrambled egg	1.49→4.76
Spaghetti sauce	0.61→5.77

the absorption of this iron may be poor (perhaps only 1 to 2 percent), but every little bit helps a person who is trying to increase iron intake.

Iron Supplementation People who are iron deficient may need supplements as well as an iron-rich, absorption-enhancing diet. Many physicians routinely recommend iron supplements to pregnant women, infants, and young children. Iron from supplements is less well absorbed than that from food, so the doses must be high. The absorption of iron taken as ferrous sulfate is better than that from other iron supplements. Absorption also improves when supplements are taken between meals, at bedtime on an empty stomach, and with liquids (other than milk, tea, or coffee, which inhibit absorption). Taking iron supplements in a single dose instead of several doses per day is equally effective and may improve a person's willingness to take it regularly.

There is no benefit to taking iron supplements with orange juice because vitamin C does not enhance absorption from supplements as it does from foods. Vitamin C enhances iron absorption by converting insoluble ferric iron in foods to the more soluble ferrous iron, and supplemental iron is already in the ferrous form. Constipation is a common side effect of iron supplementation; drinking plenty of water may help to relieve this problem. The best strategy to ensure compliance is to individualize the dose, formulation, and schedule. Most importantly, iron supplements should be taken only when prescribed by a physician who has assessed an iron deficiency.

› REVIEW IT

Most of the body's iron is in hemoglobin and myoglobin, where it carries oxygen for use in energy metabolism; some iron is also required for enzymes involved in a variety of reactions. Special proteins assist with iron absorption, transport, and storage—all helping to maintain an appropriate balance—because both too little and too much iron can be damaging. Iron deficiency is most common among infants and young children, teenagers, women of childbearing age, and pregnant women. Symptoms include fatigue and anemia. Iron overload is most common in men. Heme iron, which is found only in meat, fish, and poultry, is better absorbed than nonheme iron, which occurs in most foods. Nonheme iron absorption is improved by eating iron-containing foods with foods containing the MFP factor and vitamin C; absorption is limited by phytates and oxalates. The accompanying table provides a summary of iron.

Iron

RDA	**Significant Sources**
Men: 8 mg/day Women: 18 mg/day (19–50 yr) 8 mg/day (51+)	Red meats, fish, poultry, shellfish, eggs, legumes, dried fruits
UL	**Deficiency Symptoms**
Adults: 45 mg/day	Anemia: weakness, fatigue, headaches; impaired work performance and cognitive function; impaired immunity; pale skin, nail beds, mucous membranes, and palm creases; concave nails; inability to regulate body temperature; pica
Chief Functions in the Body	**Toxicity Symptoms**
Part of the protein hemoglobin, which carries oxygen in the blood; part of the protein myoglobin in muscles, which makes oxygen available for muscle contraction; necessary for the utilization of energy as part of the cells' metabolic machinery	GI distress Iron overload: infections, fatigue, joint pain, skin pigmentation, organ damage

Zinc

Zinc is an essential trace element required for numerous metabolic reactions.[26] Virtually all cells contain zinc, but the highest concentrations are found in muscle and bone.

Zinc Roles in the Body Zinc supports the work of hundreds of proteins in the body, such as the **metalloenzymes,** which participate in a variety of metabolic processes, and **transcription factors,** which regulate gene expression.* In addition, zinc stabilizes cell membranes and DNA, helping to strengthen antioxidant defenses against free-radical attacks. Zinc also assists in immune function and in growth and development. Zinc participates in the synthesis, storage, and release of the hormone insulin in the pancreas, although it does not appear to play a direct role in insulin's action. Zinc interacts with platelets in blood clotting, affects thyroid hormone function, and influences behavior and learning performance. It is needed to produce the active form of vitamin A (retinal) in visual pigments and the retinol-binding protein that transports vitamin A. It is essential to normal taste perception, wound healing, sperm production, and fetal development. A zinc deficiency impairs all these and other functions, underlining the vast importance of zinc in supporting the body's proteins.

Zinc Absorption The body's handling of zinc resembles that of iron in some ways and differs in others. A key difference is the circular passage of zinc from the small intestine to the body and back again.

The rate of zinc absorption varies from about 15 to 40 percent, depending on the amount of zinc consumed—as zinc intake increases, the rate of absorption decreases, and as zinc intake decreases, the rate of absorption increases.[27] Like iron, dietary factors such as phytates influence absorption, limiting its bioavailability.[28]

Upon absorption into an intestinal cell, zinc has two options. Zinc may participate in the metabolic functions of the intestinal cell itself, or it may be retained within the intestinal cells by **metallothionein** until the body needs zinc. Metallothionein plays a key role in storing and distributing zinc throughout the body.

*Among the metalloenzymes requiring zinc are carbonic anhydrase, deoxythymidine kinase, DNA and RNA polymerase, and alkaline phosphatase.

zinc: an essential trace mineral that is part of many enzymes and a constituent of insulin.

metalloenzymes (meh-TAL-oh-EN-zimes): enzymes that contain one or more minerals as part of their structures.

transcription factors: proteins that bind to specific sites in DNA and alter gene expression.

metallothionein (meh-TAL-oh-THIGH-oh-neen): a sulfur-rich protein that avidly binds with and transports metals such as zinc.

- **metallo** = containing a metal
- **thio** = containing sulfur
- **ein** = a protein

> **FIGURE 13-8 Enteropancreatic Circulation of Zinc**

Some zinc from food is absorbed by the small intestine and sent to the pancreas to be incorporated into digestive enzymes that return to the small intestine. This cycle is called the *enteropancreatic circulation* of zinc.

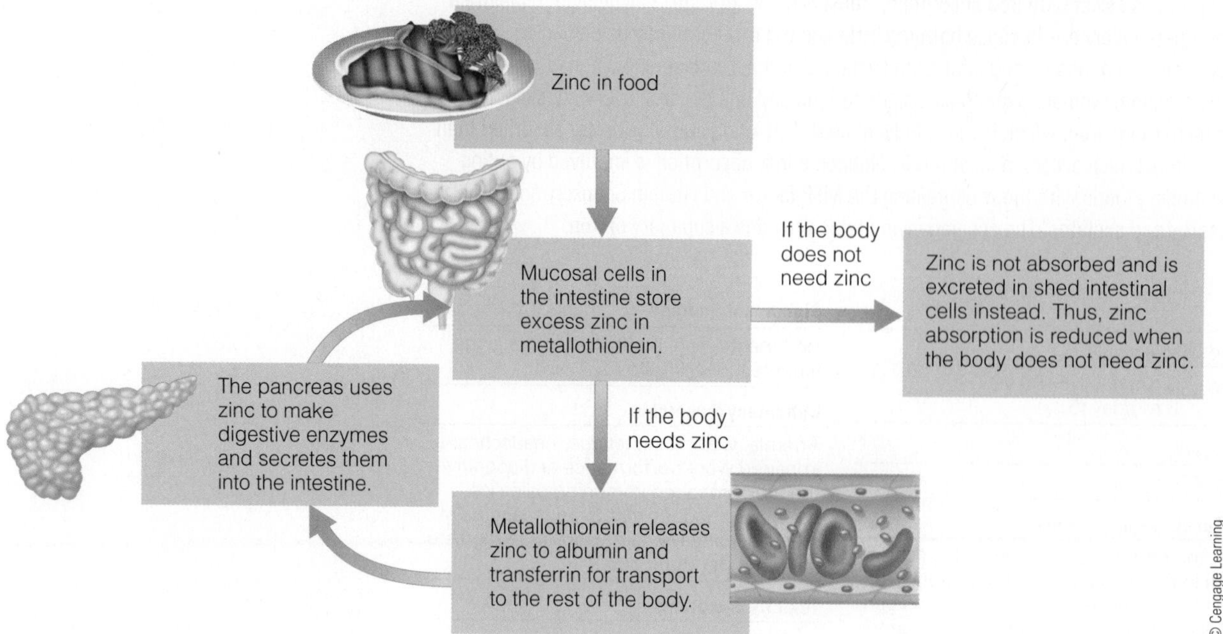

Zinc in food
Mucosal cells in the intestine store excess zinc in metallothionein.
If the body does not need zinc
Zinc is not absorbed and is excreted in shed intestinal cells instead. Thus, zinc absorption is reduced when the body does not need zinc.
The pancreas uses zinc to make digestive enzymes and secretes them into the intestine.
If the body needs zinc
Metallothionein releases zinc to albumin and transferrin for transport to the rest of the body.

enteropancreatic (EN-ter-oh-PAN-kree-AT-ik) **circulation:** the circulatory route from the pancreas to the small intestine and back to the pancreas.

> **FIGURE 13-9 Zinc-Deficiency Symptom—The Stunted Growth of Dwarfism**

The growth retardation, known as dwarfism, is rightly ascribed to zinc deficiency because it is partially reversible when zinc is restored to the diet.

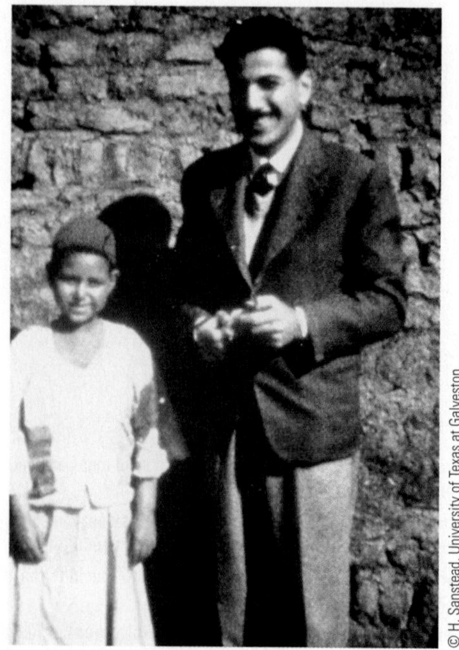

The Egyptian man on the right is an adult of average height. The Egyptian boy on the left is 17 years old but is only 4 feet tall, like a 7-year-old in the United States. His genitalia are like those of a 6-year-old.

Zinc Transport After being absorbed, some zinc eventually reaches the pancreas, where it is incorporated into many of the digestive enzymes that the pancreas releases into the small intestine at mealtimes. The small intestine thus receives two doses of zinc with each meal—one from foods and the other from the zinc-rich pancreatic juices. The recycling of zinc in the body from the pancreas to the small intestine and back to the pancreas is referred to as the **enteropancreatic circulation** of zinc. Each time zinc circulates through the small intestine, it may be excreted in shed intestinal cells or reabsorbed into the body (see Figure 13-8). The body loses zinc primarily in feces. Smaller losses occur in urine, shed skin, hair, sweat, menstrual fluids, and semen.

Numerous proteins participate in zinc transport. Zinc's main transport vehicle in the blood is the protein albumin. Some zinc also binds to transferrin—the same transferrin that carries iron in the blood.

Zinc Deficiency Severe zinc deficiency is not widespread in developed countries, but in the developing world, nearly 2 billion people are zinc deficient.[29] Human zinc deficiency was first reported in the 1960s in children and adolescent boys in Egypt, Iran, and Turkey. Children have especially high zinc needs because they are growing rapidly and synthesizing many zinc-containing proteins, and the native diets among those populations were not meeting these needs. Middle Eastern diets are traditionally low in the richest zinc source, meats. Furthermore, the staple foods in these diets are legumes, unleavened breads, and other whole-grain foods—all high in fiber and phytates, which inhibit zinc absorption.*

Figure 13-9 shows the severe growth retardation and mentions the immature sexual development characteristic of zinc deficiency. In addition, zinc deficiency hinders digestion and absorption, causing diarrhea, which worsens malnutrition not only for zinc, but for other nutrients as well. It also impairs the immune response, making infections likely—among them, pneumonia and GI tract infections, which worsen malnutrition, including zinc malnutrition (a classic downward spiral of events).[30] Chronic zinc deficiency damages the central

*Unleavened bread contains no yeast, which normally breaks down phytates during fermentation.

> **FIGURE 13-10 Zinc in Selected Foods**

Food	Serving size (kcalories)
Bread, whole wheat	1-oz slice (70 kcal)
Cornflakes, fortified	1 oz (110 kcal)
Spaghetti pasta	½ c cooked (99 kcal)
Tortilla, flour	1 10" round (234 kcal)
Broccoli	½ c cooked (22 kcal)
Carrots	½ c shredded raw (24 kcal)
Potato	1 medium baked w/skin (133 kcal)
Tomato juice	¾ c (31 kcal)
Banana	1 medium raw (109 kcal)
Orange	1 medium raw (62 kcal)
Strawberries	½ c fresh (22 kcal)
Watermelon	1 slice (92 kcal)
Milk	1 c reduced-fat 2% (121 kcal)
Yogurt, plain	1 c low-fat (155 kcal)
Cheddar cheese	1½ oz (171 kcal)
Cottage cheese	½ c low-fat 2% (101 kcal)
Pinto beans	½ c cooked (117 kcal)
Peanut butter	2 tbs (188 kcal)
Sunflower seeds	1 oz dry (165 kcal)
Tofu (soybean curd)	½ c (76 kcal)
Ground beef, lean	3 oz broiled (244 kcal)
Chicken breast	3 oz roasted (140 kcal)
Tuna, canned in water	3 oz (99 kcal)
Egg	1 hard cooked (78 kcal)
Excellent, and sometimes unusual, sources:	
Oysters	3 oz cooked (139 kcal)
Sirloin steak, lean	3 oz broiled (172 kcal)
Crab	3 oz cooked (94 kcal)

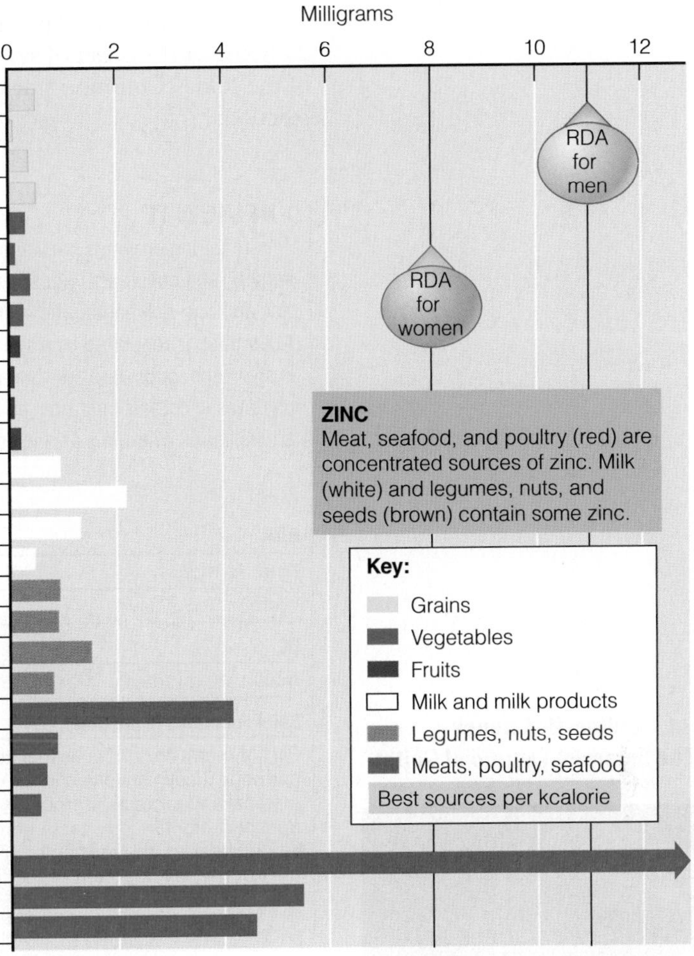

nervous system and brain and may lead to poor motor development and cognitive performance. Because zinc deficiency directly impairs vitamin A metabolism, vitamin A–deficiency symptoms often appear. Zinc deficiency also disturbs thyroid function and the metabolic rate. It alters taste, causes loss of appetite, and slows wound healing—in fact, its symptoms are so pervasive that generalized malnutrition and sickness are more likely to be the diagnosis than simple zinc deficiency.

Zinc Toxicity High doses (more than 50 milligrams) of zinc may cause vomiting, diarrhea, headaches, exhaustion, and other symptoms. The UL for adults was set at 40 milligrams based on zinc's interference in copper metabolism—an effect that, in animals, leads to degeneration of the heart muscle.

Zinc Recommendations and Sources Figure 13-10 shows zinc amounts in selected foods per serving. Zinc is highest in protein-rich foods such as shellfish (especially oysters), meats, poultry, milk, and cheese. Legumes and whole-grain products are good sources of zinc if eaten in large quantities; in typical US diets, the phytate content of grains is not high enough to impair zinc absorption. Vegetables vary in zinc content depending on the soil in which they are grown. Average zinc intakes in the United States are slightly higher than recommendations.

Zinc Supplementation In developed countries, most people obtain enough zinc from the diet without resorting to supplements. In developing countries, zinc supplementation plays a major role in effectively reducing the incidence of disease and death associated with diarrhea and pneumonia.[31]

Zinc lozenges may shorten the duration, but not the severity, of common cold symptoms.[32] Lozenges of zinc acetate or zinc gluconate are most effective,

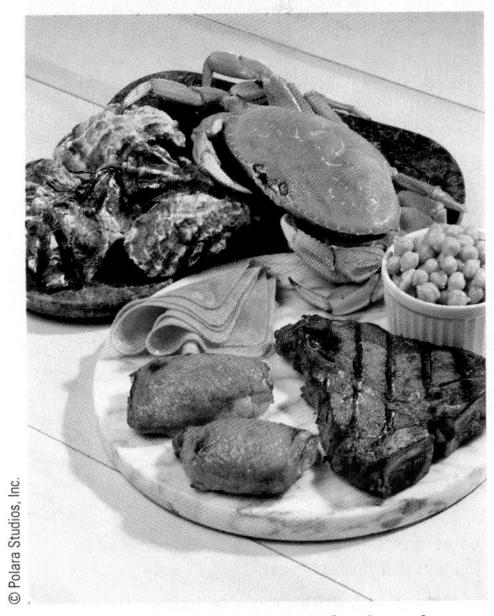

Zinc is highest in protein-rich foods such as oysters, beef, poultry, legumes, and nuts.

whereas other zinc compounds, including those with flavor enhancers, are much less effective.[33] In addition to selecting the appropriate zinc formulation, consumers need to take relatively high doses (75 milligrams) of the lozenges within 24 hours of the onset of symptoms and continue daily throughout the duration of the cold.[34] Common side effects of zinc lozenges include nausea and bad taste reactions.

› REVIEW IT

Zinc-requiring enzymes participate in a multitude of reactions affecting growth, vitamin A activity, and pancreatic digestive enzyme synthesis, among others. After a meal, both dietary zinc and zinc-rich pancreatic secretions (via enteropancreatic circulation) are absorbed. Absorption is regulated by a special binding protein (metallothionein) in the small intestine. Protein-rich foods derived from animals are the best sources of bioavailable zinc. Fiber and phytates in cereals bind zinc, limiting absorption. Growth retardation and sexual immaturity are hallmark symptoms of zinc deficiency. The accompanying table provides a summary of zinc.

Zinc

RDA	Significant Sources
Men: 11 mg/day Women: 8 mg/day	Protein-containing foods: red meats, shellfish, whole grains; some fortified cereals
UL	**Deficiency Symptoms**[a]
Adults: 40 mg/day	Growth retardation, delayed sexual maturation, impaired immune function, hair loss, eye and skin lesions, loss of appetite
Chief Functions in the Body	**Toxicity Symptoms**
Part of many enzymes; associated with the hormone insulin; involved in making genetic material and proteins, immune reactions, transport of vitamin A, taste perception, wound healing, the making of sperm, and the normal development of the fetus	Loss of appetite, impaired immunity, low HDL, copper and iron deficiencies

[a]A rare inherited disease of zinc malabsorption, *acrodermatitis* (AK-roh-der-ma-TIE-tis) *enteropathica* (EN-teroh- PATH-ick-ah), causes additional and more severe symptoms.

> FIGURE 13-11 Iodine-Deficiency Symptom—The Enlarged Thyroid of Goiter

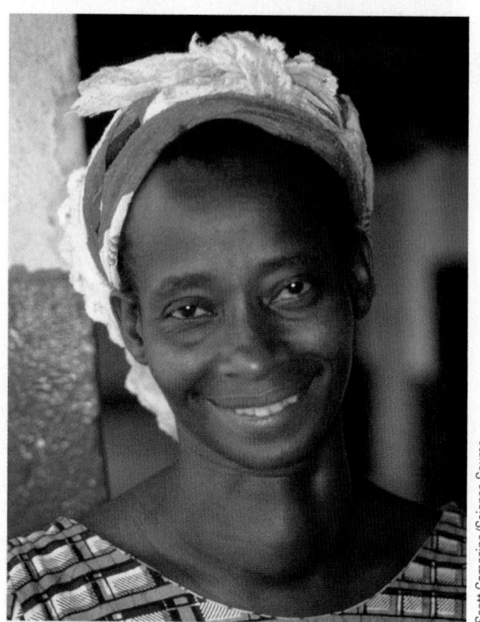

Scott Camazine/Science Source

In iodine deficiency, the thyroid gland enlarges—a condition known as simple goiter. Iodine toxicity also enlarges the thyroid gland, creating a similar-looking goiter.

Iodine

Traces of **iodine** are indispensable to life. In the GI tract, iodine from foods becomes iodide, which is readily absorbed.

Iodide Roles in the Body Iodide is an integral part of the thyroid hormones that regulate body temperature, metabolic rate, reproduction, growth, blood cell production, nerve and muscle function, and more.* By controlling the rate at which the cells use oxygen, these hormones influence the amount of energy expended during basal metabolism.

Iodine Deficiency The hypothalamus regulates thyroid hormone production by controlling the release of the pituitary's thyroid-stimulating hormone (TSH).** With iodine deficiency, thyroid hormone production declines, and the body responds by secreting more TSH in a futile attempt to accelerate iodide uptake by the thyroid gland. If a deficiency persists, the cells of the thyroid gland enlarge to trap as much iodide as possible. Sometimes the gland enlarges until it makes a visible lump in the neck, a **goiter** (shown in Figure 13-11).

Goiter afflicts about 200 million people the world over, many of them in South America, Asia, and Africa. In all but 4 percent of these cases, the cause is iodine deficiency. As for the 4 percent (8 million), most have goiter because they regularly eat excessive amounts of foods that contain an antithyroid substance

iodine: an essential trace mineral that is needed for the synthesis of thyroid hormones.

goiter (GOY-ter): an enlargement of the thyroid gland due to an iodine deficiency, malfunction of the gland, or overconsumption of a goitrogen. Goiter caused by iodine deficiency is sometimes called *simple goiter.*

*The thyroid gland releases tetraiodothyronine (T_4), commonly known as *thyroxine* (thigh-ROCKS-in), to its target tissues. Upon reaching the cells, T_4 loses one iodine, becoming triiodothyronine (T_3), which is the active form of the hormone.

**Thyroid-stimulating hormone is also called *thyrotropin*.

(goitrogen) whose effect is not counteracted by dietary iodine. Goitrogen-containing foods include vegetables such as cabbage, spinach, radishes, and rutabagas; legumes such as soybeans and peanuts; and fruits such as peaches and strawberries. The goitrogens present in plants remind us that even natural components of foods can cause harm when eaten in excess.

Goiter may be the earliest and most obvious sign of iodine deficiency, but the most tragic and prevalent damage occurs in the brain. Iodine deficiency is the most common cause of *preventable* mental retardation and brain damage in the world. Nearly one-third of the world's school-age children have iodine deficiency.[35] Children with even a mild iodine deficiency typically have goiters and perform poorly in school. With sustained treatment, however, mental performance in the classroom as well as thyroid function improves.

Even in the United States, pregnant women may not get as much iodine as they need.[36] A severe iodine deficiency during pregnancy causes the extreme and irreversible mental and physical retardation known as **cretinism.*** Cretinism affects approximately 6 million people worldwide and can be averted by the early diagnosis and treatment of maternal iodine deficiency. A worldwide effort to provide iodized salt to people living in iodine-deficient areas has been dramatically successful. An estimated 70 percent of all households in developing countries have access to iodized salt.[37] Because iron deficiency is common among people with iodine deficiency and because iron deficiency reduces the effectiveness of iodized salt, dual fortification with both iron and iodine may be most beneficial.

Iodine Toxicity Excessive intakes of iodine can interfere with thyroid function and enlarge the gland, just as deficiency can. During pregnancy, exposure to excessive iodine from foods, prenatal supplements, or medications is especially damaging to the developing infant. An infant exposed to toxic amounts of iodine during gestation may develop a goiter so severe as to block the airways and cause suffocation. The UL is 1100 micrograms per day for an adult—several times higher than average or recommended intakes (review Figure 13-1 on p. 408). For perspective, most foods provide 3 to 75 micrograms of iodine per serving.

Iodine Recommendations and Sources The ocean is the world's major source of iodine. In coastal areas, kelp, seafood, water, and even iodine-containing sea mist are dependable iodine sources. Further inland, the amount of iodine in foods is variable and generally reflects the amount present in the soil in which plants are grown or on which animals graze. Landmasses that were once under the ocean have soils rich in iodine; those in flood-prone areas where water leaches iodine from the soil are poor in iodine. In the United States, the iodization of salt provides about 60 micrograms of iodine per gram of salt. This tiny amount eliminated the widespread misery caused by iodine deficiency during the 1930s, but iodized salt is not available in many parts of the world. Some countries add iodine to bread, fish paste, or drinking water instead.

Although the average consumption of iodine in the United States exceeds recommendations, it falls below toxic levels. Some of the excess iodine in the US diet stems from fast foods, which use iodized salt liberally. Some iodine comes from bakery products and from milk. The baking industry uses iodates (iodine salts) as dough conditioners, and most dairies feed cows iodine-containing medications and use iodine to disinfect milking equipment. Processed foods in the United States use regular salt, not iodized salt.

The recommended intake of iodine for adults is a minuscule amount. The need for iodine is easily met by consuming seafood, vegetables grown in iodine-rich soil, and iodized salt. Just one-half teaspoon of iodized salt provides the RDA for iodine. In the United States, labels indicate whether salt is iodized.

*The underactivity of the thyroid gland is known as *hypothyroidism* and may be caused by iodine deficiency or any number of other causes. Without treatment, an infant with *congenital hypothyroidism* will develop the physical and mental retardation of *cretinism*.

goitrogen (GOY-troh-jen): a substance that enlarges the thyroid gland and causes *toxic goiter.* Goitrogens occur naturally in such foods as cabbage, kale, brussels sprouts, cauliflower, broccoli, and kohlrabi.

cretinism (CREE-tin-ism): a congenital disease characterized by mental and physical retardation and commonly caused by maternal iodine deficiency during pregnancy.

› REVIEW IT

Iodide, the ion of the mineral iodine, is an essential component of the thyroid hormones. An iodine deficiency can lead to simple goiter (enlargement of the thyroid gland) and can impair fetal development, causing cretinism. Iodization of salt has largely eliminated iodine deficiency in the United States. The accompanying table provides a summary of iodine.

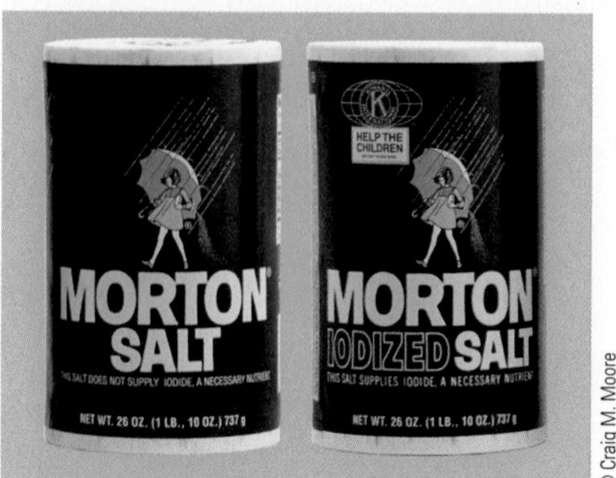

Only "iodized salt" has had iodine added.

© Craig M. Moore

Iodine

RDA	**Deficiency Disease**
Adults: 150 μg/day	Simple goiter, cretinism
UL	**Deficiency Symptoms**
1100 μg/day	Underactive thyroid gland, goiter, mental and physical retardation in infants (cretinism)
Chief Functions in the Body	**Toxicity Symptoms**
A component of two thyroid hormones that help to regulate growth, development, and metabolic rate	Underactive thyroid gland, elevated TSH, goiter
Significant Sources	
Iodized salt, seafood, bread, dairy products, plants grown in iodine-rich soil and animals fed those plants	

Selenium

The essential mineral **selenium** shares some of the chemical characteristics of the mineral sulfur. This similarity allows selenium to substitute for sulfur in the amino acids methionine, cysteine, and cystine.

Selenium Roles in the Body Selenium is one of the body's antioxidant nutrients, working primarily as a part of proteins—most notably, the glutathione peroxidase enzymes.[38] Glutathione peroxidase and vitamin E work in tandem. Glutathione peroxidase prevents free-radical formation, thus blocking the chain reaction before it begins; if free radicals do form and a chain reaction starts, vitamin E stops it. (Highlight 11 describes free-radical formation, chain reactions, and antioxidant action in detail.) Other selenium-containing enzymes selectively activate or inactivate the thyroid hormones.

Selenium Deficiency Selenium deficiency is associated with **Keshan disease**—a heart disease that is prevalent in regions of China where the soil and foods lack selenium.[39] Although the primary cause of this heart disease is probably a virus or toxin, selenium deficiency appears to predispose people to it, and adequate selenium seems to prevent it.[40] Symptoms of selenium deficiency include impaired cognition and poor immunity.[41]

Selenium and Cancer Limited research suggests that the antioxidant action of selenium may protect against some types of cancers.[42] Selenium supplements, however, have not proved effective in preventing cancer and may in fact damage DNA and cause harm.[43]

Selenium Recommendations and Sources Selenium is found in the soil, and therefore in the crops grown for consumption. People living in regions with selenium-poor soil may still get enough selenium, partly because they eat vegetables and grains transported from other regions and partly because they eat meats, milk, and eggs, which are reliable sources of selenium. Eating as few as two Brazil nuts a day effectively improves selenium status. Average intakes in the United States exceed the RDA, which is based on the amount needed to maximize glutathione peroxidase activity.

Selenium Toxicity Because high doses of selenium are toxic, a UL has been set. Selenium toxicity causes loss and brittleness of hair and nails, garlic breath odor, and nervous system abnormalities.

selenium (se-LEEN-ee-um): an essential trace mineral that is part of an antioxidant enzyme.

Keshan (KESH-an or ka-SHAWN) **disease:** the heart disease associated with selenium deficiency; named for one of the provinces of China where it was first studied. Keshan disease is characterized by heart enlargement and insufficiency; fibrous tissue replaces the muscle tissue that normally composes the middle layer of the walls of the heart.

› REVIEW IT

Selenium is an antioxidant nutrient that works closely with the glutathione peroxidase enzyme and vitamin E. Selenium is found in association with protein in foods. Deficiencies are associated with a predisposition to a type of heart abnormality known as Keshan disease. The accompanying table provides a summary of selenium.

Selenium

RDA

Adults: 55 µg/day

UL

Adults: 400 µg/day

Chief Functions in the Body

Defends against oxidation; regulates thyroid hormone

Significant Sources

Seafood, meat, whole grains, fruits, and vegetables (depending on soil content)

Deficiency Symptoms

Predisposition to heart disease characterized by cardiac tissue becoming fibrous (Keshan disease)

Toxicity Symptoms

Loss and brittleness of hair and nails; skin rash, fatigue, irritability, and nervous system disorders; garlic breath odor

Copper The body contains about 100 milligrams of **copper** in a variety of cells and tissues. Copper balance and transport depend on a system of proteins.

Copper Roles in the Body Copper serves as a constituent of several enzymes. The copper-containing enzymes have diverse metabolic roles with one common characteristic: all involve reactions that consume oxygen or oxygen radicals. For example, copper-containing enzymes catalyze the oxidation of ferrous iron to ferric iron, which allows iron to bind to transferrin. Copper's role in iron metabolism makes it a key factor in hemoglobin synthesis. Copper- and zinc-containing enzymes participate in the body's natural defenses against the oxidative damage of free radicals. Still other copper enzymes help to manufacture collagen, inactivate histamine, and degrade serotonin. Copper, like iron, is needed in many of the reactions involved in energy metabolism.

Copper Deficiency and Toxicity Typical US diets provide adequate amounts of copper, and deficiency is rare. In animals, copper deficiency raises blood cholesterol and damages blood vessels, raising questions about whether low dietary copper might contribute to cardiovascular disease in humans.

Some genetic disorders create a copper toxicity, but excessive intakes from foods are unlikely. Excessive intakes from supplements may cause liver damage, and therefore a UL has been set.

Two rare genetic disorders affect copper status in opposite directions.[44] In **Menkes disease,** the intestinal cells absorb copper, but cannot release it into circulation, causing a life-threatening deficiency. Treatment involves giving copper intravenously. In **Wilson's disease,** copper accumulates in the liver and brain, creating a life-threatening toxicity. Wilson's disease can be controlled by reducing copper intake, using chelating agents such as penicillamine, and taking zinc supplements, which interfere with copper absorption.

Copper Recommendations and Sources The richest food sources of copper are legumes, whole grains, nuts, shellfish, and seeds. More than half of the copper from foods is absorbed, and the major route of elimination appears to be bile. Water may also provide copper, depending on the type of plumbing pipe and the hardness of the water.

› REVIEW IT

Copper is a component of several enzymes, all of which are involved in some way with oxygen or oxidation. Some act as antioxidants; others are essential to iron metabolism. Legumes,

copper: an essential trace mineral that is part of many enzymes.

Menkes disease: a genetic disorder of copper transport that creates a copper deficiency and results in mental retardation, poor muscle tone, seizures, brittle kinky hair, and failure to thrive.

Wilson's disease: a genetic disorder of copper metabolism that creates a copper toxicity and results in neurologic symptoms such as tremors, impaired speech, inappropriate behaviors, and personality changes.

› REVIEW IT Copper (*continued*)

whole grains, and shellfish are good sources of copper. The accompanying table provides a summary of copper.

Copper

RDA	Significant Sources
Adults: 900 µg/day	Seafood, nuts, whole grains, seeds, legumes
UL	**Deficiency Symptoms**
Adults: 10,000 µg/day (10 mg/day)	Anemia, bone abnormalities
Chief Functions in the Body	**Toxicity Symptoms**
Necessary for the absorption and use of iron in the formation of hemoglobin; part of several enzymes	Liver damage

Manganese

The human body contains a mere 20 milligrams of **manganese**. Most of it can be found in the bones and metabolically active organs such as the liver, kidneys, and pancreas.

Manganese Roles in the Body Manganese acts as a cofactor for many enzymes that facilitate the metabolism of carbohydrate, lipids, and amino acids. In addition, manganese-containing metalloenzymes assist in bone formation and the conversion of pyruvate to a TCA cycle compound.

Manganese Deficiency and Toxicity Manganese requirements are low, and many plant foods contain significant amounts of this trace mineral, so deficiencies are rare. As is true of other trace minerals, however, dietary factors such as phytates inhibit its absorption. In addition, high intakes of iron and calcium limit manganese absorption, so people who use supplements of those minerals regularly may impair their manganese status.

Manganese toxicity is more likely to occur from a contaminated environment than from an excessive dietary intake. Miners who inhale large quantities of manganese dust on the job over prolonged periods show symptoms of a brain disease, along with abnormalities in appearance and behavior. A UL has been established based on intakes from food, water, and supplements.

Manganese Recommendations and Sources Grain products make the greatest contribution of manganese to the diet. With insufficient information to establish an RDA, an AI was set based on average intakes.

› REVIEW IT

Manganese-dependent enzymes are involved in bone formation and various metabolic processes. Because manganese is widespread in plant foods, deficiencies are rare, although regular use of calcium and iron supplements may limit manganese absorption. The accompanying table provides a summary of manganese.

Manganese

AI	Significant Sources
Men: 2.3 mg/day	Nuts, whole grains, leafy vegetables, tea
Women: 1.8 mg/day	**Deficiency Symptoms**
UL	Rare
Adults: 11 mg/day	**Toxicity Symptoms**
Chief Functions in the Body	Nervous system disorders
Cofactor for several enzymes; bone formation	

Fluoride

Fluoride is present in virtually all soils, water supplies, plants, and animals. The body contains only a trace of fluoride, but with this amount, the crystalline deposits in teeth are larger and more perfectly formed.

manganese: an essential trace mineral that acts as a cofactor for many enzymes.

fluoride: an essential trace mineral that makes teeth stronger and more resistant to decay.

Fluoride Roles in the Body As Chapter 12 explains, during the mineralization of bones and teeth, calcium and phosphorus form crystals called hydroxyapatite. Then fluoride replaces the hydroxyl (OH) portions of the hydroxyapatite crystal, forming **fluorapatite,** which makes the teeth stronger and more resistant to decay.

Dental caries ranks as the nation's most widespread public health problem: an estimated 95 percent of the population have decayed, missing, or filled teeth. These dental problems can quickly lead to a multitude of nutrition problems by interfering with a person's ability to chew and eat a wide variety of foods. Where fluoride is lacking, dental decay is common.

Drinking water is usually the best source of fluoride, and 75 percent of the US population served by community water systems receives optimal levels of fluoride (see Figure 13-12).[45] Fluoridation of drinking water (to raise the concentration to 0.7 milligram per liter of water) protects against dental caries and supports oral health.[46] By fluoridating the drinking water, a community offers its residents, particularly the children, a safe, economical, practical, and effective way to defend against dental caries. Most bottled waters lack fluoride.

Fluoride Toxicity Too much fluoride can damage the teeth, causing **fluorosis.**[47] For this reason, a UL has been established. In mild cases, the teeth develop small white flecks; in severe cases, the enamel becomes pitted and permanently stained (as shown in Figure 13-13). Fluorosis occurs only during tooth development and cannot be reversed, making its prevention during the first 3 years of life a high priority.[48] To limit fluoride ingestion, take care not to swallow fluoride-containing dental products such as toothpaste and mouthwash and use fluoride supplements only as prescribed by a physician.

Fluoride Recommendations and Sources As mentioned earlier, much of the US population has access to water with an optimal fluoride concentration, which typically delivers about 1 milligram per person per day. Fish and most teas contain appreciable amounts of natural fluoride.

> FIGURE 13-12 **US Population with Access to Fluoridated Water through Public Water Systems**

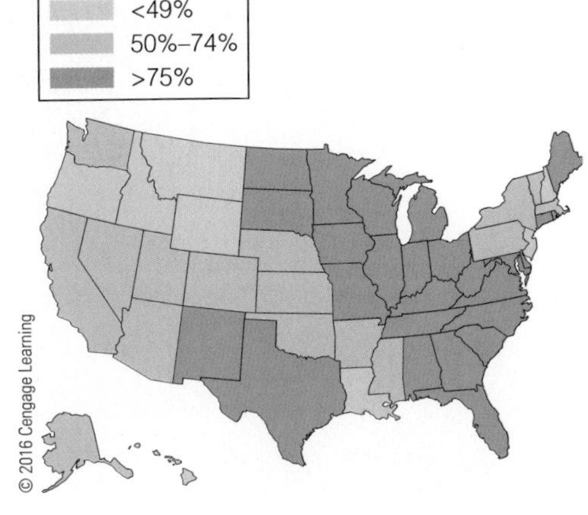

> FIGURE 13-13 **Fluoride-Toxicity Symptom—The Mottled Teeth of Fluorosis**

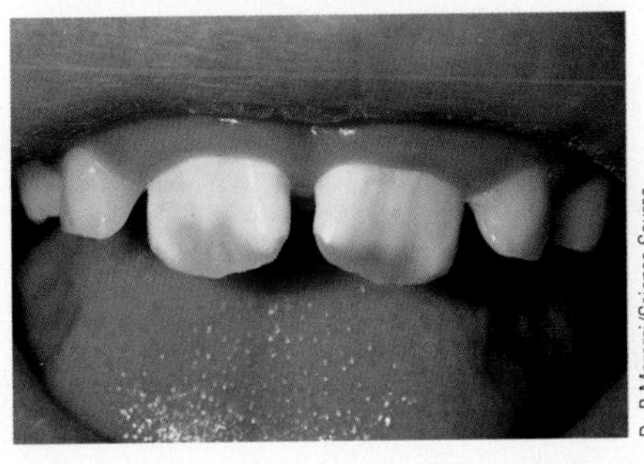

> REVIEW IT

Fluoride makes teeth stronger and more resistant to decay. Fluoridation of public water supplies can significantly reduce the incidence of dental caries, but excess fluoride during tooth development can cause fluorosis—discolored and pitted tooth enamel. The accompanying table provides a summary of fluoride.

Fluoride

AI	
Men: 4 mg/day	
Women: 3 mg/day	
UL	
Adults: 10 mg/day	
Chief Functions in the Body	
Strengthens teeth; helps to make teeth resistant to decay	

Significant Sources
Drinking water (if fluoride containing or fluoridated), tea, seafood
Deficiency Symptoms
Susceptibility to tooth decay
Toxicity Symptoms
Fluorosis (pitting and discoloration of teeth)

Chromium

Chromium is an essential mineral that participates in carbohydrate and lipid metabolism. Like iron, chromium assumes different charges. In chromium, the Cr^{+++} ion is the most stable and most commonly found in foods.

Chromium Roles in the Body Chromium helps maintain glucose homeostasis by enhancing the activity of the hormone insulin.* When chromium is lacking, a diabetes-like condition may develop, with elevated blood glucose and impaired

*Small organic compounds that enhance insulin's actions are called *glucose tolerance factors (GTF)*. Some glucose tolerance factors contain chromium.

fluorapatite (floor-APP-uh-tite): the stabilized form of tooth crystal, in which fluoride has replaced the hydroxyl groups of hydroxyapatite.

fluorosis (floor-OH-sis): discoloration and pitting of tooth enamel caused by excess fluoride during tooth development.

chromium (KRO-mee-um): an essential trace mineral that enhances the activity of insulin.

glucose tolerance, insulin response, and glucagon response. Some research suggests that chromium supplements lower blood glucose or improve insulin responses in type 2 diabetes, but findings have not been consistent.[49]

Chromium Recommendations and Sources Chromium is present in a variety of foods. The best sources are unrefined foods, particularly liver, brewer's yeast, and whole grains. The more refined foods people eat, the less chromium they ingest.

Chromium Supplements Supplement advertisements have succeeded in convincing consumers that they can lose fat and build muscle by taking chromium picolinate. Whether chromium supplements (either picolinate or plain) reduce body fat or improve muscle strength remains controversial. (Highlight 14 discusses chromium picolinate and other supplements athletes use in the hopes of improving their performance.)

› REVIEW IT

Chromium enhances insulin's action. A deficiency can impair glucose homeostasis. Chromium is widely available in unrefined foods including brewer's yeast, whole grains, and liver. The accompanying table provides a summary of chromium.

Chromium

AI	Significant Sources
Men: 35 µg/day Women: 25 µg/day	Meats (especially liver), whole grains, brewer's yeast
Chief Functions in the Body	**Deficiency Symptoms**
Enhances insulin action and may improve glucose tolerance	Diabetes-like condition
	Toxicity Symptoms
	None reported

Molybdenum

Molybdenum acts as a working part of several metalloenzymes. Dietary deficiencies of molybdenum are unknown because the amounts needed are minuscule—as little as 0.1 part per million parts of body tissue. Legumes, breads and other grain products, leafy green vegetables, milk, and liver are molybdenum-rich foods. Average daily intakes fall within the suggested range of intakes.

Molybdenum toxicity in people is rare. It has been reported in animal studies, and a UL has been established. Characteristics of molybdenum toxicity include kidney damage and reproductive abnormalities.

› REVIEW IT

Molybdenum is found in a variety of foods and participates in several metabolic reactions. The accompanying table provides a summary of molybdenum.

Molybdenum

RDA	Significant Sources
Adult: 45 µg/day	Legumes, cereals, nuts
UL	**Deficiency Symptoms**
Adults: 2 mg/day	Unknown
Chief Functions in the Body	**Toxicity Symptoms**
Cofactor for several enzymes	None reported; reproductive effects in animals

molybdenum (mo-LIB-duh-num): an essential trace mineral that acts as a cofactor for many enzymes.

13.3 Contaminant Minerals

› LEARN IT Describe how contaminant minerals disrupt body processes and impair nutrition status.

Chapter 12 and this chapter explain the many ways minerals serve the body—maintaining fluid and electrolyte balance, providing structural support to the bones, transporting oxygen, and assisting enzymes. In contrast to the essential minerals that the body requires, contaminant minerals impair the body's growth, work capacity, and general health. Contaminant minerals include the **heavy metals** lead, mercury, and cadmium, which enter the food supply by way of soil, water, and air pollution. This section focuses on lead poisoning because it is a serious environmental threat to young children and because reducing blood lead levels in children is a goal of the Healthy People initiative. Much of the information on lead applies to the other contaminant minerals as well—they all disrupt body processes and impair nutrition status similarly.

Like other minerals, lead is indestructible; the body cannot change its chemistry. Chemically similar to nutrient minerals such as iron, calcium, and zinc (cations with two positive charges), lead displaces them from some of the metabolic sites they normally occupy so they are then unable to perform their roles. For example, lead competes with iron in heme, but it cannot carry oxygen. Similarly, lead competes with calcium in the brain, but it cannot signal messages from nerve cells. Excess lead in the blood also deranges the structure of red blood cell membranes, making them leaky and fragile. Lead interacts with white blood cells, too, impairing their ability to fight infection, and it binds to antibodies, thwarting their effort to resist disease.

Children with iron deficiency are particularly vulnerable to lead toxicity. Chapter 16 examines the damaging effects of iron deficiency and lead toxicity on a child's growth and development.[50]

› REVIEW IT Describe how contaminant minerals disrupt body processes and impair nutrition status.

Lead typifies the ways all heavy metals behave in the body: they interfere with nutrients that are trying to do their jobs. The "good guy" nutrients are shoved aside by the "bad guy" contaminants. Then, when the contaminants cannot perform the roles of the nutrients, health diminishes. To safeguard our health, we must defend ourselves against contamination by eating nutrient-rich foods and preserving a clean environment.

This chapter completes the introductory lessons on the nutrients. Each nutrient from the amino acids to zinc has been described rather thoroughly—its chemistry, roles in the body, sources in the diet, symptoms of deficiency and toxicity, and influences on health and disease. Such a detailed examination is informative, but it can also be misleading. It is important to step back from the detailed study of the individual nutrients to look at them as a whole. After all, people eat foods, not nutrients, and most foods deliver dozens of nutrients. Furthermore, nutrients work cooperatively with one another in the body; their actions are most often *inter*actions. This chapter alone mentioned how iron depends on vitamin C to keep it in its active form and copper to incorporate it into hemoglobin, how zinc is needed to activate and transport vitamin A, and how both iodine and selenium are needed for the synthesis of thyroid hormones. The table on p. 430 provides a summary of the trace minerals for your review. Highlight 13 explores the benefits of phytochemicals.

heavy metals: mineral ions such as mercury and lead, so called because they are of relatively high atomic weight. Many heavy metals are poisonous.

› REVIEW IT The Trace Minerals

Mineral and Chief Functions	Deficiency Symptoms	Toxicity Symptoms[a]	Significant Sources
Iron			
Part of the protein hemoglobin, which carries oxygen in the blood; part of the protein myoglobin in muscles, which makes oxygen available for muscle contraction; necessary for energy metabolism	Anemia: weakness, fatigue, headaches; impaired work performance; impaired immunity; pale skin, nail beds, mucous membranes, and palm creases; concave nails; inability to regulate body temperature; pica	GI distress; iron overload: infections, fatigue, joint pain, skin pigmentation, organ damage	Red meats, fish, poultry, shellfish, eggs, legumes, dried fruits
Zinc			
Part of insulin and many enzymes; involved in making genetic material and proteins, immune reactions, transport of vitamin A, taste perception, wound healing, the making of sperm, and normal fetal development	Growth retardation, delayed sexual maturation, impaired immune function, hair loss, eye and skin lesions, loss of appetite	Loss of appetite, impaired immunity, low HDL, copper and iron deficiencies	Protein-containing foods: red meats, fish, shellfish, poultry, whole grains; fortified cereals
Iodine			
A component of the thyroid hormones that help to regulate growth, development, and metabolic rate	Underactive thyroid gland, goiter, mental and physical retardation (cretinism)	Underactive thyroid gland, elevated TSH, goiter	Iodized salt; seafood; plants grown in iodine-rich soil and animals fed those plants
Selenium			
Part of an enzyme that defends against oxidation; regulates thyroid hormone	Associated with Keshan disease	Nail and hair brittleness and loss; fatigue, irritability, and nervous system disorders, skin rash, garlic breath odor	Seafoods, organ meats; other meats, whole grains, fruits, and vegetables (depending on soil content)
Copper			
Helps form hemoglobin; part of several enzymes	Anemia, bone abnormalities	Liver damage	Seafood, nuts, legumes, whole grains, seeds
Manganese			
Cofactor for several enzymes; bone formation	Rare	Nervous symptom disorders	Nuts, whole grains, leafy vegetables, tea
Fluoride			
Maintains health of bones and teeth; confers decay resistance on teeth	Susceptibility to tooth decay	Fluorosis (pitting and discoloration) of teeth	Drinking water (if fluoridated), tea, seafood
Chromium			
Enhances insulin action, may improve glucose intolerance	Diabetes-like condition	None reported	Meats (liver), whole grains, brewer's yeast
Molybdenum			
Cofactor for several enzymes	Unknown	None reported	Legumes, cereals, nuts

[a]Acute toxicities of many minerals cause abdominal pain, nausea, vomiting, and diarrhea.

Nutrition Portfolio

Trace minerals from a variety of foods, especially those in the protein foods group, support many of your body's activities. Go to Diet & Wellness Plus and choose one of the days on which you tracked your diet for an entire day. Select the Intake vs. Goals report and then consider the following questions. Remember that scoring 100 percent on this report means you met your goal.

- Your Intake vs. Goals report may only display your intake for two of the trace minerals: iron and zinc. How was your intake for these two trace minerals?

Now look at the Intake Spreadsheet report and consider the following questions:

- How often do you include meats, seafood, poultry, legumes, and enriched or fortified grain products weekly? These foods often contain trace minerals.

- What are the advantages of using iodized salt?
- Does your community provide fluoridated water?

DIET & WELLNESS **PLUS** To complete this exercise, go to your Diet & Wellness Plus at www.cengagebrain.com.

› STUDY IT To review the key points of this chapter and take a practice quiz, go to the study cards at the end of the book.

REFERENCES

1. A. Kritharis, T. P. Bradley, and D. R. Budman, The evolving use of arsenic in pharmacotherapy of malignant disease, *Annals of Hematology* 92 (2013): 719–730.
2. M. Muñoz, J. A. García-Erce, and A. F. Remacha, Disorders of iron metabolism. Part 1: Molecular basis of iron homeostasis, *Journal of Clinical Pathology* 64 (2011): 281–286; M. D. Knutson, Iron-sensing proteins that regulate hepcidin and enteric iron absorption, *Annual Review of Nutrition* 30 (2010): 149–171.
3. P. A. Sharp, Intestinal iron absorption: Regulation by dietary & systematic factors, *International Journal for Vitamin and Nutrition Research* 80 (2010): 231–242.
4. R. Collings and coauthors, The absorption of iron from whole diets: A systematic review, *American Journal of Clinical Nutrition* 98 (2013): 65–81.
5. K. E. Finberg, Unraveling mechanisms regulating systemic iron homeostasis, *American Society of Hematology Education Book* 2011 (2011): 532–537; T. Ganz and E. Nemeth, Hepcidin and disorders of iron metabolism, *Annual Review of Medicine* 62 (2011): 347–360; M. Wessling-Resnick, Iron homeostasis and the inflammatory response, *Annual Review of Nutrition* 30 (2010): 105–122.
6. T. Ganz, Hepcidin and iron regulation: 10 years later, *Blood* 117 (2011): 4425–4433; J. Kaplan, D. M. Ward, and I. De Domenico, The molecular basis of iron overload disorders and iron-linked anemias, *International Journal of Hematology* 93 (2011): 14–20; A. Pietrangelo, Hereditary hemochromatosis: Pathogenesis, diagnosis, and treatment, *Gastroenterology* 139 (2010): 393–408.
7. S. R. Lynch, Why nutritional iron deficiency persists as a worldwide problem, *Journal of Nutrition* 141 (2011): 763S–768S.
8. A. C. Cepeda-Lopez and coauthors, Sharply higher rates of iron deficiency in obese Mexican women and children are predicted by obesity-related inflammation rather than by differences in dietary iron intake, *American Journal of Clinical Nutrition* 93 (2011): 975–983.
9. L. Tussing-Humphreys and coauthors, Rethinking iron regulation and assessment in iron deficiency, anemia of chronic disease, and obesity: Introducing hepcidin, *Journal of the Academy of Nutrition and Dietetics* 112 (2012): 391–400.
10. N. Milman, Anemia: Still a major health problem in many parts of the world, *Annals of Hematology* 90 (2011): 369–377.
11. D. I. Thurnham and coauthors, Adjusting plasma ferritin concentrations to remove the effects of subclinical inflammation in the assessment of iron deficiency: A meta-analysis, *American Journal of Clinical Nutrition* 92 (2010): 546–555; M. A. Ayoya and coauthors, α_1-Acid glycoprotein, hepcidin, C-reactive protein, and serum ferritin are correlated in anemic schoolchildren with *Schistosoma haematobium*, *American Journal of Clinical Nutrition* 91 (2010): 1784–1790.
12. J. P. McClung and L. E. Murray-Kolb, Iron nutrition and premenopausl women: Effects of poor iron status on physical and neuropsychological performance, *Annual Review of Nutrition* 33 (2013): 271–288.
13. P. Vaucher and coauthors, Effect of iron supplementation on fatigue in nonanemic menstruating women with low ferritin: A randomized controlled trial, *Canadian Medical Association Journal* 184 (2012): 1247–1254.
14. L. E. Murray-Kolb, Iron status and neuropsychological consequences in women of reproductive age: What do we know and where are we headed? *Journal of Nutrition* 141 (2011): 747S–755S; K. Kordas, Iron, lead, and children's behavior and cognition, *Annual Review of Nutrition* 30 (2010): 123–148.
15. B. Lozoff, Early iron deficiency has brain and behavior effects consistent with dopaminergic dysfunction, *Journal of Nutrition* 141 (2011): 740S–746S.
16. S. L. Young, Pica in pregnancy: New ideas about an old condition, *Annual Review of Nutrition* 30 (2010): 403–422.
17. G. J. Anderson and F. Wang, Essential but toxic: Controlling the flux of iron in the body, *Clinical and Experimental Pharmacology and Physiology* 39 (2012): 719–724.
18. P. Brissot and coauthors, Molecular diagnosis of genetic iron-overload disorders, *Expert Review of Molecular Diagnostics* 10 (2010): 755–763.
19. N. C. Andrews, Closing the iron gate, *New England Journal of Medicine* 366 (2012): 376–377; C. Camaschella and E. Poggiali, Inherited disorders of iron metabolism, *Current Opinion in Pediatrics* 23 (2011): 14–20.
20. G. A. Ramm and R. G. Ruddell, Iron homeostasis, hepatocellular injury, and fibrogenesis in hemochromatosis: The role of inflammation in a noninflammatory liver disease, *Seminars in Liver Disease* 30 (2010): 271–287.
21. X. Zheng and coauthors, Hepatic iron stores are increased as assessed by magnetic resonance imaging in a Chinese population with altered glucose homeostasis, *American Journal of Clinical Nutrition* 94 (2011): 1012–1019.
22. R. E. Fleming and P. Ponka, Iron overload in human disease, *New England Journal of Medicine* 366 (2012): 348–359; G. M. Brittenham, Iron-chelating therapy for transfusional iron overload, *New England Journal of Medicine* 364 (2011): 146–156.
23. C. Camaschella, Treating iron overload, *New England Journal of Medicine* 368 (2013): 2325–2327.
24. N. Ahluwalia and coauthors, Iron status is associated with carotid atherosclerotic plaques in middle-aged adults, *Journal of Nutrition* 140 (2010): 812–816.
25. A. C. Bronstein and coauthors, 2009 Annual Report of the American Association of Poison Control Centers' National Poison Data System (NPDS): 27th Annual Report, *Clinical Toxicology* 28 (2010): 979–1178.
26. J. C. King, Zinc: An essential but elusive nutrient, *American Journal of Clinical Nutrition* 94 (2011): 679S–684S.
27. J. R. Hunt, Algorithms for iron and zinc bioavailability: Are they accurate? *International Journal of Vitamin and Nutrition Research* 80 (2010): 257–262; J. C. King, Does zinc absorption reflect zinc status? *International Journal of Vitamin and Nutrition Research* 80 (2010): 300–306.
28. K. M. Hambidge and coauthors, Zinc bioavailability and homeostasis, *American Journal of Clinical Nutrition* 91 (2010): 1478S–1483S.
29. A. S. Prasad, Discovery of human zinc deficiency: Its impact on human health and disease, *Advances in Nutrition* 4 (2013): 176–190.
30. J. B. Barnett, D. H. Hamer, and S. N. Meydani, Low zinc status: A new risk factor for pneumonia in the elderly? *Nutrition Reviews* 68 (2010): 30–37.
31. M. E. Penny, Zinc supplementation in public health, *Annals of Nutrition and Metabolism* 62 (2013): 31–42.

32. M. Science and coauthors, Zinc for the treatment of the common cold: A systematic review and meta-analysis of randomized controlled trials, *Canadian Medical Association Journal* 184 (2012): E551–E561.
33. G. A. Eby, Zinc lozenges as cure for the common cold—A review and hypothesis, *Medical Hypotheses* 74 (2010): 482–492.
34. M. Singh and R. R. Das, Zinc for the common cold, *Cochrane Database of Systemic Reviews* 6 (2013): CD001364.
35. M. Andersson, V. Karumbunathan, and M. B. Zimmerman, Global iodine status in 2011 and trends over the past decade, *Journal of Nutrition* 142 (2012): 744–750.
36. A. Stagnaro-Green, S. Sullivan, and E. N. Pearce, Iodine supplementation during pregnancy and lactation, *Journal of the American Medical Association* 308 (2012): 2463–2464; C. G. Perrine and coauthors, Some subgroups of reproductive age women in the United States may be at risk for iodine deficiency, *Journal of Nutrition* 140 (2010): 1489–1494.
37. GAIN-UNICEF Universal Salt Iodization Partnership Program, www.gainhealth.org/programs/USI, accessed January 2014.
38. S. J. Fairweather-Tait and coauthors, Selenium in human health and disease, *Antioxidants and Redox Signaling* 4 (2011): 1337–1383.
39. C. Lei and coauthors, Is selenium deficiency really the cause of Keshan disease? *Environmental Geochemistry and Health* 33 (2011): 183–188; J. Yang and coauthors, Selenium level surveillance for the year 2007 of Keshan disease in endemic areas and analysis on surveillance results between 2003 and 2007, *Biological Trace Element Research* 138 (2010): 53–59.
40. S. Sun, Chronic exposure to cereal mycotoxin likely citreoviridin may be a trigger for Keshan disease mainly through oxidative stress mechanism, *Medical Hypotheses* 74 (2010): 841–842.
41. M. P. Rayman, Selenium and human health, *Lancet* 379 (2012): 1256–1268.
42. C. D. Davis, P. A. Tsuji, and J. A. Milner, Selenoproteins and cancer prevention, *Annual Review of Nutrition* 32 (2012): 73–95; R. Hurst and coauthors, Selenium and prostate cancer: Systematic review and meta-analysis, *American Journal of Clinical Nutrition* 96 (2012): 111–122; G. Dennert and coauthors, Selenium for preventing cancer, *Cochrane Database of Systematic Reviews* 5 (2011): CD005195; S. J. Fairweather-Tait and coauthors, Selenium in human health and disease, *Antioxidants and Redox Signaling* 14 (2011): 1337–1383.
43. B. K. Dunn and coauthors, A nutrient approach to prostate cancer prevention: The Selenium and Vitamin E Cancer Prevention Trial (SELECT), *Nutrition and Cancer* 62 (2010): 896–918; J. Brozmanová and coauthors, Selenium: A double-edged sword for defense and offence in cancer, *Archives of Toxicology* 84 (2010): 919–938.
44. D. L. de Romaña and coauthors, Risks and benefits of copper in light of new insights of copper homeostasis, *Journal of Trace Elements in Medicine and Biology* 25 (2011): 3–13.
45. 2012 Water Fluoridation Statistics, www.cdc.gov/fluoridation/statistics/2012stats.htm, updated November 22, 2013.
46. Position of the Academy of Nutrition and Dietetics: The impact of fluoride on health, *Journal of the Academy of Nutrition and Dietetics* 112 (2012): 1443–1453.
47. E. D. Beltrán-Aguilar, L. Barker, and B. A. Dye, Prevalence and severity of dental fluorosis in the United States, *NCHS Data Brief* 53 (2010): 1–8.
48. M. A. Buzalaf and S. M. Levy, Fluoride intake of children: Considerations for dental caries and dental fluorosis, *Monographs in Oral Science* 22 (2011): 1–19.
49. Y. Hua and coauthors, Molecular mechanisms of chromium in alleviating insulin resistance, *Journal of Nutritional Biochemistry* 23 (2012): 313–319; Z. Q. Wang and W. T. Cefalu, Current concepts about chromium supplementation in type 2 diabetes and insulin resistance, *Current Diabetes Reports* 10 (2010): 145–151.
50. C. Warniment, K. Tsang, and S. S. Galazka, Lead poisoning in children, *American Family Physician* 81 (2010): 751–757.

HIGHLIGHT > 13
Phytochemicals and Functional Foods

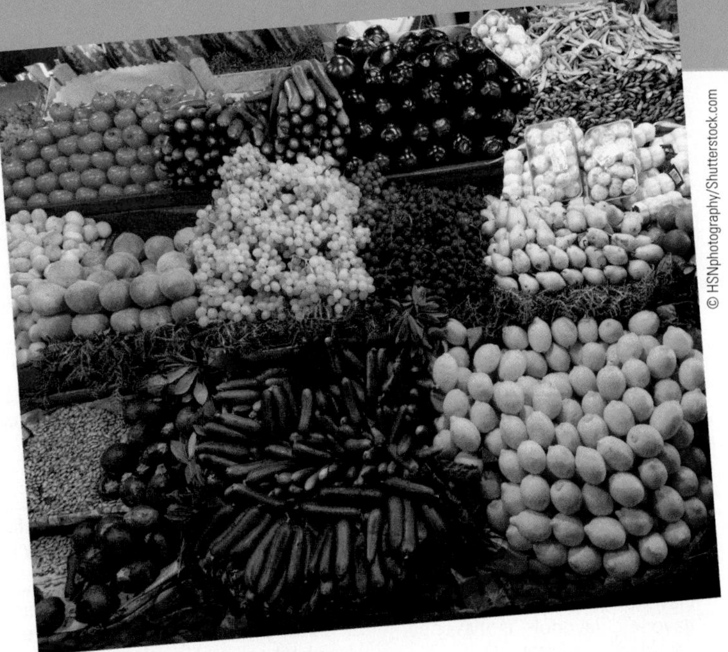
© HSNphotography/Shutterstock.com

› LEARN IT Define *phytochemicals* and explain how they might defend against chronic diseases.

Chapter 13 completes the introductory lessons on the six classes of nutrients—carbohydrates, lipids, proteins, vitamins, minerals, and water. In addition to these nutrients, foods contain thousands of other compounds, including the **phytochemicals.** Chapter 1 introduces the phytochemicals as compounds found in plant-derived foods that have biological activity in the body. Research on phytochemicals is unfolding daily, adding to our knowledge of their roles in human health, but there are still many questions and only tentative answers. Just a few of the tens of thousands of phytochemicals have been researched at all, and only a sampling are mentioned in this highlight—enough to illustrate their wide variety of food sources and roles in supporting health.

The concept that foods provide health benefits beyond those of the nutrients emerged from numerous epidemiological studies showing the protective effects of plant-based diets on cancer and heart disease. People have been using foods to maintain health and prevent disease for years, but now these foods have been given a name—they are called **functional foods.**[1] (The accompanying glossary defines this and other terms.) As Chapter 1 explains, functional foods include all foods (whole, fortified, enriched, or enhanced foods) that have a potentially beneficial effect on health.[2] Much of this text touts the benefits of nature's functional foods—whole grains rich in dietary fibers, oily fish rich in omega-3 fatty acids, and fresh fruits rich in phytochemicals, for example. This highlight begins with a look at some of these familiar functional foods, the phytochemicals they contain, and their roles in disease prevention. Then the discussion turns to examine the most controversial of functional foods—novel foods to which phytochemicals have been added to promote health. How these foods fit into a healthy diet is still unclear.

The Phytochemicals

In foods, phytochemicals impart tastes, aromas, colors, and other characteristics. They give hot peppers their burning sensation, garlic its pungent flavor, and tomatoes their red color. In the body, phytochemicals can have profound physiological effects—acting as antioxidants, mimicking hormones, stimulating enzymes, interfering with DNA replication, suppressing inflammation, destroying bacteria, and binding to cell walls. Any of these actions may prevent the development of chronic diseases, depending in part on how genetic factors interact with the phytochemicals. Phytochemicals might also have adverse effects when consumed in excess. Table H13-1 (p. 434) presents the names, possible effects, and food sources of some of the better-known phytochemicals.

Defending against Cancer

A variety of phytochemicals from a variety of foods appear to protect against DNA damage and defend the body against cancer. A few examples follow.

GLOSSARY

carotenoids (kah-ROT-eh-noyds): pigments commonly found in plants and animals, some of which have vitamin A activity. The carotenoid with the greatest vitamin A activity is beta-carotene.

flavonoids (FLAY-von-oyds): yellow pigments in foods; phytochemicals that may exert physiological effects on the body.

flaxseeds: the small brown seeds of the flax plant; valued in nutrition as a source of fiber, lignans, and omega-3 fatty acids.

functional foods: foods that have a potentially beneficial effect on health when consumed as part of a varied diet on a regular basis at effective levels.

lignans: phytochemicals present in flaxseed that are converted to phytosterols by intestinal bacteria and are under study as possible anticancer agents.

lutein (LOO-teen): a plant pigment of yellow hue; a phytochemical believed to play roles in eye functioning and health.

lycopene (LYE-koh-peen): a pigment responsible for the red color of tomatoes and other red-hued vegetables; a phytochemical that may act as an antioxidant in the body.

phytochemicals: nonnutrient compounds found in plants. Some phytochemicals have biological activity in the body.

- **phyto** = plant

phytoestrogens: phytochemicals structurally similar to human estrogen that weakly mimic or modulate estrogen's action in the body. Phytoestrogens include the isoflavones *genistein, daidzein,* and *glycitein.*

plant sterols: phytochemicals that have structural similarities to cholesterol and lower blood cholesterol by interfering with cholesterol absorption. Plant sterols include *sterol esters* and *stanol esters.*

TABLE H13-1 **Phytochemicals—Their Food Sources and Actions**

Name	Possible Effects	Food Sources
Alkylresorcinols (phenolic lipids)	May contribute to the protective effect of grains in reducing the risks of diabetes, heart disease, and some cancers.	Whole-grain wheat and rye
Allicin (organosulfur compound)	Antimicrobial that may reduce ulcers; may lower blood cholesterol.	Chives, garlic, leeks, onions, scallions
Capsaicin	Modulates blood clotting, possibly reducing the risk of fatal clots in heart and artery disease.	Hot peppers
Carotenoids (including beta-carotene, lycopene, lutein, zeaxanthin, and hundreds of related compounds)	Act as antioxidants, possibly reducing risks of cancer and other diseases.	Deeply pigmented fruits and vegetables (apricots, broccoli, cantaloupe, carrots, pink grapefruit, pumpkin, spinach, sweet potatoes, tomatoes, red peppers, watermelon)
Curcumin (polyphenol)	Acts as an antioxidant and anti-inflammatory agent; may reduce blood clot formation; may inhibit enzymes that activate carcinogens.	Turmeric, a yellow-colored spice common in curry powder
Flavonoids (including anthocyanins, flavones, flavonols, isoflavones, catechins, and others)	Act as antioxidants; scavenge carcinogens; bind to nitrates in the stomach, preventing conversion to nitrosamines; inhibit cell proliferation.	Berries, black tea, celery, citrus fruits, green tea, olives, onions, oregano, purple grapes, purple grape juice, soybeans and soy products, vegetables, whole wheat, wine
Genistein and daidzein (isoflavonoids)	Phytoestrogens that inhibit cell replication in GI tract; may reduce risk of breast, colon, ovarian, prostate, and other estrogen-sensitive cancers; may reduce cancer cell survival; may reduce risk of osteoporosis.	Soybeans, soy flour, soy milk, tofu, textured vegetable protein, other legume products
Indoles (organosulfur compound)	May trigger production of enzymes that block DNA damage from carcinogens; may inhibit estrogen action.	Cruciferous vegetables such as bok choy, broccoli, brussels sprouts, cabbage, cauliflower, collard greens, mustard greens, kale, swiss chard, watercress
Isothiocyanates (organosulfur compounds, including sulforaphane)	Act as antioxidants; inhibit enzymes that activate carcinogens; activate enzymes that detoxify carcinogens; may reduce risk of breast cancer, prostate cancer, and colorectal cancer.	Cruciferous vegetables such as bok choy, broccoli, broccoli sprouts, brussels sprouts, cabbage, cauliflower, collard greens, mustard greens, kale, swiss chard, watercress
Lignans (polyphenol)	Phytoestrogens that block estrogen activity in cells possibly reducing the risk of cancer of the breast, colon, ovaries, and prostate.	Flaxseed, whole grains
Monoterpenes (including limonene)	May trigger enzyme production to detoxify carcinogens; inhibit cancer promotion and cell proliferation.	Citrus fruits, cherries
Phenolic acids (including ellagic acid)	May trigger enzyme production to make carcinogens water soluble, facilitating excretion.	Coffee beans, fruits (apples, blueberries, cherries, grapes, oranges, pears, prunes), oats, potatoes, soybeans
Phytic acid (phenolic acid)	Binds to minerals, preventing free-radical formation, possibly reducing cancer risk.	Whole grains
Resveratrol (flavonoid)	Acts as an antioxidant; may inhibit cancer growth; reduce inflammation, LDL oxidation, and blood clot formation.	Red wine, peanuts, grapes, raspberries
Saponins (glucosides)	May interfere with DNA replication, preventing cancer cells from multiplying; stimulate immune response.	Alfalfa sprouts, other sprouts, green vegetables, potatoes, tomatoes
Tannins (flavonoid)	Act as antioxidants; may inhibit carcinogen activation and cancer promotion.	Black-eyed peas, grapes, lentils, red and white wine, tea

Soy may protect against breast and prostate cancers.[3] Soybeans—as well as other legumes, **flaxseeds,** whole grains, fruits, and vegetables—are a rich source of an array of phytochemicals, among them the **phytoestrogens.** Because the chemical structure of phytoestrogens is similar to the hormone estrogen, they can weakly mimic or modulate the effects of estrogen in the body. They also have antioxidant activity that appears to slow the growth of some cancers. Soy foods appear to be most effective when consumed in moderation early and throughout life.[4] Importantly, soy extracts and phytoestrogen supplements are ill-advised—especially for women with breast cancer and those with high risk factors—as phytoestrogens may promote the growth of estrogen-dependent tumors (such as breast cancer).[5] The American Cancer Society recommends that women with breast cancer should consume only *moderate* amounts of soy as part of a healthy plant-based diet and should not intentionally ingest high levels of soy or supplements of phytoestrogens.

Limited evidence suggests that tomatoes may offer protection against some cancers.[6] Among the phytochemicals thought to be responsible for this effect is **lycopene,** one of the many **carotenoids.**[7] Lycopene is the pigment that gives apricots, guava, papaya, pink grapefruits, and watermelon their red color—and it is especially abundant in tomatoes. Because food processing and cooking can improve carotenoid absorption, cooked tomato products, such as spaghetti sauce, provide even more lycopene. Lycopene is a powerful antioxidant that seems to inhibit the growth of cancer cells. Importantly, the benefits of lycopene have been seen when people have eaten *foods* containing lycopene; lycopene supplements may interfere with cancer treatments.[8]

Soybeans and tomatoes are only two of the many fruits and vegetables credited with providing anticancer activity. Strong and convincing evidence shows that the risk of many cancers, and perhaps of cancer in general, decreases when diets include an abundance of fruits and vegetables.[9] To that end, current recommendations urge consumers to eat five to nine servings of fruits and vegetables a day.

Defending against Heart Disease

Diets based primarily on unprocessed foods appear to support heart health better than those founded on highly refined foods—perhaps because of the abundance of nutrients, fiber, or phytochemicals such as the **flavonoids.** Flavonoids, a large group of phytochemicals known for their health-promoting qualities, are found in whole grains, legumes, soy, vegetables, fruits, herbs, spices, teas, chocolate, nuts, olive oil, and red wines.[10] Flavonoids are powerful antioxidants that may help to protect LDL cholesterol against oxidation, minimize inflammation, and reduce blood platelet stickiness, thereby slowing the progression of atherosclerosis and making blood clots less likely. Whereas an abundance of flavonoid-containing *foods* in the diet may lower the risks of chronic diseases, no claims can be made for flavonoids themselves as the protective factor, particularly when they are extracted from foods and sold as supplements. In fact, purified flavonoids may even be harmful.[11]

In addition to flavonoids, fruits and vegetables are rich in carotenoids such as beta-carotene and **lutein.** Studies suggest that a diet rich in carotenoids may lower the risk of heart disease by decreasing inflammation and oxidative stress.[12]

The **plant sterols** of soy and the **lignans** of flaxseed may also protect against heart disease. These cholesterol-like molecules are naturally found in all plants and inhibit cholesterol absorption in the body. As a result, blood cholesterol levels decline.[13] These phytochemicals also seem to protect against heart disease by reducing inflammation and lowering blood pressure.[14]

Defending against Other Diseases

Most research on phytochemicals has focused on cancer and heart disease, but phytochemicals defend against other diseases as well. The orange-yellow pigment curcumin, commonly found in curry powder, may help reverse insulin resistance, inflammation, and other symptoms associated with obesity.[15] The carotenoids lutein and zeaxanthin may protect the eyes and skin from ultraviolet light damage and the bones from mineral loss.[16]

The Phytochemicals in Perspective

Because foods deliver thousands of phytochemicals in addition to dozens of nutrients, researchers must be careful in giving credit for particular health benefits to any one compound. Diets rich in whole grains, legumes, vegetables, fruits, and nuts seem to protect against heart disease and cancer, but identifying *the* specific foods or components of foods that are responsible is difficult. Each food possesses a unique array of phytochemicals—citrus fruits provide monoterpenes; grapes, resveratrol; and flaxseed, lignans. (Review Table H13-1, p. 434, for the possible effects and other food sources of these phytochemicals.) Broccoli may contain as many as 10,000 different phytochemicals—each with the potential to influence some action in the body. Beverages such as wine, spices such as oregano, and oils such as olive oil (especially virgin olive oil) contain many phytochemicals that may explain, in part, why people who eat a traditional Mediterranean diet have reduced risks of heart disease and cancer. Phytochemicals might also explain why the DASH diet is so effective in lowering blood pressure and blood lipids. Even identifying all of the phytochemicals and their effects doesn't answer all the questions because the actions of phytochemicals may be complementary or overlapping—which reinforces the principle of variety in diet planning. For an appreciation of the array of phytochemicals offered by a variety of foods, see Figure H13-1 (p. 436).

Functional Foods

Because foods naturally contain thousands of phytochemicals that are biologically active in the body, virtually all of them have some value in supporting health.[17] In other words, even simple, whole foods, in reality, are functional foods. Cranberries may help prevent urinary tract infections; garlic may lower blood cholesterol; grapes may reduce inflammation; and green tea may protect against nonalcoholic fatty liver disease, just to name a few examples.[18] Functional foods rich in phytochemicals are easy to find in the produce section of grocery stores. Just look for the colorful fruits and vegetables (see Table H13-2, p. 437). But food manufacturers continue to create new functional foods as well.

Many processed foods become functional foods when they are fortified with nutrients or enhanced with phytochemicals or herbs (calcium-fortified orange juice, for example). Less frequently, an entirely new food is created, as in the case of a meat substitute made of mycoprotein—a protein derived from a fungus.* This functional food not only provides dietary fiber, polyunsaturated fats, and high-quality protein, but it also lowers LDL cholesterol, raises HDL cholesterol, improves glucose response, and prolongs satiety after a meal. Such a novel functional food raises the question—is it a food or a drug?

*This mycoprotein product is marketed under the trade name Quorn (pronounced KWORN).

> **FIGURE H13-1 An Array of Phytochemicals in a Variety of Foods and Beverages**

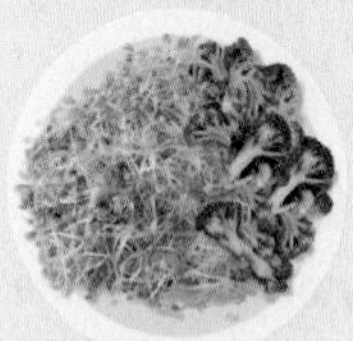
Broccoli and broccoli sprouts (and brussels sprouts, bok choy, cabbage, cauliflower, kale, collard greens, swiss chard, turnips, and watercress) contain an abundance of the cancer-fighting phytochemicals sulforaphane and indoles.

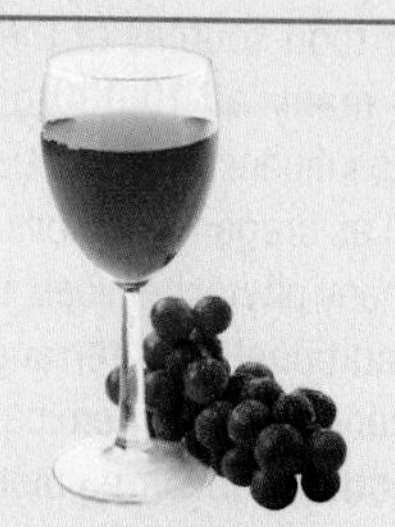
The phytochemical resveratrol found in grapes (and nuts) protects against cancer by inhibiting cell growth and against heart disease by limiting clot formation and inflammation.

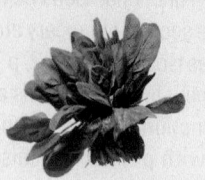

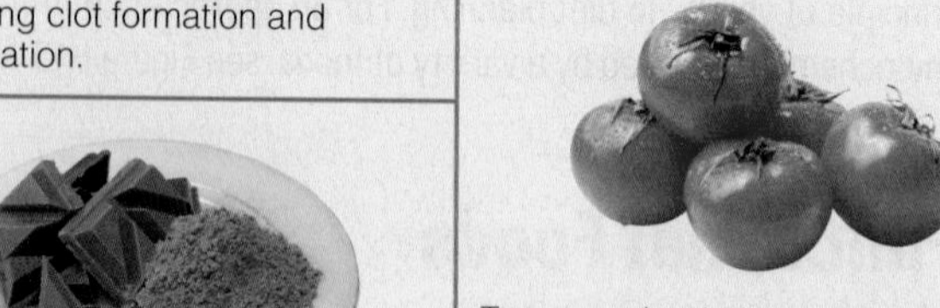
The flavonoids in cocoa and chocolate defend against oxidation and reduce the tendency of blood to clot.

Spinach (and collard greens, corn, swiss chard, and winter squash) contains the carotenoids lutein and zeaxanthin, which help protect the eyes against macular degeneration.

An apple a day—rich in phenolic acids—may protect against heart disease.

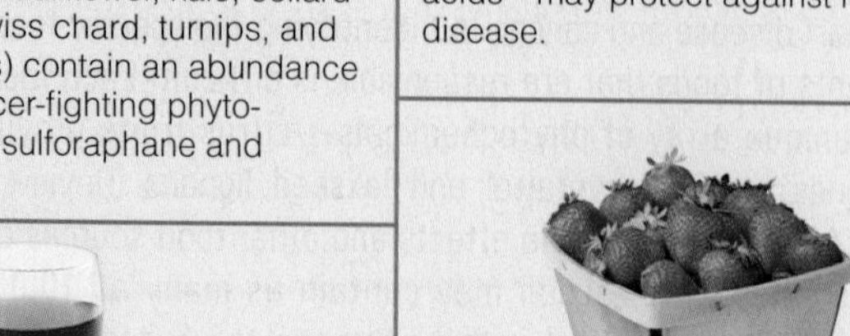
The ellagic acid of strawberries (and blackberries, blueberries, raspberries, and grapes) may inhibit certain types of cancer and decrease cholesterol levels.

Tomatoes (and pink grapefruit, red peppers, and watermelons), with their abundant lycopene, may defend against cancer and heart disease by protecting DNA from oxidative damage.

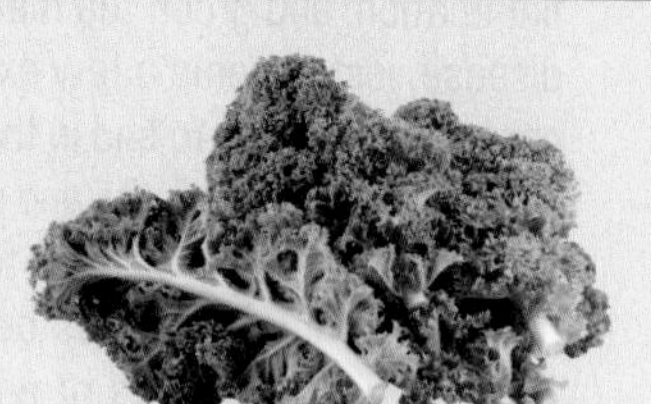
Quercetins—commonly found in kale (and onions, pears, and grapes)—reduce inflammation from allergies, inhibit tumor growth, and protect the lungs.

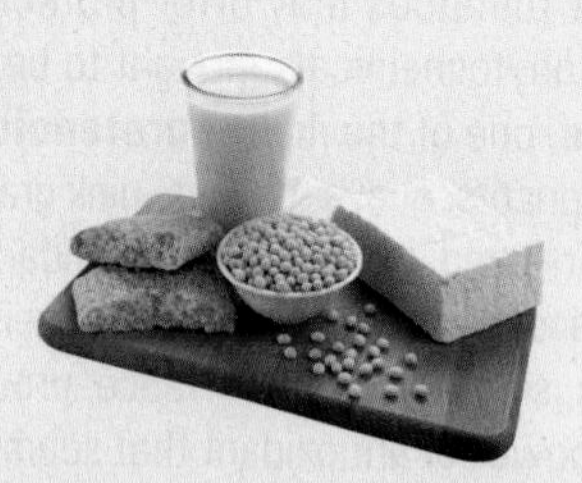
The phytoestrogens of soybeans seem to starve cancer cells and inhibit tumor growth; the plant sterols may lower blood cholesterol and protect cardiac arteries.

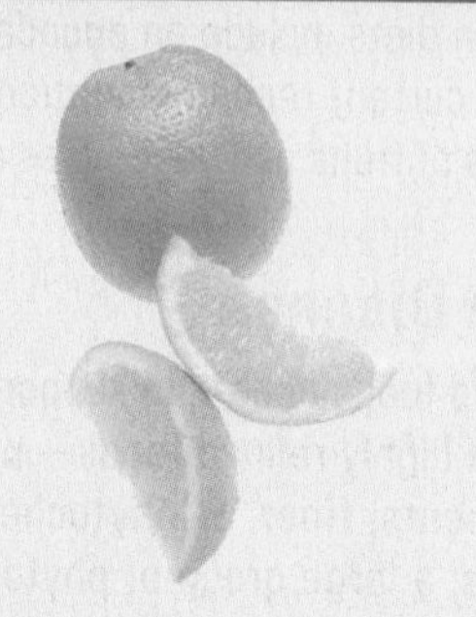
The monoterpenes of citrus fruits (and cherries) may protect the lungs.

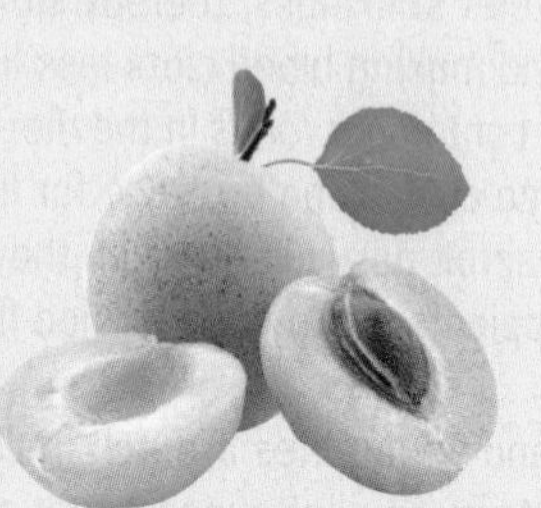
Colorful foods such as apricots (and cantaloupes, carrots, kale, kiwifruit, mangoes, papaya, pumpkins, spinach, sweet potatoes, and winter squash) contain beta-carotene, which may help slow aging, protect against some cancers, improve lung function, and reduce complications of diabetes.

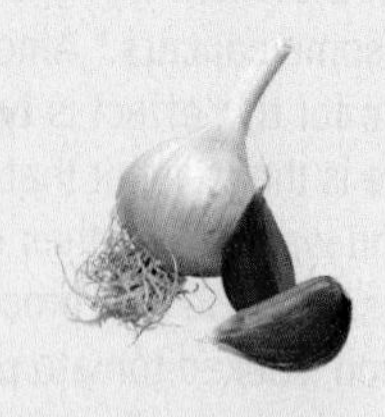
Garlic (and chives, leeks, onions, and scallions), with its abundant organosulfur compounds, may lower blood cholesterol and blood pressure and protect against stomach cancer.

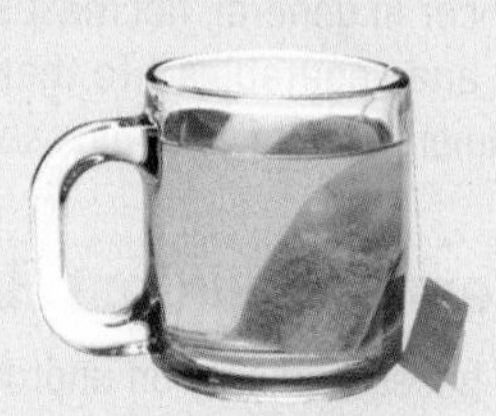
The flavonoids in black tea may protect against heart disease, whereas those in green tea may defend against cancer.

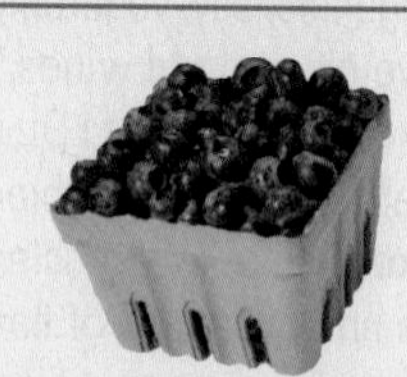
Blueberries (and cherries, plums, and strawberries), a rich source of anthocyanins, may protect against the effects of aging.

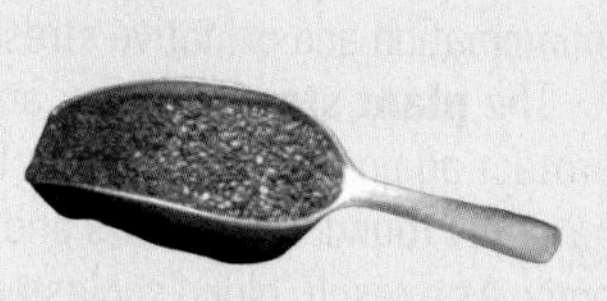
Flaxseed, the richest source of lignans, may prevent the spread of cancer.

TABLE H13-2 **The Colors of Foods Rich in Phytochemicals**

Red	White-Brown	Orange-Yellow	Blue-Purple	Green
Anthocyanins Lycopene	Allicin Allyl sulfides	Beta-carotene Limonene	Anthocyanins Ellagic acid Phenolics	Beta-carotene Lutein Indoles
Beets Cherries Cranberries Pink grapefruit Pomegranates Radicchio Radishes Raspberries Red apples Red peppers Red potatoes Rhubarb Strawberries Tomatoes Watermelon	Bananas Brown pears Cauliflower Chives Dates Garlic Ginger Leeks Mushrooms Onions Parsnips Shallots Turnips	Apricots Cantaloupe Carrots Lemons Mangoes Nectarines Oranges Papayas Peaches Persimmons Pineapple Pumpkin Rutabagas Squash Sweet potatoes Tangerines Yellow peppers	Black currants Blackberries Blueberries Dried plums Eggplant Elderberries Plums Purple figs Purple peppers Raisins Purple cabbage Purple grapes	Artichokes Arugula Asparagus Avocados Broccoli Brussels sprouts Cabbage Celery Cucumbers Endive Green apples Green beans Green grapes Green onions Green pears Green peppers Honeydew melon Kiwifruit Leafy greens Limes Okra Peas Snow peas Spinach Sugar snap peas Watercress Zucchini

Foods as Pharmacy

Hippocrates is credited with saying, "Let food be thy medicine and medicine be thy food." This simple message, uttered thousands of years ago, recognizes how good food supports good health.

Not too long ago, most of us could agree on what was a food and what was a drug. Today, functional foods blur the distinctions. They have characteristics similar to both foods and drugs, but do not fit neatly into either category. Consider margarine, for example.

Eating nonhydrogenated margarine sparingly instead of butter generously may lower blood cholesterol slightly over several months and clearly falls into the food category. Taking a statin drug, on the other hand, lowers blood cholesterol significantly within weeks and clearly falls into the drug category. But margarine enhanced with a plant sterol that lowers blood cholesterol is in a gray area between the two. The margarine looks and tastes like a food, but it acts like a drug.

The use of functional foods as drugs creates a whole new set of diet-planning challenges. Not only must foods provide an adequate intake of all the nutrients to support good health, but they must also deliver druglike ingredients to protect against disease. Like drugs used to treat chronic diseases, functional foods may need to be eaten several times a day for several months or even years to have a beneficial effect. Sporadic users may be disappointed in the results. Margarine enriched with 2 to 3 grams of plant sterols may reduce cholesterol by up to 15 percent, much more than regular margarine does, but not nearly as much as the more than 30 percent reduction seen with cholesterol-lowering drugs. For this reason, functional foods may be

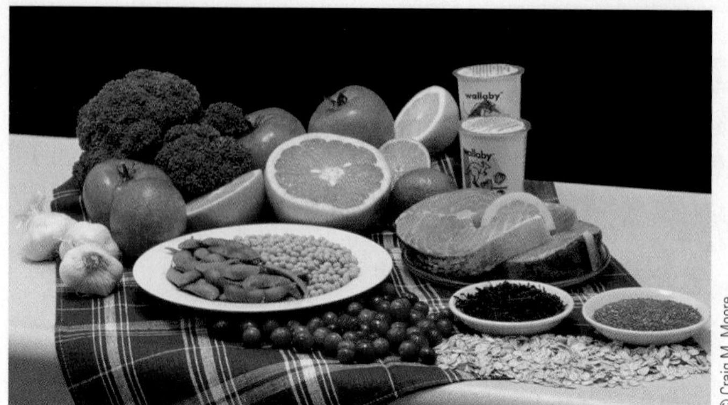

© Craig M. Moore

Nature offers a variety of functional foods that provide us with many health benefits.

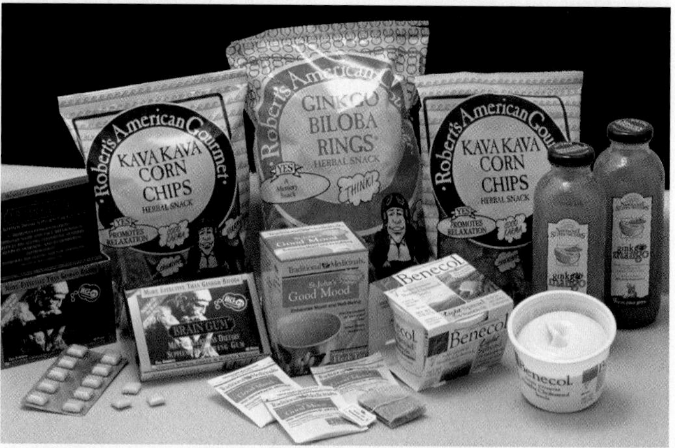

© Craig M. Moore

Functional foods currently on the market promise to "enhance mood," "promote relaxation and good karma," "increase alertness," and "improve memory," among other claims.

more useful for prevention and mild cases of disease than for intervention and more severe cases. In any case, because prescription medicines are so much more effective and because people respond to plant sterols so differently, consumers should always make treatment decisions in consultation with their health care providers.[19]

Foods and drugs differ dramatically in cost as well. Functional foods such as fruits and vegetables incur no added costs, but foods that have been manufactured with added phytochemicals can be expensive, costing up to six times as much as their conventional counterparts. The price of functional foods typically falls between that of traditional foods and medicines.

Unanswered Questions

To achieve a desired health effect, which is the better choice: to eat a novel functional food created to affect a specific body function or to adjust the diet? Does it make more sense to use a margarine enhanced with a plant sterol that lowers blood cholesterol or simply to limit the amount of butter eaten?* Is it smarter to eat eggs enriched with omega-3 fatty acids or to restrict egg consumption? Might functional foods offer a sensible solution for improving our nation's health—if done correctly? Perhaps so, but the problem is that the food industry moves faster than either scientists or the Food and Drug Administration. Consumers were able to buy soup with St. John's wort that claimed to enhance mood and fruit juice with echinacea that was supposed to fight colds while scientists were still conducting their studies on these ingredients. Research to determine the safety and effectiveness of these substances is still in progress. Until this work is complete, consumers are on their own in finding answers to the following questions:

- *Does it work?* Research is generally lacking and findings are often inconclusive.
- *How much does it contain?* Food labels are not required to list the quantities of added phytochemicals. Even if they were, consumers have no standard for comparison and cannot deduce whether the amounts listed are a little or a lot. Most importantly, until research is complete, food manufacturers do not know what amounts (if any) are most effective—or most toxic.
- *Is it safe?* Functional foods can act like drugs. They contain ingredients that can alter body functions and cause allergies, drug interactions, drowsiness, and other side effects. Yet, unlike drug labels, food labels do not provide instructions for the dosage, frequency, or duration of treatment.
- *Is it healthy?* Adding phytochemicals to a food does not magically make it a healthy choice. A candy bar fortified with phytochemicals is still made mostly of sugar and fat.

Critics suggest that the designation "functional foods" may be nothing more than a marketing tool. After all, even the most experienced researchers cannot yet identify the perfect combination of nutrients and phytochemicals to support optimal health. Yet manufacturers are freely experimenting with various concoctions as if they possessed that knowledge. Is it okay for them to sprinkle phytochemicals on fried snack foods or caramel candies and label them "functional," thus implying health benefits?

Future Foods

Nature has elegantly designed foods to provide us with a complex array of dozens of nutrients and thousands of additional compounds that may benefit health—most of which we have yet to identify or understand. Over the years, we have taken those foods, deconstructed them, and then reconstructed them in an effort to "improve" them. With new scientific understandings of how nutrients—and the myriad other compounds in foods—interact with genes, we may someday be able to design *specific* eating patterns to meet the *exact* health needs of *each* individual. Indeed, our knowledge of the human genome and of human nutrition may well merge to allow specific recommendations for individuals based on their predisposition to diet-related diseases.

*Margarine products that lower blood cholesterol contain either sterol esters from vegetable oils, soybeans, and corn or stanol esters from wood pulp.

If the present trend continues, someday physicians may be able to prescribe the perfect foods to enhance your health, and farmers will be able to grow them. As Highlight 19 explains, scientists have already developed gene technology to alter the composition of food crops. They can grow rice enriched with vitamin A and tomatoes containing a hepatitis vaccine, for example. It seems quite likely that foods can be created to meet every possible human need. But then, in a sense, that was largely true 100 years ago when we relied on the bounty of nature.

CRITICAL THINKING QUESTIONS

A. Which is the better choice—to eat processed foods that have been enhanced with phytochemicals or to eat natural foods that are rich in phytochemicals?

B. Some research suggests that cranberries may help prevent urinary tract infections, but what about cranberry supplements? Limited research suggests that *foods* rich in phytoestrogens may benefit heart, bone, breast, and menopausal health, but *phytoestrogen supplements* or *phytoestrogen-enhanced functional foods* are not recommended, particularly for women at high risk of breast cancer. How can you determine whether a phytochemical and/or functional food offers a safe and sensible solution to improving your health?

REFERENCES

1. W. R. Kapsak and coauthors, Functional foods: Consumer attitudes, perceptions, and behaviors in a growing market, *Journal of the American Dietetic Association* 111 (2011): 804–810.
2. Position of the Academy of Nutrition and Dietetics: Functional foods, *Journal of the Academy of Nutrition and Dietetics* 113 (2013): 1096–1103.
3. D. C. Vitale and coauthors, Isoflavones: Estrogenic activity, biological effect and bioavailability, *European Journal of Metabolism and Pharmacokinetics* 38 (2013): 15–25; M. Adjakly and coauthors, Genistein and daidzein: Different molecular effects on prostate cancer, *Anticancer Research* 33 (2013): 39–44; P. L. de Souza and coauthors, Clinical pharmacology of isoflavones and its relevance for potential prevention of prostate cancer, *Nutrition Reviews* 68 (2010): 542–555.
4. L. Hilakivi-Clarke, J. E. Andrade, and W. Helferich, Is soy consumption good or bad for the breast? *Journal of Nutrition* 140 (2010): 2326S–2334S.
5. S. Andres and coauthors, Risks and benefits of dietary isoflavones for cancer, *Critical Reviews in Toxicology* 41 (2011): 463–506.
6. N. P. Gullet and coauthors, Cancer prevention with natural compounds, *Seminars in Oncology* 37 (2010): 258–281.
7. J. Talvas and coauthors, Differential effects of lycopene consumed in tomato paste and lycopene in the form of a purified extract on target genes of cancer prostatic cells, *American Journal of Clinical Nutrition* 91 (2010): 1716–1724.
8. B. Cassileth, Lycopene, *Oncology* 24 (2010): 296.
9. T. J. Key, Fruit and vegetables and cancer risk, *British Journal of Cancer* 104 (2011): 6–11; J. M. Matés and coauthors, Anticancer antioxidant regulatory functions of phytochemicals, *Current Medicinal Chemistry* 18 (2011): 2315–2338.
10. O. K. Chun and coauthors, Estimation of antioxidant intakes from diet and supplements in US adults, *Journal of Nutrition* 140 (2010): 317–324.
11. S. Egert and G. Rimbach, Which sources of flavonoids: Complex diets or dietary supplements? *Advances in Nutrition* 2 (2011): 8–14.
12. G. Riccioni and coauthors, Novel phytonutrient contributors to antioxidant protection against cardiovascular disease, *Nutrition* 28 (2012): 605–610; P. Giordano and coauthors, Carotenoids and cardiovascular risk, *Current Pharmaceutical Design* 18 (2012): 5577–5589.
13. M. A. Shaghaghi, S. S. Abumweis, and P. J. H. Jones, Cholesterol-lowering efficacy of plant sterols/stanols provided in capsule and tablet formats: Results of a systematic review and meta-analysis, *Journal of the Academy of Nutrition and Dietetics* 113 (2013): 1494–1503; S. R. Eussen and coauthors, Dose-dependent cholesterol-lowering effects of phytosterol/phytostanol-enriched margarine in statin users and statin non-users under free-living conditions, *Public Health Nutrition* 14 (2011): 1823–1832; R. P. Mensink and coauthors, Plant stanols deose-dependently decrease LDL-cholesterol concentrations, but not cholesterol-standardized fat-soluble antioxidant concentrations, at intakes up to 9 g/d, *American Journal of Clinical Nutrition* 92 (2010): 24–33; S. B. Racette and coauthors, Dose effects of dietary phytosterols on cholesterol metabolism: A controlled feeding study, *American Journal of Clinical Nutrition* 91 (2010): 32–38.
14. R. A. Othman and M. H. Moghadasian, Beyond cholesterol-lowering effects of plant sterols: Clinical and experimental evidence of anti-inflammatory properties, *Nutrition Reviews* 69 (2011): 371–382.
15. B. B. Aggarwal, Targeting inflammation-induced obesity and metabolic diseases by curcumin and other nutraceuticals, *Annual Review of Nutrition* 30 (2010): 173–199; L. Alappat and A. B. Awad, Curcumin and obesity: Evidence and mechanisms, *Nutrition Reviews* 68 (2010): 729–738.
16. S. M. Abdel-Aal and coauthors, Dietary sources of lutein and zeaxanthin carotenoids and their role in eye health, *Nutrients* 5 (2013): 1169–1185.
17. A. S. Chang, B. Y. Yeong, and W. P. Koh, Symposium on plant polyphenols: Nutrition, health and innovations, June 2009, *Nutrition Reviews* 68 (2010): 246–252.
18. K. Ried, C. Toben, and P. Fakler, Effect of garlic on serum lipids: An updated meta-analysis, *Nutrition Reviews* 71 (2013): 282–299; C. Masterjohn and R. S. Bruno, Therapeutic potential of green tea in nonalcoholic fatty liver disease, *Nutrition Reviews* 70 (2012): 41–56; C. Wang and coauthors, Cranberry-containing products for prevention of urinary tract infections in susceptible populations, *Archives of Internal Medicine* 172 (2012): 988–996; C. Chuang and M. K. McIntosh, Potential mechanisms by which polyphenol-rich grapes prevent obesity-mediated inflammation and metabolic diseases, *Annual Review of Nutrition* 31 (2011): 155–176.
19. S. A. Doggrell, Lowering LDL cholesterol with margarine containing plant stanol/sterol esters: Is it still relevant in 2011? *Complementary Therapies in Medicine* 19 (2011): 37–46; T. C. Rideout and coauthors, High basal fractional cholesterol synthesis is associated with nonresponse of plasma LDL cholesterol to plant sterol therapy, *American Journal of Clinical Nutrition* 92 (2010): 41–46.

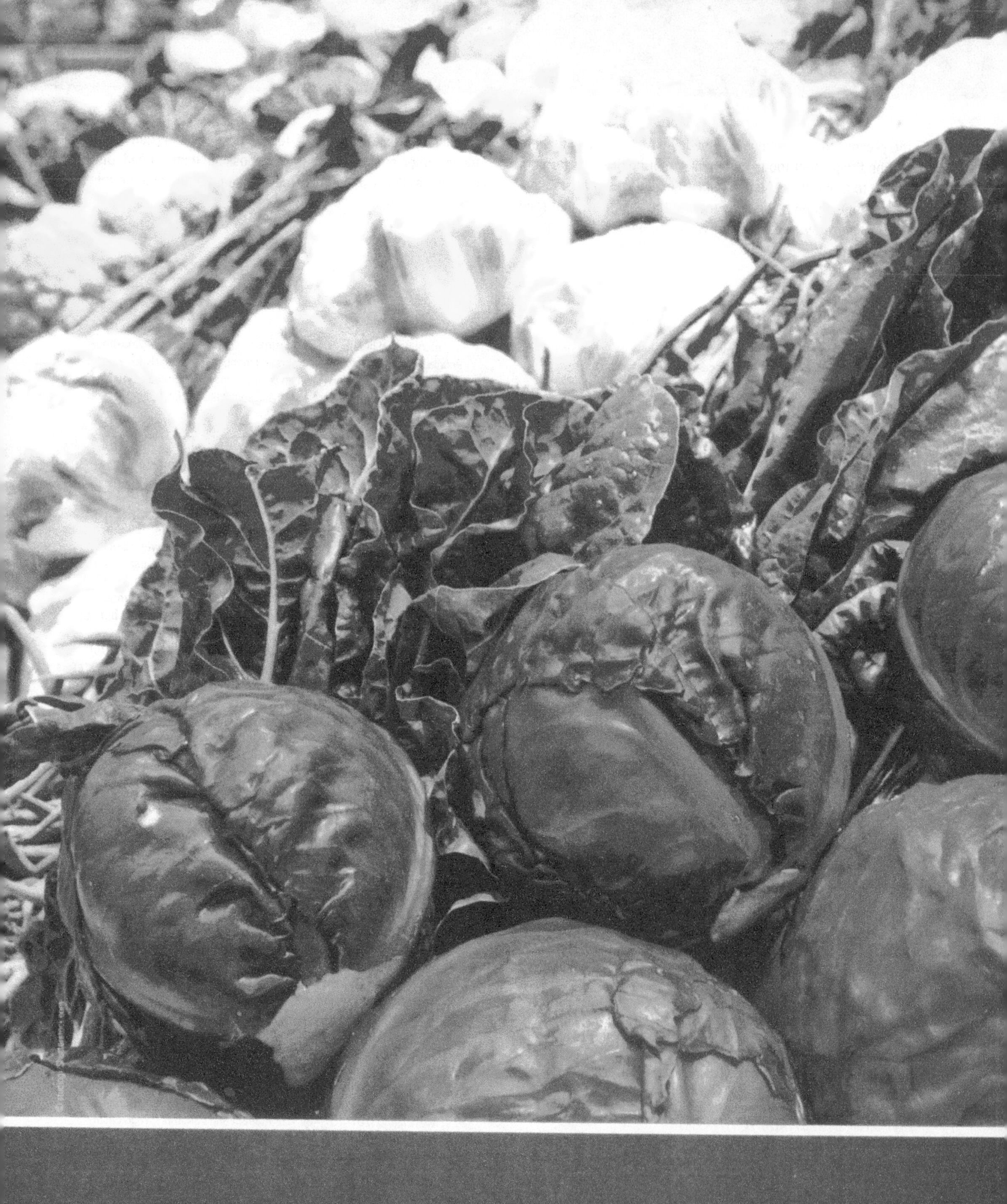

19

Consumer Concerns about Foods and Water

LEARNING GPS

Nutrition in Your Life

Do you know what causes food poisoning and how to protect yourself against it? Were you alarmed to learn that french fries contain acrylamide or that fish contain mercury? Are you concerned about the pesticides that might linger on fruits and vegetables—or the hormones and antibiotics that remain in beef and chicken? Do you wonder whether foods contain enough nutrients—or too many additives? Making informed choices and practicing a few food safety tips will allow you to enjoy a variety of foods while limiting your risks of experiencing food-related illnesses. In the Nutrition Portfolio at the end of this chapter, you can review your food-handling practices.

Take a moment to consider the task of supplying food to more than 300 million people in the United States (and millions more in all corners of the world). To feed this nation, farmers grow and harvest crops; dairy producers supply milk products; ranchers raise livestock; shippers deliver foods to manufacturers by land, sea, and air; manufacturers prepare, process, preserve, and package products for refrigerated food cases and grocery-store shelves; and grocers store the food and supply it to consumers. After much time, much labor, and extensive transport, an abundant supply of a large variety of safe foods finally reaches consumers at reasonable market prices.

The **FDA** is a large federal agency with a multitude of global responsibilities.[1] Its primary mission is to protect consumers from unsafe foods and drugs, which it does by using a network of people and sophisticated equipment.[2] More than 2000 FDA inspectors process more than 24 million shipments from more than 300,000 manufacturers representing more than 150 countries. (The glossary on p. 628 identifies the various food regulatory agencies by their abbreviations.)

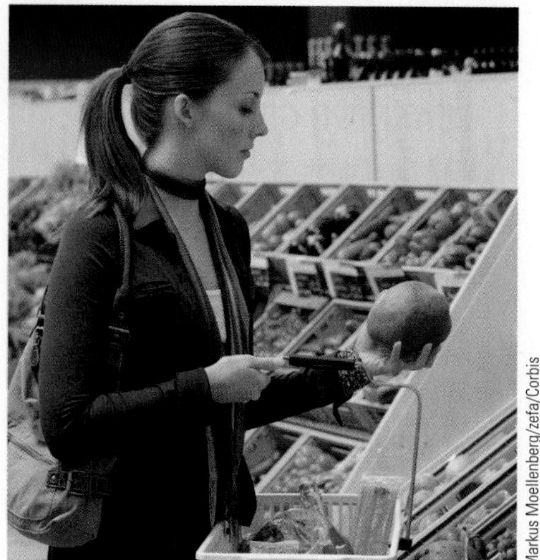
Markus Moellenberg/zefa/Corbis

With the benefits of a safe and abundant food supply comes the responsibility to select, prepare, and store foods safely.

19.1 Food Safety and Foodborne Illnesses

› LEARN IT Describe how foodborne illnesses can be prevented.

Government agencies focus on the potential **hazard** of foods, which differs from the **toxicity** of a substance—a distinction worth understanding. Anything can be toxic. Toxicity simply means that a substance *can* cause harm *if* enough is consumed. We consume many substances that are toxic, without **risk,** because the amounts are so small. The term *hazard,* on the other hand, is more relevant to our daily lives because it refers to the harm that is *likely* under real-life conditions. Consumers rely on government monitoring agencies to set **safety** standards and can learn to protect themselves from food-related illnesses by taking a few preventive measures.

This chapter focuses on the actions of individuals to promote food safety. It addresses the following food safety concerns:

- Foodborne illnesses
- Nutritional adequacy of foods
- Environmental contaminants
- Naturally occurring toxicants
- Pesticides
- Food additives
- Water safety

The chapter begins with the FDA's highest priority—the serious and prevalent threat of foodborne illnesses. The highlight that follows looks at genetically engineered foods.

Foodborne illness is the leading food safety concern because **outbreaks** of food poisoning far outnumber episodes of any other kind of food contamination. The **CDC** estimates 48 million cases of foodborne illnesses occur each year in the United States.[3] More than 100,000 people become so sick as to need hospitalization. For some 3000 people each year, the symptoms are so severe as to cause death. The following symptoms demand medical attention:

- Bloody diarrhea or diarrhea lasting more than 3 days
- Difficulty breathing or swallowing
- Double vision
- Fever lasting more than 24 hours
- Headache, muscle stiffness, and fever
- Numbness, muscle weakness, and tingling sensations in the skin
- Rapid heart rate, fainting, and dizziness

Most vulnerable are pregnant women; very young, very old, sick, or malnourished people; and those with a weakened immune system (as in AIDS).[4] By taking the proper precautions, people can minimize their chances of contracting foodborne illnesses.

hazard: a source of danger; used to refer to circumstances in which harm is possible under normal conditions of use.

toxicity: the ability of a substance to harm living organisms. All substances are toxic if high enough concentrations are used.

risk: a measure of the probability and severity of harm.

safety: the condition of being free from harm or danger.

foodborne illness: an illness transmitted to human beings through food and water, caused by either an infectious agent (foodborne infection) or a poisonous substance (food intoxication); commonly known as *food poisoning.*

outbreaks: two or more cases of a similar illness resulting from the ingestion of a common food.

GLOSSARY OF FOOD REGULATORY AGENCIES

CDC (Centers for Disease Control and Prevention): a branch of the Department of Health and Human Services that is responsible for, among other things, monitoring foodborne diseases.
www.cdc.gov

EPA (Environmental Protection Agency): a federal agency that is responsible for, among other things, regulating pesticides and establishing water quality standards.
www.epa.gov

FAO (Food and Agriculture Organization): an international agency (part of the United Nations) that has adopted standards to regulate pesticide use among other responsibilities.
www.fao.org

FDA (Food and Drug Administration): the federal agency responsible for ensuring the safety and wholesomeness of all dietary supplements and foods processed and sold in interstate commerce except meat, poultry, and eggs (which are under the jurisdiction of the USDA); inspecting food plants and imported foods; and setting standards for food composition and product labeling.
www.fda.gov

USDA (US Department of Agriculture): the federal agency responsible for enforcing standards for the wholesomeness and quality of meat, poultry, and eggs produced in the United States; conducting nutrition research; and educating the public about nutrition.
www.usda.gov

WHO (World Health Organization): an international agency concerned with promoting health and eradicating disease.
www.who.int

Foodborne Infections and Food Intoxications Foodborne illness can be caused by either an infection or an intoxication. Table 19-1 summarizes the foodborne illnesses responsible for 90 percent of illnesses, hospitalizations, and deaths, along with their food sources, general symptoms, and prevention methods.

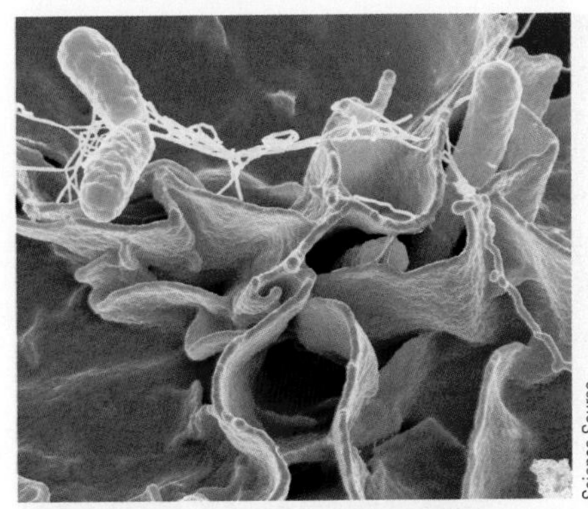

Science Source

An infection with *Salmonella* bacteria typically causes diarrhea, fever, and abdominal cramps.

pathogens (PATH-oh-jenz): microorganisms capable of producing disease.

Foodborne Infections Foodborne infections are caused by eating foods contaminated by infectious microbes. Among foodborne infections, norovirus and *Salmonella* are the leading causes of hospitalizations and deaths.[5] **Pathogens** commonly enter the GI tract in contaminated foods such as undercooked poultry and unpasteurized milk. Symptoms generally include abdominal cramps, fever, vomiting, and diarrhea.

Food Intoxications Food intoxications are caused by eating foods containing natural toxins or, more likely, microbes that produce toxins. The most common food toxin is produced by *Staphylococcus aureus;* it affects more than

TABLE 19-1 Foodborne Illnesses

Common Organism Name	Most Frequent Food Sources	Onset and General Symptoms	Prevention Methods[a]
Foodborne Infections			
Campylobacter (KAM-pee-loh-BAK-ter) bacterium	Raw and undercooked poultry, unpasturized milk, contaminated water	Onset: 2 to 5 days. Diarrhea, vomiting, abdominal cramps, fever; sometimes bloody stools; lasts 2 to 10 days.	Cook foods thoroughly; use pasteurized milk; use sanitary food-handling methods.
E.coli: (**O157:H7**) bacterium	Undercooked ground beef, unpasteurized milk and juices, raw cookie dough, raw fruits and vegetables, contaminated water, and person-to-person contact	Onset: 1 to 8 days. Severe bloody diarrhea, abdominal cramps, vomiting; lasts 5 to 10 days.	Cook ground beef thoroughly; use pasteurized milk; use sanitary food-handling methods; use treated, boiled, or bottled water.
Norovirus	Person-to-person contact; raw foods, salads, sandwiches	Onset: 1 to 2 days. Vomiting; lasts 1 to 2 days.	Use sanitary food-handling methods.
Listeria (lis-TER-ee-AH) bacterium	Unpasteurized milk; fresh soft cheeses; luncheon meats, hot dogs	Onset: 1 to 21 days. Fever, muscle aches; nausea, vomiting, blood poisoning, complications in pregnancy, and meningitis (stiff neck, severe headache, and fever).	Use sanitary food-handling methods; cook foods thoroughly; use pasteurized milk.
Clostridium (klo-STRID-ee-um) ***perfringens*** (per-FRINGE-enz) bacterium	Meats and meat products stored at between 120°F and 130°F	Onset: 8 to 16 hours. Abdominal pain, diarrhea, nausea; lasts 1 to 2 days.	Use sanitary food-handling methods; use pasteurized milk; cook foods thoroughly; refrigerate foods promptly and properly.
Salmonella (sal-moh-NEL-ah) bacteria (>2300 types)	Raw or undercooked eggs, meats, poultry, raw milk and other dairy products, shrimp, frog legs, yeast, coconut, pasta, and chocolate	Onset: 1 to 3 days. Fever, vomiting, abdominal cramps, diarrhea; lasts 4 to 7 days; can be fatal.	Use sanitary food-handling methods; use pasteurized milk; cook foods thoroughly; refrigerate foods promptly and properly.
Food Intoxications			
Botulism (BOT-chew-lizm) Botulinum toxin produced by *Clostridium botulinum* bacterium, which grows without oxygen, in low-acid foods, and at temperatures between 40°F and 120°F; the ***botulinum*** (BOT-chew-line-um) ***toxin*** responsible for botulism is called ***botulin*** (BOT-chew-lin).	Anaerobic environment of low acidity (canned corn, peppers, green beans, soups, beets, asparagus, mushrooms, ripe olives, spinach, tuna, chicken, chicken liver, liver pâté, luncheon meats, ham, sausage, stuffed eggplant, lobster, and smoked and salted fish)	Onset: 4 to 36 hours. Nervous system symptoms, including double vision, inability to swallow, speech difficulty, and progressive paralysis of the respiratory system; often fatal; leaves prolonged symptoms in survivors.	Use proper canning methods for low-acid foods; refrigerate homemade garlic and herb oils; avoid commercially prepared foods with leaky seals or with bent, bulging, or broken cans. Do not give infants honey because it may contain spores of *Clostridium botulinum,* which is a common source of infection for infants.
Staphylococcal (STAF-il-oh-KOK-al) **food poisoning** Staphylococcal toxin (produced by *Staphylococcus aureus* bacterium)	Toxin produced in improperly refrigerated meats; egg, tuna, potato, and macaroni salads; cream-filled pastries	Onset: 1 to 6 hours. Diarrhea, nausea, vomiting, abdominal cramps, fever; lasts 1 to 2 days.	Use sanitary food-handling methods; cook food thoroughly; refrigerate foods promptly and properly; use proper home-canning methods.
Toxoplasma (TOK-so-PLAZ-ma) parasite	Raw or undercooked meat; unwashed fruits and vegetables; contaminated water	Onset: 7 to 21 days. Swollen glands, fever, headache, muscle pain, stiff neck.	Use sanitary food-handling methods; cook foods thoroughly.

NOTE: Travelers' diarrhea is most commonly caused by *E. coli, Campylobacter jejuni, Shigella,* and *Salmonella.*

[a]The "How To" on pp. 632–633 provides more details on the proper handling, cooking, and refrigeration of foods.

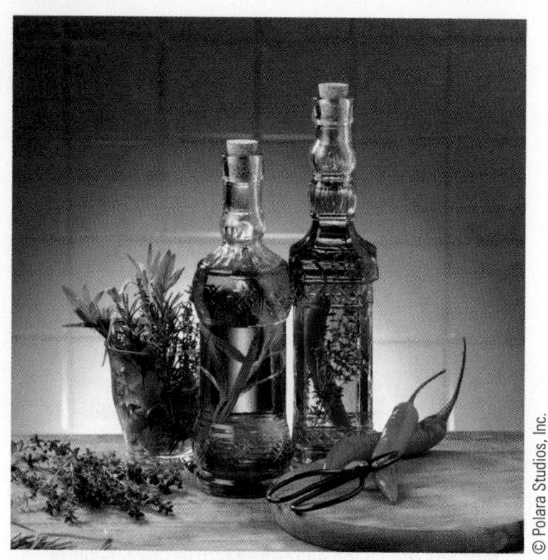
© Polara Studios, Inc.

To prevent food intoxication from homemade flavored oils, wash and dry the herbs before adding them to the oil and keep the oil refrigerated.

1 million people each year. Less common, but more infamous, is *Clostridium botulinum*, an organism that produces a deadly toxin in anaerobic conditions such as improperly canned (especially home-canned) foods and improperly stored foods (such as homemade herb-flavored oils or commercially made, chilled foods stored at room temperature). The botulinum toxin paralyzes muscles, making it difficult to see, speak, swallow, and breathe. Because death can occur within 24 hours of onset, botulism demands immediate medical attention. Even then, survivors may suffer the effects for months or years.

Other microbial toxins—called aflatoxins—are not common in the United States, but threaten the health of more than half the world's population.[6] Aflatoxins contaminate corn, grains, and nuts in tropical countries where foods are stored in warm, humid conditions that promote fungal growth. Strategies to reduce exposure in vulnerable populations need to become a worldwide priority.

Food Safety in the Marketplace

Transmission of foodborne illness has changed as our food supply and lifestyles have changed.[7] In the past, foodborne illness was caused by one person's error in a small setting, such as improperly refrigerated egg salad at a family picnic, and affected only a few victims. Today, we eat more foods that have been prepared and packaged by others. Consequently, when a food manufacturer or cruise ship chef makes an error, foodborne illness can quickly affect many people. An estimated 80 percent of reported foodborne illnesses are caused by errors in a commercial setting, such as the improper **pasteurization** of milk at a large dairy.

In 2010, a *Salmonella* outbreak led to the recall of 500 million eggs from two farms. In 2011, a cantaloupe farm had to recall more than 300,000 cases of fruit when *Listeria* poisoning killed 29 people and made 139 others sick. In 2013, *Cyclospora* from salads and fresh cilantro from Mexico infected more than 600 people in 25 states. In 2014, 1.8 million pounds of ground beef contaminated with *E. Coli* was recalled. These incidents and others focus the national spotlight on two important safety issues: disease-causing organisms are commonly found in foods, and safe food-handling practices can minimize harm from most of these foodborne pathogens.

Industry Controls

All food producers use a **Hazard Analysis Critical Control Point (HACCP)** plan to help prevent foodborne illnesses at their source. Each slaughterhouse, packer, distributor, and transporter of susceptible foods must identify "critical control points" that pose a risk of contamination and then devise and implement verifiable ways to eliminate or minimize the risk. The HACCP system has proved a remarkable success for domestic products, but such programs do not apply to imported foods.

An estimated 10 to 15 percent of all food consumed in the United States is imported from more than 230 countries each year. Many countries cooperate with the FDA and have adopted many of the safe food-handling practices used in the United States, but some imported foods come from countries with little or no regulatory oversight. To help consumers distinguish between imported and domestic foods, certain foods—including fish, shellfish, meats, fruits, vegetables, and some nuts—must display the country of origin on the label, specifying where they were produced.

Consumer Awareness

Canned and packaged foods sold in grocery stores are easily controlled, but rare accidents do happen. Batch numbering makes it possible to recall contaminated foods through public announcements via the Internet, newspapers, television, and radio. In the grocery store, consumers can buy items before the "sell by" date and inspect the safety seals and wrappers of packages. A broken seal, bulging can lid, or mangled package fails to protect the consumer against microbes, insects, spoilage, or even vandalism.

State and local health regulations provide guidelines on the cleanliness of facilities and the safe preparation of foods for restaurants, cafeterias, and

pasteurization: heat processing of food that inactivates some, but not all, microorganisms in the food; not a sterilization process. Bacteria that cause spoilage are still present.

Hazard Analysis Critical Control Points (HACCP): a systematic plan to identify and correct potential microbial hazards in the manufacturing, distribution, and commercial use of food products; commonly referred to as "HASS-ip."

fast-food establishments. Even so, consumers can also take the following actions to help prevent foodborne illnesses when dining out:

- Wash hands with hot, soapy water before meals.
- Expect clean tabletops, dinnerware, utensils, and food preparation areas.
- Expect cooked foods to be served piping hot and salads to be fresh and cold.
- Refrigerate take-home items within 2 hours and use leftovers within 3 to 4 days.

Improper handling of foods can occur anywhere along the line from commercial farms and manufacturers to supermarkets and restaurants to private homes. Maintaining a safe food supply requires everyone's efforts (see Figure 19-1).

Food Safety in the Kitchen Whether microbes multiply and cause illness depends, in part, on a few key food-handling behaviors in the kitchen—whether the kitchen is in your home, a school cafeteria, a gourmet restaurant, or a commercial canning facility. Figure 19-2 (p. 632) summarizes the four simple things that can help most to prevent foodborne illness:

- *Clean.* Keep a clean, safe kitchen by washing hands and surfaces often. Wash countertops, cutting boards, sponges, and utensils in hot, soapy water before and after each step of food preparation. To reduce bacterial contamination on hands, wash hands with soap and warm water; if soap and water are not available, use an alcohol-based sanitizing gel.[8]
- *Separate.* Avoid foodborne infections by keeping raw eggs, meat, poultry, and seafood separate from other foods. Wash all utensils and surfaces (such as cutting boards or platters) that have been in contact with these foods with hot, soapy water before using them again. Bacteria inevitably left on the surfaces from the raw meat can recontaminate the cooked meat or other foods—a problem known as **cross-contamination.** Washing raw eggs, meat, and poultry is not recommended because the extra handling increases the risk of cross-contamination.
- *Cook.* Keep hot foods hot by cooking to proper temperatures. Foods need to cook long enough to reach internal temperatures that will kill microbes and maintain adequate temperatures to prevent bacterial growth until the foods are served.

cross-contamination: the contamination of food by bacteria that occurs when the food comes into contact with surfaces previously touched by raw meat, poultry, or seafood.

> FIGURE 19-1 **Food Safety from Farm to Table**

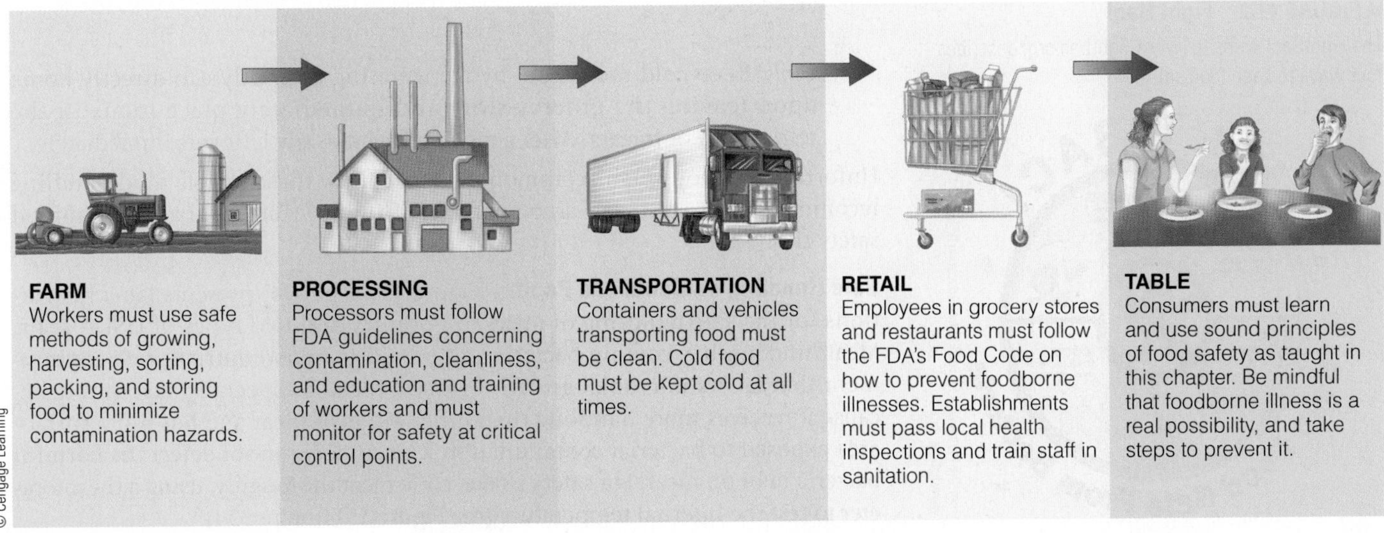

FARM
Workers must use safe methods of growing, harvesting, sorting, packing, and storing food to minimize contamination hazards.
PROCESSING
Processors must follow FDA guidelines concerning contamination, cleanliness, and education and training of workers and must monitor for safety at critical control points.
TRANSPORTATION
Containers and vehicles transporting food must be clean. Cold food must be kept cold at all times.
RETAIL
Employees in grocery stores and restaurants must follow the FDA's Food Code on how to prevent foodborne illnesses. Establishments must pass local health inspections and train staff in sanitation.
TABLE
Consumers must learn and use sound principles of food safety as taught in this chapter. Be mindful that foodborne illness is a real possibility, and take steps to prevent it.

>How To

Prevent Foodborne Illnesses

Most foodborne illnesses can be prevented by following four simple rules: clean, separate, cook, and chill.

Clean

- Wash fruits and vegetables in a clean sink with a scrub brush and warm water; store washed and unwashed produce separately.
- Use hot, soapy water to wash hands, utensils, dishes, nonporous cutting boards, and countertops before handling food and between tasks when working with different foods. Use a bleach solution on cutting boards (one capful per gallon of water).
- Cover cuts with clean bandages before food preparation; dirty bandages carry harmful microorganisms.
- Mix foods with utensils, not hands; keep hands and utensils away from mouth, nose, and hair.
- Anyone may be a carrier of bacteria and should avoid coughing or sneezing over food. A person with a skin infection or infectious disease should not prepare food.
- Clean sponges every day by microwaving wet sponges at full power for one minute or running them through the dishwasher. Wash dish cloths and dish towels regularly and use fresh, clean ones every day.
- Clean up food spills and crumb-filled crevices.

Separate

- Wash all surfaces that have been in contact with raw meats, poultry, eggs, fish, and shellfish before reusing.
- Serve cooked foods on a clean plate with a clean utensil. Separate raw foods from those that have been cooked.
- Don't use marinade that was in contact with raw meat for basting or sauces.

Cook

- When cooking meats or poultry, use a thermometer to test the internal temperature. Insert the thermometer between the thigh and the body of a turkey or into the thickest part of other meats, making sure the tip of the thermometer is not in contact with bone or the pan. Cook to the temperature indicated for that particular meat (see Figure 19-4 on p. 634); cook hamburgers to at least medium well done. If you have safety questions, call the USDA Meat and Poultry Hotline: (800) 535-4555.
- Cook stuffing separately, or stuff poultry just prior to cooking.
- Do not cook large cuts of meat or turkey in a microwave oven; it leaves some parts undercooked while overcooking others.
- Cook eggs before eating them (soft-boiled for at least 3½ minutes; scrambled until set, not runny; fried for at least 3 minutes on one side and 1 minute on the other).
- Cook seafood thoroughly. If you have safety questions about seafood, call the FDA hotline: (800) FDA-4010.
- When serving foods, maintain temperatures at 140°F or higher.
- Heat leftovers thoroughly to at least 165°F. Do not reheat leftovers in crock pots, slow cookers, or chafing dishes.
- Bring sauces, soups, and gravies to a boil.

Chill

- When running errands, stop at the grocery store last. When you get home, refrigerate the perishable groceries (such as meats and dairy products) immediately. Do not leave perishables in the car any longer than it takes for ice cream to melt.
- Put packages of raw meat, fish, or poultry on a plate before refrigerating to prevent juices from dripping on food stored below.
- Buy only foods that are solidly frozen in store freezers.
- Keep cold foods at 40°F or less; keep frozen foods at 0°F or less (keep a thermometer in the refrigerator).
- Marinate meats in the refrigerator, not on the counter.
- Look for "Keep Refrigerated" or "Refrigerate After Opening" on food labels.

(*Continued*)

> **FIGURE 19-2 Fight Bac!**

The FightBac! website (www.fightbac.org) describes four ways to keep food safe.

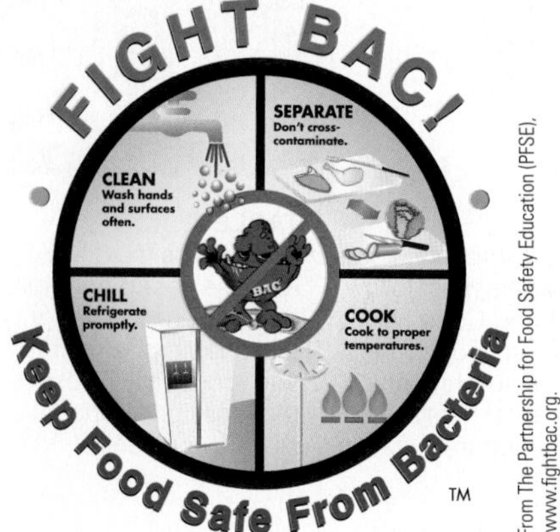

From The Partnership for Food Safety Education (PFSE). www.fightbac.org.

- *Chill.* Keep cold foods cold by refrigerating promptly. Go directly home upon leaving the grocery store and immediately place foods in the refrigerator or freezer. After a meal, refrigerate any leftovers immediately.

Unfortunately, consumers commonly fail to follow these simple food-handling recommendations.[9] See the accompanying "How To" feature for additional food safety tips.

Safe Handling of Meats and Poultry Figure 19-3 (p. 634) presents label instructions for the safe handling of meat and poultry and two types of USDA seals. Meats and poultry contain bacteria and provide a moist, nutrient-rich environment that favors microbial growth. Ground meat is especially susceptible because it receives more handling than other kinds of meat and has more surface area exposed to bacterial contamination. Consumers cannot detect the harmful bacteria in or on meat. For safety's sake, cook meat thoroughly, using a thermometer to test the internal temperature (see Figure 19-4 on p. 634).

- Refrigerate leftovers promptly; use shallow containers to cool foods faster; use leftovers within 3 to 4 days.
- Thaw meats or poultry in the refrigerator, not at room temperature. If you must hasten thawing, use cool water (changed every 30 minutes) or a microwave oven.
- Freeze meat, fish, or poultry immediately if not planning to use within a few days.

In General

- Do not reuse disposable containers; use nondisposable containers or recycle instead.
- Do not taste food that is suspect. "If in doubt, throw it out."
- Throw out foods with danger-signaling odors. Be aware, though, that most food-poisoning bacteria are odorless, colorless, and tasteless.
- Do not buy or use items that have broken seals or mangled packaging; such containers cannot protect against microbes, insects, spoilage, or even vandalism. Check safety seals, buttons, and expiration dates.
- Follow label instructions for storing and preparing packaged and frozen foods; throw out foods that have been thawed or refrozen.
- Discard foods that are discolored, moldy, or decayed or that have been contaminated by insects or rodents.

For Specific Food Items

- *Canned goods.* Carefully discard food from cans that leak or bulge so that other people and animals will not accidentally ingest it; before canning, seek professional advice from the USDA Extension Service (find information and local offices at the USDA website).
- *Milk and cheeses.* Use only pasteurized milk and milk products. Aged cheeses, such as cheddar and Swiss, do well for an hour or two without refrigeration, but they should be refrigerated or stored in an ice chest for longer periods.
- *Eggs.* Use clean eggs with intact shells. Do not eat eggs, even pasteurized eggs, raw; raw eggs are commonly found in Caesar salad dressing, eggnog, cookie dough, hollandaise sauce, and key lime pie. Cook eggs until whites are firmly set and yolks begin to thicken.
- *Honey.* Honey may contain dormant bacterial spores, which can awaken in the human body to produce botulism. In adults, this poses little hazard, but infants younger than 1 year of age should never be fed honey. Honey can accumulate enough toxin to kill an infant; it has been implicated in several cases of sudden infant death. (Honey can also be contaminated with environmental pollutants picked up by the bees.)
- *Mayonnaise.* Commercial mayonnaise may actually help a food to resist spoilage because of the acid content. Still, keep it refrigerated after opening.
- *Mixed salads.* Mixed salads of chopped ingredients spoil easily because they have extensive surface area for bacteria to invade, and they have been in contact with cutting boards, hands, and kitchen utensils that easily transmit bacteria to food (regardless of their mayonnaise content). Chill them well before, during, and after serving.
- *Picnic foods.* Choose foods that last without refrigeration, such as fresh fruits and vegetables, breads and crackers, and canned spreads and cheeses that can be opened and used immediately. Pack foods cold, layer ice between foods, and keep foods out of water.
- *Seafood.* Buy only fresh seafood that has been properly refrigerated or iced. Cooked seafood should be stored separately from raw seafood to avoid cross-contamination.

NOTE: Learn more about food safety at www.HomeFoodSafety.org or by downloading *Is My Food Safe?*, a free phone app sponsored by the Academy of Nutrition and Dietetics.

› TRY IT After cutting the fat from a pork loin, you rinse the wooden cutting board under warm water before using it to chop vegetables. Discuss whether this precaution is adequate to protect against cross-contamination.

Unrelated to safe handling practices, **bovine spongiform encephalopathy (BSE)** is a slowly progressive, fatal disease that affects the central nervous system of cattle and wild game such as deer and elk.[10] A similar disease develops in people who have eaten contaminated beef from infected cows (milk products appear to be safe).* The USDA has taken numerous steps to prevent the transmission of BSE in cattle, and consequently, the risks from US cattle are extremely low.

Safe Handling of Seafood Most seafood available in the United States is safe, but eating it undercooked or raw can cause severe illnesses—hepatitis, worms, parasites, viral intestinal disorders, and other diseases.** Rumor has it that freezing fish will make it safe to eat raw, but this is only partly true. Commercial freezing kills mature parasitic worms, but only cooking can

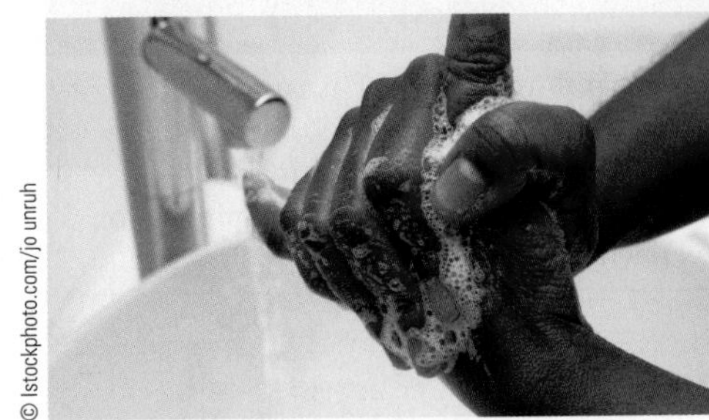

Wash your hands with warm water and soap for at least 20 seconds before preparing or eating food to reduce the chance of microbial contamination.

bovine spongiform encephalopathy (BOH-vine SPON-jih-form in-SEF-eh-LOP-eh-thee) or **BSE:** an often fatal illness of cattle and wild game that affects the nervous system and is transmitted to people by eating infected meats; commonly called *mad cow disease.*

*The human form of BSE is called *variant Creutzfeldt-Jakob Disease (vCJD).*

**Diseases caused by toxins from the sea include ciguatera poisoning, scombroid poisoning, and paralytic and neurotoxic shellfish poisoning.

> **FIGURE 19-3 Meat and Poultry Safety, Grading, and Inspection Seals**

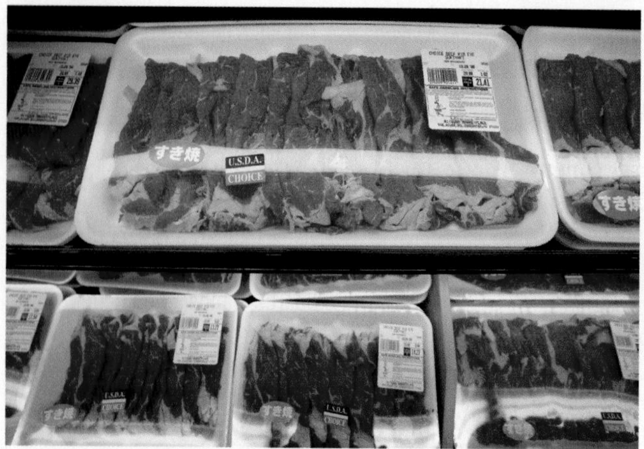

James Leynse/Corbis News/Corbis

Neither inspection nor grading guarantees that the product will not cause foodborne illnesses, but consumers can help to prevent foodborne illnesses by following the safe handling instructions.

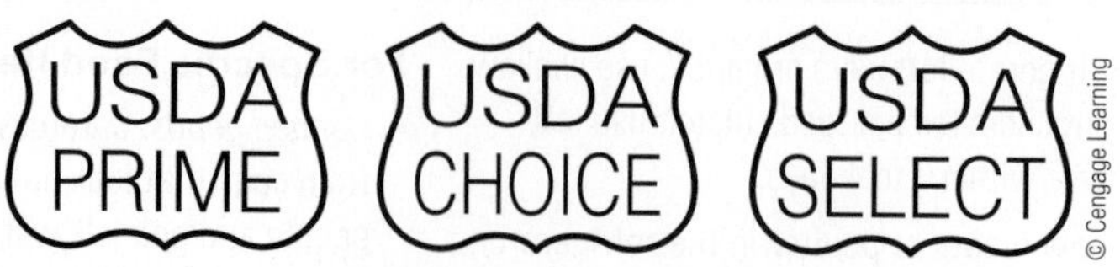

© Cengage Learning

The voluntary "Graded by USDA" seal indicates that the product has been graded for tenderness, juiciness, and flavor. Beef is graded Prime (abundant marbling of the meat muscle), Choice (less marbling), or Select (lean). Similarly, poultry is graded A, B, or C.

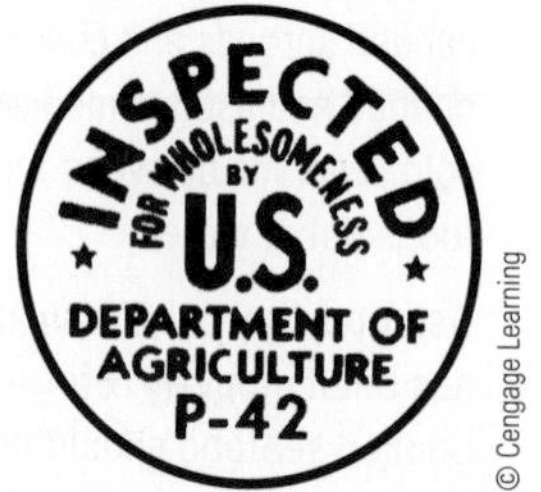

© Cengage Learning

The mandatory "Inspected and Passed by the USDA" seal ensures that meat and poultry products are safe, wholesome, and correctly labeled. Inspection does not guarantee that the meat is free of potentially harmful bacteria.

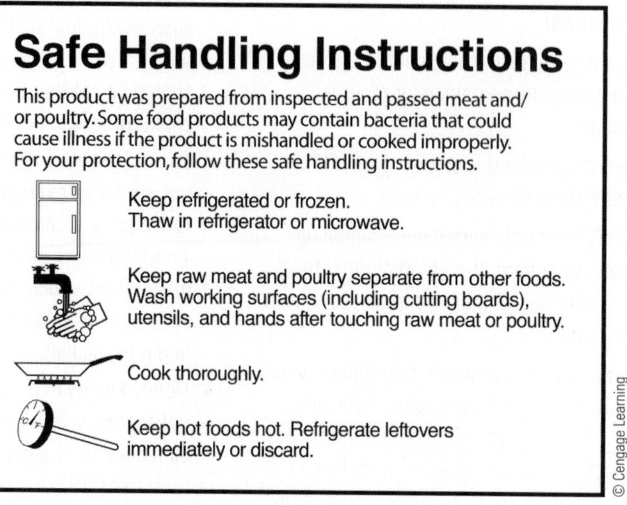

Safe Handling Instructions
This product was prepared from inspected and passed meat and/or poultry. Some food products may contain bacteria that could cause illness if the product is mishandled or cooked improperly. For your protection, follow these safe handling instructions.
Keep refrigerated or frozen. Thaw in refrigerator or microwave.
Keep raw meat and poultry separate from other foods. Wash working surfaces (including cutting boards), utensils, and hands after touching raw meat or poultry.
Cook thoroughly.
Keep hot foods hot. Refrigerate leftovers immediately or discard.

© Cengage Learning

The USDA requires that safe handling instructions appear on all packages of meat and poultry.

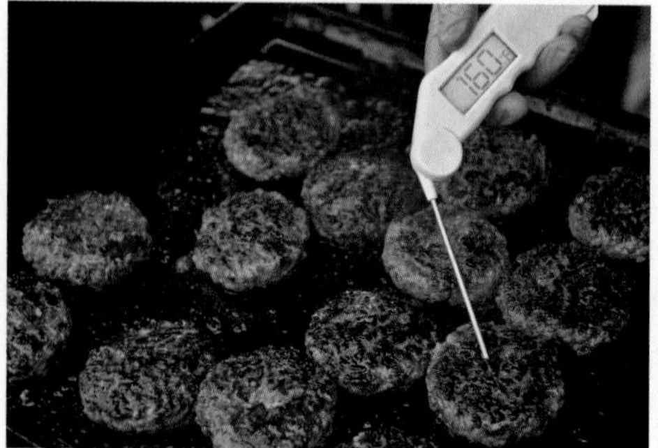

© Charles Stirling/Alamy

Cook hamburgers to 160°F; color alone cannot determine doneness. Some burgers will turn brown before reaching 160°F, whereas others may retain some pink color, even when cooked to 175°F.

> **FIGURE 19-4 Recommended Safe Temperatures (Fahrenheit)**

Bacteria multiply rapidly at temperatures between 40°F and 140°F. Cook foods to the minimum internal temperatures shown on this thermometer and hold them at 140°F or higher. Place the thermometer in the thickest part of the meat; for whole cuts of meat, allow the meat to rest for 3 minutes before carving or consuming.

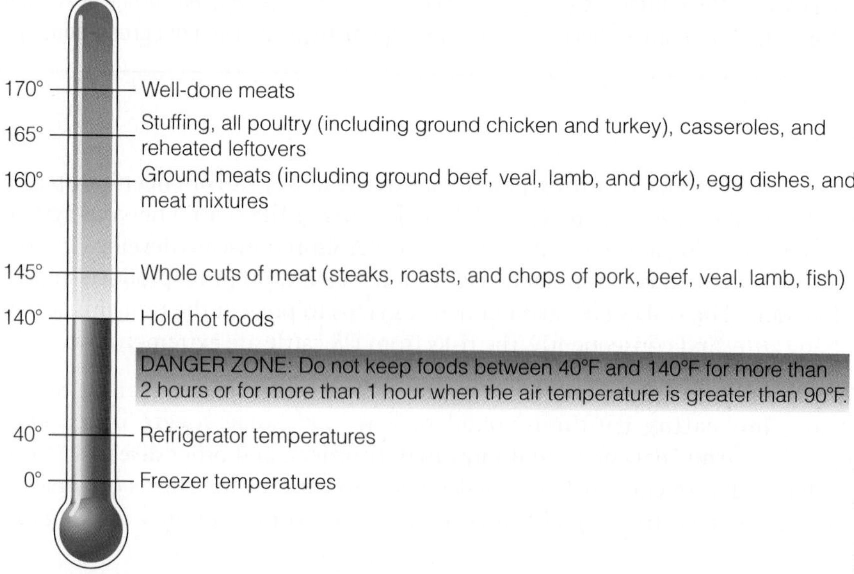

170° Well-done meats
165° Stuffing, all poultry (including ground chicken and turkey), casseroles, and reheated leftovers
160° Ground meats (including ground beef, veal, lamb, and pork), egg dishes, and meat mixtures

140° Hold hot foods
DANGER ZONE: Do not keep foods between 40°F and 140°F for more than 2 hours or for more than 1 hour when the air temperature is greater than 90°F.

© Cengage Learning

NOTE: To reduce the risk of foodborne illnesses, the *Dietary Guidelines for Americans* suggest that consumers heed this temperature danger zone. Professionals in the food industry must adhere to more specific guidelines as published in the FDA Food Code, available at www.fda.gov/FoodCode.

kill all worm eggs and other microorganisms that can cause illness. For safety's sake, all seafood should be cooked until it is opaque.

As for **sushi,** even a master chef cannot detect harmful microbes that may occur in even the best-quality, freshest fish. The marketing term *sushi grade* implies wholesomeness, but is not legally defined and does not guarantee quality, purity, or freshness. Sushi can be safe to eat when chefs combine cooked seafood and other ingredients into these delicacies.

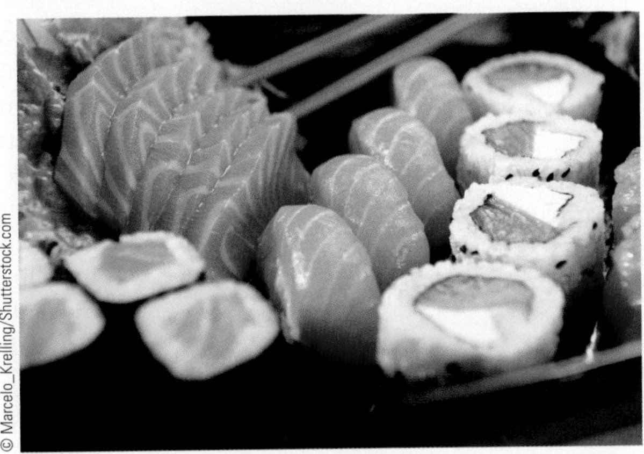

Eating raw seafood is a risky proposition.

Eating raw oysters can be dangerous for anyone, but people with liver disease and weakened immune systems are most vulnerable. At least 10 species of bacteria found in raw oysters can cause serious illness and even death. Raw oysters may also carry the hepatitis A virus, which can cause liver disease. Some hot sauces can kill many of these bacteria, but not the virus; alcohol inactivates some bacteria, but not enough to guarantee protection (or to recommend drinking alcohol). Pasteurization of raw oysters—holding them at a specified temperature for a specified time—holds promise for killing bacteria without cooking the oyster or altering its texture or flavor.

As population density increases along the shores of seafood-harvesting waters, pollution inevitably invades the sea life there. Preventing seafood-borne illness is in large part a task of controlling water pollution. To help ensure a safe seafood market, the FDA requires processors to adopt food safety practices based on the HACCP system mentioned earlier.

Chemical pollution and microbial contamination lurk not only in the water, but also in the boats and warehouses where seafood is cleaned, prepared, and refrigerated. Because seafood is one of the most perishable foods, time and temperature are critical to its freshness, flavor, and safety. To keep seafood as fresh as possible, people in the industry must "keep it cold, keep it clean, and keep it moving." Wise consumers eat it cooked.

Other Precautions and Procedures Fresh food generally smells fresh. Not all types of food poisoning are detectable by odor, but some bacterial wastes produce "off" odors—and food with an abnormal odor is spoiled. Throw it out or, if it was recently purchased, return it to the grocery store. Do not taste it. Table 19-2 lists safe refrigerator storage times for selected foods.

Local health departments and the USDA and FDA websites can provide additional information about food safety. If precautions fail and a mild foodborne illness develops, drink clear liquids to replace fluids lost through vomiting and diarrhea. If serious foodborne illness is suspected, first call a physician. Then wrap the remainder of the suspected food and label the container so that the food cannot be mistakenly eaten, place it in the refrigerator, and hold it for possible inspection by health authorities.

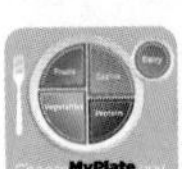

> DIETARY GUIDELINES FOR AMERICANS

Follow food safety recommendations when preparing and eating foods to reduce the risk of foodborne illnesses. To avoid microbial foodborne illness:

- Clean hands, food contact surfaces, and fruits and vegetables.
- Separate raw, cooked, and ready-to-eat foods while shopping, preparing, or storing foods.
- Cook foods to a safe temperature to kill microorganisms.
- Chill (refrigerate) perishable foods promptly and defrost foods properly.
- Do *not* wash or rinse meat or poultry.
- Avoid raw (unpasteurized) milk or any products made from unpasteurized milk, raw or partially cooked eggs or foods containing raw eggs, raw or undercooked meat and poultry, unpasteurized juices, and raw sprouts.

TABLE 19-2 **Safe Refrigerator Storage Times (≤40°F)**

1 to 2 Days
Raw ground meats, breakfast or other raw sausages, raw fish or poultry; gravies
3 to 5 Days
Raw steaks, roasts, or chops; cooked meats, poultry, vegetables, and mixed dishes; lunchmeats (packages opened); mayonnaise salads (chicken, egg, pasta, tuna); fresh vegetables (spinach, green beans, tomatoes)
1 Week
Hard-cooked eggs, bacon or hot dogs (opened packages); smoked sausages or seafood; milk, cottage cheese
1 to 2 Weeks
Yogurt; carrots, celery, lettuce
2 to 4 Weeks
Fresh eggs (in shells); lunchmeats, bacon, or hot dogs (packages unopened); dry sausages (pepperoni, hard salami); most aged and processed cheeses (Swiss, brick)
2 Months
Mayonnaise (opened jar); most dry cheeses (Parmesan, Romano)

sushi: vinegar-flavored rice and seafood, typically wrapped in seaweed and stuffed with colorful vegetables. Some sushi is stuffed with raw fish; other varieties contain cooked seafood.

Food Safety while Traveling People who travel to other countries have a 50–50 chance of contracting a foodborne illness, commonly described as **travelers' diarrhea.** Like many other foodborne illnesses, travelers' diarrhea is a sometimes serious, always annoying bacterial infection of the digestive tract. The risk is high because, for one thing, some countries' cleanliness standards for food and water are lower than those in the United States. For another, every region's microbes are different, and although people are immune to the microbes in their own neighborhoods, they have had no chance to develop immunity to the pathogens in places they are visiting for the first time. In addition to the food safety tips outlined on pp. 632–633, precautions while traveling include:

- Wash hands frequently with soap and hot water, especially before handling food or eating. Use sanitizing gel or hand wipes regularly.
- Eat only well-cooked and hot or canned foods. Eat raw fruits or vegetables only if washed in purified water and peeled with clean hands.
- Use purified, bottled water for drinking, making ice cubes, and brushing teeth. Alternatively, use disinfecting tablets or boil water.
- Refuse dairy products that have not been pasteurized and refrigerated properly.
- Travel with antidiarrheal medication in case efforts to avoid illness fail.

To sum up these recommendations, "Boil it, cook it, peel it, or forget it."

Advances in Food Safety

Advances in technology have dramatically improved the quality and safety of foods available on the market. From pasteurization in the early 1900s to irradiation in the early 2000s, these advances offer numerous benefits, but they also raise consumer concerns.*

Irradiation The use of low-dose **irradiation** protects consumers from foodborne illnesses by:

- Controlling mold in grains
- Sterilizing spices and teas for storage at room temperature
- Controlling insects and extending shelf life in fresh fruits and vegetables (inhibits the growth of sprouts on potatoes and onions and delays ripening in some fruits such as strawberries and mangoes)
- Destroying harmful bacteria in fresh and frozen beef, poultry, lamb, and pork

Some foods, however, are not candidates for irradiation. For example, when irradiated, high-fat meats develop off-odors, egg whites turn milky, grapefruits become mushy, and milk products change flavor. Incidentally, the milk in those boxes kept at room temperature on grocery-store shelves is *not* irradiated; it is sterilized with an **ultrahigh temperature (UHT) treatment.**

The use of food irradiation has been extensively evaluated over the past 50 years; approved for use in more than 40 countries; and supported by numerous health agencies, including the **FAO, WHO,** and the American Medical Association. Irradiation does not make foods radioactive, nor does it noticeably change the taste, texture, or appearance of approved foods. Vitamin loss is minimal and comparable to amounts lost in other food-processing methods such as canning. Because irradiation kills bacteria without the use of heat, it is sometimes called "cold pasteurization."

Consumer Concerns about Irradiation Many consumers associate the term *radiation* with cancer, birth defects, and mutations, and consequently have strong negative emotions about using irradiation on foods. Some may mistakenly fear that irradiated food has been contaminated by radioactive particles, such as occurs in

*During the past century, pasteurization of milk helped to control typhoid fever, tuberculosis, scarlet fever, diphtheria, and other infectious diseases.

travelers' diarrhea: nausea, vomiting, and diarrhea caused by consuming food or water contaminated by any of several organisms, most commonly, *E. coli, Shigella, Campylobacter jejuni,* and *Salmonella.*

irradiation: sterilizing a food by exposure to energy waves, similar to ultraviolet light and microwaves; sometimes called *ionizing radiation.*

ultrahigh temperature (UHT) treatment: sterilizing a food by brief exposure to temperatures above those normally used.

the aftermath of a nuclear accident. Some balk at the idea of irradiating, and thus sterilizing, contaminated foods and prefer instead the elimination of unsanitary slaughtering and food preparation conditions. Food producers, on the other hand, are eager to use irradiation, but they hesitate to do so until consumers are ready to accept it and willing to pay for it. Once consumers understand the benefits of irradiation, about half are willing to use irradiated foods, but most are not willing to pay more.

Regulation of Irradiation The FDA has established regulations governing the specific uses of irradiation and allowed doses. Each food that has been treated with irradiation must say so on its label (see Figure 19-5). Labels can be misleading, however. Products that use irradiated foods as ingredients are not required to say so on the label. Furthermore, consumers may interpret the *absence* of the irradiation symbol to mean that the food was produced without any kind of treatment. This is not true; it is just that the FDA does not require label statements for other treatments used for the same purpose, such as postharvest fumigation with pesticides.

Other Pasteurizing Systems Other technologies using high-intensity pulsed light or electron beams have also been approved by the FDA. Like irradiation, these technologies kill microorganisms and extend the shelf life of foods without diminishing their nutrient content.

> FIGURE 19-5 Irradiation symbol

This international symbol, called the radura, identifies retail foods that have been irradiated. The phrases "Treated by irradiation" or "Treated with radiation" must accompany the symbol. The irradiation label is not required on commercially prepared foods that contain irradiated ingredients, such as spices. Foods approved for irradiation include eggs; fresh fruit (strawberries, citrus, papaya); oysters, clams, mussels, scallops, crabs, lobsters, shrimp; raw beef, lamb, poultry, pork; spices, tea; vegetables (iceberg lettuce, fresh spinach, potatoes, tomatoes, onions); wheat.

> REVIEW IT Describe how foodborne illnesses can be prevented.

Millions of people suffer mild to life-threatening symptoms caused by foodborne illnesses (review Table 19-1, p. 629). As the "How To" feature on pp. 632–633 describes, most of these illnesses can be prevented by storing and cooking foods at their proper temperatures and by preparing them in sanitary conditions. Irradiation of certain foods protects consumers from foodborne illnesses, but it also raises some concerns.

19.2 Nutritional Adequacy of Foods and Diets

> LEARN IT Explain how to minimize nutrient losses in the kitchen.

In years past, when most foods were whole and farm fresh, the task of meeting nutrient needs primarily involved balancing servings from the various food groups. Today, however, foods have changed. Advances in food production over the past century have set the stage for the widespread dissemination of ultra-processed products—new creations that have little to do with natural foods and contain highly processed ingredients. Many of these "new" foods appeal to consumers' demands for convenience and flavor, but do not necessarily deliver a balanced assortment of needed nutrients. In fact, most lack fiber, vitamins, minerals, and phytochemicals, but deliver excessive amounts of sugar, salt, and *trans* and saturated fats—the perfect combination of dietary factors to promote obesity and chronic diseases.[11] Advertisers spend much effort and money encouraging consumers to buy their products quickly, frequently, and abundantly, not on promoting healthy eating habits—unless that would increase sales too. For health's sake, consumers will want to buy fewer processed foods, prepare more meals at home using whole fresh foods, and dine at restaurants that prepare meals from scratch.

Obtaining Nutrient Information To help consumers find their way among the abundance of available foods, the FDA has developed extensive nutrition labeling regulations, as Chapter 2 describes. In addition, the USDA's *Dietary Guidelines for Americans* help consumers combine foods into healthful eating patterns, and MyPlate helps them to put those guidelines into practice (see Chapter 2).

Minimizing Nutrient Losses In addition to selecting nutritious foods and preparing them safely, consumers can improve their nutrition health by learning to store and cook foods in ways that minimize nutrient losses. Water-soluble vitamins are the most vulnerable of the nutrients, but both vitamins and minerals can be lost when they dissolve in water that is then discarded.

Fruits and vegetables contain enzymes that both synthesize and degrade vitamins. After a fruit or vegetable has been picked, vitamin synthesis stops, but degradation continues. To slow the degradation of vitamins, most fruits and vegetables should be kept refrigerated until used. Because many vitamins are easily destroyed by oxygen, fruits and vegetables that have been cut and juice that has been opened should be stored in airtight containers and refrigerated. (Degradative enzymes are most active at warmer temperatures.)

Water-soluble vitamins readily dissolve in water. To prevent losses during washing, rinse fruits and vegetables before cutting. To minimize losses during cooking, steam, griddle, or microwave vegetables; pressure cooking and boiling cause the greatest nutrient losses. Alternatively, use the cooking water when preparing meals such as casseroles and soups.

Finally, keep in mind that most vitamin losses are not catastrophic and that a law of diminishing returns operates. Do not fret over small losses or waste time that may be valuable in improving your health in other ways. Be assured that if you start with plenty of fruits and vegetables and are reasonably careful in their storage and preparation, you will receive a sufficient supply of all the nutrients they provide.

› REVIEW IT Explain how to minimize nutrient losses in the kitchen.
In the marketplace, food labels, the *Dietary Guidelines for Americans*, and MyPlate all help consumers learn about nutrition and how to plan healthy diets. At home, consumers can minimize nutrient losses from fruits and vegetables by refrigerating them, washing them before cutting them, storing them in airtight containers, and cooking them for short times in minimal water.

19.3 Environmental Contaminants

› LEARN IT Explain how environmental contaminants get into foods and how people can protect themselves against contamination.

Concern about environmental contamination of foods is growing as the world becomes more populated and more industrialized. Industrial processes pollute the air, water, and soil. Plants absorb the **contaminants,** and people consume the plants (grains, vegetables, legumes, and fruits) or the meat and milk products from livestock that have eaten the plants. Similarly, polluted water contaminates the fish and other seafood that people eat. Environmental contaminants in air, water, and foods find their way into our bodies and have the potential to cause numerous health problems.

Harmfulness of Environmental Contaminants The potential harmfulness of a contaminant depends in part on its **persistence**—the extent to which it lingers in the environment or in the body. Some contaminants in the environment are short-lived because microorganisms or agents such as sunlight or oxygen can break them down. Some contaminants in the body may linger for only a short time because the body rapidly excretes them or metabolizes them to harmless compounds. These contaminants present little cause for concern. Some contaminants, however, resist breakdown and can accumulate. Each level of the **food chain,** then, has a greater concentration than the one below **(bioaccumulation).** Figure 19-6 shows how bioaccumulation leads to high concentrations of toxins in animals and in people at the top of the food chain.

Contaminants enter the environment in various ways. Accidental spills are rare but can have devastating effects. More commonly, small amounts are released over long periods. The following paragraphs describe how contaminants can enter the food supply.

Methylmercury A classic example of acute contamination occurred in 1953 when a number of people in Minamata, Japan, became ill with a disease no one had seen before. By 1960, 121 cases had been reported, including 23 in infants. Mortality

contaminants: substances that make a food impure and unsuitable for ingestion.

persistence: stubborn or enduring continuance; with respect to food contaminants, the quality of persisting, rather than breaking down, in the bodies of animals and human beings.

food chain: the sequence in which living things depend on other living things for food.

bioaccumulation: the accumulation of contaminants in the flesh of animals high on the food chain.

> **FIGURE 19-6 Bioaccumulation of Toxins in the Food Chain**

This example features fish as the food for human consumption, but bioaccumulation of toxins occurs on land as well when cows, pigs, and chickens eat or drink contaminated foods or water.

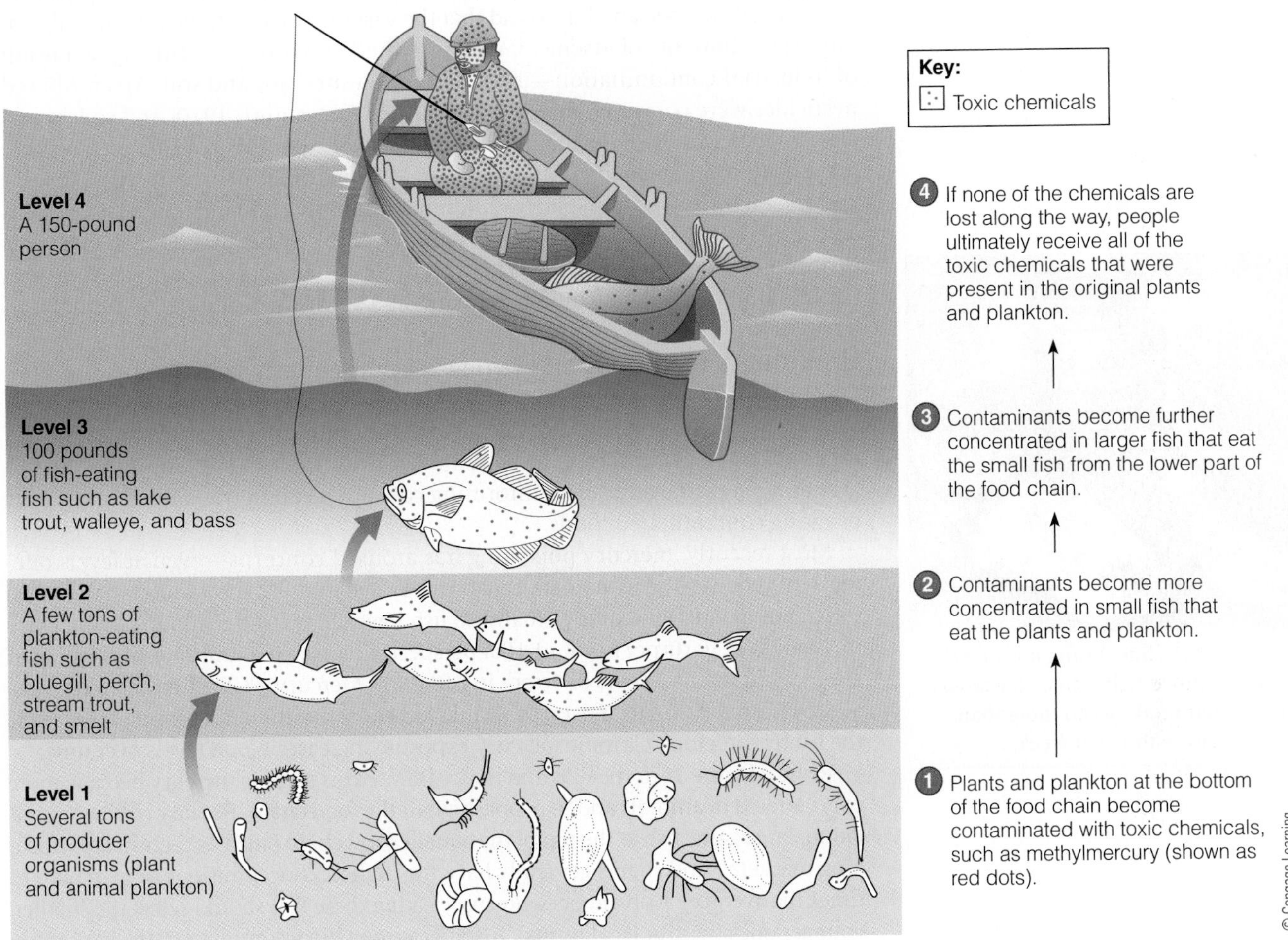

Key:
Toxic chemicals
Level 4
A 150-pound person
Level 3
100 pounds of fish-eating fish such as lake trout, walleye, and bass
Level 2
A few tons of plankton-eating fish such as bluegill, perch, stream trout, and smelt
Level 1
Several tons of producer organisms (plant and animal plankton)
4 If none of the chemicals are lost along the way, people ultimately receive all of the toxic chemicals that were present in the original plants and plankton.
3 Contaminants become further concentrated in larger fish that eat the small fish from the lower part of the food chain.
2 Contaminants become more concentrated in small fish that eat the plants and plankton.
1 Plants and plankton at the bottom of the food chain become contaminated with toxic chemicals, such as methylmercury (shown as red dots).
© Cengage Learning

was high; 46 died, and the survivors suffered blindness, deafness, lack of coordination, and intellectual deterioration. The cause was ultimately revealed to be methylmercury contamination of fish from the bay where these people lived. The infants who contracted the disease had not eaten any fish, but their mothers had, and even though the mothers exhibited no symptoms during their pregnancies, the poison affected their unborn babies. Manufacturing plants in the region were discharging mercury-containing waste into the waters of the bay, the mercury was turning into methylmercury, and the fish in the bay were accumulating this poison in their bodies. Some of the affected families had been eating fish from the bay every day.

PBB and PCB In 1973, half a ton of **PBB (polybrominated biphenyls),** toxic **organic halogens**, were accidentally mixed into some livestock feed that was distributed throughout the state of Michigan. The PBB found its way into millions of animals and then into the people who ate the meat. The seriousness of the accident came to light when dairy farmers reported that their cows were going dry, aborting their calves, and developing abnormal growths on their hooves. Although more than 30,000 cattle, sheep, and swine and more than a million chickens were destroyed, an estimated 97 percent of Michigan's residents had been exposed to PBB. Some of the exposed farm residents suffered nervous system aberrations and liver disorders.

A similar accident occurred in 1979 when **PCB (polychlorinated biphenyls)** contaminated rice oil in Taiwan. Women who had eaten the tainted rice oil gave birth to children with developmental problems. Decades later, young men who were exposed to PCB during gestation had reduced fertility. The interactive

PBB (polybrominated biphenyl) and **PCB (polychlorinated biphenyl):** toxic organic halogens used in pesticides, paints, and flame retardants.

organic halogens: an organic compound containing one or more atoms of a halogen—fluorine, chlorine, iodine, or bromine.

effects of PCB and mercury—two environmental contaminants found in fish—are especially damaging to brain functions such as balance and coordination.

Arsenic The FDA routinely tests apple juice and other fruit juices, looking for harmful substances, and has found that the vast majority of apple juice tested contains trace amounts of arsenic.[12] Arsenic—whether naturally occurring or a result of industrial contamination—is found in the water, air, and soil. Arsenic-based pesticides were commonly used in the United States until 1970, and so low levels of arsenic can be detected in agricultural fields. For this reason, even organic juices may contain arsenic. After assessing the quantities of arsenic in apple juice and the quantities of apple juice children commonly consume, the FDA is confident about the overall safety of apple juice. The FDA will take action when arsenic in apple juice is detected at 10 parts per billion, or greater. (For perspective, 1 part per billion is equivalent to about 1 second in 32 years or 1 cent in $10 million.)

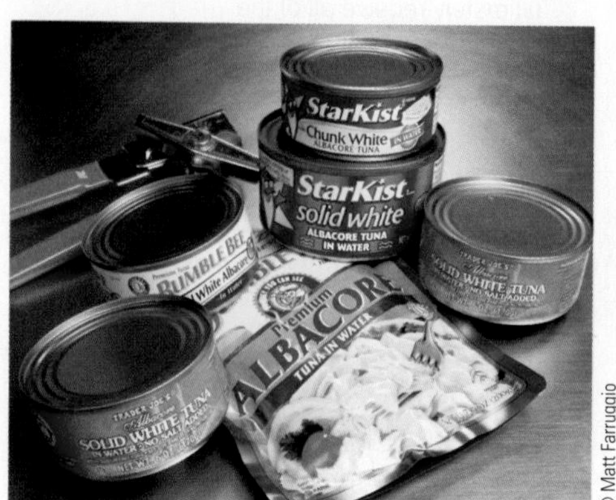

© Matt Farruggio

Because albacore ("white") tuna has more mercury than canned light tuna, consumers should limit their intake to no more than 6 ounces of albacore tuna per week.

Guidelines for Consumers How much of a threat do environmental contaminants pose to the food supply? For the most part, the hazards appear to be small. The FDA regulates the presence of contaminants in foods and requires foods with unsafe amounts to be removed from the market. Similarly, health agencies may issue advisories informing consumers about the potential dangers of eating contaminated foods.

Most recently, mercury poisoning has aroused concerns—even at levels one-tenth of those in the Minamata catastrophe. Fish and other seafood are the main sources of dietary mercury. Virtually all fish have at least trace amounts of mercury (median, 0.17 parts per million). (For perspective, 1 part per million is equivalent to about 1 minute in 2 years or 1 cent in $10,000.) Mercury, PCB, chlordane, dioxins, and DDT are the toxins most responsible for fish contamination, but mercury leads the list by threefold. Chronic mercury exposure increases blood levels over time.

Review Figure 19-6 (p. 639) and notice how toxins such as mercury become more concentrated in animals and in people high in the food chain. Because of bioaccumulation, large game fish at the top of the aquatic food chain (such as tilefish, swordfish, king mackerel, and shark) generally have the highest concentrations of mercury (10 times the average). Consumers who enjoy eating these fish should select the smaller, younger ones (within legal limits). Also because of bioaccumulation, the concentrations in fish may be a million times higher than the concentrations in the water itself.

The **EPA** regulates commercial fishing to help ensure that fish destined for consumption in the United States meet safety standards for mercury and other contaminants. Farm-raised fish usually have lower concentrations of mercury than fish caught in the wild. Consequently, most consumers in the United States are not in danger of receiving harmful levels of mercury from fish.

The potential harm from contaminants must be balanced against the potential benefits from nutrients.[13] Pregnant and lactating women and young children are most vulnerable because mercury toxicity damages the developing brain. Yet they are also likely to benefit from consuming seafood rich in omega-3 fatty acids. To receive the benefits and minimize the risks, the FDA advises that pregnant and lactating women and young children can safely consume up to 12 ounces of a variety of seafood per week. Commonly eaten choices that are relatively low in mercury include shrimp, canned light tuna, salmon, pollock, and catfish. In addition, albacore ("white") tuna should be limited to 6 ounces per week and large predatory fish (tilefish, swordfish, king mackerel, and shark) should be avoided altogether. Although limiting seafood during pregnancy is advisable, such a strategy may have a relatively small effect on prenatal blood mercury levels.[14]

What about the noncommercial fish a person catches from a local lake, river, or ocean? After all, it's almost impossible to tell whether water is contaminated without sophisticated equipment. Each state monitors its waters and issues advisories to inform the public if chemical contaminants have been found in the local fish. To find out whether a fish advisory has been posted in your region, call the local or state environmental health department.

All things considered, fish continue to support a healthy diet, providing valuable protein, omega-3 fatty acids, and minerals. For most adults, the benefits of protecting against heart disease outweigh the risks of consuming seafood regularly.[15] Ideally, consumers would select fish with high levels of omega-3 fatty acids and low levels of mercury, such as anchovies, herring, lake trout, mackerel, pollock, salmon, sardines, smelt, and tilapia.[16] In addition, they should select a variety of seafood to reduce the risk of exposure to contaminants from a single source.

› REVIEW IT Explain how environmental contaminants get into foods and how people can protect themselves against contamination.

Foods may become contaminated as pollutants enter the air, land, and sea. So far, the hazards appear relatively small. In all cases, two principles apply. First, remain alert to the possibility of contamination of foods and keep an ear open for public health announcements and advice. Second, eat a variety of foods. Varying food choices is an effective defensive strategy against the accumulation of toxins in the body. Each food eaten dilutes contaminants that may be present in other components of the diet.

19.4 Natural Toxicants in Foods

› LEARN IT Identify natural toxicants and determine whether they are hazardous.

Consumers concerned about food contamination may think that they can eliminate all poisons from their diets by eating only "natural" foods. On the contrary, nature has provided plants with an abundant array of toxicants. A few examples will show how even "natural" foods may contain potentially harmful substances. They also show that although the *potential* for harm exists, *actual* harm rarely occurs.

Poisonous mushrooms are a familiar example of plants that can be harmful when eaten. Few people know, though, that other commonly eaten foods contain substances that can cause illnesses. Cabbage, bok choy, turnips, mustard greens, kale, brussels sprouts, cauliflower, broccoli, kohlrabi, and radishes contain small quantities of goitrogens—compounds that can enlarge the thyroid gland. Eating exceptionally large amounts of goitrogen-containing vegetables can aggravate a preexisting thyroid problem, but it usually does not initiate one. Problems may develop when exceptionally large amounts (2 to 3 pounds a day) of these vegetables are eaten raw; cooking deactivates the enzyme that normally inhibits the uptake of iodine in the thyroid.[17]

Lima beans and fruit seeds such as apricot pits contain cyanogens—inactive compounds that produce the deadly poison cyanide upon activation by a specific plant enzyme. For this reason, many countries restrict commercially grown lima beans to those varieties with the lowest cyanogen contents. As for fruit seeds, they are seldom deliberately eaten. An occasional swallowed seed or two presents no danger, but a couple of dozen seeds can be fatal to a small child. Perhaps the most infamous cyanogen in seeds is laetrile—a compound erroneously represented as a cancer cure. True, laetrile kills cancer, but only at doses that kill the person too. The combination of cyanide poisoning and lack of medical attention is life-threatening.

The humble potato contains many natural poisons, including **solanine,** a powerful narcotic-like substance. Most of a potato's solanine is found in the sprouts and in the green layer that develops just beneath the skin. Solanine poisoning is extremely rare, however, because the small amounts of solanine (8 milligrams per 100 grams of potato) normally found in potatoes are harmless—even when the potato skin is eaten. Solanine can be toxic, however, and presents a hazard when consumed in large quantities (20 to 25 milligrams per 100 grams of potato). Cooking does not destroy solanine, but it can be removed by peeling the potato. Symptoms of solanine poisoning include gastrointestinal disturbances and neurological disorders.

solanine (SOH-lah-neen): a poisonous narcotic-like substance present in potato skins and sprouts.

› REVIEW IT Identify natural toxicants and determine whether they are hazardous.
Natural toxicants include the goitrogens in cabbage, cyanogens in lima beans, and solanine in potatoes. These examples of naturally occurring toxicants illustrate two familiar principles. First, any substance can be toxic when consumed in excess. Second, poisons are poisons, whether made by people or by nature. Remember, it is not the source of a chemical that makes it hazardous, but its chemical structure and the quantity consumed.

19.5 Pesticides

› LEARN IT Debate the risks and benefits of using pesticides.

The use of **pesticides** in agriculture is controversial. They help to ensure the survival of crops, but they leave **residues** in the environment and on some of the foods we eat. Balancing the benefits of pesticides to agriculture and food production against the risks to the environment and human health is an ongoing challenge.[18]

pesticides: chemicals used to control insects, weeds, fungi, and other pests on plants, vegetables, fruits, and animals. Used broadly, the term includes herbicides (to kill weeds), insecticides (to kill insects), and fungicides (to kill fungi).

residues: whatever remains. In the case of pesticides, those amounts that remain on or in foods when people buy and use them.

tolerance level: the maximum amount of a residue permitted in a food when a pesticide is used according to label directions.

Hazards and Regulation of Pesticides

Ideally, a pesticide destroys the pest and quickly degenerates to nontoxic products without accumulating in the food chain. Then, by the time consumers eat the food, no harmful residues remain. Unfortunately, no such perfect pesticide exists. As new pesticides are developed, government agencies assess their risks and benefits and vigilantly monitor their use.

Hazards of Pesticides Pesticides applied in the field may linger on foods. Health risks from pesticide exposure are probably small for healthy adults, but children, the elderly, and people with weakened immune systems may be vulnerable to some types of pesticide poisoning. Studies report associations between pesticides and childhood cancers, decreased cognitive function, and behavioral problems.[19] To protect infants and children, government agencies set a **tolerance level** for each pesticide by first identifying foods that children commonly eat in large amounts and then considering the effects of pesticide exposure during each developmental stage. Research shows that estimates of dietary pesticide intakes in children are similar to actual measured intakes.[20]

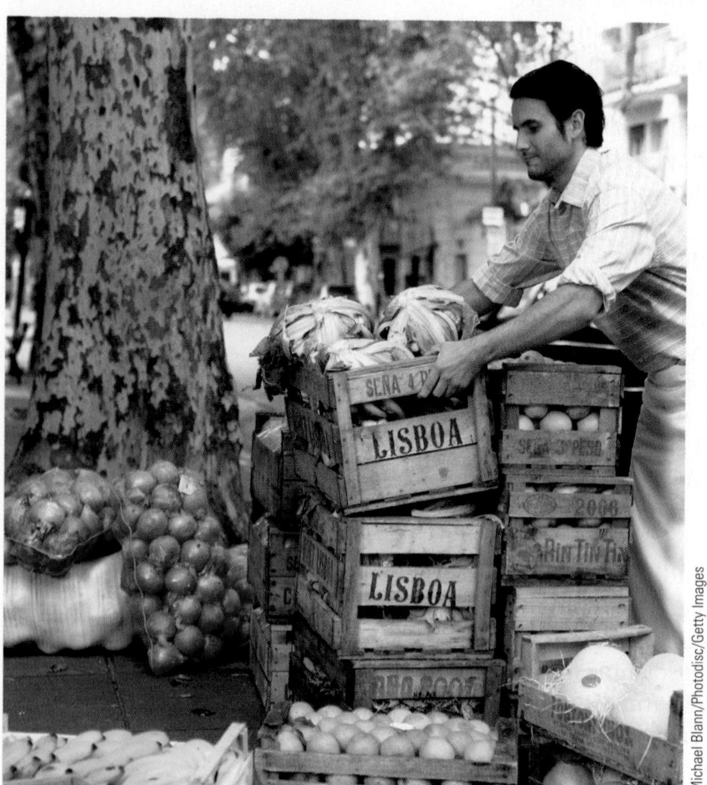

Michael Blann/Photodisc/Getty Images

As many as 400 varieties of fruits and vegetables are imported from other countries.

Regulation of Pesticides Consumers depend on the EPA and the FDA to keep pesticide use within safe limits. These agencies evaluate the risks and benefits of a pesticide's use by asking such questions as: How dangerous is it? How much residue is left on the crop? How much harm does the pesticide do to the environment? How necessary is it? What are the alternatives to its use?

If the pesticide is approved, the EPA establishes a tolerance level for its presence in foods, well below the level at which it could cause any conceivable harm. Tolerance regulations also state the specific crops to which each pesticide can be applied. If a pesticide is misused, growers risk fines, lawsuits, and destruction of their crops.

Once tolerances are set, the FDA enforces them by monitoring foods and livestock feeds for the presence of pesticides. Over the past several decades of testing, the FDA has seldom found residues above tolerance levels, so it appears that pesticides are generally used according to regulations. Minimal pesticide use means lower costs for growers. In addition to costs, many farmers are also concerned about the environment, the quality of their farmland, and a safe food supply. Where violations are found, they are usually due to unusual weather conditions, use of unapproved pesticides, or misuse—for example, application of a particular pesticide to a crop for which it has not been approved.

Pesticides from Other Countries A substantial and increasing amount of the fruits and vegetables consumed in the United States are imported from other countries. These countries have their own pesticide regulations—some more, and others less, stringent than those in the United States. To export into the United States, countries are required to comply with US pesticide tolerance limits, but FDA testing of imported produce is fairly limited.[21] Consequently, the extent to which US consumers are exposed to elevated levels of pesticide residues from imported foods compared with domestic crops is relatively unknown.

Monitoring Pesticides The FDA collects and analyzes samples of both domestic and imported foods. If the agency finds samples in violation of regulations, it can seize the products or order them destroyed. Individual states also scan for pesticides (as well as for industrial chemicals) and provide information to the FDA.

Food in the Fields In addition to its ongoing surveillance, the FDA conducts focused sampling to determine the presence of particular pesticides in specific crops. For example, the agency might search for aldicarb in potatoes, captan in cherries, and diaminozide (the chemical name for Alar) in apples, among others.

Food on the Plate In addition to monitoring crops in the field for pesticides, the FDA also monitors people's actual intakes. The agency conducts the Total Diet Study (sometimes called the "Market Basket Survey") to estimate the dietary intakes of pesticide residues by eight age and gender groups from infants to senior citizens. Four times a year, FDA surveyors buy almost 300 foods from US grocery stores, each time in several cities. They prepare the foods table ready and then analyze them not only for pesticides, but also for essential minerals, industrial chemicals, **heavy metals**, and radioactive materials. In all, the survey reports on more than 6000 samples a year, including samples imported from 100 countries. Most heavily sampled are fresh vegetables, fruits, and dairy products.

The Total Diet Study provides a direct estimate of the amounts of pesticide residues that remain in foods as they are usually eaten—after they have been washed, peeled, and cooked. Analyses reveal that almost all samples fall well below the amounts considered acceptable. The amount considered acceptable is "the daily intake of a chemical, which, if ingested over a lifetime, appears to be without appreciable risk." *Without appreciable risk* means "practical certainty that injury will not result even after a lifetime of exposure." All in all, these findings confirm the safety of the US food supply.

Consumer Concerns Despite these reassuring reports, consumers still worry that food monitoring may not be adequate. For one thing, manufacturers develop new pesticides all the time. For another, as described earlier, other countries use different pesticides and follow less stringent guidelines. For still another, although US regulations may protect crops adequately, they may not necessarily protect the environment or the people who work in the fields. Concerns over poisoning of soil, waterways, wildlife, and workers may well be valid. In addition to harming workers, occupational exposure to pesticides is associated with brain tumors in their children.[22]

The FDA does not sample *all* food shipments or test for *all* pesticides in each sample. In fact, the FDA inspects only about 1 percent of the food that enters the United States. The FDA is a *monitoring* agency, and as such, it cannot, nor can it be expected to, guarantee 100 percent safety in the food supply. Instead, it sets standards so that substances do not become a hazard, checks enough samples to adequately assess average food safety, and acts promptly when problems or suspicions arise.

Minimizing Risks Whether consumers ingest pesticide residues depends on a number of factors. How much of a given food does the consumer eat? What pesticide was used on it? How much was used? How long ago was the food last sprayed? Did environmental conditions promote pest growth or pesticide breakdown? How well was the produce washed? Was it peeled or cooked? With so

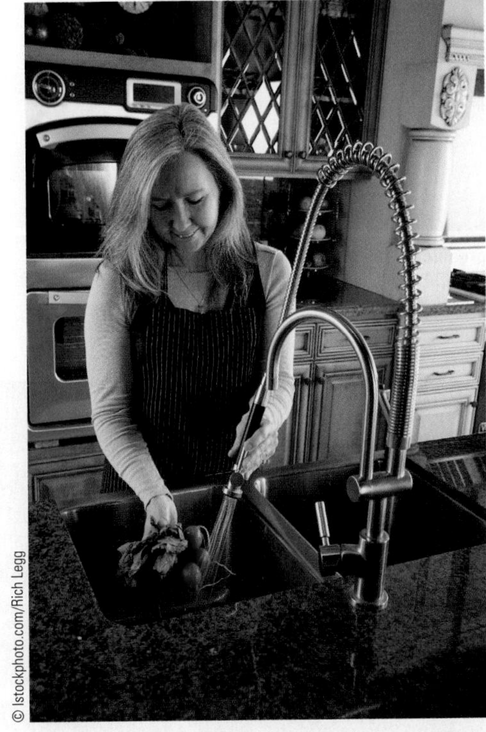

Washing fresh fruits and vegetables removes most, if not all, of the pesticide residues that might have been present.

heavy metals: mineral ions such as mercury or lead, so called because of their relatively high atomic weight; many heavy metals are poisonous.

TABLE 19-3 Tips to Minimize Pesticide Residues and Bacteria Contamination

When Shopping for Foods
• Select fruits and vegetables that do not have holes.
• Select a variety of foods to minimize exposure to any one pesticide.
• Consider buying certified organic foods when shopping for produce most likely to be contaminated (see Table 19-4).
When Preparing Foods
• Wash your hands for 20 seconds with warm water and soap before and after preparing foods.
• Trim the fat from meat, and remove the skin from poultry and fish; discard fats and oils in broths and pan drippings (pesticide residues concentrate in the animal's fat).
• Wash fresh produce in warm running water, gently rub soft produce or use a scrub brush on firm produce, and rinse thoroughly.
• Use a knife to peel an orange and grapefruit; do not bite into the peel.
• Discard the outer leaves of leafy vegetables such as cabbage and lettuce.
• Cut away damaged or bruised areas.
• Wash fruits and vegetables before peeling to avoid transferring dirt and bacteria from the knife onto the produce. Peel waxed fruits and vegetables; waxes don't wash off and can seal in pesticide residues.
• Peel vegetables such as carrots and fruits such as apples when possible (peeling removes dirt, bacteria, and pesticides that remain in or on the peel, but also removes fibers, vitamins, and minerals).

many factors, consumers cannot know for sure whether pesticide residues remain on foods, but they can minimize their risks by following the guidelines offered in Table 19-3; washing, peeling, and cooking fruits and vegetables reduces pesticide residue levels.[23] The food supply is protected well enough that consumers who take these precautions can feel secure that the foods they eat are safe.

Alternatives to Pesticides The use of pesticides has helped to generate higher crop yields that feed the world and protect against diseases transmitted by insects. Still, many consumers are leery. To feed a nation while using fewer pesticides requires creative farming methods. Highlight 19 describes how scientists can genetically alter plants to enhance their production of natural pesticides, and Chapter 20 presents alternative, or sustainable, agriculture methods. These methods include such practices as rotating crops, releasing organisms into fields to destroy pests, and planting nonfood crops nearby to kill pests or attract them away from the food crops. For example, releasing sterile male fruit flies into orchards helps to curb the population growth of these pests; some flowers, such as marigolds, release natural insecticides and are often planted near crops such as tomatoes. Such alternative farming methods are more labor-intensive and may produce smaller yields than conventional methods, at least initially. Over time, though, by eliminating expensive pesticides, fertilizers, and fuels, these alternatives may actually cut costs more than they cut yields.

organic: in agriculture, crops grown and processed according to USDA regulations defining the use of fertilizers, herbicides, insecticides, fungicides, preservatives, and other chemical ingredients.

Organically Grown Crops Alternative methods are especially useful for farmers who want to produce and market **organic** crops that are grown and processed according to USDA regulations defining the use of synthetic fertilizers, herbicides, insecticides, fungicides, preservatives, and other chemical ingredients. Similarly, meat, poultry, eggs, and dairy products may be called organic if the livestock has been raised according to USDA regulations defining the grazing conditions and the use of organic feed, hormones, and antibiotics. In addition, producers may *not* claim products are organic if they have been irradiated, genetically engineered, or grown with fertilizer made from sewer sludge. Figure 19-7 shows examples of food labels for products using organic ingredients.

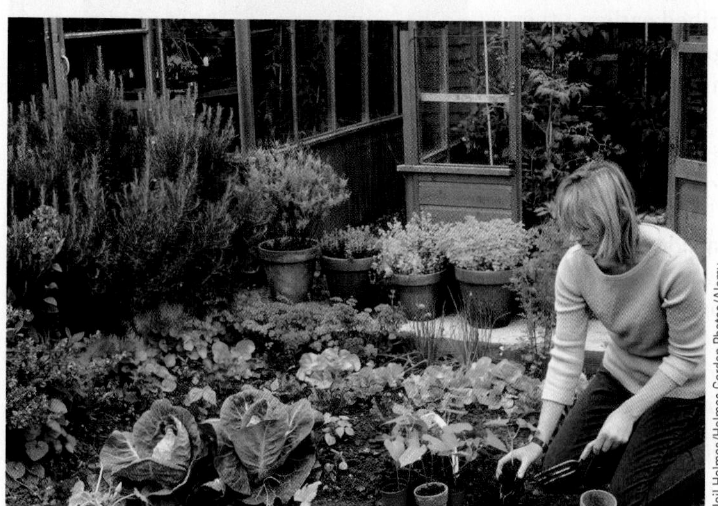

People can grow organic crops when their gardens or farms are relatively small.

Most organic foods are marked as such, but consumers can also determine whether fruits and vegetables are organic by reading the product code on produce stickers. Codes for conventionally grown produce are four digits. Regular bananas, for example, have the code 4011. Codes for organic produce are five digits and begin with 9. (Thus the product code for organic bananas is 94011.) Codes for genetically modified produce are also five digits and begin with 8. (Genetically modified bananas are given the product code 84011.)

Consumers spend more than $25 billion a year on organic foods. Reasons for buying organic include avoiding pesticides, benefiting the environment, protecting animals, improving worker safety, and obtaining safer and more nutritious foods.

> FIGURE 19-7 **Food Labels for Organic Products**

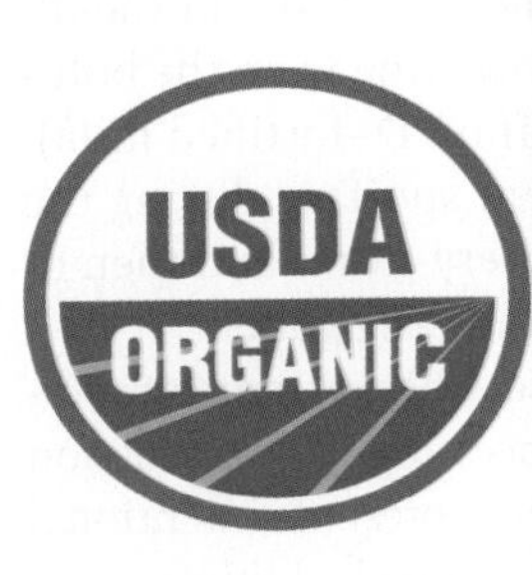

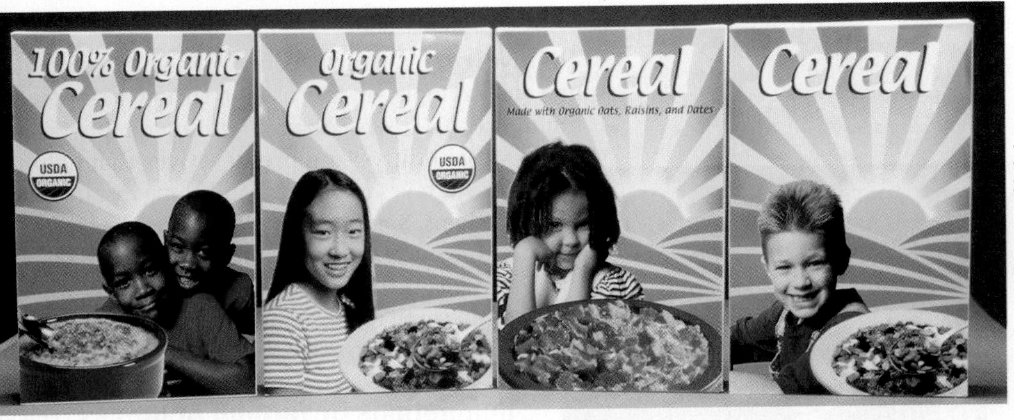

Source: United States Department of Agriculture

Organic foods that have met USDA standards may use this seal on their labels.

Foods made with 100 percent organic ingredients may claim "100% organic" and use the seal.

Foods made with at least 95 percent organic ingredients may claim "organic" and use the seal.

Foods made with at least 70 percent organic ingredients may list up to three of those ingredients on the front panel.

Foods made with less than 70 percent organic ingredients may list them on the side panel, but cannot make any claims on the front.

Eating organic foods does reduce exposure to pesticide residues.[24] In as little as five days, eating organic foods can reduce urinary pesticide metabolites to nondetectable levels; this relatively simple and quick way to reduce pesticide exposure may be especially valuable to children.[25] Each year, an environmental advocacy group publishes a list of the most popular fruits and vegetables that are most and least likely to have pesticide residues (see Table 19-4).[26] The suggestion is that because pesticide residues in conventionally grown foods are higher than in organic foods, consumers may want to pay attention to these lists when considering whether to make organic purchases. Some research contradicts such advice and indicates that the pesticide residues on even the most contaminated fruits and vegetables pose negligible risks and that using organic products does not reduce risks.[27] Whether buying conventionally grown or organically grown produce, consumers benefit most from eating at least five servings of fruits and vegetables daily.

Are organic foods nutritionally superior to conventional foods? For the most part, nutrient differences are relatively small and within the range that normally occurs in crops. Some research suggests that organic crops may have a longer shelf life and better flavor, perhaps due to differences in soil type, soil nutrients, or environmental conditions.[28] Limited research suggests that foods produced organically have increased amounts of some phytochemicals.[29] Researchers disagree about whether eating organic foods offers any real health benefits.[30]

Interestingly, organic has intense meanings for many consumers. In one study, participants tasting foods, such as two yogurts, rated the one labeled "organic" as more nutritious, lower in fat, and worth more money and the one labeled "regular" as more flavorful—even though both yogurts were organic and identical (only their labels differed).[31]

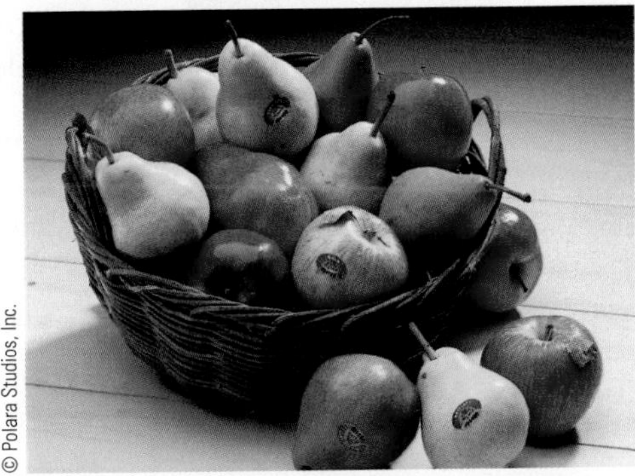

© Polara Studios, Inc.

Many consumers are willing to pay a little more for organic produce.

TABLE 19-4 Most and Least Pesticide-Contaminated Fruits and Vegetables

Most Contaminated	Least Contaminated
Apples	Corn
Strawberries	Onions
Grapes	Pineapples
Celery	Avocados
Peaches	Cabbage
Spinach	Peas
Bell peppers	Papayas
Nectarines (imported)	Mangoes
Cucumbers	Asparagus
Potatoes	Eggplant
Cherry tomatoes	Kiwi
Hot peppers	Grapefruit
Blueberries	Cantaloupe
Lettuce	Sweet potatoes
Snap peas (imported)	Mushrooms

NOTE: These fruits and vegetables are ranked in order of their pesticide load.

> REVIEW IT Debate the risks and benefits of using pesticides.

Pesticides can safely improve crop yields when used according to regulations, but they can also be hazardous when used inappropriately. The FDA tests both domestic and imported foods for pesticide residues in the fields and in market basket surveys of foods prepared table ready. Consumers can minimize their ingestion of pesticide residues on foods by following the suggestions in Table 19-3. Alternative farming methods may allow farmers to grow crops with few or no pesticides.

19.6 Food Additives

› LEARN IT List common food additives, their purposes, and examples.

Additives confer many benefits on foods. Some reduce the risk of foodborne illness (for example, nitrites used in curing meat prevent poisoning from the botulinum toxin). Others enhance nutrient quality (as in vitamin D–fortified milk). Most additives are **preservatives** that help prevent spoilage during the time it takes to deliver foods long distances to grocery stores and then to kitchens. Some additives simply make foods look and taste good.

Intentional additives are put into foods on purpose, whereas indirect additives may get in unintentionally before or during processing. This discussion begins with the regulations that govern additives, then presents intentional additives class by class, and finally says a word about indirect additives.

Without additives, bread would quickly get moldy, and salad dressing would go rancid.

Regulations Governing Additives

The FDA's regulation of additives focuses primarily on safety.[32] To receive permission to use a new additive in food products, a manufacturer must satisfy the FDA that the additive is:

- Effective (it does what it is supposed to do)
- Detectable and measurable in the final food product
- Safe (when fed in large doses to animals under strictly controlled conditions, it causes no cancer, birth defects, or other injury)

On approving an additive's use, the FDA writes a regulation stating in what amounts and in what foods the additive may be used. No additive receives permanent approval, and all must undergo periodic review.

The GRAS List Many familiar substances are exempted from complying with the FDA's approval process because they are **generally recognized as safe (GRAS),** based either on their extensive, long-term use in foods or on current scientific evidence. Several hundred substances are on the GRAS list, including such items as salt, sugar, caffeine, and many spices. Whenever substantial scientific evidence or public outcry has questioned the safety of any substance on the GRAS list, it has been reevaluated. If a legitimate question has been raised about a substance, it has been removed or reclassified. Meanwhile, the entire GRAS list is subjected to ongoing review.

The Delaney Clause One risk that the US law on additives refuses to tolerate at any level is the risk of cancer. To remain on the GRAS list, an additive must not have been found to be a **carcinogen** in any test on animals or human beings. The **Delaney Clause** (the part of the law that states this criterion) is uncompromising in addressing carcinogens in foods and drugs; in fact, it has been under fire for many years for being too strict and inflexible.

The Delaney Clause is best understood as a product of a different historical era. It was adopted decades ago, at a time when scientists knew less about the relationships between carcinogens and cancer development. At that time, most substances were detectable in foods only in relatively large amounts, such as parts per thousand. Today, scientific understanding of cancer has progressed, and technology has advanced so that carcinogens in foods can be detected even when they are present only in parts per billion or even per trillion. (For perspective, one part per trillion is equivalent to about 1 inch in 16 million miles; or 1 second in 32,000 years.) Earlier, "zero risk" may have seemed attainable, but today we know it is not: all substances, no matter how pure, can be shown to be contaminated at some level with one carcinogen or another. For these reasons, the FDA prefers to deem additives (and pesticides and other contaminants) safe if lifetime use presents no more than a one-in-a-million risk of cancer to human beings. Thus, instead of the "zero-risk" policy of the Delaney Clause, the FDA uses a "negligible-risk" standard, sometimes referred to as the ***de minimis* rule.**

Margin of Safety Whatever risk level is permitted, actual risks must be determined by research. To determine risks posed by an additive, researchers feed test

additives: substances not normally consumed as foods but added to food either intentionally or by accident.

preservatives: antimicrobial agents, antioxidants, and other additives that retard spoilage or maintain desired qualities, such as softness in baked goods.

generally recognized as safe (GRAS): food additives that have long been in use and are believed to be safe. First established by the FDA in 1958, the GRAS list is subject to revision as new facts become known.

carcinogen: a substance that can cause cancer; the adjective is *carcinogenic*.

Delaney Clause: a 1958 amendment to the Food, Drugs, and Cosmetic Act of 1938, named after Congressman James Delaney of New York that states that no substance known to cause cancer in animals or human beings at any dose level shall be added to foods.

***de minimis* rule:** a guideline that defines risk as a cancer rate of less than one cancer per million people exposed to a contaminant over a 70-year lifetime.

animals the additive at several concentrations throughout their lives. The additive is then permitted in foods in amounts 100 times *below* the lowest level that is found to cause any harmful effect—that is, at a 1/100 **margin of safety.** In many foods, *naturally* occurring substances occur with narrower margins of safety. Even nutrients pose risks at dose levels above those recommended and normally consumed: for older adults, the RDA for vitamin D is only 1/5 of the Upper Level.

Risks versus Benefits Of course, additives would not be added to foods if they only presented risks. In general, additives are used in foods when they offer benefits that outweigh the risks or make the risks worth taking. No amount of risk may be worth taking in the case of color additives that only enhance appearance but do not improve health or safety. In contrast, the FDA finds it worth taking the small risks associated with the use of nitrites on meat products, for example, because nitrites inhibit the formation of the deadly botulinum toxin. The choice involves a compromise between the risks of using additives and the risks of doing without them.

It is the manufacturers' responsibility to use only the amounts of additives that are necessary to achieve the needed effect, and no more. The FDA also requires that additives *not* be used:

- To disguise faulty or inferior products
- To deceive the consumer
- If use would significantly destroy nutrients
- If effects can be achieved by economical, sound manufacturing processes instead

Intentional Food Additives

Intentional food additives are added to foods to give them some desirable characteristic: resistance to spoilage, color, flavor, texture, stability, or nutritional value. Some food additives derive from natural sources (for example, beets may provide food coloring); others are not found in nature, but can be synthesized as artificial ingredients. In addition, some natural ingredients can also be synthesized as artificial ingredients (for example, vitamin C may be derived from an orange or manufactured in a laboratory). All additives—whether natural or artificial—are subject to the same FDA safety standards. This section describes additives people most often ask about.

Foods can go bad in many ways. One way is by becoming contaminated with microbes that cause foodborne illnesses, a hazard that justifies the use of antimicrobial agents.

Antimicrobials The most widely used antimicrobial agents are ordinary salt and sugar. Salt has been used throughout history to preserve meat and fish; sugar serves the same purpose in canned and frozen fruits and in jams and jellies. Both exert their protective effect primarily by capturing water and making it unavailable to microbes.

Other antimicrobial agents, the **nitrites,** are added to foods for three main purposes: to preserve color, especially the pink color of hot dogs and other cured meats; to enhance flavor by inhibiting rancidity, especially in cured meats and poultry; and to protect against bacterial growth. In amounts smaller than those needed to confer color, nitrites prevent the growth of the bacteria that produce the deadly botulinum toxin.

Nitrites clearly prevent food spoilage and bacterial contamination, but their use has been controversial. During the curing process and in the human body, nitrites can be converted to **nitrosamines.** Some nitrosamines are known to cause cancer in animals, but evidence is lacking in humans.[33] In fact, limited evidence suggests that nitrites may actually be beneficial to human health.[34] The USDA and FDA regulate and monitor the use of nitrites in foods and beverages.

Another food additive used in ready-to-eat meat and poultry products—such as sausages, hot dogs, and bologna—is a mixture of viruses known as **bacteriophages.** Bacteriophages destroy the bacterium *Listeria monocytogenes,* thus protecting consumers from the potentially life-threatening foodborne illness listeriosis. These additives are included in the ingredients list on food labels as a "bacteriophage preparation."

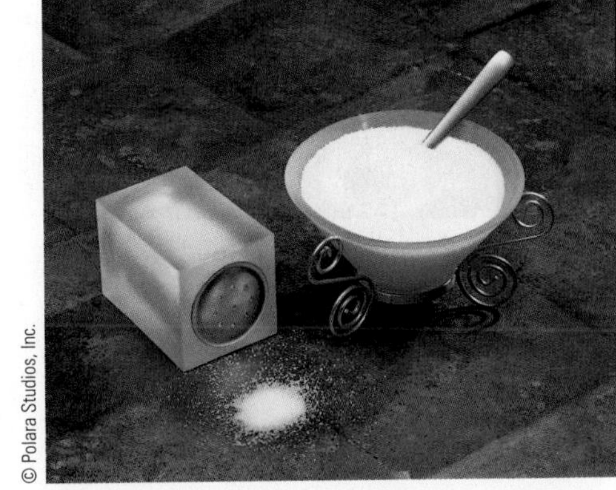

Both salt and sugar act as preservatives by extracting water from food; microbes cannot grow without water.

margin of safety: when speaking of food additives, a zone between the concentration normally used and that at which a hazard exists. For common table salt, for example, the margin of safety is 1/5 (five times the amount normally used would be hazardous).

intentional food additives: additives intentionally added to foods, such as nutrients, colors, and preservatives.

nitrites (NYE-trites): salts added to food to prevent botulism. One example is sodium nitrite, which is used to preserve meats.

nitrosamines (nye-TROHS-uh-meens): derivatives of nitrites that may be formed in the stomach when nitrites combine with amines. Nitrosamines are carcinogenic in animals.

bacteriophages (bak-TIR-ee-oh-fayjz): viruses that infect bacteria.

- **bacterio** = bacteria
- **phage** = eat

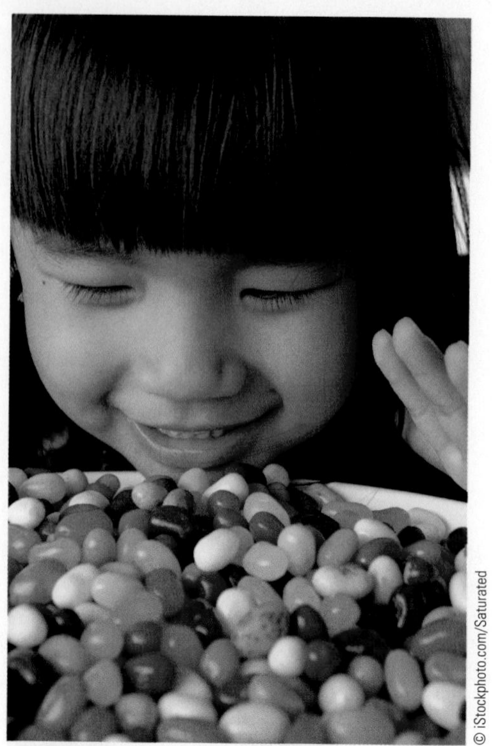
© iStockphoto.com/Saturated

Color additives not only make foods attractive, but they identify flavors as well. Everyone agrees that yellow jellybeans should taste lemony and black ones should taste like licorice.

Antioxidants Another way food can go bad is by exposure to oxygen (oxidation). Often, these changes involve no hazard to health, but they damage the food's appearance, flavor, and nutritional quality. Oxidation is easy to detect when sliced apples or potatoes turn brown or when oil goes rancid. Antioxidants prevent these reactions. Among the antioxidants approved for use in foods are vitamin C (ascorbate) and vitamin E (tocopherol).

Another group of antioxidants, the **sulfites,** cost less than the vitamins. Sulfites prevent oxidation in many processed foods and alcoholic beverages (especially wine). Because some people experience adverse reactions, the FDA prohibits sulfite use on foods intended to be consumed raw, with the exception of grapes, and requires foods and drugs that contain sulfite additives to declare it on their labels. For most people, sulfites pose no hazard in the amounts used in products, but there is one more consideration—sulfites destroy the B vitamin thiamin. For this reason, the FDA prohibits their use in foods that are important sources of the vitamin, such as enriched grain products.

Two other antioxidants in wide use are **BHA** and **BHT,** which prevent rancidity in baked goods and snack foods. Several tests have shown that animals fed large amounts of BHT develop *less* cancer when exposed to carcinogens and live *longer* than controls. Apparently, BHT protects against cancer through its antioxidant effect, which is similar to that of the antioxidant nutrients. The amount of BHT ingested daily from the US diet, however, contributes little to the body's antioxidant defense system. A caution: at intakes higher than those that protect against cancer, BHT *causes* cancer. Vitamins E and C remain the most important dietary antioxidants to strengthen defenses against cancer. (See Highlight 11 for a full discussion.)

Colors Only a few artificial colors remain on the FDA's list of additives approved for use in foods—a highly select group that has survived considerable testing. Colors derived from the natural pigments of plants must meet standards of purity and safety, just as artificial colors do. Examples of natural pigments commonly used by the food industry are the caramel that tints cola beverages and baked goods and the carotenoids that color margarine, cheeses, and pastas. Carotenoids are also added to the feed for farm-raised salmon, which deepens the pink flesh color.

Flavors Myriad natural flavors, artificial flavors, and flavor enhancers are among the most often used food additives. Many foods taste delicious because manufacturers have added the natural flavors of spices, herbs, essential oils, fruits, and fruit juices. Some spices, notably those used in Mediterranean cooking, provide antioxidant protection as well as flavors. Often, natural flavors are used in combination with artificial flavors.

One of the best-known flavor enhancers is **monosodium glutamate,** or **MSG**—a sodium salt of the amino acid glutamic acid. MSG is used widely in a number of foods, especially Asian foods, canned vegetables, soups, and processed meats. Besides enhancing the well-known sweet, salty, bitter, and sour tastes, MSG itself may possess a unique flavor. Adverse reactions to MSG—known as the **MSG symptom complex**—may occur in people with asthma and in sensitive individuals who consume large amounts of MSG, especially on an empty stomach. Otherwise, MSG is considered safe for adults. It is not allowed in foods designed for infants, however. Food labels require ingredient lists to itemize all additives, including MSG.

Sugar Alternatives The sugar alternatives, introduced in Chapter 4, are among the most widely used artificial flavor additives. Table 4-8 (p. 119) provides a summary of alternative sweeteners. This section presents safety issues surrounding a few of the most controversial ones.

Questions about the safety of the artificial sweetener saccharin surfaced in 1977, when experiments suggested that large doses of saccharin (equivalent to hundreds of cans of diet soda daily for a lifetime) increased the risk of bladder cancer in rats. As a result, the FDA proposed banning saccharin. Public outcry in favor of saccharin was so loud, however, that Congress imposed a moratorium on the ban while additional safety studies were conducted. Products containing

sulfites: salts containing sulfur that are added to foods to prevent spoilage.

BHA and **BHT:** preservatives commonly used to slow the development of off-flavors, odors, and color changes caused by oxidation. BHA is butylated hydroxyanisole, and BHT is butylated hydroxytoluene.

monosodium glutamate (MSG): a sodium salt of the amino acid glutamic acid commonly used as a flavor enhancer. The FDA classifies MSG as a "generally recognized as safe" ingredient.

MSG symptom complex: an acute, temporary intolerance reaction that may occur after the ingestion of the additive MSG (monosodium glutamate). Symptoms include burning sensations, chest and facial flushing and pain, and throbbing headaches.

saccharin were required to carry a warning label until 2001, when studies concluded that saccharin did not cause cancer in humans. Common sense dictates that consuming large amounts of any substance is probably not wise, but at current, moderate intake levels, saccharin appears to be safe for most people.

Aspartame—a simple chemical compound made of two amino acids (phenylalanine and aspartic acid) and a methyl group (CH_3)—must bear a warning label for people with the inherited disease phenylketonuria (PKU). People with PKU are unable to dispose of any excess phenylalanine. The accumulation of phenylalanine and its by-products is toxic to the developing nervous system, causing irreversible brain damage. The little extra phenylalanine from aspartame poses only a small risk, even in heavy aspartame users, but people with PKU need to get all their required phenylalanine from protein- and nutrient-rich foods instead of from an artificial sweetener.

During metabolism in the body, the methyl group of aspartame temporarily becomes methyl alcohol (methanol)—a potentially toxic compound. This breakdown also occurs in aspartame-sweetened beverages when they are stored at warm temperatures over time. The amount of methanol produced may be safe to consume, but a person may not want to, considering that the beverage has lost its sweetness. In the body, enzymes convert methanol to formaldehyde, another toxic compound. Finally, formaldehyde is broken down to carbon dioxide. Before aspartame could be approved, the quantities of these products generated during metabolism had to be determined, and they were found to fall below the threshold at which they would cause harm. In fact, ounce for ounce, tomato juice yields six times as much methanol as a diet soda.

The amount of artificial sweetener considered safe is called the **Acceptable Daily Intake (ADI)** and represents the amount of consumption that, if maintained every day throughout a person's life, would still be considered safe by a wide margin. It usually reflects an amount 100 times less than the level at which no observed effects occur in animal research studies. The ADI for aspartame, for example, is 50 milligrams per kilogram of body weight. For a 150-pound adult, the ADI is equivalent to 97 packets of Equal or 20 cans of soft drinks sweetened only with aspartame every day for a lifetime. Most people who use aspartame consume less than 5 milligrams per kilogram of body weight per day. Table 4-8 (p. 119) includes the ADI for approved sweeteners.

Texture and Stability Some additives help to maintain a desirable consistency in foods. Emulsifiers keep mayonnaise stable, control crystallization in syrups, disperse spices in salad dressings, and allow powdered coffee creamer to dissolve easily. Gums are added to thicken foods and help form gels. Yeast may be added to provide leavening, and bicarbonates and acids may be used to control acidity.

Nutrients As mentioned earlier, nutrients are sometimes added as antioxidants (vitamins C and E) or for color (beta-carotene and other carotenoids). In addition, manufacturers sometimes add nutrients to fortify or maintain the nutritional quality of foods. Included among nutrient additives are the five nutrients added to grains (thiamin, riboflavin, niacin, folate, and iron), the iodine added to salt, the vitamins A and D added to milk, and the nutrients added to fortified breakfast cereals. Appropriate uses of nutrient additives are to:

- Correct dietary deficiencies known to result in diseases
- Restore nutrients to levels found in the food before storage, handling, and processing
- Balance the vitamin, mineral, and protein contents of a food in proportion to the energy content
- Correct nutritional inferiority in a food that replaces a more nutritious traditional food

A nutrient-poor food with nutrients added may appear to be nutrient-rich, but it is rich only in those nutrients chosen for addition. Table 19-5 (p. 650) summarizes intentional food additives.

Acceptable Daily Intake (ADI): the estimated amount of a sweetener that individuals can safely consume each day over the course of a lifetime without adverse effect.

TABLE 19-5 Intentional Food Additives

Food Additive	Purpose	Common Examples
Antimicrobials	Prevent food spoilage from microorganisms	Salt, sugar, nitrites and nitrates (such as sodium nitrate), bacteriophages
Antioxidants	Prevent oxidative changes in color, flavor, or texture and delay rancidity and other damage to foods caused by oxygen	Vitamin C (erythorbic acid, sodium ascorbate), vitamin E (tocopherol), sulfites (sulfur dioxide, sodium sulfite, sodium bisulfite, potassium bisulfite, sodium metabisulfite, potassium metabisulfite), BHA and BHT
Colors	Enhance appearance	Artificial: indigotine, erythrosine, tartrazine Natural: annatto (yellow), caramel (yellowish brown), carotenoids (yellowish orange), dehydrated beets (reddish brown), grape skins (red, green)
Flavors	Enhance taste	Salt, sugar, spices, artificial sweeteners, MSG
Emulsifiers and gums	Thicken, stabilize, or otherwise improve consistency and texture	Emulsifiers: lecithin, alginates, mono- and diglycerides Gums: agar, alginates, carrageenan, guar, locust bean, psyllium, pectin, xanthan gum, gum arabic, cellulose derivatives
Nutrients (vitamins and minerals)	Improve the nutritive value by replacing vitamins and minerals lost in processing (enrichment) or adding vitamins or minerals that may be lacking in the diet (fortification)	Thiamin, niacin, riboflavin, folate, iron (in grain products); iodine (in salt); vitamins A and D (in milk); vitamin C and calcium (in fruit drinks); vitamin B_{12} (in vegetarian foods)

Indirect Food Additives **Indirect** or **incidental additives** find their way into foods during harvesting, production, processing, storage, or packaging. Incidental additives may include tiny bits of plastic, glass, paper, tin, and other substances from packages as well as chemicals from processing, such as the solvent used to decaffeinate coffee. The following paragraphs discuss six different types of indirect additives that sometimes make headline news.

Acrylamide Raw potatoes don't have it, but french fries do—acrylamide, a compound that forms when carbohydrate-rich foods containing sugars and the amino acid asparagine are cooked at high temperatures. Apparently, acrylamide has been in foods ever since we started baking, frying, and roasting, but only recently has its presence been analyzed. At high doses, acrylamide causes cancer in animals and nerve damage in people. As such, scientists classify it as both a carcinogen and a **genotoxicant.** Quantities commonly found in foods such as french fries, potato chips, breakfast cereals, and cookies, however, appear to be well below the amounts that cause such damage. The FDA is investigating how acrylamide is formed in foods, how its formation can be limited, and whether its presence is harmful.

Food Packaging The FDA ensures the safety of food packaging and assesses whether packaging materials might migrate into foods. These materials include coatings on can interiors, plastics, papers, and sealants.

Some microwave products are sold in "active packaging" that helps to cook the food; for example, pizzas are often heated on a metalized film laminated to paperboard. This film absorbs the microwave energy in the oven and reaches temperatures as high as 500°F. At such temperatures, packaging components migrate into the food. For this reason, manufacturers must perform specific tests to determine whether materials are migrating into foods. If they are, their safety must be confirmed by strict procedures similar to those governing intentional additives.

Most microwave products are sold in "passive packaging" that is transparent to microwaves and simply holds the food as it cooks. These containers don't get much hotter than the foods, but materials still migrate at high temperatures. Consumers should not reuse these containers in the microwave oven. Instead they should use only glass or ceramic containers labeled as microwave safe; tiny air bubbles in some glass may expand when microwaved, causing the glass to break and glazes on some ceramics to leach, contaminating the food. In the United States, these ceramic containers cannot be sold without a permanent marking stating "Not for food use." Similarly, use only plastic wraps labeled as microwave-safe. Avoid using disposable styrofoam or plastic containers such as those used for carryout or margarine.

Similarly, a chemical known as bisphenol A (BPA) can leach from hard-plastic bottles and coatings of some food cans into food and beverages. The FDA has some concern about the potential health effects of BPA and is taking steps to

indirect or **incidental additives:** substances that can get into food as a result of contact during growing, processing, packaging, storing, cooking, or some other stage before the foods are consumed; sometimes called *accidental additives.*

genotoxicant: a substance that mutates or damages genetic material.

reduce exposure in the food supply, including banning its use in baby bottles and sippy cups.[35] Consumers who want to limit their exposure to BPA should know that plastic containers marked with recycle codes 3 or 7 may be made with BPA. In addition, consumers should not expose plastic containers made with BPA to heat, including hot liquids, microwaves, or dishwashers.

To limit contamination and waste from packaging, some manufacturers are creating food wrappers and containers that are edible and soluble. For example, coatings similar to those used to cover pills might encase powdered cocoa; when dropped into hot water, the casing dissolves.

Dioxins Coffee filters, milk cartons, paper plates, and frozen food packages, if made from bleached paper, can contaminate foods with small quantities of **dioxins**—compounds formed during chlorine treatment of wood pulp during paper manufacture. Dioxin contamination of foods from such products appears only in trace quantities—in the parts-per-trillion range (recall, for perspective, that one part per trillion is equal to 1 second in 32,000 years). Such levels appear to present no health risks to people, but scientists recognize that dioxins are extremely toxic and are likely to cause cancer in humans. Accordingly, the paper industry has reduced its use of chlorine to cut dioxin exposure. In the meantime, the FDA has concluded that drinking milk from bleached-paper cartons presents no health hazard. Contrary to e-mail warnings, plastics do not yield dioxins when broken down, and dioxins are not released from plastic wrap when microwaved. Human exposure to dioxins comes primarily from foods such as beef, milk products, pork, fish, and shellfish.

Decaffeinated Coffee Many consumers have tried to eliminate caffeine from their diets by selecting decaffeinated coffee. To remove caffeine from coffee beans, manufacturers often use methylene chloride in a process that leaves traces of the chemical in the final product. The FDA estimates that the average cup of coffee decaffeinated this way contains about 0.1 part per million of methylene chloride, which seems to pose no significant threat. A person drinking decaffeinated coffee containing 100 times as much methylene chloride every day for a lifetime has a one-in-a-million chance of developing cancer from it. People are exposed to much more methylene chloride from other sources such as hair sprays and paint-stripping solutions. Still, some consumers prefer either to return to caffeine or to select coffee decaffeinated in another way, perhaps by steam. Unfortunately, manufacturers are not required to state on their labels the type of decaffeination process used in their products. Many labels provide consumer-information telephone numbers for those who have such questions.

Hormones Hormones are a unique type of incidental additive in that their use is intentional, but their presence in the final food product is not. The FDA has approved about a dozen hormones for use in food-producing animals, and the USDA has established limits for residues allowed in meat products.

Some ranchers in the United States treat cattle with **bovine growth hormone (BGH).** All cows make BGH naturally, but when given higher doses, animals produce leaner meats, and dairy cows produce more milk. Scientists can genetically alter bacteria to produce BGH, which allows laboratories to harvest huge quantities of the hormone and sell it to farmers as a drug.

Indeed, traces of BGH do remain in the meat and milk of both hormone-treated and untreated cows. BGH residues have not been tested for safety in human beings because residues of the natural hormone have always been present in milk and meat, and the amount found in treated cows is within the range that can occur naturally. Furthermore, BGH, being a peptide hormone, is denatured by the heat used in processing milk and cooking meat, and it is also digested by enzymes in the GI tract. The FDA has determined that BGH absorption does not occur in humans and that BGH is biologically inactive in humans even if injected. According to the National Institutes of Health, "As currently used in the United States, meat and milk from [hormone] treated cows are as safe as those from untreated cows." Whether hormones that have passed through the animals into feces and then contaminated the soil and water interfere with plants or animals in the environment remains controversial.

dioxins (dye-OCK-sins): a class of chemical pollutants created as by-products of chemical manufacturing, incineration, chlorine bleaching of paper pulp, and other industrial processes. Dioxins persist in the environment and accumulate in the food chain.

bovine growth hormone (BGH): a hormone produced naturally in the pituitary gland of a cow that promotes growth and milk production; now produced for agricultural use by bacteria.

- **bovine** = of cattle

Antibiotics Like hormones, antibiotics are also intentionally given to livestock, and residues may remain in the meats and milks. Consequently, people consuming these foods receive tiny doses of antibiotics regularly, and those with sensitivity to antibiotics may suffer allergic reactions. To minimize drug residues in foods, the FDA requires a specified time between the time of medication and the time of slaughter to allow for drug metabolism and excretion.

Of greater concern to the public's health is the widespread use of antibiotics in food animal production and the consequent development of antibiotic resistance.[36] Physicians and veterinarians use an estimated 5 million pounds of antibiotics to treat infections in people and animals, but farmers add five times as much to livestock feed to enhance growth. Not surprisingly, meat from these animals contains resistant bacteria. Such indiscriminate use of antibiotics can be catastrophic to the treatment of disease in human beings. Antibiotics are less effective in treating people who are infected with resistant bacteria. The FDA continues to monitor the use of antibiotics in the food industry with the goal of ensuring that antibiotics remain effective in treating human disease. Antibiotic resistance is immediately and significantly reduced when conventional farms remove antibiotics in their transition to becoming organic farms.[37]

› REVIEW IT List common food additives, their purposes, and examples.
On the whole, the benefits of food additives seem to justify the risks associated with their use. The FDA regulates the use of the intentional additives (summarized in Table 19-5, p. 650). Incidental additives sometimes get into foods during processing, but rarely present a hazard, although some processes such as treating livestock with hormones and antibiotics raise consumer concerns.

19.7 Consumer Concerns about Water

› LEARN IT Discuss consumer concerns about water.

Foods are not alone in transmitting diseases; water is guilty too.[38] In fact, *Cryptosporidium* and *Cyclospora*, commonly found in fresh fruits and vegetables, and *Vibrio vulnificus*, found in raw oysters, are commonly transmitted through contaminated water. In addition to microorganisms, water may contain many of the same impurities that foods do: environmental contaminants, pesticides, and additives such as chlorine used to kill pathogenic microorganisms and fluoride used to protect against dental caries. A glass of "water" is more than just H_2O. This discussion examines the sources of drinking water, harmful contaminants, and ways to ensure water safety.

Sources of Drinking Water Water that is suitable for drinking is called **potable.** Only 1 percent of all the earth's water is potable. Drinking water comes from two sources—surface water and groundwater. In the United States, each source supplies water for about half of the population.

Most major cities obtain their drinking water from surface water—the water in lakes, rivers, and reservoirs. Surface water is readily contaminated because it is directly exposed to acid rain, runoff from highways and urban areas, pesticide runoff from agricultural areas, and industrial wastes that are dumped directly into it. Surface water contamination is reversible, however, because fresh rain constantly replaces the water. It is also cleansed to some degree by aeration, sunlight, and plants and microorganisms that live in it.

Groundwater is the water in underground aquifers—rock formations that are saturated with and yield usable water. People who live in rural areas rely mostly on groundwater pumped up from private wells. Groundwater is contaminated more slowly than surface water, but also more permanently. Contaminants deposited on the ground migrate slowly through the soil before reaching groundwater. Once there, the contaminants break down less rapidly than in surface water because of the lack of aeration, sunlight, and aerobic microorganisms. The slow replacement of groundwater also helps contaminants remain for a long time. Groundwater is especially susceptible to contamination from hazardous waste sites, dumps and landfills,

potable (POH-tah-bul): suitable for drinking.

underground tanks storing gasoline and other chemicals, and improperly discarded household chemicals and solvents.

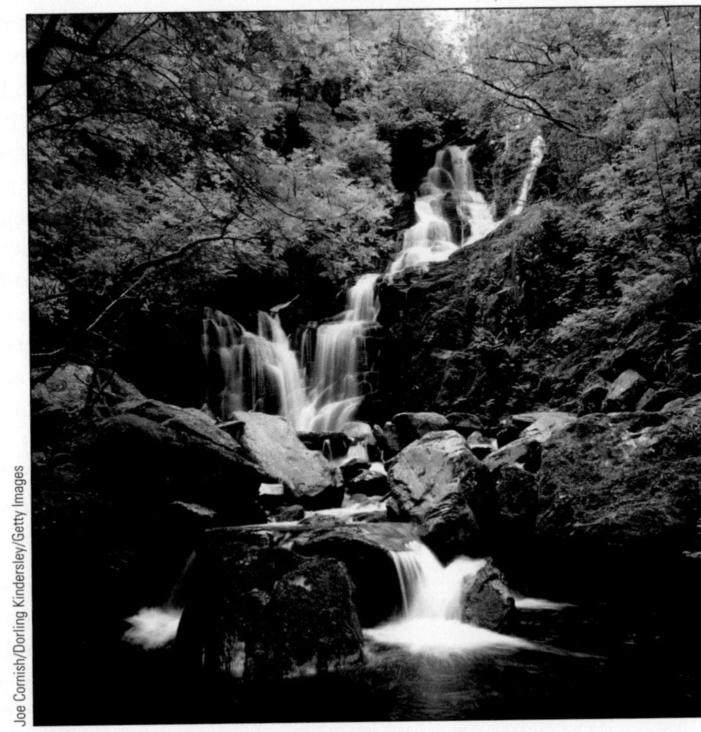
Joe Cornish/Dorling Kindersley/Getty Images

Clean rivers represent irreplaceable water resources.

Water Systems and Regulations Public water systems treat water to remove contaminants that have been detected above acceptable levels. During treatment, a disinfectant (usually, chlorine) is added to kill bacteria. The addition of chlorine to public water is an important public health measure that appears to offer great benefits and small risks. On the one hand, chlorinated water has eliminated such waterborne diseases as typhoid fever, which once ravaged communities, killing thousands of people. On the other hand, it has been associated with an increase in bladder cancer and dioxin contamination of the environment. The EPA is responsible for ensuring that public water systems meet minimum standards for protecting public health.*

Even safe water may have characteristics that some consumers find unpleasant. Most of these problems reflect the mineral content of the water. For example, manganese and copper give water a metallic taste, and sulfur produces a "rotten egg" odor. Iron leaves a rusty brown stain on plumbing fixtures and laundry. Calcium and magnesium (commonly found in "hard water") build up in coffeemakers and hot water heaters. Similarly, soap is not easily rinsed away in hard water, leaving bathtubs and laundry looking dingy. For these and other reasons, some consumers have adopted alternatives to the public water system.

Home Water Treatments To ease concerns about the quality of drinking water, some people purchase home water-treatment systems. Because the EPA does not certify or endorse these water-treatment systems, consumers must shop carefully. Manufacturers offer a variety of units for removing contaminants from drinking water. None of them removes all contaminants, and each has its own advantages and disadvantages. Choosing the right treatment unit depends on the kinds of contaminants in the water. For example, activated carbon filters are particularly effective in removing chlorine, heavy metals such as mercury, and organic contaminants from sediment. Reverse osmosis forces pressurized water through a membrane, flushing out minerals such as sodium and some microorganisms such as *Giardia*. Ozonation uses ozone gas to disinfect water. And distillation systems, which boil water and condense the steam to water, kill microorganisms but leave behind minerals such as lead. Therefore, before purchasing a home water-treatment unit, a consumer must first determine the quality of the water. In some cases, a state or county health department will test water samples or can refer the consumer to a certified laboratory. Consumers need to be aware that unscrupulous vendors may use scare tactics during home inspections to prompt sales.

Bottled Water Despite the higher cost, many people turn to bottled water as an alternative to tap water. Almost 10 billion gallons of bottled water are sold in the United States annually—an average of more than 30 gallons per person.[39] The FDA regulates bottled drinking water and has established quality and safety standards compatible with those set by the EPA for public water systems. In addition, all bottled waters must be processed, packaged, and labeled in accordance with FDA regulations. Water quality may vary among brands because of variations in the source water used and company practices, but bottled water is neither safer nor healthier than tap water.

As Chapter 14 discusses, some bottled waters are marketed as "enhanced water"—water that has been enhanced with sweeteners, juices, coloring, flavors, vitamins, minerals, protein, or extra oxygen. Consumers perceive these bottled waters as healthful and sales have skyrocketed.

Labels on bottled water must identify the water's source. Approximately 75 percent of bottled waters derive from protected groundwater (from springs

*The EPA's safe drinking water hotline: (800) 426–4791.

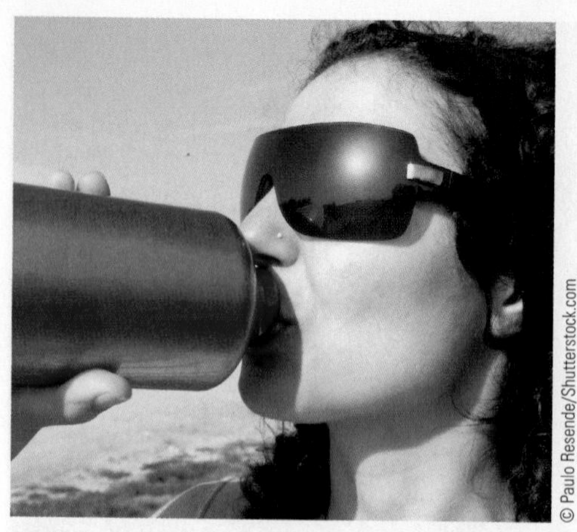
© Paulo Resende/Shutterstock.com

Realizing that fossil fuels and many gallons of water are used to create and transport plastic water bottles, concerned consumers use refillable bottles to save money and the environment.

or wells)—the same as tap water. This water is usually treated before being bottled. For example, it may be disinfected with ozone gas rather than chlorine. Ozone kills microorganisms, then disintegrates spontaneously into water and oxygen, leaving behind no toxic by-products. Other bottled waters may be treated by filtration to remove pathogens and other particles. Bottled waters may also be treated by reverse osmosis or ion exchange to remove minerals. Alternatively, the water may be distilled into a vapor and then condensed again into water, thus removing any dissolved solids. These processes allow the bottle to be labeled "purified water." Most bottled waters do not contain fluoride; consequently, they do not provide the tooth protection of fluoridated water from community public water systems.

Despite government regulations, some contamination has been detected in some bottled waters.[40] Although the amounts of most contaminants found in bottled waters are probably insignificant, consumers should be aware that bottled water is not necessarily purer than the water from their taps. In fact, some bottled waters come from the same municipal water sources as that for consumers' home taps. As a safeguard, the FDA recommends that bottled water be handled like other foods and be refrigerated after opening.

Protection of drinking water is a subject of ongoing concern and controversy. It may soon become a source of conflict between the world's nations as the population continues to grow and the renewable water supply remains constant. Estimates are that within the next 50 years, half of the world's people will not have enough clean water to meet their needs. To avert this potential calamity, we must take active steps to conserve water, clean polluted water, desalinate seawater, and curb population growth.

› REVIEW IT Discuss consumer concerns about water.
Like foods, water may contain infectious microorganisms, environmental contaminants, pesticide residues, and additives. The EPA monitors the safety of the public water system, but many consumers choose home water-treatment systems or bottled water instead of tap water.

As this chapter said at the start, supplying food safely to hundreds of millions of people is an incredible challenge—one that is met, for the most part, with incredible efficiency. The following chapter describes a contrasting situation—that of the food supply not reaching the people.

Nutrition Portfolio

Practicing food safety allows you to eat a variety of foods, with little risk of foodborne illnesses.

- Review your food-handling practices and describe how effectively you wash your hands, utensils, and kitchen surfaces when preparing foods.
- Describe the steps you take to separate raw and cooked foods while storing and preparing them.
- Describe how you can ensure that you cook foods to a safe temperature and refrigerate perishable foods promptly.

Go to Diet & Wellness Plus and choose one of the days on which you tracked your diet and activity for an entire day. Select the Intake Spreadsheet report to help you answer the following questions:

- Imagine for a moment that you got a foodborne illness on this particular day. Which food would you most suspect to have contained the illness-causing organism or toxin? Why would you suspect that food more than the other foods you ate that day?

DIET & WELLNESS PLUS To complete this exercise, go to your Diet & Wellness Plus at **www.cengagebrain.com**.

› STUDY IT To review the key points of this chapter and take a practice quiz, go to the study cards at the end of the book.

REFERENCES

1. K. Stewart and L. O. Gostin, Food and Drug Administration regulation of food safety, *Journal of the American Medical Association* 306 (2011): 88–89; J. M. Sharfstein, The FDA—A misunderstood agency, *Journal of the American Medical Association* 306 (2011): 1250–1251.
2. J. E. Riviere and G. J. Buckely, eds., *Ensuring Safe Foods and Medical Products through Stronger Regulatory Systems Abroad* (Washington, DC: National Academies Press), 2012.
3. M. T. Osterholm, Foodborne disease in 2011: The rest of the story, *New England Journal of Medicine* 364 (2011): 889–891; Centers for Disease Control and Prevention, Press release: New estimates more precise, December 15, 2010.
4. B. M. Lund and S. J. O'Brien, The occurrence and prevention of foodborne disease in vulnerable people, *Foodborne Pathogens and Disease* 8 (2011): 961–973.
5. S. J. Chai and coauthors, Salmonella enterica serotype enteritidis: Increasing incidence of domestically acquired infections, *Clinical Infectious Diseases* 54 (2012): S488–S497; A. J. Hall and coauthors, Updated norovirus outbreak management and disease prevention guidelines, *Morbidity and Mortality Weekly Report* 60 (2011): 1–15; E. Scallan and coauthors, Foodborne illness acquired in the United States—Major pathogens, *Emerging Infectious Diseases* 17 (2011): 7–15; L. H. Gould and coauthors, Surveillance for foodborne disease outbreaks: United States, 2008, *Morbidity and Mortality Weekly Report* 60 (2011): 1197–1202.
6. C. P. Wild and Y. Y. Gong, Mycotoxins and human disease: A largely ignored global health issue, *Carcinogenesis* 31 (2010): 71–82.
7. Position of the American Dietetic Association: Food and water safety, *Journal of the American Dietetic Association* 109 (2009): 1449–1460.
8. Centers for Disease Control and Prevention, Handwashing: Clean hands save lives, www.cdc.gov/handwashing, December 11, 2013.
9. K. Stein, The results of an international germ study: Should registered dietitians be surprised by the surprise? *Journal of the Academy of Nutrition and Dietetics* 113 (2013): 1288–1294.
10. J. Y. Abrams and coauthors, Travel history, hunting, and venison consumption related to prion disease exposure, 2006–2007 FoodNet Population Survey, *Journal of the American Dietetic Association* 111 (2011): 858–863; US Food and Drug Administration, All about BSE, www.fda.gov/animalveterinary, April 20, 2010.
11. D. S. Ludwig, Technology, diet, and the burden of chronic disease, *Journal of the American Medical Association* 305 (2011): 1352–1353.
12. US Food and Drug Administration, Questions and answers: Arsenic in apple juice, www.fda.gov/Food/ResourcesForYou/Consumers/ucm271595.htm, July 15, 2013.
13. S. K. Sagiv and coauthors, Prenatal exposure to mercury and fish consumption during pregnancy and attention-deficity/hyperactivity disorder-related behavior in children, *Archives of Pediatrics and Adolescent Medicine* 166 (2012): 1123–1131.
14. J. Golding and coauthors, Dietary predictors of maternal prenatal blood mercury levels in the ALSPAC Birth Cohort Study, *Environmental Health Perspectives* 121 (2013): 1214–1218.
15. M. Wennberg and coauthors, Myocardial infarction in relation to mercury and fatty acids from fish: A risk-benefit analysis based on pooled Finnish and Swedish data in men, *American Journal of Clinical Nutrition* 96 (2012): 706–713.
16. K. R. Mahaffey and coauthors, Balancing the benefits of n-3 polyunsaturated fatty acids and the risks of methylmercury exposure from fish consumption, *Nutrition Reviews* 69 (2011): 493–508.
17. M. Chu and T. F. Seltzer, Myxedema coma induced by ingestion of raw bok choy, *New England Journal of Medicine* 362 (2010): 1945–1946.
18. C. A. Damalas and I. G. Eleftherohorinos, Pesticide exposure, safety issues, and risk assessment indicators, *International Journal of Environmental Research and Public* Health 8 (2011): 1402–1419.
19. Council on Environmental Health, Pesticide exposure in children, *Pediatrics* 130 (2012): e1757–e1763; R. Vogt and coauthors, Cancer and non-cancer health effects from food contaminant exposures for children and adults in California: A risk assessment, *Environmental Health* 11 (2012): 83–97.
20. A. M. Riederer and C. Lu, Measured versus simulated dietary pesticide intakes in children, *Food Additives and Contaminants* 29 (2012): 1922–1937.
21. R. A. Neff and coauthors, A comparative study of allowable pesticide residue levels on produce in the United States, *Globalization and Health* 8 (2012): 2–16.
22. G. van Maele-Fabry, P. Hoet, and D. Lison, Parental occupational exposure to pesticides as risk factor for brain tumors in children and young adults: A systematic review and meta-analysis, *Environment International* 56 (2013): 19–31.
23. B. M. Keikotlhaile, P. Spanoghe, and W. Steurbaut, Effects of food processing on pesticide residues in fruits and vegetables: A meta-analysis approach, *Food and Chemical Toxicology* 48 (2010): 1–6.
24. C. Smith-Spangler and coauthors, Are organic foods safer or healthier than conventional alternatives? *Annals of Internal Medicine* 157 (2012): 348–366; C. K. Winter, Pesticide residues in imported, organic, and "suspect" fruits and vegetables, *Journal of Agricultural and Food Chemistry* 60 (2012): 4425–4429.
25. L. Oates and M. Cohen, Assessing diet as a modifiable risk factor for pesticide exposure, *International Journal of Environmental Research and Public* Health 8 (2011): 1792–1804.
26. Environmental Working Group, "EWG's Shoppers Guides to Pesticides in Produce," www.ewg.org/foodnews/summary.php, 2013.
27. C. K. Winter and J. M. Katz, Dietary exposure to pesticide residues from commodities alleged to contain the highest contamination levels, *Journal of Toxicology* 2011 (2011): 589–674.
28. J. P. Reganold and coauthors, Fruit and soil quality of organic and conventional strawberry agroecosystems, *PLoS ONE* 5 (2010): e12346.
29. A. Vallverdú-Queralt and coauthors, Is there any difference between the phenolic content of organic and conventional tomato juices? *Food Chemistry* 130 (2012): 222–227.
30. W. J. Crinnion, Organic foods contain higher levels of certain nutrients, lower levels of pesticides, and may provide health benefits for the consumer, *Alternative Medicine Review* 15 (2010): 4–12; A. D. Dangour and coauthors, Nutrition-related health effects of organic foods: A systematic review, *American Journal of Clinical Nutrition* 92 (2010): 203–210.
31. J. L. Wan-chen and coauthors, You taste what you see: Do organic labels bias taste perceptions? *Food Quality and Preference* 29 (2013): 33–39.
32. T. G. Neltner and coauthors, Navigating the US food additive regulatory program, *Comprehensive Reviews in Food Science and Food Safety* 10 (2011): 342–368.
33. N. S. Bryan and coauthors, Ingested nitrate and nitrite and stomach cancer risk: An updated review, *Food and Cheimcal Toxicology* 50 (2012): 3646–3665; B. Aschebrook-Kilfoy and coauthors, Pancreatic cancer and exposure to dietary nitrate and nitrite in the NIH-AARP Diet and Health Study, *American Journal of Epidemiology* 174 (2011): 305–315.
34. D. K. Parthasarathy and N. S. Bryan, Sodium nitrite: The "cure" for nitric oxide insufficiency, *Meat Science* 92 (2012): 274–279.
35. Food and Drug Administration, Update on bisphenol A for use in food contact applications, www.fda.gov, revised March 2010.
36. L. B. Price and coauthors, *Staphylococcus aureus* CC398: Host adaptation and emergence of methicillin resistance in livestock, *mBio* 3 (2012): e00305–e00311.
37. A. R. Sapkota and coauthors, Lower prevalence of antibiotic-resistant enterococci on U.S. conventional poultry farms that transitioned to organic practices, *Environmental Health Perspectives* 119 (2011): 1622–1628.
38. M. C. Hlavsa and coauthors, Surveillance for waterborne disease and outbreaks and other health events associated with recreational water: United States, 2007–2008, *Morbidity and Mortality Weekly Report* 60 (2011): 1–75.
39. International Bottled Water Association, U.S. consumption of bottled water shows continued growth, increasing 6.2 percent in 2012; sales up 6.7 percent, www.bottledwater.org, April 25, 2013.
40. M. Diduch, Z. Polkowska, and J. Namiesnik, Chemical quality of bottled waters: A review, *Journal of Food Science* 76 (2011): R178–R196.

HIGHLIGHT > 19
Food Biotechnology

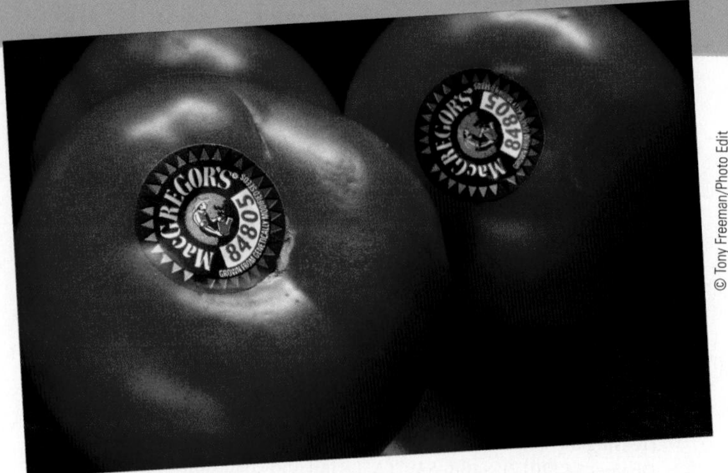

© Tony Freeman/Photo Edit

› LEARN IT Debate the pros and cons surrounding genetically engineered foods.

Advances in food **biotechnology** promise just about everything from the frivolous (a tear-free onion) to the profound (a hunger-free world). Already biotechnology has produced leaner meats, longer shelf lives, better nutrient composition, and greater crop yields grown with fewer pesticides. Overall, biotechnology offers numerous opportunities to overcome food shortages, improve the environment, and eliminate disease. But it also raises concerns about possible risks to the environment and human health. Critics assert that biotechnology will exacerbate world hunger, destroy the environment, and endanger health. This highlight presents some of the many issues surrounding genetically engineered foods, and the accompanying glossary defines key terms.

The Promises of Genetic Engineering

For centuries, farmers have been selectively breeding plants and animals to shape the characteristics of their crops and livestock. They have created prettier flowers, hardier vegetables, and leaner animals. Consider the success of selectively breeding corn. Early farmers in Mexico began with a wild, native plant called teosinte (tay-oh-SEEN-tay) that bears only five or six kernels on each small spike. Many years of patient selective breeding have produced large ears filled with hundreds of plump kernels aligned in perfect formation, row after row.

Such genetic improvements, together with the use of irrigation, fertilizers, and pesticides, were responsible for more than half of the increases in US crop yields in the 20th century. Farmers still use selective breeding, but now, in the 21st century, advances in **genetic engineering** have brought rapid and dramatic changes to agriculture and food production.

Although selective breeding works, it is slow and imprecise because it involves mixing thousands of genes from two plants and hoping for the best. With genetic engineering, scientists can improve crops (or livestock) by introducing a copy of the specific gene needed to produce the desired trait. Figure H19-1 illustrates the difference. Once introduced, the selected gene acts like any other gene—it provides instructions for making a protein. The protein then determines a characteristic in the genetically modified plant or animal. In short, the process is now faster and more refined. Farmers no longer need to wait patiently for breeding to yield improved crops and animals, nor must they even respect natural lines of reproduction among species. Laboratory scientists can copy genes from one organism and insert them into almost any other organism—plant, animal, or microbe. Their work is changing not only the way farmers plant, fertilize, and harvest their crops, but also the ways the food industry processes food and consumers receive nutrients, phytochemicals, and drugs.

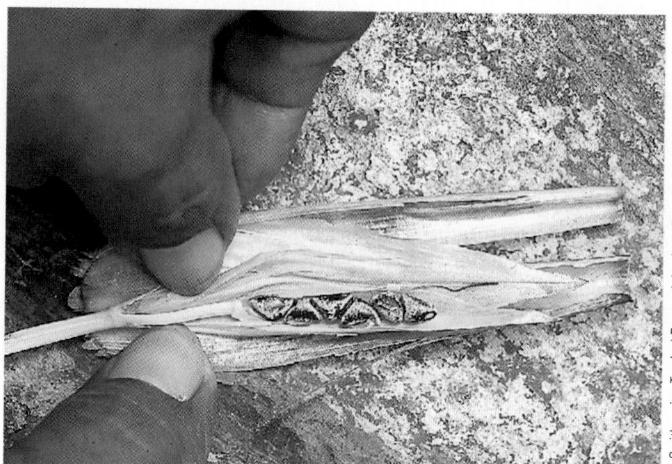
© Smithsonian Tropical Research Institute/Antonio Montaner, photographer

This wild predecessor of corn, with its sparse five or six kernels, bears little resemblance to today's large, full, sweet ears.

GLOSSARY

biotechnology: the use of biological systems or organisms to create or modify products. Examples include the use of bacteria to make yogurt, yeast to make beer, and cross-breeding to enhance crop production.

clone: a genetic copy of an organism created without sexual reproduction; similar to identical twins, but born at different times.

genetic engineering: the use of biotechnology to modify the genetic material of living cells so that they will produce new substances or perform new functions. Foods produced via this technology are called *genetically modified (GM)* or *genetically engineered (GE) foods.*

plant-pesticides: pesticides made by the plants themselves.

rennin: an enzyme that coagulates milk; found in the gastric juice of cows, but not human beings.

> FIGURE H19-1 **Selective Breeding and Genetic Engineering Compared**

Traditional Selective Breeding

Traditional selective breeding combines many genes from two varieties of the same species to produce one with the desired characteristics.

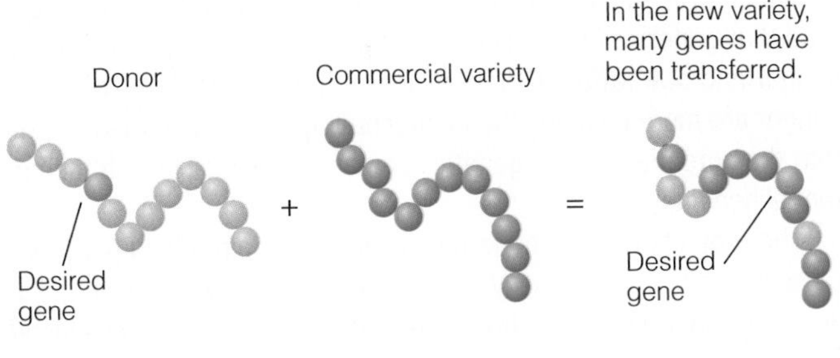

Genetic Engineering

Through genetic engineering, a single gene is (or several are) transferred from the same or different species to produce one with the desired characteristics.

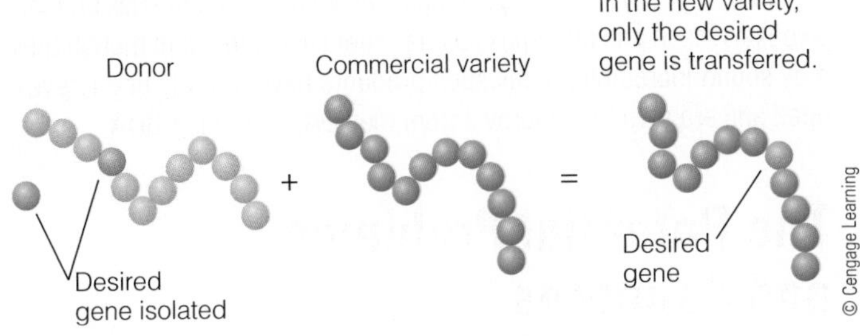

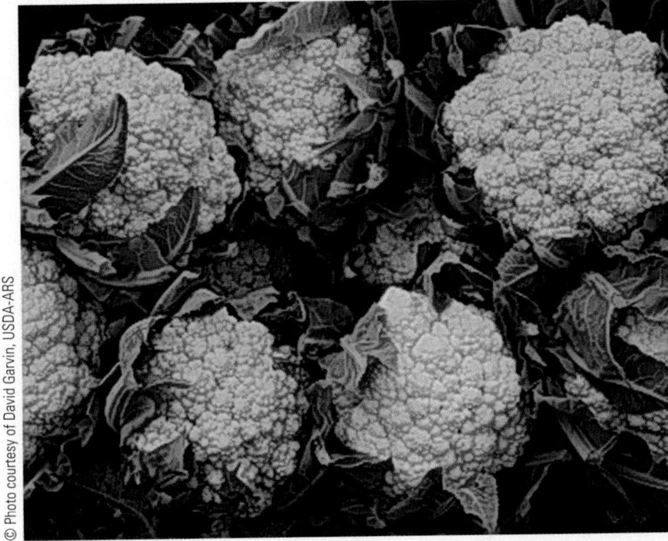

Genetically modified cauliflower is orange, reflecting a change in a single gene that increases its production of beta-carotene 100-fold.

Extended Shelf Life

Among the first products of genetic engineering to hit the market were tomatoes that stay firm and ripe longer than regular tomatoes that are typically harvested green and ripened in the stores. These genetically modified tomatoes promise less waste and higher profits. Normally, tomatoes produce an enzyme (remember that enzymes are proteins) that softens them after they have been picked. Scientists can now introduce into a tomato plant a gene that is a mirror image of the one that codes for the "softening" enzyme. This gene blocks synthesis of the softening enzyme. Without this enzyme, the genetically altered tomato softens more slowly than a regular tomato, allowing growers to harvest it at its most flavorful and nutritious vine-ripe stage.

Improved Nutrient Composition

Genetic engineering can also improve the nutrient composition of foods.[1] Instead of manufacturers adding nutrients to foods during processing, plants can be genetically altered to do the fortification work—a strategy called *biofortification.* Biofortification of staple crops with key vitamins and minerals can effectively combat the nutrient deficiency diseases that claim so many lives worldwide. Genetically modifying cassava, one of the world's major staple crops, can improve its protein and iron content.[2] Soybeans may be implanted with a gene that upgrades soy protein to a quality approaching that of milk. Corn has been modified to contain twice the amount of lysine and tryptophan, its two limiting amino acids.[3] Soybean and canola plants can be genetically modified to alter the composition of their oils, making them richer in the heart-healthy monounsaturated fatty acids. "Golden rice," which has received genes from a daffodil and a bacterium that enable it to make beta-carotene, offers promise in treating vitamin A deficiency worldwide.[4] (Chapter 11 describes how vitamin A deficiency contributes to the deaths of 2 million children and the blindness of a half million each year.) Of course, increasing nutrients in crops may have unintended consequences as well. For example, when broccoli is manipulated to increase its selenium content, production of the cancer-fighting phytochemical sulforaphane declines.

In addition to enhancing the nutrient composition, genetically modified crops can also produce more of the phytochemicals that help maintain health and reduce the risks of chronic diseases (see Highlight 13). They can also be coaxed to produce less phytate, which allows more zinc to be absorbed. The possibilities seem endless.

Efficient Food Processing

Genetic engineering also helps to process foods more efficiently, which saves money. For example, the protein **rennin**, which is used to coagulate milk in the production of cheese, has traditionally been harvested from the stomachs of calves, a costly process. Now scientists can insert a copy of the rennin gene into bacteria and then use bacterial cultures to mass-produce rennin—saving time, money, space, and animals.

Genetic engineering can also help to bypass costly food-processing steps. At present, people who are lactose intolerant can buy milk that has been processed to include the lactase enzyme. Wouldn't it be more convenient, and less expensive, if scientists could genetically modify cows to make lactose-free milk directly? They've done it. Decaffeinated coffee beans are another real possibility.

Genetic research today has progressed well beyond tweaking a gene here and there to produce a desired trait. Scientists can now **clone** animals. By cloning animals, scientists have the ability to produce both needed food and pharmaceutical products. The FDA has declared that food from cloned livestock is safe to eat, but the USDA has asked farmers to keep cloned animals off the market. Because cloning an animal costs tens of thousands of dollars, it would be incredibly unprofitable to slaughter it for meat. For this reason, cloned animals are used primarily for breeding and their natural-born offspring are used primarily for food. Because the FDA does not distinguish between foods from cloned animals or their offspring and foods from conventional animals, food labels are not required to provide this information.

Efficient Drug Delivery

Using cloned animals and other organisms in the development of pharmaceuticals is whimsically called "biopharming." For example, a goat that has been genetically modified to produce a malaria vaccine in its milk could provide both nourishment and immunization to a whole village of people now left unprotected because they lack food and medical help. Similarly, researchers have figured out how to induce hens to produce eggs with a drug to treat multiple sclerosis. Bananas and potatoes have been designed to make hepatitis vaccines, and tobacco leaves to make AIDS drugs. Researchers can also harvest vaccines by genetically altering hydroponically grown tomato plants to secrete a protein through their root systems into the water. Using foods to deliver drugs is only a small part of the promise and potential that biotechnology offers the field of medicine.

Genetically Assisted Agriculture

Genetic engineering has helped farmers to increase yields, extend growing seasons, and grow crops that resist herbicides. More than 90 percent of the soybean crops in the United States have been genetically engineered to withstand a potent herbicide. As a result, farmers can spray whole fields with this herbicide and kill the weeds without harming the soybeans.

Similarly, farmers can grow crops that produce their own pesticides—substances known as **plant-pesticides.** Corn, broccoli, and potatoes have received a gene from a bacterium that produces a protein that is toxic to leaf-chewing caterpillars (but not to humans). Yellow squash has been given two genes that confer resistance to the most common viral diseases. Potatoes can now produce a beetle-killing toxin in their leaves. These crops and many others like them are currently being grown or tested in fields around the United States. Growing crops that make their own pesticides allows farmers to save time, increase yields, and use fewer, or less harmful, pesticides. Genetically modified crops have decreased the environmental impact associated with pesticide use.

Other Possibilities

Many other biotechnology possibilities are envisioned for the near future. Shrimp may be empowered to fight diseases with genetic ammunition borrowed from sea urchins. Milk may be produced without its major allergen.[5] Plants may be given special molecules to help them grow in polluted soil. With these and other advances, farmers may reliably produce bumper crops of food every year on far fewer acres of land, with less loss of water and topsoil, and far less use of toxic pesticides and herbicides. Supporters of biotechnology predict that these efforts will enhance food production and help meet the challenge of feeding an ever-increasing world population. They contend that genetically modified crops have the potential to eliminate hunger and starvation. Others suggest that the problems of world hunger are more complex than biotechnology alone can resolve and that the potential risks of genetic engineering may outweigh the potential benefits.

The projects mentioned in this highlight are already in progress. Close on their heels are many more ingenious ideas. What if salt tolerance could be transplanted from a coastal marsh plant into crop plants? Could crops then be irrigated with seawater, thus conserving dwindling freshwater supplies? Or could crops be genetically designed to use less water? Would the world food supply increase if rice farmers could grow plants that were immune to disease? What if consumers could dictate which traits scientists insert into food plants? Would they choose to add phytochemicals to fight cancer or reduce the risk of heart disease? These and other possibilities seem unlimited, and though they may sound incredible, many such products have already been developed and are awaiting approval from the FDA, EPA, and USDA.

The Potential Problems and Concerns

Consumers accept or reject foods and technology depending on their perceptions of the associated benefits and risks.[6] For the most part, when something is perceived as being beneficial, it is also perceived as having low risk. Perceptions of risk and rejection increase when conditions are unfamiliar, uncertain, unknown, or uncontrollable or consequences are severe, whereas perceptions of benefits and acceptance increase when conditions are traditional, well known, and familiar. In the case of genetically modified foods, many consumers are understandably suspicious of an unfamiliar and complicated processing technique; they haven't accepted that the benefits might outweigh the risks.

Although many scientists hail biotechnology with confidence, others have reservations. Most consumers know little about biotechnology or the extent to which their foods contain genetically modified foods. Some consumers have concerns about what they call "Frankenfoods." Those who oppose biotechnology fear for the safety of a world where genetic tampering produces effects that are not yet fully understood. They suspect that the food industry may be driven by potential profits, without ethical considerations or laws to harness the effects. They point out that even the scientists who developed the techniques cannot predict the ultimate outcomes of their discoveries. These consumers don't want to eat a scientific experiment or interfere with natural systems. Genetic decisions, they say, are best left to the powers of nature.

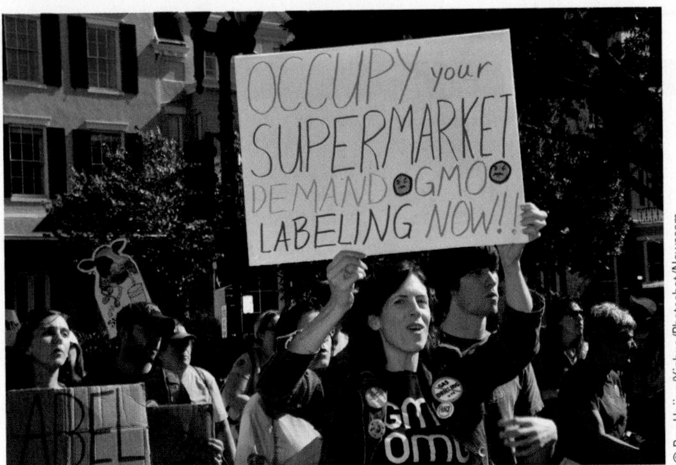

© Ren Haijun/Xinhua/Photoshot/Newscom

Many consumers believe that genetically modified foods should be labeled as such.

If science and the marketplace are allowed to drive biotechnology without restraint, critics fear that the following problems may result:

- *Disruption of natural ecosystems.* New, genetically unique organisms that have no natural place in the food chain or evolutionary biological systems could escape into the environment and reproduce.
- *Introduction of diseases.* Newly created viruses may mutate to cause deadly diseases that may attack plants, animals, or human beings. Genetically modified bacteria may develop resistance to antibiotics, making the drugs useless in fighting infections.
- *Introduction of allergens and toxins.* Genetically modified crops may contain new substances that have consequences, such as causing allergies.
- *Creation of biological weapons.* Fatal bacterial and viral diseases may be developed for use as weapons.
- *Ethical dilemmas.* Critics pose the question "How many human genes does an organism have to contain before it is considered human? For instance, how many human genes would a green pepper have to contain before one would have qualms about eating it?"

Proponents of biotechnology respond that evidence to date does not justify these concerns. Opponents counter that the lack of evidence showing harm does not provide evidence showing safety. These opposing views illustrate the tension between the forward thrust of science and the hesitation of consumers. Some would argue for more research on the safety of genetically modified food, while others assert that more research is a waste of resources and that it is time to embrace biotechnology with enthusiasm.[7] In addition to evaluating the potential risks and benefits, genetically modified crops need international oversight. Table H19-1 (p. 660) summarizes the issues.

From another perspective, some argue that the concerns expressed by those protesting genetically engineered foods reflect prejudices acquired in an elitist world of fertile land and abundant food. Those living in poverty-stricken areas of the world do not have the luxury of determining how to grow crops and process foods. They cannot afford the delays created when protesters destroy test crops and disrupt scientific meetings. They need solutions now. People are starving, and genetic engineering holds great promise for increasing crop yields and providing those people with food.[8]

The work of Nobel Peace Prize Laureate Dr. Norman Borlaug and his team over the past four decades attests to the benefits of using technology to defend against hunger. By developing grains that resist pests and diseases, they have been able to increase yields and provide real solutions to global hunger problems. When Mexico used Borlaug's special breed of dwarf wheat, yields increased threefold compared with traditional varieties. India increased wheat production tenfold and became self-sufficient in its grain production. Pakistan increased its wheat production fivefold and sub-Saharan Africa more than tripled crop yields by changing farming practices. The combination of improved conventional systems and biotechnology produces more food to meet the nutritional needs of more people.[9]

At a minimum, critics of biotechnology have made a strong case for rigorous safety testing and labeling of new products. They contend, for example, that when a new gene has been introduced into a food, tests should ensure that other, unwanted genes have not accompanied it. If a disease-producing microorganism has donated genetic material, scientists must prove that no dangerous characteristic from the microorganism has also entered the food. If the inserted genetic material comes from a source to which some people develop allergies, such as nuts, then the new product should be labeled to alert them. Furthermore, if the newly altered genetic material creates proteins that have never before been encountered by the human body, their effects should be rigorously studied to ensure that people can eat them safely.

FDA Regulations

The FDA has taken the position that foods produced through biotechnology and cloning are not substantially different from others and require no special testing, regulations, or labeling. After all, most foods available today have already been genetically altered by years of selective breeding. The new vegetable broccoflower, a product of sophisticated cross-breeding of broccoli with cauliflower, met no testing or approval barriers on its way to the dinner plate. When the vegetable became available on the market, scientists studied its nutrient contents, but they did not question its safety.

In most cases, the new genetically modified food differs from the old conventional one only by a gene or two. The rennin produced by bacteria is structurally and functionally the same as the rennin produced by calves, for example. For that reason, the FDA considers it and other genetically engineered foods "generally recognized as safe (GRAS)."

A product such as the tomato described earlier need not be tested because its new gene *prevents* synthesis of a protein and adds nothing but a tiny fragment of genetic material. Nor does this tomato require special labeling because it is not significantly different from the many other varieties of tomatoes on the market. On the other hand, any substance introduced into a food (such as a hormone or protein) by way of bioengineering must meet the same safety standards applied to all additives. A tomato plant with a gene that, for example, produces a pesticide cannot be marketed until tests prove it safe for consumption.

HIGHLIGHT > 19

TABLE H19-1 Food Biotechnology: Point, Counterpoint

Arguments in Opposition to Genetic Engineering	Arguments in Support of Genetic Engineering
1. **Ethical and moral issues.** It's immoral to "play God" by mixing genes from organisms unable to do so naturally. Religious and vegetarian groups object to genes from prohibited species occurring in their allowable foods.	1. **Ethical and moral issues.** Scientists throughout history have been persecuted and even put to death by fearful people who accuse them of playing God. Yet, today many of the world's citizens enjoy a long and healthy life of comfort and convenience because of once-feared scientific advances put to practical use.
2. **Imperfect technology.** The technology is young and imperfect—genes rarely function in just one way, their placement is imprecise ("shotgun"), and all of their potential effects are impossible to predict. Toxins are as likely to be produced as the desired trait. More than 95 percent of DNA is called "junk" because scientists have not yet determined its function.	2. **Advanced technology.** Recombinant DNA technology is precise and reliable. Many of the most exciting recent advances in medicine, agriculture, and technology were made possible by the application of this technology.
3. **Environmental concerns.** Environmental side effects are unknown. The power of a genetically modified organism to change the world's environments is unknown until such changes actually occur—then the "genie is out of the bottle." Once out, insects, birds, and the wind distribute genetically altered seed and pollen to points unknown.	3. **Environmental protection.** Genetic engineering may be the only hope of saving rain forest and other habitats from destruction. Through genetic engineering, farmers can make use of previously unproductive lands such as salt-rich soils and arid areas.
4. **"Genetic pollution."** Other kinds of pollution can often be cleaned up with money, time, and effort. Once genes are spliced into living things, those genes forever bear the imprint of human tampering.	4. **Genetic improvements.** Genetic side effects are more likely to benefit the environment than to harm it.
5. **Crop vulnerability.** Pests and diseases can quickly adapt to overtake genetically identical plants or animals around the world. Diversity is key to defense.	5. **Improved crop resistance.** Pests and diseases can be specifically fought on a case-by-case basis. Biotechnology is the key to defense.
6. **Loss of gene pool.** Loss of genetic diversity threatens to deplete valuable gene banks from which scientists can develop new agricultural crops.	6. **Gene pool preserved.** Thanks to advances in genetics, laboratories around the world are able to stockpile the genetic material of millions of species that, without such advances, would have been lost forever.
7. **Profit motive.** Genetic engineering will profit industry more than the world's poor and hungry.	7. **Everyone profits.** Industries benefit from genetic engineering, and a thriving food industry benefits the nation and its people, as witnessed by countries lacking such industries. Genetic engineering promises to provide adequate nutritious food for millions who lack such food today. Developed nations gain cheaper, more attractive, more delicious foods with greater variety and availability year round.
8. **Unproven safety for people.** Human safety testing of genetically altered products is generally lacking. The population is an unwitting experimental group in a nationwide laboratory study for the benefit of industry.	8. **Safe for people.** Human safety testing of genetically altered products is unneeded because the products are essentially the same as the original foodstuffs.
9. **Increased allergens.** Allergens can be unwittingly transferred into foods.	9. **Control of allergens.** A few allergens can be transferred into foods, but these are known. Also, foods likely to contain them are clearly labeled to warn consumers. Some foods are being designed to eliminate the allergen.
10. **Decreased nutrients.** A fresh-looking tomato or other produce held for several weeks may have lost substantial nutrients.	10. **Increased nutrients.** Genetic modifications can easily enhance the nutrients in foods.
11. **No product tracking.** Without labeling, the food industry cannot track problems to the source.	11. **Excellent product tracking.** The identity and location of genetically altered foodstuffs are known, and they can be tracked should problems arise.
12. **Overuse of herbicides.** Farmers, knowing that their crops resist herbicide effects, will use them liberally.	12. **Conservative use of herbicides.** Farmers will not waste expensive herbicides in second or third applications when the prescribed amount gets the job done the first time.
13. **Increased consumption of pesticides.** When a pesticide is produced by the flesh of produce, consumers cannot wash it off the skin of the produce with running water as they can with ordinary sprays.	13. **Reduced pesticides on foods.** Pesticides produced by plants in tiny amounts known to be safe for consumption are more predictable than applications by agricultural workers who make mistakes. Because other genetic manipulations will eliminate the need for postharvest spraying, fewer pesticides will reach the dinner table.
14. **Lack of oversight.** Government oversight is run by industry people for the benefit of industry—no one is watching out for the consumer.	14. **Sufficient regulation and rapid response.** Government agencies are efficient in identifying and correcting problems as they occur in the industry.

The FDA assures consumers that all bioengineered foods on the market today are as safe as their traditional counterparts.

Foods produced through biotechnology that are substantially different from others must be labeled to identify that difference. For example, if the nutrient composition of the new product differs from its traditional counterpart, as in the soybean and canola oils mentioned earlier, then labeling is required. Similarly, if an allergy-causing protein has been introduced to a nonallergenic food, then labeling must warn consumers.

Most consumers want all genetically altered products clearly labeled. Consumer advocacy groups claim that by not requiring such labeling, the FDA forces millions of consumers to be guinea pigs, unwittingly testing genetically engineered foods. Additionally, they say, people who have religious objections to consuming foods to which genes of prohibited organisms have been added have no way of identifying those foods. For example, someone keeping a kosher kitchen may unknowingly use a food containing genes from a pig. Currently, labeling is voluntary. Manufacturers may state that a product has been "genetically engineered." Those who do would be wise to explain its purpose and benefit. When consumers recognize a personal health benefit, most tend to accept genetically engineered foods.

Speaking in defense of the FDA's position are the FDA itself, recognized as the nation's leading expert and advocate for food safety, and the Academy of Nutrition and Dietetics, which represents current scientific thinking in nutrition.[10] Many other scientific organizations agree, contending that biotechnology can deliver an improved food supply if we give it a fair chance to do so.

Will these new technologies provide foods to meet the needs of the future? Some would say yes. Biotechnology holds a world of promise, and with proper safeguards and controls, it may yield products that meet the needs of consumers almost perfectly.

CRITICAL THINKING QUESTIONS

A. How might people from different countries view the risks and benefits of biotechnology?

B. Controversy surrounds the safety and use of food biotechnology. Genetically modified foods raise concerns about long-term health and environmental consequences. Even though most scientists agree that these foods are safe and perhaps even beneficial to consumers, many consumers still express uncertainty. What is your position on food biotechnology and genetically modified foods? What could be done to minimize any associated risks and alleviate fears?

REFERENCES

1. M. N. McGloughlin, Modifying agricultural crops for improved nutrition, *Nature Biotechnology* 30 (2010): 494–504.
2. E. Leyva-Guerrero and coauthors, Iron and protein biofortification of cassava: Lessons learned, *Current Opinion in Biotechnology* 23 (2012): 257–264.
3. E. T. Nuss and S. A. Tanumihardjo, Quality protein maize for Africa: Closing the protein inadequacy gap in vulnerable populations, *Advanced Nutrition* 2 (2011): 217–224.
4. G. Tang and coauthors, β-Carotene in Golden Rice is as good as β-carotene in oil at providing vitamin A to children, *American Journal of Clinical Nutrition* 96 (2012): 658–664.
5. A. Jabed and coauthors, Targeted microRNA expression in dairy cattle directs production of β-lactoglobulin-free, high-casein milk, *Proceedings of the National Academy of Sciences* 109 (2012): 16811–16816.
6. Ø. Ureland and coauthors, State of the art in benefit-risk analysis: Consumer perception, *Food and Chemical Toxicology* 50 (2012): 67–76.
7. H. I. Miller, The regulation of agricultural biotechnology: Science shows a better way, *Nature Biotechnology* 27 (2010): 628–634.
8. M. A. Parry and M. J. Hawkesford, Food security: Increasing yield and improving resource use efficiency, *Proceedings of the Nutrition Society* 69 (2010): 592–600.
9. M. S. Swaminathan, Achieving food security in times of crisis, *Nature Biotechnology* 27 (2010): 453–460.
10. Position of the American Dietetic Association: Agricultural and food biotechnology, *Journal of the American Dietetic Association* 106 (2006): 285–293.

Appendixes

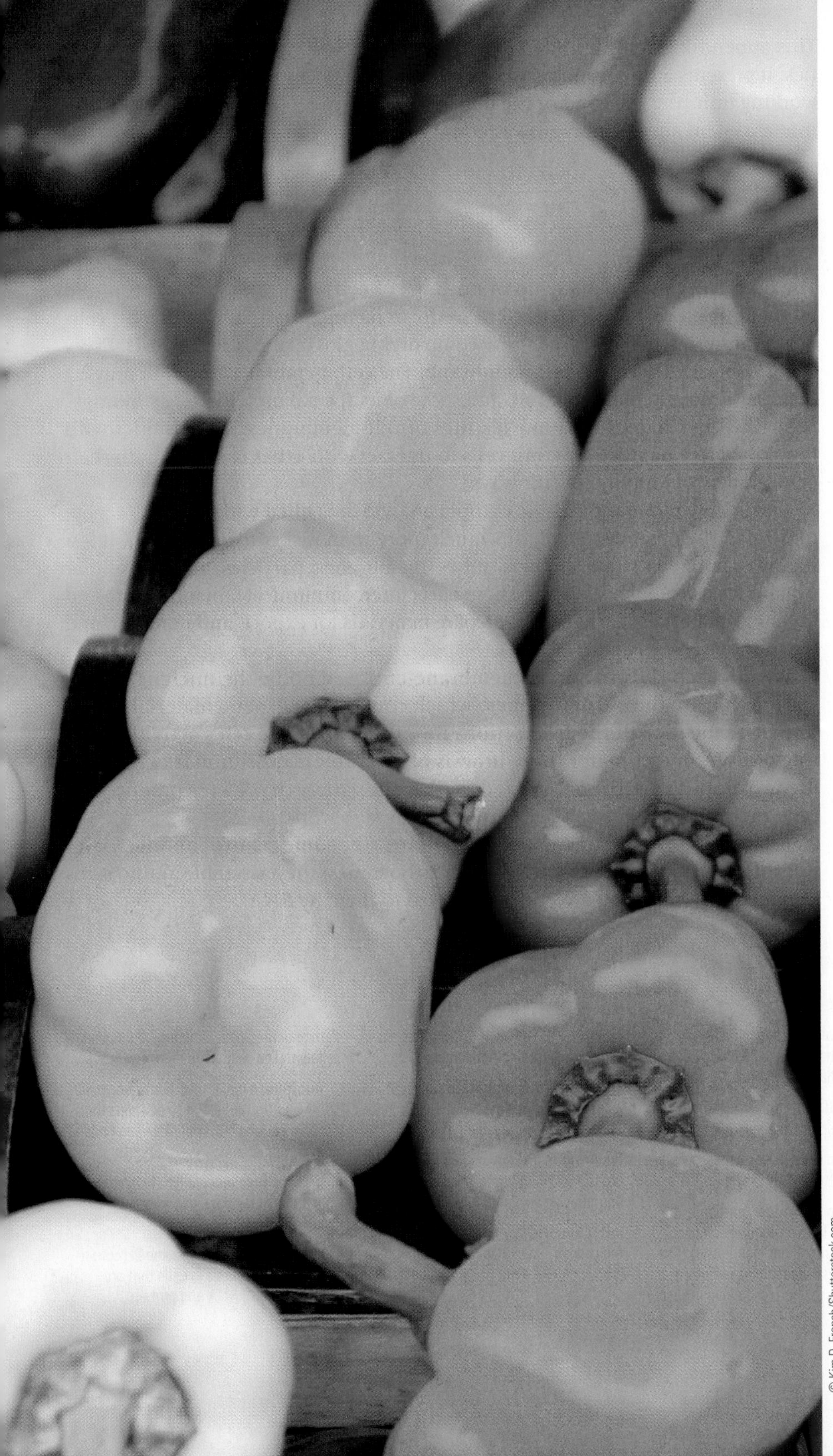

Appendix A Cells, Hormones, and Nerves

CONTENTS

This appendix offers an understanding of how the body coordinates its activities. It presents a brief summary of the structure and function of the body's basic working unit (the cell) and of the body's two major regulatory systems (the hormonal system and the nervous system).

Cells

The body's organs are made up of millions of cells and of materials produced by them. Each **cell** is specialized to perform its organ's functions, but all cells have common structures (see the accompanying glossary and Figure A-l). Every cell is contained within a **cell membrane.** The cell membrane assists in moving materials into and out of the cell, and some of its special proteins act as "pumps" (described in Chapter 6). Some features of cell membranes, such as microvilli (described in Chapter 3), permit cells to interact with other cells and with their environments in highly specific ways.

Inside the membrane lies the **cytoplasm,** which is filled with **cytosol,** a jelly-like fluid. The cytoplasm contains much more than just cytosol, though. It is a highly organized system of fibers, tubes, membranes, particles, and subcellular **organelles** as complex as a city. These parts intercommunicate, manufacture and exchange materials, package and prepare materials for export, and maintain and repair themselves.

Within each cell is another membrane-enclosed body, the **nucleus.** Inside the nucleus are the **chromosomes,** which contain the genetic material, DNA. The DNA encodes all the instructions for carrying out the cell's activities. The role of DNA in coding for the synthesis of cell proteins is summarized in Figure 6-7 on p. 178. Chapter 6 also describes the variety of proteins produced by cells and some of the ways they perform the body's work.

Among the organelles within a cell are ribosomes, mitochondria, and lysosomes. Figure 6-7 briefly refers to the **ribosomes;** they assemble amino acids into proteins, following directions conveyed to them by RNA.

GLOSSARY OF CELL STRUCTURES

cell: the basic structural unit of all living things.

cell membrane: the thin layer of tissue that surrounds the cell and encloses its contents, made primarily of lipid and protein.

chromosomes: structures within the nucleus of a cell made of DNA and associated proteins. Human beings have 46 chromosomes in 23 pairs. Each chromosome has many genes.

cytoplasm (SIGH-toh-plazm): the cell contents, except for the nucleus.

cytosol: the fluid of cytoplasm that contains water, ions, nutrients, and enzymes.

endoplasmic reticulum (en-doh-PLAZ-mic reh-TIC-you-lum): a complex network of intracellular membranes. The *rough endoplasmic reticulum* is dotted with ribosomes, where protein synthesis takes place. The *smooth endoplasmic reticulum* bears no ribosomes.

Golgi (GOAL-gee) **apparatus:** a set of membranes within the cell where secretory materials are packaged for export.

lysosomes (LYE-so-zomes): cellular organelles; membrane-enclosed sacs of degradative enzymes.

mitochondria (my-toh-KON-dree-uh): the cellular organelles responsible for producing ATP aerobically; made of membranes with enzymes mounted on them. (The singular is *mitochondrion.*)

nucleus: a major membrane-enclosed body within cells, which contains the cell's genetic material (DNA) embedded in chromosomes.

organelles: subcellular structures such as ribosomes, mitochondria, and lysosomes.

ribosomes (RYE-boh-zomes): protein-making organelles in cells that are composed of RNA and protein.

> **FIGURE A-1 The Structure of a Typical Cell**

The cell shown might be one in a gland (such as the pancreas) that produces secretory products (enzymes) for export (to the intestine). The rough endoplasmic reticulum with its ribosomes produces the enzymes; the smooth reticulum conducts them to the Golgi region; the Golgi membranes merge with the cell membrane, where the enzymes can be released into the extracellular fluid.

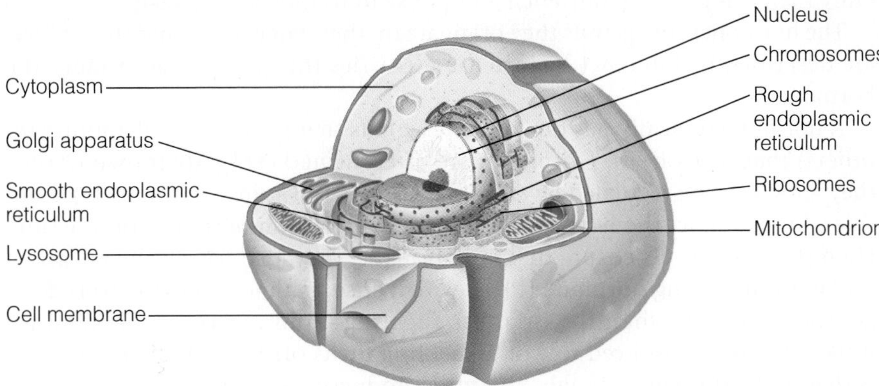

The **mitochondria** are made of intricately folded membranes that bear thousands of highly organized sets of enzymes on their inner and outer surfaces. Mitochondria are crucial to energy metabolism (described in Chapter 7) and muscles conditioned to work aerobically are packed with them. Their presence is implied whenever the TCA cycle and electron transport chain are mentioned because the mitochondria house the needed enzymes.*

The **lysosomes** are membrane-enclosed sacs of degradative enzymes. When a cell needs to self-destruct or to digest materials in its surroundings, its lysosomes release their enzymes. Lysosomes are active when tissue repair or remodeling is taking place—for example, in cleaning up infections, healing wounds, shaping embryonic organs, and remodeling bones.

In addition to these and other cellular organelles, the cell's cytoplasm contains a highly organized system of membranes, the **endoplasmic reticulum.** The ribosomes, mentioned earlier, may either float freely in the cytoplasm or be mounted on the endoplasmic reticulum. A surface dotted with ribosomes looks speckled under the microscope and is called "rough" endoplasmic reticulum; such a surface without ribosomes is called "smooth." Some intracellular membranes are organized into tubules that collect cellular materials, merge with the cell membrane, and discharge their contents to the outside of the cell; these membrane systems are named the **Golgi apparatus,** after the scientist who first described them. The rough and smooth endoplasmic reticula and the Golgi apparatus are continuous with one another, so secretions produced deep in the interior of the cell can be efficiently transported and released to the outside. These and other cell structures enable cells to perform a multitude of specialized functions.

The actions of cells are coordinated by both hormones and nerves. Among the types of cellular organelles are receptors for the hormones delivering instructions that originate elsewhere in the body. Some hormones penetrate the cell and its nucleus and attach to receptors on chromosomes, where they activate certain genes to initiate, stop, speed up, or slow down synthesis of certain proteins as needed. Other hormones attach to receptors on the cell surface and transmit their messages from there. The hormones are described in the next section; the nerves, in the one following.

---

*For the reactions of glycolysis, the TCA cycle, and the electron transport chain, see Chapter 7 and Appendix C. The reactions of glycolysis take place in the cytoplasm; the conversion of pyruvate to acetyl CoA takes place in the mitochondria, as do the TCA cycle and electron transport chain reactions. The mitochondria then release carbon dioxide, water, and ATP as their end products.

Hormones

Hormones are chemical messengers secreted by a variety of glands in response to altered conditions in the body. Each hormone travels in the blood to all parts of the body, but only its specific target cells possess receptors to accept it. Only then can the hormone elicit a response to restore homeostasis.

The hormones, the glands they originate in, their target cells, and their effects are described in Table A-1. Figure A-2 identifies the glands that produce the hormones.

A hormone typically has one or more signals that turn it on and another (or others) that turns it off. Hormones are often turned off by their own effects; they are said to be regulated by *negative feedback* (see Figure 3-12 on p. 86). Consider, for example, the hormone prolactin, which promotes milk production. High prolactin levels ensure that milk is made; they also trigger the release of prolactin-inhibiting hormone (PIH), which ensures that prolactin levels don't get too high. But when the infant is suckling—and creating a demand for milk—PIH is not allowed to work (suckling turns off PIH). The consequence is that prolactin remains high, and milk production continues. Demand from the infant thus directly adjusts the supply of milk. The need is met through the interaction of the nerves and hormones.

Every body part is affected by hormones. Each different hormone has unique effects, and hormones that oppose each other are produced in carefully regulated amounts, so each can respond to the exact degree that is appropriate to the condition.

As Table A-1 summarizes, hormones have an enormous impact on body processes. The body's other overall regulating agency is the nervous system.

> **FIGURE A-2 The Endocrine System**

These organs and glands release hormones that regulate body processes. An *endocrine gland* secretes its product directly into *(endo)* the blood; for example, the pancreas cells that secrete insulin into the blood. An *exocrine gland* secretes its product(s) out *(exo)* to an epithelial surface either directly or through a duct; the sweat glands of the skin and the pancreas cells that secrete digestive enzymes into the gastrointestinal tract are both examples. The pancreas is therefore both an endocrine and an exocrine gland.

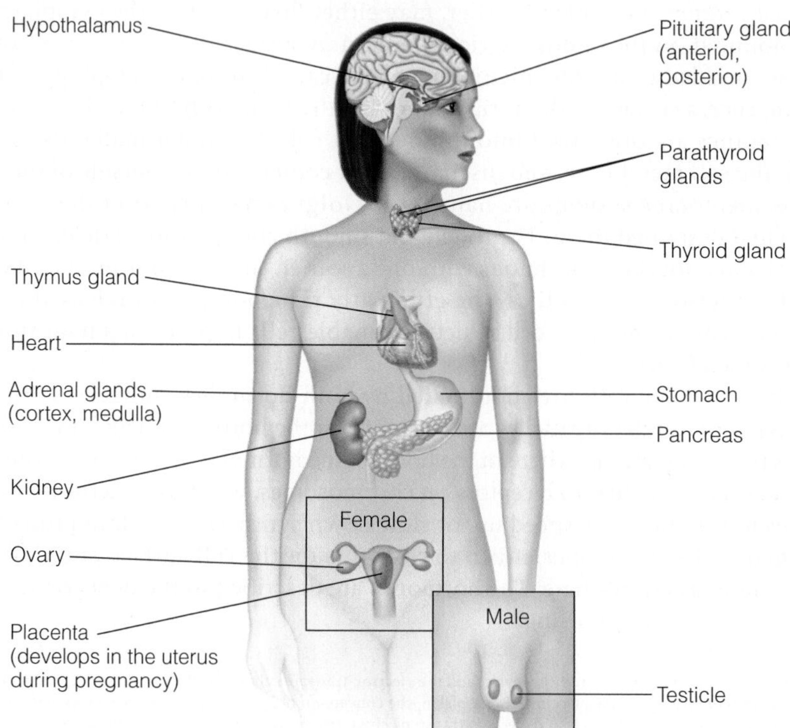

hormones: chemical messengers. Hormones are secreted by a variety of endocrine glands in response to altered conditions in the body. Each hormone travels to one or more specific target tissues or organs, where it elicits a specific response to maintain homeostasis. The study of hormones and their actions is called *endocrinology*.

TABLE A-1 Summary of Major Hormones

Gland	Hormone	Target Cells	Action
Anterior pituitary	Adrenocorticotropin (ACTH)	Adrenal cortex	Stimulates secretion of glucocorticoids and androgens
Adrenal cortex	Aldosterone	Kidneys	Stimulates sodium reabsorption, thereby regulating acid-base balance, blood volume, and blood pressure
Posterior pituitary	Antidiuretic hormone (ADH); also called vasopressin	Arteries	Causes vasoconstriction
		Kidneys	Promotes water retention
Thyroid gland	Calcitonin	Bones	Lowers blood calcium by moving calcium from the bloodstream into the bones whenever blood calcium rises above normal
		Kidneys	Increases excretion of calcium and phosphorus
Duodenum	Cholecystokinin	Gallbladder	Releases bile into the intestine
		Pancreas	Releases pancreatic juices into the intestine
Hypothalamus	Corticotropin-releasing hormone (CRH)	Anterior pituitary	Controls release of adrenocorticotropin (ACTH)
Kidneys	Erythropoietin	Bone marrow	Stimulates red blood cell production
Ovaries	Estrogens	Female sexual tissues	Promotes growth, development, and health of all tissues involved in female sexuality
Anterior pituitary	Follicle-stimulating hormone (FSH)	Ovaries (female)	Stimulates follicular development and ovulation
		Testicles (male)	Stimulates sperm production
Stomach, duodenum	Gastrin	Stomach	Stimulates gastric acid secretion; slows motility
Hypothalamus	Growth hormone releasing hormone (GHRH) and growth hormone inhibiting hormone (GHIH or somatostatin)	Anterior pituitary	Controls release of growth hormone (GH)
Pancreas (alpha cells)	Glucagon	Liver	Promotes the breakdown of glycogen to glucose
		Most cells	Increases use of fat and amino acids for energy
Adrenal cortex	Glucocorticoids	Most cells	Protects against stress; raises blood glucose
Hypothalamus	Gonadotropin-releasing hormone (GnRH)	Anterior pituitary	Controls release of follicle-stimulating hormone (FSH) and luteinizing hormone (LH)
Anterior pituitary	Growth hormone (GH); also called somatotropin	All tissues	Stimulates growth; regulates metabolism
Pancreas (beta cells)	Insulin	Most cells	Stimulates nutrient uptake into cells
Anterior pituitary	Luteinizing hormone (LH)	Ovaries (female)	Stimulates follicular development and ovulation
		Testicles (male)	Stimulates testosterone production
Adrenal medulla	Norepinephrine and epinephrine; formerly called noradrenalin and adrenalin, respectively	Many cells	Facilitates the body's readiness for fight or flight: maintains blood pressure, increases cardiac output, constricts blood vessels, keeps airways open, raises blood glucose levels
Posterior pituitary	Oxytocin	Uterus (female in late pregnancy)	Induces muscle contractions during childbirth
		Mammary glands (female in lactation)	Causes milk ejection during lactation
Parathyroid gland	Parathyroid hormone (PTH); also called parathormone	Bones	Releases stored calcium into the blood
		Kidneys	Slows calcium excretion
		Intestines	Increases calcium absorption
Corpus luteum, placenta	Progesterone	Uterus	Facilitates implantation at the start of pregnancy
		Mammary glands	Stimulates mammary gland development for lactation
Anterior pituitary	Prolactin	Mammary glands (female in lactation)	Stimulates milk production
Hypothalamus	Prolactin-inhibiting hormone (PIH)	Anterior pituitary	Controls release of prolactin
Duodenum	Secretin	Pancreas	Stimulates bicarbonate secretion into the intestine; slows stomach motility
Testicles	Testosterone	Male sexual tissues	Promotes growth, development, and health of all tissues involved in male sexuality
Anterior pituitary	Thyroid-stimulating hormone (TSH)	Thyroid gland	Stimulates synthesis and release of thyroid hormones (thyroxine and triiodothyronine)
Thyroid gland	Thyroxine	Many cells	Regulates metabolic rate, growth, and heat production
Hypothalamus	TSH-releasing hormone (TRH)	Anterior pituitary	Controls release of thyroid-stimulating hormone (TSH)
Skin	Vitamin D	Intestines	Increases calcium absorption

Nerves

The nervous system has a central control system that can evaluate information about conditions within and outside the body, and an expansive communication system that receives information and sends instructions. The control system is the brain and spinal cord, called the **central nervous system;** and the communication system between the center and the parts is the **peripheral nervous system.** The smooth functioning that results from the systems' adjustments to changing conditions is homeostasis.

The nervous system is best understood as two systems that use the same or similar pathways to receive and transmit their messages. The **somatic nervous system** controls the voluntary muscles; the **autonomic nervous system** controls the involuntary, internal muscles and organs.

When scientists were first studying the autonomic nervous system, they noticed that when something hurt one organ of the body, some of the other organs reacted as if in sympathy for the afflicted one. They therefore named the nerve network they were studying the **sympathetic nervous system.** The term is still used today to refer to the branch of the autonomic nervous system that responds to stressful conditions. The other branch that supports normal conditions is called the **parasympathetic nervous system.** (Think of the sympathetic branch as the emergency responder when homeostasis needs prompt restoring and the parasympathetic branch as the steady commander during normal times.) Both systems transmit their messages through the brain and spinal cord. Nerves of the two branches travel side by side along the same pathways to transmit their messages, but they oppose each other's actions (see Figure A-3).

An example will show how the sympathetic and parasympathetic nervous systems work to maintain homeostasis. When you go outside in cold weather, your skin's temperature receptors send "cold" messages to the spinal cord and brain. Your conscious mind may intervene at this point to tell you to zip your jacket, but let's say you have no jacket. Your sympathetic nervous system reacts to the external stressor, the cold. It signals your skin-surface capillaries to shut down so that your blood will circulate deeper in your tissues, where it will conserve heat. Your sympathetic nervous system also signals involuntary contractions of the small muscles just under the skin surface. The product of these muscle contractions is heat, and the visible result is goose bumps. If these measures do not raise your body temperature enough, then the sympathetic nerves signal your large muscle groups to shiver; the contractions of these large muscles produce still more heat. All of this activity helps to maintain your homeostasis (with respect to temperature) under conditions of external extremes (cold) that would throw it off balance. The cold was a stressor; the body's response was resistance.

Now let's say you come in and sit by a fire and drink hot cocoa. You are warm and no longer need all that sympathetic activity. At this point, your parasympathetic nerves take over; they signal your skin-surface capillaries to dilate again, your goose bumps to subside, and your muscles to relax. Your body is back to normal. This is recovery.

GLOSSARY OF NERVOUS SYSTEM

autonomic nervous system: the division of the nervous system that controls the body's automatic responses. Its two branches are the *sympathetic* branch, which helps the body respond to stressors from the outside environment, and the *parasympathetic* branch, which regulates normal body activities between stressful times.

central nervous system: the central part of the nervous system; the brain and spinal cord.

parasympathetic nervous system: the part of the autonomic nervous system that dominates during nonstressful conditions and includes such effects as normal heart rate, pupil dilation, and peristalsis.

peripheral (puh-RIFF-er-ul) **nervous system:** the peripheral (outermost) part of the nervous system; the vast complex of wiring that extends from the central nervous system to the body's outermost areas. It contains both *somatic* and *autonomic* components.

somatic (so-MAT-ick) **nervous system:** the division of the nervous system that controls the voluntary muscles, as distinguished from the autonomic nervous system, which controls involuntary functions.

sympathetic nervous system: the part of the autonomic nervous system that dominates during stressful conditions and includes such effects as increased heart rate, dilated pupils, slowed peristalsis, and secretion of epinephrine and norepinephrine.

> **FIGURE A-3 The Organization of the Nervous System**

The brain and spinal cord evaluate information about conditions within and outside the body, and the peripheral nerves receive information and send instructions.

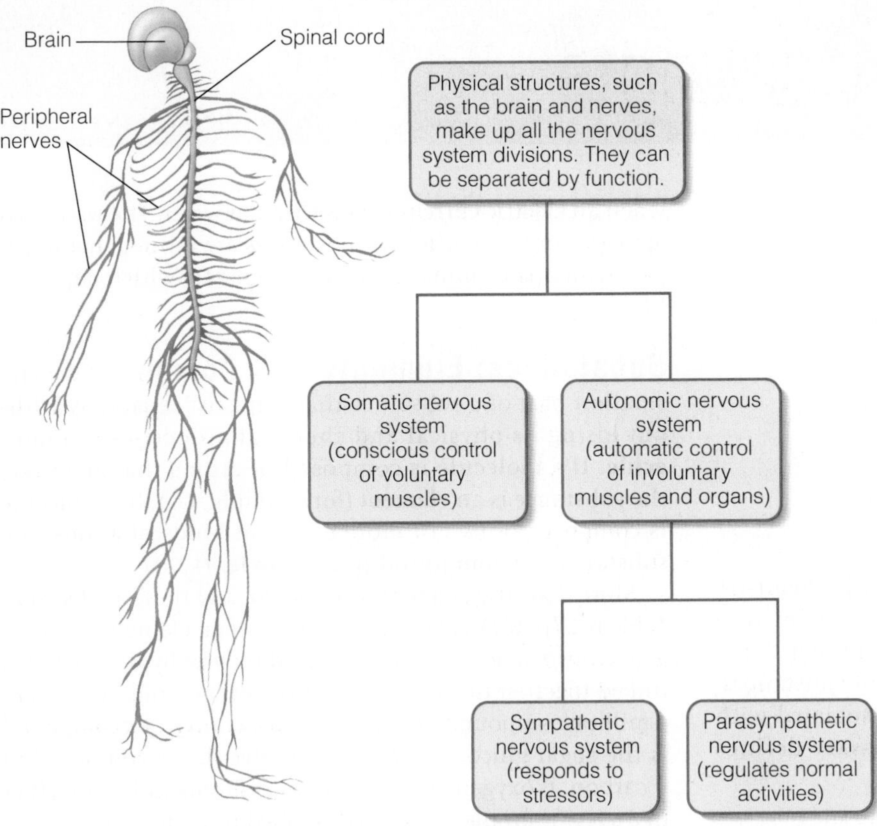

Putting It Together

The hormonal and nervous systems coordinate body functions by transmitting and receiving messages. The point-to-point messages of the nervous system travel through the spinal cord and brain, whereas the messages of the hormonal system are sent through the bloodstream, and any organ with the appropriate receptors can pick them up. Nerve impulses travel faster than hormonal messages do—although both are remarkably swift. Whereas your brain's command to wiggle your toes reaches the toes within a fraction of a second and stops as quickly, a gland's message to alter a body condition may take several seconds or minutes to get started and may fade away equally slowly.

Together, the two systems possess every characteristic a superb communication network needs: varied speeds of transmission, along with private communication lines or public broadcasting systems, depending on the needs of the moment. The hormonal system, together with the nervous system, integrates the whole body's functioning so that all parts act smoothly together.

Appendix B Basic Chemistry Concepts

CONTENTS

This appendix provides the background in basic chemistry needed to understand the nutrition concepts presented in this book. Chemistry is the branch of natural science that deals with the composition and properties of substances, how substances interact, and the **energy** associated with these interactions. The accompanying glossary defines related terms.

The Properties of Atoms

Every substance has physical and chemical properties that distinguish it from all other substances and thus give it a unique identity. The physical properties include such characteristics as color, taste, texture, and odor, as well as the temperatures at which a substance changes its state (from a solid to a liquid or from a liquid to a gas) and the weight of a unit volume (its density). The chemical properties of a substance have to do with how it reacts with other substances or responds to a change in its environment.

A physical change does not change a substance's chemical composition. The three physical states—ice, water, and steam—all consist of two hydrogen atoms and one oxygen atom bound together. In contrast, a chemical change occurs when an electric current passes through water. The water disappears, and two different substances are formed: hydrogen gas, which is flammable, and oxygen gas, which supports life.

Substances: Elements and Compounds The smallest part of a substance that can exist separately without losing its physical and chemical properties is a **molecule**. If a molecule is composed of **atoms** that are alike, the substance is an **element** (for example, O_2). If a molecule is composed of two or more different kinds of atoms, the substance is a **compound** (for example, H_2O).

More than 100 elements are known, and these are listed in Table B-1 (p. B-1). A familiar example of an element is hydrogen, whose molecules are composed only of hydrogen atoms linked together in pairs (H_2). On the other hand, more than a million compounds are known. An example of a compound is the sugar glucose. Each of its molecules is composed of 6 carbon, 6 oxygen, and 12 hydrogen atoms linked together in a specific arrangement (as described in Chapter 4).

The Nature of Atoms Atoms themselves are made of smaller particles. Within an atom's nucleus are protons (positively charged particles), and surrounding the nucleus are an equal number of electrons (negatively charged particles). The number of protons in the nucleus of an atom determines the atomic number. The positive charge on a proton is equal to the negative charge on an electron, so the charges cancel each other out and leave the atom neutral to its surroundings.

The nucleus may also include neutrons, subatomic particles that have no charge. Protons and neutrons are of equal mass, and together they give an atom its atomic mass. Electrons bond atoms together to make molecules, and they are involved in chemical reactions.

GLOSSARY

anions (AN-eye-uns)**:** negatively changed ions.

atoms: the smallest components of an element that have all of the properties of the element.

cations (CAT-eye-uns)**:** positively changed ions.

compound: a substance composed of two or more different atoms—for example, water (H_2O).

covalent bonds: strong chemical bonds formed between atoms by sharing electrons.

element: a substance composed of atoms that are alike—for example, iron (Fe).

energy: the capacity to do work. The energy in food is chemical energy. The body can convert this chemical energy to mechanical, electrical, or heat energy.

ions (EYE-uns)**:** atoms or molecules that have gained or lost one or more electrons and therefore have electrical charges. Examples include the positively charged sodium ion (Na^+) and the negatively charged chloride ion (Cl^-).

molecule: two or more atoms of the same or different elements joined by chemical bonds. Examples are molecules of the element oxygen, composed of two oxygen atoms (O_2), and molecules of the compound water, composed of two hydrogen atoms and one oxygen atom (H_2O).

TABLE B-1 The Elements

Number of Protons (Atomic Number)	Element	Number of Electrons in Outer Shell
1	Hydrogen (H)	1
2	Helium (He)	2
3	Lithium (Li)	1
4	Beryllium (Be)	2
5	Boron (B)	3
6	Carbon (C)	4
7	Nitrogen (N)	5
8	Oxygen (O)	6
9	Fluorine (F)	7
10	Neon (Ne)	8
11	Sodium (Na)	1
12	Magnesium (Mg)	2
13	Aluminum (Al)	3
14	Silicon (Si)	4
15	Phosphorus (P)	5
16	Sulfur (S)	6
17	Chlorine (Cl)	7
18	Argon (Ar)	8
19	Potassium (K)	1
20	Calcium (Ca)	2
21	Scandium (Sc)	2
22	Titanium (Ti)	2
23	Vanadium (V)	2
24	Chromium (Cr)	1
25	Manganese (Mn)	2
26	Iron (Fe)	2
27	Cobalt (Co)	2
28	Nickel (Ni)	2
29	Copper (Cu)	1
30	Zinc (Zn)	2
31	Gallium (Ga)	3
32	Germanium (Ge)	4
33	Arsenic (As)	5
34	Selenium (Se)	6
35	Bromine (Br)	7
36	Krypton (Kr)	8
37	Rubidium (Rb)	1
38	Strontium (Sr)	2
39	Yttrium (Y)	2
40	Zirconium (Zr)	2
41	Niobium (Nb)	1
42	Molybdenum (Mo)	1
43	Technetium (Tc)	1
44	Ruthenium (Ru)	1
45	Rhodium (Rh)	1
46	Palladium (Pd)	—
47	Silver (Ag)	1
48	Cadmium (Cd)	2
49	Indium (In)	3
50	Tin (Sn)	4
51	Antimony (Sb)	5
52	Tellurium (Te)	6
53	Iodine (I)	7
54	Xenon (Xe)	8
55	Cesium (Cs)	1
56	Barium (Ba)	2
57	Lanthanum (La)	2
58	Cerium (Ce)	2
59	Praseodymium (Pr)	2
60	Neodymium (Nd)	2
61	Promethium (Pm)	2
62	Samarium (Sm)	2
63	Europium (Eu)	2
64	Gadolinium (Gd)	2
65	Terbium (Tb)	2
66	Dysprosium (Dy)	2
67	Holmium (Ho)	2
68	Erbium (Er)	2
69	Thulium (Tm)	2
70	Ytterbium (Yb)	2
71	Lutetium (Lu)	2
72	Hafnium (Hf)	2
73	Tantalum (Ta)	2
74	Tungsten (W)	2
75	Rhenium (Re)	2
76	Osmium (Os)	2
77	Iridium (Ir)	2
78	Platinum (Pt)	1
79	Gold (Au)	1
80	Mercury (Hg)	2
81	Thallium (Tl)	3
82	Lead (Pb)	4
83	Bismuth (Bi)	5
84	Polonium (Po)	6
85	Astatine (At)	7
86	Radon (Rn)	8
87	Francium (Fr)	1
88	Radium (Ra)	2
89	Actinium (Ac)	2
90	Thorium (Th)	2
91	Protactinium (Pa)	2
92	Uranium (U)	2
93	Neptunium (Np)	2
94	Plutonium (Pu)	2
95	Americium (Am)	2
96	Curium (Cm)	2
97	Berkelium (Bk)	2
98	Californium (Cf)	2
99	Einsteinium (Es)	2
100	Fermium (Fm)	2
101	Mendelevium (Md)	2
102	Nobelium (No)	2
103	Lawrencium (Lr)	2
104	Rutherfordium (Rf)	2
105	Dubnium (Db)	2
106	Seaborgium (Sg)	2
107	Bohrium (Bh)	2
108	Hassium (Hs)	2
109	Meitnerium (Mt)	2
110	Darmstadtium (Ds)	2

Key
Elements found in energy-yielding nutrients, vitamins, and water
Major minerals
Trace minerals

Each element has a characteristic number of protons in its atom's nucleus. For example, the hydrogen atom (the simplest of all) possesses a single proton, with a single electron associated with it:

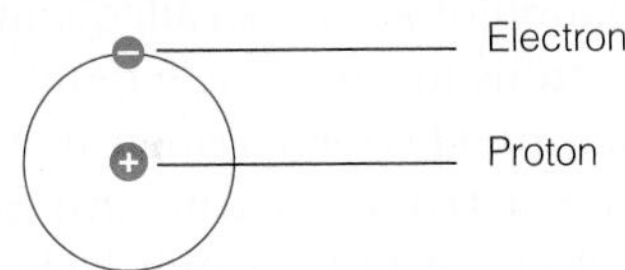

Hydrogen atom (H), atomic number 1

Just as hydrogen always has one proton, helium always has two, lithium three, and so on. The atomic number of each element is the number of protons in the nucleus of that atom, and this never changes in a chemical reaction; it gives the atom its identity. The atomic numbers for the known elements are listed in Table B-1.

In addition to hydrogen, the atoms most common in living things are carbon (C), nitrogen (N), and oxygen (O), whose atomic numbers are 6, 7, and 8, respectively. Their structures are more complicated than that of hydrogen, but each of them possesses the same number of electrons as there are protons in the nucleus. These electrons are found in orbits, or shells (shown below).

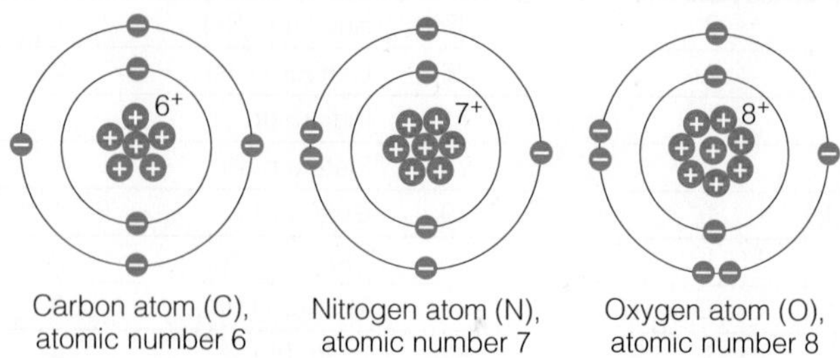

In these and all diagrams of atoms that follow, only the protons and electrons are shown. The neutrons, which contribute only to atomic weight, not to charge, are omitted.

The most important structural feature of an atom for determining its chemical behavior is the number of electrons in its outermost shell. The first, or innermost, shell is full when it is occupied by two electrons; so an atom with two or more electrons has a filled first shell. When the first shell is full, electrons begin to fill the second shell.

The second shell is completely full when it has eight electrons. A substance that has a full outer shell tends not to enter into chemical reactions. Atomic number 10, neon, is a chemically inert substance because its outer shell is complete. Fluorine, atomic number 9, has a great tendency to attract an electron from other substances to complete its outer shell, and thus it is highly reactive. Carbon has a half-full outer shell, which helps explain its great versatility; it can combine with many other elements in a variety of ways to form a large number of compounds.

Atoms seek to reach a state of maximum stability or of lowest energy in the same way that a ball will roll down a hill until it reaches the lowest place. An atom achieves a state of maximum stability:

- By gaining or losing electrons to either fill or empty its outer shell.
- By sharing its electrons with other atoms and thereby completing its outer shell.

The number of electrons determines how the atom will chemically react with other atoms.

Chemical Bonding

Atoms often complete their outer shells by sharing electrons with other atoms. In order to complete its outer shell, a carbon atom requires four electrons. A hydrogen atom requires one. Thus, when a carbon atom shares electrons with four hydrogen atoms, each completes its outer shell (as shown in the next drawing). Electron sharing binds the atoms together and satisfies the conditions of maximum stability for the molecule. The outer shell of each atom is complete because hydrogen effectively has the required 2 electrons in its first (outer) shell, and carbon has 8 electrons in its second (outer) shell; and the molecule is electrically neutral, with a total of 10 protons and 10 electrons.

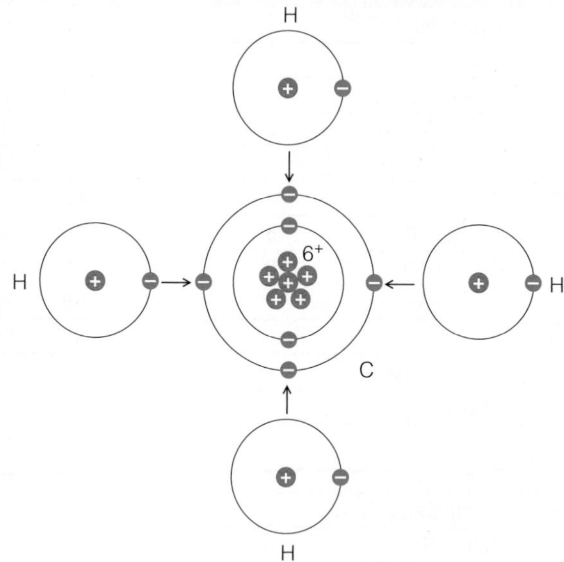

When a carbon atom shares electrons with four hydrogen atoms, a methane molecule is made.

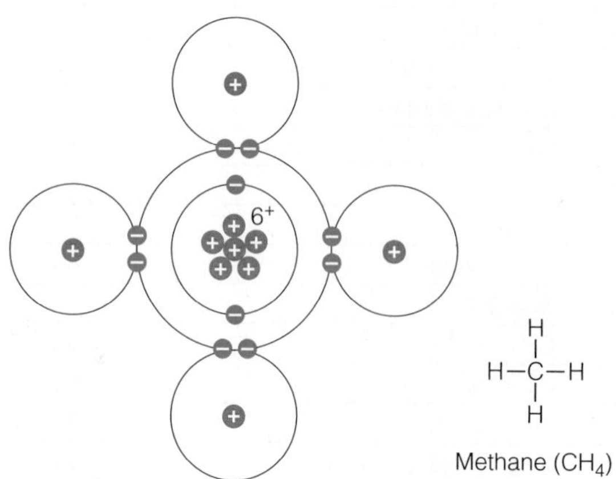

The chemical formula for methane is CH_4. Note that by sharing electrons, every atom achieves a filled outer shell.

Bonds that involve the sharing of electrons, like the bonds in methane between the one carbon and the four hydrogens, are the most stable kind of association that atoms can form with one another. These bonds are called **covalent bonds,** and the resulting combination of atoms is called a molecule. A single pair of shared electrons forms a single bond. A simplified way to represent a single bond is with a single line.

Similarly, one nitrogen atom and three hydrogen atoms can share electrons to form one molecule of ammonia (NH_3):

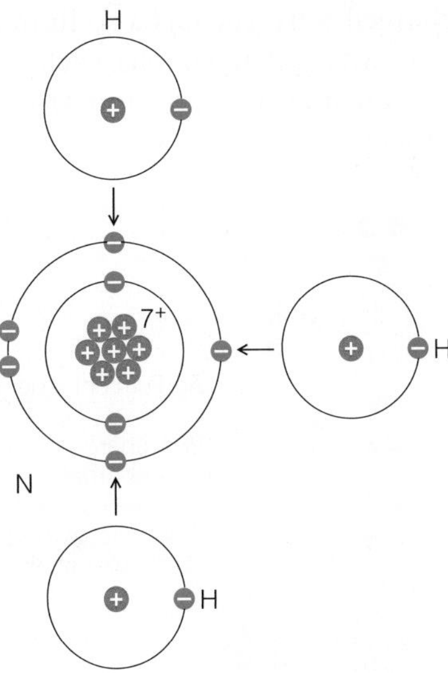

When a nitrogen atom shares electrons with three hydrogen atoms, an ammonia molecule is made.

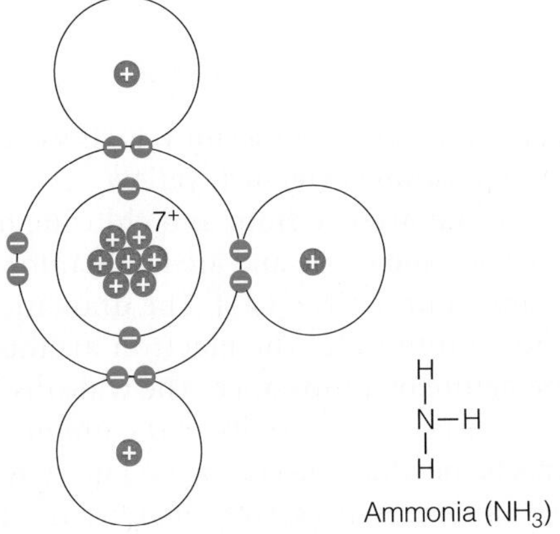

The chemical formula for ammonia is NH_3. Count the electrons in each atom's outer shell to confirm that it is filled.

One oxygen atom may be bonded to two hydrogen atoms to form one molecule of water (H_2O):

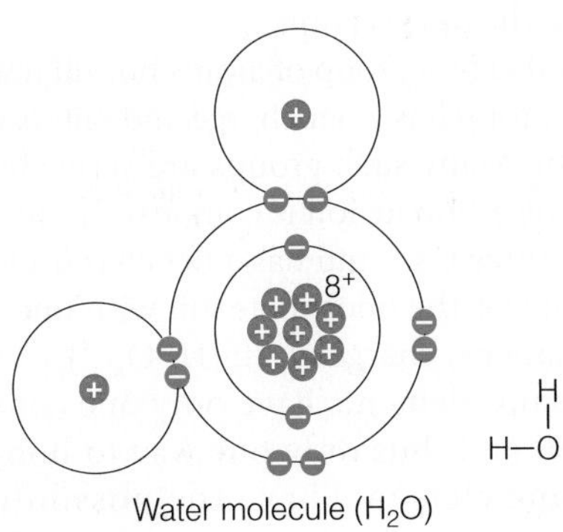

When two oxygen atoms form a molecule of oxygen, they must share two pairs of electrons. This double bond may be represented as two lines:

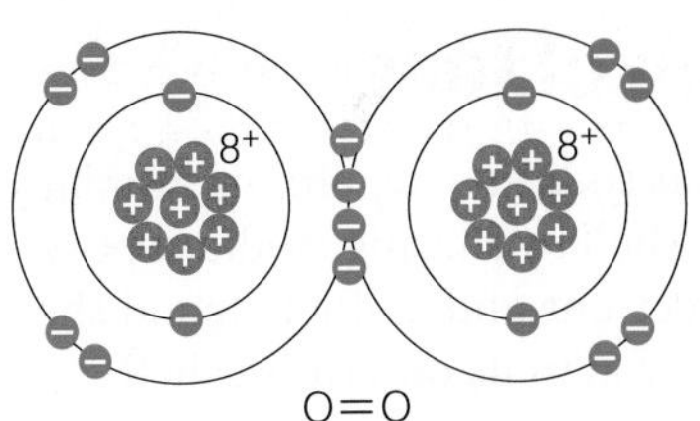

Small atoms form the tightest, most stable bonds. H, O, N, and C are the smallest atoms capable of forming one, two, three, and four electron-pair bonds, respectively. This is the basis for the statement in Chapter 4 that in drawings of compounds containing these atoms, hydrogen must always have one, oxygen two, nitrogen three, and carbon four bonds radiating to other atoms:

H—   —O—   —N—   —C—

The stability of the associations between these small atoms (hydrogen, carbon, nitrogen, and oxygen) and the versatility with which they can combine make them very common in living things. Interestingly all cells—whether they come from animals, plants, or bacteria—contain the same elements in very nearly the same proportions. The elements commonly found in living things are shown in Table B-2.

TABLE B-2 Elemental Composition of the Human Body

Element	Chemical Symbol	By Weight (%)
Oxygen	O	65.0
Carbon	C	18.0
Hydrogen	H	10.0
Nitrogen	N	3.0
Calcium	Ca	1.5
Phosphorus	P	1.0
Potassium	K	0.4
Sulfur	S	0.3
Sodium	Na	0.2
Chloride	Cl	0.1
Magnesium	Mg	0.1
Total		99.6[a]

[a]The remaining 0.4 percent by weight is contributed by the trace elements: chromium (Cr), copper (Cu), zinc (Zn), selenium (Se), molybdenum (Mo), fluorine (F), iodine (I), manganese (Mn), and iron (Fe). Cells may also contain variable traces of some of the following: boron (B), cobalt (Co), Lithium (Li), strontium (Sr), aluminum (AL), silicon (Si), Lead (Pb), vanadium (V), arsenic (As), bromine (Br), and others.

Formation of Ions

An atom such as sodium (Na, atomic number 11) cannot easily fill its outer shell by sharing. Sodium possesses a filled first shell of two electrons and a filled second shell of eight; there is only one electron in its outermost shell:

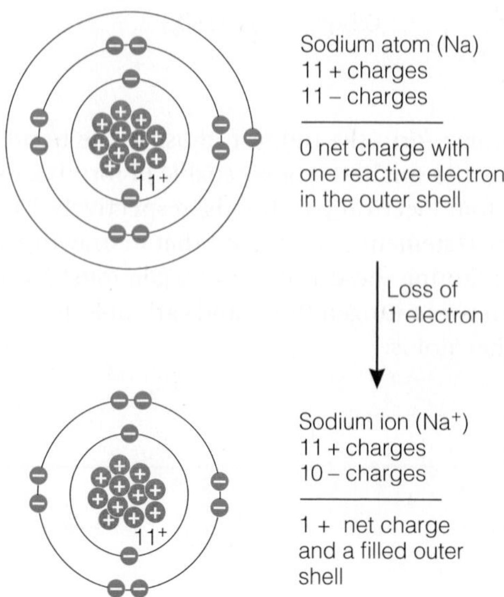

If sodium loses this electron, it satisfies one condition for stability: a filled outer shell (now its second shell counts as the outer shell). However, it is not electrically neutral. It has 11 protons (positive) and only 10 electrons (negative). It therefore has a net positive charge. An atom or molecule that has lost or gained one or more electrons and so is electrically charged is called an **ion**.

An atom such as chlorine (Cl, atomic number 17), with seven electrons in its outermost shell, can share electrons to fill its outer shell, or it can gain one electron to complete its outer shell and thus give it a negative charge:

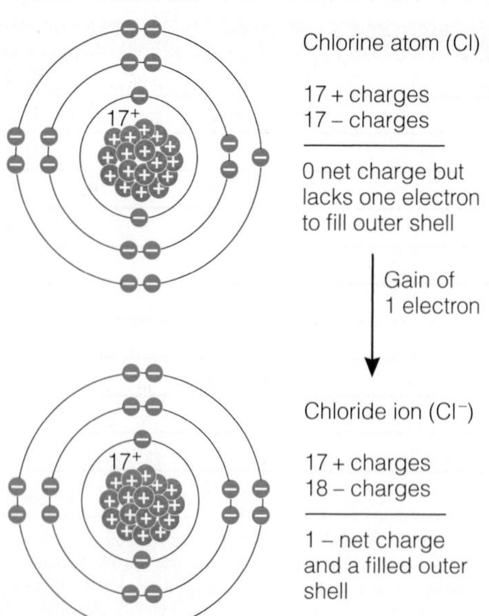

Positively charged ions, such as a sodium ion (Na^+), are called **cations**; negatively charged ions, such as a chloride ion (Cl^-), are called **anions**. Cations and anions attract one another to form salts:

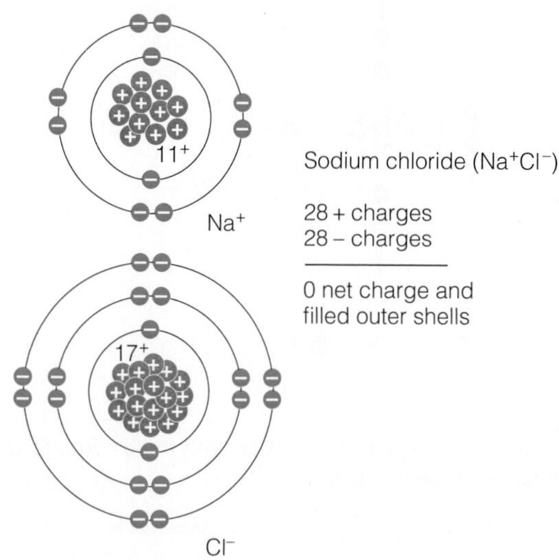

With all its electrons, sodium is a shiny, highly reactive metal; chlorine is the poisonous greenish yellow gas that was used in World War I. But after sodium and chlorine have shared electrons, they become stable and are familiar to you as table salt, or sodium chloride (Na^+Cl^-). The dramatic difference illustrates how profoundly the electron arrangement can influence the nature of a substance. The wide distribution of salt in nature attests to the stability of the union between the ions. Each meets the other's needs (a good marriage).

When dry, salt exists as crystals; its ions are stacked very regularly into a lattice, with positive and negative ions alternating in a three-dimensional checkerboard structure. In water, however, the salt quickly dissolves, and its ions separate from one another, forming an electrolyte solution in which they move about freely. Covalently bonded molecules rarely dissociate like this in a water solution. The most common exception is when they behave like acids and release H^+ ions, as discussed in the next section.

An ion can also be a group of atoms bound together in such a way that the group has a net charge and enters into reactions as a single unit. Many such groups are active in the fluids of the body. The bicarbonate ion is composed of five atoms—one H, one C, and three Os—and has a net charge of −1 (HCO_3^-). Another example is the phosphate ion with one H, one P, and four O, that has a net charge of −2 (HPO_4^{-2}).

Whereas many elements have only one configuration in the outer shell and thus only one way to bond with other elements, some elements have the possibility of varied configurations. Iron is such an element. Under some conditions iron loses two electrons, and under other circumstances it loses three. If iron loses two electrons, it then has a net charge of +2 and is called ferrous iron (Fe^{++}). If it loses three electrons, it becomes the +3 ion called ferric iron (Fe^{+++}).

Ferrous iron (Fe^{++})	Ferric iron (Fe^{+++})
(lost 2 outer-shell electrons)	(lost 3 outer-shell electrons)
26 + charges	26 + charges
24 − charges	23 − charges
2 + net charge	3 + net charge

Remember that a positive charge on an ion means that negative charges—electrons—have been lost and not that positive charges have been added to the nucleus.

Water, Acids, and Bases

Water The water molecule is electrically neutral, having equal numbers of protons and electrons. When a hydrogen atom shares its electron with oxygen, however, that electron will spend most of its time closer to the positively charged oxygen nucleus. This leaves the positive proton (nucleus of the hydrogen atom) exposed on the outer part of the water molecule. We know, too, that the two hydrogens both bond toward the same side of the oxygen. These two facts explain why water molecules are polar: they have regions that are more positively and more negatively charged.

Polar molecules like water are attracted to one another by the forces between the positive areas of one and the negative areas of another. These attractive forces, sometimes known as polar bonds or hydrogen bonds, occur among many molecules and also within different parts of the same molecule. Although very weak in comparison with covalent bonds, polar bonds may occur in such abundance that they become exceedingly important in determining the structure of large molecules such as proteins and DNA.

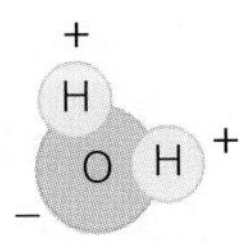

This diagram of a polar water molecule shows the negative area near the O and the positive area near the H atoms.

Water molecules have a slight tendency to ionize, separating into positive (H^+) and negative (OH^-) ions. In pure water, a small but constant number of these ions is present, and the number of positive ions exactly equals the number of negative ions.

Acids An acid is a substance that releases H^+ ions (protons) in a water solution. Hydrochloric acid (HCl^-) is such a substance because it dissociates in a water solution into H^+ and Cl^- ions. Acetic acid is also an acid because it dissociates in water to acetate ions and free H^+:

```
   H  O              H  O
   |  ‖              |  ‖
H–C– C–O–H  →  H–C– C–O⁻ + H⁺
   |                 |
   H                 H
```

Acetic acid dissociates into an acetate ion and a hydrogen ion.

The more H^+ ions released, the stronger the acid. Chemists define degrees of acidity by means of the pH scale, which runs from 0 to 14. The pH expresses the concentration of H^+ ions: a pH of 1 is extremely acidic, 7 is neutral, and 13 is very basic. There is a tenfold difference in the concentration of H^+ ions between points on this scale. A solution with pH 3, for example, has 10 times as many H^+ ions as a solution with pH 4. Figure 3-6 on p. 77 presents the pH of common substances.

Bases A base is a substance that can combine with H^+ ions, thus reducing the acidity of a solution. The compound ammonia is such a substance. The ammonia molecule has two electrons that are not shared with any other atom; a hydrogen ion (H^+) is a proton without an outer shell of electrons. The proton readily combines with the ammonia molecule to form an ion; thus a free H^+ is withdrawn from the solution and no longer contributes to its acidity. Many nitrogen-containing compounds are important bases in living systems. Acids and bases neutralize each other to produce substances that are neither acid nor base.

Chemical Reactions

A chemical reaction results in the breakdown or formation of substances. Almost all such reactions involve a change in the bonding of atoms. Old bonds are broken, and new ones are formed. The nuclei of atoms are never involved in chemical reactions—only the outer-shell electrons participate. At the end of a chemical reaction, the number of atoms of each type is always the same as at the beginning. For example, two hydrogen molecules ($2H_2$) can react with one oxygen molecule (O_2) to form two water molecules ($2H_2O$). In this reaction two substances (hydrogen and oxygen) disappear, and a new one (water) is formed, but at the end of the reaction there are still four H atoms and two O atoms, just as there were at the beginning. Because the atoms are now linked in a different way, their characteristics and properties have changed.

In many instances chemical reactions involve the exchange of electrons or protons between molecules. In such reactions the molecule that gains one or more electrons (or loses one or more protons) is said to be reduced; the molecule that loses electrons (or gains protons) is oxidized. A hydrogen ion is equivalent to a proton.

Oxidation and reduction reactions take place simultaneously because an electron or proton that is lost by one molecule is accepted by another. The addition of an atom of oxygen is also oxidation because oxygen (with six electrons in the outer shell) accepts two electrons in becoming bonded. Oxidation occurs, then, with the loss of electrons, the gain of protons, or the addition of oxygen (with six electrons); reduction occurs with the opposite—a gain of electrons, a loss of protons, or a loss of oxygen. The addition of hydrogen atoms to oxygen to form water can thus be described as the reduction of oxygen *or* the oxidation of hydrogen.

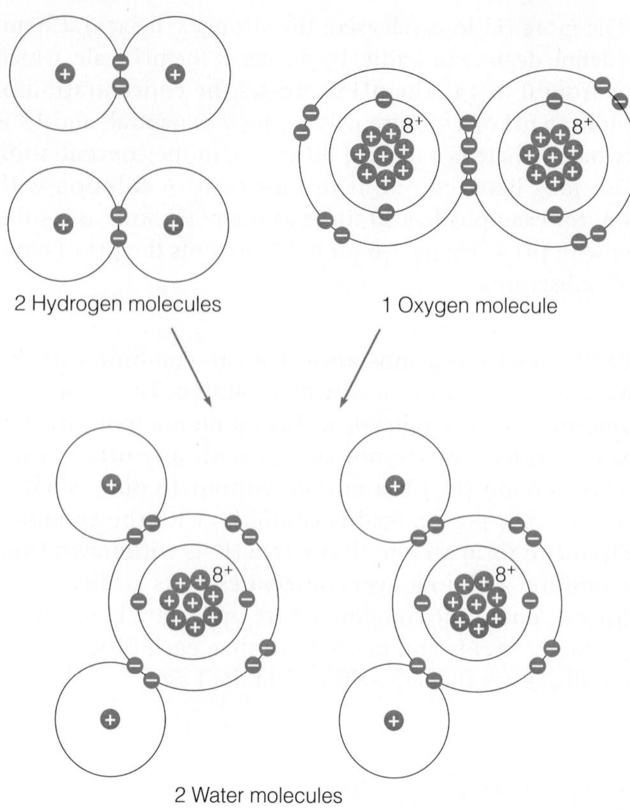

Structures:

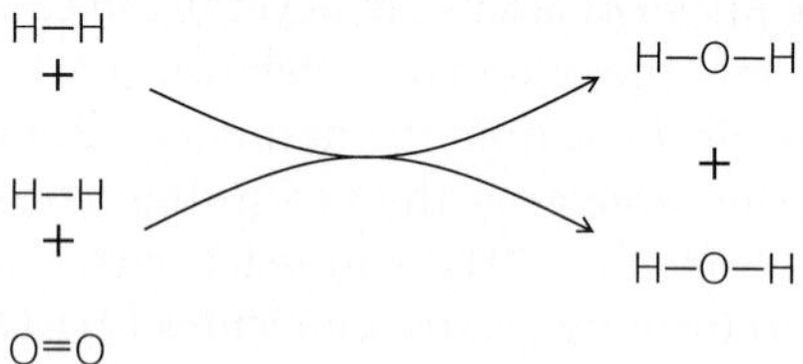

Formulas:

$$2H_2 + O_2 \longrightarrow 2H_2O$$

Hydrogen and oxygen react to form water.

Reactions in which the end products contain more energy than the reacting compounds started with are called endergonic, or "uphill," reactions and do not occur until an energy source is provided. An example of such an energy source is the sunlight used in photosynthesis reactions that combine carbon dioxide and water (low-energy compounds) to form glucose (a higher-energy compound). Conversely, the oxidation of glucose to carbon dioxide and water is an exergonic, or "downhill," reaction because the end products have less energy than the starting product. Oftentimes, but not always, reduction reactions are endergonic, resulting in an increase in the energy of the end products. Oxidation reactions often, but not always, are exergonic.

Chemical reactions tend to occur spontaneously if the end products are in a lower energy state and therefore are more stable than the reacting compounds. These reactions often give off energy in the form of heat as they occur. The generation of heat by wood burning in a fireplace and the maintenance of warmth in the human body both depend on energy-yielding chemical reactions. These downhill reactions occur easily although they may require some activation energy to get them started, just as a ball requires a push to start rolling.

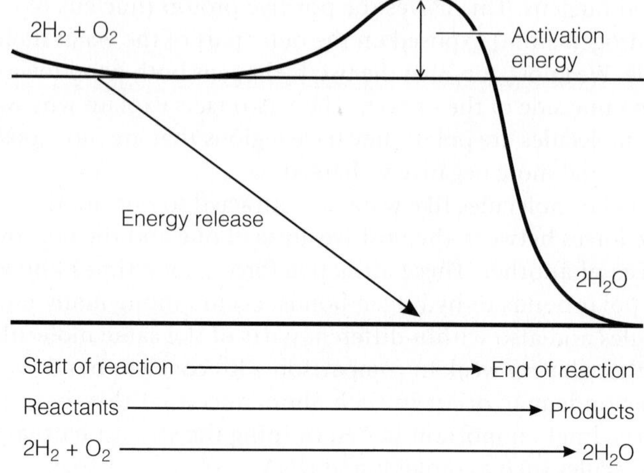

Formation of Free Radicals

Normally, when a chemical reaction takes place, bonds break and re-form to create new, stable compounds. Occasionally, bonds break in such a way as to create a free radical—a molecule with one or more unpaired electrons. When they do, free radicals are formed. Free radicals are highly unstable and quickly react with other compounds, forming more free radicals in a chain reaction. A cascade may ensue in which many highly reactive radicals are generated, resulting in damage that contributes to the development of many chronic diseases (see Highlight 11 for more details). Free radicals are of special interest in nutrition because the antioxidant properties of vitamins C and E as well as those of beta-carotene and the mineral selenium protect against the destructive effects of these free radicals.

Appendix C Biochemical Structures and Pathways

This appendix describes the biochemical structures and pathways most important to the study of nutrition. It begins by presenting diagrams of nutrients commonly found in the human diet. Following the diagrams of nutrients are sections on the major metabolic pathways mentioned in Chapter 7—glycolysis, fatty acid oxidation, amino acid degradation, the TCA cycle, and the electron transport chain—and a description of how alcohol interferes with these pathways. Discussions of the urea cycle and the formation of ketone bodies complete the appendix.

CONTENTS

Carbohydrates

Monosaccharides

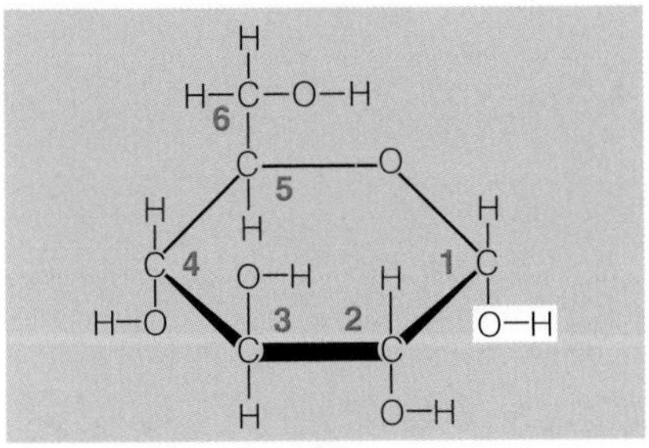

Glucose (alpha form). The ring would be at right angles to the plane of the paper. The bonds directed upward are above the plane; those directed downward are below the plane. This molecule is considered an alpha form because the OH on carbon 1 points downward.

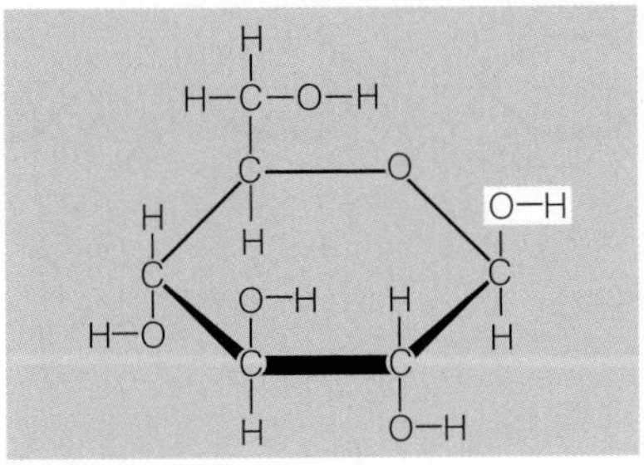

Glucose (beta form). The OH on carbon 1 points upward.
Fructose, galactose: see Chapter 4.

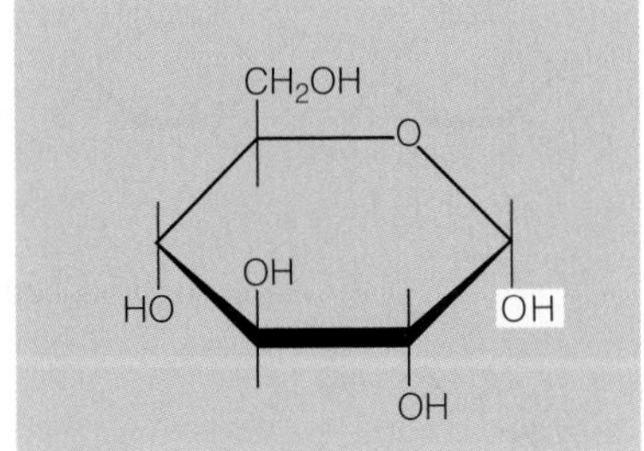

Glucose (alpha form) shorthand notation. This notation, in which the carbons in the ring and single hydrogens have been eliminated, will be used throughout this appendix.

Disaccharides

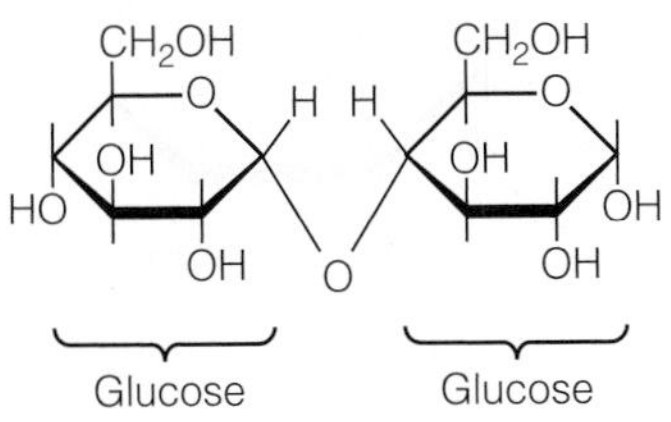

Glucose Glucose

Maltose.

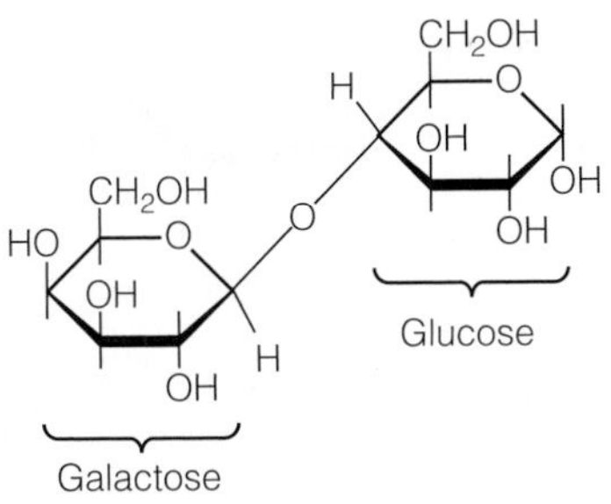

Galactose Glucose

Lactose (alpha form).

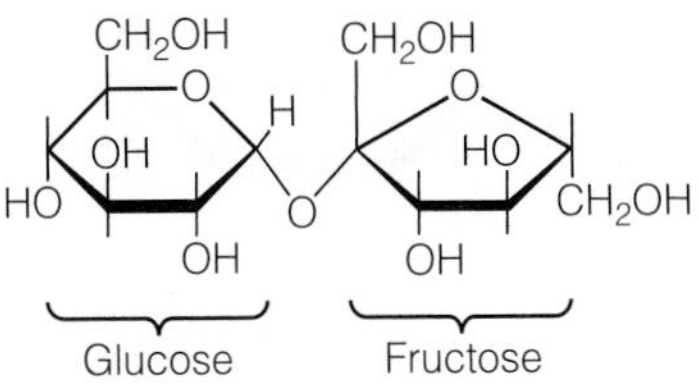

Glucose Fructose

Sucrose.

Polysaccharides: Starches As described in Chapter 4, starch, glycogen, and cellulose are all long chains of glucose molecules covalently linked together. (Appendix B discusses covalent bonding.)

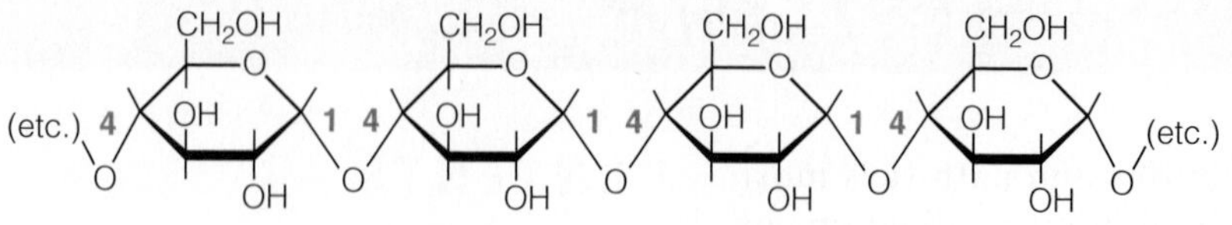

Amylose (unbranched starch)

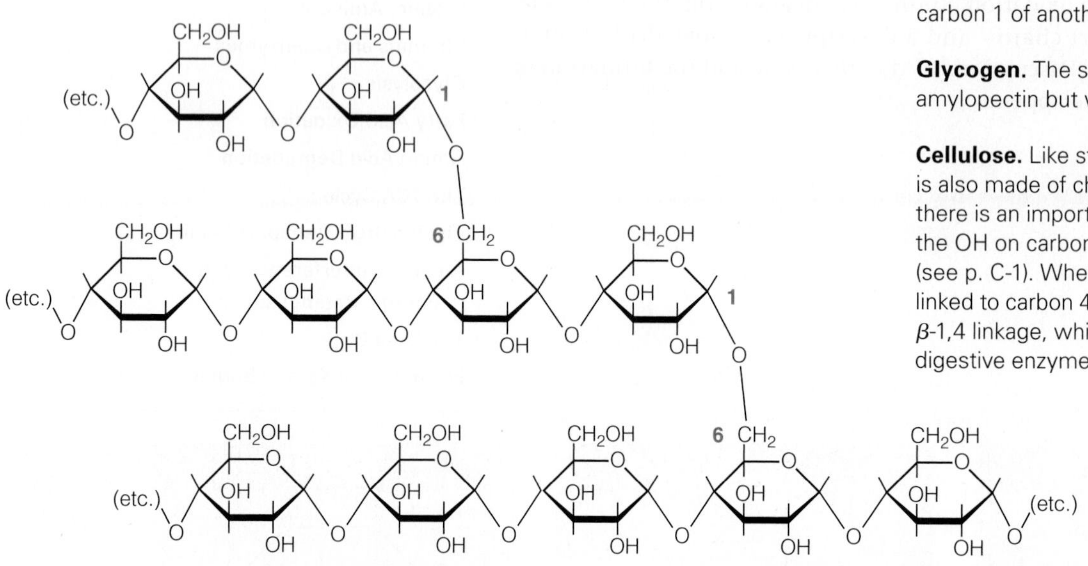

Amylopectin (branched starch)

Starch. Two kinds of covalent bonds link the glucose molecules in starch, giving rise to two kinds of chains. Amylose is composed of straight chains, with carbon 1 of one glucose linked to carbon 4 of the next (α-1,4 linkage). Amylopectin is made up of straight chains like amylose, but has occasional branches where the carbon 6 of a glucose is also linked to the carbon 1 of another glucose (α-1,6 linkage).

Glycogen. The structure of glycogen is like amylopectin but with many more branches.

Cellulose. Like starch and glycogen, cellulose is also made of chains of glucose units, but there is an important difference: in cellulose, the OH on carbon 1 is in the beta position (see p. C-1). When carbon 1 of one glucose is linked to carbon 4 of the next, it forms a β-1,4 linkage, which cannot be broken by digestive enzymes in the human GI tract.

Polysaccharides: Fibers Fibers, such as hemicelluloses, consist of long chains of various monosaccharides.

Monosaccharides common in the backbone chain of hemicelluloses:*

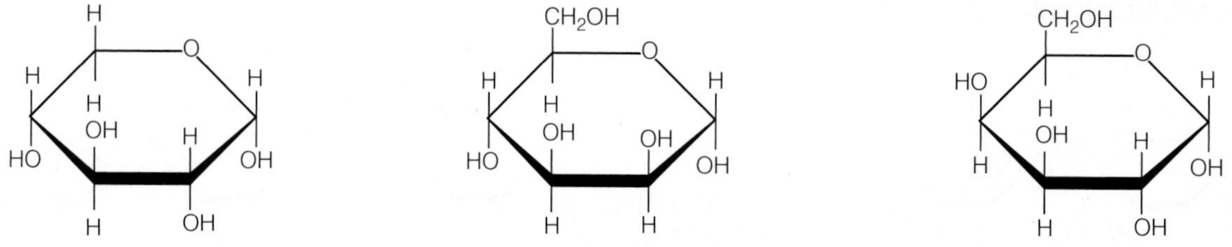

Xylose

Mannose

Galactose

*These structures are shown in the alpha form with the H on the carbon pointing upward and the OH pointing downward, but they may also appear in the beta form with the H pointing downward and the OH upward.

Monosaccharides common in the side chains of hemicelluloses:

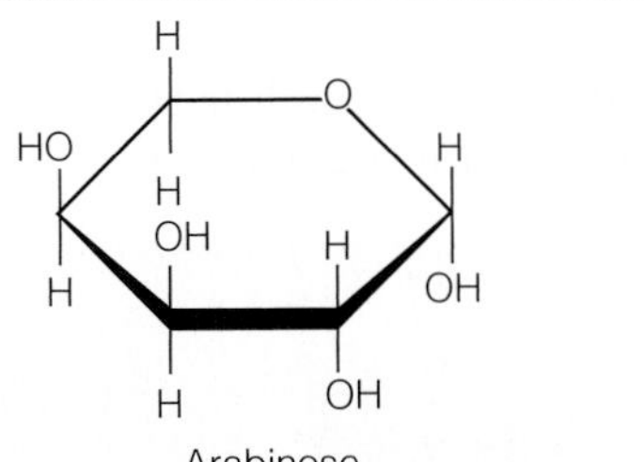

Arabinose

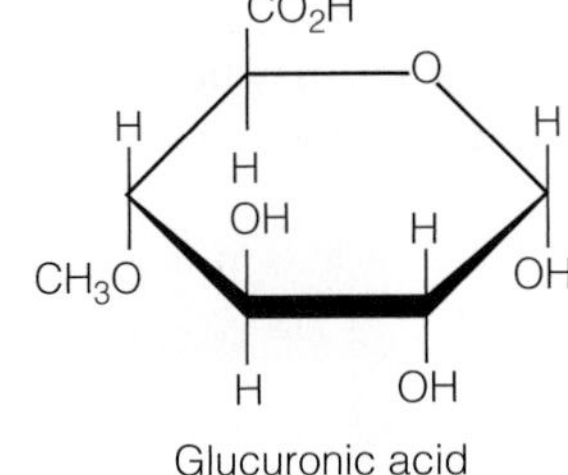

Glucuronic acid

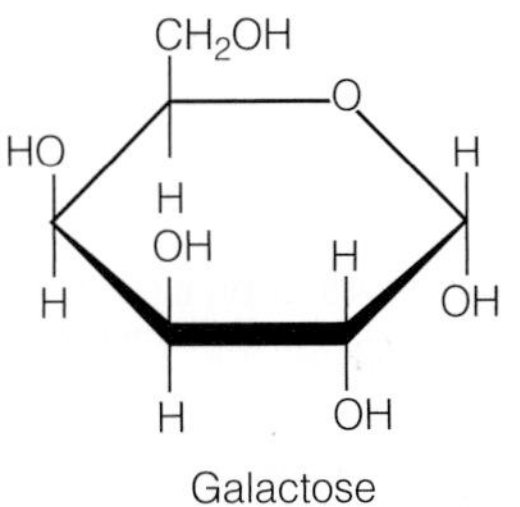

Galactose

Hemicelluloses. The most common hemicelluloses are composed of a backbone chain of xylose, mannose, and galactose, with branching side chains of arabinose, glucuronic acid, and galactose.

Lipids

TABLE C-1 Saturated Fatty Acids Found in Natural Fats

Saturated Fatty Acids	Chemical Formulas	Number of Carbons	Major Food Sources
Butyric	C_3H_7COOH	4	Butterfat
Caproic	$C_5H_{11}COOH$	6	Butterfat
Caprylic	$C_7H_{15}COOH$	8	Coconut oil
Capric	$C_9H_{19}COOH$	10	Palm oil
Lauric	$C_{11}H_{23}COOH$	12	Coconut oil, palm oil
Myristic	$C_{13}H_{27}COOH$	14	Coconut oil, palm oil
Palmitic	$C_{15}H_{31}COOH$	16	Palm oil
Stearic	$C_{17}H_{35}COOH$	18	Most animal fats
Arachidic	$C_{19}H_{39}COOH$	20	Peanut oil
Behenic	$C_{21}H_{43}COOH$	22	Seeds
Lignoceric	$C_{23}H_{47}COOH$	24	Peanut oil

NOTE: The most common fatty acids are myristic, palmitic, and stearic.

TABLE C-2 Unsaturated Fatty Acids Found in Natural Fats

Unsaturated Fatty Acids	Chemical Formulas	Number of Carbons	Number of Double Bonds	Standard Notation[a]	Omega Notation[b]	Major Food Sources
Palmitoleic	$C_{15}H_{29}COOH$	16	1	16:1;9	16:1ω7	Seafood, beef
Oleic	$C_{17}H_{33}COOH$	18	1	18:1;9	18:1ω9	Olive oil, canola oil
Linoleic	$C_{17}H_{31}COOH$	18	2	18:2;9,12	18:2ω6	Sunflower oil, safflower oil
Linolenic	$C_{17}H_{29}COOH$	18	3	18:3;9,12,15	18:3ω3	Soybean oil, canola oil
Arachidonic	$C_{19}H_{31}COOH$	20	4	20:4;5,8,11,14	20:4ω6	Eggs, most animal fats
Eicosapentaenoic	$C_{19}H_{29}COOH$	20	5	20:5;5,8,11,14,17	20:5ω3	Seafood
Docosahexaenoic	$C_{21}H_{31}COOH$	20	6	22:6;4,7,10,13,16,19	22:6ω3	Seafood

NOTE: A fatty acid has two ends; designated the methyl (CH_3) end and the carboxyl, or acid (COOH), end.

[a]Standard chemistry notation begins counting carbons at the acid end. The number of carbons the fatty acid contains comes first, followed by a colon and another number that indicates the number of double bonds; next comes a semicolon followed by a number or numbers indicating the positions of the double bonds. Thus the notation for linoleic acid, an 18-carbon fatty acid with two double bonds between carbons 9 and 10 and between carbons 12 and 13, is 18:2;9,12.

[b]Because fatty acid chains are lengthened by adding carbons at the acid end of the chain, chemists use the omega system of notation to ease the task of identifying them. The omega system begins counting carbons at the methyl end. The number of carbons the fatty acid contains comes first, followed by a colon and the number of double bonds; next come the omega symbol (ω) and a number indicating the position of the double bond nearest the methyl end. Thus linoleic acid with its first double bond at the sixth carbon from the methyl end would be noted 18:2ω6 in the omega system.

APPENDIX C

Protein: Amino Acids

The common amino acids may be classified into the seven groups listed below based on their structural similarities. Amino acids marked with an asterisk (*) are essential.

1. Amino acids with aliphatic side chains, which consist of hydrogen and carbon atoms (hydrocarbons):

```
   H O
   | ‖
 H-C-C-OH
   |
   NH2
```
Glycine (Gly)

```
     H O
     | ‖
 H3C-C-C-OH
     |
     NH2
```
Alanine (Ala)

```
 H3C     H O
    \    | ‖
     CH-C-C-OH
    /    |
 H3C     NH2
```
Valine* (Val)

```
 H3C         H O
    \        | ‖
     CH-CH2-C-C-OH
    /        |
 H3C         NH2
```
Leucine* (Leu)

```
             H O
             | ‖
 H3C-CH2-CH-C-C-OH
          |  |
         CH3 NH2
```
Isoleucine* (Ile)

2. Amino acids with hydroxyl (OH) side chains:

```
         H O
         | ‖
 HO-CH2-C-C-OH
         |
         NH2
```
Serine (Ser)

```
        H O
        | ‖
 H3C-CH-C-C-OH
     |  |
     OH NH2
```
Threonine* (Thr)

3. Amino acids with side chains containing acidic groups or their amides, which contain the group NH_2:

```
    O       H O
    ‖       | ‖
 HO-C-CH2-C-C-OH
            |
            NH2
```
Aspartic acid (Asp)

```
    O           H O
    ‖           | ‖
 HO-C-CH2-CH2-C-C-OH
                |
                NH2
```
Glutamic acid (Glu)

```
             H O
             | ‖
 NH2-C-CH2-C-C-OH
     ‖       |
     O       NH2
```
Asparagine (Asn)

```
                 H O
                 | ‖
 NH2-C-CH2-CH2-C-C-OH
     ‖           |
     O           NH2
```
Glutamine (Gln)

4. Amino acids with basic side chains:

```
                             H O
                             | ‖
 NH2-CH2-CH2-CH2-CH2-C-C-OH
                             |
                             NH2
```
Lysine* (Lys)

```
                        H O
                        | ‖
 NH2-C-NH-CH2-CH2-CH2-C-C-OH
     ‖                  |
     NH                 NH2
```
Arginine (Arg)

```
              H O
              | ‖
 H-C=C-CH2-C-C-OH
   | |        |
   N N        NH2
    \ /\
     C  H
     |
     H
```
Histidine* (His)

5. Amino acids with aromatic side chains, which are characterized by the presence of at least one ring structure:

```
  H   H
   \ /
   C-C         H O
  /   \\       | ‖
H-C     C-CH2-C-C-OH
  \\   /       |
   C=C         NH2
  /   \
 H     H
```
Phenylalanine* (Phe)

```
   H   H
    \ /
    C-C         H O
   /   \\       | ‖
HO-C     C-CH2-C-C-OH
   \\   /       |
    C=C         NH2
   /   \
  H     H
```
Tyrosine (Tyr)

```
      H
      |              H O
 H    C              | ‖
  \  // \           
   C     C---C-CH2-C-C-OH
   |     ‖   ‖       |
   C     C   C       NH2
  / \\  /  \ / \
 H    C     N   H
      |     |
      H     H
```
Tryptophan* (Trp)

6. Amino acids with side chains containing sulfur atoms:

```
         H O
         | ‖
 HS-CH2-C-C-OH
         |
         NH2
```
Cysteine (Cys)

```
                    H O
                    | ‖
 CH3-S-CH2-CH2-C-C-OH
                    |
                    NH2
```
Methionine* (Met)

7. Imino acid:

```
   H H
   | |/H
 H-C-C    O
   |  \   ‖
   |   C-C-OH
   |  / |
 H-C-N  H
   | |
   H H
```
Proline (Pro)

Proline has the same chemical structure as the other amino acids, but its amino group has given up a hydrogen to form a ring.

Vitamins and Coenzymes

Vitamin A: retinol. Retinol is the alcohol form of vitamin A.

Vitamin A: retinal. Retinal is the aldehyde form of vitamin A.

Vitamin A: retinoic acid. Retinoic acid is the acid form of vitamin A.

Vitamin A precursor: beta-carotene. Beta-carotene is the carotenoid with the most vitamin A activity.

Thiamin. Thiamin is part of the coenzyme thiamin pyrophosphate (TPP).

Thiamin pyrophosphate (TPP). TPP is a coenzyme that includes the thiamin molecule as part of its structure.

Riboflavin. Riboflavin is a part of two coenzymes—flavin mononucleotide (FMN) and flavin adenine dinucleotide (FAD).

Flavin mononucleotide (FMN). FMN is a coenzyme that includes the riboflavin molecule as part of its structure.

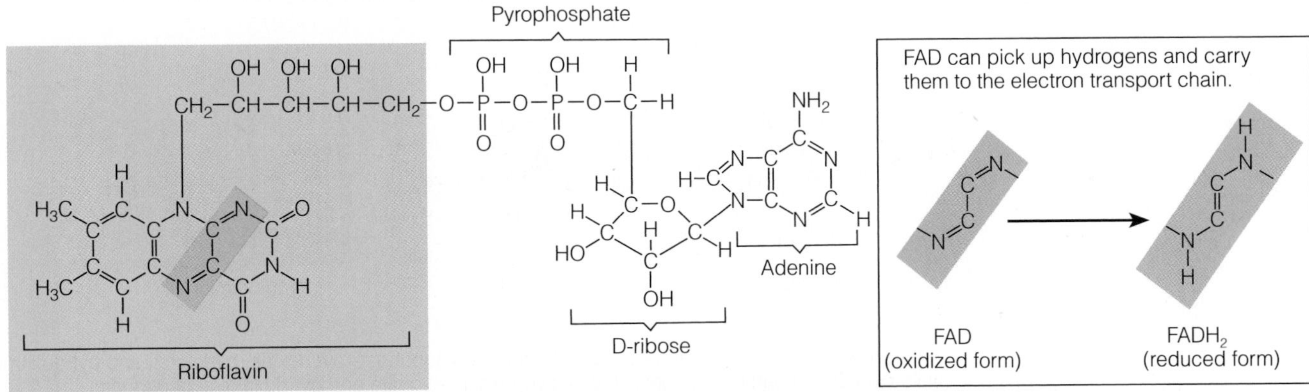

Flavin adenine dinucleotide (FAD). FAD is a coenzyme that includes the riboflavin molecule as part of its structure.

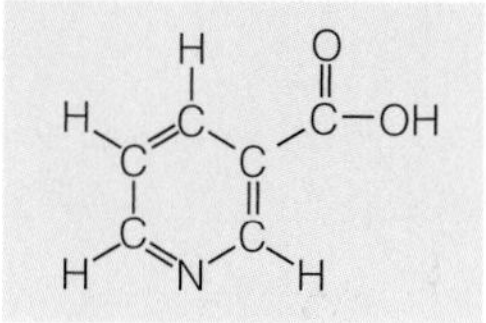

Nicotinic acid

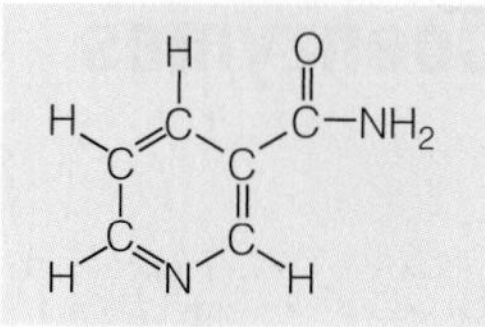

Nicotinamide

Niacin (nicotinic acid and nicotinamide). Niacin is a part of two coenzymes—nicotinamide adenine dinucleotide (NAD^+) and nicotinamide adenine dinucleotide phosphate ($NADP^+$).

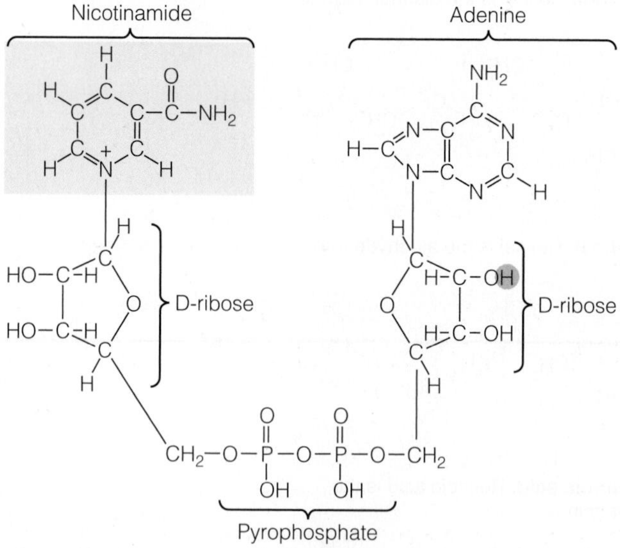

Nicotinamide

Adenine

D-ribose

D-ribose

Pyrophosphate

Nicotinamide adenine dinucleotide (NAD^+). NAD is a coenzyme that includes niacin as part of its structure. NADP has the same structure as NAD but with a phosphate group attached to the O instead of the H.

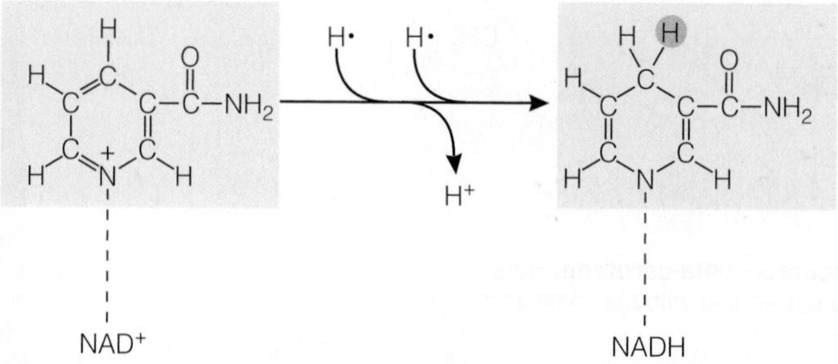

NAD^+

NADH

Reduced NAD^+ (NADH). When NAD^+ is reduced by the addition of H^+ and two electrons, it becomes the coenzyme NADH. (The dots on the H entering this reaction represent electrons—see Appendix B.)

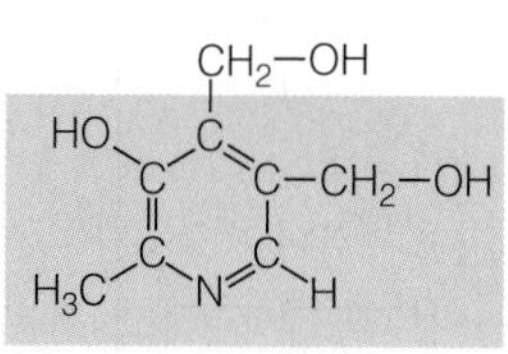

Pyridoxine

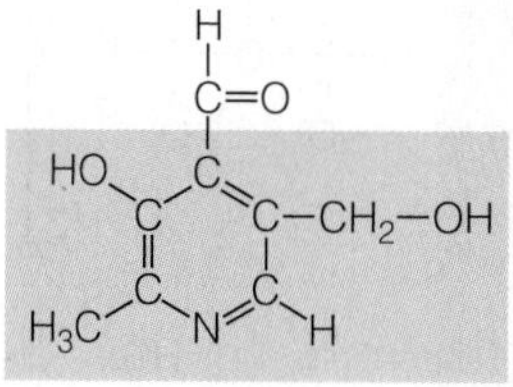

Pyridoxal

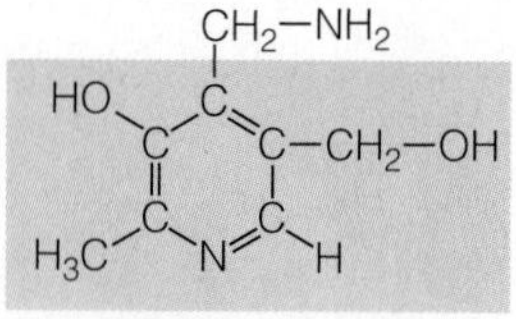

Pyridoxamine

Vitamin B_6. Vitamin B_6 is a general name for three compounds—pyridoxine, pyridoxal, and pyridoxamine, which become a part of two coenzymes—pyridoxal phosphate and pyridoxamine phosphate.

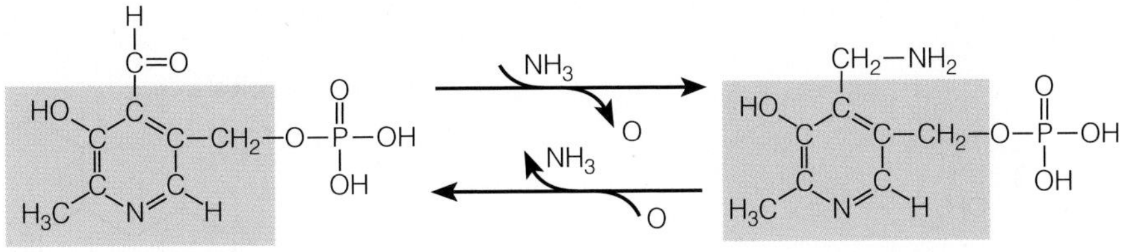

Pyridoxal phosphate

Pyridoxamine phosphate

Pyridoxal phosphate (PLP) and pyridoxamine phosphate. These coenzymes include vitamin B_6 as part of their structures.

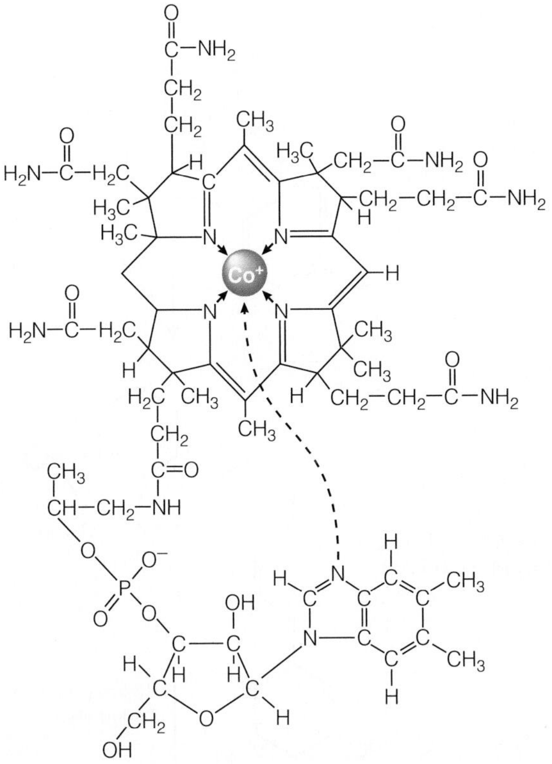

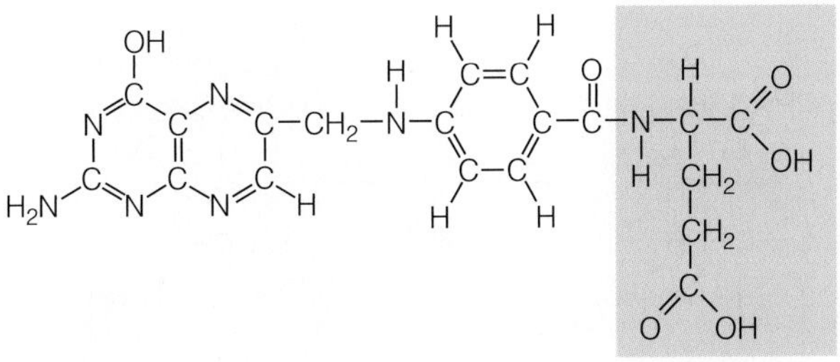

Folate (folacin or folic acid). Folate consists of a double ring combined with a single ring and at least one glutamate (a nonessential amino acid highlighted in color). Folate is a part of the coenzyme tetrahydrofolate (THF).

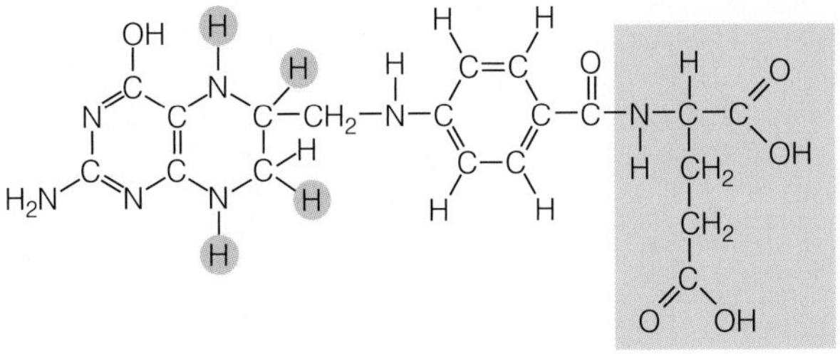

Vitamin B_{12} (cyanocobalamin). The arrows in this diagram indicate that the spare electron pairs on the nitrogens attract them to the cobalt.

Tetrahydrofolate (THF). THF is the active coenzyme form of folate and has four added hydrogens. An intermediate form, dihydrofolate, has two added hydrogens.

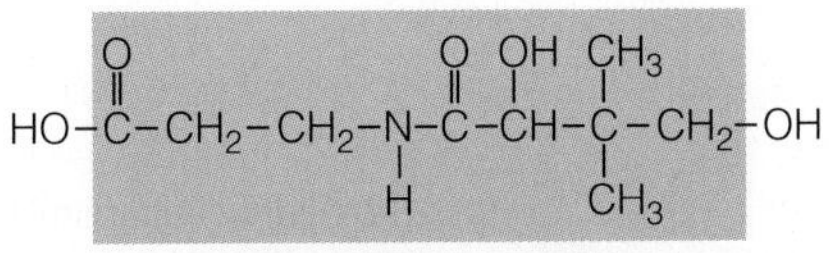

Pantothenic acid. Pantothenic acid is part of coenzyme A (CoA).

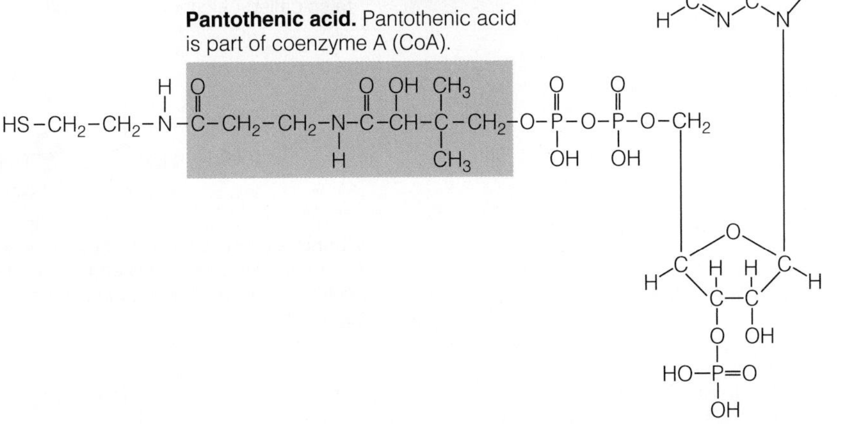

Coenzyme A (CoA). Coenzyme A is a coenzyme that includes pantothenic acid as part of its structure.

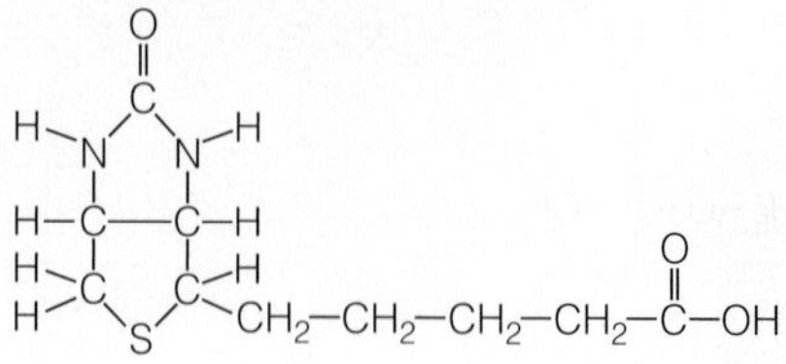

Biotin.

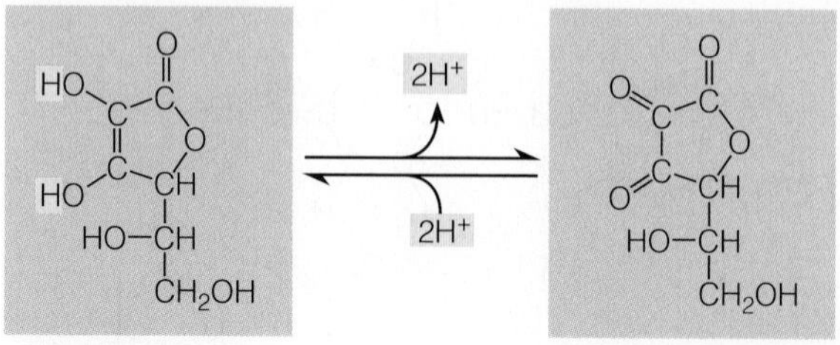

2H⁺

Ascorbic acid
(reduced form)

Dehydroascorbic acid
(oxidized form)

Vitamin C. Two hydrogen atoms with their electrons are lost when ascorbic acid is oxidized and gained when it is reduced again.

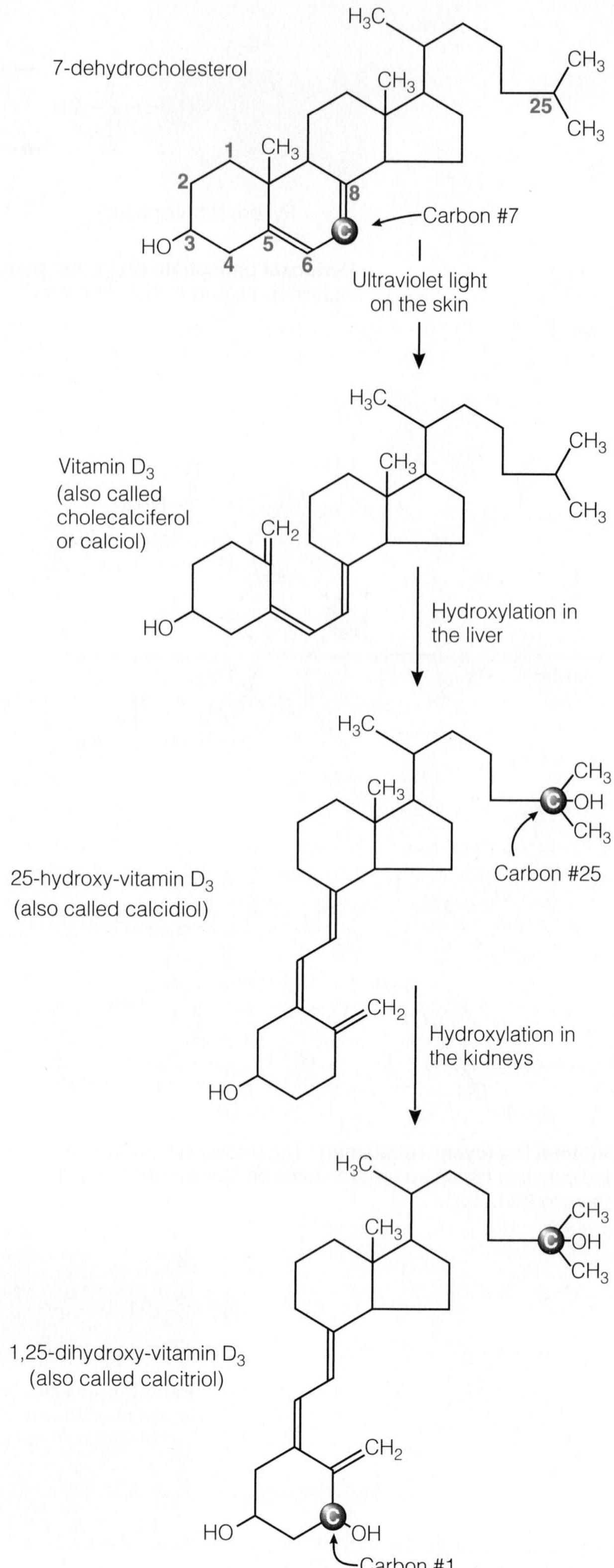

Vitamin D. The synthesis of active vitamin D begins with 7-dehydrocholesterol, a precursor made in the liver from cholesterol. (The carbon atoms at which changes occur are numbered.)

APPENDIX C

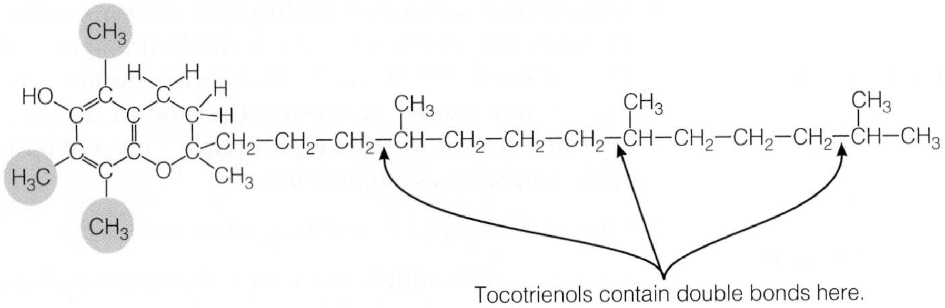

Tocotrienols contain double bonds here.

Vitamin E (alpha-tocopherol). Vitamin E consists of two subgroups—the tocopherols and the tocotrienols. All are made up of a complex ring structure with a long saturated (in tocopherols) or unsaturated (in tocotrienols) side chain. The number and positions of methyl groups (CH_3) distinguish the members within each subgroup.

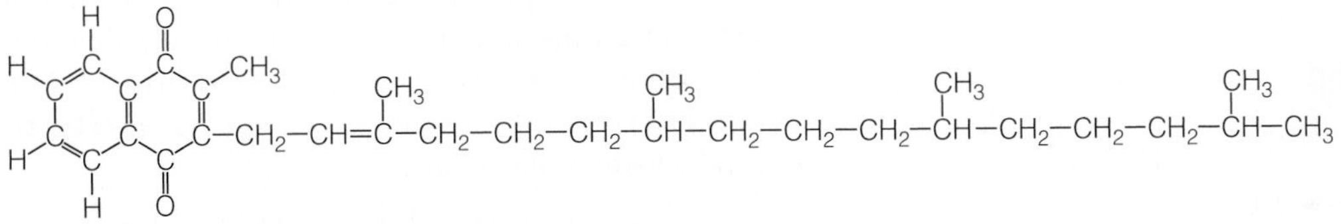

Vitamin K (phylloquinone). Naturally occurring compounds with vitamin K activity include phylloquinones (from plants) and menaquinones (from bacteria). The chemical structure of menaquinones differs only slightly from that of phylloquinones.

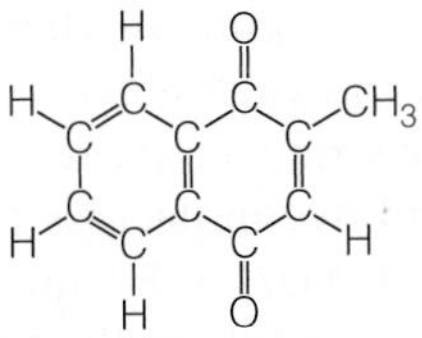

Vitamin K (menadione). Menadione is a synthetic compound that has the same activity as natural vitamin K.

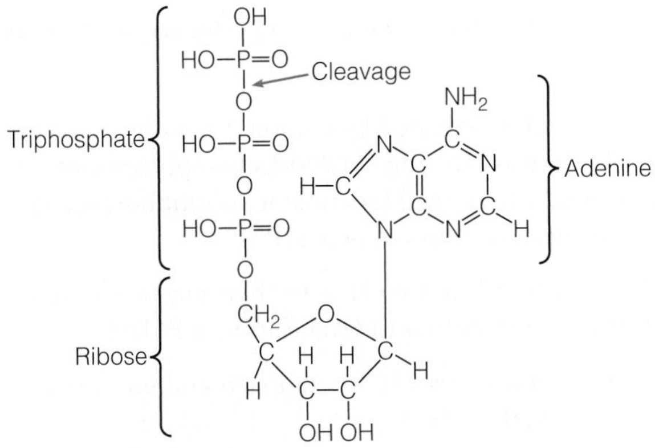

Triphosphate

Cleavage

Adenine

Ribose

Adenosine triphosphate (ATP). The high-energy compound ATP releases energy when one or two phosphate groups split off. The cleavage point marks the bond that is broken when ATP splits to become ADP + P.

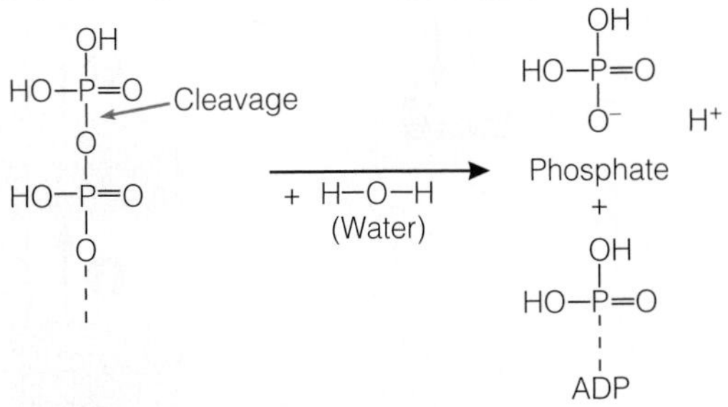

Cleavage

+ H–O–H (Water)

Phosphate + ADP

Adenosine diphosphate (ADP).

APPENDIX C

Glycolysis

Figure C-1 depicts glycolysis. The following text describes key steps as numbered on the figure.

> **FIGURE C-1 Glycolysis**

Notice that galactose and fructose enter at different places but continue on the same pathway.

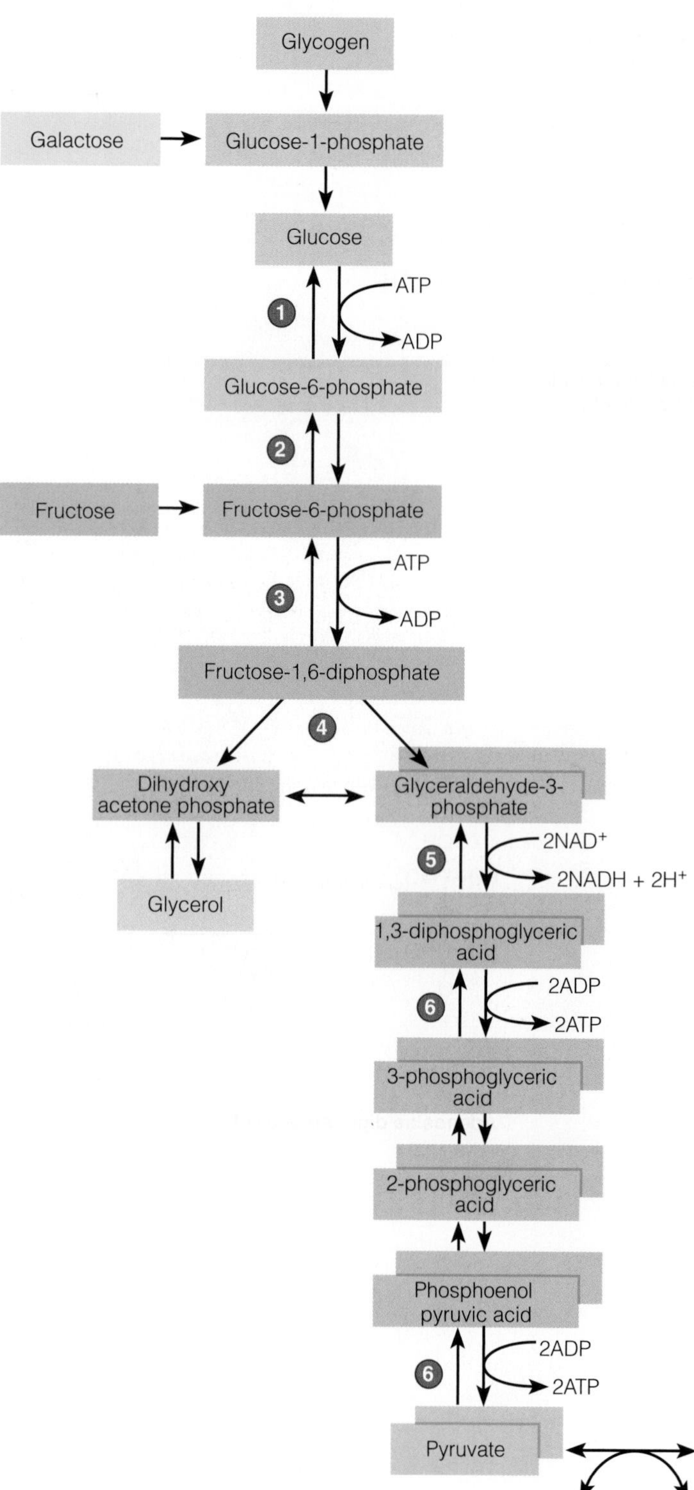

1. A phosphate is attached to glucose at the carbon that chemists call number 6 (review the first diagram of glucose on p. C-1 to see how chemists number the carbons in a glucose molecule). The product is called, logically enough, glucose-6-phosphate. One ATP molecule is used to accomplish this.
2. Glucose-6-phosphate is rearranged by an enzyme.
3. A phosphate is added in another reaction that uses another molecule of ATP. The resulting product is fructose-1,6-diphosphate. At this point the 6-carbon sugar has a phosphate group on its first and sixth carbons and is ready to break apart.
4. When fructose-1,6-diphosphate breaks in half, the two 3-carbon compounds are not identical. Each has a phosphate group attached, but only glyceraldehyde-3-phosphate converts directly to pyruvate. The other compound, however, converts easily to glyceraldehyde-3-phosphate.
5. In the next step, NAD^+ is reduced to $NADH + H^+$.
6. In two of the following steps ATP is regenerated.

Remember that in effect two molecules of glyceraldehyde-3-phosphate are produced from glucose; therefore, four ATP molecules are generated from each glucose molecule. Two ATP were needed to get the sequence started, so the net gain at this point is two ATP and two molecules of $NADH + H^+$. As you will see later, each $NADH + H^+$ moves to the electron transport chain to unload its hydrogens, producing more ATP.

Fatty Acid Oxidation

Figure C-2 presents fatty acid oxidation. The sequence is as follows.

1. The fatty acid is activated by combining with coenzyme A (CoA). In this reaction, ATP loses two phosphorus atoms and becomes AMP (adenosine monophosphate)—the equivalent of a loss of two ATP.
2. In the next reaction, two H with their electrons are removed and transferred to FAD, forming $FADH_2$.
3. In a later reaction, two H are removed and go to NAD^+ (forming $NADH + H^+$).
4. The fatty acid is cleaved at the "beta" carbon, the second carbon from the carboxyl (COOH) end. This break results in a fatty acid that is two carbons shorter than the previous one and a 2-carbon molecule of

> **FIGURE C-2 Fatty Acid Oxidation**

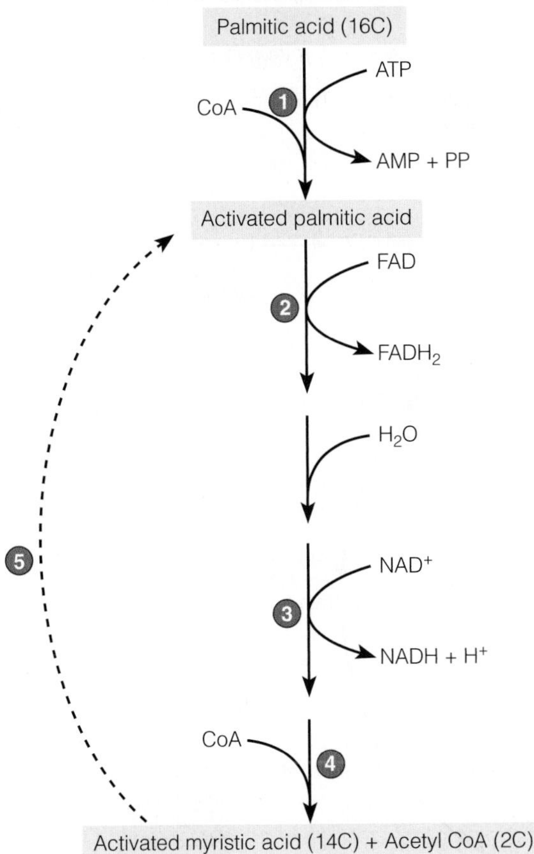

acetyl CoA. At the same time, another CoA is attached to the fatty acid, thus activating it for its turn through the series of reactions.

5. The sequence is repeated with each cycle producing an acetyl CoA and a shorter fatty acid until only a 2-carbon fatty acid remains—acetyl CoA.

In the example shown in Figure C-2, palmitic acid (a 16-carbon fatty acid) will go through this series of reactions seven times, using the equivalent of two ATP for the initial activation and generating seven $FADH_2$, seven NADH + H^+, and eight acetyl CoA. As you will see later, each of the seven $FADH_2$ will enter the electron transport chain, yielding two ATP (for a total of 14). Similarly, each NADH + H^+ will enter the electron transport chain, yielding three ATP (for a total of 21). Thus the oxidation of a 16-carbon fatty acid uses 2 ATP and generates 35 ATP. When the eight acetyl CoA enter the TCA cycle, even more ATP will be generated, as a later section describes.

Amino Acid Degradation

The first step in amino acid degradation is the removal of the nitrogen-containing amino group through either deamination (Figure 6-11 on p. 183) or transamination (Figure 6-12 on p. 183) reactions. Then the remaining carbon skeletons may enter the metabolic pathways at different places, as shown in Figure C-3 (p. C-12).

The TCA Cycle

The tricarboxylic acid, or TCA, cycle is the set of reactions that break down acetyl CoA to carbon dioxide and hydrogen atoms. Pyruvate derived from glycolysis does not enter the TCA cycle directly; instead pyruvate enters the mitochondrion, loses a carbon group, and bonds with a molecule of CoA to become acetyl CoA. The TCA cycle uses any substance that can be converted to acetyl CoA directly or indirectly through pyruvate.

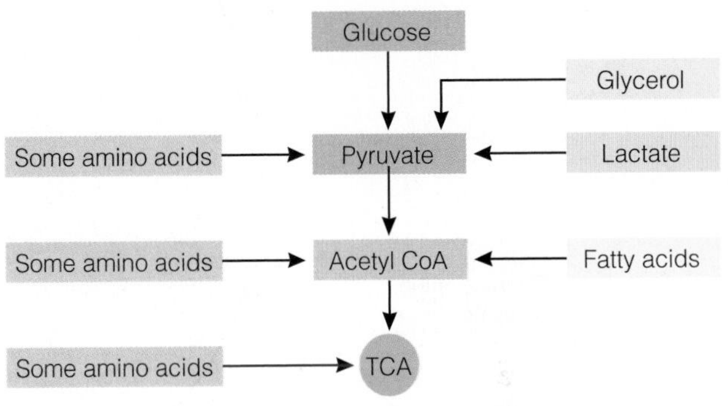

Any substance that can be converted to acetyl CoA directly, or indirectly through pyruvate, may enter the TCA cycle.

The pathway from pyruvate to acetyl CoA is complex. We have included only those steps that will help you understand the transfer of energy from the nutrients. Pyruvate loses a carbon to carbon dioxide and is attached to a molecule of CoA. In the process, NAD^+ picks up two hydrogens with their associated electrons, becoming NADH + H^+.

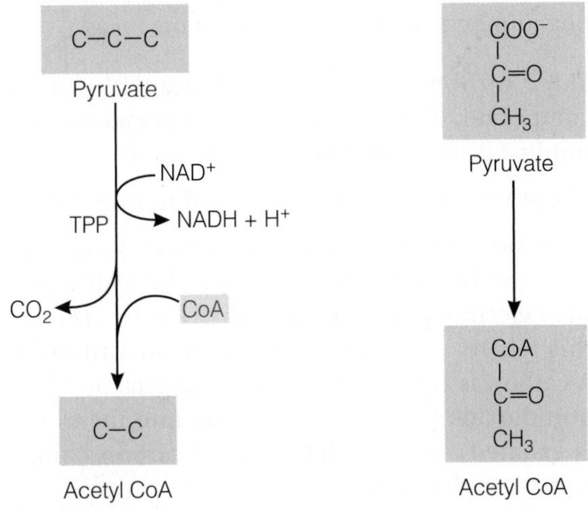

The step from pyruvate to acetyl CoA. (TPP and NAD are coenzymes containing the B vitamins thiamin and niacin, respectively.)

> FIGURE C-3 Amino Acids Enter the Metabolic Pathways

After losing their amino groups, carbon skeletons can be converted to one of seven molecules that can enter the TCA cycle (presented in Figure C-4).

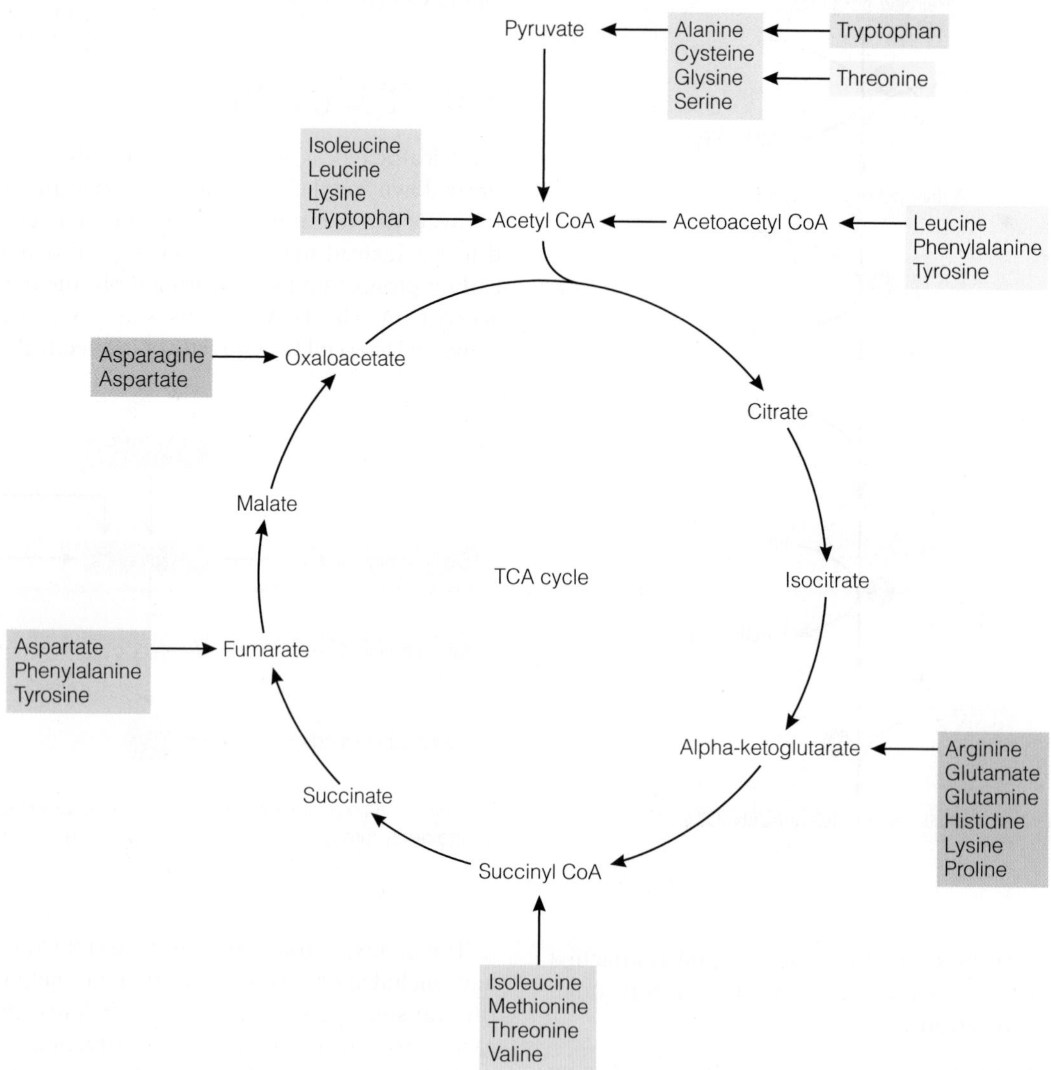

Let's follow the steps of the TCA cycle (see the corresponding numbers in Figure C-4 on the next page).

1. The 2-carbon acetyl CoA combines with a 4-carbon compound, oxaloacetate. The CoA comes off, and the product is a 6-carbon compound, citrate.
2. The atoms of citrate are rearranged to form isocitrate.
3. Now two H (with their two electrons) are removed from the isocitrate. NAD^+ accepts the hydrogens with their electrons and becomes $NADH + H^+$. (Remember this $NADH + H^+$, but let's follow the carbons first.) A carbon is combined with two oxygens, forming carbon dioxide (which diffuses away into the blood and is exhaled). What is left is the 5-carbon compound alpha-ketoglutarate.
4. Now two compounds interact with alpha-ketoglutarate—a molecule of CoA and a molecule of NAD^+. In this complex reaction, a carbon and two oxygens are removed (forming carbon dioxide); two hydrogens are removed and go to NAD^+ (forming $NADH + H^+$); and the remaining 4-carbon compound is attached to the CoA, forming succinyl CoA. (Remember this $NADH + H^+$ also. You will see later what happens to it.)
5. Now two molecules react with succinyl CoA—a molecule called GDP and one of phosphate (P). The CoA comes off, the GDP and P combine to form the high-energy compound GTP (similar to ATP), and succinate remains. (Remember this GTP.)
6. In the next reaction, two H with their electrons are removed from succinate and are transferred to a molecule of FAD (a coenzyme like NAD^+) to form $FADH_2$. The product that remains is fumarate. (Remember this $FADH_2$.)
7. Next a molecule of water is added to fumarate, forming malate.

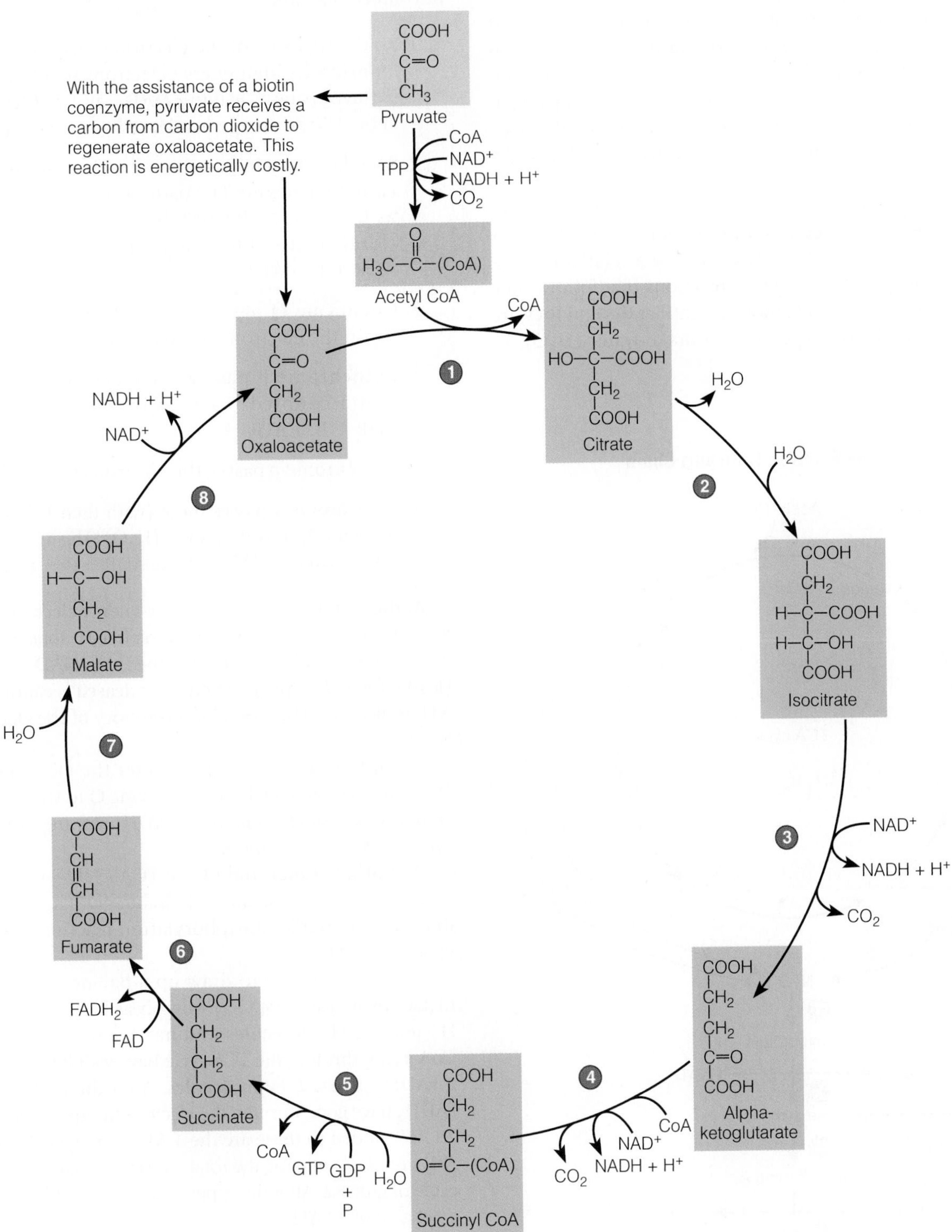

8. A molecule of NAD^+ accepts two H with their associated electrons and forms NADH + H^+. The product that remains is the 4-carbon compound oxaloacetate. (Remember this NADH + H^+.)

The cycle is complete and we are back where we started. The oxaloacetate can combine with another molecule of acetyl CoA (step 1), and the cycle can begin again.

So far, we have seen two carbons brought in with acetyl CoA and two carbons ending up in carbon dioxide. But where are the energy and the ATP that were promised?

A review of the eight steps of the TCA cycle shows that the compounds NADH + H^+ (three molecules), $FADH_2$, and GTP captured energy along the way. To see how this energy ends up in ATP, we must follow the electrons further—into the electron transport chain.

The Electron Transport Chain

The six reactions described here are a highly simplified overview of the electron transport chain, which is shown below the TCA cycle in Figure C-5. Since oxygen is required for these reactions, and ADP and P are combined to form ATP in several of them (ADP is phosphorylated), the reactions of the electron transport chain are also called *oxidative phosphorylation*.

An important concept to remember at this point is that an electron is not a fixed amount of energy. The electrons that bond the H to NAD^+ in NADH have a relatively large amount of energy. In the series of reactions that follow, they release this energy in small amounts, until at the end they are attached (with H) to oxygen (O) to make water (H_2O). In some of the steps, the energy they release is captured into ATP in coupled reactions.

1. In the first step of the electron transport chain, NADH transfers its high-energy electrons to a molecule called a flavoprotein, leaving NAD^+ and reduced flavoprotein. A little energy is released as heat in this reaction.
2. The flavoprotein passes on the electrons to a molecule called coenzyme Q. Again a little energy is released as heat, but ADP and P bond together and form ATP, storing much of the energy. This is a coupled reaction: ADP + P → ATP.
3. Coenzyme Q passes the electrons to cytochrome *b*. Again the electrons release energy.
4. Cytochrome *b* passes the electrons to cytochrome *c* in a coupled reaction in which ATP is formed: ADP + P → ATP.
5. Cytochrome *c* passes the electrons to cytochrome *a*.
6. Cytochrome *a* passes them (with their H) to an atom of oxygen (O), forming water (H_2O). This is a coupled reaction in which ATP is formed: ADP + P → ATP.

> **FIGURE C-5 The Electron Transport Chain**

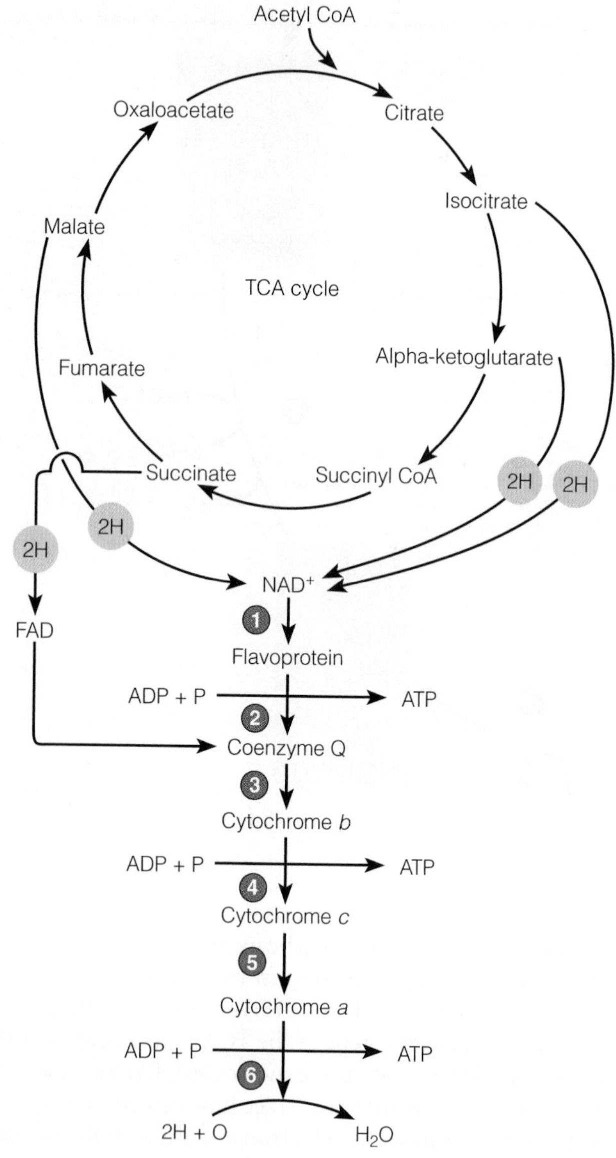

At the end of the chain, the low-energy electrons are passed to oxygen, which combines with the free H^+ ions to form water. As Figure C-5 shows, each time the three NADH are oxidized (losing their electrons), the energy released is captured in three ATP molecules. This completes the story of the electrons from NADH.

As for $FADH_2$, its electrons enter the electron transport chain at coenzyme Q. From coenzyme Q to water, ATP is generated in two steps. Therefore, $FADH_2$ coming out of the TCA cycle yields two ATP molecules.

One other compound of the TCA cycle—GTP—does not enter the electron transport chain but gives its energy directly to ADP in a simple phosphorylation reaction. This reaction yields one ATP.

It is now possible to draw up a balance sheet of glucose metabolism (see Table C-3). Glycolysis has yielded 4 NADH + H^+ and 4 ATP molecules and has spent 2 ATP. The 2 acetyl CoA going through the TCA cycle have yielded 6 NADH + H^+, 2 $FADH_2$, and 2 GTP molecules. After the NADH + H^+ and $FADH_2$ have gone through the electron transport chain, there are 28 ATP. Added to these are the 4 ATP from glycolysis and the 2 ATP from GTP, making the total 34 ATP generated from one molecule of glucose. After the expense of 2 ATP is subtracted, there is a net gain of 32 ATP.*

A similar balance sheet from the complete breakdown of one 16-carbon fatty acid would show a net gain of 129 ATP.

---

*The total may sometimes be 30 ATP. The NADH + H^+ generated in the cytoplasm during glycolysis pass their electrons on to shuttle molecules, which move them into the mitochondria. One shuttle, malate, contributes its electrons to the electron transport chain before the first site of ATP synthesis, yielding 5 ATP. Another, glycerol phosphate, adds its electrons into the chain beyond that first site, yielding 3 ATP. Thus sometimes 5, and sometimes 3, ATP result from the NADH + H^+ that arise from glycolysis. The amount depends on the cell.

TABLE C-3 Balance Sheet for Glucose Metabolism

		ATP
Glycolysis:	4 ATP − 2 ATP	2
1 glucose to 2 pyruvate	2 NADH + H^+	3–5[a]
2 pyruvate to 2 acetyl CoA	2 NADH + H^+	5
TCA cycle and electron transport chain:		
2 isocitrate	2 NADH + H^+	5
2 alpha-ketoglutarate	2 NADH + H^+	5
2 succinyl CoA	2 GTP	2
2 succinate	2 $FADH_2$	3
2 malate	2 NADH + H^+	5
Total ATP collected from one molecule glucose:		30–32

[a]Each NADH + H^+ from glycolysis can yield 1.5 or 2.5 ATP. See the accompanying text.

As mentioned earlier, 35 ATP were generated from the 7 $FADH_2$ and 7 NADH + H^+ produced during fatty acid oxidation. The 8 acetyl CoA produced will each generate 12 ATP as they go through the TCA cycle and the electron transport chain, for a total of 96 more ATP. After subtracting the 2 ATP needed to activate the fatty acid initially, the net yield from one 16-carbon fatty acid: 35 + 96 − 2 = 129 ATP.

These calculations help explain why fat yields more energy (measured as kcalories) per gram than carbohydrate or protein. The more hydrogen atoms a fuel contains, the more ATP will be generated during oxidation. The 16-carbon fatty acid molecule, with its 32 hydrogen atoms, generates 129 ATP, whereas glucose, with its 12 hydrogen atoms, yields only 32 ATP.

The TCA cycle and the electron transport chain are the body's major means of capturing the energy from nutrients in ATP molecules. Other means, such as anaerobic glycolysis, contribute energy quickly, but the aerobic processes are the most efficient.

Alcohol's Interference with Energy Metabolism

Highlight 7 provides an overview of how alcohol interferes with energy metabolism. With an understanding of the TCA cycle, a few more details may be appreciated. During alcohol metabolism, the enzyme alcohol dehydrogenase oxidizes alcohol to acetaldehyde while it simultaneously reduces a molecule of NAD^+ to NADH + H^+. The related enzyme acetaldehyde dehydrogenase reduces another NAD^+ to NADH + H^+ while it oxidizes acetaldehyde to acetyl CoA, the compound that enters the TCA cycle to generate energy. Thus, whenever alcohol is being metabolized in the body, NAD^+ diminishes, and NADH + H^+ accumulates, thus altering the body's "redox state." NAD^+ can oxidize, and NADH + H^+ can reduce, many other compounds as well. During alcohol metabolism, however, NAD^+ becomes unavailable for the multitude of reactions for which it is required.

As the previous sections just explained, for glucose to be completely metabolized, the TCA cycle must be operating, and NAD^+ must be present. If these conditions are not met (and when alcohol is present, they may not be), the pathway will be blocked, and traffic will back up—or an alternate route will be taken. Think about this as you follow the pathway shown in Figure C-6.

In each step of alcohol metabolism in which NAD^+ is converted to NADH + H^+, hydrogen ions accumulate, resulting in a dangerous shift of the acid-base balance toward acid (Chapter 12 explains acid-base balance). The accumulation of NADH + H^+ slows TCA cycle activity, so pyruvate and acetyl CoA build up. This condition favors the conversion of

> **FIGURE C-6 Ethanol Enters the Metabolic Pathways**

This is a simplified version of the glucose-to-energy pathway showing the entry of ethanol. The coenzyme NAD (which is the active form of the B vitamin niacin) is the only one shown here; however, many others are involved.

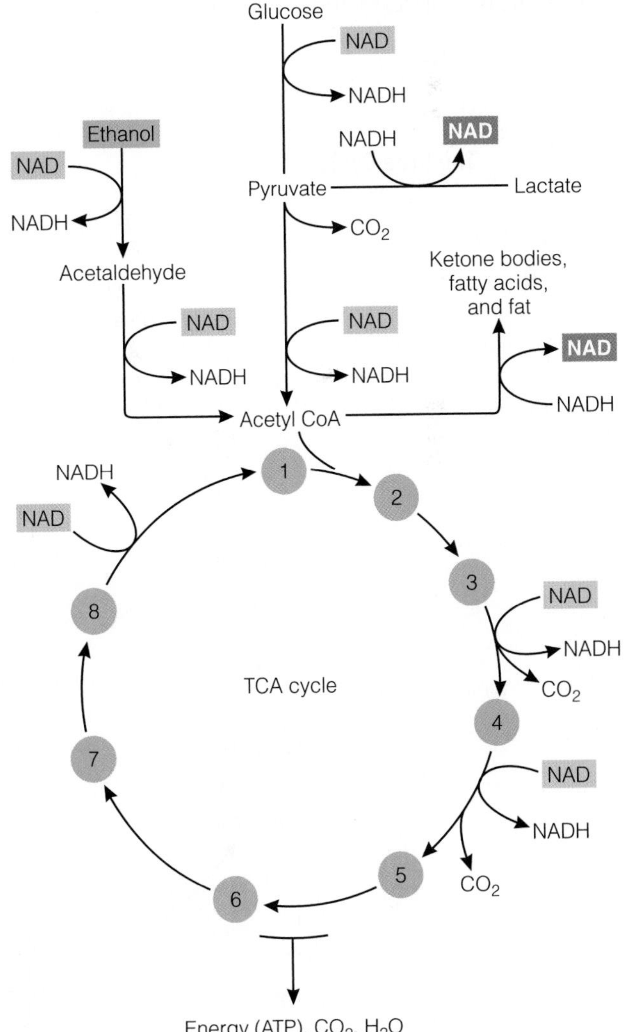

pyruvate to lactate, which serves as a temporary storage place for hydrogens from NADH + H^+. The conversion of pyruvate to lactate restores some NAD^+, but a lactate buildup has serious consequences of its own. It adds to the body's acid burden and interferes with the excretion of uric acid, causing goutlike symptoms. Molecules of acetyl CoA become building blocks for fatty acids or ketone bodies. The making of ketone bodies consumes acetyl CoA and generates NAD^+; but some ketone bodies are acids, so they push the acid-base balance further toward acid.

Thus alcohol cascades through the metabolic pathways, wreaking havoc along the way. These consequences have physical effects, as Highlight 7 describes.

The Urea Cycle

Chapter 6 sums up the process by which waste nitrogen is eliminated from the body by stating that ammonia molecules combine with carbon dioxide to produce urea. This is true, but it is not the whole story. Urea is produced in a multistep process within the cells of the liver.

Ammonia, freed from an amino acid or other compound during metabolism anywhere in the body, arrives at the liver by way of the bloodstream and is taken into a liver cell. There, it is first combined with carbon dioxide and a phosphate group from ATP to form carbamyl phosphate:

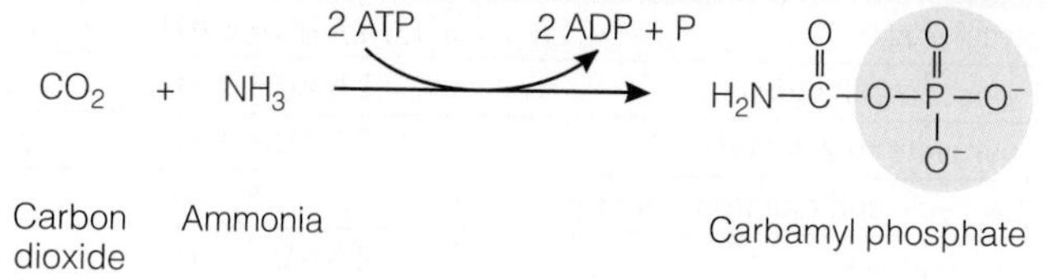

$$\underset{\text{Carbon dioxide}}{CO_2} + \underset{\text{Ammonia}}{NH_3} \xrightarrow{\text{2 ATP} \rightarrow \text{2 ADP + P}} \underset{\text{Carbamyl phosphate}}{H_2N{-}\overset{\displaystyle O}{\overset{\|}{C}}{-}O{-}\overset{\displaystyle O}{\overset{\|}{P}}{-}O^-} \quad (\text{with } O^- \text{ on P})$$

Figure C-7 shows the cycle of four reactions that follow.

1. Carbamyl phosphate combines with the amino acid ornithine, losing its phosphate group. The compound formed is citrulline.
2. Citrulline combines with the amino acid aspartic acid, to form argininosuccinate. The reaction requires energy from ATP. (In this reaction, ATP loses two phosphorus atoms, and becomes adenosine monophosphate, AMP.)
3. Argininosuccinate is split, forming another acid, fuma-rate, and the amino acid arginine.
4. Arginine loses its terminal carbon with two attached amino groups and picks up an oxygen from water. The

> FIGURE C-7 **The Urea Cycle**

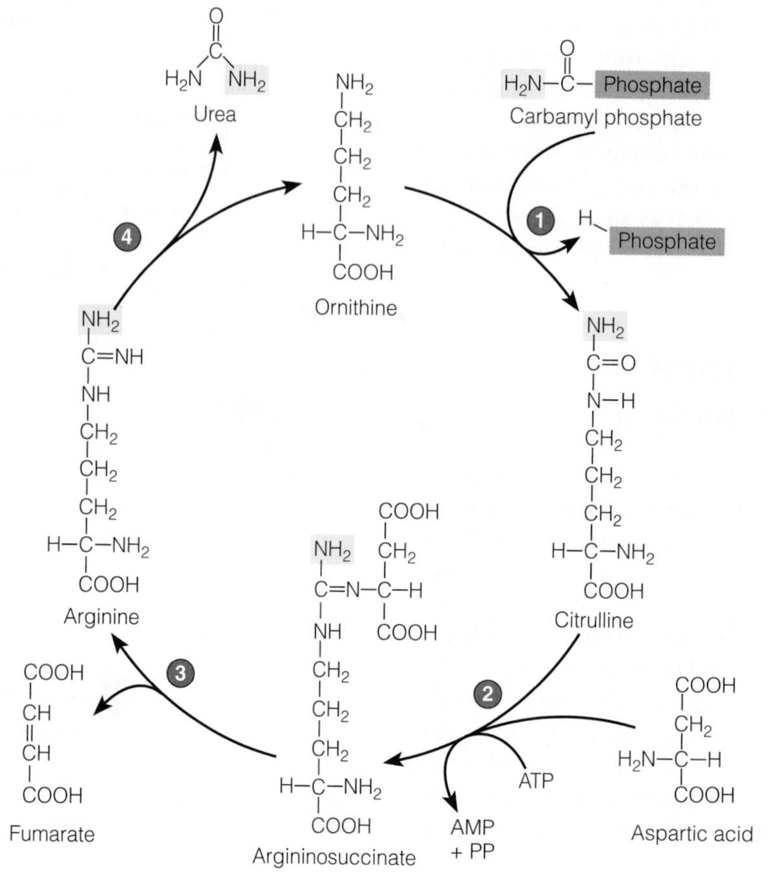

APPENDIX C

end product is urea, which the kidneys excrete in the urine. The compound that remains is ornithine, identical to the ornithine with which this series of reactions began, ready to react with another molecule of carbamyl phosphate and turn the cycle again.

Formation of Ketone Bodies

Normally, fatty acid oxidation proceeds all the way to carbon dioxide and water. In ketosis, however, an intermediate is formed from the condensation of two molecules of acetyl CoA: acetoacetyl CoA. Figure C-8 shows the formation of ketone bodies from that intermediate.

1. Acetoacetyl CoA condenses with acetyl CoA to form a 6-carbon intermediate, beta-hydroxy-beta-methylglutaryl CoA.
2. This intermediate is cleaved to acetyl CoA and acetoacetate.
3. Acetoactate can be metabolized either to beta-hydroxybutyrate acid (step 3a) or to acetone (3b).

Acetoacetate, beta-hydroxybutyrate, and acetone are the ketone bodies of ketosis. Two are real ketones (they have a C=O group between two carbons); the other is an alcohol that has been produced during ketone formation—hence the term *ketone bodies,* rather than ketones, to describe the three of them. There are many other ketones in nature; these three are characteristic of ketosis in the body.

> FIGURE C-8 **The Formation of Ketone Bodies**

$H_3C-\overset{O}{\overset{\|}{C}}-CH_2-\overset{O}{\overset{\|}{C}}-CoA$ + $H_3C-\overset{O}{\overset{\|}{C}}-CoA$ + H_2O

Acetoacetyl CoA | Acetyl CoA | Water

1

$HOOC-CH_2-C(CH_3)(OH)-CH_2-\overset{O}{\overset{\|}{C}}-CoA$ + CoA

Beta-hydroxy-beta-methylglutaryl CoA | Coenzyme A

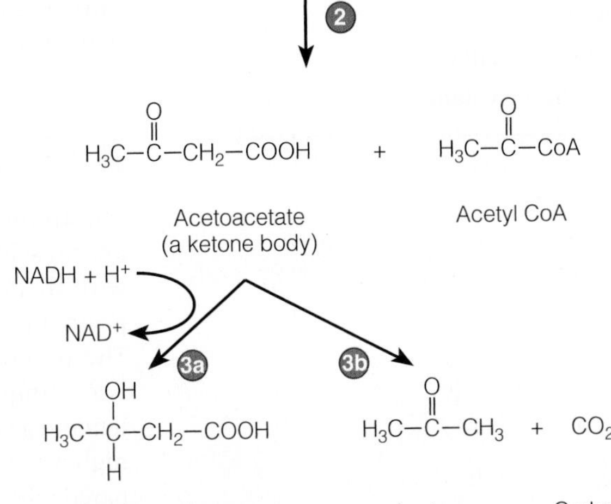

Appendix D Measures of Protein Quality

CONTENTS

In a world where food is scarce and many people's diets contain marginal or inadequate amounts of protein, it is important to know which foods contain the highest-quality protein. Chapter 6 describes protein quality, and this appendix presents different measures researchers use to assess the quality of a food protein. Measures of protein quality aim to determine how well a food protein supports the body's normal metabolism and growth. The accompanying glossary defines related terms.

Amino Acid Score

The **amino acid score** predicts protein quality based on the pattern of essential amino acids. It compares the essential amino acid composition of a food protein with that of a reference protein (egg). The score of each amino acid in the food protein is described as a percentage of the amino acid in the reference protein. The amino acid with the lowest percentage score is the most limiting amino acid. For example, results might find that compared with the reference amino acids, leucine gets a 93, lysine gets an 80, and all the other essential amino acids get higher scores. Lysine is the limiting amino acid (the one that falls shortest compared with egg). If the protein's limiting amino acid is 80 percent of the amount found in the reference protein, it receives an amino acid score of 80. The advantages of amino acid scoring are that it is simple and inexpensive, it easily identifies the limiting amino acid, and it can be used to score mixtures of different proportions of multiple proteins mathematically without having to create a mixture to test. Its chief weakness is that it fails to estimate the digestibility of a protein, which may strongly affect the protein's quality.

PDCAAS

The **protein digestibility-corrected amino acid score,** or **PDCAAS,** is a widely used measurement of protein quality.[1] The PDCAAS compares the amino acid composition of a food protein with human amino acid requirements and corrects for digestibility. First the protein's essential amino acid composition is

GLOSSARY

amino acid score: a measure of protein quality assessed by comparing a protein's amino acid pattern with that of a reference protein; also called the *chemical score.*

biological value (BV): a measure of protein quality assessed by measuring the amount of protein nitrogen that is retained from a given amount of protein nitrogen absorbed.

DIAAS (digestible indispensable amino acid score): a measure of protein quality similar to PDCAAS, except it determines protein digestibility at the end of the small intestine, which more accurately reflects the extent of amino acid absorption.

net protein utilization (NPU): a measure of protein quality assessed by measuring the amount of protein nitrogen that is retained from a given amount of protein nitrogen eaten.

PDCAAS (protein digestibility-corrected amino acid score): a measure of protein quality assessed by comparing the amino acid score of a food protein with the amino acid requirements of preschool-age children and then correcting for the true digestibility of the protein.

protein efficiency ratio (PER): a measure of protein quality assessed by determining how well a given protein supports weight gain in growing rats; used to establish the protein quality for infant formulas and baby foods.

determined, and then it is compared against the amino acid requirements of preschool-aged children.[2] This comparison reveals the most limiting amino acid—the one that falls shortest compared with the reference. If a food protein's limiting amino acid is 70 percent of the amount found in the reference protein, it receives a score of 70. The amino acid score is multiplied by the food's protein digestibility percentage to determine the PDCAAS. The accompanying "How To" provides an example of how to calculate the PDCAAS, and Table D-1 lists the PDCAAS values of selected foods.

TABLE D-1 PDCAAS Values of Selected Foods

Food	PDCAAS
Casein (milk protein)	1.00
Egg white	1.00
Soybean (isolate)	.99
Beef	.92
Pea flour	.69
Kidney beans (canned)	.68
Chickpeas (canned)	.66
Pinto beans (canned)	.66
Rolled oats	.57
Lentils (canned)	.52
Peanut meal	.52
Whole wheat	.40

NOTE: 1.0 is the maximum PDCAAS a food protein can receive.

DIAAS

Recently, the Food and Agriculture Organization of the United Nations recommended that a new method, known as Digestible Indispensable Amino Acid Score (DIAAS), should replace PDCAAS as the preferred method to determine protein quality.[3] The DIAAS overcomes some of the weaknesses of the current PDCAAS method. Whereas PDCAAS estimates protein digestibility over the entire intestine and uses a single digestibility score, the DIAAS determines amino acid digestibility at the end of the small intestine, which more accurately reflects the extent of amino acids absorption, and considers the digestibility of individual amino acids, as opposed to the protein as a whole.

>How To

Measure Protein Quality Using PDCAAS

To calculate the PDCAAS (protein digestibility-corrected amino acid score), researchers first determine the amino acid profile of the test protein (in this example, pinto beans). The second column of the table below presents the essential amino acid profile for pinto beans. The third column presents the amino acid reference pattern.

To determine how well the food protein meets human needs, researchers calculate the ratio by dividing the second column by the third column (for example, $30 \div 18 = 1.67$). The amino acid with the lowest percentage is the most limiting amino acid—in this case, methionine. Its percentage is the amino acid score for the protein—in this case, 0.84.

The amino acid score alone, however, does not account for digestibility. Protein digestibility, as determined by animal studies, yields a value of 79 percent for pinto beans. Together, the amino acid score and the digestibility value determine the PDCAAS:

$$\text{PDCAAS} = \text{protein digestibility} \times \text{amino acid score}$$

$$\text{PDCAAS for pinto beans} = 0.79 \times 0.84 = 0.66$$

Thus the PDCAAS for pinto beans is 0.66 as Table D-1 shows.

Essential Amino Acids	Amino Acid Profile of Pinto Beans (mg/g protein)	Amino Acid Reference Pattern (mg/g protein)	Amino Acid Score
Histidine	30.0	18	1.67
Isoleucine	42.5	25	1.70
Leucine	80.4	55	1.46
Lysine	69.0	51	1.35
Methionine (+ cystine)	21.1	25	0.84
Phenylalanine (+ tyrosine)	90.5	47	1.93
Threonine	43.7	27	1.62
Tryptophan	8.8	7	1.26
Valine	50.1	32	1.57

Biological Value

The **biological value (BV)** of a food protein measures its efficiency in supporting the body's growth and maintenance. In a test of biological value, two nitrogen balance studies are done. In the first, no protein is fed, and nitrogen (N) excretions in the urine and feces are measured. It is assumed that under these conditions, N lost in the urine is the amount the body loses each day, regardless of food protein; this endogenous N is "urinary N on a zero-protein diet." The N lost in the feces is the amount the body loses each day, regardless of food protein; this metabolic N is "fecal N on a zero-protein diet."

In the second study, a diet containing the test protein in an amount equal to the requirement is fed. Intakes and losses are measured; then the BV is derived using this formula:

$$\text{BV} = \frac{\text{N retained}}{\text{N absorbed}} \times 100$$

The more nitrogen retained, the higher the protein quality. (Recall that when an essential amino acid is missing, protein synthesis stops, and the remaining amino acids are deaminated and the nitrogen excreted.)

Egg protein has a BV of 100, indicating that 100 percent of the nitrogen absorbed is retained. Supplied in adequate quantity, a protein with a BV of 70 or greater can support human growth as long as energy intake is adequate. Table D-2 presents the BV for selected foods.

TABLE D-2 Biological Values (BV) of Selected Foods

Food	BV
Egg	100
Milk	93
Beef	75
Fish	75
Corn	72

NOTE: 100 is the maximum BV a food protein can receive.

Net Protein Utilization

Like BV, **net protein utilization (NPU)** measures how efficiently a protein is used by the body and involves two balance studies. The difference is that NPU measures retention of food nitrogen consumed rather than food nitrogen absorbed (as in BV). The formula for NPU is:

$$\text{NPU} = \frac{\text{N retained}}{\text{N intake}} \times 100$$

The numerator is the same as for BV, but the denominator represents food N intake only—not N absorbed.

Protein Efficiency Ratio

The **protein efficiency ratio (PER)** measures the weight gain of a growing animal and compares it to the animal's protein intake. To determine the PER of a food protein, young, growing animals are given a standard diet containing about 10 percent (by weight) of the test protein. After a specified period of time, weight gain is measured and compared to the amount of test protein consumed. The PER is expressed as:

$$\text{PER} = \frac{\text{weight gain (g)}}{\text{protein intake (g)}}$$

Table D-3 presents PER values for selected foods.

TABLE D-3 Protein Efficiency Ratio (PER) Values of Selected Proteins

Protein	PER
Casein (milk)	2.8
Soy	2.4
Glutein (wheat)	0.4

REFERENCES

1. G. Schaafsma, Advantages and limitations of the protein digestibility-corrected amino acid score (PDCAAS) as a method for evaluating protein quality in human diets, *British Journal of Nutrition* 108 (2012): S333–S336.
2. D. J. Millward, Amino acid scoring patterns for protein quality assessment, *British Journal of Nutrition* 108 (2012): S31–S43.
3. S. Leser, The 2013 FAO report on dietary protein quality evaluation in human nutrition: Recommendations and implications, *Nutrition Bulletin* 38 (2013): 421–428.

Appendix E Nutrition Assessment

Nutrition assessment evaluates a person's health from a nutrition perspective. Many factors influence or reflect nutrition status. Consequently, the assessor, usually a registered dietitian assisted by other qualified health-care professionals, gathers information from many sources, including:

- Historical information.
- Anthropometric measurements.
- Physical examinations.
- Biochemical analyses (laboratory tests).

Each of these methods involves collecting data in a variety of ways and interpreting each finding in relation to the others to create a total picture.

The accurate gathering of this information and its careful interpretation are the basis for a meaningful evaluation. The more information gathered about a person, the more accurate the assessment will be. Gathering information is a time-consuming process, however, and time is often a rare commodity in the health care setting. Nutrition care is only one part of total care. It may not be practical or essential to collect detailed information on each person.

A strategic compromise is to screen patients by collecting preliminary data. Data such as height-weight and hematocrit are easy to obtain and can alert health-care workers to potential problems. **Nutrition screening** identifies patients who will require additional nutrition assessment. This appendix provides a sample of the procedures, standards, and charts commonly used in nutrition assessment.

CONTENTS

Historical Information

Clues about a person's nutrition status and nutrient requirements become evident with a careful review of a person's historical information (see Table E-1). A thorough history identifies risk factors associated with poor nutrition status (see Table E-2) and reveals personal preferences that need consideration when developing a nutrition care plan. Historical information is obtained from the medical record and interviews with the patient or caregiver.

TABLE E-1 **Historical Information Used in Nutrition Assessments**

Type of History	What It Identifies
Medical history	Current and previous mental and physical health problems and surgeries, chronic disease risks, and family medical history that affect nutrient needs, nutrition status, or the need for intervention to prevent or alleviate health problems
Personal and social history	Personal, cultural, financial, and environmental influences on food intake, nutrient needs, and diet therapy options
Medication and supplement history	Medications (prescription and over-the-counter), illicit drugs, dietary supplements, and alternative therapies that affect nutrition status
Food and nutrition history	Nutrient intake excesses or deficiencies and reasons for imbalances

nutrition screening: the use of preliminary nutrition assessment techniques to identify people who are malnourished or are at risk for malnutrition.

APPENDIX E

TABLE E-2 Risk Factors for Malnutrition

Medical History

- Acquired immune deficiency syndrome (AIDS)
- Alcoholism
- Anorexia (lack of appetite)
- Anorexia nervosa
- Bulimia nervosa
- Burns (extensive or severe)
- Cancer
- Celiac disease
- Chewing or swallowing difficulties (including poorly fitted dentures, dental caries, missing teeth, and mouth ulcers)
- Chronic obstructive pulmonary disease
- Circulatory problems
- Constipation
- Crohn's disease
- Cystic fibrosis
- Decubitus ulcers (pressure sores)
- Dementia
- Depleted blood proteins
- Depression
- Diabetes mellitus
- Diarrhea, prolonged or severe
- Drug addiction
- Dysphagia
- Failure to thrive
- Feeding disabilities
- Fever
- GI tract disorders or surgery
- Heart disease
- HIV infection
- Hormonal imbalance
- Hyperlipidemia
- Hypertension
- Infections
- Inflammatory bowel diseases
- Kidney disease
- Liver disease
- Lung disease
- Malabsorption
- Mental illness
- Mental retardation
- Multiple pregnancies
- Nausea
- Neurologic disorders
- Organ failure
- Overweight
- Pancreatic insufficiency
- Paralysis
- Physical disability
- Pneumonia
- Pregnancy
- Radiation therapy
- Surgery (recent or major)
- Tobacco use
- Trauma
- Ulcerative colitis
- Ulcers
- Underweight
- Vomiting (prolonged or severe)

Personal and Social History

- Access to groceries
- Activities
- Age
- Cognitive abilities
- Economic status
- Education
- Employment
- Ethnic/cultural identity
- Home and family situation
- Kitchen facilities
- Religious beliefs

Medication and Supplement History

- Dietary and herbal supplements
- Illicit drug use
- Over-the-counter drugs
- Prescription medicines

Food and Nutrition History

- Deficient or excessive food intakes
- Food allergies or intolerances
- Food insecurity
- Frequently eating out
- Intravenous fluids (other than total parenteral nutrition) for 7 or more days
- Monotonous diet (lacking variety)
- Nutrition knowledge
- Poor appetite
- Restricted or fad diets
- Unbalanced diet (omitting any food group)
- Weight gains or losses (recent)

An adept history taker uses the interview both to gather facts and to establish a rapport with the patient. This section briefly reviews the major areas of nutrition concern in a person's history.

Medical History The assessor can obtain a **medical history** from records completed by the attending physician, nurse, or other health-care professional. In addition, conversations with the patient can uncover valuable information previously overlooked because no one thought to ask or because the patient was not thinking clearly when asked.

An accurate, complete medical history includes the family medical history as well and can reveal conditions that increase a patient's risk for malnutrition (review Table E-2). Diseases and their therapies can have either immediate or long-term effects on nutrition status by interfering with ingestion, digestion, absorption, metabolism, or excretion of nutrients.

Personal and Social History A **personal and social history** reveals factors that influence food choices and a person's ability to manage health

medical history: an account of a patient's current and past health status and disease risks.

personal and social history: a record of a person's social and economic background, including such factors as education, income, and ethnic identity.

and nutrition problems. The ethnic background and religious beliefs of both the patient and the other members of the household influence food choices. Financial concerns influence access to healthy food choices. In general, the quality of the diet declines as income falls. At some point, the ability to purchase the foods required to meet nutrient needs is lost; an inadequate income puts an adequate diet out of reach. Agencies use poverty indexes to identify people at risk for poor nutrition and to qualify people for government food assistance programs.

Low income affects not only the power to purchase foods but also the ability to shop for, store, and cook them; some individuals depend on others to procure and prepare meals. A skilled assessor will note whether a person has transportation to a grocery store that sells a sufficient variety of low-cost foods, and whether the person has access to a refrigerator and stove.

Medication and Supplement History The many interactions of foods and drugs require that healthcare professionals take a **medication and supplement history** and pay special attention to any patient who takes drugs routinely. If a person is taking any drug, the assessor records the name of the drug; the dose, frequency, and duration of intake; the reason for taking the drug; and signs of any adverse effects.

The interactions of drugs and nutrients may take many forms:

- Drugs can alter food intake and the absorption, metabolism, and excretion of nutrients.
- Foods and nutrients can alter the absorption, metabolism, and excretion of drugs.

Highlight 17 discusses nutrient-drug interactions in more detail, and Table H17-1 (p. 580) summarizes the mechanisms by which these interactions occur and provides specific examples.

Food and Nutrition History A **food and nutrition history** (often called a *diet history*) provides a record of a person's eating habits and food intake and can help identify possible nutrient imbalances. Food choices are an important part of lifestyle. The assessor who asks nonjudgmental questions about eating habits and food intake encourages trust and enhances the likelihood of obtaining accurate information.

Besides identifying possible nutrient imbalances, food and nutrition histories provide valuable clues about how a person will accept diet changes should they be necessary. Information about what and how a person eats provides the background for realistic and attainable nutrition goals. The following section describes the most common methods of gathering food intake information.

Food Intake Data Assessors evaluate food intake using various tools such as the 24-hour recall, the food record, the food frequency questionnaire, and direct observation. Food models or photos and measuring devices can help patients identify the types of foods and quantities consumed. The assessor also needs to know how the foods are prepared and when they are eaten. In addition to asking about foods, assessors will ask about beverage consumption, including beverages containing alcohol or caffeine.

24-Hour Dietary Recall The **24-hour dietary recall** provides data for one day only and is commonly used in nutrition surveys to obtain estimates of the typical food intakes for a population. The assessor asks an individual to recount all the foods and beverages consumed in the past 24 hours or for the previous day. The interview includes questions about the times of meals and snacks, amounts consumed, and methods of food preparation.

medication and supplement history: a record of all the drugs, over-the-counter and prescribed, as well as dietary and herbal supplements that a person takes routinely.

food and nutrition history: a record of eating behaviors and the foods a person eats.

24-hour dietary recall: a record of foods eaten by a person for one 24-hour period.

The multiple-pass method is the most effective approach for obtaining an accurate list of foods consumed. In this procedure, the interview includes four or five separate passes through the 24-hour period of interest. In the first pass, the person provides a "quick list" of foods consumed without being prompted by the interviewer. The second pass helps the person remember foods that are often forgotten, such as beverages, bread, additions to foods (such as butter on toast), savory snacks, and sweets. Third and fourth passes elicit additional details about the foods consumed, such as the amounts eaten, preparation methods, and places where foods were obtained or consumed. A final pass provides an opportunity to recall foods and to probe for additional details. The entire multiple-pass interview can be conducted in about 30 to 45 minutes.

An advantage of the 24-hour recall is that it is relatively easy to obtain. It does not, however, provide enough information to allow accurate generalizations about an individual's usual food intake. The previous day's intake may not be typical, for example, or the person may be unable to report portion sizes accurately or may conceal or forget information about foods eaten. This limitation is partially overcome when 24-hour dietary recalls are collected on several nonconsecutive days.

Food Record Another tool for history taking is the **food record,** in which the person records food and beverages consumed, including the quantity and method of preparation. Chapter 9 (Figure 9-8, p. 286) provides an example. A food record can help both the assessor and the patient to determine factors associated with eating that may affect dietary balance and adequacy.

Food records work especially well with cooperative people but require considerable time and effort on their part. A prime advantage is that the record keeper assumes an active role and may for the first time become aware of personal food habits and assume responsibility for them. It also provides the assessor with an accurate picture of the person's lifestyle and factors that affect food intake. For these reasons, a food record can be particularly useful in outpatient counseling for such nutrition problems as overweight, underweight, or food allergy. The major disadvantages stem from poor compliance in recording the data and conscious or unconscious changes in eating habits that may occur while the person is keeping the record.

Food Frequency Questionnaire An assessor uses a **food frequency questionnaire** to survey the foods and beverages regularly consumed during a specific time period. Some questionnaires are qualitative only: food lists contain common foods, organized by food group, with check boxes to indicate frequency of consumption. Other types of questionnaires can collect semiquantitative information by including portion sizes as well. This information helps pinpoint foods and food groups, and therefore nutrients, that may be excessive or deficient in the diet. That a person ate no vegetables yesterday may not seem particularly significant, but never eating vegetables is a warning of possible nutrient deficiencies. When used with the usual intake or 24-hour recall approach, the food frequency questionnaire enables the assessor to double-check the accuracy of the information obtained.

Direct Observation In facilities that serve meals, food intakes can be directly observed and analyzed. This method can also reveal a person's food preferences, changes in appetite, and any problems with a prescribed diet. Health practitioners use direct observation to estimate a patient's intake of food energy (and often, protein) during a single day or on several consecutive days. To estimate food and nutrient intakes, the clinician records the dietary items that a patient is given at meals and subtracts the amounts remaining after meals are completed; this procedure allows an estimate of the amounts of foods and beverages actually consumed. Although a useful means of discerning patients' intakes, direct observation requires regular and careful documentation and can be labor-intensive and costly.

Analysis of Food Intake Data After collecting food intake data, the assessor estimates nutrient intakes, either informally by using food guides or formally by

food record: an extensive, accurate log of all foods eaten over a period of several days or weeks. A food record that includes associated information such as when, where, and with whom each food is eaten is sometimes called a *food diary.*

food frequency questionnaire: a checklist of foods on which a person can record the frequency with which he or she eats each food.

using diet analysis programs. The assessor compares intakes with standards, usually nutrient recommendations or dietary guidelines, to determine how closely the person's diet meets the standards. Are the types and amounts of proteins, carbohydrates (including fiber), and fats (including cholesterol) appropriate? Are all food groups included in appropriate amounts? Is caffeine or alcohol consumption excessive? Are intakes of any vitamins or minerals (including sodium and iron) excessive or deficient? An informal evaluation is possible only if the assessor has enough prior experience with formal calculations to "see" nutrient amounts in reported food intakes without calculations. Even then, such an informal analysis is best followed by a spot check for key nutrients by actual calculation.

Formal calculations can be performed either manually (by looking up each food in a table of food composition, recording its nutrients, and adding them up) or by using a diet analysis program. The assessor then compares the intakes with standards such as the RDA.

Limitations of Food Intake Analysis Diet histories can be most informative, but the skillful assessor also keeps their limitations in mind. For example, a diet analysis program tends to imply greater accuracy than is possible to obtain from data as uncertain as the starting information. Nutrient contents of foods listed in tables of food composition or stored in computer databases are averages and, for some nutrients, incomplete. In addition, the available data on nutrient contents of foods do not reflect the amounts of nutrients a person actually absorbs. Iron is a case in point: its availability from a given meal may vary depending on the person's iron status; the relative amounts of heme iron, nonheme iron, vitamin C, meat, fish, and poultry eaten at the meal; and the presence of inhibitors of iron absorption such as tea, coffee, and nuts. (Chapter 13 describes the many factors that influence iron absorption from a meal.)

Furthermore, reported portion sizes may not be correct. The person who reports eating "a serving" of greens may not distinguish between ¼ cup and 2 cups; only individuals who have practice measuring food quantities can accurately report serving sizes. Children tend to remember the serving sizes of foods they like as being larger than serving sizes of foods they dislike.

An estimate of nutrient intakes from a food and nutrition history, combined with other sources of information, allows the assessor to confirm or eliminate the possibility of suspected nutrition problems. The assessor must constantly remember that nutrient intakes in adequate amounts do not guarantee adequate nutrient status for an individual. Likewise, insufficient intakes do not always indicate deficiencies, but instead alert the assessor to possible problems. Each person digests, absorbs, metabolizes, and excretes nutrients in a unique way; individual needs vary. Intakes of nutrients identified by diet histories are only pieces of a puzzle that must be put together with other indicators of nutrition status in order to extract meaning.

Anthropometric Measurements

Anthropometrics are physical measurements that reflect body composition and development (see Table E-3). They serve three main purposes: first, to evaluate the progress of growth in pregnant women, infants, children, and adolescents; second, to detect undernutrition and overnutrition in all age groups; and third, to measure changes in body composition over time.

Health-care professionals compare anthropometric measurements taken on an individual with population standards specific for gender and age or with previous measures of the individual. Measurements taken periodically and compared with previous measurements reveal changes in an individual's status.

Mastering the techniques for taking anthropometric measurements requires proper instruction and practice to ensure reliability. Once the correct techniques are learned, taking measurements is easy and requires minimal equipment.

anthropometrics (AN-throw-poe-MET-ricks): measurements of the physical characteristics of the body, such as height and weight.
- **anthropos** = human
- **metric** = measuring

> **FIGURE E-1 Length Measurement of an Infant**

An infant is measured lying down on a measuring board with a fixed headboard and a movable footboard. Note that two people are needed to measure the infant's length.

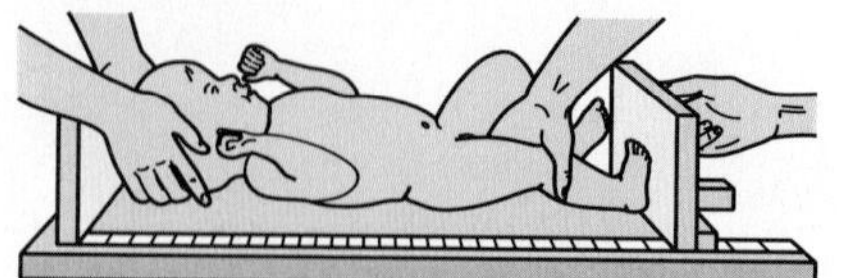

TABLE E-3 Anthropometric Measurements Used in Nutrition Assessments

Type of Measurement	What It Reflects
Abdominal girth measurement	Abdominal fluid retention and abdominal organ size
Height-weight	Overnutrition and undernutrition; growth in children
Head circumference	Brain growth and development in infants and children under age 2
Skinfold	Subcutaneous and total body fat
Waist circumference	Body fat distribution

Height and weight are well-recognized anthropometrics; other anthropometrics include skinfold measurements and various measures of lean tissue. Other measures are useful in specific situations. For example, a head circumference measurement may help to assess brain development in an infant, and an abdominal girth measurement supplies information about abdominal fluid retention in individuals with liver disease.

Measures of Growth and Development

Height and weight are among the most common and useful anthropometric measurements. Length measurements for infants and children up to age 3 and height measurements for children over 3 are particularly valuable in assessing growth and therefore nutrition status. For adults, height measurements alone are not critical, but help to estimate healthy weight and to interpret other assessment data. Once adult height has been reached, changes in body weight provide useful information in assessing overnutrition and undernutrition.

Height For infants and children younger than 3, health-care professionals may use special equipment to measure length. The assessor lays the barefoot infant on a measuring board that has a fixed headboard and movable footboard attached at right angles to the surface (see Figure E-1). Often two people are needed to obtain an accurate measurement: one to gently hold the infant's head against the headboard, and the other to straighten the infant's legs and move the footboard to the bottom of the infant's feet.

The procedure for measuring a child who can stand erect and cooperate is the same as for an adult. The best way to measure standing height is with the person's back against a flat wall to which a nonstretchable measuring tape or stick has been fixed (see Figure E-2). The person stands erect, without shoes, with heels together. The person's line of sight should be horizontal, with the heels, buttocks, shoulders, and head touching the wall. The assessor places a ruler or other inflexible object on top of the head at a right angle to the wall; carefully checks the height measurement; and records it immediately in either inches or centimeters so that the correct measurement will not be forgotten.

The measuring rod of a scale is commonly used, but is less accurate because it bends easily. The assessor follows the same general procedure, asking the person to face away from the scale and to take extra care to stand erect.

Unfortunately, many health-care professionals merely ask patients how tall they are rather than measuring their height. Self-reported height is often inaccurate and should be used only as a last resort when measurement is impractical (in the case of an uncooperative patient, an emergency admission, or the like).

Weight Valid weight measurements require scales that have been carefully maintained, calibrated, and checked for accuracy at regular intervals. Beam balance and electronic scales are the most accurate. To measure infants' weight, assessors use special scales that allow infants to lie or sit (see Figure E-3). Weighing infants naked, without diapers, is standard procedure. Children who can stand are weighed in the same way as adults (see Figure E-4). To make repeated measures useful, standardized conditions are necessary. Each weighing should take

> **FIGURE E-2 Height Measurement of an Older Child or Adult**

Height is measured most accurately when the person stands against a flat wall to which a measuring tape has been affixed.

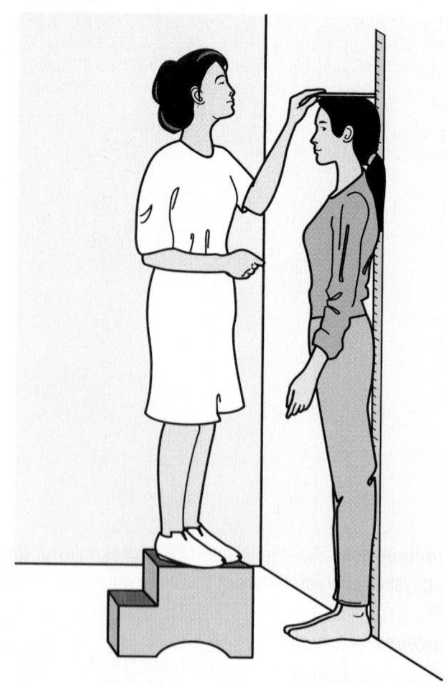

place at the same time of day (preferably before breakfast), in the same amount of clothing (without shoes), after the person has voided, and on the same scale. Special scales and hospital beds with built-in scales are available for weighing people who are bedridden. Bathroom scales are inaccurate and inappropriate in a professional setting. As with all measurements, the assessor records the observed weight immediately in either pounds or kilograms.

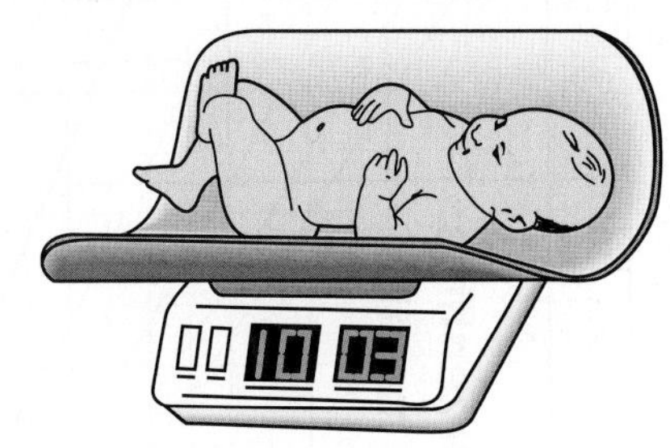

> **FIGURE E-3 Weight Measurement of an Infant**
Infants sit or lie down on scales that are designed to hold them while they are being weighed.

Head Circumference Assessors may also measure head circumference to confirm that infant growth is proceeding normally or to help detect malnutrition and evaluate the extent of its impact on brain size. To measure head circumference, the assessor places a nonstretchable tape so that it encircles the largest part of the infant's or child's head: just above the eyebrow ridges, just above the point where the ears attach, and around the occipital prominence at the back of the head. To ensure accurate recording, the assessor immediately notes the measure in either inches or centimeters.

Analysis of Measures in Infants and Children Growth retardation is a sign of poor nutrition status. Obesity is also a sign that dietary intervention may be needed.

Health professionals generally evaluate physical development by monitoring the growth rate of a child and comparing this rate with standard charts. Standard charts compare weight to age, height to age, and weight to height; ideally, height and weight are in roughly the same percentile. Although individual growth patterns may vary, a child's growth curve will generally stay at about the same percentile throughout childhood. In children whose growth has been retarded, nutrition rehabilitation will ideally induce height and weight to increase to higher percentiles. In overweight children, the goal is for weight to remain stable as height increases, until weight becomes appropriate for height.

To evaluate growth in infants, an assessor uses charts such as those in Figures E-5 (A and B) through E-10 (A and B). The assessor follows these steps to plot a weight measurement on a percentile graph:

- Select the appropriate chart based on age and gender.
- Locate the child's age along the horizontal axis on the bottom of the chart.
- Locate the child's weight in pounds or kilograms along the vertical axis.
- Mark the chart where the age and weight lines intersect, and read off the percentile.

To assess length, height, or head circumference, the assessor follows the same procedure, using the appropriate chart. (When length is measured, use the chart for birth to 36 months; when height is measured, use the chart for 2 to 20 years.) Head circumference percentile should be similar to the child's height and weight percentiles. With height, weight, and head circumference measures plotted on growth percentile charts, a skilled clinician can begin to interpret the data.

Percentile charts divide the measures of a population into 100 equal divisions. Thus half of the population falls above the 50th percentile, and half falls below. The use of percentile measures allows for comparisons among people of the same age and gender. For example, a 6-month-old female infant whose weight is at the 75 percentile weighs more than 75 percent of the female infants her age.

Head circumference is generally measured in children under 2 years of age. Because the brain grows rapidly before birth and during early infancy, extreme and chronic malnutrition during these times can impair brain development, curtailing the number of brain cells and the size of head circumference. Nonnutritional factors, such as certain disorders and genetic variation, can also influence head circumference.

Analysis of Measures in Adults For adults, health-care professionals typically compare weights with weight-for-height standards. One such standard is the body mass index (BMI), described in Chapter 8, which is useful for estimating the risk to health associated with overnutrition. The inside back cover shows BMI for various heights and weights.

> **FIGURE E-4 Weight Measurement of an Older Child or Adult**
Whenever possible, children and adults are measured on beam balance or electronic scales to ensure accuracy.

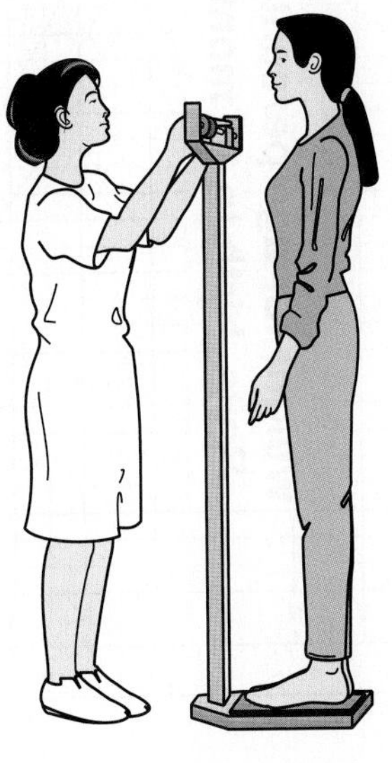

> FIGURE E-5A **Weight-for-Age Percentiles: Boys, Birth to 36 Months**

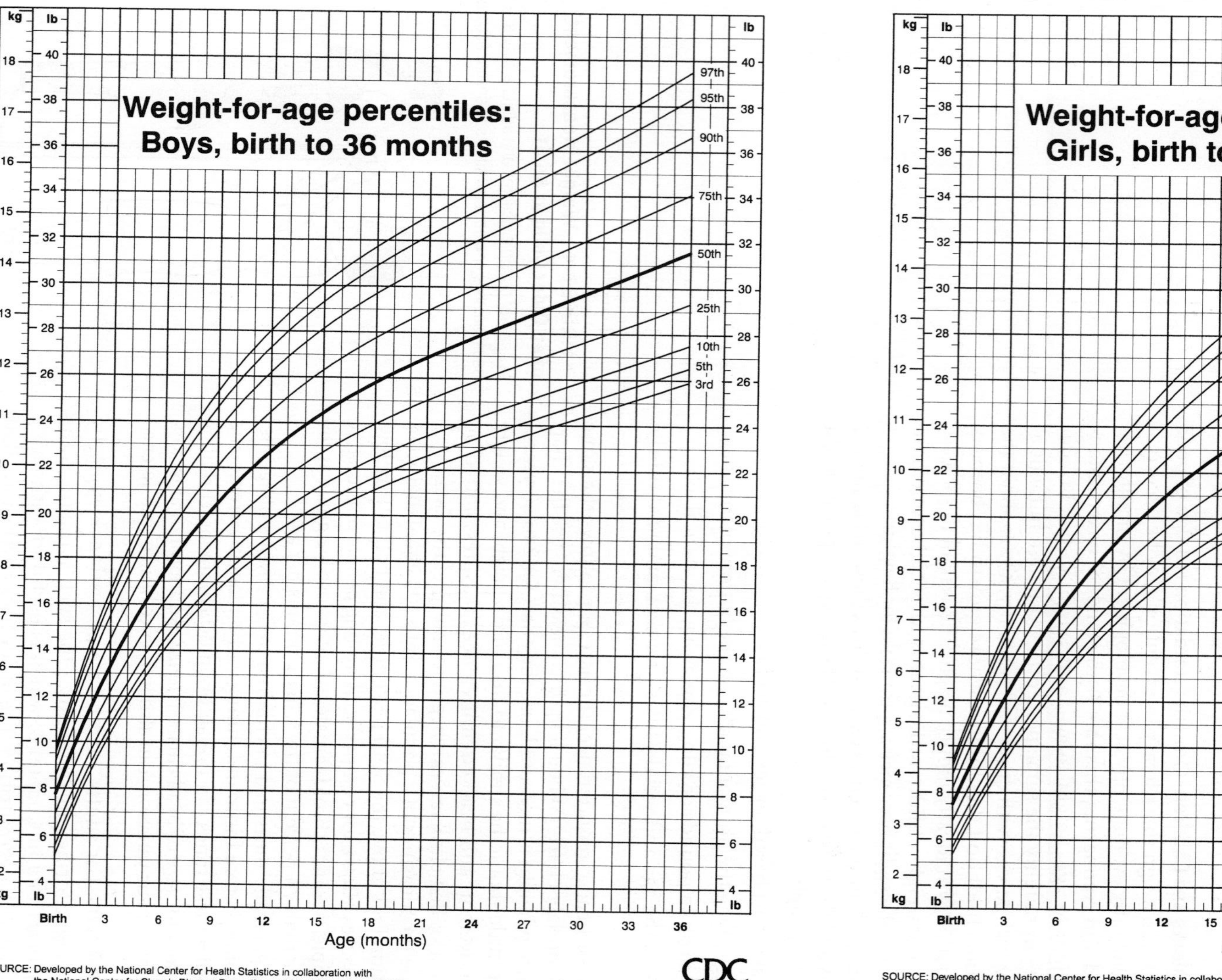

SOURCE: Developed by the National Center for Health Statistics in collaboration with the National Center for Chronic Disease Prevention and Health Promotion (2000).

Figure 1. Weight-for-age percentiles, boys, birth to 36 months, CDC growth charts: United States

> FIGURE E-5B **Weight-for-Age Percentiles: Girls, Birth to 36 Months**

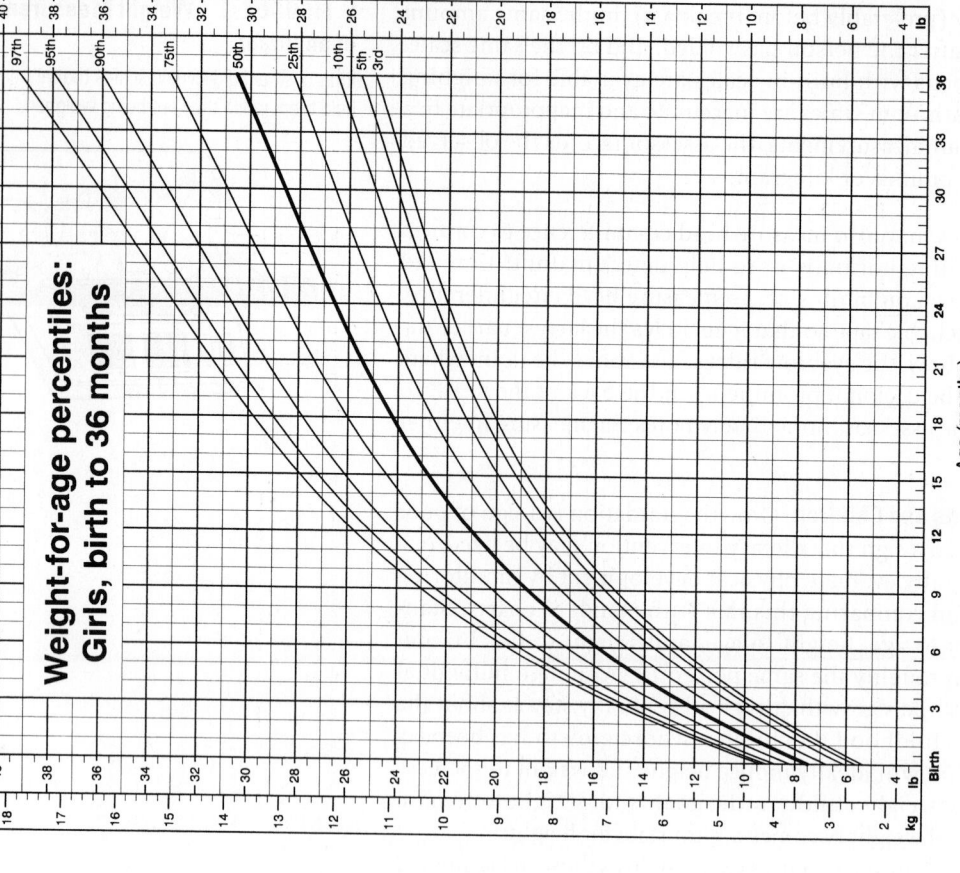

Weight-for-age percentiles:
Girls, birth to 36 months

Age (months)

SOURCE: Developed by the National Center for Health Statistics in collaboration with the National Center for Chronic Disease Prevention and Health Promotion (2000).

Figure 2. Weight-for-age percentiles, girls, birth to 36 months, CDC growth charts: United States

> FIGURE E-6A Length-for-Age Percentiles: Boys, Birth to 36 Months

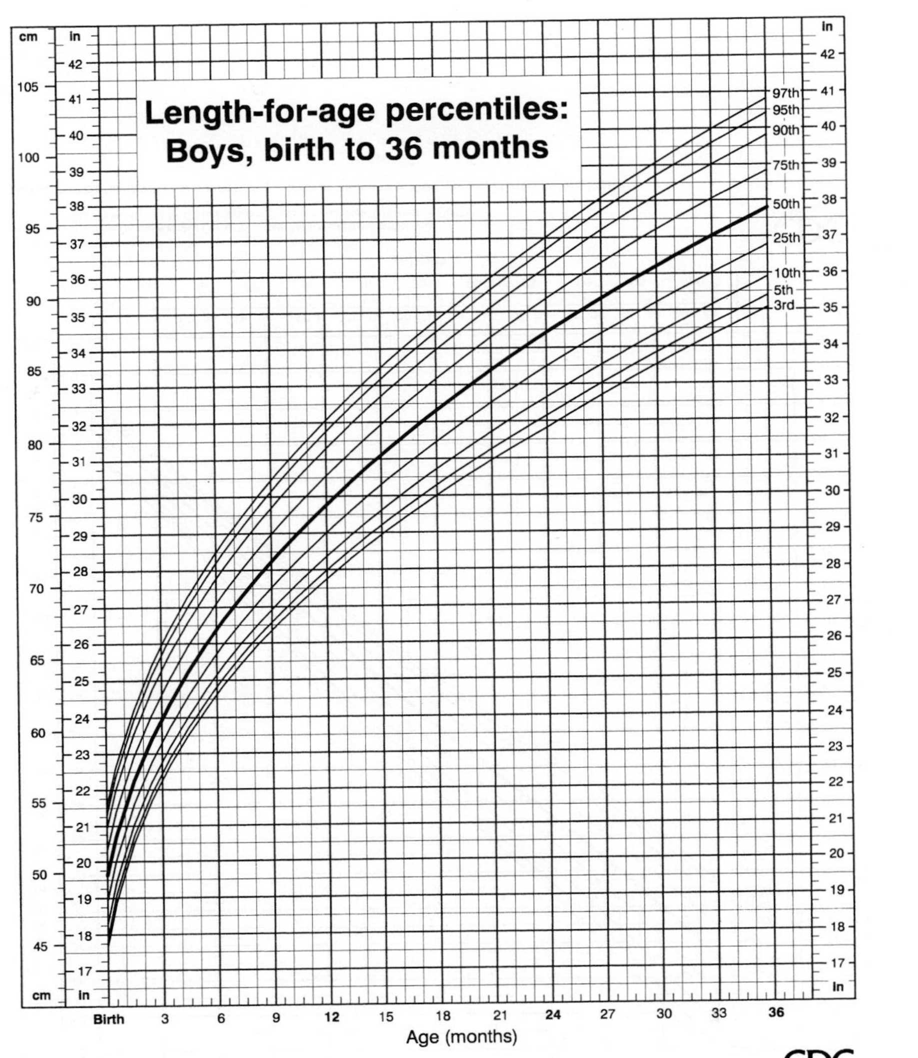

SOURCE: Developed by the National Center for Health Statistics in collaboration with the National Center for Chronic Disease Prevention and Health Promotion (2000).

Figure 3. Length-for-age percentiles, boys, birth to 36 months, CDC growth charts: United States

> FIGURE E-6B Length-for-Age Percentiles: Girls, Birth to 36 Months

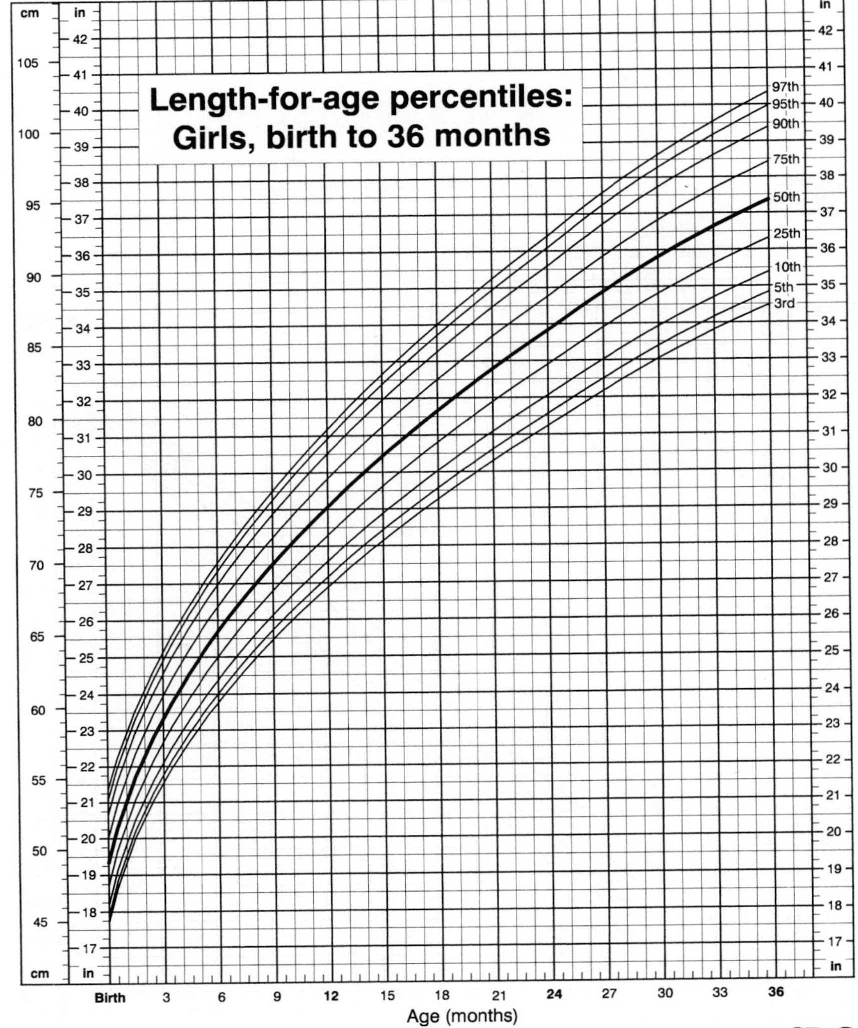

SOURCE: Developed by the National Center for Health Statistics in collaboration with the National Center for Chronic Disease Prevention and Health Promotion (2000).

Figure 4. Length-for-age percentiles, girls, birth to 36 months, CDC growth charts: United States

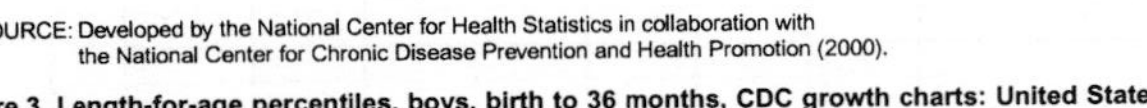

> **FIGURE E-7A** Weight-for-Length Percentiles: Boys, Birth to 36 Months

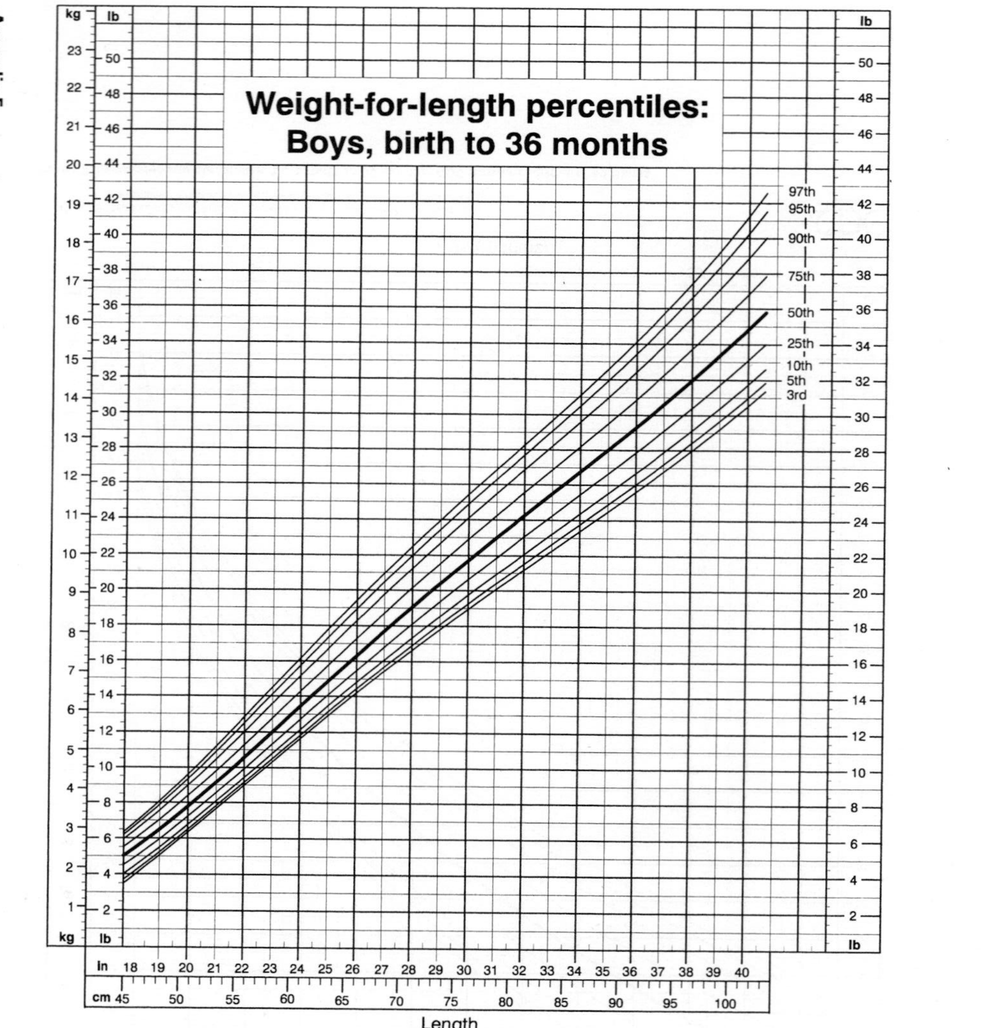

Revised and corrected June 8, 2000.
SOURCE: Developed by the National Center for Health Statistics in collaboration with the National Center for Chronic Disease Prevention and Health Promotion (2000).

Figure 5. Weight-for-length percentiles, boys, birth to 36 months, CDC growth charts: United States

> **FIGURE E-7B** Weight-for-Length Percentiles: Girls, Birth to 36 Months

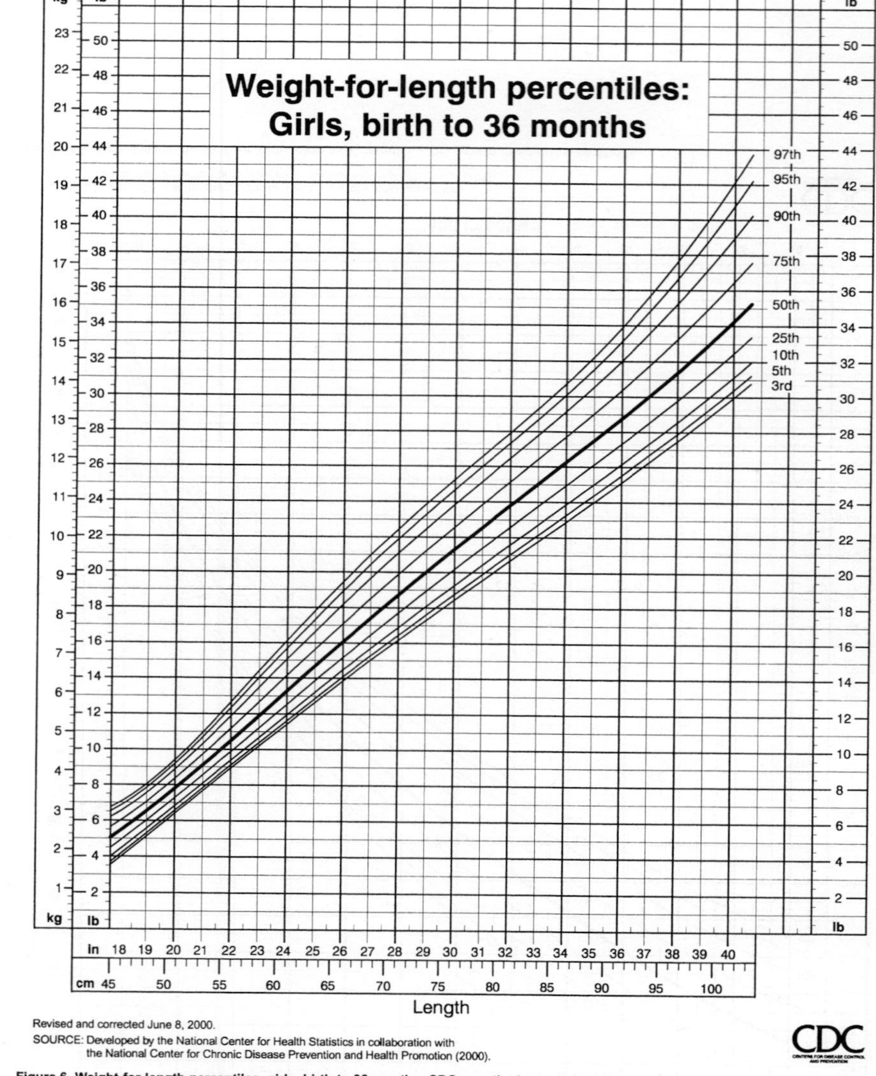

Revised and corrected June 8, 2000.
SOURCE: Developed by the National Center for Health Statistics in collaboration with the National Center for Chronic Disease Prevention and Health Promotion (2000).

Figure 6. Weight-for-length percentiles, girls, birth to 36 months, CDC growth charts: United States

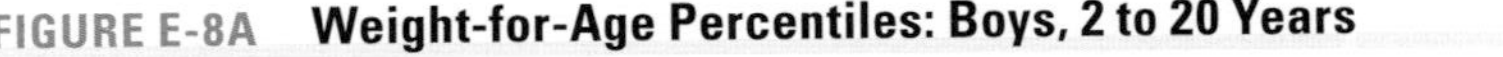

> FIGURE E-8A Weight-for-Age Percentiles: Boys, 2 to 20 Years

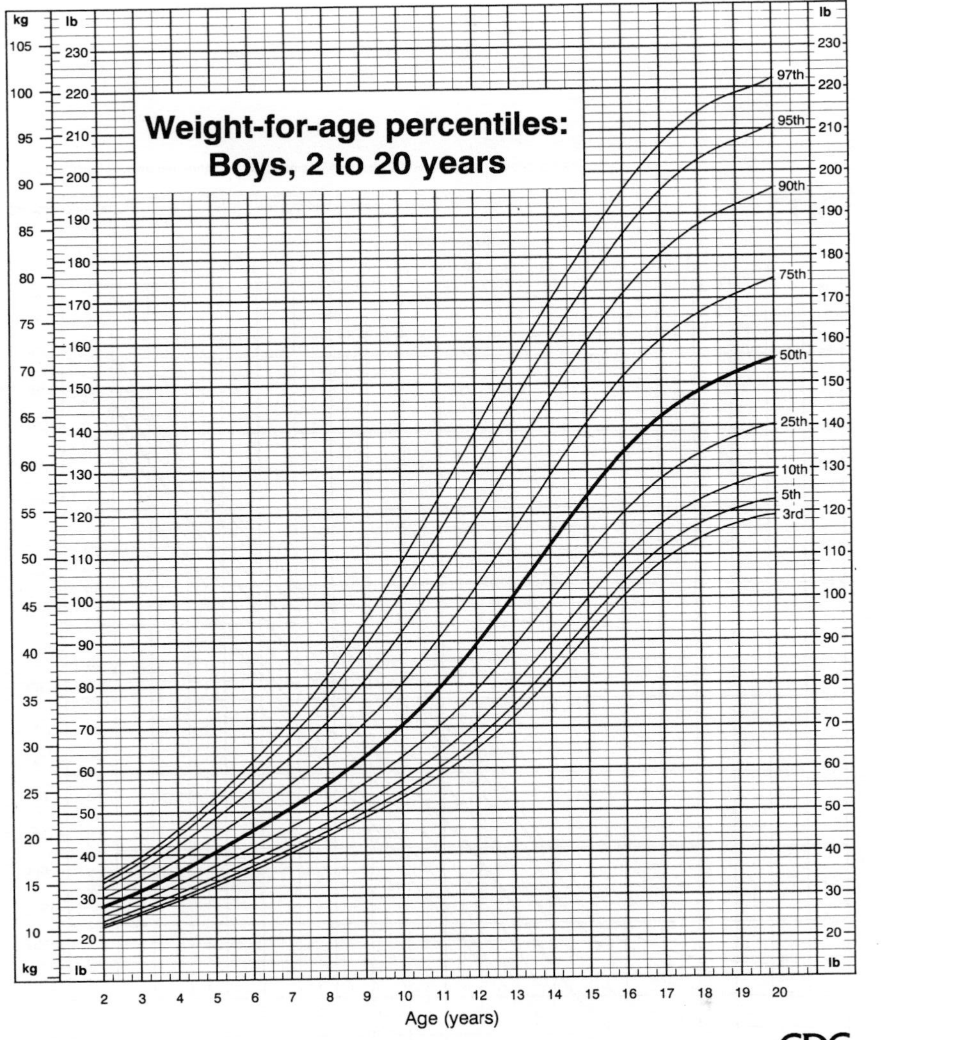

SOURCE: Developed by the National Center for Health Statistics in collaboration with the National Center for Chronic Disease Prevention and Health Promotion (2000).

Figure 9. Weight-for-age percentiles, boys, 2 to 20 years, CDC growth charts: United States

> FIGURE E-8B Weight-for-Age Percentiles: Girls, 2 to 20 Years

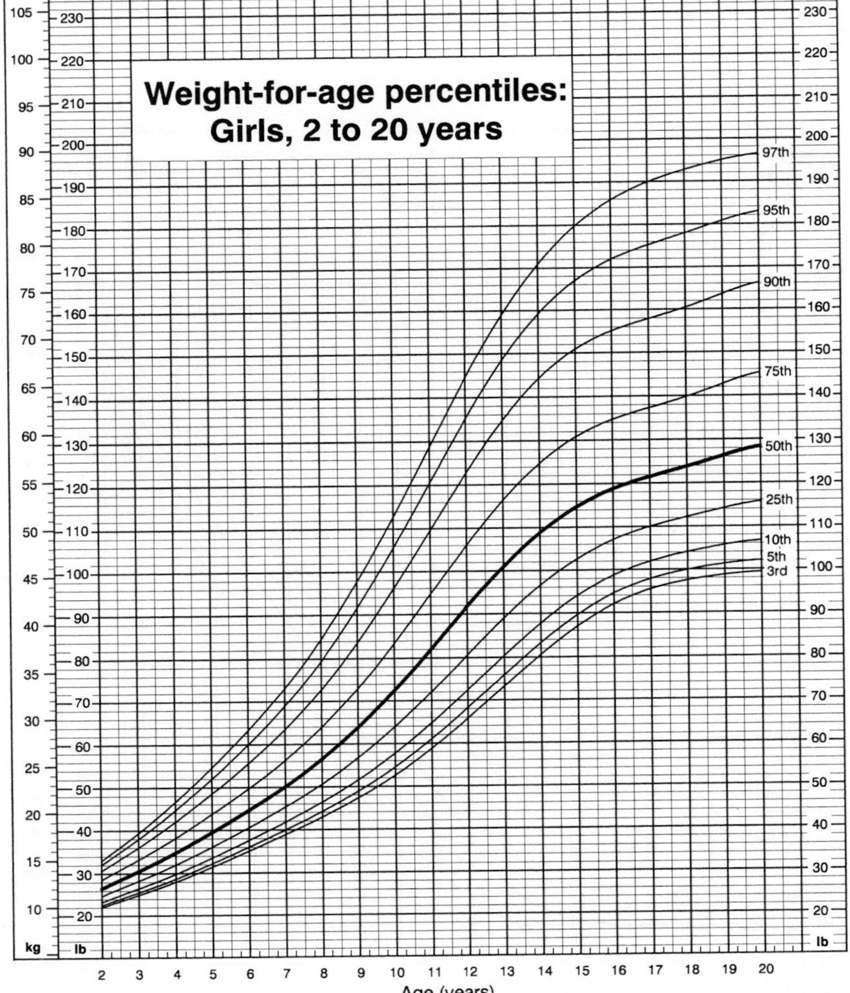

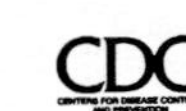

SOURCE: Developed by the National Center for Health Statistics in collaboration with the National Center for Chronic Disease Prevention and Health Promotion (2000).

Figure 10. Weight-for-age percentiles, girls, 2 to 20 years, CDC growth charts: United States

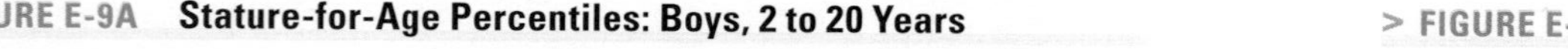

> FIGURE E-9A **Stature-for-Age Percentiles: Boys, 2 to 20 Years**

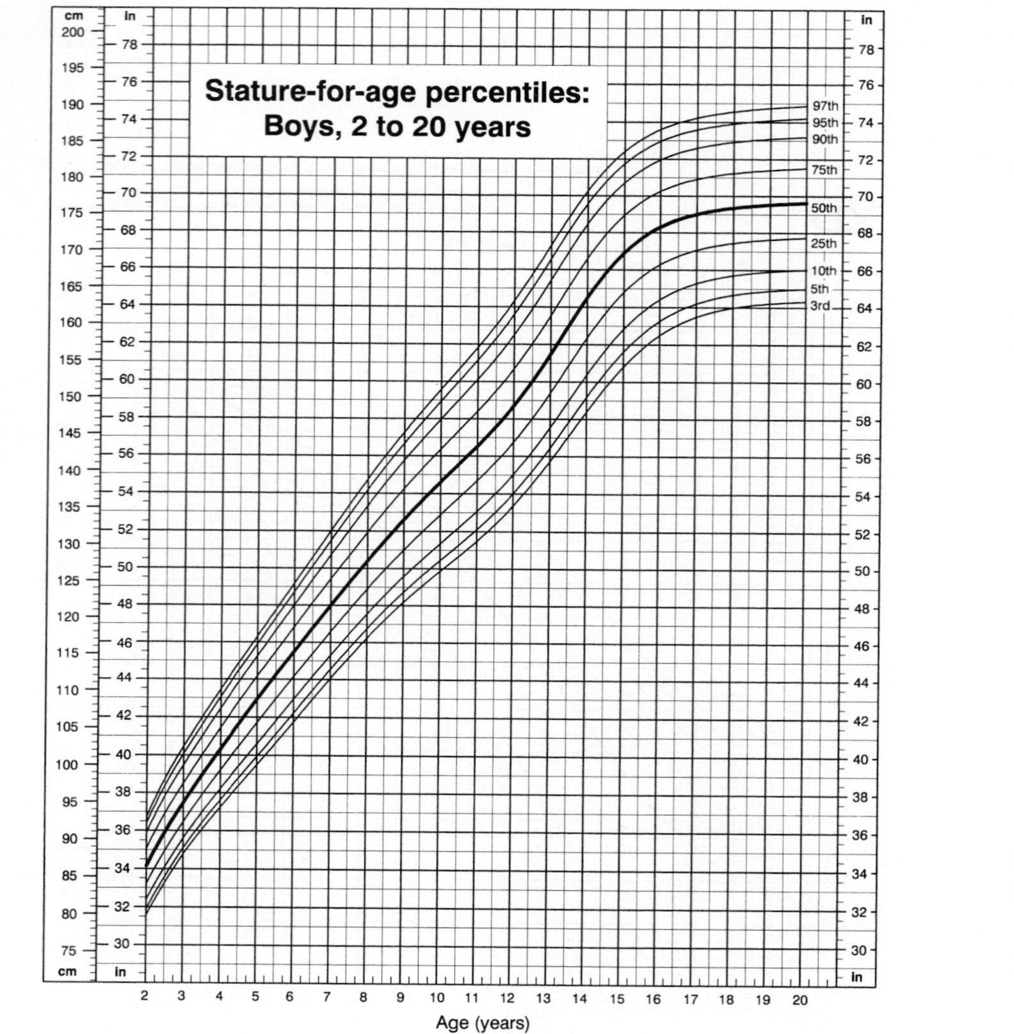

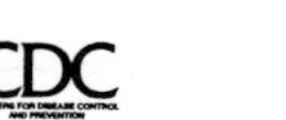

SOURCE: Developed by the National Center for Health Statistics in collaboration with the National Center for Chronic Disease Prevention and Health Promotion (2000).

Figure 11. Stature-for-age percentiles, boys, 2 to 20 years, CDC growth charts: United States

> FIGURE E-9B **Stature-for-Age Percentiles: Girls, 2 to 20 Years**

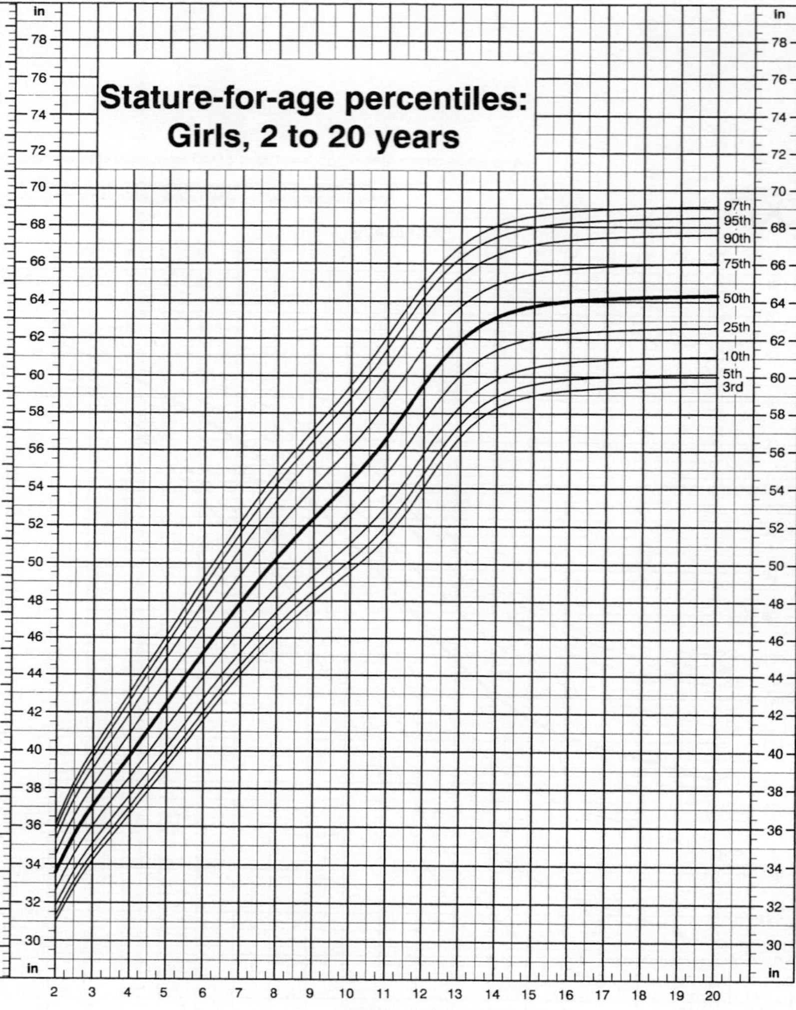

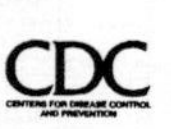

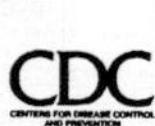

SOURCE: Developed by the National Center for Health Statistics in collaboration with the National Center for Chronic Disease Prevention and Health Promotion (2000).

Figure 12. Stature-for-age percentiles, girls, 2 to 20 years, CDC growth charts: United States

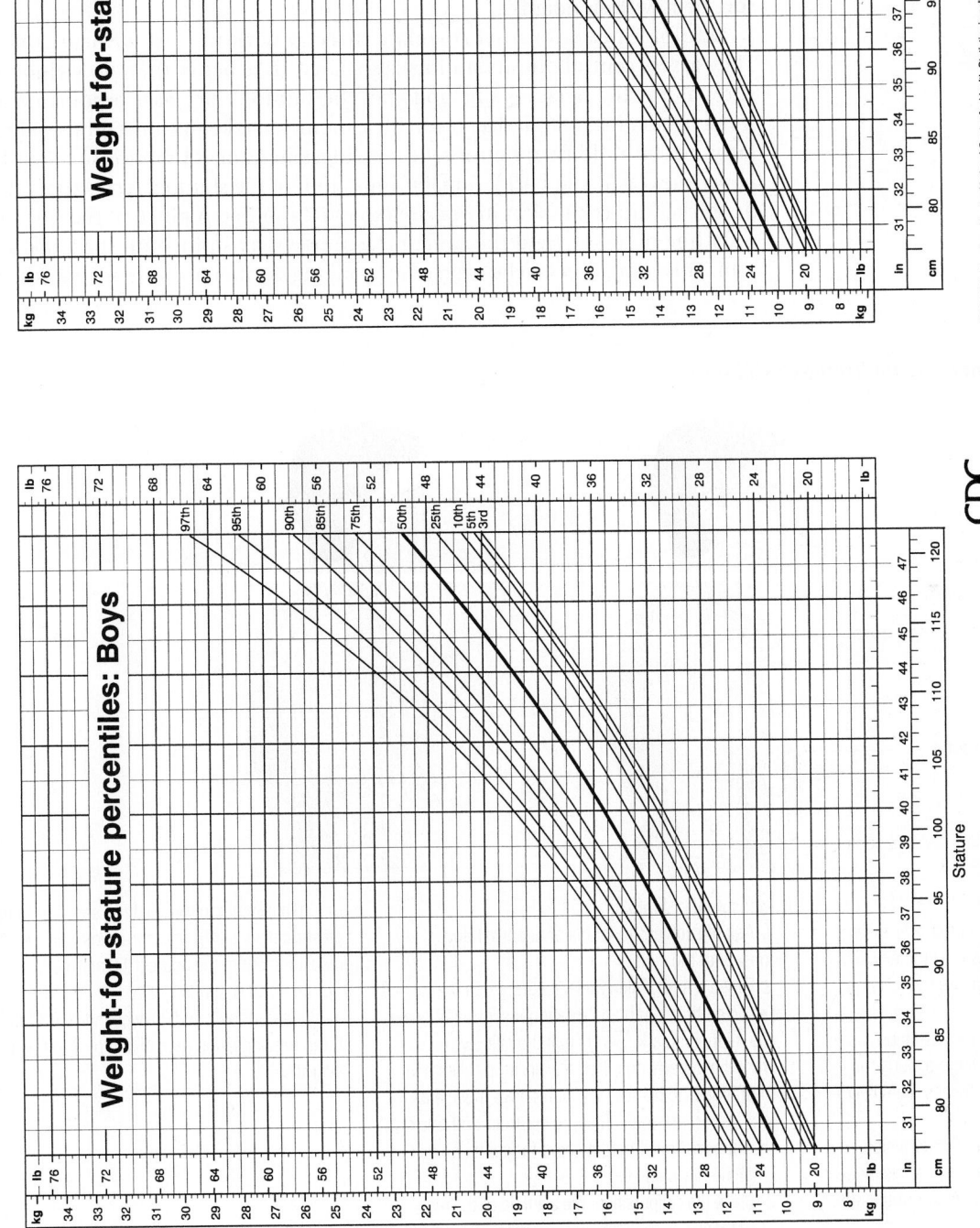

> FIGURE E-10A Weight-for-Stature Percentiles: Boys, 2 to 20 Years

> FIGURE E-10B Weight-for-Stature Percentiles: Girls, 2 to 20 Years

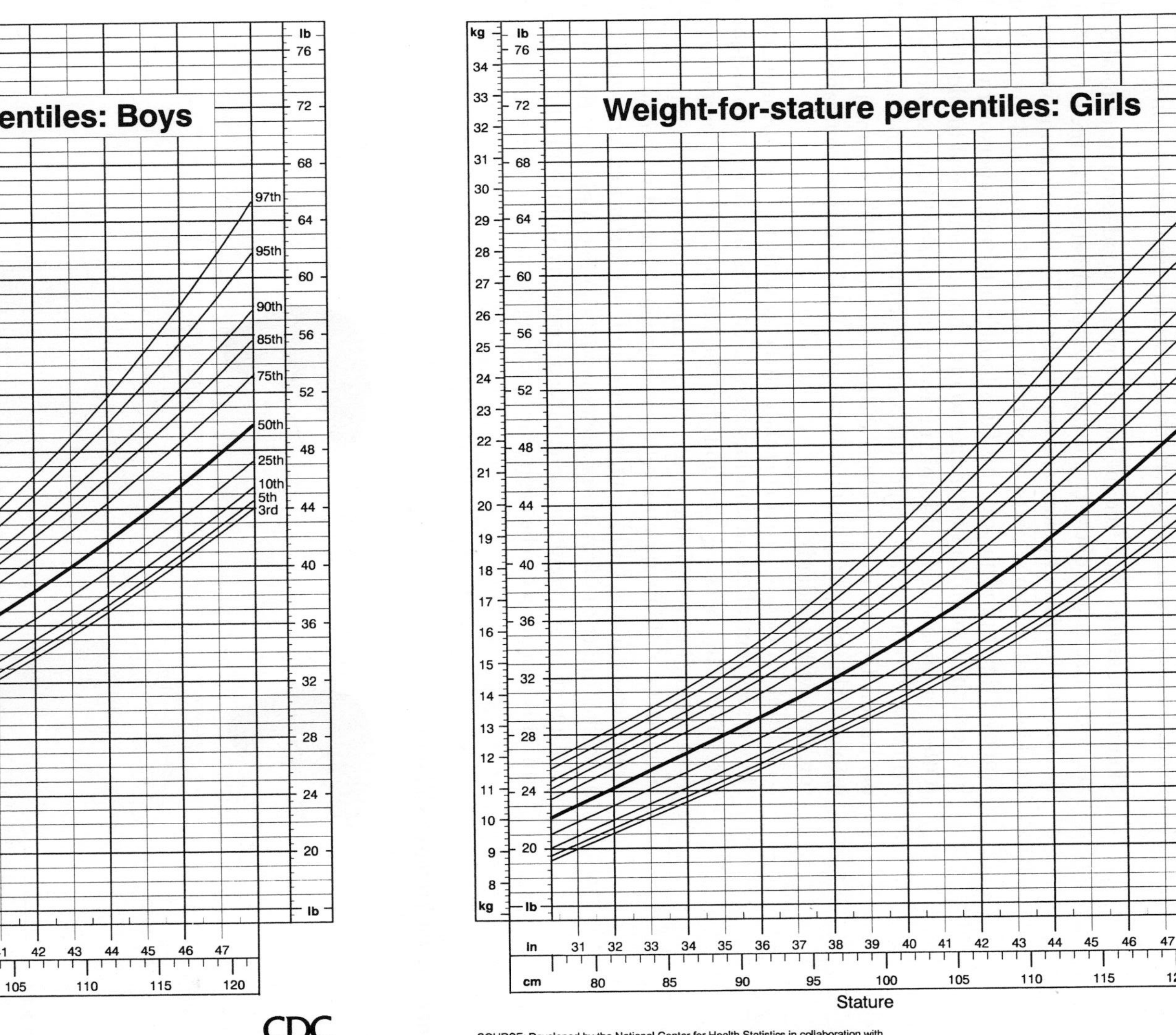

SOURCE: Developed by the National Center for Health Statistics in collaboration with the National Center for Chronic Disease Prevention and Health Promotion (2000).

Figure 13. Weight-for-stature percentiles, boys, CDC growth charts: United States

SOURCE: Developed by the National Center for Health Statistics in collaboration with the National Center for Chronic Disease Prevention and Health Promotion (2000).

Figure 14. Weight-for-stature percentiles, girls, CDC growth charts: United States

Measures of Body Fat and Lean Tissue Significant weight changes in both children and adults can reflect overnutrition and undernutrition. To estimate the degree to which fat stores or lean tissues are affected by overnutrition or malnutrition, several anthropometric measurements are useful (review Table E-3 on p. E-6).

Skinfold Measures Skinfold measures provide a good estimate of total body fat and a fair assessment of the fat's location. Approximately half the fat in the body lies directly beneath the skin, and the thickness of this subcutaneous fat reflects total body fat. In some parts of the body, such as the back and the back of the arm over the triceps muscle, this fat is loosely attached; a person can pull it up between the thumb and forefinger to obtain a measure of skinfold thickness. (Other common sites for skinfold measures include the biceps, subscapular area below the shoulder blade, suprailiac area above the hip bone, abdomen, and upper thigh.) To measure skinfold, a skilled assessor follows a standard procedure using reliable calipers (illustrated in Figure E-11) and then compares the measurement with standards.

Skinfold measurements correlate directly with the risk of heart disease. They assess central obesity and its associated risks better than do weight measures alone. If a person gains body fat, the skinfold increases proportionately; if the person loses fat, it decreases. Measurements taken from central-body sites (around the abdomen) better reflect changes in fatness than those taken from upper sites (arm and back). A major limitation of the skinfold test is that fat may be thicker under the skin in one area than in another. A pinch at the side of the waistline may not yield the same measurement as a pinch on the back of the arm. This limitation can be overcome by taking skinfold measurements at several

> **FIGURE E-11 How to Measure the Triceps Skinfold**

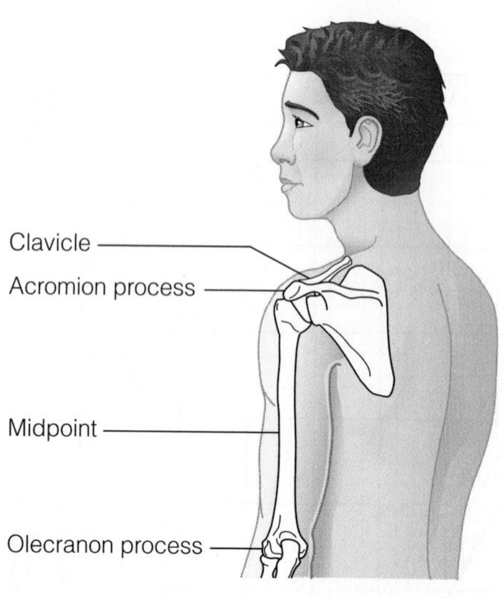

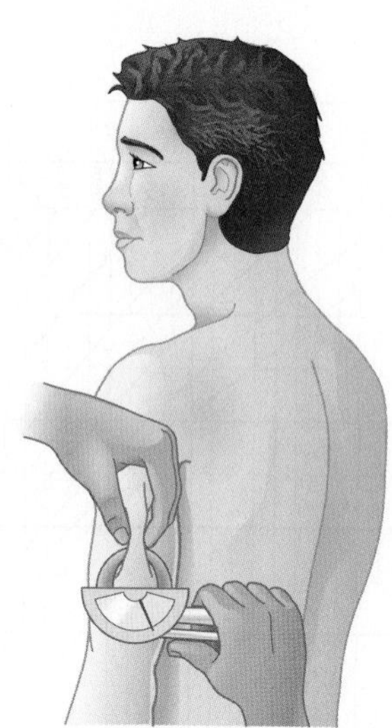

A. Find the midpoint of the arm:

1. Ask the subject to bend his or her arm at the elbow and lay the hand across the stomach. (If he or she is right-handed, measure the left arm, and vice versa.)
2. Feel the shoulder to locate the acromion process. It helps to slide your fingers along the clavicle to find the acromion process. The olecranon process is the tip of the elbow.
3. Place a measuring tape from the acromion process to the tip of the elbow. Divide this measurement by 2, and mark the midpoint of the arm with a pen.

B. Measure the skinfold:

1. Ask the subject to let his or her arm hang loosely to the side.
2. Grasp a fold of skin and subcutaneous fat between the thumb and forefinger slightly above the midpoint mark. Gently pull the skin away from the underlying muscle. (This step takes a lot of practice. To be sure you don't have muscle as well as fat, ask the subject to contract and relax the muscle. You should be able to feel if you are pinching muscle.)
3. Place the calipers over the skinfold at the midpoint mark, and read the measurement to the nearest 1.0 millimeter in two to three seconds. (If using plastic calipers, align pressure lines, and read the measurement to the nearest 1.0 millimeter in two to three seconds.)
4. Repeat steps 2 and 3 twice more. Add the three readings, and then divide by 3 to find the average.

(often three) different places on the body (including upper-, central-, and lower-body sites) and comparing each measurement with standards for that site. Multiple measures are not always practical in clinical settings, however, and most often, the triceps skinfold measurement alone is used because it is easily accessible. Skinfold measures are not useful in assessing changes in body fat over time.

Waist Circumference Chapter 8 describes how fat distribution correlates with health risks and mentioned that the waist circumference is a valuable indicator of fat distribution. To measure waist circumference, the assessor places a nonstretchable tape around the person's body, crossing just above the upper hip bones and making sure that the tape remains on a level horizontal plane on all sides (see Figure E-12). The tape is tightened slightly, but without compressing the skin.

Waist-to-Hip Ratio Alternatively, some clinicians measure both the waist and the hips. To calculate the waist-to-hip ratio, divide the waistline measurement by the hip measurement. For example, a woman with a 28-inch waist and 38-inch hips would have a ratio of 28 ÷ 38 = 0.74. Like the waist circumference, the waist-to-hip ratio also assesses abdominal obesity, but provides no more information than using the waist circumference alone. In general, women with a waist-to-hip ratio of 0.80 or greater and men with a waist-to-hip ratio of 0.90 or greater have a high risk of health problems.

Hydrodensitometry To estimate body density using hydrodensitometry, the person is weighed twice—first on land and then again when submerged under water. Underwater weighing usually generates a good estimate of body fat and is useful in research, although the technique has drawbacks: it requires bulky, expensive, and

> FIGURE E-12 **How to Measure Waist Circumference**

Place the measuring tape around the waist just above the bony crest of the hip. The tape runs parallel to the floor and is snug (but does not compress the skin). The measurement is taken at the end of normal expiration.

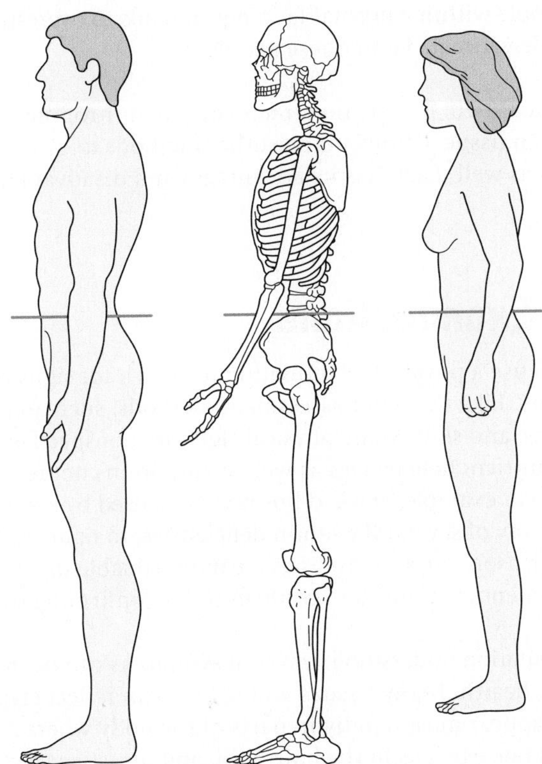

SOURCE: National Institutes of Health Obesity Education Initiative, *Clinical Guidelines on the Identification, Evaluation, and Treatment of Overweight and Obesity in Adults* (Washington, D.C.: U.S. Department of Health and Human Services, 1998), p. 59.

TABLE E-4 **Methods of Estimating Body Fat and Its Distribution**

Method	Cost	Ease of Use	Accuracy	Measures Fat Distribution
Height and weight	Low	Easy	High	No
Skinfolds	Low	Easy	Low	Yes
Circumferences	Low	Easy	Moderate	Yes
Ultrasound	Moderate	Moderate	Moderate	Yes
Hydrodensitometry	Low	Moderate	High	No
Heavy water tritiated	Moderate	Moderate	High	No
Deuterium oxide, or heavy oxygen	High	Moderate	High	No
Potassium isotope (^{40}K)	Very high	Difficult	High	No
Total body electrical conductivity (TOBEC)	High	Moderate	High	No
Bioelectric impedance (BIA)	Moderate	Easy	High	No
Dual-energy X-ray absorptiometry (DEXA)	High	Easy	High	No
Computed tomography (CT)	Very high	Difficult	High	Yes
Magnetic resonance imaging (MRI)	Very high	Difficult	High	Yes

SOURCE: Adapted from G. A. Bray, a handout presented at the North American Association for the Study of Obesity and Emory University School of Medicine Conference on Obesity. Update: Pathophysiology, Clinical Consequences, and Therapeutic Options, Atlanta, Georgia, August 31–September 2, 1992.

nonportable equipment. Furthermore, submerging some people (especially those who are very young, very old, ill, or fearful) under water is not always practical.

Bioelectric Impedance To measure body fat using the bioelectric impedance technique, a very-low-intensity electrical current is briefly sent through the body by way of electrodes placed on the wrist and ankle. As is true of other anthropometric techniques, bioelectrical impedance requires standardized procedures and calibrated instruments to provide reliable results. Recent food intake and hydration status, for example, influence results. Bioelectrical impedance is most accurate for people within a normal fat range; it tends to overestimate fat in lean people and underestimate fat in obese people.

Chapter 8 (Figure 8-10, p. 251) illustrates several anthropometric measures of body fat and lean tissue. Clinicians use other methods to estimate body fat and its distribution as well. Each has its advantages and disadvantages as Table E-4 summarizes.

Physical Examinations

An assessor can use a physical examination to search for signs of nutrient deficiency or toxicity. Like the other assessment methods, such an examination requires knowledge and skill. Many physical signs are nonspecific; they can reflect any of several nutrient deficiencies as well as conditions not related to nutrition (see Table E-5). For example, cracked lips may be caused by sunburn, windburn, dehydration, or any of several B vitamin deficiencies, to name just a few possible causes. For this reason, physical findings are most valuable in revealing problems for other assessment techniques to confirm or for confirming other assessment measures.

With this limitation understood, physical symptoms can be most informative about nutrition health. Many tissues and organs can reflect signs of malnutrition. The signs appear most rapidly in parts of the body where cell replacement occurs at a high rate, such as in the hair, skin, and digestive tract (including the mouth and tongue). The summary tables in Chapters 10, 11, 12, and 13 list additional physical signs of vitamin and mineral malnutrition.

TABLE E-5 Physical Findings Used in Nutrition Assessments

Body System	Signs of Good Health	Signs of Malnutrition	Other Possible Causes
Hair	Shiny, firm in the scalp	Dull, brittle, dry, loose; falls out (severe acute malnutrition); corkscrew hair (vitamin C)	Excessive hair bleaching; hair loss from aging, chemotherapy, or radiation therapy
Eyes	Bright, clear, pink, moist membranes; adjust easily to light	Pale membranes (iron); spots, dryness, night blindness (vitamin A); redness at corners of eyes (B vitamins)	Anemia unrelated to nutrition; eye disorders; allergies; aging
Mouth	No sores, swelling, or bleeding; red tongue; normal sense of taste; no caries; ability to chew and swallow; smooth lips	Bleeding gums (vitamin C); smooth or magenta tongue (B vitamins); poor taste sensation (zinc); dry, cracked, or sores in the corners of the lips (B vitamins)	Sunburn, windburn, excessive salivation from ill-fitting dentures or various disorders, medications, periodontal diseases, poor dental hygiene
Skin	Smooth, firm, good color	Poor wound healing (severe acute malnutrition, vitamin C, zinc); dry, rough, lack of fat under skin (essential fatty acids, vitamin A, B vitamins); bruising or bleeding under skin (vitamin C and vitamin K); pale (iron)	Poor skin hygiene, diabetes mellitus, aging, medications
Nails	Firm, pink, smooth	Spoon-shaped, brittle, pale (iron); rigid (protein malnutrition)	

Biochemical Analyses

All of the approaches to nutrition assessment discussed so far are external approaches. Biochemical analyses or laboratory tests help to determine what is happening to the body internally. Common tests are based on analysis of blood and urine samples, which contain nutrients, enzymes, and metabolites that reflect nutrition status. Other tests, such as blood glucose, help pinpoint disease-related problems with nutrition implications. Tests that define fluid and electrolyte balance, acid-base balance, and organ function also have nutrition implications. Table E-6 lists biochemical tests most useful for assessing vitamin and mineral status.

The interpretation of biochemical data requires skill. Long metabolic sequences lead to the production of the end-products and metabolites seen in blood and urine. No single test can reveal nutrition status because many factors influence test results. The low blood concentration of a nutrient may reflect a primary deficiency of that nutrient, but it may also be secondary to the deficiency of one or several other nutrients or to a disease. Taken together with other assessment data, however, laboratory test results help to create a picture that becomes clear with careful interpretation. They are especially useful in helping to detect subclinical malnutrition by uncovering early signs of malnutrition before the clinical signs of a classic deficiency disease appear.

Laboratory tests used to assess vitamin and mineral status (review Table E-6) are particularly useful when combined with diet histories and physical findings. Vitamin and mineral levels present in the blood and urine sometimes reflect recent rather than long-term intakes. This makes detecting subclinical deficiencies difficult. Furthermore, many nutrients interact; therefore, the amounts of other nutrients in the body can affect a lab value for a particular nutrient. It is also important to remember that nonnutrient conditions such as diseases influence biochemical measures.

It is beyond the scope of this text to describe all lab tests and their relations to nutrition status. Instead, the emphasis is on lab tests used to detect protein malnutrition and nutritional anemias.

Protein Malnutrition No single biochemical analysis can adequately evaluate protein malnutrition. This discussion focuses on the measures commonly used today—transthyretin, retinol-binding protein, serum transferrin, and IGF-1 (insulin-like growth factor 1). Table E-7 provides standards for these indicators.

TABLE E-6 Biochemical Tests Useful for Assessing Vitamin and Mineral Status

Nutrient	Assessment Tests
Vitamins	
Vitamin A	Serum retinol, retinol-binding protein
Thiamin[a]	Erythrocyte (red blood cell) transketolase activity, erythrocyte thiamin pyrophosphate
Riboflavin[a]	Erythrocyte glutathione reductase activity
Vitamin B_6[a]	Urinary xanthurenic acid excretion after tryptophan load test, erythrocyte transaminase activity, plasma pyridoxal 5′-phosphate (PLP)
Niacin	Plasma or urinary metabolites NMN (N-methyl nicotinamide) or 2-pyridone, or preferably both expressed as a ratio
Folate[b]	Serum folate, erythrocyte folate (reflects liver stores)
Vitamin B_{12}[b]	Serum vitamin B_{12}, serum and urinary methylmalonic acid, Schilling test
Biotin	Urinary biotin, urinary 3-hydroxyisovaleric acid
Vitamin C	Plasma vitamin C[c], leukocyte vitamin C
Vitamin D	Serum vitamin D
Vitamin E	Serum α-tocopherol, erythrocyte hemolysis
Vitamin K	Serum vitamin K, plasma prothrombin; blood-clotting time (prothrombin time) is not an adequate indicator
Minerals	
Phosphorus	Serum phosphate
Sodium	Serum sodium
Chloride	Serum chloride
Potassium	Serum potassium
Magnesium	Serum magnesium, urinary magnesium
Iron	Hemoglobin, hematocrit, serum ferritin, total iron-binding capacity (TIBC), erythrocyte protoporphyrin, serum iron, transferrin saturation
Iodine	Serum thyroxine or thyroid-stimulating hormone (TSH), urinary iodine
Zinc	Plasma zinc, hair zinc
Copper	Erythrocyte superoxide dismutase, serum copper, serum ceruloplasmin
Selenium	Erythrocyte selenium, glutathione peroxidase activity

[a]Urinary measurements for these vitamins are common, but may be of limited use. Urinary measurements reflect recent dietary intakes and may not provide reliable information concerning the severity of a deficiency.
[b]Folate assessments should always be conducted in conjunction with vitamin B_{12} assessments (and vice versa) to help distinguish the cause of common deficiency symptoms.
[c]Vitamin C shifts between the plasma and the white blood cells known as leukocytes; thus a plasma determination may not accurately reflect the body's pool. A measurement of leukocyte vitamin C can provide information about the body's stores of vitamin C. A combination of both tests may be more reliable than either one alone.
SOURCE: Adapted from H. E. Sauberlich, *Laboratory Tests for the Assessment of Nutritional Status* (Boca Raton, FIA.: CRC Press, 1999).

Although serum albumin is easily and routinely measured, it lacks the sensitivity to assess protein malnutrition because of its long turnover rate.*

Transthyretin and Retinol-Binding Protein Transthyretin and retinol-binding protein occur as a complex in the plasma.** They have a rapid turnover and thus respond quickly to dietary protein inadequacy and therapy.*** Conditions other than malnutrition that lower transthyretin include metabolic stress, hemodialysis, and hypothyroidism; those that raise transthyretin include kidney disease and corticosteroid use. Conditions other than protein malnutrition that lower retinol-binding protein include vitamin A deficiency, metabolic stress, hyperthyroidism, liver disease, and cystic fibrosis; kidney disease raises retinol-binding protein levels.

TABLE E-7 Normal Values for Serum Proteins

Test	Normal Values
Albumin (g/dL)	3.5–5.0
Transferrin (mg/dL)	200–400
Transthyretin (mg/dL)	16–40
Retinol-binding protein (mg/dL)	3–7
IGF-1 (μg/L)	300

NOTE: Levels less than normal suggest compromised protein status.

*The half-life of albumin is 14 to 20 days, an indication of a slow degradation rate.
**Transthyretin is also known as *prealbumin* or *thyroxine-binding prealbumin*.
***The half-lives of transthyretin and retinol-binding protein are 2 days and 12 hours, respectively.

Serum Transferrin Serum transferrin transports iron; consequently, its concentrations reflect both protein and iron status. Using transferrin as an indicator of protein status is complicated when an iron deficiency is present. Transferrin rises as iron deficiency grows worse and falls as iron status improves. Markedly reduced transferrin levels indicate severe protein malnutrition; in mild-to-moderate protein malnutrition, transferrin levels may vary, limiting their usefulness. Conditions other than protein malnutrition that lower transferrin include liver disease, kidney disease, and metabolic stress; those that raise transferrin include pregnancy, iron deficiency, hepatitis, blood loss, and oral contraceptive use. Although transferrin breaks down in the body more quickly than albumin, it is still relatively slow to respond to changes in protein intake and is not a sensitive indicator of the response to therapy.*

IGF-1 (Insulin-like Growth Factor 1) IGF-1 (insulin-like growth factor 1) declines in protein malnutrition. IGF-1 has a relatively short half-life and responds specifically to dietary protein rather than energy.** For these reasons, it is a sensitive indicator of protein status and response to therapy. Conditions that decrease IGF-1 include anorexia nervosa, inflammatory bowel disease, celiac disease, HIV infection, and fasting.

Nutritional Anemias

Anemia, a symptom of a wide variety of nutrition- and nonnutrition-related disorders, is characterized by a reduced number of red blood cells. Iron, folate, and vitamin B_{12} deficiencies caused by inadequate intake, poor absorption, or abnormal metabolism of these nutrients are the most common nutritional anemias. The remainder of this appendix describes laboratory tests that distinguish among the various nutrition-related anemias. Some nonnutrition-related causes of anemia include massive blood loss, infections, hereditary blood disorders such as sickle-cell anemia, and chronic liver or kidney disease.

Assessment of Iron-Deficiency Anemia

Iron deficiency, a common mineral deficiency, develops in stages. First, iron stores diminish, then transport iron decreases, and finally hemoglobin production falls. Chapter 13 describes iron deficiency in detail. This section describes tests used to uncover iron deficiency as it progresses. Table E-8 (p. E-20) provides values used for assessing iron status. Although other tests are more specific in detecting early deficiencies, hemoglobin and hematocrit are the most commonly available tests.

Hemoglobin Iron forms an integral part of the hemoglobin molecule that transports oxygen to the cells. In iron deficiency, the body cannot synthesize hemoglobin. Low hemoglobin values signal depleted iron stores. Table E-8 provides normal hemoglobin values. Hemoglobin's usefulness in evaluating iron status is limited, however, because hemoglobin concentrations drop fairly late in the development of iron deficiency, and other nutrient deficiencies and medical conditions can also alter hemoglobin concentrations.

Hematocrit Hematocrit is commonly used to diagnose iron-deficiency anemia, even though it is an inconclusive measure of iron status. The hematocrit is the percentage of red blood cells in the total blood volume. Table E-8 on p. E-20 includes normal values for hematocrit. Low values indicate microcytic (abnormally small-celled), hypochromic (abnormally lacking in color) red blood cells.

Low hemoglobin and hematocrit values alert the assessor to the possibility of iron deficiency. However, many nutrients and other conditions can affect hemoglobin and hematocrit. The following tests of iron status help pinpoint true iron deficiency.

Serum Ferritin In the first stage of iron deficiency, iron stores diminish. Measures of serum ferritin provide an estimate of iron stores. Serum ferritin is

*The half-life of transferrin is 8 to 10 days.

**The half-life of IGF-1 is 12 to 15 hours.

TABLE E-8 **Normal Values for Iron**

Test	Normal Values
Hemoglobin (g/dL)	12–16 (female)
	13–17 (male)
Hematocrit (%)	35–45 (female)
	39–49 (male)
Serum ferritin (ng/mL)	30–300
Total iron-binding capacity (μg/dL)	250–450
Serum iron (mg/dL)	50–180
Mean corpuscualr volume (fL)	80–100
Transferrin (mg/dL)	200–360
Transferrin saturation (%)	20–50
Erythrocyte protoporphyrin (μg/dL RBC)	<70

not a reliable indicator of iron deficiency, however, because its concentrations are increased by infection, inflammation, alcohol consumption, and liver disease.

The second stage of iron deficiency is characterized by a decrease in transport iron. This is revealed by an increase in the iron-binding capacity of the protein transferrin and a decrease in serum iron. These changes are reflected by the transferrin saturation, which is calculated from the ratio of the other two values as described in the following paragraphs.

Total Iron-Binding Capacity (TIBC) Iron travels through the blood bound to the protein transferrin. TIBC is a measure of the total amount of iron that transferrin can carry. Lab technicians measure iron-binding capacity directly. Table E-8 includes the normal values for TIBC.

Serum Iron Lab technicians can also measure serum iron directly. Elevated values indicate iron overload; reduced values indicate iron deficiency. Table E-8 shows the normal values for serum iron.

Transferrin Saturation The percentage of transferrin that is saturated with iron is an indirect measure that is derived from the serum iron and total iron-binding capacity measures as follows:

$$\% \text{ Transferrin} = \frac{\text{serum iron}}{\text{total iron-binding capacity}} \times 100$$

Table E-8 shows normal values for transferrin saturation. During iron deficiency, transferrin saturation decreases. The transferrin saturation value is a useful indicator of iron status because it includes information about both the iron and transferrin content of the blood.

The third stage of iron deficiency occurs when the supply of transport iron diminishes to the point that it limits hemoglobin production. It is characterized by increases in erythrocyte protoporphyrin, a decrease in mean corpuscular volume, and decreased hemoglobin and hematocrit.

Erythrocyte Protoporphyrin The iron-containing portion of the hemoglobin molecule is heme. Heme is a combination of iron and protoporphyrin. Protoporphyrin accumulates in the blood when iron supplies are inadequate for the formation of heme. Protoporphyrin may also increase when hemoglobin synthesis is impaired for other reasons, such as lead poisoning or inflammation. Lab technicians can measure erythrocyte protoporphyrin directly in a blood sample. The normal values of erythrocyte protoporphyrin are shown in Table E-8.

Mean Corpuscular Volume (MCV) The hematocrit value divided by the red blood cell count provides a measure of the average size of a red blood cell, referred to as the mean corpuscular volume (MCV). Such a measure helps to classify the type of nutrient anemia. In iron deficiency, the red blood cells are smaller than average.

Assessment of Folate and Vitamin B_{12} Anemias

Folate deficiency and vitamin B_{12} deficiency present a similar clinical picture—an anemia characterized by abnormally large red blood cell precursors (megaloblasts) in the bone marrow and abnormally large, mature red blood cells (macrocytic cells) in the blood. Distinguishing between these two deficiencies is essential because their treatments differ. Giving folate to a person with vitamin B_{12} deficiency improves many of the lab test results indicative of vitamin B_{12} deficiency, but this is a dangerous error because vitamin B_{12} deficiency causes nerve damage that folate cannot correct. Thus inappropriate folate administration masks vitamin B_{12}-deficiency anemia, and nerve damage worsens. For this reason, it is critical to determine whether the anemia results from a folate deficiency or from a vitamin B_{12} deficiency. The following biochemical assessment measures help to make this distinction.

Mean Corpuscular Volume (MCV) As previously mentioned, the MCV is a measure of red blood cell size. In folate and vitamin B_{12} deficiencies, the red blood cells are larger than average (macrocytic). Additional tests must be performed to differentiate folate deficiency from vitamin B_{12} deficiency. Macrocytic cells may also result from a high alcohol intake, liver disease, and various medications.

Serum Folate and Vitamin B_{12} Levels Analyses of serum folate and vitamin B_{12} levels are usually among the first tests conducted to determine the cause of macrocytic red blood cells. Low serum levels of either nutrient is consistent with a deficiency, whereas adequate levels can help rule out deficiency. Folate levels are not a specific measure of folate status, however; they increase with folate consumption and decrease with alcohol consumption, pregnancy, or use of anticonvulsant medications. Folate depletion is characterized by a fall in the folate concentrations of red blood cells (erythrocytes). As erythrocyte folate levels diminish, folate-deficiency anemia develops. Because low erythrocyte folate concentrations also occur with vitamin B_{12} deficiency, serum vitamin B_{12} concentrations must also be measured. Table E-9 shows standards for folate and vitamin B_{12} assessment.

Methylmalonic Acid and Homocysteine Levels To determine whether a nutrient is deficient, measures are taken of substances that accumulate when the functions of the nutrient are impaired. For example, the amino acid homocysteine

TABLE E-9 Normal Values for Folate and Vitamin B_{12}

Test	Normal Values
Serum folate (ng/mL)[a]	3–16
Serum homocysteine (µmol/L)	5–14
Erythrocyte folate (ng/mL)[a]	140–628
Serum vitamin B_{12} (pg/mL)	200–835
Serum methylmalonic acid (nmol/L)	70–270

NOTE: A nanogram (ng) is one-billionth of a gram; a picogram (pg) is one-trillionth of a gram.
[a]To convert folate values (ng/mL) to international standard units (nmol/L), multiply by 2.266.

usually increase in both folate and vitamin B_{12} deficiencies because both nutrients are needed for its metabolism. Methylmalonic acid is a breakdown product of several amino acids and requires vitamin B_{12} for its metabolism; its concentrations are elevated in vitamin B_{12} deficiency, but not in folate deficiency. Thus this measure is useful in distinguishing between the two.

Schilling Test Vitamin B_{12} deficiency usually arises from malabsorption, not from poor intake. To determine whether malabsorption is the cause, a small oral dose of radioactive vitamin B_{12} is given, and urinary excretion is measured. This test is rarely performed, but it measures vitamin B_{12} absorption and is called a Schilling test.

Antibodies to Intrinsic Factor Serum antibodies for intrinsic factor can help confirm a diagnosis of pernicious anemia, an autoimmune disease characterized by destruction of the cells that produce intrinsic factor. Intrinsic factor is a protein required for vitamin B_{12} absorption, as Chapter 10 explains.

Cautions about Nutrition Assessment

The tests outlined here yield information that becomes meaningful only when conducted and interpreted by a skilled clinician. Potential sources of error may be introduced at any step, from the collection of samples and data to their reporting and analyses. Equipment must be regularly calibrated to ensure accuracy of measurements. In addition, the assessor must keep in mind that each assessment method and measure is useful to confirm or eliminate the possibility of suspected nutrition problems. For example, the assessor must constantly remember that a sufficient intake of a nutrient does not guarantee adequate nutrient status for an individual. Conversely, the apparent inadequate intake of a nutrient does not, by itself, establish that a deficiency exists.

Appendix F Estimated Energy Needs

Chapter 8 described how to calculate estimated energy requirements (EER) by using an equation that accounts for gender, age, weight, height, and physical activity level. This appendix presents tables that provide a shortcut to estimating daily energy requirements, as developed by the *Dietary Guidelines for Americans*, and based on the EER equations of the Dietary Reference Intakes.

Table F-1 describes three activity levels: sedentary, moderately active, and active. Table F-2 presents estimated daily energy needs by age, gender, and these three levels of physical activity. Keep in mind that these values are estimates that have been rounded to the nearest 200 kcalories; an individual's energy needs may be higher or lower than these average estimates. EER equations for this table use reference heights and weights. For children and adolescents, reference heights and weights vary. For adults, the reference man is 5 feet 10 inches tall and weighs 154 pounds and the reference woman is 5 feet 4 inches tall and weighs 126 pounds. Estimates for women do not include women who are pregnant or breastfeeding.

TABLE F-1 Sedentary, Moderately Active, and Active People

Sedentary	A lifestyle that includes only the light physical activity associated with typical day-to-day life.
Moderately active	A lifestyle that includes physical activity equivalent to walking about 1.5 to 3 miles per day at 3 to 4 miles per hour in addition to the light physical activity associated with typical day-to-day life.
Active	A lifestyle that includes physical activity equivalent to walking more than 3 miles per day at 3 to 4 miles per hour in addition to the light physical activity associated with typical day-to-day life.

TABLE F-2 Estimated Daily kCalorie Needs by Age, Gender, and Physical Activity Level

Age (years)	Gender/Activity Level					
	Male/Sedentary	Male/Moderately Active	Male/Active	Female/Sedentary	Female/Moderately Active	Female/Active
2	1000	1000	1000	1000	1000	1000
3	1200	1400	1400	1000	1200	1400
4	1200	1400	1600	1200	1400	1400
5	1200	1400	1600	1200	1400	1600
6	1400	1600	1800	1200	1400	1600
7	1400	1600	1800	1200	1600	1800
8	1400	1600	2000	1400	1600	1800
9	1600	1800	2000	1400	1600	1800
10	1600	1800	2200	1400	1800	2000

Continued

TABLE F-2 Estimated Daily kCalorie Needs by Age, Gender, and Physical Activity Level *(continued)*

Age (years)	Gender/Activity Level					
	Male/Sedentary	Male/Moderately Active	Male/Active	Female/Sedentary	Female/Moderately Active	Female/Active
11	1800	2000	2200	1600	1800	2000
12	1800	2200	2400	1600	2000	2200
13	2000	2200	2600	1600	2000	2200
14	2000	2400	2800	1800	2000	2400
15	2200	2600	3000	1800	2000	2400
16–18	2400	2800	3200	1800	2000	2400
19–20	2600	2800	3000	2000	2200	2400
21–25	2400	2800	3000	2000	2200	2400
26–30	2400	2600	3000	1800	2000	2400
31–35	2400	2600	3000	1800	2000	2200
36–40	2400	2600	2800	1800	2000	2200
41–45	2200	2600	2800	1800	2000	2200
46–50	2200	2400	2800	1800	2000	2200
51–55	2200	2400	2800	1600	1800	2200
56–60	2200	2400	2600	1600	1800	2200
61–65	2000	2400	2600	1600	1800	2000
66–75	2000	2200	2600	1600	1800	2000
76+	2000	2200	2400	1600	1800	2000

SOURCE: U.S. Department of Agriculture and U.S. Department of Health and Human Services, *Dietary Guidelines for Americans 2010*, www.dietaryguidelines.gov.

Appendix G Exchange Lists for Diabetes

Chapter 2 introduces the exchange system, and this appendix provides details from the *2008 Choose Your Foods: Exchange Lists for Diabetes*. Exchange lists can help people with diabetes to manage their blood glucose levels by controlling the amount and kinds of carbohydrates they consume. These lists can also help in planning diets for weight management by controlling kcalorie and fat intake.*

CONTENTS

The Exchange System

The exchange system sorts foods into groups by their proportions of carbohydrate, fat, and protein (Table G-1). These groups may be organized into several exchange lists of foods (Tables G-2 through G-12 on pp. G-3–G-16). For example, the carbohydrate group includes these exchange lists:

- Starch
- Fruits
- Milk (fat-free, reduced-fat, and whole)
- Sweets, Desserts, and Other Carbohydrates
- Nonstarchy Vegetables

TABLE G-1 The Food Lists

Lists	Typical Item/Portion Size	Carbohydrate (g)	Protein (g)	Fat (g)	Energy[a] (kcal)
Carbohydrates					
Starch[b]	1 slice bread	15	0–3	0–1	80
Fruits	1 small apple	15	—	—	60
Milk					
Fat-free, low-fat, 1%	1 c fat-free milk	12	8	0–3	100
Reduced-fat, 2%	1 c reduced-fat milk	12	8	5	120
Whole	1 c whole milk	12	8	8	160
Sweets, desserts, and other carbohydrates[c]	2 small cookies	15	varies	varies	varies
Nonstarchy vegetables	½ c cooked carrots	5	2	—	25
Meat and Meat Substitutes					
Lean	1 oz chicken (no skin)	—	7	0–3	45
Medium-fat	1 oz ground beef	—	7	4–7	75
High-fat	1 oz pork sausage	—	7	8+	100
Plant-based proteins	½ c tofu	varies	7	varies	varies
Fats	1 tsp butter	—	—	5	45
Alcohol	12 oz beer	varies	—	—	100

[a]The energy value for each exchange list represents an approximate average for the group and does not reflect the precise number of grams of carbohydrate, protein, and fat. For example, a slice of bread contains 15 grams of carbohydrate (60 kcalories), 3 grams protein (12 kcalories), and a little fat—rounded to 80 kcalories for ease in calculating. A ½ cup of vegetables (not including starchy vegetables) contains 5 grams carbohydrate (20 kcalories) and 2 grams protein (8 more), which has been rounded down to 25 kcalories.

[b]The Starch list includes cereals, grains, breads, crackers, snacks, starchy vegetables (such as corn, peas, and potatoes), and legumes (dried beans, peas, and lentils).

[c]The Sweets, Desserts, and Other Carbohydrates list includes foods that contain added sugars and fats such as sodas, candy, cakes, cookies, doughnuts, ice cream, pudding, syrup, and frozen yogurt.

*The Exchange Lists are the basis of a meal planning system designed by a committee of the American Diabetes Association and The Academy of Nutrition and Dietetics. While designed primarily for people with diabetes and others who must follow special diets, the Exchange Lists are based on principles of good nutrition that apply to everyone.

Then any food on a list can be "exchanged" for any other on that same list. Another group for alcohol has been included as a reminder that these beverages often deliver substantial carbohydrate and kcalories, and therefore warrant their own list.

Serving Sizes

The serving sizes have been carefully adjusted and defined so that a serving of any food on a given list provides roughly the same amount of carbohydrate, fat, and protein, and, therefore, total energy. Any food on a list can thus be exchanged, or traded, for any other food on the same list without significantly affecting the diet's energy-nutrient balance or total kcalories. For example, a person may select 17 small grapes or ½ large grapefruit as one fruit exchange, and either choice would provide roughly 15 grams of carbohydrate and 60 kcalories. A whole grapefruit, however, would count as 2 fruit exchanges.

To apply the system successfully, users must become familiar with the specified serving sizes. A convenient way to remember the serving sizes and energy values is to keep in mind a typical item from each list (review Table G-1).

The Foods on the Lists

Foods do not always appear on the exchange list where you might first expect to find them. They are grouped according to their energy-nutrient contents rather than by their source (such as milks), their outward appearance, or their vitamin and mineral contents. For example, cheeses are grouped with meats (not milk) because, like meats, cheeses contribute energy from protein and fat but provide negligible carbohydrate.

For similar reasons, starchy vegetables such as corn, green peas, and potatoes are found on the Starch list with breads and cereals, not with the vegetables. Likewise, bacon is grouped with the fats and oils, not with the meats.

Diet planners learn to view mixtures of foods, such as casseroles and soups, as combinations of foods from different exchange lists. They also learn to interpret food labels with the exchange system in mind.

Controlling Energy, Fat, and Sodium

The exchange lists help people control their energy intakes by paying close attention to serving sizes. People wanting to lose weight can limit foods from the Sweets, Desserts, and Other Carbohydrates and Fats lists, and they might choose to avoid the Alcohol list altogether. The Free Foods list provide low-kcalorie choices.

By assigning items like bacon to the Fats list, the exchange lists alert consumers to foods that are unexpectedly high in fat. Even the Starch list specifies which grain products contain added fat (such as biscuits, cornbread, and waffles) by marking them with a symbol to indicate added fat (the symbols are explained in the table keys). In addition, the exchange lists encourage users to think of fat-free milk as milk and of whole milk as milk with added fat, and to think of lean meats as meats and of medium-fat and high-fat meats as meats with added fat. To that end, foods on the milk and meat lists are separated into categories based on their fat contents (review Table G-1). The Milk list is subdivided for fat-free, reduced fat, and whole; the meat list is subdivided for lean, medium fat, and high fat. The meat list also includes plant-based proteins, which tend to be rich in fiber. Notice that many of these foods (p. G-11) bear the symbol for "high fiber."

People wanting to control the sodium in their diets can begin by eliminating any foods bearing the "high sodium" symbol. In most cases, the symbol identifies foods that, in one serving, provide 480 milligrams or more of sodium. Foods on the Combination Foods or Fast Foods lists that bear the symbol provide more than 600 milligrams of sodium. Other foods may also contribute substantially to sodium (consult Chapter 12 for details).

Planning a Healthy Diet

To obtain a daily variety of foods that provide healthful amounts of carbohydrate, protein, and fat, as well as vitamins, minerals, and fiber, the meal plan for adults and teenagers should include at least:

- Two to three servings of nonstarchy vegetables
- Two servings of fruits
- Six servings of grains (at least three of whole grains), beans, and starchy vegetables
- Two servings of low-fat or fat-free milk
- About 6 ounces of meat or meat substitutes
- *Small* amounts of fat and sugar

The actual amounts are determined by age, gender, activity levels, and other factors that influence energy needs.

APPENDIX G

TABLE G-2 Starch

The Starch list includes bread, cereals and grains, starchy vegetables, crackers and snacks, and legumes (dried beans, peas, and lentils).
1 starch choice = 15 grams carbohydrate, 0–3 grams protein, 0–1 grams fat, and 80 kcalories.

NOTE: In general, one starch exchange is ½ cup cooked cereal, grain, or starchy vegetable; ⅓ cup cooked rice or pasta; 1 ounce of bread product; ¾ ounce to 1 ounce of most snack foods.

Bread

Food	Serving Size
Bagel, large (about 4 oz)	¼ (1 oz)
(!) Biscuit, 2½ inches across	1
Bread	
(☺) reduced-kcalorie	2 slices (1½ oz)
white, whole-grain, pumpernickel, rye, unfrosted raisin	1 slice (1 oz)
Chapatti, small, 6 inches across	1
(!) Cornbread, 1¾ inch cube	1 (1½ oz)
English muffin	½
Hot dog bun or hamburger bun	½ (1 oz)
Naan, 8 inches by 2 inches	¼
Pancake, 4 inches across, ¼ inch thick	1
Pita, 6 inches across	½
Roll, plain, small	1 (1 oz)
(!) Stuffing, bread	⅓ cup
(!) Taco shell, 5 inches across	2
Tortilla, corn, 6 inches across	1
Tortilla, flour, 6 inches across	1
Tortilla, flour, 10 inches across	⅓
(!) Waffle, 4-inch square or 4 inches across	1

Cereals and Grains

Food	Serving Size
Barley, cooked	⅓ cup
Bran, dry	
(☺) oat	¼ cup
(☺) wheat	½ cup
(☺) Bulgur (cooked)	½ cup
Cereals	
(☺) bran	½ cup
cooked (oats, oatmeal)	½ cup
puffed	1½ cups
shredded wheat, plain	½ cup
sugar-coated	½ cup
unsweetened, ready-to-eat	¾ cup
Couscous	⅓ cup
Granola	
low-fat	¼ cup
(!) regular	¼ cup
Grits, cooked	½ cup
Kasha	½ cup
Millet, cooked	⅓ cup

(continued)

KEY

(☺) = More than 3 grams of dietary fiber per serving.

(!) = Extra fat, or prepared with added fat. (Count as 1 starch + 1 fat.)

(salt shaker) = 480 milligrams or more of sodium per serving.

TABLE G-2 **Starch (*continued*)**

Cereals and Grains—continued

Food	Serving Size
Muesli	¼ cup
Pasta, cooked	⅓ cup
Polenta, cooked	⅓ cup
Quinoa, cooked	⅓ cup
Rice, white or brown, cooked	⅓ cup
Tabbouleh (tabouli), prepared	½ cup
Wheat germ, dry	3 Tbsp
Wild rice, cooked	½ cup

Starchy Vegetables

Food	Serving Size
Cassava	⅓ cup
Corn	½ cup
on cob, large	½ cob (5 oz)
☺ Hominy, canned	¾ cup
☺ Mixed vegetables with corn, peas, or pasta	1 cup
☺ Parsnips	½ cup
☺ Peas, green	½ cup
Plantain, ripe	⅓ cup
Potato	
baked with skin	¼ large (3 oz)
boiled, all kinds	½ cup or ½ medium (3 oz)
▽ mashed, with milk and fat	½ cup
french fried (oven-baked)[a]	1 cup (2 oz)
☺ Pumpkin, canned, no sugar added	1 cup
Spaghetti/pasta sauce	½ cup
☺ Squash, winter (acorn, butternut)	1 cup
☺ Succotash	½ cup
Yam, sweet potato, plain	½ cup

Crackers and Snacks[b]

Food	Serving Size
Animal crackers	8
Crackers	
▽ round-butter type	6
saltine-type	6
▽ sandwich-style, cheese or peanut butter filling	3
▽ whole-wheat regular	2–5 (¾ oz)
☺ whole-wheat lower fat or crispbreads	2–5 (¾ oz)
Graham cracker, 2½-inch square	3
Matzoh	¾ oz
Melba toast, about 2-inch by 4-inch piece	4
Oyster crackers	20
Popcorn	3 cups
▽ ☺ with butter	3 cups
☺ no fat added	3 cups
☺ lower fat	3 cups
Pretzels	¾ oz
Rice cakes, 4 inches across	2
Snack chips	
fat-free or baked (tortilla, potato), baked pita chips	15–20 (¾ oz)
▽ regular (tortilla, potato)	9–13 (¾ oz)

Beans, Peas, and Lentils[c]

The choices on this list count as 1 starch + 1 lean meat.

Food	Serving Size
☺ Baked beans	⅓ cup
☺ Beans, cooked (black, garbanzo, kidney, lima, navy, pinto, white)	½ cup
☺ Lentils, cooked (brown, green, yellow)	½ cup
☺ Peas, cooked (black-eyed, split)	½ cup
🧂 ☺ Refried beans, canned	½ cup

KEY

☺ = More than 3 grams of dietary fiber per serving.

▽ = Extra fat, or prepared with added fat. (Count as 1 starch + 1 fat.)

🧂 = 480 milligrams or more of sodium per serving.

[a]Restaurant-style french fries are on the Fast Foods list.

[b]For other snacks, see the Sweets, Desserts, and Other Carbohydrates list. For a quick estimate of serving size, an open handful is equal to about 1 cup or 1 to 2 ounces of snack food.

[c]Beans, peas, and lentils are also found on the Meat and Meat Substitutes list.

TABLE G-3 Fruits

Fruit[a]

The Fruits list includes fresh, frozen, canned, and dried fruits and fruit juices. 1 fruit choice = 15 grams carbohydrate, 0 grams protein, 0 grams fat, and 60 kcalories.

NOTE: In general, one fruit exchange is ½ cup canned or fresh fruit or unsweetened fruit juice; 1 small fresh fruit (4 ounces); 2 tablespoons dried fruit.

Food	Serving Size
Apple, unpeeled, small	1 (4 oz)
Apples, dried	4 rings
Applesauce, unsweetened	½ cup
Apricots	
canned	½ cup
dried	8 halves
☺ fresh	4 whole (5½ oz)
Banana, extra small	1 (4 oz)
☺ Blackberries	¾ cup
Blueberries	¾ cup
Cantaloupe, small	⅓ melon or 1 cup cubed (11 oz)
Cherries	
sweet, canned	½ cup
sweet fresh	12 (3 oz)
Dates	3
Dried fruits (blueberries, cherries, cranberries, mixed fruit, raisins)	2 Tbsp
Figs	
dried	1½
☺ fresh	1½ large or 2 medium (3½ oz)
Fruit cocktail	½ cup
Grapefruit	
large	½ (11 oz)
sections, canned	¾ cup
Grapes, small	17 (3 oz)
Honeydew melon	1 slice or 1 cup cubed (10 oz)
☺ Kiwi	1 (3½ oz)
Mandarin oranges, canned	¾ cup
Mango, small	½ (5½ oz) or ½ cup
Nectarine, small	1 (5 oz)
☺ Orange, small	1 (6½ oz)
Papaya	½ or 1 cup cubed (8 oz)
Peaches	
canned	½ cup
fresh, medium	1 (6 oz)
Pears	
canned	½ cup
fresh, large	½ (4 oz)
Pineapple	
canned	½ cup
fresh	¾ cup
Plums	
canned	½ cup
dried (prunes)	3
small	2 (5 oz)
☺ Raspberries	1 cup
☺ Strawberries	1¼ cup whole berries
☺ Tangerines, small	2 (8 oz)
Watermelon	1 slice or 1¼ cups cubes (13½ oz)

Fruit Juice

Food	Serving Size
Apple juice/cider	½ cup
Fruit juice blends, 100% juice	⅓ cup
Grape juice	⅓ cup
Grapefruit juice	½ cup
Orange juice	½ cup
Pineapple juice	½ cup
Prune juice	⅓ cup

KEY

☺ = More than 3 grams of dietary fiber per serving.

▽ = Extra fat, or prepared with added fat. (Count as 1 starch + 1 fat.)

🧂 = 480 milligrams or more of sodium per serving.

[a]The weight listed includes skin, core, seeds, and rind.

TABLE G-4 Milk

The Milk list groups milks and yogurts based on the amount of fat they have (fat-free/low fat, reduced fat, and whole). Cheeses are found on the Meat and Meat Substitutes list and cream and other dairy fats are found on the Fats list.

NOTE: In general, one milk choice is 1 cup (8 fluid ounces or ½ pint) milk or yogurt.

Milk and Yogurts

Food	Serving Size
Fat-free or low-fat (1%)	
1 fat-free/low-fat milk choice = 12 g carbohydrate, 8 g protein, 0–3 g fat, and 100 kcal.	
Milk, buttermilk, acidophilus milk, Lactaid	1 cup
Evaporated milk	½ cup
Yogurt, plain or flavored with an artificial sweetener	⅔ cup (6 oz)
Reduced-fat (2%)	
1 reduced-fat milk choice = 12 g carbohydrate, 8 g protein, 5 g fat, and 120 kcal.	
Milk, acidophilus milk, kefir, Lactaid	1 cup
Yogurt, plain	⅔ cup (6 oz)
Whole	
1 whole milk choice = 12 g carbohydrate, 8 g protein, 8 g fat, and 160 kcal.	
Milk, buttermilk, goat's milk	1 cup
Evaporated milk	½ cup
Yogurt, plain	8 oz

Dairy-Like Foods

Food	Serving Size	Count as
Chocolate milk		
fat-free	1 cup	1 fat-free milk + 1 carbohydrate
whole	1 cup	1 whole milk + 1 carbohydrate
Eggnog, whole milk	½ cup	1 carbohydrate + 2 fats
Rice drink		
flavored, low fat	1 cup	2 carbohydrates
plain, fat-free	1 cup	1 carbohydrate
Smoothies, flavored, regular	10 oz	1 fat-free milk + 2½ carbohydrates
Soy milk		
light	1 cup	1 carbohydrate + ½ fat
regular, plain	1 cup	1 carbohydrate + 1 fat
Yogurt		
and juice blends	1 cup	1 fat-free milk + 1 carbohydrate
low carbohydrate (less than 6 grams carbohydrate per choice)	⅔ cup (6 oz)	½ fat-free milk
with fruit, low-fat	⅔ cup (6 oz)	1 fat-free milk + 1 carbohydrate

TABLE G-5 Sweets, Desserts, and Other Carbohydrates

1 other carbohydrate choice = 15 grams carbohydrate, variable grams protein, variable grams fat, and variable kcalories.

NOTE: In general, one choice from this list can substitute for foods on the Starch, Fruits, or Milk lists.

Beverages, Soda, and Energy/Sports Drinks

Food	Serving Size	Count as
Cranberry juice cocktail	½ cup	1 carbohydrate
Energy drink	1 can (8.3 oz)	2 carbohydrates
Fruit drink or lemonade	1 cup (8 oz)	2 carbohydrates

TABLE G-5 Sweets, Desserts, and Other Carbohydrates (*continued*)

Food	Serving Size	Count as
Beverages, Soda, and Energy/Sports Drinks—continued		
Hot chocolate		
regular	1 envelope added to 8 oz water	1 carbohydrate + 1 fat
sugar-free or light	1 envelope added to 8 oz water	1 carbohydrate
Soft drink (soda), regular	1 can (12 oz)	2½ carbohydrates
Sports drink	1 cup (8 oz)	1 carbohydrate

Food	Serving Size	Count as
Brownies, Cake, Cookies, Gelatin, Pie, and Pudding		
Brownie, small, unfrosted	1¼-inch square, ⅞ inch high (about 1 oz)	1 carbohydrate + 1 fat
Cake		
angel food, unfrosted	1⁄12 of cake (about 2 oz)	2 carbohydrates
frosted	2-inch square (about 2 oz)	2 carbohydrates + 1 fat
unfrosted	2-inch square (about 2 oz)	1 carbohydrate + 1 fat
Cookies		
chocolate chip	2 cookies (2¼ inches across)	1 carbohydrate + 2 fats
gingersnap	3 cookies	1 carbohydrate
sandwich, with crème filling	2 small (about ⅔ oz)	1 carbohydrate + 1 fat
sugar-free	3 small or 1 large (¾-1 oz)	1 carbohydrate + 1–2 fats
vanilla wafer	5 cookies	1 carbohydrate + 1 fat
Cupcake, frosted	1 small (about 1¾ oz)	2 carbohydrates + 1–1½ fats
Fruit cobbler	½ cup (3½ oz)	3 carbohydrates + 1 fat
Gelatin, regular	½ cup	1 carbohydrate
Pie		
commercially prepared fruit, 2 crusts	⅙ of 8-inch pie	3 carbohydrates + 2 fats
pumpkin or custard	⅛ of 8-inch pie	1½ carbohydrates + 1½ fats
Pudding		
regular (made with reduced-fat milk)	½ cup	2 carbohydrates
sugar-free or sugar- and fat-free (made with fat-free milk)	½ cup	1 carbohydrate

Food	Serving Size	Count as
Candy, Spreads, Sweets, Sweeteners, Syrups, and Toppings		
Candy bar, chocolate/peanut	2 "fun size" bars (1 oz)	1½ carbohydrates + 1½ fats
Candy, hard	3 pieces	1 carbohydrate
Chocolate "kisses"	5 pieces	1 carbohydrate + 1 fat
Coffee creamer		
dry, flavored	4 tsp	½ carbohydrate + ½ fat
liquid, flavored	2 Tbsp	1 carbohydrate
Fruit snacks, chewy (pureed fruit concentrate)	1 roll (¾ oz)	1 carbohydrate
Fruit spreads, 100% fruit	1½ Tbsp	1 carbohydrate
Honey	1 Tbsp	1 carbohydrate
Jam or jelly, regular	1 Tbsp	1 carbohydrate
Sugar	1 Tbsp	1 carbohydrate
Syrup		
chocolate	2 Tbsp	2 carbohydrates
light (pancake type)	2 Tbsp	1 carbohydrate
regular (pancake type)	1 Tbsp	1 carbohydrate

(*continued*)

TABLE G-5 Sweets, Desserts, and Other Carbohydrates (*continued*)

Condiments and Sauces[a]		
Food	Serving Size	Count as
Barbeque sauce	3 Tbsp	1 carbohydrate
Cranberry sauce, jellied	¼ cup	1½ carbohydrates
🧂 Gravy, canned or bottled	½ cup	½ carbohydrate + ½ fat
Salad dressing, fat-free, low-fat, cream-based	3 Tbsp	1 carbohydrate
Sweet and sour sauce	3 Tbsp	1 carbohydrate
Doughnuts, Muffins, Pastries, and Sweet Breads		
Food	Serving Size	Count as
Banana nut bread	1-inch slice (1 oz)	2 carbohydrates + 1 fat
Doughnut		
cake, plain	1 medium (1½ oz)	1½ carbohydrates + 2 fats
yeast type, glazed	3¾ inches across (2 oz)	2 carbohydrates + 2 fats
Muffin (4 oz)	¼ muffin (1 oz)	1 carbohydrate + ½ fat
Sweet roll or Danish	1 (2½ oz)	2½ carbohydrates + 2 fats
Frozen Bars, Frozen Desserts, Frozen Yogurt, and Ice Cream		
Food	Serving Size	Count as
Frozen pops	1	½ carbohydrate
Fruit juice bars, frozen, 100% juice	1 bar (3 oz)	1 carbohydrate
Ice cream		
fat-free	½ cup	1½ carbohydrates
light	½ cup	1 carbohydrate + 1 fat
no sugar added	½ cup	1 carbohydrate + 1 fat
regular	½ cup	1 carbohydrate + 2 fats
Sherbet, sorbet	½ cup	2 carbohydrates
Yogurt, frozen		
fat-free	⅓ cup	1 carbohydrate
regular	½ cup	1 carbohydrate + 0–1 fat
Granola Bars, Meal Replacement Bars/Shakes, and Trail Mix		
Food	Serving Size	Count as
Granola or snack bar, regular or low-fat	1 bar (1 oz)	1½ carbohydrates
Meal replacement bar	1 bar (1⅓ oz)	1½ carbohydrates + 0–1 fat
Meal replacement bar	1 bar (2 oz)	2 carbohydrates + 1 fat
Meal replacement shake, reduced kcalorie	1 can (10–11 oz)	1½ carbohydrates + 0–1 fat
Trail mix		
candy/nut-based	1 oz	1 carbohydrate + 2 fats
dried fruit-based	1 oz	1 carbohydrate + 1 fat

KEY

🧂 = 480 milligrams or more of sodium per serving.

[a]You can also check the Fats list and Free Foods list for other condiments.

TABLE G-6 Nonstarchy Vegetables

The Nonstarchy Vegetables list includes vegetables that have few grams of carbohydrates or kcalories; starchy vegetables are found on the Starch list. 1 nonstarchy vegetable choice = 5 grams carbohydrate, 2 grams protein, 0 grams fat, and 25 kcalories.

NOTE: In general, one nonstarchy vegetable choice is ½ cup cooked vegetables or vegetable juice or 1 cup raw vegetables. Count 3 cups of raw vegetables or 1½ cups of cooked vegetables as one carbohydrate choice.

Nonstarchy Vegetables[a]
Amaranth or Chinese spinach
Artichoke
Artichoke hearts
Asparagus
Baby corn
Bamboo shoots
Beans (green, wax, Italian)
Bean sprouts
Beets
🧂 Borscht
Broccoli
☺ Brussels sprouts
Cabbage (green, bok choy, Chinese)
☺ Carrots
Cauliflower
Celery
☺ Chayote
Coleslaw, packaged, no dressing
Cucumber
Eggplant
Gourds (bitter, bottle, luffa, bitter melon)
Green onions or scallions
Greens (collard, kale, mustard, turnip)
Hearts of palm
Jicama
Kohlrabi
Leeks
Mixed vegetables (without corn, peas, or pasta)
Mung bean sprouts
Mushrooms, all kinds, fresh
Okra
Onions
Oriental radish or daikon
Pea pods
☺ Peppers (all varieties)
Radishes
Rutabaga
🧂 Sauerkraut
Soybean sprouts
Spinach
Squash (summer, crookneck, zucchini)
Sugar pea snaps
☺ Swiss chard
Tomato
Tomatoes, canned
🧂 Tomato sauce
🧂 Tomato/vegetable juice
Turnips
Water chestnuts
Yard-long beans

KEY

☺ = More than 3 grams of dietary fiber per serving.

🧂 = 480 milligrams or more of sodium per serving.

[a]Salad greens (like chicory, endive, escarole, lettuce, romaine, spinach, arugula, radicchio, watercress) are on the Free Foods list.

TABLE G-7 Meat and Meat Substitutes

The Meat and Meat Substitutes list groups foods based on the amount of fat they have (lean meat, medium-fat meat, high-fat meat, and plant-based proteins).

Lean Meats and Meat Substitutes

1 lean meat choice = 0 grams carbohydrate, 7 grams protein, 0–3 grams fat, and 45 kcalories.

Food	Amount
Beef: Select or Choice grades trimmed of fat: ground round, roast (chuck, rib, rump), round, sirloin, steak (cubed, flank, porterhouse, T-bone), tenderloin	1 oz
🧂 Beef jerky	1 oz
Cheeses with 3 grams of fat or less per oz	1 oz
Cottage cheese	¼ cup
Egg substitutes, plain	¼ cup
Egg whites	2
Fish, fresh or frozen, plain: catfish, cod, flounder, haddock, halibut, orange roughy, salmon, tilapia, trout, tuna	1 oz
🧂 Fish, smoked: herring or salmon (lox)	1 oz
Game: buffalo, ostrich, rabbit, venison	1 oz
🧂 Hot dog with 3 grams of fat or less per oz (8 dogs per 14 oz package) *Note: May be high in carbohydrate.*	1
Lamb: chop, leg, or roast	1 oz
Organ meats: heart, kidney, liver *Note: May be high in cholesterol.*	1 oz
Oysters, fresh or frozen	6 medium
Pork, lean	
🧂 Canadian bacon	1 oz
rib or loin chop/roast, ham, tenderloin	1 oz
Poultry, without skin: Cornish hen, chicken, domestic duck or goose (well-drained of fat), turkey	1 oz
Processed sandwich meats with 3 grams of fat or less per oz: chipped beef, deli thin-sliced meats, turkey ham, turkey kielbasa, turkey pastrami	1 oz
Salmon, canned	1 oz
Sardines, canned	2 medium
🧂 Sausage with 3 grams of fat or less per oz	1 oz
Shellfish: clams, crab, imitation shellfish, lobster, scallops, shrimp	1 oz
Tuna, canned in water or oil, drained	1 oz
Veal, lean chop, roast	1 oz

Medium-Fat Meat and Meat Substitutes

1 medium-fat meat choice = 0 grams carbohydrate, 7 grams protein, 4–7 grams fat, and 75 kcalories.

Food	Amount
Beef: corned beef, ground beef, meatloaf, Prime grades trimmed of fat (prime rib), short ribs, tongue	1 oz

Medium-Fat Meat and Meat Substitutes—*continued*

Food	Amount
Cheeses with 4–7 grams of fat per oz: feta, mozzarella, pasteurized processed cheese spread, reduced-fat cheeses, string	1 oz
Egg *Note: High in cholesterol, so limit to 3 per week.*	1
Fish, any fried product	1 oz
Lamb: ground, rib roast	1 oz
Pork: cutlet, shoulder roast	1 oz
Poultry: chicken with skin; dove, pheasant, wild duck, or goose; fried chicken; ground turkey	1 oz
Ricotta cheese	2 oz or ¼ cup
🧂 Sausage with 4–7 grams of fat per oz	1 oz
Veal, cutlet (no breading)	1 oz

High-Fat Meat and Meat Substitutes

1 high-fat meat choice = 0 grams carbohydrate, 7 grams protein, 8+ grams fat, and 100 kcalories. These foods are high in saturated fat, cholesterol, and kcalories and may raise blood cholesterol levels if eaten on a regular basis. Try to eat 3 or fewer servings from this group per week.

Food	Amount
Bacon	
🧂 pork	2 slices (16 slices per lb or 1 oz each, before cooking)
🧂 turkey	3 slices (½ oz each before cooking)
Cheese, regular: American, bleu, brie, cheddar, hard goat, Monterey jack, queso, and Swiss	1 oz
▽ 🧂 Hot dog: beef, pork, or combination (10 per lb-sized package)	1
🧂 Hot dog: turkey or chicken (10 per lb-sized package)	1
Pork: ground, sausage, spareribs	1 oz
Processed sandwich meats with 8 grams of fat or more per oz: bologna, pastrami, hard salami	1 oz
🧂 Sausage with 8 grams fat or more per oz: bratwurst, chorizo, Italian, knockwurst, Polish, smoked, summer	1 oz

(*continued*)

KEY

☺ = More than 3 grams of dietary fiber per serving.

▽ = Extra fat, or prepared with added fat. (Count as 1 starch + 1 fat.)

🧂 = 480 milligrams or more of sodium per serving.

TABLE G-7 Meat and Meat Substitutes (*continued*)

Plant-Based Proteins[a]

1 plant-based protein choice = variable grams carbohydrate, 7 grams protein, variable grams fat, and variable kcalories.
Because carbohydrate content varies among plant-based proteins, you should read the food label.

Food	Serving Size	Count as
"Bacon" strips, soy-based	3 strips	1 medium-fat meat
☺ Baked beans	⅓ cup	1 starch + 1 lean meat
☺ Beans, cooked: black, garbanzo, kidney, lima, navy, pinto, white[a]	½ cup	1 starch + 1 lean meat
☺ "Beef" or "sausage" crumbles, soy-based	2 oz	½ carbohydrate + 1 lean meat
"Chicken" nuggets, soy-based	2 nuggets (1½ oz)	½ carbohydrate + 1 medium-fat meat
☺ Edamame	½ cup	½ carbohydrate + 1 lean meat
Falafel (spiced chickpea and wheat patties)	3 patties (about 2 inches across)	1 carbohydrate + 1 high-fat meat
Hot dog, soy-based	1 (1½ oz)	½ carbohydrate + 1 lean meat
☺ Hummus	⅓ cup	1 carbohydrate + 1 high-fat meat
☺ Lentils, brown, green, or yellow	½ cup	1 carbohydrate + 1 lean meat
☺ Meatless burger, soy-based	3 oz	½ carbohydrate + 2 lean meats
☺ Meatless burger, vegetable- and starch-based	1 patty (about 2½ oz)	1 carbohydrate + 2 lean meats
Nut spreads: almond butter, cashew butter, peanut butter, soy nut butter	1 Tbsp	1 high-fat meat
☺ Peas, cooked: black-eyed and split peas	½ cup	1 starch + 1 lean meat
🧂 ☺ Refried beans, canned	½ cup	1 starch + 1 lean meat
"Sausage" patties, soy-based	1 (1½ oz)	1 medium-fat meat
Soy nuts, unsalted	¾ oz	½ carbohydrate + 1 medium-fat meat
Tempeh	¼ cup	1 medium-fat meat
Tofu	4 oz (½ cup)	1 medium-fat meat
Tofu, light	4 oz (½ cup)	1 lean meat

KEY

☺ = More than 3 grams of dietary fiber per serving.

⚠ = Extra fat, or prepared with added fat. (Add an additional fat choice to this food.)

🧂 = 480 milligrams or more of sodium per serving (based on the sodium content of a typical 3-oz serving of meat, unless 1 or 2 oz is the normal serving size).

[a]Beans, peas, and lentils are also found on the Starch list; nut butters in smaller amounts are found in the Fats list.

APPENDIX G

TABLE G-8 Fats

Fats and oils have mixtures of unsaturated (polyunsaturated and monounsaturated) and saturated fats. Foods on the Fats list are grouped together based on the major type of fat they contain. 1 fat choice = 0 grams carbohydrate, 0 grams protein, 5 grams fat, and 45 kcalories.

NOTE: In general, one fat exchange is 1 teaspoon of regular margarine, vegetable oil, or butter; 1 tablespoon of regular salad dressing.
When used in large amounts, bacon and peanut butter are counted as high-fat meat choices (see Meat and Meat Substitutes list). Fat-free salad dressings are found on the Sweets, Desserts, and Other Carbohydrates list. Fat-free products such as margarines, salad dressings, mayonnaise, sour cream, and cream cheese are found on the Free Foods list.

Monounsaturated Fats

Food	Serving Size
Avocado, medium	2 Tbsp (1 oz)
Nut butters (trans fat-free): almond butter, cashew butter, peanut butter (smooth or crunchy)	1½ tsp
Nuts	
almonds	6 nuts
Brazil	2 nuts
cashews	6 nuts
filberts (hazelnuts)	5 nuts
macadamia	3 nuts
mixed (50% peanuts)	6 nuts
peanuts	10 nuts
pecans	4 halves
pistachios	16 nuts
Oil: canola, olive, peanut	1 tsp
Olives	
black (ripe)	8 large
green, stuffed	10 large

Polyunsaturated Fats

Food	Serving Size
Margarine: lower-fat spread (30%–50% vegetable oil, *trans* fat-free)	1 Tbsp
Margarine: stick, tub (*trans* fat-free) or squeeze (*trans* fat-free)	1 tsp
Mayonnaise	
reduced-fat	1 Tbsp
regular	1 tsp
Mayonnaise-style salad dressing	
reduced-fat	1 Tbsp
regular	2 tsp
Nuts	
Pignolia (pine nuts)	1 Tbsp
walnuts, English	4 halves
Oil: corn, cottonseed, flaxseed, grape seed, safflower, soybean, sunflower	1 tsp
Oil: made from soybean and canola oil—Enova	1 tsp
Plant stanol esters	
light	1 Tbsp
regular	2 tsp

Polyunsaturated Fats—continued

Food	Serving Size
Salad dressing	
🧂 reduced-fat *Note: May be high in carbohydrate.*	2 Tbsp
🧂 regular	1 Tbsp
Seeds	
flaxseed, whole	1 Tbsp
pumpkin, sunflower	1 Tbsp
sesame seeds	1 Tbsp
Tahini or sesame paste	2 tsp

Saturated Fats

Food	Serving Size
Bacon, cooked, regular or turkey	1 slice
Butter	
reduced-fat	1 Tbsp
stick	1 tsp
whipped	2 tsp
Butter blends made with oil	
reduced-fat or light	1 Tbsp
regular	1½ tsp
Chitterlings, boiled	2 Tbsp (½ oz)
Coconut, sweetened, shredded	2 Tbsp
Coconut milk	
light	⅓ cup
regular	1½ Tbsp
Cream	
half and half	2 Tbsp
heavy	1 Tbsp
light	1½ Tbsp
whipped	2 Tbsp
whipped, pressurized	¼ cup
Cream cheese	
reduced-fat	1½ Tbsp (¾ oz)
regular	1 Tbsp (½ oz)
Lard	1 tsp
Oil: coconut, palm, palm kernel	1 tsp
Salt pork	¼ oz
Shortening, solid	1 tsp
Sour cream	
reduced-fat or light	3 Tbsp
regular	2 Tbsp

KEY

🧂 = 480 milligrams or more of sodium per serving.

TABLE G-9 Free Foods

A "free" food is any food or drink choice that has less than 20 kcalories and 5 grams or less of carbohydrate per serving.

- Most foods on this list should be limited to 3 servings (as listed here) per day. Spread out the servings throughout the day. If you eat all 3 servings at once, it could raise your blood glucose level.
- Food and drink choices listed here without a serving size can be eaten whenever you like.

Low Carbohydrate Foods

Food	Serving Size
Cabbage, raw	½ cup
Candy, hard (regular or sugar-free)	1 piece
Carrots, cauliflower, or green beans, cooked	¼ cup
Cranberries, sweetened with sugar substitute	½ cup
Cucumber, sliced	½ cup
Gelatin	
dessert, sugar-free	
unflavored	
Gum	
Jam or jelly, light or no sugar added	2 tsp
Rhubarb, sweetened with sugar substitute	½ cup
Salad greens	
Sugar substitutes (artificial sweeteners)	
Syrup, sugar-free	2 Tbsp

Modified Fat Foods with Carbohydrate

Food	Serving Size
Cream cheese, fat-free	1 Tbsp (½ oz)
Creamers	
nondairy, liquid	1 Tbsp
nondairy, powdered	2 tsp
Margarine spread	
fat-free	1 Tbsp
reduced-fat	1 tsp
Mayonnaise	
fat-free	1 Tbsp
reduced-fat	1 tsp
Mayonnaise-style salad dressing	
fat-free	1 Tbsp
reduced-fat	1 tsp
Salad dressing	
fat-free or low-fat	1 Tbsp
fat-free, Italian	2 Tbsp
Sour cream, fat-free or reduced-fat	1 Tbsp
Whipped topping	
light or fat-free	2 Tbsp
regular	1 Tbsp

Condiments

Food	Serving Size
Barbecue sauce	2 tsp
Catsup (ketchup)	1 Tbsp
Honey mustard	1 Tbsp
Horseradish	
Lemon juice	
Miso	1½ tsp
Mustard	
Parmesan cheese, freshly grated	1 Tbsp
Pickle relish	1 Tbsp
Pickles	
🧂 dill	1½ medium
sweet, bread and butter	2 slices
sweet, gherkin	¾ oz
Salsa	¼ cup
🧂 Soy sauce, light or regular	1 Tbsp
Sweet and sour sauce	2 tsp
Sweet chili sauce	2 tsp
Taco sauce	1 Tbsp
Vinegar	
Yogurt, any type	2 Tbsp

Drinks/Mixes

Any food on the list—without a serving size listed—can be consumed in any moderate amount.

- 🧂 Bouillon, broth, consommé
- Bouillon or broth, low-sodium
- Carbonated or mineral water
- Club soda
- Cocoa powder, unsweetened (1 Tbsp)
- Coffee, unsweetened or with sugar substitute
- Diet soft drinks, sugar-free
- Drink mixes, sugar-free
- Tea, unsweetened or with sugar substitute
- Tonic water, diet
- Water
- Water, flavored, carbohydrate free

Seasonings

Any food on this list can be consumed in any moderate amount.

- Flavoring extracts (for example, vanilla, almond, peppermint)
- Garlic
- Herbs, fresh or dried
- Nonstick cooking spray
- Pimento
- Spices
- Hot pepper sauce
- Wine, used in cooking
- Worcestershire sauce

KEY

🧂 = 480 milligrams or more of sodium per serving.

TABLE G-10 Combination Foods

Many foods are eaten in various combinations, such as casseroles. Because "combination" foods do not fit into any one choice list, this list of choices provides some typical combination foods.

Entrees

Food	Serving Size	Count as
🧂 Casserole type (tuna noodle, lasagna, spaghetti with meatballs, chili with beans, macaroni and cheese)	1 cup (8 oz)	2 carbohydrates + 2 medium-fat meats
🧂 Stews (beef/other meats and vegetables)	1 cup (8 oz)	1 carbohydrate + 1 medium-fat meat + 0–3 fats
Tuna salad or chicken salad	½ cup (3½ oz)	½ carbohydrate + 2 lean meats + 1 fat

Frozen Meals/Entrees

Food	Serving Size	Count as
🧂 ☺ Burrito (beef and bean)	1 (5 oz)	3 carbohydrates + 1 lean meat + 2 fats
🧂 Dinner-type meal	generally 14–17 oz	3 carbohydrates + 3 medium-fat meats + 3 fats
🧂 Entrée or meal with less than 340 kcalories	about 8–11 oz	2–3 carbohydrates + 1–2 lean meats
Pizza		
🧂 cheese/vegetarian, thin crust	¼ of a 12 inch (4½–5 oz)	2 carbohydrates + 2 medium-fat meats
🧂 meat topping, thin crust	¼ of a 12 inch (5 oz)	2 carbohydrates + 2 medium-fat meats + 1½ fats
🧂 Pocket sandwich	1 (4½ oz)	3 carbohydrates + 1 lean meat + 1–2 fats
🧂 Pot pie	1 (7 oz)	2½ carbohydrates + 1 medium-fat meat + 3 fats

Salads (Deli-Style)

Food	Serving Size	Count as
Coleslaw	½ cup	1 carbohydrate + 1½ fats
Macaroni/pasta salad	½ cup	2 carbohydrates + 3 fats
🧂 Potato salad	½ cup	1½–2 carbohydrates + 1–2 fats

Soups

Food	Serving Size	Count as
🧂 Bean, lentil, or split pea	1 cup	1 carbohydrate + 1 lean meat
🧂 Chowder (made with milk)	1 cup (8 oz)	1 carbohydrate + 1 lean meat + 1½ fats
🧂 Cream (made with water)	1 cup (8 oz)	1 carbohydrate + 1 fat
🧂 Instant	6 oz prepared	1 carbohydrate
🧂 with beans or lentils	8 oz prepared	2½ carbohydrates + 1 lean meat
🧂 Miso soup	1 cup	½ carbohydrate + 1 fat
🧂 Oriental noodle	1 cup	2 carbohydrates + 2 fats
Rice (congee)	1 cup	1 carbohydrate
🧂 Tomato (made with water)	1 cup (8 oz)	1 carbohydrate
🧂 Vegetable beef, chicken noodle, or other broth-type	1 cup (8 oz)	1 carbohydrate

KEY

☺ = More than 3 grams of dietary fiber per serving.

▽ = Extra fat, or prepared with added fat.

🧂 = 600 milligrams or more of sodium per serving (for combination food main dishes/meals).

TABLE G-11 Fast Foods

The choices on the Fast Foods list are not specific fast-food meals or items, but are estimates based on popular foods. Ask the restaurant or check its website for nutrition information about your favorite fast foods.

Food	Serving Size	Count as
Breakfast Sandwiches		
Food	**Serving Size**	**Count as**
🧂 Egg, cheese, meat, English muffin	1 sandwich	2 carbohydrates + 2 medium-fat meats
🧂 Sausage biscuit sandwich	1 sandwich	2 carbohydrates + 2 high-fat meats + 3½ fats
Main Dishes/Entrees		
Food	**Serving Size**	**Count as**
🧂 ☺ Burrito (beef and beans)	1 (about 8 oz)	3 carbohydrates + 3 medium-fat meats + 3 fats
🧂 Chicken breast, breaded and fried	1 (about 5 oz)	1 carbohydrate + 4 medium-fat meats
Chicken drumstick, breaded and fried	1 (about 2 oz)	2 medium-fat meats
🧂 Chicken nuggets	6 (about 3½ oz)	1 carbohydrate + 2 medium-fat meats + 1 fat
🧂 Chicken thigh, breaded and fried	1 (about 4 oz)	½ carbohydrate + 3 medium-fat meats + 1½ fats
🧂 Chicken wings, hot	6 (5 oz)	5 medium-fat meats + 1½ fats
Oriental		
Food	**Serving Size**	**Count as**
🧂 Beef/chicken/shrimp with vegetables in sauce	1 cup (about 5 oz)	1 carbohydrate + 1 lean meat + 1 fat
🧂 Egg roll, meat	1 (about 3 oz)	1 carbohydrate + 1 lean meat + 1 fat
Fried rice, meatless	½ cup	1½ carbohydrates + 1½ fats
🧂 Meat and sweet sauce (orange chicken)	1 cup	3 carbohydrates + 3 medium-fat meats + 2 fats
🧂 ☺ Noodles and vegetables in sauce (chow mein, lo mein)	1 cup	2 carbohydrates + 1 fat
Pizza		
Food	**Serving Size**	**Count as**
Pizza		
🧂 cheese, pepperoni, regular crust	⅛ of a 14 inch (about 4 oz)	2½ carbohydrates + 1 medium-fat meat + 1½ fats
🧂 cheese/vegetarian, thin crust	¼ of a 12 inch (about 6 oz)	2½ carbohydrates + 2 medium-fat meats + 1½ fats
Sandwiches		
Food	**Serving Size**	**Count as**
🧂 Chicken sandwich, grilled	1	3 carbohydrates + 4 lean meats
🧂 Chicken sandwich, crispy	1	3½ carbohydrates + 3 medium-fat meats + 1 fat
Fish sandwich with tartar sauce	1	2½ carbohydrates + 2 medium-fat meats + 2 fats
Hamburger		
🧂 large with cheese	1	2½ carbohydrates + 4 medium-fat meats + 1 fat
regular	1	2 carbohydrates + 1 medium-fat meat + 1 fat
🧂 Hot dog with bun	1	1 carbohydrate + 1 high-fat meat + 1 fat
Submarine sandwich		
🧂 less than 6 grams fat	6-inch sub	3 carbohydrates + 2 lean meats
🧂 regular	6-inch sub	3½ carbohydrates + 2 medium-fat meats + 1 fat
Taco, hard or soft shell (meat and cheese)	1 small	1 carbohydrate + 1 medium-fat meat + 1½ fats

(continued)

KEY

☺ = More than 3 grams of dietary fiber per serving.

▽ = Extra fat, or prepared with added fat.

🧂 = 600 milligrams or more of sodium per serving (for fast-food main dishes/meals).

TABLE G-11 **Fast Foods (*continued*)**

Salads		
Food	**Serving Size**	**Count as**
Salad, main dish (grilled chicken type, no dressing or croutons)		1 carbohydrate + 4 lean meats
Salad, side, no dressing or cheese	Small (about 5 oz)	1 vegetable
Sides/Appetizers		
Food	**Serving Size**	**Count as**
French fries, restaurant style	small	3 carbohydrates + 3 fats
	medium	4 carbohydrates + 4 fats
	large	5 carbohydrates + 6 fats
Nachos with cheese	small (about 4½ oz)	2½ carbohydrates + 4 fats
Onion rings	1 serving (about 3 oz)	2½ carbohydrates + 3 fats
Desserts		
Food	**Serving Size**	**Count as**
Milkshake, any flavor	12 oz	6 carbohydrates + 2 fats
Soft-serve ice cream cone	1 small	2½ carbohydrates + 1 fat

KEY

☺ = More than 3 grams of dietary fiber per serving.

! = Extra fat, or prepared with added fat.

Salt shaker = 600 milligrams or more of sodium per serving (for fast-food main dishes/meals).

TABLE G-12 **Alcohol**

1 alcohol equivalent = variable grams carbohydrate, 0 grams protein, 0 grams fat, and 100 kcalories.

NOTE: In general, one alcohol choice (½ ounce absolute alcohol) has about 100 kcalories. For those who choose to drink alcohol, guidelines suggest limiting alcohol intake to 1 drink or less per day for women, and 2 drinks or less per day for men. To reduce your risk of low blood glucose (hypoglycemia), especially if you take insulin or a diabetes pill that increases insulin, always drink alcohol with food. While alcohol, by itself, does not directly affect blood glucose, be aware of the carbohydrate (for example, in mixed drinks, beer, and wine) that may raise your blood glucose.

Alcoholic Beverage	Serving Size	Count as
Beer		
light (4.2%)	12 fl oz	1 alcohol equivalent + ½ carbohydrate
regular (4.9%)	12 fl oz	1 alcohol equivalent + 1 carbohydrate
Distilled spirits: vodka, rum, gin, whiskey, 80 or 86 proof	1½ fl oz	1 alcohol equivalent
Liqueur, coffee (53 proof)	1 fl oz	1 alcohol equivalent + 1 carbohydrate
Sake	1 fl oz	½ alcohol equivalent
Wine		
dessert (sherry)	3½ fl oz	1 alcohol equivalent + 1 carbohydrate
dry, red or white (10%)	5 fl oz	1 alcohol equivalent

Appendix H Table of Food Composition

This edition of the table of food composition includes a wide variety of foods. It is updated with each edition to reflect current nutrient data for foods, to remove outdated foods, and to add foods that are new to the marketplace.* The nutrient database for this appendix is compiled from a variety of sources, including the USDA Nutrient Database and manufacturers' data. The USDA database provides data for a wider variety of foods and nutrients than other sources. Because laboratory analysis for each nutrient can be quite costly, manufacturers tend to provide data only for those nutrients mandated on food labels. Consequently, data for their foods are often incomplete; any missing information on this table is designated as a dash. Keep in mind that a dash means only that the information is unknown and should not be interpreted as a zero. A zero means that the nutrient is not present in the food.

Whenever using nutrient data, remember that many factors influence the nutrient contents of foods. These factors include the mineral content of the soil, the diet fed to the animal or the fertilizer used on the plant, the season of harvest, the method of processing, the length and method of storage, the method of cooking, the method of analysis, and the moisture content of the sample analyzed. With so many influencing factors, users should view nutrient data as a close approximation of the actual amount.

Diet & Wellness Plus, the dietary analysis software that accompanies this text, contains a database of 55,000 foods. The following comments will help in using that program and this appendix.

- ***Fats*** Total fats, as well as the breakdown of total fats to saturated, monounsaturated, and polyunsaturated are listed in the table. The fatty acids seldom add up to the total in part due to rounding but also because values may include some non-fatty acids, such as glycerol, phosphate, or sterols. *Trans*-fatty acids are not listed separately in this edition because newer hydrogenated fats generally add less than 0.5 grams *trans* fat to a serving of food, an amount often reported as 0.
- ***Vitamin A, Vitamin E, and Folate*** In keeping with the RDA for vitamin A, this appendix presents data for vitamin A in micrograms (µg) RAE. Similarly because the RDA for vitamin E is based only on the alpha-tocopherol form of vitamin E, this appendix reports vitamin E data in milligrams alpha-tocopherol, listed on the table as Vit E (mg α). Folate values are listed in µg DFE, a measure that adjusts for lower bioavailability of naturally occurring folate from foods compared to that from fortified foods or supplements.
- ***Bioavailability*** Keep in mind that the availability of nutrients from foods depends not only on the quantity provided by a food, but also on the amount absorbed and used by the body—the bioavailability. Chapters 10–13 provide conversion factors and additional details.

*This food composition table has been prepared by Cengage Learning. The nutritional data are supplied by Axxya Systems.

- *Using the Table* The foods and beverages in this table are organized into several categories, which are listed at the head of each right-hand page. Page numbers are provided, and each group is color-coded to make it easier to find individual foods.
- *Caffeine Sources* Caffeine occurs in several plants, including the familiar coffee bean, the tea leaf, and the cocoa bean from which chocolate is made. Most human societies use caffeine regularly, most often in beverages, for its stimulant effect and flavor. Caffeine contents of beverages vary depending on the plants they are made from, the climates and soils where the plants are grown, the grind or cut size, the method and duration of brewing, and the amounts served. The accompanying table shows that, in general, a cup of coffee contains the most caffeine; a cup of tea, less than half as much; and cocoa or chocolate, less still. As for cola beverages, they are made from kola nuts, which contain caffeine, but most of their caffeine is added, using the purified compound obtained from decaffeinated coffee beans. The FDA lists caffeine as a multipurpose GRAS (generally recognized as safe) substance that may be added to foods and beverages. Drug manufacturers also use caffeine in many products.

TABLE Caffeine Content of Selected Beverages, Foods, and Medications

Beverages and Foods	Serving Size	Average (mg)
Coffee		
Brewed	8 oz	95
Decaffeinated	8 oz	2
Expresso	1 oz	64
Instant	8 oz	64
Tea		
Brewed, green	8 oz	30
Brewed, herbal	8 oz	0
Brewed, leaf or bag	8 oz	47
Instant	8 oz	26
Lipton, Nestea, bottled iced tea	12 oz	10
Snapple iced tea (all flavors)	16 oz	42

Beverages and Foods	Serving Size	Average (mg)
Soft Drinks		
A&W Creme Soda	12 oz	29
Barq's Root Beer	12 oz	18
Colas, Dr. Pepper, Mr. Pibb, Sunkist Orange	12 oz	30–40
A&W Root Beer, club soda, Fresca, ginger ale, 7-Up, Sierra Mist, Sprite, Squirt, tonic water, caffeine-free soft drinks	12 oz	0
Mello Yello, Mountain Dew	12 oz	45–55

TABLE Caffeine Content of Selected Beverages, Foods, and Medications (*continued*)

Beverages and Foods	Serving Size	Average (mg)
Energy Drinks		
Amp	16 oz	145
Full Throttle	16 oz	200
Monster	16 oz	160
NOS	16 oz	160
Red Bull	8.3 oz	75
Rockstar	16 oz	160
Xyience Xenergy	16 oz	185
Other Beverages		
Chocolate milk or hot cocoa	8 oz	5
Coffee liqueur	1 oz	50
Starbucks Frappuccino Mocha	9.5 oz	72
Starbucks Frappuccino Vanilla	9.5 oz	64
Yoohoo chocolate drink	9 oz	3
Candies		
Baker's chocolate	1 oz	26
Dark chocolate covered coffee beans	1 oz	235
Dark chocolate	1 oz	20
Gum, caffeinated	1 piece	95
Java pops	1 pop	60
Milk chocolate	1 oz	6
Milk chocolate covered coffee beans	1 oz	224
White chocolate	1 oz	0

Beverages and Foods	Serving Size	Average (mg)
Foods		
Frozen yogurt, Ben & Jerry's coffee fudge	1 cup	85
Frozen yogurt, Häagen-Dazs coffee	1 cup	40
Frozen yogurt, chocolate	1 cup	5
Ice cream, Starbucks coffee	1 cup	50
Ice cream, Starbucks Frappuccino bar	1 bar	15
Puddings, chocolate	1 cup	5
Yogurt, Dannon coffee flavored	1 cup	45

Drugs[a]	Serving Size	Average (mg)
Cold Remedies		
Coryban-D, Dristan	1 tablet	30
Diuretics		
Aqua-Ban	1 tablet	100
Pre-Mens Forte	1 tablet	100
Pain Relievers		
Anacin, BC Fast Pain Reliever	1 tablet	32
Excedrin, Midol, Midol Max Strength	1 tablet	65
Stimulants		
Awake, NoDoz	1 tablet	100
Awake Maximum Strength, Caffedrine, NoDoz Maximum Strength, Stay Awake, Vivarin	1 tablet	200
Weight-Control Aids		
Dexatrim	1 tablet	200

[a]A pharmacologically active dose of caffiene is defined as 200 milligrams.

NOTE: The FDA suggests a maximum of 65 milligrams per 12-ounce cola beverage but does not regulate the caffeine contents of other beverages. Because products change, contact the manufacturer for an update on products you use regularly.

SOURCE: Adapted from USDA database Release 18 (www.nal.usda.gov/fnic/foodcomp/Data/), Caffeine content of foods and drugs, Center for Science and the Public Interest (www.cspinet.org/new/cafchart.htm), and R. R. McCusker, B. A. Goldberger, and E. J. Cone, Caffeine content of energy drinks, carbonated sodas, and other beverages, *Journal of Analytical Toxicology* 30(2006): 112–114.

TABLE H-1 Table of Food Composition (Computer code is for Cengage Diet Analysis program) (For purposes of calculations, use "0" for t, <1, <0.1, 0.01)

DA+ Code	Food Description	Quantity	Measure	Wt (g)	H_2O (g)	Ener (kcal)	Prot (g)	Carb (g)	Fiber (g)	Fat (g)	Fat Breakdown (g)		
											Sat	Mono	Poly
Breads, Baked Goods, Cakes, Cookies, Crackers, Chips, Pies													
	Bagels												
8534	Cinnamon and raisin	1	item(s)	71	22.7	195	7.0	39.2	1.6	1.2	0.2	0.1	0.5
8538	Oat bran	1	item(s)	71	23.4	181	7.6	37.8	2.6	0.9	0.1	0.2	0.3
4910	Plain, enriched	1	item(s)	71	25.8	182	7.1	35.9	1.6	1.2	0.3	0.4	0.5
4911	Plain, enriched, toasted	1	item(s)	66	18.7	190	7.4	37.7	1.7	1.1	0.2	0.3	0.6
72275	Whole wheat	1	item(s)	94	—	210	10.0	41.0	6.0	1.5	0	0	0.5
	Biscuits												
25008	Biscuits	1	item(s)	41	15.8	121	2.6	16.4	0.5	4.9	1.4	1.4	1.8
16729	Scone	1	item(s)	42	11.5	149	3.8	19.0	0.6	6.3	2.0	2.5	1.4
25166	Wheat biscuits	1	item(s)	55	21.0	162	3.6	21.9	1.4	6.7	1.9	1.9	2.5
	Bread												
325	Boston brown, canned	1	slice(s)	45	21.2	88	2.3	19.5	2.1	0.7	0.1	0.1	0.3
8716	Bread sticks, plain	4	item(s)	24	1.5	99	2.9	16.4	0.7	2.3	0.3	0.9	0.9
25176	Cornbread	2	piece(s)	55	25.9	141	4.6	18.4	0.6	5.4	2.1	1.5	1.4
327	Cracked wheat	1	slice(s)	25	8.9	65	2.2	12.4	1.4	1.0	0.2	0.5	0.2
9079	Croutons, plain	¼	cup(s)	8	0.4	31	0.9	5.5	0.4	0.5	0.1	0.2	0.1
8582	Egg	1	slice(s)	40	13.9	115	3.8	19.1	0.9	2.4	0.6	0.9	0.4
8585	Egg, toasted	1	slice(s)	37	10.5	117	3.9	19.5	0.9	2.4	0.6	1.1	0.4
329	French	1	slice(s)	32	8.9	92	3.8	18.1	0.8	0.6	0.2	0.1	0.3
8591	French, toasted	1	slice(s)	23	4.7	73	3.0	14.2	0.7	0.5	0.1	0.1	0.2
42096	Indian fry, made with lard (Navajo)	3	ounce(s)	85	26.9	281	5.7	41.0	—	10.4	3.9	3.8	0.9
332	Italian	1	slice(s)	30	10.7	81	2.6	15.0	0.8	1.0	0.3	0.2	0.4
1393	Mixed grain	1	slice(s)	26	9.6	69	3.5	11.3	1.9	1.1	0.2	0.2	0.5
8604	Mixed grain, toasted	1	slice(s)	24	7.6	69	3.5	11.3	1.9	1.1	0.2	0.2	0.5
8605	Oat bran	1	slice(s)	30	13.2	71	3.1	11.9	1.4	1.3	0.2	0.5	0.5
8608	Oat bran, toasted	1	slice(s)	27	10.4	70	3.1	11.8	1.3	1.3	0.2	0.5	0.5
8609	Oatmeal	1	slice(s)	27	9.9	73	2.3	13.1	1.1	1.2	0.2	0.4	0.5
8613	Oatmeal, toasted	1	slice(s)	25	7.8	73	2.3	13.2	1.1	1.2	0.2	0.4	0.5
1409	Pita	1	item(s)	60	19.3	165	5.5	33.4	1.3	0.7	0.1	0.1	0.3
7905	Pita, whole wheat	1	item(s)	64	19.6	170	6.3	35.2	4.7	1.7	0.3	0.2	0.7
338	Pumpernickel	1	slice(s)	32	12.1	80	2.8	15.2	2.1	1.0	0.1	0.3	0.4
334	Raisin, enriched	1	slice(s)	26	8.7	71	2.1	13.6	1.1	1.1	0.3	0.6	0.2
8625	Raisin, toasted	1	slice(s)	25	6.9	74	2.1	14.2	1.2	1.2	0.3	0.6	0.2
10168	Rice, white, gluten free, wheat free	1	slice(s)	38	—	100	1.0	17.0	1.0	3.5	0	—	—
8653	Rye	1	slice(s)	32	11.9	83	2.7	15.5	1.9	1.1	0.2	0.4	0.3
74338	Rye, light	1	slice(s)	43	—	100	3.0	20.0	1.0	0.5	0	—	—
8654	Rye, toasted	1	slice(s)	29	9.0	82	2.7	15.4	1.9	1.0	0.2	0.4	0.3
8588	Sourdough	1	slice(s)	25	7.0	72	2.9	14.1	0.6	0.5	0.1	0.1	0.2
8592	Sourdough, toasted	1	slice(s)	23	4.7	73	3.0	14.2	0.7	0.5	0.1	0.1	0.2
8596	Vienna, toasted	1	slice(s)	23	4.7	73	3.0	14.2	0.7	0.5	0.1	0.1	0.2
8670	Wheat	1	slice(s)	25	8.6	68	2.6	12.4	1.0	0.9	0.2	0.2	0.4
8671	Wheat, toasted	1	slice(s)	23	5.6	72	3.0	12.8	1.1	1.0	0.2	0.2	0.4
340	White	1	slice(s)	25	9.1	66	2.3	12.3	0.7	0.8	0.2	0.1	0.4
1395	Whole wheat	1	slice(s)	46	15.0	128	3.9	23.6	2.8	2.5	0.4	0.5	1.4
	Cakes												
386	Angel food, prepared from mix	1	piece(s)	50	16.5	129	3.0	29.4	0.1	0.2	0	0	0.1
8772	Butter pound, ready to eat, commercially prepared	1	slice(s)	75	18.5	291	4.1	36.6	0.4	14.9	8.7	4.4	0.8
28517	Carrot	1	slice(s)	131	56.4	340	4.8	56.8	1.8	11.1	1.0	6.1	3.6
4931	Chocolate with chocolate icing, commercially prepared	1	slice(s)	64	14.7	235	2.6	34.9	1.8	10.5	3.1	5.6	1.2
8756	Chocolate, prepared from mix	1	slice(s)	95	23.2	352	5.0	50.7	1.5	14.3	5.2	5.7	2.6
8757	Fruitcake, ready to eat, commercially prepared	1	piece(s)	43	10.9	139	1.2	26.5	1.6	3.9	0.5	1.8	1.4
14284	Lemon, prepared from mix	1	slice(s)	80	—	250	3.0	36.0	0.5	11.1	2.6	—	—
1397	Pineapple upside down, prepared from mix	1	slice(s)	115	37.1	367	4.0	58.1	0.9	13.9	3.4	6.0	3.8
411	Sponge, prepared from mix	1	slice(s)	63	18.5	187	4.6	36.4	0.3	2.7	0.8	1.0	0.4
8817	White with coconut frosting, prepared from mix	1	slice(s)	112	23.2	399	4.9	70.8	1.1	11.5	4.4	4.1	2.4
8819	Yellow with chocolate frosting, ready to eat, commercially prepared	1	slice(s)	64	14.3	243	2.0	35.4	1.0	11.4	3.7	4.6	3.0
8822	Yellow with vanilla frosting, ready to eat, commercially prepared	1	slice(s)	64	14.1	239	2.2	37.6	0.2	9.3	1.5	3.9	3.3

KEY: H-4 = Breads/Baked Goods H-8 = Cereal/Rice/Pasta H-14 = Fruit H-18 = Vegetables/Legumes H-28 = Nuts/Seeds H-30 = Vegetarian H-32 = Dairy H-40 = Eggs H-40 = Seafood H-42 = Meats H-46 = Poultry
8 = Processed Meats H-50 = Beverages H-52 = Fats/Oils H-54 = Sweets H-56 = Spices/Condiments/Sauces H-60 = Mixed Foods/Soups/Sandwiches H-66 = Fast Food H-84 = Convenience H-86 = Baby Foods

Chol (mg)	Calc (mg)	Iron (mg)	Magn (mg)	Pota (mg)	Sodi (mg)	Zinc (mg)	Vit A (μg)	Thia (mg)	Vit E (mg α)	Ribo (mg)	Niac (mg)	Vit B_6 (mg)	Fola (μg)	Vit C (mg)	Vit B_{12} (μg)	Sele (μg)
0	13	2.70	19.9	105.1	244.2	0.80	14.9	0.27	0.22	0.20	2.19	0.04	123.5	0.5	0	22.0
0	9	2.19	22.0	81.7	418.9	0.64	0.7	0.24	0.23	0.24	2.10	0.03	95.1	0.1	0	24.3
0	63	4.30	15.6	53.3	338.7	1.35	0	0.43	0.07	0.18	2.82	0.05	160.5	0.7	0	16.2
0	65	2.97	15.8	56.1	354.4	0.86	0	0.40	0.08	0.18	2.89	0.05	134.0	0	0	16.6
0	40	2.70	—	—	420.0	—	0	—	—	—	—	—	—	0	—	—
0	37	0.94	6.0	45.9	204.5	0.20	0	0.16	0.05	0.13	1.20	0.01	59.3	0	0.1	7.3
43	79	1.34	7.1	49.1	281.8	0.31	66.4	0.15	0.55	0.16	1.20	0.03	49.1	0.1	0.1	10.8
0	57	1.22	16.1	81.2	321.2	0.42	0	0.20	0.12	0.15	1.65	0.04	63.2	0.1	0.1	12.2
0	32	0.94	28.4	143.1	284.0	0.22	11.3	0.01	0.14	0.05	0.50	0.04	6.3	0	0	9.9
0	5	1.03	7.7	29.8	171.1	0.21	0	0.14	0.24	0.13	1.27	0.02	61.2	0	0	9.0
21	94	0.94	10.1	69.2	208.8	0.49	0	0.14	0.40	0.16	1.06	0.04	61.7	1.5	0.2	6.8
0	11	0.70	13.0	44.3	134.5	0.31	0	0.09	—	0.06	0.92	0.08	19.0	0	0	6.3
0	6	0.31	2.3	9.3	52.3	0.07	0	0.05	—	0.02	0.41	0	15.7	0	0	2.8
20	37	1.22	7.6	46.0	152.0	0.32	25.2	0.18	0.10	0.17	1.94	0.03	52.0	0	0	12.0
21	38	1.24	7.8	46.6	154.3	0.32	25.5	0.14	0.11	0.16	1.77	0.02	47.4	0	0	12.2
0	14	1.16	9.0	41.0	164.2	0.30	0	0.14	0.06	0.09	1.52	0.03	73.6	0.1	0	8.7
0	11	0.89	7.1	32.2	165.6	0.24	0	0.10	0.04	0.09	1.24	0.02	49.9	0	0	6.8
6	48	3.44	15.3	65.5	279.8	0.30	—	0.37	0	0.18	3.91	0.03	166.7	—	0	15.8
0	23	0.88	8.1	33.0	183.9	0.26	0	0.14	0.09	0.09	1.31	0.01	91.2	0	0	8.2
0	27	0.65	20.3	59.8	99.1	0.44	0	0.07	0.10	0.03	1.05	0.07	19.5	0	0	8.6
0	27	0.65	20.4	60.0	99.4	0.44	0	0.06	0.10	0.03	1.05	0.07	16.8	0	0	8.6
0	20	0.94	10.5	44.1	105.9	0.27	0.6	0.15	0.13	0.10	1.45	0.02	36.0	0	0	9.0
0	19	0.93	9.2	33.2	104.5	0.28	0.5	0.12	0.13	0.09	1.29	0.01	28.1	0	0	8.9
0	18	0.73	10.0	38.3	120.7	0.28	1.4	0.11	0.13	0.06	0.85	0.02	23.5	0	0	6.6
0	18	0.74	10.3	38.5	121.5	0.28	1.3	0.09	0.13	0.06	0.77	0.02	18.8	0.1	0	6.7
0	52	1.57	15.6	72.0	321.6	0.50	0	0.36	0.18	0.20	2.78	0.02	99.0	0	0	16.3
0	10	1.96	44.2	108.8	284.2	0.97	0	0.22	0.39	0.05	1.82	0.17	22.4	0	0	28.2
0	22	0.92	17.3	66.6	190.7	0.47	0	0.10	0.13	0.10	0.99	0.04	42.9	0	0	7.8
0	17	0.75	6.8	59.0	90.2	0.19	0	0.09	0.07	0.10	0.90	0.02	40.6	0	0	5.2
0	18	0.79	7.0	61.5	94.3	0.19	0	0.07	0.08	0.10	0.85	0.02	37.0	0.1	0	5.4
0	20	0.72	—	—	120.0	—	0	0.15	—	0.07	1.20	—	—	0	—	—
0	23	0.91	12.8	53.1	193.0	0.36	0	0.14	0.11	0.11	1.22	0.02	48.3	0.1	0	9.9
0	0	1.08	—	—	220.0	—	0	—	—	—	—	—	—	1.2	—	—
0	23	0.90	12.5	53.1	192.6	0.36	0	0.11	0.11	0.10	1.09	0.02	42.9	0.1	0	9.9
0	11	0.91	7.0	32.0	128.3	0.23	0	0.11	0.05	0.07	1.19	0.03	57.5	0.1	0	6.8
0	11	0.89	7.1	32.2	165.6	0.24	0	0.10	0.04	0.09	1.24	0.02	49.9	0	0	6.8
0	11	0.89	7.1	32.2	165.6	0.24	0	0.10	0.04	0.09	1.24	0.02	49.9	0	0	6.8
0	35	0.88	11.5	45.5	129.8	0.29	0	0.12	0.05	0.07	1.48	0.03	24.8	0.1	0	7.2
0	38	0.94	13.6	51.3	138.2	0.34	0	0.10	0.06	0.09	1.44	0.04	23.0	0	0	7.7
0	65	0.90	6.3	28.8	122.8	0.21	0	0.13	0.05	0.06	1.20	0.02	42.8	0	0	5.5
0	15	1.43	37.3	144.4	159.2	0.69	0	0.14	0.35	0.10	1.83	0.09	35.9	0	0	17.8
0	42	0.12	4.0	67.5	255.5	0.06	0	0.05	0	0.10	0.09	0	14.5	0	0	7.7
166	26	1.03	8.3	89.3	298.5	0.34	111.8	0.10	—	0.17	0.98	0.03	46.5	0	0.2	6.6
0	64	1.87	19.2	250.5	370.2	0.44	0	0.24	1.96	0.21	1.74	0.11	77.7	4.8	0	14.6
27	28	1.41	21.8	128.0	213.8	0.44	16.6	0.02	0.63	0.09	0.37	0.03	14.9	0.1	0.1	2.1
55	57	1.53	30.4	133.0	299.3	0.66	38.0	0.13	—	0.20	1.08	0.04	37.0	0.2	0.2	11.3
2	14	0.89	6.9	65.8	43.4	0.12	3.0	0.02	0.39	0.04	0.34	0.02	13.8	0.2	0	0.9
54	40	0.72	—	—	312.0	—	0	0.12	—	0.14	0.80		—	0	—	—
25	138	1.70	14.9	128.8	366.9	0.36	71.3	0.18	—	0.18	1.37	0.04	44.8	1.4	0.1	10.8
107	26	1.00	5.7	88.8	143.6	0.37	48.5	0.10	—	0.19	0.76	0.04	33.4	0	0.2	11.7
1	101	1.30	13.4	110.9	318.1	0.37	13.4	0.14	0.13	0.21	1.19	0.03	57.1	0.1	0.1	12.0
10	20	1.30	12.8	119.7	198.4	0.27	21.1	0.03	2.88	0.06	0.51	0	20.5	0	0	3.8
35	40	0.68	3.8	33.9	220.2	0.16	12.2	0.06	—	0.04	0.32	0.02	25.6	0	0.1	3.5

APPENDIX H

TABLE H-1 Table of Food Composition (*continued*) (Computer code is for Cengage Diet Analysis program) (For purposes of calculations, use "0" for t, <1, <0.1, 0.01)

DA+ Code	Food Description	Quantity	Measure	Wt (g)	H_2O (g)	Ener (kcal)	Prot (g)	Carb (g)	Fiber (g)	Fat (g)	Fat Breakdown (g) Sat	Mono	Poly
Breads, Baked Goods, Cakes, Cookies, Crackers, Chips, Pies—*continued*													
	Snack cakes												
8791	Chocolate snack cake, creme filled, with frosting	1	item(s)	50	9.3	200	1.8	30.2	1.6	8.0	2.4	4.3	0.9
25010	Cinnamon coffee cake	1	piece(s)	72	22.6	231	3.6	35.9	0.7	8.3	2.2	2.6	3.0
16777	Funnel cake	1	item(s)	90	37.7	275	7.3	29.2	0.9	14.3	2.7	5.5	5.4
8794	Sponge snack cake, creme filled	1	item(s)	43	8.3	159	1.5	27.2	0.4	4.9	1.8	2.1	0.8
	Snacks, chips, pretzels												
57179	Bagel chips, plain	1	ounce(s)	28	—	132	4.1	19.2	1.0	4.6	0.5	3.5	0.5
57180	Bagel chips, toasted garlic	1	ounce(s)	28	—	132	4.1	19.2	1.0	4.6	0.5	3.5	0.5
38192	Chex traditional snack mix	1	cup(s)	52	—	220	4.0	38.0	1.0	6.0	1.0	—	—
654	Potato chips, salted	1	ounce(s)	28	0.6	154	1.9	14.4	1.2	10.3	1.1	4.5	4.5
8816	Potato chips, unsalted	1	ounce(s)	28	0.5	152	2.0	15.0	1.4	9.8	3.1	2.8	3.5
5096	Pretzels, plain, hard, twists	5	item(s)	30	1.0	114	3.1	23.9	0.9	0.8	0.2	0.4	0.3
4632	Pretzels, whole wheat	1	ounce(s)	28	1.1	103	3.1	23.0	2.2	0.7	0.2	0.3	0.2
4641	Tortilla chips, plain	6	item(s)	11	0.2	53	0.8	7.1	0.6	2.5	0.3	0.7	1.2
	Cookies												
8859	Animal crackers	12	item(s)	30	1.2	134	2.1	22.2	0.3	4.1	1.0	2.3	0.6
8876	Brownie, prepared from mix	1	item(s)	24	3.0	112	1.5	12.0	0.5	7.0	1.8	2.6	2.3
25207	Chocolate chip cookies	1	item(s)	30	3.7	140	2.0	16.2	0.6	7.9	2.1	3.3	2.1
8915	Chocolate sandwich cookie with extra creme filling	1	item(s)	13	0.2	65	0.6	8.9	0.4	3.2	0.7	2.1	0.3
14145	Fig Newtons cookies	1	item(s)	16	—	55	0.5	11.0	0.5	1.0	0	—	—
8920	Fortune cookie	1	item(s)	8	0.6	30	0.3	6.7	0.1	0.2	0.1	0.1	0.0
25208	Oatmeal cookies	1	item(s)	69	12.5	234	5.4	45.3	3.2	4.2	0.7	1.3	1.8
25213	Peanut butter cookies	1	item(s)	35	4.1	162	4.2	16.9	0.9	9.2	1.7	4.7	2.4
33095	Sugar cookies	1	item(s)	16	4.1	61	1.1	7.4	0.1	3.0	0.6	1.4	0.8
9002	Vanilla sandwich cookie with creme filling	1	item(s)	10	0.2	48	0.5	7.2	0.1	2.0	0.3	0.8	0.8
	Crackers												
9012	Cheese cracker sandwich with peanut butter	4	item(s)	28	0.9	139	3.5	15.9	1.0	7.0	1.2	3.6	1.4
9008	Cheese crackers (mini)	30	item(s)	30	1.1	147	3.3	17.8	0.7	6.8	1.6	1.7	3.0
33362	Cheese crackers, low sodium	1	serving(s)	30	0.9	151	3.0	17.5	0.7	7.6	2.9	3.6	0.7
8928	Honey graham crackers	4	item(s)	28	1.2	118	1.9	21.5	0.8	2.8	0.4	1.1	1.1
9016	Matzo crackers, plain	1	item(s)	28	1.2	112	2.8	23.8	0.9	0.4	0.1	0	0.2
9024	Melba toast	3	item(s)	15	0.8	59	1.8	11.5	0.9	0.5	0.1	0.1	0.2
9028	Melba toast, rye	3	item(s)	15	0.7	58	1.7	11.6	1.2	0.5	0.1	0.1	0.2
14189	Ritz crackers	5	item(s)	16	0.5	80	1.0	10.0	0	4.5	1.0	1.0	1.7
9014	Rye crispbread crackers	1	item(s)	10	0.6	37	0.8	8.2	1.6	0.1	0	0	0.1
9040	Rye wafer	1	item(s)	11	0.6	37	1.1	8.8	2.5	0.1	0	0	0
432	Saltine crackers	5	item(s)	15	0.6	63	1.4	11.2	0.4	1.3	0.3	0.3	0.6
9046	Saltine crackers, low salt	5	item(s)	15	0.6	63	1.4	11.2	0.4	1.3	0.3	0.3	0.6
9052	Snack cracker sandwich with cheese filling	4	item(s)	28	1.1	134	2.6	17.3	0.5	5.9	1.7	3.2	0.7
9054	Snack cracker sandwich with peanut butter filling	4	item(s)	28	0.8	138	3.2	16.3	0.6	6.9	1.4	3.9	1.3
9048	Snack crackers, round	10	item(s)	30	1.0	151	2.0	18.4	0.6	7.7	1.6	2.0	3.8
9050	Snack crackers, round, low salt	10	item(s)	30	1.0	151	2.2	18.3	0.5	7.6	1.1	3.2	2.9
9044	Soda crackers	5	item(s)	15	0.6	63	1.4	11.2	0.4	1.3	0.3	0.3	0.6
9059	Wheat cracker sandwich with cheese filling	4	item(s)	28	0.9	139	2.7	16.3	0.9	7.0	1.2	2.9	2.6
9061	Wheat cracker sandwich with peanut butter filling	4	item(s)	28	1.0	139	3.8	15.1	1.2	7.5	1.3	3.3	2.5
9055	Wheat crackers	10	item(s)	30	1.0	137	2.7	20.2	1.1	5.2	0.8	1.3	2.8
9057	Wheat crackers, low salt	10	item(s)	30	0.9	142	2.6	19.5	1.4	6.2	1.6	3.4	0.8
9022	Whole wheat crackers	7	item(s)	28	0.8	120	3.0	19.5	2.9	4.0	0.6	0.9	1.9
	Pastry												
16754	Apple fritter	1	item(s)	17	6.4	61	1.0	5.5	0.2	3.9	1.0	1.6	1.1
41565	Cinnamon rolls with icing, refrigerated dough	1	serving(s)	44	12.3	145	1.9	23.5	0.6	5.0	1.4	—	—
4945	Croissant, butter	1	item(s)	57	13.2	231	4.7	26.1	1.5	12.0	6.6	3.1	0.6
9096	Danish, nut	1	item(s)	65	13.3	280	4.6	29.7	1.3	16.4	3.8	8.9	2.8
9115	Doughnut with creme filling	1	item(s)	85	32.5	307	5.4	25.5	0.7	20.8	4.6	10.3	2.6
9117	Doughnut with jelly filling	1	item(s)	85	30.3	289	5.0	33.2	0.8	15.9	4.1	8.7	2.0
4947	Doughnut, cake	1	item(s)	47	10.8	196	2.8	21.4	0.8	11.1	3.3	6.0	1.2
9105	Doughnut, cake, chocolate glazed	1	item(s)	42	6.8	175	1.9	24.1	0.9	8.4	2.2	4.7	1.0

Chol (mg)	Calc (mg)	Iron (mg)	Magn (mg)	Pota (mg)	Sodi (mg)	Zinc (mg)	Vit A (µg)	Thia (mg)	Vit E (mg α)	Ribo (mg)	Niac (mg)	Vit B_6 (mg)	Fola (µg)	Vit C (mg)	Vit B_{12} (µg)	Sele (µg)
0	58	1.80	18.0	88.0	166.0	0.52	0.5	0.02	0.55	0.04	0.46	0.07	17.5	0.9	0	1.7
26	54	1.20	8.3	72.6	275.8	0.30	0	0.18	0.35	0.17	1.30	0.03	66.1	0	0.1	9.8
55	127	1.90	16.2	147.6	271.8	0.69	56.7	0.24	1.58	0.33	1.86	0.05	75.6	0	0.3	17.5
17	10	0.58	3.4	30.2	199.8	0.25	2.1	0.08	0.26	0.07	0.66	0	23.0	0	0.1	1.5
0	0	1.09	—	—	313.9	—	0	—	—	—	—	—	—	0	—	—
0	0	1.09	—	—	303.8	—	0	—	—	—	—	—	—	0	—	—
0	0	0.72	—	—	480.0	—	0	—	—	—	—	—	—	0	—	—
0	7	0.46	19.8	465.5	136.1	0.68	0	0.02	1.91	0.07	1.19	0.20	21.3	5.3	0	2.3
0	7	0.46	19.0	361.5	2.3	0.31	0	0.05	2.58	0.06	1.08	0.19	12.8	8.8	0	2.3
0	5	1.56	8.7	40.8	407.1	0.43	0	0.15	0.10	0.10	1.54	0.01	85.6	0	0	1.8
0	8	0.76	8.5	121.9	57.6	0.18	0	0.12	—	0.08	1.85	0.08	15.3	0.3	0	
0	19	0.25	15.8	23.2	45.5	0.27	0	0	0.46	0.01	0.14	0.02	2.2	0	0	0.7
0	13	0.82	5.4	30.0	122.1	0.19	0	0.10	0.04	0.10	1.04	0.01	49.5	0	0	2.1
18	14	0.44	12.7	42.2	82.3	0.23	42.2	0.03	—	0.05	0.24	0.02	9.4	0.1	0	2.8
13	11	0.64	11.4	51.3	108.6	0.24	0	0.08	0.60	0.06	0.87	0.02	29.8	0	0	4.2
0	2	1.01	4.7	17.8	45.6	0.10	0	0.01	0.25	0.02	0.25	0	9.0	0	0	1.1
0	10	0.36	—	—	62.5	—	—	—	—	—	—	—	—	0	—	—
0	1	0.12	0.6	3.3	2.5	0.01	0.1	0.01	0	0.01	0.15	0	8.4	0	0	0.2
0	26	1.83	45.5	157.5	310.3	1.49	0	0.23	1.02	0.13	1.40	0.09	46.4	0.3	0	16.7
13	27	0.65	20.3	107.2	153.7	0.46	0	0.09	1.45	0.09	1.86	0.06	34.7	0.1	0.1	4.7
18	5	0.32	1.7	12.8	50.0	0.08	0	0.04	0.32	0.05	0.31	0.01	17.1	0	0	3.1
0	3	0.22	1.4	9.1	34.9	0.04	0	0.03	0.16	0.02	0.27	0	8.2	0	0	0.3
0	14	0.76	15.7	61.0	232.1	0.29	0.3	0.15	0.66	0.08	1.63	0.04	39.8	0	0.1	2.3
1	41	1.46	7.5	46.8	291.9	0.36	5.1	0.17	0.66	0.10	1.83	0.05	72.3	0	0.1	4.1
4	45	1.43	10.8	31.8	137.4	0.34	5.1	0.17	0.09	0.13	1.40	0.17	40.2	0	0.1	2.6
0	7	1.04	8.4	37.8	133.6	0.23	0	0.06	0.09	0.09	1.15	0.02	18.5	0	0	2.9
0	4	0.90	7.1	31.8	0	0.19	0	0.11	0.02	0.08	1.11	0.03	4.8	0	0	10.5
0	14	0.56	8.9	30.3	89.7	0.30	0	0.06	0.06	0.04	0.62	0.01	29.0	0	0	5.2
0	12	0.55	5.8	29.0	134.9	0.20	0	0.07	—	0.04	0.71	0.01	19.4	0	0	5.8
0	20	0.36	3.0	19.0	135.0	0.10	—	0.07	0.56	0.04	0.78	0.01	17.8	0	—	0.7
0	3	0.24	7.8	31.9	41.0	0.24	0	0.02	0.08	0.01	0.10	0.02	6.5	0	0	3.7
0	4	0.65	13.3	54.5	61.3	0.31	0	0.05	0.09	0.03	0.17	0.03	4.9	0	0	2.6
0	3	0.77	3.8	23.9	153.1	0.12	0	0.09	0.17	0.05	0.79	0.01	33.2	0	0	1.0
0	18	0.77	3.8	108.6	29.7	0.12	0	0.09	0.17	0.05	0.79	0.01	33.2	0	0	1.0
1	72	0.67	10.1	120.1	273.8	0.17	4.8	0.12	0.06	0.19	1.05	0.01	44.8	0	0	6.0
0	23	0.78	15.4	60.2	224.3	0.32	0.3	0.14	0.58	0.08	1.71	0.04	34.2	0	0	3.0
0	29	1.14	5.4	33.3	224.4	0.17	0	0.13	1.07	0.07	1.25	0.02	55.8	0	0	1.1
0	36	1.08	8.1	106.5	64.8	0.20	0	0.12	0.61	0.10	1.21	0.02	42.6	0	0	2.0
0	3	0.77	3.8	23.9	153.1	0.12	0	0.09	0.17	0.05	0.79	0.01	33.2	0	0	1.0
2	57	0.73	15.1	85.7	234.9	0.24	5.9	0.10	—	0.12	0.89	0.07	26.9	0.4	0	6.8
0	48	0.75	10.6	83.2	226.0	0.23	0	0.11	—	0.08	1.65	0.04	26.0	0	0	6.1
0	24	1.41	13.8	62.1	236.1	0.52	0	0.18	0.33	0.09	1.49	0.04	56.1	0	0.1	3.8
0	15	1.32	18.6	60.9	57.0	0.48	0	0.15	0.15	0.10	1.49	0.04	21.6	0	0	10.1
0	10	0.94	30.8	96.6	197.1	0.74	0	0.05	0.39	0.01	1.30	0.05	7.8	0	0	2.8
13	9	0.26	2.2	22.3	7.3	0.10	8.2	0.03	0.25	0.04	0.23	0.01	9.2	0.2	0	2.6
0	12	0.85	—	—	343.2	—	0	—	—	—	—	—	—	0	—	—
38	21	1.16	9.1	67.3	424.1	0.43	117.4	0.22	0.48	0.14	1.25	0.03	74.1	0.1	0.1	12.9
30	61	1.17	20.8	61.8	193.7	0.57	5.8	0.14	0.53	0.16	1.50	0.07	79.3	1.1	0.1	9.2
20	21	1.56	17.0	68.0	262.8	0.68	9.4	0.29	0.25	0.13	1.91	0.06	92.7	0	0.1	9.2
22	21	1.50	17.0	67.2	387.0	0.64	14.5	0.27	0.37	0.12	1.82	0.09	88.5	0	0.2	10.6
4	12	1.41	7.5	53.1	261.8	0.32	1.4	0.11	0.89	0.07	0.93	0.01	54.0	0.6	0	4.8
24	89	0.95	14.3	44.5	90.3	0.24	5.0	0.02	0.09	0.03	0.20	0.01	26.9	0	0	1.7

APPENDIX H

DA+ Code	Food Description	Quantity	Measure	Wt (g)	H_2O (g)	Ener (kcal)	Prot (g)	Carb (g)	Fiber (g)	Fat (g)	Fat Breakdown (g) Sat	Mono	Poly
	Breads, Baked Goods, Cakes, Cookies, Crackers, Chips, Pies—*continued*												
437	Doughnut, glazed	1	item(s)	60	15.2	242	3.8	26.6	0.7	13.7	3.5	7.7	1.7
10617	Toaster pastry, brown sugar cinnamon	1	item(s)	50	5.3	210	2.0	34.0	0.5	8.0	2.5	—	—
30928	Toaster pastry, cream cheese	1	item(s)	54	—	200	3.0	24.0	0.5	11.0	4.0	—	—
	Muffins												
25015	Blueberry	1	item(s)	63	29.8	160	3.4	23.0	0.8	6.0	0.9	1.6	3.0
9189	Corn, ready to eat	1	item(s)	57	18.6	174	3.4	29.0	1.9	4.8	0.8	1.2	1.8
9121	English muffin, plain, enriched	1	item(s)	57	24.0	134	4.4	26.2	1.5	1.0	0.1	0.2	0.5
29582	English muffin, toasted	1	item(s)	50	16.5	135	5.2	26.3	1.4	1.0	0.3	0.2	0.5
9145	English muffin, wheat	1	item(s)	57	24.1	127	5.0	25.5	2.6	1.1	0.2	0.2	0.5
8894	Oat bran	1	item(s)	57	20.0	154	4.0	27.5	2.6	4.2	0.6	1.0	2.4
	Granola bars												
34783	Kudos milk chocolate with M&Ms granola bar	1	item(s)	24	—	100	1.0	17.0	1.0	2.5	1.5	—	—
38187	Nature Valley fruit 'n' nut trail mix bar	1	item(s)	35	—	140	3.0	25.0	2.0	4.0	0.5	—	—
3436	Nature Valley oats 'n honey crunchy granola bars	2	item(s)	42	—	180	4.0	29.0	2.0	6.0	0.5	—	—
1383	Plain, hard	1	item(s)	25	1.0	115	2.5	15.8	1.3	4.9	0.6	1.1	3.0
4606	Plain, soft	1	item(s)	28	1.8	126	2.1	19.1	1.3	4.9	2.1	1.1	1.5
	Pies												
454	Apple pie, prepared from home recipe	1	slice(s)	155	73.3	411	3.7	57.5	2.3	19.4	4.7	8.4	5.2
470	Pecan pie, prepared from home recipe	1	slice(s)	122	23.8	503	6.0	63.7	—	27.1	4.9	13.6	7.0
33356	Pie crust mix, prepared, baked	1	slice(s)	20	2.1	100	1.3	10.1	0.4	6.1	1.5	3.5	0.8
9007	Pie crust, ready to bake, frozen, enriched, baked	1	slice(s)	16	1.1	81	1.0	9.0	0.5	4.6	1.5	2.2	0.6
472	Pumpkin pie, prepared from home recipe	1	slice(s)	155	90.7	316	7.0	40.9	—	14.4	4.9	5.7	2.8
	Rolls												
8555	Crescent dinner roll	1	item(s)	28	9.6	78	2.8	14.0	0.6	1.1	0.2	0.3	0.4
489	Hamburger roll or bun, plain	1	item(s)	43	14.7	120	4.2	21.6	0.9	1.6	0.4	0.4	0.7
490	Hard roll	1	item(s)	57	17.7	167	5.6	30.0	1.3	2.5	0.3	0.6	1.0
5127	Kaiser roll	1	item(s)	57	17.7	167	5.6	30.0	1.3	2.5	0.3	0.6	1.0
5130	Whole wheat roll or bun	1	item(s)	28	9.4	75	2.5	14.5	2.1	1.3	0.2	0.3	0.6
	Sport bars												
37026	Balance original chocolate bar	1	item(s)	50	—	200	14.0	21.0	2.0	7.0	4.0	—	—
37024	Balance original peanut butter bar	1	item(s)	50	—	200	15.0	21.0	0.5	7.0	3.0	—	—
36580	Clif Bar chocolate brownie energy bar	1	item(s)	68	—	240	10.0	44.0	5.0	5.0	1.5	—	—
36583	Clif Bar crunchy peanut butter energy bar	1	item(s)	68	—	250	11.0	42.0	5.0	6.0	1.0	—	—
36589	Clif Luna Nutz over Chocolate energy bar	1	item(s)	48	—	180	9.0	25.0	4.0	6.0	2.0	—	—
12005	PowerBar apple cinnamon	1	item(s)	65	—	230	8.0	45.0	2.0	3.5	0.5	—	—
16078	PowerBar banana	1	item(s)	65	—	240	8.0	46.0	1.0	3.5	0.5	—	—
16080	PowerBar chocolate	1	item(s)	65	—	240	8.0	45.0	3.0	3.0	1.0	—	—
29092	PowerBar peanut butter	1	item(s)	65	—	240	9.0	44.0	1.0	4.0	1.0	—	—
	Tortillas												
1391	Corn tortillas, soft	1	item(s)	24	11.0	52	1.4	10.7	1.5	0.7	0.1	0.2	0.3
1669	Flour tortilla	1	item(s)	30	9.5	90	2.4	15.4	0.7	2.0	0.5	1.1	0.4
1390	Taco shells, hard	1	item(s)	13	0.9	63	0.9	8.5	0.9	2.8	0.8	0.8	0.9
	Pancakes, waffles												
8926	Pancakes, blueberry, prepared from recipe	3	item(s)	114	60.6	253	7.0	33.1	0.8	10.5	2.3	2.6	4.7
13402	Pancakes, frozen	3	item(s)	105	—	240	5.0	41.0	1.0	6.0	1.0	—	—
9221	Waffle plain, frozen, toasted	1	item(s)	33	10.1	103	2.4	16.3	0.8	3.2	0.5	1.6	0.7
30311	Waffle, 100% whole grain	1	item(s)	182	85.2	426	16.1	60.7	4.2	14.2	3.5	5.5	4.1
500	Waffle, plain, prepared from recipe	1	item(s)	75	31.5	218	5.9	24.7	1.7	10.6	2.1	2.6	5.1
	Cereal, Flour, Grain, Pasta, Noodles, Popcorn												
	Grain												
2861	Amaranth, dry	½	cup(s)	98	11.0	362	13.2	63.6	6.5	6.8	1.4	1.6	2.7
1953	Barley, pearled, cooked	½	cup(s)	79	54.0	97	1.8	22.2	3.0	0.3	0.1	0	0.2

Chol (mg)	Calc (mg)	Iron (mg)	Magn (mg)	Pota (mg)	Sodi (mg)	Zinc (mg)	Vit A (μg)	Thia (mg)	Vit E (mg α)	Ribo (mg)	Niac (mg)	Vit B_6 (mg)	Fola (μg)	Vit C (mg)	Vit B_{12} (μg)	Sele (μg)
4	26	0.36	13.2	64.8	205.2	0.46	2.4	0.53	—	0.04	0.39	0.03	13.2	0.1	0.1	5.0
0	0	1.80	8.0	67.5	190.0	0.61	150.1	0.15	—	0.17	2.00	0.20	—	0	0	—
10	0	0.72	—	—	210.0	—	0	—	—	—	—	—	—	0	—	—
20	56	1.04	7.9	68.6	287.8	0.29	0	0.17	0.85	0.16	1.26	0.03	62.5	0.2	0.2	9.0
15	42	1.60	18.2	39.3	118.6	0.31	29.6	0.16	0.46	0.19	1.16	0.05	63.8	0	0.1	8.7
0	30	1.42	12.0	74.7	264.5	0.40	0	0.25	—	0.16	2.21	0.02	57.0	0	0	
0	99	2.33	14.0	64.5	238.5	0.70	0	0.27	0.18	0.14	2.49	0.03	90.0	0.9	0	13.1
0	101	1.64	21.1	106.0	201.2	0.61	0	0.25	0.26	0.17	1.91	0.05	46.2	0	0	16.6
0	36	2.39	89.5	289.0	224.0	1.05	0	0.15	0.38	0.05	0.24	0.09	79.2	0	0	6.3
0	300	0.36	—	—	105.0	—	0	—	—	—	—	—	—	0	—	—
0	0	0.36	—	—	100.0	—	0	—	—	—	—	—	—	0	—	—
0	0	1.08	—	95.0	160.0	—	0	—	—	—	—	—	—	0	—	—
0	15	0.72	23.8	82.3	72.0	0.50	0.5	0.06	0.51	0.03	0.39	0.02	5.6	0.2	0	4.0
0	30	0.73	21.0	92.3	79.0	0.43	0	0.08	—	0.05	0.15	0.03	6.8	0	0.1	4.6
0	11	1.74	10.9	122.4	327.0	0.29	17.0	0.23	—	0.17	1.91	0.05	58.9	2.6	0	12.1
106	39	1.81	31.7	162.3	319.6	1.24	100.0	0.23	—	0.22	1.03	0.07	41.5	0.2	0.2	14.6
0	12	0.43	3.0	12.4	145.8	0.08	0	0.06	—	0.04	0.47	0.01	22.2	0	0	4.4
0	3	0.45	2.7	18.2	74.7	0.08	0	0.05	0.09	0.02	0.55	0.01	16.3	0	0	1.1
65	146	1.97	29.5	288.3	348.8	0.71	660.3	0.14	—	0.31	1.21	0.07	43.4	2.6	0.1	11.0
0	48	0.96	6.7	35.6	140.0	0.24	0	0.18	0.02	0.06	1.33	0.02	47.9	0.4	0.1	6.4
0	74	1.47	10.3	54.6	215.0	0.37	0	0.28	0.03	0.09	2.05	0.03	73.5	0.6	0.1	9.8
0	54	1.87	15.4	61.6	310.1	0.54	0	0.27	0.24	0.19	2.42	0.02	86.1	0	0	22.3
0	54	1.87	15.4	61.6	310.1	0.54	0	0.27	0.24	0.19	2.42	0.02	86.1	0	0	22.3
0	30	0.69	24.1	77.1	135.5	0.57	0	0.07	0.26	0.04	1.04	0.06	8.5	0	0	14.0
0	150	2.70	—	260.0	160.0	2.25	—	0.22	—	0.25	3.00	0.30	102.0	60.0	0.9	10.5
0	150	2.70	—	150.0	170.0	2.25	—	0.22	—	0.25	3.00	0.30	102.0	60.0	0.9	10.5
0	250	4.50	100.0	340.0	150.0	3.00	—	0.38	—	0.25	3.00	0.40	—	60.0	0.9	14.0
0	250	4.50	100.0	270.0	230.0	3.00	—	0.38	—	0.25	3.00	0.40	—	60.0	0.9	14.0
0	350	5.40	40.0	160.0	190.0	5.25	—	0.15	—	0.68	8.00	1.50	—	12.0	4.5	24.5
0	250	4.50	—	105.0	200.0	—	0	0.22	—	0.17	—	0.50	—	42.0	—	—
0	150	2.70	—	105.0	200.0	—	0	0.22	—	0.17	—	0.50	—	42.0	—	—
0	150	2.70	—	260.0	200.0	—	0	0.22	—	0.17	—	0.50	—	42.0	—	—
0	20	0.72	—	105.0	200.0	—	0	—	—	—	—	—	—	0	—	—
0	19	0.30	17.3	44.6	10.8	0.31	0	0.02	0.07	0.02	0.36	0.05	1.2	0	0	1.5
0	32	1.00	6.0	45.9	205.8	0.16	0	0.15	0.06	0.04	1.09	0.01	60.3	0	0	7.2
0	13	0.24	11.4	31.0	32.3	0.21	0.1	0.03	0.09	0.01	0.25	0.03	11.3	0	0	0.6
64	235	1.96	18.2	157.3	469.7	0.62	57.0	0.22	—	0.31	1.74	0.06	60.4	2.5	0.2	16.0
35	40	1.80	—	—	500.0	—	0	0.30	—	0.17	2.00	—	—	0	—	—
5	101	2.28	7.9	47.5	240.9	0.17	131.3	0.17	0.32	0.23	2.93	0.34	39.3	0	1.0	4.2
4	460	3.15	69.2	424.1	910.0	1.60	3.6	0.38	1.04	0.60	3.20	0.17	80.1	0	0.6	41.3
52	191	1.73	14.3	119.3	383.3	0.51	48.8	0.20	—	0.26	1.55	0.04	51.0	0.3	0.2	34.7
0	155	7.42	241.8	495.3	3.9	2.80	0	0.11	1.16	0.19	0.90	0.58	79.9	4.1	0	18.2
0	9	1.04	17.3	73.0	2.4	0.64	0	0.07	0.01	0.05	1.62	0.09	12.6	0	0	6.8

TABLE H-1 Table of Food Composition (*continued*)

(Computer code is for Cengage Diet Analysis program) (For purposes of calculations, use "0" for t, <1, <0.1, 0.01)

DA+ Code	Food Description	Quantity	Measure	Wt (g)	H_2O (g)	Ener (kcal)	Prot (g)	Carb (g)	Fiber (g)	Fat (g)	Fat Breakdown (g) Sat	Mono	Poly
Cereal, Flour, Grain, Pasta, Noodles, Popcorn—*continued*													
1956	Buckwheat groats, cooked, roasted	½	cup(s)	84	63.5	77	2.8	16.7	2.3	0.5	0.1	0.2	0.2
1957	Bulgur, cooked	½	cup(s)	91	70.8	76	2.8	16.9	4.1	0.2	0	0	0.1
1963	Couscous, cooked	½	cup(s)	79	57.0	88	3.0	18.2	1.1	0.1	0	0	0.1
1967	Millet, cooked	½	cup(s)	120	85.7	143	4.2	28.4	1.6	1.2	0.2	0.2	0.6
1969	Oat bran, dry	½	cup(s)	47	3.1	116	8.1	31.1	7.2	3.3	0.6	1.1	1.3
1972	Quinoa, dry	½	cup(s)	85	11.3	313	12.0	54.6	6.0	5.2	0.6	1.4	2.8
	Rice												
129	Brown, long grain, cooked	½	cup(s)	98	71.3	108	2.5	22.4	1.8	0.9	0.2	0.3	0.3
2863	Brown, medium grain, cooked	½	cup(s)	98	71.1	109	2.3	22.9	1.8	0.8	0.2	0.3	0.3
37488	Jasmine, saffroned, cooked	½	cup(s)	79	—	85	2.0	19.5	0	0	0	0	0
30280	Pilaf, cooked	½	cup(s)	103	73.4	135	2.1	22.2	0.6	4.1	0.6	1.6	1.7
28066	Spanish, cooked	½	cup(s)	113	85.2	114	2.9	23.5	1.5	1.0	0.2	0.3	0.3
2867	White glutinous, cooked	½	cup(s)	87	66.7	84	1.8	18.3	0.9	0.2	0	0.1	0.1
484	White, long grain, boiled	½	cup(s)	79	54.1	103	2.1	22.3	0.3	0.2	0.1	0.1	0.1
482	White, long grain, enriched, instant, boiled	½	cup(s)	83	59.4	97	1.8	20.7	0.5	0.4	0	0.1	0
486	White, long grain, enriched, parboiled, cooked	½	cup(s)	79	55.6	97	2.3	20.6	0.7	0.3	0.1	0.1	0.1
1994	Wild brown, cooked	½	cup(s)	82	60.6	83	3.3	17.5	1.5	0.3	0	0	0.2
	Flour & grain fractions												
505	All-purpose flour, self rising, enriched	½	cup(s)	63	6.6	221	6.2	46.4	1.7	0.6	0.1	0.1	0.3
503	All-purpose flour, white, bleached, enriched	½	cup(s)	63	7.4	228	6.5	47.7	1.7	0.6	0.1	0.1	0.3
53271	Barley flour	½	cup(s)	74	9.0	255	7.8	55.1	7.5	1.2	0.2	0.2	0.6
383	Buckwheat flour, whole groat	½	cup(s)	60	6.7	201	7.6	42.4	6.0	1.9	0.4	0.6	0.6
504	Cake wheat flour, enriched	½	cup(s)	69	8.6	248	5.6	53.5	1.2	0.6	0.1	0.1	0.3
426	Cornmeal, degermed, enriched	½	cup(s)	69	7.7	255	4.9	54.8	2.7	1.2	0.1	0.2	0.4
424	Cornmeal, yellow whole grain	½	cup(s)	61	6.3	221	5.0	46.9	4.5	2.2	0.3	0.6	1.0
1978	Dark rye flour	½	cup(s)	64	6.9	208	10.2	43.9	15.2	1.4	0.2	0.2	0.7
1644	Masa corn flour, enriched	½	cup(s)	57	5.2	208	5.3	43.5	3.6	2.2	0.3	0.6	1.0
1976	Rice flour, brown	½	cup(s)	79	9.5	287	5.7	60.4	3.6	2.2	0.4	0.8	0.8
1645	Rice flour, white	½	cup(s)	79	9.4	289	4.7	63.3	1.9	1.1	0.3	0.3	0.3
1980	Semolina, enriched	½	cup(s)	84	10.6	301	10.6	60.8	3.3	0.9	0.1	0.1	0.4
2827	Soy flour, raw	½	cup(s)	42	2.2	185	14.7	14.9	4.1	8.8	1.3	1.9	4.9
1990	Wheat germ, crude	2	tablespoon(s)	14	1.6	52	3.3	7.4	1.9	1.4	0.2	0.2	0.9
506	Whole-wheat flour	½	cup(s)	60	6.4	204	7.9	43.2	6.4	1.5	0.3	0.2	0.7
	Breakfast bars												
39230	Atkins Day Break apple crisp bar	1	item(s)	35	—	130	10.0	17.0	7.0	5.0	2.0	—	—
10571	Nutri-Grain apple cinnamon cereal bar	1	item(s)	37	—	130	2.0	24.0	2.0	3.0	0.5	—	—
10647	Nutri-Grain blueberry cereal bar	1	item(s)	37	—	130	2.0	24.0	2.0	3.0	0.5	—	—
10648	Nutri-Grain raspberry cereal bar	1	item(s)	37	—	130	2.0	24.0	2.0	3.0	0.5	—	—
10649	Nutri-Grain strawberry cereal bar	1	item(s)	37	—	130	2.0	24.0	2.0	3.0	0.5	—	—
	Breakfast cereals, hot												
41046	Cream of Wheat, instant, prepared	½	cup(s)	121	101.8	75	2.2	15.8	0.7	0.3	0	0	0.2
365	Farina, enriched, cooked with water and salt	½	cup(s)	117	100.8	62	2.1	12.7	0.9	0.4	0.1	0	0.1
363	Grits, white corn, regular and quick, enriched, cooked with water and salt	½	cup(s)	121	100.3	86	2.1	17.9	1.0	0.6	0.1	0.1	0.2
8636	Grits, yellow corn, regular and quick, enriched, cooked with salt	½	cup(s)	121	102.1	79	1.5	16.8	0.8	0.5	0.1	0.1	0.2
8657	Oatmeal, cooked with water	½	cup(s)	117	97.8	83	3.0	14.0	2.0	1.8	0.4	0.5	0.7
5500	Oatmeal, maple and brown sugar, instant, prepared	1	item(s)	198	147.3	208	4.8	41.9	3.7	2.5	0.4	0.7	0.9
5510	Oatmeal, ready to serve, packet, prepared	1	item(s)	186	152.2	143	4.8	25.2	3.8	2.5	0.4	0.8	0.9
	Breakfast cereals, ready to eat												
1197	All-Bran	1	cup(s)	62	1.3	160	8.0	46.0	20.0	2.0	0	0.4	—
1200	All-Bran Buds	1	cup(s)	91	2.7	242	9.1	72.7	39.4	3.0	0	0.5	1.1

Chol (mg)	Calc (mg)	Iron (mg)	Magn (mg)	Pota (mg)	Sodi (mg)	Zinc (mg)	Vit A (µg)	Thia (mg)	Vit E (mg α)	Ribo (mg)	Niac (mg)	Vit B_6 (mg)	Fola (µg)	Vit C (mg)	Vit B_{12} (µg)	Sele (µg)
0	6	0.67	42.8	73.9	3.4	0.51	0	0.03	0.08	0.03	0.79	0.06	11.8	0	0	1.8
0	9	0.87	29.1	61.9	4.6	0.52	0	0.05	0.01	0.03	0.91	0.08	16.4	0	0	0.5
0	6	0.30	6.3	45.5	3.9	0.20	0	0.05	0.10	0.02	0.77	0.04	11.8	0	0	21.6
0	4	0.76	52.8	74.4	2.4	1.09	0	0.13	0.02	0.10	1.60	0.13	22.8	0	0	1.1
0	27	2.54	110.4	266.0	1.9	1.46	0	0.55	0.47	0.10	0.44	0.08	24.4	0	0	21.2
0	40	3.89	167.5	478.8	4.3	2.64	0.9	0.31	2.08	0.27	1.29	0.41	156.5	—	0	7.2
0	10	0.41	41.9	41.9	4.9	0.61	0	0.09	0.03	0.02	1.49	0.14	3.9	0	0	9.6
0	10	0.52	42.9	77.0	1.0	0.60	0	0.10	—	0.01	1.30	0.15	3.9	0	0	38.0
0	—	0.54	—	—	195.0	—	—	—	—	—	—	—	—	—	—	—
0	12	1.15	9.3	53.6	366.7	0.37	0	0.13	0.50	0.02	1.24	0.06	73.1	0.4	0	4.3
0	17	0.73	44.1	157.6	14.7	0.65	126.7	0.13	0.28	0.03	1.72	0.18	8.8	6.3	0	6.8
0	2	0.12	4.3	8.7	4.3	0.36	0	0.02	0.03	0.01	0.25	0.02	0.9	0	0	4.9
0	8	0.95	9.5	27.6	0.8	0.39	0	0.13	0.03	0.01	1.17	0.07	76.6	0	0	5.9
0	7	1.46	4.1	7.4	3.3	0.40	0	0.06	0.01	0.01	1.43	0.04	97.3	0	0	4.0
0	15	1.43	7.1	44.2	1.6	0.29	0	0.17	0.01	0.02	1.82	0.12	107.4	0	0	7.3
0	2	0.49	26.2	82.8	2.5	1.10	0	0.04	0.20	0.07	1.06	0.11	21.3	0	0	0.7
0	211	2.92	11.9	77.5	745.6	0.39	0	0.42	0.03	0.26	3.64	0.03	191.9	0	0	21.5
0	9	2.90	13.8	66.9	1.3	0.44	0	0.49	0.04	0.31	3.69	0.03	181.9	0	0	21.2
0	24	1.98	71.0	228.6	3.0	1.48	0	0.27	0.42	0.08	4.64	0.29	5.9	0	0	27.9
0	25	2.44	150.6	346.2	6.6	1.87	0	0.25	0.19	0.11	3.69	0.35	32.4	0	0	3.4
0	10	5.01	11.0	71.9	1.4	0.42	0	0.61	0.01	0.29	4.65	0.02	193.2	0	0	3.4
0	2	3.01	22.1	98.0	4.8	0.46	7.6	0.38	0.08	0.26	3.43	0.13	231.1	0	0	7.2
0	4	2.10	77.5	175.1	21.4	1.11	6.7	0.23	0.26	0.12	2.22	0.19	15.3	0	0	9.5
0	24	3.18	102.4	458.9	1.3	3.23	0.6	0.20	1.75	0.16	2.73	0.28	21.1	0	0	11.5
0	78	4.27	53.0	149.9	2.8	1.03	0	0.84	0.07	0.46	5.66	0.27	190.9	0	0	8.0
0	9	1.56	88.5	228.3	6.3	1.94	0	0.35	0.95	0.06	5.01	0.58	12.6	0	0	—
0	8	0.28	27.6	60.0	0.0	0.63	0	0.11	0.09	0.02	2.05	0.34	3.2	0	0	11.9
0	14	3.64	39.2	155.3	0.8	0.88	0	0.68	0.22	0.48	5.00	0.09	217.9	0	0	74.6
0	87	2.70	182.0	1066.9	5.5	1.66	2.5	0.25	0.83	0.49	1.83	0.20	146.3	0	0	3.2
0	6	0.90	34.4	128.3	1.7	1.77	0	0.27	—	0.07	0.98	0.19	40.4	0	0	11.4
0	20	2.16	82.2	217.8	1.2	1.56	0	0.30	0.43	0.10	2.97	0.24	26.4	0	0	37.1
0	200	1.44	—	35.0	140.0	—	—	0.15	—	0.17	2.00	—	68.0	12.0	—	—
0	200	1.80	—	—	105.0	1.50	225.0	0.22	—	0.43	5.00	0.50	—	0	—	—
0	200	1.80	—	—	105.0	1.50	225.0	0.22	—	0.43	5.00	0.50	—	0	—	—
0	200	1.80	—	—	100.0	1.50	225.0	0.22	—	0.43	5.00	0.50	—	0	—	—
0	200	1.80	—	—	120.0	1.50	225.0	0.22	—	0.43	5.00	0.50	—	0	—	—
0	77	5.99	7.2	24.1	123.1	0.21	280.0	0.28	0.02	0.25	3.73	0.37	121.9	0	0	4.2
0	113	6.21	8.2	26.8	146.8	0.27	0	0.15	0.05	0.08	1.74	0.11	138.6	0	0	3.5
0	1	0.69	8.5	32.7	269.8	0.22	0	0.10	0.04	0.07	0.97	0.06	46.0	0	0	3.8
0	1	0.69	6.1	26.6	269.8	0.17	0	0.12	0.02	0.07	0.92	0.04	44.8	0	0	3.3
0	11	1.05	31.6	81.9	4.7	1.17	0	0.09	0.09	0.02	0.26	0.01	7.0	0	0	6.3
0	99	7.40	48.1	136.7	272.2	1.09	0	1.12	—	0.05	2.55	0.33	56.5	0	0	11.1
0	109	4.79	48.9	138.5	242.7	1.11	0	0.78	—	0.05	1.78	0.22	40.2	0	0	3.8
0	200	9.00	200.0	700.0	160.0	3.00	300.5	0.75	0.77	0.85	10.00	4.00	1362.8	12.4	12.0	5.8
0	0	13.64	186.4	—	636.4	4.55	455.0	1.14	0.65	1.27	15.15	6.06	2052.7	18.2	18.2	26.3

APPENDIX H

TABLE H-1 Table of Food Composition (*continued*) (Computer code is for Cengage Diet Analysis program) (For purposes of calculations, use "0" for t, <1, <0.1, 0.01)

DA+ Code	Food Description	Quantity	Measure	Wt (g)	H_2O (g)	Ener (kcal)	Prot (g)	Carb (g)	Fiber (g)	Fat (g)	Fat Breakdown (g)		
											Sat	Mono	Poly
	Cereal, Flour, Grain, Pasta, Noodles, Popcorn—*continued*												
1199	Apple Jacks	1	cup(s)	28	0.8	100	1.0	25.0	3.0	0.5	0	0.1	0.2
1204	Cap'n Crunch	1	cup(s)	36	0.9	147	1.3	30.7	1.3	2.0	1.3	0	0
1205	Cap'n Crunch Crunchberries	1	cup(s)	35	0.9	133	1.3	29.3	1.3	2.0	1.3	0.2	0.3
1206	Cheerios	1	cup(s)	28	1.1	100	3.0	20.0	3.0	2.0	0	0.5	0.5
3415	Cocoa Puffs	1	cup(s)	36	0.6	147	1.3	30.7	1.3	2.0	0	0.7	0.7
1207	Cocoa Rice Krispies	1	cup(s)	41	1.2	160	1.3	36.0	0.7	1.3	0.7	0.2	0.1
5522	Complete wheat bran flakes	1	cup(s)	39	1.1	120	4.0	30.7	6.7	0.7	0	0	0
1211	Corn Flakes	1	cup(s)	28	1.1	100	2.0	24.0	1.0	0	0	0	0
1247	Corn Pops	1	cup(s)	32	1.0	120	1.0	29.0	3.0	0	0	0	0
1937	Cracklin' Oat Bran	1	cup(s)	65	1.8	267	5.3	46.7	8.0	9.3	4.0	3.1	2.0
58208	Fiber One Honey Clusters	1	cup(s)	52	—	160	5.0	42.0	13.0	1.5	0	0	0.5
1220	Froot Loops	1	cup(s)	29	0.9	110	1.0	25.0	3.0	1.0	0.5	0.1	0.2
38214	Frosted Cheerios	1	cup(s)	37	0.8	147	2.7	30.7	2.7	1.3	0	0	0.7
372	Frosted Flakes	1	cup(s)	40	1.3	147	1.3	36.0	1.3	0	0	0	0
1221	Frosted Mini-Wheats	1	cup(s)	47	2.6	158	4.7	37.9	4.7	0.8	0	0	0.4
1223	Granola, prepared	½	cup(s)	61	3.3	298	9.1	32.5	5.5	14.7	2.5	5.8	5.6
2415	Honey Bunches of Oats honey roasted	1	cup(s)	40	1.2	160	2.7	33.3	2.7	2.0	0	1.3	0
1227	Honey Nut Cheerios	1	cup(s)	37	0.8	147	2.7	29.3	2.7	2.0	0	0.7	0.7
1248	Honey Smacks	1	cup(s)	36	0.6	133	2.7	32.0	1.3	0.7	0	0.2	0.3
2424	Honeycomb	1	cup(s)	21	0.3	87	1.3	18.7	0.7	0.7	0	0	0
10286	Kashi Whole Grain Puffs	1	cup(s)	19	0.6	70	2.0	15.0	1.0	0.5	0	0.2	0.2
41142	Kellogg's Mueslix	1	cup(s)	82	7.2	294	7.5	60.2	6.8	4.5	0.5	2.1	1.1
1231	Kix	1	cup(s)	24	0.7	88	1.6	20.0	2.4	0.8	0	0	0
30569	Life	1	cup(s)	43	1.8	160	4.0	33.3	2.7	2.0	0	0.7	0.7
1233	Lucky Charms	1	cup(s)	36	1.1	147	2.7	29.3	1.3	1.3	0	0	0
38220	Multi Grain Cheerios	1	cup(s)	29	0.7	110	2.0	24.0	3.0	1.0	0	0	0.5
1201	Multi-Bran Chex	1	cup(s)	63	1.6	213	4.0	52.0	8.0	2.0	0	0	0.7
13633	Post Bran Flakes	1	cup(s)	40	1.1	133	4.0	32.0	6.7	0.7	0	0	0
1241	Product 19	1	cup(s)	30	0.9	100	2.0	25.0	1.0	0	0	0	0
32432	Puffed rice, fortified	1	cup(s)	14	0.4	56	0.9	12.6	0.2	0.1	0	—	—
32433	Puffed wheat, fortified	1	cup(s)	12	0.4	44	1.8	9.6	0.5	0.1	0	—	—
5584	Quaker Oatmeal Squares, brown sugar	1	cup(s)	55	1.1	210	6.0	44.0	5.0	2.5	0.5	1.0	1.0
41095	Quaker Oatmeal Squares, cinnamon	1	cup(s)	60	1.6	227	6.7	46.8	5.2	2.9	0.5	1.0	0.9
2420	Raisin Bran	1	cup(s)	59	4.8	190	4.0	46.0	8.0	1.0	0	0	0.5
1244	Rice Chex	1	cup(s)	27	0.7	100	2.0	23.0	0.0	0.5	0	0	0
1245	Rice Krispies	1	cup(s)	26	0.9	104	1.6	23.2	0.4	0	0	0	0
13648	Shredded Wheat	1	cup(s)	54	0.9	184	5.7	46.0	6.9	1.1	0	0	0.6
1246	Special K	1	cup(s)	31	0.9	120	6.0	23.0	0.5	0.5	0	0.1	0.2
41119	Total Raisin Bran	1	cup(s)	55	4.6	172	3.1	42.2	5.0	0.9	0.2	0.2	0.4
1253	Total whole grain	1	cup(s)	40	1.1	133	2.7	30.7	4.0	0.7	0	0	0
1254	Trix	1	cup(s)	32	0.6	120	1.0	28.0	1.0	1.5	0	0.5	0.5
41030	Wheat Chex	1	cup(s)	30	0.8	104	2.9	24.7	3.7	0.5	0.1	0.1	0.3
382	Wheat germ, toasted	2	tablespoon(s)	14	0.8	54	4.1	7.0	2.1	1.5	0.3	0.2	0.9
1257	Wheaties	1	cup(s)	36	0.9	133	4.0	29.3	4.0	0.7	0	0	0
	Pasta, noodles												
449	Chinese chow mein noodles, cooked	½	cup(s)	23	0.3	103	2.4	15.1	0.6	4.0	0.4	1.2	2.4
1995	Corn pasta, cooked	½	cup(s)	70	47.8	88	1.8	19.5	3.4	0.5	0.1	0.1	0.2
448	Egg noodles, enriched, cooked	½	cup(s)	80	54.2	110	3.6	20.1	1.0	1.7	0.3	0.5	0.4
1563	Egg noodles, spinach, enriched, cooked	½	cup(s)	80	54.8	106	4.0	19.4	1.8	1.3	0.3	0.4	0.3
440	Macaroni, enriched, cooked	½	cup(s)	70	43.5	111	4.1	21.6	1.3	0.7	0.1	0.1	0.2
2000	Macaroni, tricolor vegetable, enriched, cooked	½	cup(s)	67	45.8	86	3.0	17.8	2.9	0.1	0	0	0
1996	Plain pasta, fresh-refrigerated, cooked	½	cup(s)	64	43.9	84	3.3	16.0		0.7	0.1	0.1	0.3
1725	Ramen noodles, cooked	½	cup(s)	114	90.9	104	3.0	15.4	1.0	4.3	0.2	0.2	0.2
2878	Soba noodles, cooked	½	cup(s)	95	69.4	94	4.8	20.4	—	0.1	0	0	0
2879	Somen noodles, cooked	½	cup(s)	88	59.8	115	3.5	24.2	—	0.2	0	0	0.1
2881	Spaghetti, enriched, cooked	½	cup(s)	70	43.5	111	4.1	21.6	1.3	0.7	0.1	0.1	0.2
2884	Spaghetti, whole wheat, cooked	½	cup(s)	70	47.0	87	3.7	18.6	3.2	0.4	0.1	0.1	0.1

Chol (mg)	Calc (mg)	Iron (mg)	Magn (mg)	Pota (mg)	Sodi (mg)	Zinc (mg)	Vit A (μg)	Thia (mg)	Vit E (mg α)	Ribo (mg)	Niac (mg)	Vit B_6 (mg)	Fola (μg)	Vit C (mg)	Vit B_{12} (μg)	Sele (μg)
0	0	4.50	5.9	35.0	130.0	1.50	146.8	0.38	0.04	0.43	5.00	0.50	184.5	15.0	1.5	1.6
0	0	6.00	19.4	66.7	266.7	5.00	0	0.51	0.26	0.57	6.68	0.67	906.7	0	0	2.3
0	0	6.00	18.7	66.7	253.4	5.00	0	0.51	0.22	0.57	6.68	0.67	906.8	0	0	0
0	100	8.10	40.0	170.0	190.0	3.75	150.1	0.38	0.19	0.43	5.00	0.50	460.3	6.0	1.5	8.0
0	133	6.00	10.7	80.0	200.0	5.00	23.8	0.50	0.28	0.57	6.67	0.67	199.1	8.0	2.0	2.3
0	53	6.00	15.7	80.0	200.0	1.98	203.3	0.50	0.11	0.57	6.61	0.67	446.4	20.0	2.0	6.7
0	0	24.00	53.3	226.7	280.0	20.00	300.5	2.00	17.92	2.27	26.67	2.67	901.4	80.0	8.0	4.1
0	0	8.12	2.5	25.0	200.0	0.05	127.3	0.38	0.04	0.43	5.00	0.50	221.8	6.0	1.5	2.3
0	0	1.80	2.2	45.0	125.0	1.57	143.1	0.38	0.02	0.43	5.00	0.50	174.7	6.0	1.5	2.1
0	27	2.40	80.0	293.3	200.0	2.03	300.5	0.50	0.37	0.57	6.66	0.65	218.2	20.0	2.0	7.0
0	100	4.50	32.0	320.0	280.0	3.75	0	0.38	—	0.43	5.00	0.50		0	1.5	—
0	0	4.50	6.7	35.0	135.0	1.50	144.7	0.38	0.03	0.43	5.00	0.50	150.5	15.0	1.5	1.7
0	133	6.00	19.9	73.3	226.6	5.00	200.1	0.50	0.16	0.57	6.67	0.67	448.3	8.0	2.0	5.8
0	0	6.00	2.8	26.7	186.7	0.06	200.2	0.50	0.04	0.57	6.67	0.67	254.0	8.0	2.0	1.8
0	0	12.80	47.4	158.1	4.0	1.19	0	0.30	0	0.34	3.95	0.40	149.2	0	1.2	1.9
0	48	2.58	106.8	329.4	15.3	2.46	0.6	0.45	6.78	0.18	1.31	0.18	50.0	0.7	0	17.0
0	0	14.40	21.3	73.3	200.0	0.40	300.3	0.50	0.59	0.57	6.67	0.67	549.6	0	2.0	3.3
0	133	6.00	42.7	153.3	253.3	5.00	200.1	0.50	0.36	0.57	6.67	0.67	448.3	8.0	2.0	8.8
0	0	0.48	21.2	53.3	66.7	0.47	200.2	0.50	0.17	0.58	6.66	0.67	224.6	8.0	2.0	17.5
0	0	1.80	10.7	33.3	120.0	1.00	150.1	0.25	0.04	0.28	3.33	0.33	122.2	0	1.0	4.3
0	0	0.36	29.3	60.0	0	0.58	0	0.02	0.17	0.03	0.61	0.06	6.1	0	0	6.8
0	48	6.76	73.4	256.5	207.8	5.61	135.2	0.66	5.94	0.66	8.25	3.05	1023.3	0.3	9.1	14.3
0	120	6.48	12.2	36.0	168.0	3.00	116.3	0.30	0.06	0.34	4.00	0.40	317.8	4.8	1.2	2.0
0	133	10.80	40.5	120.0	213.4	5.00	0	0.50	0.26	0.57	6.67	0.67	544.0	0	0	1.4
0	133	6.00	10.7	60.0	253.3	5.00	201.2	0.50	0.10	0.57	6.67	0.67	451.1	8.0	2.0	5.9
0	97	18.00	16.0	85.0	200.0	15.00	150.2	1.50	13.50	1.70	20.00	2.00	676.3	15.0	6.0	4.9
0	133	21.60	80.0	253.3	413.4	5.00	184.2	0.50	0.19	0.57	6.67	0.67	888.7	8.0	2.0	5.0
0	0	10.80	80.0	240.0	293.3	2.00	300.3	0.50	0.93	0.57	6.67	0.67	453.3	0	2.0	3.2
0	0	18.00	15.9	50.0	210.0	15.00	225.0	1.50	20.10	1.70	20.01	2.00	675.9	60.0	6.0	3.6
0	1	4.44	3.5	15.8	0.4	0.14	0	0.36	—	0.25	4.94	0.01	2.7	0	0	1.5
0	3	3.80	17.4	41.8	0.5	0.28	0	0.31	—	0.22	4.24	0.02	3.8	0	0	14.8
0	100	16.20	60.0	210.0	250.0	3.75	150.4	0.38	1.35	0.43	5.00	0.50	680.0	6.0	0	3.8
0	127	17.71	69.6	218.4	204.6	4.51	180.6	0.45	1.85	0.51	6.01	0.60	732.6	7.2	0	3.8
0	20	10.80	100.0	310.0	250.0	2.25	225.2	0.38	0.48	0.43	5.00	0.50	333.9	0	1.5	3.5
0	100	9.00	24.0	45.0	250.0	3.75	150.1	0.38	0.18	0.43	5.00	0.50	339.1	6.0	1.5	1.1
0	0	7.20	6.9	24.0	176.0	0.33	300.2	0.30	0.03	0.34	4.00	0.40	241.0	12.0	1.2	4.8
0	23	1.24	68.9	218.3	0	1.72	0	0.14	0	0.07	3.45	0.62	23.2	0	0	1.5
0	0	8.10	19.2	50.0	220.0	0.60	225.2	0.53	4.74	0.59	7.00	2.00	675.8	21.0	6.0	7.0
0	1038	18.70	33.0	277.2	186.4	15.56	154.6	1.54	14.01	1.76	20.74	2.08	698.5	0	6.2	3.8
0	1333	24.00	42.7	120.0	253.3	20.00	200.4	2.00	18.00	2.27	26.67	2.67	901.2	80.0	8.0	1.6
0	100	4.50	8.0	40.0	180.0	3.75	150.1	0.38	0.38	0.43	5.00	0.50	165.8	6.0	1.5	2.1
0	64	9.18	25.5	110.7	171.0	3.36	95.1	0.24	0.20	0.27	3.18	0.32	429.9	3.8	1.0	1.5
0	6	1.28	45.2	133.7	0.6	2.35	0.7	0.24	2.26	0.12	0.79	0.14	49.7	0.8	0	9.2
0	27	10.80	32.0	126.7	253.3	10.00	200.4	1.00	0.43	1.13	13.33	1.33	403.6	8.0	4.0	1.7
0	5	1.06	11.7	27.0	190.6	0.31	0	0.13	0.53	0.09	1.34	0.03	38.0	0	0	9.7
0	1	0.17	25.2	21.7	0	0.44	2.1	0.04	—	0.02	0.39	0.04	4.2	0	0	2.0
23	10	1.18	16.8	30.4	4.0	0.52	4.8	0.23	0.14	0.11	1.66	0.04	110.4	0	0.1	19.1
26	15	0.87	19.2	29.6	9.6	0.50	8.0	0.20	0.44	0.10	1.18	0.09	75.2	0	0.1	17.4
0	5	0.90	12.6	30.8	0.7	0.36	0	0.19	0.04	0.10	1.18	0.03	83.3	0	0	18.5
0	7	0.33	12.7	20.8	4.0	0.29	3.3	0.08	0.14	0.04	0.72	0.02	71.0	0	0	13.3
21	4	0.73	11.5	15.4	3.8	0.36	3.8	0.13	—	0.10	0.63	0.02	66.6	0	0.1	—
18	9	0.89	8.5	34.5	414.5	0.31	—	0.08	0.11	0.05	0.71	0.03	—	0.1	0	—
0	4	0.46	8.5	33.3	57.0	0.11	0	0.09	—	0.02	0.48	0.04	6.7	0	0	
0	7	0.46	1.8	25.5	141.7	0.19	0	0.02	—	0.03	0.09	0.01	1.8	0	0	
0	5	0.90	12.6	30.8	0.7	0.36	0	0.19	0.04	0.10	1.18	0.03	83.3	0	0	18.5
0	11	0.74	21.0	30.8	2.1	0.57	0	0.08	0.21	0.03	0.49	0.06	3.5	0	0	18.1

DA+ Code	Food Description	Quantity	Measure	Wt (g)	H_2O (g)	Ener (kcal)	Prot (g)	Carb (g)	Fiber (g)	Fat (g)	Fat Breakdown (g)		
											Sat	Mono	Poly
Cereal, Flour, Grain, Pasta, Noodles, Popcorn—*continued*													
	Popcorn												
476	Air popped	1	cup(s)	8	0.3	31	1.0	6.2	1.2	0.4	0	0.1	0.2
4619	Caramel	1	cup(s)	35	1.0	152	1.3	27.8	1.8	4.5	1.3	1.0	1.6
4620	Cheese flavored	1	cup(s)	35	0.9	185	3.3	18.2	3.5	11.7	2.3	3.4	5.4
477	Popped in oil	1	cup(s)	11	0.1	64	0.8	5.0	0.9	4.8	0.8	1.1	2.6
Fruit and Fruit Juices													
	Apples												
226	Applesauce, sweetened, canned	½	cup(s)	123	100.8	84	0.2	21.5	1.5	0.2	0	0	0.1
227	Applesauce, unsweetened, canned	½	cup(s)	122	107.6	51	0.2	13.7	1.3	0.1	0	0	0
38492	Crabapples	1	item(s)	35	27.6	27	0.1	7.0	0.9	0.1	0	0	0
948	Dried, sulfured	¼	cup(s)	22	6.8	52	0.2	14.2	1.9	0.1	0	0	0
952	Juice, prepared from frozen concentrate	½	cup(s)	120	105.0	56	0.2	13.8	0.1	0.1	0	0	0
225	Juice, unsweetened, canned	½	cup(s)	124	109.4	57	0.1	14.0	0.2	0.2	0	0	0
223	Raw medium, with peel	1	item(s)	182	155.7	95	0.5	25.1	4.4	0.3	0.1	0	0.1
224	Slices	½	cup(s)	55	46.6	28	0.1	7.5	1.3	0.1	0	0	0
946	Slices without skin, boiled	½	cup(s)	86	73.1	45	0.2	11.7	2.1	0.3	0	0	0.1
	Apricot												
228	Fresh without pits	4	item(s)	140	120.9	67	2.0	15.6	2.8	0.5	0	0.2	0.1
229	Halves with skin, canned in heavy syrup	½	cup(s)	129	100.1	107	0.7	27.7	2.1	0.1	0	0	0
230	Halves, dried, sulfured	¼	cup(s)	33	10.1	79	1.1	20.6	2.4	0.2	0	0	0
	Avocado												
233	California, whole, without skin or pit	½	cup(s)	115	83.2	192	2.3	9.9	7.8	17.7	2.4	11.3	2.1
234	Florida, whole, without skin or pit	½	cup(s)	115	90.6	138	2.6	9.0	6.4	11.6	2.3	6.3	1.9
2998	Pureed	½	cup(s)	115	84.2	184	2.3	9.8	7.7	16.9	2.4	11.3	2.1
	Banana												
4580	Dried chips	¼	cup(s)	18	0.8	93	0.4	10.5	1.4	6.0	5.2	0.4	0.1
235	Fresh whole, without peel	1	item(s)	118	88.4	105	1.3	27.0	3.1	0.4	0.1	0	0.1
	Blackberries												
958	Frozen, unsweetened	½	cup(s)	76	62.1	48	0.9	11.8	3.8	0.3	0	0	0.2
237	Raw	½	cup(s)	72	63.5	31	1.0	6.9	3.8	0.4	0	0	0.2
	Blueberries												
959	Canned in heavy syrup	½	cup(s)	128	98.3	113	0.8	28.2	2.0	0.4	0	0.1	0.2
960	Frozen, unsweetened	½	cup(s)	78	67.1	40	0.3	9.4	2.1	0.5	0	0.1	0.2
238	Raw	½	cup(s)	74	62.3	42	0.5	10.7	1.8	0.2	0	0	0.1
	Boysenberries												
961	Canned in heavy syrup	½	cup(s)	128	97.6	113	1.3	28.6	3.3	0.2	0	0	0.1
962	Frozen, unsweetened	½	cup(s)	66	56.7	33	0.7	8.0	3.5	0.2	0	0	0.1
35576	Breadfruit	1	item(s)	384	271.3	396	4.1	104.1	18.8	0.9	0.2	0.1	0.3
	Cherries												
967	Sour red, canned in water	½	cup(s)	122	109.7	44	0.9	10.9	1.3	0.1	0	0	0
3000	Sour red, raw	½	cup(s)	78	66.8	39	0.8	9.4	1.2	0.2	0.1	0.1	0.1
3004	Sweet, canned in heavy syrup	½	cup(s)	127	98.2	105	0.8	26.9	1.8	0.2	0	0.1	0.1
969	Sweet, canned in water	½	cup(s)	124	107.9	57	1.0	14.6	1.9	0.2	0	0	0
240	Sweet, raw	½	cup(s)	77	63.3	49	0.8	12.3	1.6	0.2	0	0	0
	Cranberries												
3007	Chopped, raw	½	cup(s)	55	47.9	25	0.2	6.7	2.5	0.1	0	0	0
1717	Cranberry apple juice drink	½	cup(s)	123	102.6	77	0	19.4	0	0.1	0	0	0.1
1638	Cranberry juice cocktail	½	cup(s)	127	109.0	68	0	17.1	0	0.1	0	0	0.1
241	Cranberry juice cocktail, low calorie, with saccharin	½	cup(s)	119	112.8	23	0	5.5	0	0	0	0	0
242	Cranberry sauce, sweetened, canned	¼	cup(s)	69	42.0	105	0.1	26.9	0.7	0.1	0	0	0
	Dates												
244	Domestic, chopped	¼	cup(s)	45	9.1	125	1.1	33.4	3.6	0.2	0	0	0
243	Domestic, whole	¼	cup(s)	45	9.1	125	1.1	33.4	3.6	0.2	0	0	0
	Figs												
975	Canned in heavy syrup	½	cup(s)	130	98.8	114	0.5	29.7	2.8	0.1	0	0	0.1
974	Canned in water	½	cup(s)	124	105.7	66	0.5	17.3	2.7	0.1	0	0	0.1
973	Raw, medium	2	item(s)	100	79.1	74	0.8	19.2	2.9	0.3	0.1	0.1	0.1

GE KEY: H-4 = Breads/Baked Goods H-8 = Cereal/Rice/Pasta H-14 = Fruit H-18 = Vegetables/Legumes H-28 = Nuts/Seeds H-30 = Vegetarian H-32 = Dairy H-40 = Eggs H-40 = Seafood H-42 = Meats H-46 = Poultry
48 = Processed Meats H-50 = Beverages H-52 = Fats/Oils H-54 = Sweets H-56 = Spices/Condiments/Sauces H-60 = Mixed Foods/Soups/Sandwiches H-66 = Fast Food H-84 = Convenience H-86 = Baby Foods

Chol (mg)	Calc (mg)	Iron (mg)	Magn (mg)	Pota (mg)	Sodi (mg)	Zinc (mg)	Vit A (µg)	Thia (mg)	Vit E (mg α)	Ribo (mg)	Niac (mg)	Vit B_6 (mg)	Fola (µg)	Vit C (mg)	Vit B_{12} (µg)	Sele (µg)
0	1	0.26	11.5	26.3	0.6	0.25	0.8	0.01	0.02	0.01	0.18	0.01	2.5	0	0	0
2	15	0.61	12.3	38.4	72.5	0.20	0.7	0.02	0.42	0.02	0.77	0.01	1.8	0	0	1.3
4	40	0.79	32.0	91.9	312.9	0.71	13.4	0.04	—	0.08	0.51	0.08	3.9	0.2	0.2	4.2
0	0	0.22	8.7	20.0	116.4	0.34	0.9	0.01	0.27	0.01	0.13	0.01	2.8	0	0	0.2
0	4	0.15	3.7	92.3	2.5	0.04	0	0.02	0.22	0.03	0.09	0.03	1.2	2.1	0	0.4
0	5	0.28	3.7	90.3	2.4	0.04	1.2	0.03	0.20	0.04	0.10	0.03	3.7	1.2	0	0.4
0	6	0.13	2.5	67.9	0.3	—	0.7	0.01	0.21	0.01	0.04	—	2.0	2.8	0	—
0	3	0.30	3.4	96.8	18.7	0.04	0	0	0.11	0.03	0.20	0.03	0	0.8	0	0.3
0	7	0.31	6.0	150.6	8.4	0.05	0	0	0.01	0.02	0.05	0.04	0	0.7	0	0.1
0	10	0.15	6.2	125.2	5.0	0.02	0	0.03	0.01	0.02	0.09	0.02	0	1.1	0	0.1
0	11	0.22	9.1	194.7	1.8	0.07	5.5	0.03	0.33	0.05	0.17	0.07	5.5	8.4	0	0
0	3	0.07	2.7	58.3	0.5	0.02	1.6	0.01	0.10	0.01	0.05	0.02	1.6	2.5	0	0
0	4	0.16	2.6	75.2	0.9	0.03	1.7	0.01	0.04	0.01	0.08	0.04	0.9	0.2	0	0.3
0	18	0.55	14.0	362.6	1.4	0.28	134.4	0.04	1.25	0.06	0.84	0.08	12.6	14.0	0	0.1
0	12	0.39	9.0	180.6	5.2	0.14	80.0	0.03	0.77	0.03	0.49	0.07	2.6	4.0	0	0.1
0	18	0.87	10.5	381.5	3.3	0.13	59.1	0	1.42	0.02	0.85	0.05	3.3	0.3	0	0.7
0	15	0.70	33.4	583.1	9.2	0.78	8.1	0.09	2.27	0.16	2.20	0.33	102.4	10.1	0	0.5
0	12	0.20	27.6	403.7	2.3	0.46	8.1	0.02	3.06	0.06	0.77	0.09	40.2	20.0	0	—
0	14	0.63	33.4	557.8	8.1	0.74	8.0	0.08	2.38	0.15	2.00	0.30	93.2	11.5	0	0.5
0	3	0.22	13.7	96.4	1.1	0.13	0.7	0.02	0.04	0	0.13	0.05	2.5	1.1	0	0.3
0	6	0.31	31.9	422.4	1.2	0.18	3.5	0.04	0.12	0.09	0.78	0.43	23.6	10.3	0	1.2
0	22	0.60	16.6	105.7	0.8	0.19	4.5	0.02	0.88	0.03	0.91	0.05	25.7	2.3	0	0.3
0	21	0.45	14.4	116.6	0.7	0.38	7.9	0.01	0.84	0.02	0.47	0.02	18.0	15.1	0	0.3
0	6	0.42	5.1	51.2	3.8	0.09	2.6	0.04	0.49	0.07	0.14	0.05	2.6	1.4	0	0.1
0	6	0.14	3.9	41.8	0.8	0.05	1.5	0.02	0.37	0.03	0.40	0.05	5.4	1.9	0	0.1
0	4	0.21	4.4	57.0	0.7	0.12	2.2	0.03	0.42	0.03	0.31	0.04	4.4	7.2	0	0.1
0	23	0.55	14.1	115.2	3.8	0.24	2.6	0.03	—	0.04	0.29	0.05	43.5	7.9	0	0.5
0	18	0.56	10.6	91.7	0.7	0.15	2.0	0.03	0.57	0.02	0.51	0.04	41.6	2.0	0	0.1
0	65	2.07	96.0	1881.6	7.7	0.46	7.7	0.42	0.38	0.12	3.46	0.38	53.8	111.4	0	2.3
0	13	1.67	7.3	119.6	8.5	0.09	46.4	0.02	0.28	0.05	0.22	0.05	9.8	2.6	0	0
0	12	0.25	7.0	134.1	2.3	0.08	49.6	0.02	0.05	0.03	0.31	0.03	6.2	7.8	0	0
0	11	0.44	11.4	183.4	3.8	0.13	10.1	0.03	0.22	0.05	0.50	0.03	5.1	4.6	0	0
0	14	0.45	11.2	162.4	1.2	0.10	9.9	0.03	0.29	0.05	0.51	0.04	5.0	2.7	0	0
0	10	0.28	8.5	170.9	0	0.05	2.3	0.02	0.05	0.03	0.12	0.04	3.1	5.4	0	0
0	4	0.14	3.3	46.8	1.1	0.05	1.6	0.01	0.66	0.01	0.06	0.03	0.6	7.3	0	0.1
0	4	0.09	1.2	20.8	2.5	0.02	0	0	0.15	0	0	0	0	48.4	0	0
0	4	0.13	1.3	17.7	2.5	0.04	0	0	0.28	0	0.05	0	0	53.5	0	0.3
0	11	0.05	2.4	29.6	3.6	0.02	0	0	0.06	0	0	0	0	38.2	0	0
0	3	0.15	2.1	18.0	20.1	0.03	1.4	0.01	0.57	0.01	0.07	0.01	0.7	1.4	0	0.2
0	17	0.45	19.1	291.9	0.9	0.13	0	0.02	0.02	0.03	0.57	0.07	8.5	0.2	0	1.3
0	17	0.45	19.1	291.9	0.9	0.13	0	0.02	0.02	0.03	0.57	0.07	8.5	0.2	0	1.3
0	35	0.36	12.9	128.2	1.3	0.14	2.6	0.03	0.16	0.05	0.55	0.09	2.6	1.3	0	0.3
0	35	0.36	12.4	127.7	1.2	0.15	2.5	0.03	0.10	0.05	0.55	0.09	2.5	1.2	0	0.1
0	35	0.37	17.0	232.0	1.0	0.15	7.0	0.06	0.11	0.05	0.40	0.11	6.0	2.0	0	0.2

DA+ Code	Food Description	Quantity	Measure	Wt (g)	H_2O (g)	Ener (kcal)	Prot (g)	Carb (g)	Fiber (g)	Fat (g)	Fat Breakdown (g)		
											Sat	Mono	Poly
Fruit and Fruit Juices—*continued*													
	Fruit cocktail & salad												
245	Fruit cocktail, canned in heavy syrup	½	cup(s)	124	99.7	91	0.5	23.4	1.2	0.1	0	0	0
978	Fruit cocktail, canned in juice	½	cup(s)	119	103.6	55	0.5	14.1	1.2	0	0	0	0
977	Fruit cocktail, canned in water	½	cup(s)	119	107.6	38	0.5	10.1	1.2	0.1	0	0	0
979	Fruit salad, canned in water	½	cup(s)	123	112.1	37	0.4	9.6	1.2	0.1	0	0	0
	Gooseberries												
982	Canned in light syrup	½	cup(s)	126	100.9	92	0.8	23.6	3.0	0.3	0	0	0.1
981	Raw	½	cup(s)	75	65.9	33	0.7	7.6	3.2	0.4	0	0	0.2
	Grapefruit												
251	Juice, pink, sweetened, canned	½	cup(s)	125	109.1	57	0.7	13.9	0.1	0.1	0	0	0
249	Juice, white	½	cup(s)	124	111.2	48	0.6	11.4	0.1	0.1	0	0	0
3022	Pink or red, raw	½	cup(s)	114	100.8	48	0.9	12.2	1.8	0.2	0	0	0
247	Raw, white	½	cup(s)	115	104.1	38	0.8	9.7	1.3	0.1	0	0	0
248	Sections, canned in light syrup	½	cup(s)	127	106.2	76	0.7	19.6	0.5	0.1	0	0	0
983	Sections, canned in water	½	cup(s)	122	109.6	44	0.7	11.2	0.5	0.1	0	0	0
	Grapes												
255	American, slip skin	½	cup(s)	46	37.4	31	0.3	7.9	0.4	0.2	0.1	0	0
256	European, red or green, adherent skin	½	cup(s)	76	60.8	52	0.5	13.7	0.7	0.1	0	0	0
3159	Juice drink, canned	½	cup(s)	125	106.6	71	0	18.2	0.1	0	0	0	0
259	Juice, sweetened, with added vitamin C, prepared from frozen concentrate	½	cup(s)	125	108.6	64	0.2	15.9	0.1	0.1	0	0	0
3060	Raisins, seeded, packed	¼	cup(s)	41	6.8	122	1.0	32.4	2.8	0.2	0.1	0	0.1
987	**Guava, raw**	1	item(s)	55	44.4	37	1.4	7.9	3.0	0.5	0.1	0	0.2
35593	**Guava, strawberry**	1	item(s)	6	4.8	4	0	1.0	0.3	0	0	0	0
3027	**Jackfruit**	½	cup(s)	83	60.6	78	1.4	19.2	1.2	0.5	0.2	0.1	0.1
990	**Kiwi fruit or Chinese gooseberries**	1	item(s)	76	63.1	46	0.9	11.1	2.3	0.4	0	0	0.2
	Lemon												
262	Juice	1	tablespoon(s)	15	14.1	3	0.1	1.1	0	0	0	0	0
993	Peel	1	teaspoon(s)	2	1.6	1	0	0.3	0.2	0	0	0	0
992	Raw	1	item(s)	108	94.4	22	1.3	11.6	5.1	0.3	0	0	0.1
	Lime												
269	Juice	1	tablespoon(s)	15	14.0	4	0.1	1.3	0.1	0	0	0	0
994	Raw	1	item(s)	67	59.1	20	0.5	7.1	1.9	0.1	0	0	0
995	**Loganberries, frozen**	½	cup(s)	74	62.2	40	1.1	9.6	3.9	0.2	0	0	0.1
	Mandarin orange												
1038	Canned in juice	½	cup(s)	125	111.4	46	0.8	11.9	0.9	0	0	0	0
1039	Canned in light syrup	½	cup(s)	126	104.7	77	0.6	20.4	0.9	0.1	0	0	0
999	**Mango**	½	cup(s)	83	68.9	49	0.7	12.4	1.3	0.3	0.1	0.1	0.1
1005	**Nectarine, raw, sliced**	½	cup(s)	69	60.4	30	0.7	7.3	1.2	0.2	0	0.1	0.1
	Melons												
271	Cantaloupe	½	cup(s)	80	72.1	27	0.7	6.5	0.7	0.2	0	0	0.1
1000	Casaba melon	½	cup(s)	85	78.1	24	0.9	5.6	0.8	0.1	0	0	0
272	Honeydew	½	cup(s)	89	79.5	32	0.5	8.0	0.7	0.1	0	0	0.1
318	Watermelon	½	cup(s)	76	69.5	23	0.5	5.7	0.3	0.1	0	0	0
	Orange												
14412	Juice with calcium and vitamin D	½	cup(s)	120	105.5	55	1.0	13.0	0	0	0	0	0
29630	Juice, fresh squeezed	½	cup(s)	124	109.5	56	0.9	12.9	0.2	0.2	0	0	0
14411	Juice, not from concentrate	½	cup(s)	120	105.5	55	1.0	13.0	0	0	0	0	0
278	Juice, unsweetened, prepared from frozen concentrate	½	cup(s)	125	109.7	56	0.8	13.4	0.2	0.1	0	0	0
3040	Peel	1	teaspoon(s)	2	1.5	2	0	0.5	0.2	0	0	0	0
273	Raw	1	item(s)	131	113.6	62	1.2	15.4	3.1	0.2	0	0	0
274	Sections	½	cup(s)	90	78.1	42	0.8	10.6	2.2	0.1	0	0	0
	Papaya												
16830	Dried, strips	2	item(s)	46	9.6	131	1.4	33.0	5.2	0.8	0.2	0.2	0.2
282	Raw	½	cup(s)	70	61.6	30	0.3	7.6	1.2	0.2	0.1	0.1	0
35640	**Passion fruit, purple**	1	item(s)	18	13.1	17	0.4	4.2	1.9	0.1	0	0	0.1
	Peach												
285	Halves, canned in heavy syrup	½	cup(s)	131	103.9	97	0.6	26.1	1.7	0.1	0	0	0.1

GE KEY: H-4 = Breads/Baked Goods H-8 = Cereal/Rice/Pasta H-14 = Fruit H-18 = Vegetables/Legumes H-28 = Nuts/Seeds H-30 = Vegetarian H-32 = Dairy H-40 = Eggs H-40 = Seafood H-42 = Meats H-46 = Poultry
48 = Processed Meats H-50 = Beverages H-52 = Fats/Oils H-54 = Sweets H-56 = Spices/Condiments/Sauces H-60 = Mixed Foods/Soups/Sandwiches H-66 = Fast Food H-84 = Convenience H-86 = Baby Foods

Chol (mg)	Calc (mg)	Iron (mg)	Magn (mg)	Pota (mg)	Sodi (mg)	Zinc (mg)	Vit A (µg)	Thia (mg)	Vit E (mg α)	Ribo (mg)	Niac (mg)	Vit B_6 (mg)	Fola (µg)	Vit C (mg)	Vit B_{12} (µg)	Sele (µg)
0	7	0.36	6.2	109.1	7.4	0.10	12.4	0.02	0.50	0.02	0.46	0.06	3.7	2.4	0	0.6
0	9	0.25	8.3	112.6	4.7	0.11	17.8	0.01	0.47	0.02	0.48	0.06	3.6	3.2	0	0.6
0	6	0.30	8.3	111.4	4.7	0.11	15.4	0.02	0.47	0.01	0.43	0.06	3.6	2.5	0	0.6
0	9	0.37	6.1	95.6	3.7	0.10	27.0	0.02	—	0.03	0.46	0.04	3.7	2.3	0	1.0
0	20	0.42	7.6	97.0	2.5	0.14	8.8	0.03	—	0.07	0.19	0.02	3.8	12.6	0	0.5
0	19	0.23	7.5	148.5	0.8	0.09	11.3	0.03	0.28	0.02	0.22	0.06	4.5	20.8	0	0.4
0	10	0.45	12.5	202.2	2.5	0.07	0	0.05	0.05	0.03	0.40	0.02	12.5	33.6	0	0.1
0	11	0.25	14.8	200.1	1.2	0.06	1.2	0.05	0.27	0.02	0.25	0.05	12.4	46.9	0	0.1
0	25	0.09	10.3	154.5	0	0.08	66.4	0.05	0.15	0.04	0.23	0.06	14.9	35.7	0	0.1
0	14	0.07	10.3	170.2	0	0.08	2.3	0.04	0.15	0.02	0.31	0.05	11.5	38.3	0	1.6
0	18	0.51	12.7	163.8	2.5	0.10	0	0.05	0.11	0.03	0.31	0.03	11.4	27.1	0	1.1
0	18	0.50	12.2	161.0	2.4	0.11	0	0.05	0.11	0.03	0.30	0.02	11.0	26.6	0	1.1
0	6	0.13	2.3	87.9	0.9	0.02	2.3	0.04	0.09	0.03	0.14	0.05	1.8	1.8	0	0
0	8	0.27	5.3	144.2	1.5	0.05	2.3	0.05	0.14	0.05	0.14	0.06	1.5	2.4	0	0.1
0	9	0.16	7.5	41.3	11.3	0.04	0	0.28	0	0.44	0.18	0.04	1.3	33.1	0	0.1
0	5	0.13	5.0	26.3	2.5	0.05	0	0.02	0	0.03	0.16	0.05	1.3	29.9	0	0.1
0	12	1.07	12.4	340.3	11.6	0.07	0	0.05	—	0.08	0.46	0.08	1.2	2.2	0	0.2
0	10	0.14	12.1	229.4	1.1	0.13	17.0	0.04	0.40	0.02	0.60	0.06	27.0	125.6	0	0.3
0	1	0.01	1.0	17.5	2.2	—	0.3	0		0	0.04	0.00		2.2	0	
0	20	0.19	23.9	369.6	1.6	0.11	4.1	0.09	0.28	0.05	0.76	0.27	19.8	11.3	0	0.5
0	26	0.24	12.9	237.1	2.3	0.11	3.0	0.02	1.11	0.02	0.26	0.05	19.0	70.5	0	0.2
0	1	0.01	0.9	15.7	0.2	0.01	0	0	0.02	0	0.01	0.01	3.0	5.9	0	0
0	3	0.02	0.3	3.2	0.1	0	0.1	0	0	0	0.01	0.0	0.3	2.6	0	0
0	66	0.76	13.0	156.6	3.2	0.11	2.2	0.05	—	0.04	0.22	0.12	—	83.2	0	1.0
0	2	0.01	1.2	18.0	0.3	0.01	0.3	0	0.03	0	0.02	0.01	1.5	4.6	0	0
0	22	0.40	4.0	68.3	1.3	0.07	1.3	0.02	0.15	0.01	0.13	0.03	5.4	19.5	0	0.3
0	19	0.47	15.4	106.6	0.7	0.25	1.5	0.04	0.64	0.02	0.62	0.05	19.1	11.2	0	0.1
0	14	0.34	13.7	165.6	6.2	0.63	53.5	0.10	0.12	0.04	0.55	0.05	6.2	42.6	0	0.5
0	9	0.47	10.1	98.3	7.6	0.30	52.9	0.07	0.13	0.06	0.56	0.05	6.3	24.9	0	0.5
0	9	0.13	8.3	138.6	0.8	0.07	44.5	0.02	0.74	0.03	0.55	0.10	35.5	30.0	0	0.5
0	4	0.19	6.2	138.7	0	0.12	11.7	0.02	0.53	0.02	0.78	0.02	3.5	3.7	0	0
0	7	0.17	9.6	213.6	12.8	0.14	135.2	0.03	0.04	0.02	0.59	0.06	16.8	29.4	0	0.3
0	9	0.29	9.4	154.8	7.7	0.06	0.0	0.01	0.04	0.03	0.20	0.14	6.8	18.5	0	0.3
0	5	0.15	8.8	201.8	15.9	0.08	2.7	0.03	0.02	0.01	0.37	0.08	16.8	15.9	0	0.6
0	5	0.18	7.6	85.1	0.8	0.08	21.3	0.03	0.04	0.02	0.14	0.03	2.3	6.2	0	0.3
0	175	0	12.0	225.0	0	0.06	0	0.08	0.24	0.03	0.40	0.06	—	36.0	0	0.1
0	14	0.25	13.6	248.0	1.2	0.06	12.4	0.11	0.05	0.04	0.50	0.05	37.2	62.0	0	0.1
0	10	0	12.4	225.0	0	0.06	0	0.08	0.24	0.03	0.40	0.06	—	36.0	0	0.1
0	11	0.12	12.4	236.6	1.2	0.06	6.2	0.10	0.25	0.02	0.25	0.05	54.8	48.4	0	0.1
0	3	0.02	0.4	4.2	0.1	0	0.4	0	0	0	0.02	0.00	0.6	2.7	0	0
0	52	0.13	13.1	237.1	0	0.09	14.4	0.11	0.24	0.05	0.37	0.08	39.3	69.7	0	0.7
0	36	0.09	9.0	162.9	0	0.06	9.9	0.08	0.16	0.04	0.25	0.05	27.0	47.9	0	0.5
0	61	0.76	63.9	554.3	24.4	0.24	71.8	0.05	0.92	0.07	0.98	0.10	56.6	37.1	0	1.8
0	14	0.17	14.7	127.4	5.6	0.06	32.9	0.02	0.21	0.02	0.25	0.03	25.9	42.6	0	0.4
0	2	0.29	5.2	62.6	5.0	0.02	11.5	0	0	0.02	0.27	0.02	2.5	5.4	0	0.1
0	4	0.35	6.6	120.5	7.9	0.12	22.3	0.01	0.64	0.03	0.80	0.02	3.9	3.7	0	0.4

DA+ Code	Food Description	Quantity	Measure	Wt (g)	H_2O (g)	Ener (kcal)	Prot (g)	Carb (g)	Fiber (g)	Fat (g)	Fat Breakdown (g) Sat	Mono	Poly
	Fruit and Fruit Juices—*continued*												
286	Halves, canned in water	½	cup(s)	122	113.6	29	0.5	7.5	1.6	0.1	0	0	0
283	Raw, medium	1	item(s)	150	133.3	59	1.4	14.3	2.3	0.4	0	0.1	0.1
290	Slices, sweetened, frozen	½	cup(s)	125	93.4	118	0.8	30.0	2.3	0.2	0	0.1	0.1
	Pear												
8672	Asian	1	item(s)	122	107.7	51	0.6	13.0	4.4	0.3	0	0.1	0.1
80684	Bartlett	1	item(s)	177	148.9	112	0.7	26.6	5.5	0.3	—	—	—
294	Halves, canned in heavy syrup	½	cup(s)	133	106.9	98	0.3	25.5	2.1	0.2	0	0	0
1012	Halves, canned in juice	½	cup(s)	124	107.2	62	0.4	16.0	2.0	0.1	0	0	0
291	Raw	1	item(s)	166	139.4	95	0.6	25.3	5.1	0.2	0	0.1	0.2
1017	**Persimmon**	1	item(s)	25	16.1	32	0.2	8.4	—	0.1	0	0	0
	Pineapple												
3053	Canned in extra heavy syrup	½	cup(s)	130	101.0	108	0.4	28.0	1.0	0.1	0	0	0
1019	Canned in juice	½	cup(s)	125	104.0	75	0.5	19.5	1.0	0.1	0	0	0
296	Canned in light syrup	½	cup(s)	126	108.0	66	0.5	16.9	1.0	0.2	0	0	0.1
1018	Canned in water	½	cup(s)	123	111.7	39	0.5	10.2	1.0	0.1	0	0	0
299	Juice, unsweetened, canned	½	cup(s)	125	108.0	66	0.4	16.1	0.3	0.2	0	0	0.1
295	Raw, diced	½	cup(s)	78	66.7	39	0.4	10.2	1.1	0.1	0	0	0
1024	**Plantain, cooked**	½	cup(s)	77	51.8	89	0.6	24.0	1.8	0.1	0.1	0	0
300	**Plum, raw, large**	1	item(s)	66	57.6	30	0.5	7.5	0.9	0.2	0	0.1	0
1027	**Pomegranate**	1	item(s)	282	219.8	234	4.7	52.7	11.3	3.3	0.3	0.3	0.2
	Prunes												
5644	Dried	2	item(s)	17	5.2	40	0.4	10.7	1.2	0.1	0	0	0
305	Dried, stewed	½	cup(s)	124	86.5	133	1.2	34.8	3.8	0.2	0	0.1	0
306	Juice, canned	1	cup(s)	256	208.0	182	1.6	44.7	2.6	0.1	0	0.1	0
	Raspberries												
309	Raw	½	cup(s)	62	52.7	32	0.7	7.3	4.0	0.4	0	0	0.2
310	Red, sweetened, frozen	½	cup(s)	125	90.9	129	0.9	32.7	5.5	0.2	0	0	0.1
39793	**Rhubarb, frozen, cooked with sugar**	½	cup(s)	120	81.3	139	0.5	37.4	2.4	0.1	0	0	0
	Strawberries												
313	Raw	½	cup(s)	72	65.5	23	0.5	5.5	1.4	0.2	0	0	0.1
315	Sweetened, frozen, thawed	½	cup(s)	128	99.5	99	0.7	26.8	2.4	0.2	0	0	0.1
16828	**Tangelo**	1	item(s)	95	82.4	45	0.9	11.2	2.3	0.1	0	0	0
	Tangerine												
1040	Juice	½	cup(s)	124	109.8	53	0.6	12.5	0.2	0.2	0	0	0
316	Raw	1	item(s)	88	74.9	47	0.7	11.7	1.6	0.3	0	0.1	0.1
	Vegetables, Legumes												
	Amaranth												
1043	Leaves, boiled, drained	½	cup(s)	66	60.4	14	1.4	2.7	—	0.1	0	0	0.1
1042	Leaves, raw	1	cup(s)	28	25.7	6	0.7	1.1	—	0.1	0	0	0
8683	**Arugula leaves, raw**	1	cup(s)	20	18.3	5	0.5	0.7	0.3	0.1	0	0	0.1
	Artichoke												
1044	Boiled, drained	1	item(s)	120	100.9	64	3.5	14.3	10.3	0.4	0.1	0	0.2
2885	Hearts, boiled, drained	½	cup(s)	84	70.6	45	2.4	10.0	7.2	0.3	0.1	0.0	0.1
	Asparagus												
566	Boiled, drained	½	cup(s)	90	83.4	20	2.2	3.7	1.8	0.2	0	0	0.1
568	Canned, drained	½	cup(s)	121	113.7	23	2.6	3.0	1.9	0.8	0.2	0	0.3
40162	Frozen, boiled, drained	½	cup(s)	90	84.7	16	2.7	1.7	1.4	0.4	0.1	0	0.2
	Bamboo shoots												
1048	Boiled, drained	½	cup(s)	60	57.6	7	0.9	1.2	0.6	0.1	0	0	0.1
1049	Canned, drained	½	cup(s)	66	61.8	12	1.1	2.1	0.9	0.3	0.1	0	0.1
	Beans												
1801	Adzuki beans, boiled	½	cup(s)	87	57.7	111	6.5	21.5	6.4	0.1	0	0	0
511	Baked beans with franks, canned	½	cup(s)	130	89.8	184	8.7	19.9	8.9	8.5	3.0	3.7	1.1
513	Baked beans with pork in sweet sauce, canned	½	cup(s)	127	89.5	140	6.6	26.7	5.4	1.7	0.4	0.4	0.7
512	Baked beans with pork in tomato sauce, canned	½	cup(s)	127	93.0	119	6.5	23.6	5.1	1.2	0.4	0.4	0.2
1805	Black beans, boiled	½	cup(s)	86	56.5	114	7.6	20.4	7.5	0.5	0.1	0	0.2
14597	Chickpeas, garbanzo beans or bengal gram, boiled	½	cup(s)	82	49.4	134	7.3	22.5	6.2	2.1	0.2	0.5	0.9
569	Fordhook lima beans, frozen, boiled, drained	½	cup(s)	85	62.1	88	5.2	16.4	4.9	0.3	0.1	0	0.1
1806	French beans, boiled	½	cup(s)	89	58.9	114	6.2	21.3	8.3	0.7	0.1	0	0.4
2773	Great northern beans, boiled	½	cup(s)	89	61.1	104	7.4	18.7	6.2	0.4	0.1	0	0.2

GE KEY: H-4 = Breads/Baked Goods H-8 = Cereal/Rice/Pasta H-14 = Fruit H-18 = Vegetables/Legumes H-28 = Nuts/Seeds H-30 = Vegetarian H-32 = Dairy H-40 = Eggs H-40 = Seafood H-42 = Meats H-46 = Poultry
48 = Processed Meats H-50 = Beverages H-52 = Fats/Oils H-54 = Sweets H-56 = Spices/Condiments/Sauces H-60 = Mixed Foods/Soups/Sandwiches H-66 = Fast Food H-84 = Convenience H-86 = Baby Foods

Chol (mg)	Calc (mg)	Iron (mg)	Magn (mg)	Pota (mg)	Sodi (mg)	Zinc (mg)	Vit A (µg)	Thia (mg)	Vit E (mg α)	Ribo (mg)	Niac (mg)	Vit B_6 (mg)	Fola (µg)	Vit C (mg)	Vit B_{12} (µg)	Sele (µg)
0	2	0.39	6.1	120.8	3.7	0.11	32.9	0.01	0.60	0.02	0.64	0.02	3.7	3.5	0	0.4
0	9	0.38	13.5	285.0	0	0.25	24.0	0.04	1.10	0.05	1.21	0.04	6.0	9.9	0	0.2
0	4	0.46	6.3	162.5	7.5	0.06	17.5	0.02	0.77	0.04	0.82	0.02	3.8	117.8	0	0.5
0	5	0	9.8	147.6	0	0.02	0	0.01	0.15	0.01	0.27	0.03	9.8	4.6	0	0.1
—	16	0.34	10.6	178.8	1.8	0.14	1.8	0.02	0.21	0.05	0.29	0.05	—	7.8	—	0.2
0	7	0.29	5.3	86.4	6.7	0.11	0	0.01	0.11	0.03	0.32	0.02	1.3	1.5	0	0
0	11	0.36	8.7	119.0	5.0	0.11	0	0.01	0.10	0.01	0.25	0.02	1.2	2.0	0	0
0	15	0.30	11.6	192.6	1.7	0.17	1.7	0.02	0.20	0.04	0.27	0.05	11.6	7.1	0	0.2
0	7	0.63	—	77.5	0.3	—	—	—	—	—	—	—	—	16.5	0	—
0	18	0.49	19.5	132.6	1.3	0.14	1.3	0.12	—	0.03	0.37	0.10	6.5	9.5	0	—
0	17	0.35	17.4	151.9	1.2	0.12	2.5	0.12	0.01	0.02	0.35	0.09	6.2	11.8	0	0.5
0	18	0.49	20.2	132.3	1.3	0.15	2.5	0.11	0.01	0.03	0.37	0.09	6.3	9.4	0	0.5
0	18	0.49	22.1	156.2	1.2	0.15	2.5	0.11	0.01	0.03	0.37	0.09	6.2	9.5	0	0.5
0	16	0.39	15.0	162.5	2.5	0.14	0	0.07	0.03	0.03	0.25	0.13	22.5	12.5	0	0.1
0	10	0.22	9.3	84.5	0.8	0.09	2.3	0.06	0.02	0.02	0.39	0.09	13.9	37.0	0	0.1
0	2	0.45	24.6	358.0	3.8	0.10	34.7	0.04	0.10	0.04	0.58	0.18	20.0	8.4	0	1.1
0	4	0.11	4.6	103.6	0	0.07	11.2	0.02	0.17	0.02	0.28	0.02	3.3	6.3	0	0
0	28	0.85	33.8	665.5	8.5	0.99	0	0.19	1.69	0.15	0.83	0.21	107.2	28.8	0	1.4
0	7	0.16	6.9	123.0	0.3	0.07	6.6	0.01	0.07	0.03	0.32	0.03	0.7	0.1	0	0.1
0	24	0.51	22.3	398.0	1.2	0.24	21.1	0.03	0.24	0.12	0.90	0.27	0	3.6	0	0.1
0	31	3.02	35.8	706.6	10.2	0.54	0	0.04	0.31	0.18	2.01	0.56	0	10.5	0	1.5
0	15	0.42	13.5	92.9	0.6	0.26	1.2	0.02	0.54	0.02	0.37	0.03	12.9	16.1	0	0.1
0	19	0.81	16.3	142.5	1.3	0.22	3.8	0.02	0.90	0.06	0.29	0.04	32.5	20.6	0	0.4
0	174	0.25	14.4	115.2	1.2	0.10	4.8	0.02	0.23	0.03	0.24	0.02	6.0	4.0	0	1.1
0	12	0.30	9.4	110.2	0.7	0.10	0.7	0.02	0.21	0.02	0.28	0.03	17.3	42.3	0	0.3
0	14	0.60	7.7	124.9	1.3	0.06	1.3	0.02	0.31	0.10	0.37	0.04	5.1	50.4	0	0.9
0	38	0.09	9.5	171.9	0	0.07	10.4	0.08	0.17	0.04	0.27	0.06	28.5	50.5	0	0.5
0	22	0.25	9.9	219.8	1.2	0.04	16.1	0.07	0.16	0.02	0.12	0.05	6.2	38.3	0	0.1
0	33	0.13	10.6	146.1	1.8	0.06	29.9	0.05	0.18	0.03	0.33	0.07	14.1	23.5	0	0.1
0	138	1.49	36.3	423.1	13.9	0.58	91.7	0.01	—	0.09	0.37	0.12	37.6	27.1	0	0.6
0	60	0.65	15.4	171.1	5.6	0.25	40.9	0.01	—	0.04	0.18	0.05	23.8	12.1	0	0.3
0	32	0.29	9.4	73.8	5.4	0.09	23.8	0.01	0.09	0.02	0.06	0.01	19.4	3.0	0	0.1
0	25	0.73	50.4	343.2	72.0	0.48	1.2	0.06	0.23	0.11	1.33	0.10	106.8	8.9	0	0.2
0	18	0.51	35.3	240.2	50.4	0.34	0.8	0.04	0.16	0.07	0.93	0.07	74.8	6.2	0	0.2
0	21	0.82	12.6	201.6	12.6	0.54	45.0	0.15	1.35	0.13	0.98	0.07	134.1	6.9	0	5.5
0	19	2.21	12.1	208.1	347.3	0.48	49.6	0.07	1.48	0.12	1.15	0.13	116.2	22.3	0	2.1
0	16	0.50	9.0	154.8	2.7	0.37	36.0	0.06	1.08	0.09	0.93	0.02	121.5	22.0	0	3.5
0	7	0.14	1.8	319.8	2.4	0.28	0	0.01	—	0.03	0.18	0.06	1.2	0	0	0.2
0	5	0.21	2.6	52.4	4.6	0.43	0.7	0.02	0.41	0.02	0.09	0.09	2.0	0.7	0	0.3
0	24	1.74	45.2	462.8	7.0	1.54	0	0.10	—	0.06	0.62	0.08	105.3	0	0	1.0
8	62	2.24	36.3	304.3	556.8	2.42	5.2	0.08	0.21	0.07	1.17	0.06	38.8	3.0	0.4	8.4
1	72	2.09	40.5	322.6	426.3	1.02	1.3	0.06	0.06	0.07	0.44	0.07	10.1	3.4	0	6.3
9	71	4.10	43.0	373.2	552.8	6.93	5.1	0.07	0.13	0.06	0.62	0.08	19.0	3.8	0	5.9
0	23	1.81	60.2	305.3	0.9	0.96	0	0.21	—	0.05	0.43	0.06	128.1	0	0	1.0
0	40	2.37	39.4	238.6	5.7	1.25	0.8	0.10	0.29	0.05	0.43	0.11	141.0	1.1	0	3.0
0	26	1.55	35.7	258.6	58.7	0.63	8.5	0.06	0.25	0.05	0.91	0.10	17.9	10.9	0	0.5
0	56	0.96	49.6	327.5	5.3	0.57	0	0.12	—	0.05	0.48	0.09	66.4	1.1	0	1.1
0	60	1.89	44.3	346.0	1.8	0.78	0	0.14	—	0.05	0.60	0.10	90.3	1.2	0	3.6

DA+ Code	Food Description	Quantity	Measure	Wt (g)	H_2O (g)	Ener (kcal)	Prot (g)	Carb (g)	Fiber (g)	Fat (g)	Fat Breakdown (g)		
											Sat	Mono	Poly
Vegetables, Legumes—*continued*													
2736	Hyacinth beans, boiled, drained	½	cup(s)	44	37.8	22	1.3	4.0	—	0.1	0.1	0.1	0
570	Lima beans, baby, frozen, boiled, drained	½	cup(s)	90	65.1	95	6.0	17.5	5.4	0.3	0.1	0	0.1
515	Lima beans, boiled, drained	½	cup(s)	85	57.1	105	5.8	20.1	4.5	0.3	0.1	0	0.1
579	Mung beans, sprouted, boiled, drained	½	cup(s)	62	57.9	13	1.3	2.6	0.5	0.1	0	0	0
510	Navy beans, boiled	½	cup(s)	91	58.1	127	7.5	23.7	9.6	0.6	0.1	0.1	0.4
32816	Pinto beans, boiled, drained, no salt added	½	cup(s)	63	58.8	14	1.2	2.6	—	0.2	0	0	0.1
1052	Pinto beans, frozen, boiled, drained	½	cup(s)	47	27.3	76	4.4	14.5	4.0	0.2	0	0	0.1
514	Red kidney beans, canned	½	cup(s)	128	99.8	104	6.7	19.0	6.8	0.5	0.1	0.1	0.3
71879	Red kidney beans, canned, reduced sodium	½	cup(s)	130	—	105	7.0	22.0	8.0	0.0	0	—	—
1810	Refried beans, canned	½	cup(s)	119	90.6	108	6.4	18.2	6.1	1.4	0.5	0.5	0.4
1053	Shell beans, canned	½	cup(s)	123	111.1	37	2.2	7.6	4.2	0.2	0	0	0.1
1670	Soybeans, boiled	½	cup(s)	86	53.8	149	14.3	8.5	5.2	7.7	1.1	1.7	4.4
1108	Soybeans, green, boiled, drained	½	cup(s)	90	61.7	127	11.1	9.9	3.8	5.8	0.7	1.1	2.7
1807	White beans, small, boiled	½	cup(s)	90	56.6	127	8.0	23.1	9.3	0.6	0.1	0.1	0.2
575	Yellow snap, string or wax beans, boiled, drained	½	cup(s)	63	55.8	22	1.2	4.9	2.1	0.2	0	0	0.1
576	Yellow snap, string or wax beans, frozen, boiled, drained	½	cup(s)	68	61.7	19	1.0	4.4	2.0	0.1	0	0	0.1
	Beets												
584	Beet greens, boiled, drained	½	cup(s)	72	64.2	19	1.9	3.9	2.1	0.1	0	0	0.1
2730	Pickled, canned with liquid	½	cup(s)	114	92.9	74	0.9	18.5	3.0	0.1	0	0	0
581	Sliced, boiled, drained	½	cup(s)	85	74.0	37	1.4	8.5	1.7	0.2	0	0	0.1
583	Sliced, canned, drained	½	cup(s)	85	77.4	26	0.8	6.1	1.5	0.1	0	0	0
580	Whole, boiled, drained	2	item(s)	100	87.1	44	1.7	10.0	2.0	0.2	0	0	0.1
585	**Cowpeas or black-eyed peas, boiled, drained**	½	cup(s)	83	62.3	80	2.6	16.8	4.1	0.3	0.1	0	0.1
	Broccoli												
588	Chopped, boiled, drained	½	cup(s)	78	69.6	27	1.9	5.6	2.6	0.3	0.1	0	0.1
590	Frozen, chopped, boiled, drained	½	cup(s)	92	83.5	26	2.9	4.9	2.8	0.1	0	0	0.1
587	Raw, chopped	½	cup(s)	46	40.6	15	1.3	3.0	1.2	0.2	0	0	0
16848	**Broccoflower, raw, chopped**	½	cup(s)	32	28.7	10	0.9	1.9	1.0	0.1	0	0	0
	Brussels sprouts												
591	Boiled, drained	½	cup(s)	78	69.3	28	2.0	5.5	2.0	0.4	0.1	0	0.2
592	Frozen, boiled, drained	½	cup(s)	78	67.2	33	2.8	6.4	3.2	0.3	0.1	0	0.2
	Cabbage												
595	Boiled, drained, no salt added	1	cup(s)	150	138.9	35	1.9	8.3	2.8	0.1	0	0	0
35611	Chinese (pak choi or bok choy), boiled with salt, drained	1	cup(s)	170	162.4	20	2.7	3.0	1.7	0.3	0	0	0.1
16869	Kim chee	1	cup(s)	150	137.6	32	2.4	5.9	1.8	0.3	0	0	0.2
594	Raw, shredded	1	cup(s)	70	64.5	18	0.9	4.1	1.8	0.1	0	0	0
596	Red, shredded, raw	1	cup(s)	70	63.3	22	1.0	5.2	1.5	0.1	0	0	0.1
597	Savoy, shredded, raw	1	cup(s)	70	63.7	19	1.4	4.3	2.2	0.1	0	0	0
35417	**Capers**	1	teaspoon(s)	4	—	2	0	0	0	0	0	0	0.0
	Carrots												
8691	Baby, raw	8	item(s)	80	72.3	28	0.5	6.6	2.3	0.1	0	0	0.1
601	Grated	½	cup(s)	55	48.6	23	0.5	5.3	1.5	0.1	0	0	0.1
1055	Juice, canned	½	cup(s)	118	104.9	47	1.1	11.0	0.9	0.2	0	0	0.1
600	Raw	½	cup(s)	61	53.9	25	0.6	5.8	1.7	0.1	0	0	0.1
602	Sliced, boiled, drained	½	cup(s)	78	70.3	27	0.6	6.4	2.3	0.1	0	0	0.1
32725	**Cassava or manioc**	½	cup(s)	103	61.5	165	1.4	39.2	1.9	0.3	0.1	0.1	0
	Cauliflower												
606	Boiled, drained	½	cup(s)	62	57.7	14	1.1	2.5	1.4	0.3	0	0	0.1
607	Frozen, boiled, drained	½	cup(s)	90	84.6	17	1.4	3.4	2.4	0.2	0	0	0.1
605	Raw, chopped	½	cup(s)	50	46.0	13	1.0	2.5	1.0	0.1	0	0	0
	Celery												
609	Diced	½	cup(s)	51	48.2	8	0.3	1.5	0.8	0.1	0	0	0
608	Stalk	2	item(s)	80	76.3	13	0.6	2.4	1.3	0.1	0	0	0.1
	Chard												
1057	Swiss chard, boiled, drained	½	cup(s)	88	81.1	18	1.6	3.6	1.8	0.1	0	0	0
1056	Swiss chard, raw	1	cup(s)	36	33.4	7	0.6	1.3	0.6	0.1	0	0	0

Chol (mg)	Calc (mg)	Iron (mg)	Magn (mg)	Pota (mg)	Sodi (mg)	Zinc (mg)	Vit A (µg)	Thia (mg)	Vit E (mg α)	Ribo (mg)	Niac (mg)	Vit B_6 (mg)	Fola (µg)	Vit C (mg)	Vit B_{12} (µg)	Sele (µg)
0	18	0.33	18.3	114.0	0.9	0.17	3.0	0.02	—	0.04	0.21	0.01	20.4	2.2	0	0.7
0	25	1.76	50.4	369.9	26.1	0.50	7.2	0.06	0.58	0.05	0.69	0.10	14.4	5.2	0	1.5
0	27	2.08	62.9	484.8	14.5	0.67	12.8	0.12	0.12	0.08	0.88	0.16	22.1	8.6	0	1.7
0	7	0.40	8.7	62.6	6.2	0.29	0.6	0.03	0.04	0.06	0.51	0.03	18.0	7.1	0	0.4
	63	2.15	48.2	354.0	0	0.94	0	0.22	0.01	0.06	0.59	0.13	127.4	0.8	0	2.6
0	9	0.42	11.3	61.7	32.1	0.11	0	0.04	—	0.04	0.46	0.03	18.3	3.8	0	0.4
0	24	1.27	25.4	303.6	39.0	0.32	0	0.13	—	0.05	0.30	0.09	16.0	0.3	0	0.7
0	37	1.60	38.4	332.8	327.7	0.79	0	0.14	0.03	0.09	0.63	0.10	33.3	1.0	0	1.4
0	80	1.80	—	400.0	130.0	—	0	—	—	—	—	—	—	0	0	—
0	39	1.99	45.2	399.8	534.3	0.77	0	0.04	0.06	0.02	0.50	0.13	13.1	7.1	0	7.7
0	36	1.21	18.4	133.5	409.1	0.33	13.5	0.04	0.04	0.07	0.25	0.06	22.0	3.8	0	2.6
0	88	4.42	74.0	442.9	0.9	0.99	0	0.13	0.30	0.25	0.34	0.20	46.4	1.5	0	6.3
0	131	2.25	54.0	485.1	12.6	0.82	7.2	0.23	—	0.14	1.13	0.05	99.9	15.3	0	1.3
0	65	2.54	60.9	414.4	1.8	0.98	0	0.21	—	0.05	0.24	0.11	122.6	0	0	1.2
0	29	0.80	15.6	186.9	1.9	0.22	2.5	0.05	0.28	0.06	0.38	0.04	20.6	6.1	0	0.3
0	33	0.59	16.2	85.1	6.1	0.32	4.1	0.02	0.03	0.06	0.26	0.04	15.5	2.8	0	0.3
0	82	1.37	49.0	654.5	173.5	0.36	275.8	0.08	1.30	0.21	0.36	0.10	10.1	17.9	0	0.6
0	12	0.47	17.0	168.0	299.6	0.30	2.3	0.01	0.07	0.05	0.28	0.06	30.6	2.6	0	1.1
0	14	0.67	19.6	259.4	65.5	0.30	1.7	0.02	0.03	0.03	0.28	0.06	68.0	3.1	0	0.6
0	13	1.55	14.5	125.9	165.0	0.18	0.9	0.01	0.03	0.03	0.13	0.05	25.5	3.5	0	0.4
0	16	0.79	23.0	305.0	77.0	0.35	2.0	0.03	0.04	0.04	0.33	0.07	80.0	3.6	0	0.7
0	106	0.92	42.9	344.9	3.3	0.85	33.0	0.08	0.18	0.12	1.16	0.05	104.8	1.8	0	2.1
0	31	0.52	16.4	228.5	32.0	0.35	60.1	0.05	1.13	0.10	0.43	0.16	84.2	50.6	0	1.2
0	30	0.56	12.0	130.6	10.1	0.26	46.9	0.05	1.21	0.07	0.42	0.12	51.5	36.9	0	0.6
0	21	0.33	9.6	143.8	15.0	0.19	14.1	0.03	0.35	0.05	0.29	0.08	28.7	40.6	0	1.1
0	11	0.23	6.4	96.0	7.4	0.20	2.6	0.03	0.01	0.03	0.23	0.07	18.2	28.2	0	0.2
0	28	0.94	15.6	247.3	16.4	0.26	30.4	0.08	0.34	0.06	0.47	0.14	46.8	48.4	0	1.2
0	20	0.37	13.9	224.8	11.6	0.19	35.7	0.08	0.40	0.09	0.42	0.22	78.3	35.4	0	0.5
0	72	0.25	22.5	294.0	12.0	0.30	6.0	0.09	0.21	0.06	0.37	0.17	45.0	56.3	0	0.9
0	158	1.77	18.7	630.7	459.0	0.29	360.4	0.05	0.15	0.11	0.73	0.28	69.7	44.2	0	0.7
0	137	1.23	27.0	367.5	936.0	0.36	274.5	0.07	0.41	0.10	0.78	0.33	85.5	68.1	0	1.5
0	28	0.33	8.4	119.0	12.6	0.13	3.5	0.04	0.10	0.03	0.16	0.09	30.1	25.6	0	0.2
0	32	0.56	11.2	170.1	18.9	0.15	39.2	0.04	0.08	0.05	0.29	0.15	12.6	39.9	0	0.4
0	25	0.28	19.6	161.0	19.6	0.19	35.0	0.05	0.12	0.02	0.21	0.13	56.0	21.7	0	0.6
0	0	0	—	—	140.0	—	0	—	—	—	—	—	—	0	—	—
0	26	0.71	8.0	189.6	62.4	0.14	552.0	0.02	—	0.03	0.44	0.08	21.6	2.1	0	0.7
0	18	0.17	6.6	176.0	37.9	0.13	459.3	0.04	0.36	0.03	0.54	0.08	10.5	3.2	0	0.1
0	28	0.54	16.5	344.6	77.9	0.21	1128.1	0.11	1.37	0.06	0.46	0.26	4.7	10.0	0	0.7
0	20	0.18	7.3	195.2	42.1	0.15	509.4	0.04	0.40	0.04	0.60	0.08	11.6	3.6	0	0.1
0	23	0.27	7.8	183.3	45.2	0.16	664.6	0.05	0.80	0.03	0.50	0.12	10.9	2.8	0	0.5
0	16	0.28	21.6	279.1	14.4	0.35	1.0	0.09	0.20	0.05	0.88	0.09	27.8	21.2	0	0.7
0	10	0.20	5.6	88.0	9.3	0.11	0.6	0.03	0.04	0.03	0.25	0.11	27.3	27.5	0	0.4
0	15	0.37	8.1	125.1	16.2	0.12	0	0.03	0.05	0.05	0.28	0.08	36.9	28.2	0	0.5
0	11	0.21	7.5	149.5	15.0	0.14	0	0.03	0.04	0.03	0.25	0.09	28.5	24.1	0	0.3
0	20	0.10	5.6	131.3	40.4	0.07	11.1	0.01	0.14	0.03	0.16	0.04	18.2	1.6	0	0.2
0	32	0.16	8.8	208.0	64.0	0.10	17.6	0.02	0.22	0.05	0.26	0.06	28.8	2.5	0	0.3
0	51	1.98	75.3	480.4	156.6	0.29	267.8	0.03	1.65	0.08	0.31	0.07	7.9	15.8	0	0.8
0	18	0.65	29.2	136.4	76.7	0.13	110.2	0.01	0.68	0.03	0.14	0.04	5.0	10.8	0	0.3

DA+ Code	Food Description	Quantity	Measure	Wt (g)	H_2O (g)	Ener (kcal)	Prot (g)	Carb (g)	Fiber (g)	Fat (g)	Fat Breakdown (g)		
											Sat	Mono	Poly
Vegetables, Legumes—*continued*													
	Collard greens												
610	Boiled, drained	½	cup(s)	95	85.7	31	2.6	5.4	3.8	0.7	0	0	0.2
611	Frozen, chopped, boiled, drained	½	cup(s)	85	75.2	31	2.5	6.0	2.4	0.3	0.1	0	0.2
	Corn												
29614	Yellow corn, fresh, cooked	1	item(s)	100	73.0	95	3.4	20.9	2.4	1.5	0.2	0.4	0.6
615	Yellow creamed sweet corn, canned	½	cup(s)	128	100.8	92	2.2	23.2	1.5	0.5	0.1	0.2	0.3
612	Yellow sweet corn, boiled, drained	½	cup(s)	82	60.2	79	2.8	17.2	2.0	1.2	0.2	0.3	0.5
614	Yellow sweet corn, frozen, boiled, drained	½	cup(s)	82	63.2	66	2.1	15.8	2.0	0.5	0.1	0.2	0.3
	Cucumber												
703	Pickled, dill	¼	cup(s)	39	36.6	5	0.2	1.0	0.4	0.1	0	0	0
2755	Pickled, dill, low sodium	¼	cup(s)	39	35.5	7	0.2	1.6	0.5	0.1	0	0	0
618	Raw	¼	item(s)	75	71.7	11	0.5	2.7	0.4	0.1	0	0	0
	Dandelion greens												
620	Chopped, boiled, drained	½	cup(s)	53	47.1	17	1.0	3.4	1.5	0.3	0.1	0	0.1
2734	Raw	1	cup(s)	55	47.1	25	1.5	5.1	1.9	0.4	0.1	0	0.2
1066	**Eggplant, boiled, drained**	½	cup(s)	50	44.4	17	0.4	4.3	1.2	0.1	0	0	0
621	**Endive or escarole, chopped, raw**	1	cup(s)	50	46.9	9	0.6	1.7	1.6	0.1	0	0	0
8784	**Jicama or yambean**	½	cup(s)	67	60.1	25	0.5	5.9	3.3	0.1	0	0	0.0
	Kale												
623	Frozen, chopped, boiled, drained	½	cup(s)	65	58.8	20	1.8	3.4	1.3	0.3	0	0	0.2
29313	Raw	1	cup(s)	67	56.3	33	2.9	5.9	1.3	0.6	0.1	0	0.2
	Kohlrabi												
1072	Boiled, drained	½	cup(s)	83	74.5	24	1.5	5.5	0.9	0.1	0	0	0
1071	Raw	1	cup(s)	135	122.8	36	2.3	8.4	4.9	0.1	0	0	0.1
	Leeks												
1074	Boiled, drained	½	cup(s)	52	47.2	16	0.4	4.0	0.5	0.1	0	0	0.1
1073	Raw	1	cup(s)	89	73.9	54	1.3	12.6	1.6	0.3	0	0	0.1
	Lentils												
522	Boiled	¼	cup(s)	50	34.5	57	4.5	10.0	3.9	0.2	0	0	0.1
1075	Sprouted	1	cup(s)	77	51.9	82	6.9	17.0	—	0.4	0	0.1	0.2
	Lettuce												
625	Butterhead leaves	11	piece(s)	83	78.9	11	1.1	1.8	0.9	0.2	0	0	0.1
624	Butterhead, Boston or Bibb	1	cup(s)	55	52.6	7	0.7	1.2	0.6	0.1	0	0	0.1
626	Iceberg	1	cup(s)	72	68.9	10	0.6	2.1	0.9	0.1	0	0	0.1
628	Iceberg, chopped	1	cup(s)	55	52.6	8	0.5	1.6	0.7	0.1	0	0	0
629	Looseleaf	1	cup(s)	36	34.2	5	0.5	1.0	0.5	0.1	0	0	0
1665	Romaine, shredded	1	cup(s)	47	44.5	8	0.6	1.5	1.0	0.1	0	0	0.1
	Mushrooms												
15585	Crimini (about 6)	3	ounce(s)	85	—	28	3.7	2.8	1.9	0	0	0	0
8700	Enoki	30	item(s)	90	79.5	33	2.4	7.0	2.4	0.3	0	0	0.1
1079	Mushrooms, boiled, drained	½	cup(s)	78	71.0	22	1.7	4.1	1.7	0.4	0	0	0.1
1080	Mushrooms, canned, drained	½	cup(s)	78	71.0	20	1.5	4.0	1.9	0.2	0	0	0.1
630	Mushrooms, raw	½	cup(s)	48	44.4	11	1.5	1.6	0.5	0.2	0	0	0.1
35465	Portabella, raw	1	item(s)	84	78.0	18	1.8	3.3	1.1	0.3	0.1	0	0.1
2743	Shiitake, cooked	½	cup(s)	73	60.5	41	1.1	10.4	1.5	0.2	0	0.1	0
	Mustard greens												
2744	Frozen, boiled, drained	½	cup(s)	75	70.3	14	1.7	2.3	2.1	0.2	0	0.1	0
29319	Raw	1	cup(s)	56	50.8	15	1.6	2.6	1.8	0.2	0	0.1	0
	Okra												
16866	Batter coated, fried	11	piece(s)	83	50.3	159	4.0	20.1	2.3	7.1	1.4	2.8	2.4
32742	Frozen, boiled, drained, no salt added	½	cup(s)	92	83.8	27	1.5	5.9	1.9	0.2	0.1	0	0.1
632	Sliced, boiled, drained	½	cup(s)	80	74.1	18	1.5	3.6	2.0	0.2	0	0	0
	Onions												
635	Chopped, boiled, drained	½	cup(s)	105	92.3	46	1.4	10.7	1.5	0.2	0	0	0.1
2748	Frozen, boiled, drained	½	cup(s)	106	97.8	30	0.8	7.0	1.9	0.1	0	0	0
1081	Onion rings, breaded and pan fried, frozen, heated	10	piece(s)	71	20.2	289	3.8	27.1	0.9	19.0	6.1	7.7	3.6
633	Raw, chopped	½	cup(s)	80	71.3	32	0.9	7.5	1.4	0.1	0	0	0
16850	Red onions, sliced, raw	½	cup(s)	58	51.2	23	0.6	5.4	1.0	0.1	0	0	0
636	Scallions, green or spring onions	2	item(s)	30	26.9	10	0.5	2.2	0.8	0.1	0	0	0

ǃE KEY: H-4 = Breads/Baked Goods H-8 = Cereal/Rice/Pasta H-14 = Fruit H-18 = Vegetables/Legumes H-28 = Nuts/Seeds H-30 = Vegetarian H-32 = Dairy H-40 = Eggs H-40 = Seafood H-42 = Meats H-46 = Poultry
ǃ8 = Processed Meats H-50 = Beverages H-52 = Fats/Oils H-54 = Sweets H-56 = Spices/Condiments/Sauces H-60 = Mixed Foods/Soups/Sandwiches H-66 = Fast Food H-84 = Convenience H-86 = Baby Foods

Chol (mg)	Calc (mg)	Iron (mg)	Magn (mg)	Pota (mg)	Sodi (mg)	Zinc (mg)	Vit A (μg)	Thia (mg)	Vit E (mg α)	Ribo (mg)	Niac (mg)	Vit B_6 (mg)	Fola (μg)	Vit C (mg)	Vit B_{12} (μg)	Sele (μg)
0	134	1.07	20.0	111.2	14.3	0.22	361.0	0.04	0.84	0.10	0.55	0.12	15.2	17.3	0	0.5
0	179	0.95	25.5	213.5	42.5	0.23	489.0	0.04	1.06	0.10	0.54	0.10	64.6	22.5	0	1.3
0	3	0.45	26.0	217.0	227.0	0.62	13.0	0.09	0.09	0.06	1.67	0.14	23.0	5.5	0	0.2
0	4	0.49	21.8	171.5	364.8	0.68	5.1	0.03	0.09	0.07	1.23	0.08	57.6	5.9	0	0.5
0	2	0.37	21.3	178.8	0.8	0.51	10.7	0.08	0.07	0.05	1.38	0.11	18.9	4.5	0	0.2
0	2	0.39	23.0	191.1	0.8	0.52	8.2	0.02	0.06	0.05	1.08	0.08	28.7	2.9	0	0.6
0	16	0.14	2.7	35.7	339.1	0.04	3.5	0.01	0.03	0.01	0.04	0.01	0.4	0.3	0	0
0	3	0.21	4.3	45.0	7.0	0.05	5.0	0.01	—	0.01	0.02	0.01	0.4	0.7	0	0
0	12	0.21	9.8	110.6	1.5	0.15	3.8	0.02	0.02	0.02	0.07	0.03	5.3	2.1	0	0.2
0	74	0.94	12.6	121.8	23.1	0.15	179.6	0.07	1.28	0.09	0.27	0.08	6.8	9.4	0	0.2
0	103	1.70	19.8	218.3	41.8	0.23	279.4	0.10	1.89	0.14	0.44	0.14	14.8	19.3	0	0.3
0	3	0.12	5.4	60.9	0.5	0.06	1.0	0.04	0.20	0.01	0.30	0.04	6.9	0.6	0	0
0	26	0.41	7.5	157.0	11.0	0.40	54.0	0.04	0.22	0.04	0.20	0.01	71.0	3.3	0	0.1
0	8	0.40	8.0	100.0	2.7	0.11	0.7	0.01	0.31	0.02	0.13	0.03	8.0	13.5	0	0.5
0	90	0.61	11.7	208.6	9.8	0.12	477.8	0.03	0.60	0.07	0.44	0.06	9.1	16.4	0	0.6
0	101	0.98	31.5	329.0	25.5	0.38	335.0	0.07	—	0.09	0.67	0.18	20.8	80.4	0	0.6
0	21	0.33	15.7	280.5	17.3	0.26	1.6	0.03	0.43	0.02	0.32	0.13	9.9	44.5	0	0.7
0	32	0.54	25.6	472.5	27.0	0.04	2.7	0.07	0.65	0.03	0.54	0.20	21.6	83.7	0	0.9
0	16	0.57	7.3	45.2	5.2	0.03	21.3	0.01	0.26	0.01	0.10	0.06	12.5	2.2	0	0.3
0	53	1.87	24.9	160.2	17.8	0.11	73.9	0.05	0.82	0.03	0.36	0.21	57.0	10.7	0	0.9
0	9	1.65	17.8	182.7	1.0	0.63	0	0.08	0.05	0.04	0.52	0.09	89.6	0.7	0	1.4
0	19	2.47	28.5	247.9	8.5	1.16	1.5	0.18	—	0.10	0.87	0.15	77.0	12.7	0	0.5
0	29	1.02	10.7	196.4	4.1	0.17	136.9	0.05	0.15	0.05	0.29	0.07	60.2	3.1	0	0.5
0	19	0.68	7.2	130.9	2.8	0.11	91.3	0.03	0.10	0.03	0.20	0.05	40.1	2.0	0	0.3
0	13	0.30	5.0	101.5	7.2	0.11	18.0	0.03	0.13	0.02	0.09	0.03	20.9	2.0	0	0.1
0	10	0.23	3.9	77.5	5.5	0.08	13.8	0.02	0.10	0.01	0.07	0.02	15.9	1.5	0	0.1
0	13	0.31	4.7	69.8	10.1	0.06	133.2	0.03	0.08	0.03	0.14	0.03	13.7	3.3	0	0.2
0	16	0.46	6.6	116.1	3.8	0.11	204.9	0.03	0.06	0.03	0.15	0.03	63.9	1.9	0	0.2
0	0	0.67	—	—	32.6	—	0	—	—	—	—	—	—	0	0	—
0	0	1.03	14.4	323.1	2.7	0.58	—	0.20	0.01	0.18	6.33	0.09	43.2	0	0	2.0
0	5	1.36	9.4	277.7	1.6	0.68	0	0.06	0.01	0.23	3.48	0.07	14.0	3.1	0	9.3
0	9	0.62	11.7	100.6	331.5	0.56	0	0.07	0.01	0.02	1.24	0.05	9.4	0	0	3.2
0	1	0.24	4.3	152.6	2.4	0.25	0	0.04	0	0.19	1.73	0.05	8.2	1.0	0	4.5
0	3	0.26	9.2	305.8	7.6	0.45	0	0.05	0.02	0.11	3.77	0.12	23.5	0	0	15.6
0	2	0.32	10.1	84.8	2.9	0.96	0	0.03	0	0.12	1.09	0.12	15.2	0.2	0	18.0
0	76	0.84	9.8	104.3	18.8	0.15	265.5	0.03	1.01	0.04	0.19	0.08	52.5	10.4	0	0.4
0	64	0.92	17.9	215.0	11.2	0.14	84.6	0.04	1.13	0.06	0.45	0.10	6.7	39.2	0	0.5
40	47	1.54	34.7	190.6	142.7	0.57	28.9	0.21	0.69	0.16	1.52	0.14	95.7	8.6	0.1	7.3
0	68	0.48	36.8	169.3	2.8	0.45	13.8	0.07	0.29	0.09	0.57	0.03	92.0	8.8	0	0.6
0	62	0.22	28.8	108.0	4.8	0.34	11.2	0.11	0.22	0.04	0.70	0.15	36.8	13.0	0	0.3
0	23	0.25	11.5	174.3	3.1	0.22	0	0.04	0.02	0.02	0.17	0.14	15.8	5.5	0	0.6
0	17	0.32	6.4	114.5	12.7	0.07	0	0.02	0.01	0.03	0.15	0.07	13.8	2.8	0	0.4
0	22	1.20	13.5	91.6	266.3	0.30	7.8	0.20	—	0.10	2.56	0.05	73.1	1.0	0	2.5
0	18	0.17	8.0	116.8	3.2	0.14	0	0.04	0.02	0.02	0.09	0.10	15.2	5.9	0	0.4
0	13	0.12	5.8	83.9	2.3	0.10	0	0.03	0.01	0.02	0.07	0.07	10.9	4.3	0	0.3
0	22	0.44	6.0	82.8	4.8	0.12	15.0	0.02	0.17	0.02	0.16	0.02	19.2	5.6	0	0.2

DA+ Code	Food Description	Quantity	Measure	Wt (g)	H_2O (g)	Ener (kcal)	Prot (g)	Carb (g)	Fiber (g)	Fat (g)	Fat Breakdown (g) Sat	Mono	Poly
	Vegetables, Legumes—*continued*												
16860	**Palm hearts, cooked**	½	cup(s)	73	50.7	84	2.0	18.7	1.1	0.1	0	0	0.1
637	**Parsley, chopped**	1	tablespoon(s)	4	3.3	1	0.1	0.2	0.1	0	0	0	0
638	**Parsnips, sliced, boiled, drained**	½	cup(s)	78	62.6	55	1.0	13.3	2.8	0.2	0	0.1	0
	Peas												
639	Green peas, canned, drained	½	cup(s)	88	72.0	60	3.9	9.9	4.3	0.7	0.1	0.1	0.3
641	Green peas, frozen, boiled, drained	½	cup(s)	80	63.6	62	4.1	11.4	4.4	0.2	0	0	0.1
35694	Pea pods, boiled with salt, drained	½	cup(s)	80	71.1	32	2.6	5.2	2.2	0.2	0	0	0.1
1082	Peas and carrots, canned with liquid	½	cup(s)	128	112.4	48	2.8	10.8	2.5	0.3	0.1	0	0.2
1083	Peas and carrots, frozen, boiled, drained	½	cup(s)	80	68.6	38	2.5	8.1	2.5	0.3	0.1	0	0.2
2750	Snow or sugar peas, frozen, boiled, drained	½	cup(s)	80	69.3	42	2.8	7.2	2.5	0.3	0.1	0	0.1
640	Snow or sugar peas, raw	½	cup(s)	32	28.0	13	0.9	2.4	0.8	0.1	0	0	0
29324	Split peas, sprouted	½	cup(s)	60	37.4	74	5.3	16.3	—	0.4	0.1	0	0.2
	Peppers												
644	Green bell or sweet, boiled, drained	½	cup(s)	68	62.5	19	0.6	4.6	0.8	0.1	0	0	0.1
643	Green bell or sweet, raw	½	cup(s)	75	69.9	15	0.6	3.5	1.3	0.1	0	0	0
1664	Green hot chili	1	item(s)	45	39.5	18	0.9	4.3	0.7	0.1	0	0	0
1663	Green hot chili, canned with liquid	½	cup(s)	68	62.9	14	0.6	3.5	0.9	0.1	0	0	0
1086	Jalapeno, canned with liquid	½	cup(s)	68	60.4	18	0.6	3.2	1.8	0.6	0.1	0	0.3
8703	Yellow bell or sweet	1	item(s)	186	171.2	50	1.9	11.8	1.7	0.4	0.1	0	0.2
1087	**Poi**	½	cup(s)	120	86.0	134	0.5	32.7	0.5	0.2	0	0	0.1
	Potatoes												
1090	Au gratin mix, prepared with water, whole milk and butter	½	cup(s)	122	96.3	113	2.8	15.7	1.1	5.0	3.2	1.4	0.2
1089	Au gratin, prepared with butter	½	cup(s)	123	90.7	162	6.2	13.8	2.2	9.3	5.8	2.6	0.3
5791	Baked, flesh and skin	1	item(s)	202	151.3	188	5.1	42.7	4.4	0.3	0.1	0	0.1
645	Baked, flesh only	½	cup(s)	61	46.0	57	1.2	13.1	0.9	0.1	0	0	0
1088	Baked, skin only	1	item(s)	58	27.4	115	2.5	26.7	4.6	0.1	0	0	0
5795	Boiled in skin, flesh only, drained	1	item(s)	136	104.7	118	2.5	27.4	2.1	0.1	0	0	0.1
5794	Boiled, drained, skin and flesh	1	item(s)	150	115.9	129	2.9	29.8	2.5	0.2	0	0	0.1
647	Boiled, flesh only	½	cup(s)	78	60.4	67	1.3	15.6	1.4	0.1	0	0	0
648	French fried, deep fried, prepared from raw	14	item(s)	113	47.9	335	4.6	39.5	5.0	18.3	2.4	7.3	7.9
649	French fried, frozen, heated	14	item(s)	70	43.7	115	1.9	19.4	2.0	3.7	0.7	2.3	0.2
1091	Hashed brown	½	cup(s)	78	36.9	207	2.3	27.4	2.5	9.8	1.5	4.1	3.7
652	Mashed with margarine and whole milk	½	cup(s)	105	79.0	119	2.1	17.8	1.6	4.4	1.0	2.0	1.2
653	Mashed, prepared from dehydrated granules with milk, water, and margarine	½	cup(s)	105	79.8	122	2.2	16.9	1.4	5.0	1.2	2.2	1.4
2759	Microwaved	1	item(s)	202	145.5	212	4.9	49.0	4.6	0.2	0.1	0	0.1
2760	Microwaved in skin, flesh only	½	cup(s)	78	57.1	78	1.6	18.1	1.2	0.1	0	0	0
5804	Microwaved, skin only	1	item(s)	58	36.8	77	2.5	17.2	4.2	0.1	0	0	0
1097	Potato puffs, frozen, heated	½	cup(s)	64	38.2	122	1.3	17.8	1.6	5.5	1.2	3.9	0.3
1094	Scalloped mix, prepared with water, whole milk and butter	½	cup(s)	124	98.6	116	2.6	15.9	1.4	5.4	3.3	1.5	0.2
1093	Scalloped, prepared with butter	½	cup(s)	123	99.2	108	3.5	13.2	2.3	4.5	2.8	1.3	0.2
	Pumpkin												
656	Canned	½	cup(s)	123	110.2	42	1.3	9.9	3.6	0.3	0.2	0	0
1773	Boiled, drained	½	cup(s)	123	114.8	25	0.9	6.0	1.3	0.1	0	0	0
	Radicchio												
8731	Leaves, raw	1	cup(s)	40	37.3	9	0.6	1.8	0.4	0.1	0	0	0
2498	Raw	1	cup(s)	40	37.3	9	0.6	1.8	0.4	0.1	0	0	0
657	**Radishes**	6	item(s)	27	25.7	4	0.2	0.9	0.4	0	0	0	0
1099	**Rutabaga, boiled, drained**	½	cup(s)	85	77.9	26	0.8	5.8	1.5	0.2	0	0	0.1
658	**Sauerkraut, canned**	½	cup(s)	118	109.2	22	1.1	5.1	3.4	0.2	0	0	0.1
	Seaweed												
1102	Kelp	½	cup(s)	40	32.6	17	0.7	3.8	0.5	0.2	0.1	0	0
1104	Spirulina, dried	½	cup(s)	56	2.6	162	32.2	13.4	2.0	4.3	1.5	0.4	1.2
1106	**Shallots**	3	tablespoon(s)	30	23.9	22	0.8	5.0	1.0	0	0	0	0

E KEY: H-4 = Breads/Baked Goods H-8 = Cereal/Rice/Pasta H-14 = Fruit H-18 = Vegetables/Legumes H-28 = Nuts/Seeds H-30 = Vegetarian H-32 = Dairy H-40 = Eggs H-40 = Seafood H-42 = Meats H-46 = Poultry
8 = Processed Meats H-50 = Beverages H-52 = Fats/Oils H-54 = Sweets H-56 = Spices/Condiments/Sauces H-60 = Mixed Foods/Soups/Sandwiches H-66 = Fast Food H-84 = Convenience H-86 = Baby Foods

Chol (mg)	Calc (mg)	Iron (mg)	Magn (mg)	Pota (mg)	Sodi (mg)	Zinc (mg)	Vit A (μg)	Thia (mg)	Vit E (mg α)	Ribo (mg)	Niac (mg)	Vit B_6 (mg)	Fola (μg)	Vit C (mg)	Vit B_{12} (μg)	Sele (μg)
0	13	1.23	7.3	1318.4	10.2	2.72	2.2	0.03	0.37	0.13	0.62	0.53	14.6	5.0	0	0.5
0	5	0.24	1.9	21.1	2.1	0.04	16.0	0	0.03	0	0.05	0	5.8	5.1	0	0
0	29	0.45	22.6	286.3	7.8	0.20	0	0.06	0.78	0.04	0.56	0.07	45.2	10.1	0	1.3
0	20	1.03	15.8	92.8	238.9	0.58	37.6	0.09	0.33	0.05	0.86	0.05	27.1	3.7	0	1.5
0	19	1.22	17.6	88.0	57.6	0.54	84.0	0.23	0.02	0.08	1.18	0.09	47.2	7.9	0	0.8
0	34	1.58	20.8	192.0	192.0	0.30	41.6	0.10	0.31	0.06	0.43	0.12	23.2	38.3	0	0.6
0	29	0.96	17.9	127.5	331.5	0.74	368.5	0.09	—	0.07	0.74	0.11	23.0	8.4	0	1.1
0	18	0.75	12.8	126.4	54.4	0.36	380.8	0.18	0.42	0.05	0.92	0.07	20.8	6.5	0	0.9
0	47	1.92	22.4	173.6	4.0	0.39	52.8	0.05	0.38	0.10	0.45	0.14	28.0	17.6	0	0.6
0	14	0.66	7.6	63.0	1.3	0.09	17.0	0.05	0.12	0.03	0.19	0.05	13.2	18.9	0	0.2
0	22	1.36	33.6	228.6	12.0	0.63	4.8	0.14	—	0.09	1.85	0.16	86.4	6.2	0	0.4
0	6	0.31	6.8	112.9	1.4	0.08	15.6	0.04	0.34	0.02	0.32	0.16	10.9	50.6	0	0.2
0	7	0.25	7.4	130.4	2.2	0.10	13.4	0.04	0.28	0.02	0.36	0.17	7.4	59.9	0	0
0	8	0.54	11.3	153.0	3.2	0.14	26.5	0.04	0.31	0.04	0.43	0.13	10.4	109.1	0	0.2
0	5	0.34	9.5	127.2	797.6	0.12	24.5	0.01	0.47	0.03	0.54	0.10	6.8	46.2	0	0.2
0	16	1.28	10.2	131.2	1136.3	0.23	57.8	0.03	0.47	0.03	0.27	0.13	9.5	6.8	0	0.3
0	20	0.86	22.3	394.3	3.7	0.32	18.6	0.05	—	0.05	1.66	0.31	48.4	341.3	0	0.6
0	19	1.06	28.8	219.6	14.4	0.26	3.6	0.16	2.76	0.05	1.32	0.33	25.2	4.8	0	0.8
18	101	0.39	18.3	267.2	535.5	0.29	63.4	0.02	—	0.10	1.15	0.05	8.5	3.8	0	3.3
28	146	0.78	24.5	485.1	530.4	0.85	78.4	0.08	—	0.14	1.22	0.21	15.9	12.1	0	3.3
0	30	2.18	56.6	1080.7	20.2	0.73	2.0	0.13	0.08	0.10	2.85	0.63	56.6	19.4	0	0.8
0	3	0.21	15.3	238.5	3.0	0.18	0	0.06	0.02	0.01	0.85	0.18	5.5	7.8	0	0.2
0	20	4.08	24.9	332.3	12.2	0.28	0.6	0.07	0.02	0.06	1.78	0.36	12.8	7.8	0	0.4
0	7	0.42	29.9	515.4	5.4	0.41	0	0.14	0.01	0.03	1.96	0.41	13.6	17.7	0	0.4
0	13	1.27	34.1	572.0	7.4	0.47	0	0.15	0.01	0.03	2.13	0.44	15.0	18.4	0	—
0	6	0.24	15.6	255.8	3.9	0.21	0	0.08	0.01	0.01	1.02	0.21	7.0	5.8	0	0.2
0	27	1.78	52.2	952.6	276.7	0.66	0	0.15	2.25	0.07	2.27	0.63	27.2	35.6	0	0.7
0	8	0.52	18.2	315.7	271.6	0.27	0	0.09	0.08	0.02	1.55	0.13	19.6	9.3	0	0.1
0	11	0.43	27.3	449.3	266.8	0.37	0	0.13	0.01	0.03	1.80	0.37	12.5	10.1	0	0.4
1	22	0.27	20.0	342.3	349.6	0.31	46.2	0.10	0.44	0.04	1.23	0.26	9.5	11.0	0.1	0.8
2	37	0.21	21.0	162.7	180.6	0.25	53.5	0.09	0.54	0.09	0.90	0.17	8.4	6.8	0.1	5.9
0	22	2.50	54.5	902.9	16.2	0.73	0	0.24	—	0.06	3.46	0.69	24.2	30.5	0	0.8
0	4	0.32	19.4	319.0	5.4	0.26	0	0.10	—	0.02	1.26	0.25	9.3	11.7	0	0.3
0	27	3.45	21.5	377.0	9.3	0.30	0	0.04	0.01	0.04	1.29	0.29	9.9	8.9	0	0.3
0	9	0.41	10.9	199.7	295.7	0.20	0	0.08	0.15	0.02	0.97	0.08	9.0	4.0	0	0.4
14	45	0.47	17.4	252.7	424.5	0.31	43.6	0.02	—	0.07	1.28	0.05	12.4	4.1	0	2.0
15	70	0.70	23.3	463.0	410.4	0.49	—	0.08	—	0.11	1.29	0.22	15.9	13.0	0	2.0
0	32	1.70	28.2	252.4	6.1	0.21	953.0	0.03	1.30	0.07	0.45	0.07	14.7	5.1	0	0.5
0	18	0.70	11.0	281.8	1.2	0.28	352.8	0.04	0.98	0.10	0.51	0.05	11.0	5.8	0	0.2
0	8	0.23	5.2	120.8	8.8	0.25	0.4	0.01	0.90	0.01	0.10	0.02	24.0	3.2	0	0.4
0	8	0.23	5.2	120.8	8.8	0.25	0.4	0.01	0.90	0.01	0.10	0.02	24.0	3.2	0	0.4
0	7	0.09	2.7	62.9	10.5	0.08	0	0	0.00	0.01	0.07	0.02	6.8	4.0	0	0.2
0	15	0.15	8.5	183.7	4.3	0.10	0	0.07	0.20	0.03	0.61	0.09	12.8	16.0	0	0.6
0	35	1.73	15.3	200.6	780.0	0.22	1.2	0.02	0.17	0.03	0.17	0.15	28.3	17.3	0	0.7
0	67	1.14	48.4	35.6	93.2	0.49	2.4	0.02	0.35	0.06	0.19	0	72.0	1.2	0	0.3
0	67	15.96	109.2	763.3	586.9	1.12	16.2	1.33	2.80	2.06	7.18	0.20	52.6	5.7	0	4.0
0	11	0.36	6.3	100.2	3.6	0.12	0	0.02	0.01	0.01	0.06	0.10	10.2	2.4	0	0.4

TABLE H-1 Table of Food Composition (*continued*) (Computer code is for Cengage Diet Analysis program) (For purposes of calculations, use "0" for t, <1, <0.1, 0.01)

DA+ Code	Food Description	Quantity	Measure	Wt (g)	H_2O (g)	Ener (kcal)	Prot (g)	Carb (g)	Fiber (g)	Fat (g)	Fat Breakdown (g)		
											Sat	Mono	Poly
Vegetables, Legumes—*continued*													
	Soybeans												
1670	Boiled	½	cup(s)	86	53.8	149	14.3	8.5	5.2	7.7	1.1	1.7	4.4
2825	Dry roasted	½	cup(s)	86	0.7	388	34.0	28.1	7.0	18.6	2.7	4.1	10.5
2824	Roasted, salted	½	cup(s)	86	1.7	405	30.3	28.9	15.2	21.8	3.2	4.8	12.3
8739	Sprouted, stir fried	½	cup(s)	62	41.7	77	8.1	5.8	0.5	4.4	0.6	1.0	2.5
	Soy products												
1813	Soy milk	1	cup(s)	240	211.3	130	7.8	15.1	1.4	4.2	0.5	1.0	2.3
2838	Tofu, dried, frozen (koyadofu)	3	ounce(s)	85	4.9	408	40.8	12.4	6.1	25.8	3.7	5.7	14.6
13844	Tofu, extra firm	3	ounce(s)	85	68.8	86	8.6	2.2	1.1	4.3	0.5	1.1	2.7
13843	Tofu, firm	3	ounce(s)	85	70.9	75	7.5	2.2	0.5	3.2	0	1.1	2.2
1816	Tofu, firm, with calcium sulfate and magnesium chloride (nigari)	3	ounce(s)	85	72.2	60	7.0	1.4	0.8	3.5	0.7	1.0	1.5
1817	Tofu, fried	3	ounce(s)	85	43.0	230	14.6	8.9	3.3	17.2	2.5	3.8	9.7
13841	Tofu, silken	3	ounce(s)	85	77.0	42	3.7	0.9	0	1.9	0	0.5	0.9
13842	Tofu, soft	3	ounce(s)	85	73.0	65	6.5	1.1	0.5	3.2	0	0.5	2.2
1671	Tofu, soft, with calcium sulfate and magnesium chloride (nigari)	3	ounce(s)	85	74.2	52	5.6	1.5	0.2	3.1	0.5	0.7	1.8
	Spinach												
663	Canned, drained	½	cup(s)	107	98.2	25	3.0	3.6	2.6	0.5	0.1	0	0.2
660	Chopped, boiled, drained	½	cup(s)	90	82.1	21	2.7	3.4	2.2	0.2	0	0	0.1
661	Chopped, frozen, boiled, drained	½	cup(s)	95	84.5	32	3.8	4.6	3.5	0.8	0.1	0	0.4
662	Leaf, frozen, boiled, drained	½	cup(s)	95	84.5	32	3.8	4.6	3.5	0.8	0.1	0	0.4
659	Raw, chopped	1	cup(s)	30	27.4	7	0.9	1.1	0.7	0.1	0	0	0
	Squash												
1662	Acorn winter, baked	½	cup(s)	102	87.0	58	1.2	15.3	4.6	0.1	0	0	0.1
29702	Acorn winter, boiled, mashed	½	cup(s)	170	152.5	58	1.1	14.9	4.4	0.1	0	0	0.1
1661	Butternut winter, baked	½	cup(s)	103	90.0	41	0.9	10.8	3.3	0.1	0	0	0
32773	Butternut winter, frozen, boiled, mashed, no salt added	½	cup(s)	121	106.4	47	1.5	12.2	—	0.1	0	0	0
29451	Butternut, frozen, boiled	½	cup(s)	120	105.4	47	1.5	12.1	1.8	0.1	0	0	0
29700	Crookneck and straightneck summer, boiled, drained	½	cup(s)	65	61.0	12	0.7	2.5	0.6	0.2	0.1	0	0.1
29703	Hubbard winter, baked	½	cup(s)	102	86.8	51	2.5	11.0	5.0	0.6	0.1	0	0.3
1660	Hubbard winter, boiled, mashed	½	cup(s)	118	107.5	35	1.7	7.6	3.4	0.4	0.1	0	0.2
29704	Spaghetti winter, boiled, drained, or baked	½	cup(s)	78	71.5	21	0.5	5.0	1.1	0.2	0	0	0.1
664	Summer, all varieties, sliced, boiled, drained	½	cup(s)	90	84.3	18	0.8	3.9	1.3	0.3	0.1	0	0.1
665	Winter, all varieties, baked, mashed	½	cup(s)	103	91.4	38	0.9	9.1	2.9	0.4	0.1	0	0.2
1112	Zucchini summer, boiled, drained	½	cup(s)	90	85.7	14	1.0	2.4	0.9	0.3	0.1	0	0.1
1113	Zucchini summer, frozen, boiled, drained	½	cup(s)	112	105.6	19	1.3	4.0	1.4	0.1	0	0	0.1
	Sweet potatoes												
666	Baked, peeled	½	cup(s)	100	75.8	90	2.0	20.7	3.3	0.2	0	0	0.1
667	Boiled, mashed	½	cup(s)	164	131.4	125	2.2	29.1	4.1	0.2	0.1	0	0.1
668	Candied, home recipe	½	cup(s)	91	57.3	150	0.8	29.3	1.9	3.2	2.0	0.8	0.2
670	Canned, vacuum pack	½	cup(s)	100	76.0	91	1.6	21.1	1.8	0.2	0	0	0.1
2765	Frozen, baked	½	cup(s)	88	64.5	88	1.5	20.5	1.6	0.1	0	0	0
1136	Yams, baked or boiled, drained	½	cup(s)	68	47.7	79	1.0	18.7	2.7	0.1	0	0	0
32785	**Taro shoots, cooked, no salt added**	½	cup(s)	70	66.7	10	0.5	2.2	—	0.1	0	0	0
	Tomatillo												
8774	Raw	2	item(s)	68	62.3	22	0.7	4.0	1.3	0.7	0.1	0.1	0.3
8777	Raw, chopped	½	cup(s)	66	60.5	21	0.6	3.9	1.3	0.7	0.1	0.1	0.3
	Tomato												
16846	Cherry, fresh	5	item(s)	85	80.4	15	0.7	3.3	1.0	0.2	0	0	0.1
671	Fresh, ripe, red	1	item(s)	123	116.3	22	1.1	4.8	1.5	0.2	0	0	0.1
675	Juice, canned	½	cup(s)	122	114.1	21	0.9	5.2	0.5	0.1	0	0	0
75	Juice, no salt added	½	cup(s)	122	114.1	21	0.9	5.2	0.5	0.1	0	0	0
1699	Paste, canned	2	tablespoon(s)	33	24.1	27	1.4	6.2	1.3	0.2	0	0	0.1
1123	Paste, canned, no salt added	2	tablespoon(s)	32	23.5	26	1.4	6.1	1.3	0.2	0	0	0.1
1700	Puree, canned	¼	cup(s)	63	54.9	24	1.0	5.6	1.2	0.1	0	0	0.1
1124	Puree, canned, no salt added	¼	cup(s)	63	54.9	24	1.0	5.6	1.2	0.1	0	0	0.1
1118	Red, boiled	½	cup(s)	120	113.2	22	1.1	4.8	0.8	0.1	0	0	0.1

GE KEY: H-4 = Breads/Baked Goods H-8 = Cereal/Rice/Pasta H-14 = Fruit H-18 = Vegetables/Legumes H-28 = Nuts/Seeds H-30 = Vegetarian H-32 = Dairy H-40 = Eggs H-40 = Seafood H-42 = Meats H-46 = Poultry
48 = Processed Meats H-50 = Beverages H-52 = Fats/Oils H-54 = Sweets H-56 = Spices/Condiments/Sauces H-60 = Mixed Foods/Soups/Sandwiches H-66 = Fast Food H-84 = Convenience H-86 = Baby Foods

Chol (mg)	Calc (mg)	Iron (mg)	Magn (mg)	Pota (mg)	Sodi (mg)	Zinc (mg)	Vit A (µg)	Thia (mg)	Vit E (mg α)	Ribo (mg)	Niac (mg)	Vit B_6 (mg)	Fola (µg)	Vit C (mg)	Vit B_{12} (µg)	Sele (µg)
0	88	4.42	74.0	442.9	0.9	0.99	0	0.13	0.30	0.25	0.34	0.20	46.4	1.5	0	6.3
0	120	3.40	196.1	1173.0	1.7	4.10	0	0.37	—	0.65	0.91	0.19	176.3	4.0	0	16.6
0	119	3.35	124.7	1264.2	140.2	2.70	8.6	0.09	0.78	0.12	1.21	0.18	181.5	1.9	0	16.4
0	51	0.25	59.5	351.5	8.7	1.30	0.6	0.26	—	0.12	0.68	0.10	78.7	7.4	0	0.4
0	60	1.54	60.0	283.2	122.4	0.29	0	0.14	0.26	0.17	1.23	0.18	43.2	0	0	11.5
0	310	8.27	50.2	17.0	5.1	4.17	22.1	0.42	—	0.27	1.01	0.24	78.2	0.6	0	46.2
0	65	1.55	—	—	0	—	0	—	—	—	—	—	—	0	—	—
0	108	1.16	—	—	0	—	0	—	—	—	—	—	—	0	—	—
0	171	1.37	31.5	125.9	10.2	0.71	0	0.05	0.01	0.05	0.09	0.06	16.2	0.2	0	8.4
0	316	4.14	51.0	124.2	13.6	1.69	0.9	0.14	0.03	0.04	0.09	0.08	23.0	0	0	24.2
0	56	0.67	—	—	0	—	0	—	—	—	—	—	—	0	—	—
0	108	1.16	—	—	0	—	0	—	—	—	—	—	—	0	—	—
0	94	0.94	23.0	102.0	6.8	0.54	0	0.04	0.01	0.03	0.45	0.04	37.4	0.2	0	7.6
0	136	2.46	81.3	370.2	344.5	0.49	524.3	0.02	2.08	0.15	0.42	0.11	104.9	15.3	0	1.5
0	122	3.21	78.3	419.4	63.0	0.68	471.6	0.09	1.87	0.21	0.44	0.22	131.4	8.8	0	1.4
0	145	1.86	77.9	286.9	92.2	0.47	572.8	0.07	3.36	0.17	0.42	0.13	114.9	2.1	0	5.2
0	145	1.86	77.9	286.9	92.2	0.47	572.8	0.07	3.36	0.17	0.42	0.13	114.9	2.1	0	5.2
0	30	0.81	23.7	167.4	23.7	0.16	140.7	0.02	0.61	0.06	0.22	0.06	58.2	8.4	0	0.3
0	46	0.98	45.2	459.0	4.2	0.18	22.1	0.18	—	0.01	0.93	0.20	20.0	11.4	0	0.7
0	44	0.95	44.2	447.1	5.1	0.19	69.7	0.17	—	0.01	0.90	0.20	18.7	11.1	0	0.7
0	42	0.62	29.7	291.1	4.1	0.13	572.0	0.07	1.32	0.02	0.99	0.13	19.5	15.5	0	0.5
0	23	0.70	10.9	161.2	2.4	0.15	202.4	0.06	—	0.05	0.56	0.08	19.4	4.2	0	0.6
0	23	0.70	10.8	159.6	2.4	0.14	200.4	0.06	0.14	0.05	0.56	0.08	19.2	4.2	0	0.6
0	14	0.28	12.9	143.6	1.3	0.19	5.2	0.03	0.08	0.03	0.29	0.07	12.3	12.5	0	0.1
0	17	0.48	22.4	365.1	8.2	0.15	341.7	0.08	0.20	0.05	0.57	0.18	16.3	9.7	0	0.6
0	12	0.33	15.3	252.5	5.9	0.12	236.0	0.05	0.14	0.03	0.39	0.12	11.8	7.7	0	0.4
0	16	0.26	8.5	90.7	13.9	0.16	4.7	0.03	0.09	0.02	0.63	0.08	6.2	2.7	0	0.2
0	24	0.32	21.6	172.8	0.9	0.35	9.9	0.04	0.13	0.04	0.46	0.06	18.0	4.9	0	0.2
0	23	0.45	13.3	247.0	1.0	0.23	267.5	0.02	0.12	0.07	0.51	0.17	20.5	9.8	0	0.4
0	16	0.33	17.1	237.6	2.7	0.30	50.4	0.03	0.11	0.02	0.46	0.07	25.2	11.6	0	0.2
0	19	0.54	14.5	216.3	2.2	0.22	10.0	0.05	0.13	0.04	0.43	0.05	8.9	4.1	0	0.2
0	38	0.69	27.0	475.0	36.0	0.32	961.0	0.11	0.71	0.11	1.49	0.29	6.0	19.6	0	0.2
0	44	1.18	29.5	377.2	44.3	0.33	1290.7	0.09	1.54	0.08	0.88	0.27	9.8	21.0	0	0.3
8	24	0.72	11.9	162.6	108.7	0.15	318.7	0.02	0.82	0.04	0.37	0.05	5.5	8.2	0	0.7
0	22	0.89	22.0	312.0	53.0	0.18	399.0	0.04	1.00	0.06	0.74	0.19	17.0	26.4	0	0.7
0	31	0.47	18.4	330.1	7.0	0.26	913.3	0.06	0.67	0.05	0.49	0.16	19.3	8.0	0	0.5
0	10	0.35	12.2	455.6	5.4	0.14	4.1	0.06	0.23	0.02	0.38	0.16	10.9	8.2	0	0.5
0	10	0.29	5.6	240.8	1.4	0.38	2.1	0.03	—	0.04	0.57	0.08	2.1	13.2	0	0.7
0	5	0.42	13.6	182.2	0.7	0.15	4.1	0.03	0.26	0.02	1.26	0.04	4.8	8.0	0	0.3
0	5	0.41	13.2	176.9	0.7	0.15	4.0	0.03	0.25	0.02	1.22	0.04	4.6	7.7	0	0.3
0	9	0.23	9.4	201.6	4.3	0.15	35.7	0.03	0.46	0.02	0.51	0.07	12.8	11.7	0	0
0	12	0.33	13.5	291.5	6.2	0.21	51.7	0.05	0.66	0.02	0.73	0.10	18.5	16.9	0	0
0	12	0.52	13.4	278.2	326.8	0.18	27.9	0.06	0.39	0.04	0.82	0.13	24.3	22.2	0	0.4
0	12	0.52	13.4	278.2	12.1	0.18	27.9	0.06	0.39	0.04	0.82	0.13	24.3	22.2	0	0.4
0	12	0.98	13.8	332.6	259.1	0.21	24.9	0.02	1.41	0.05	1.01	0.07	3.9	7.2	0	1.7
0	12	0.95	13.4	324.5	18.9	0.20	24.3	0.02	1.38	0.05	0.98	0.07	3.8	7.0	0	1.7
0	11	1.11	14.4	274.4	249.4	0.22	16.3	0.02	1.23	0.05	0.92	0.08	6.9	6.6	0	0.4
0	11	1.11	14.4	274.4	17.5	0.22	16.3	0.02	1.23	0.05	0.92	0.08	6.9	6.6	0	0.4
0	13	0.82	10.8	261.6	13.2	0.17	28.8	0.04	0.67	0.03	0.64	0.09	15.6	27.4	0	0.6

APPENDIX H

(Computer code is for Cengage Diet Analysis program) (For purposes of calculations, use "0" for t, <1, <0.1, 0.01)

DA+ Code	Food Description	Quantity	Measure	Wt (g)	H_2O (g)	Ener (kcal)	Prot (g)	Carb (g)	Fiber (g)	Fat (g)	Fat Breakdown (g)		
											Sat	Mono	Poly
	Vegetables, Legumes—*continued*												
3952	Red, diced	½	cup(s)	90	85.1	16	0.8	3.5	1.1	0.2	0	0	0.1
1120	Red, stewed, canned	½	cup(s)	128	116.7	33	1.2	7.9	1.3	0.2	0	0	0.1
1125	Sauce, canned	¼	cup(s)	61	55.6	15	0.8	3.3	0.9	0.1	0	0	0
8778	Sun dried	½	cup(s)	27	3.9	70	3.8	15.1	3.3	0.8	0.1	0.1	0.3
8783	Sun dried in oil, drained	¼	cup(s)	28	14.8	59	1.4	6.4	1.6	3.9	0.5	2.4	0.6
	Turnips												
678	Turnip greens, chopped, boiled, drained	½	cup(s)	72	67.1	14	0.8	3.1	2.5	0.2	0	0	0.1
679	Turnip greens, frozen, chopped, boiled, drained	½	cup(s)	82	74.1	24	2.7	4.1	2.8	0.3	0.1	0	0.1
677	Turnips, cubed, boiled, drained	½	cup(s)	78	73.0	17	0.6	3.9	1.6	0.1	0	0	0
	Vegetables, mixed												
1132	Mixed vegetables, canned, drained	½	cup(s)	82	70.9	40	2.1	7.5	2.4	0.2	0	0	0.1
680	Mixed vegetables, frozen, boiled, drained	½	cup(s)	91	75.7	59	2.6	11.9	4.0	0.1	0	0	0.1
7489	V8 100% vegetable juice	½	cup(s)	122	114.1	25	1.0	5.0	1.0	0	0	0	0
7490	V8 low-sodium vegetable juice	½	cup(s)	122	114.1	25	1.0	5.0	1.0	0	0	0	0
7491	V8 Spicy Hot vegetable juice	½	cup(s)	122	114.2	25	1.0	5.0	1.0	0	0	0	0
	Water chestnuts												
31073	Sliced, drained	½	cup(s)	75	—	20	0	5.0	1.0	0	0	0	0
31087	Whole	½	cup(s)	75	—	20	0	5.0	1.0	0	0	0	0
1135	Watercress	1	cup(s)	34	32.3	4	0.8	0.4	0.2	0	0	0	0
	Nuts, Seeds, and Products												
	Almonds												
32940	Almond butter with salt added	1	tablespoon(s)	16	0.3	98	3.4	3.0	1.6	8.9	1.0	5.2	2.2
1137	Almond butter, no salt added	1	tablespoon(s)	16	0.3	98	3.4	3.0	1.6	8.9	0.7	5.2	2.2
32886	Blanched	¼	cup(s)	36	1.6	214	7.8	6.8	3.6	19.0	1.4	12.1	4.5
32887	Dry roasted, no salt added	¼	cup(s)	35	0.9	205	7.3	7.3	3.8	18.0	1.4	11.2	4.5
29724	Dry roasted, salted	¼	cup(s)	35	0.9	205	7.3	7.3	3.8	18.0	1.4	11.2	4.5
29725	Oil roasted, salted	¼	cup(s)	39	1.1	238	8.3	6.9	4.1	21.7	1.7	13.7	5.3
508	Slivered	¼	cup(s)	27	1.3	155	5.7	5.9	3.3	13.3	1.0	8.3	3.3
1138	**Beechnuts, dried**	¼	cup(s)	57	3.8	328	3.5	19.1	5.3	28.5	3.3	12.5	11.5
517	**Brazil nuts, dried, unblanched**	¼	cup(s)	33	1.2	218	4.8	4.1	2.5	22.1	5.0	8.2	6.8
1166	**Breadfruit seeds, roasted**	¼	cup(s)	57	28.3	118	3.5	22.9	3.4	1.5	0.4	0.2	0.8
1139	**Butternuts, dried**	¼	cup(s)	30	1.0	184	7.5	3.6	1.4	17.1	0.4	3.1	12.8
	Cashews												
32931	Cashew butter with salt added	1	tablespoon(s)	16	0.5	94	2.8	4.4	0.3	7.9	1.6	4.7	1.3
32889	Cashew butter, no salt added	1	tablespoon(s)	16	0.5	94	2.8	4.4	0.3	7.9	1.6	4.7	1.3
1140	Dry roasted	¼	cup(s)	34	0.6	197	5.2	11.2	1.0	15.9	3.1	9.4	2.7
518	Oil roasted	¼	cup(s)	32	1.1	187	5.4	9.6	1.1	15.4	2.7	8.4	2.8
	Coconut												
32896	Dried, not sweetened	¼	cup(s)	23	0.7	150	1.6	5.4	3.7	14.6	13.0	0.6	0.2
1153	Dried, shredded, sweetened	¼	cup(s)	23	2.9	116	0.7	11.1	1.0	8.3	7.3	0.4	0.1
520	Shredded	¼	cup(s)	20	9.4	71	0.7	3.0	1.8	6.7	5.9	0.3	0.1
	Chestnuts												
1152	Chinese, roasted	¼	cup(s)	71	28.7	171	3.2	37.4	—	0.9	0.1	0.4	0.2
32895	European, boiled and steamed	¼	cup(s)	45	30.9	59	0.9	12.6		0.6	0.1	0.2	0.2
32911	European, roasted	¼	cup(s)	36	14.5	88	1.1	18.9	1.8	0.8	0.1	0.3	0.3
32922	Japanese, boiled and steamed	¼	cup(s)	35	30.5	20	0.3	4.5	—	0.1	0	0	0
32923	Japanese, roasted	¼	cup(s)	36	17.8	72	1.1	16.1	—	0.3	0	0.1	0.1
4958	**Flax seeds or linseeds**	¼	cup(s)	28	2.2	150	5.5	8.1	7.8	11.6	1.0	2.1	8.0
32904	**Ginkgo nuts, dried**	¼	cup(s)	39	4.8	134	4.0	27.9	—	0.8	0.1	0.3	0.3
	Hazelnuts or filberts												
32901	Blanched	¼	cup(s)	45	2.6	285	6.2	7.7	5.0	27.7	2.1	21.9	2.5
32902	Dry roasted, no salt added	¼	cup(s)	29	0.7	185	4.3	5.0	2.7	17.8	1.3	13.3	2.4
1156	**Hickorynuts, dried**	¼	cup(s)	30	0.8	197	3.8	5.5	1.9	19.3	2.1	9.8	6.6
	Macadamias												
32905	Dry roasted, no salt added	¼	cup(s)	34	0.5	241	2.6	4.5	2.7	25.5	4.0	19.9	0.5
32932	Dry roasted, with salt added	¼	cup(s)	34	0.5	240	2.6	4.3	2.7	25.5	4.0	19.9	0.5
1157	Raw	¼	cup(s)	34	0.5	241	2.6	4.6	2.9	25.4	4.0	19.7	0.5
	Mixed nuts												
1159	With peanuts, dry roasted	¼	cup(s)	34	0.6	203	5.9	8.7	3.1	17.6	2.4	10.8	3.7
32933	With peanuts, dry roasted, with salt added	¼	cup(s)	34	0.6	203	5.9	8.7	3.1	17.6	2.2	10.8	3.7

KEY: H-4 = Breads/Baked Goods H-8 = Cereal/Rice/Pasta H-14 = Fruit H-18 = Vegetables/Legumes H-28 = Nuts/Seeds H-30 = Vegetarian H-32 = Dairy H-40 = Eggs H-40 = Seafood H-42 = Meats H-46 = Poultry H-48 = Processed Meats H-50 = Beverages H-52 = Fats/Oils H-54 = Sweets H-56 = Spices/Condiments/Sauces H-60 = Mixed Foods/Soups/Sandwiches H-66 = Fast Food H-84 = Convenience H-86 = Baby Foods

Chol (mg)	Calc (mg)	Iron (mg)	Magn (mg)	Pota (mg)	Sodi (mg)	Zinc (mg)	Vit A (µg)	Thia (mg)	Vit E (mg α)	Ribo (mg)	Niac (mg)	Vit B_6 (mg)	Fola (µg)	Vit C (mg)	Vit B_{12} (µg)	Sele (µg)
0	9	0.24	9.9	213.3	4.5	0.15	37.8	0.03	0.49	0.02	0.53	0.07	13.5	12.3	0	0
0	43	1.70	15.3	263.9	281.8	0.22	11.5	0.06	1.06	0.04	0.91	0.02	6.4	10.1	0	0.8
0	8	0.62	9.8	201.9	319.6	0.12	13.4	0.01	0.87	0.04	0.59	0.06	6.7	4.3	0	0.1
0	30	2.45	52.4	925.3	66.7	0.54	11.9	0.14	0	0.13	2.44	0.09	18.4	10.6	0	1.5
0	13	0.74	22.3	430.4	73.2	0.21	17.6	0.05	—	0.11	1.00	0.09	6.3	28.0	0	0.8
0	99	0.58	15.8	146.2	20.9	0.10	274.3	0.03	1.35	0.05	0.30	0.13	85.0	19.7	0	0.6
0	125	1.59	21.3	183.7	12.3	0.34	441.2	0.04	2.18	0.06	0.38	0.05	32.0	17.9	0	1.0
0	26	0.14	7.0	138.1	12.5	0.09	0	0.02	0.02	0.02	0.23	0.05	7.0	9.0	0	0.2
0	22	0.86	13.0	237.2	121.4	0.33	475.1	0.04	0.24	0.04	0.47	0.06	19.6	4.1	0	0.2
0	23	0.75	20.0	153.8	31.9	0.45	194.7	0.06	0.35	0.11	0.77	0.07	17.3	2.9	0	0.3
0	20	0.36	—	235.0	210.0	—	50.0	0	0	0	0	0	—	36.0	0	—
0	10	0.18	—	450.0	70.0	—	50.0	0	—	0	0	0	—	36.0	0	—
0	20	0.54	—	325.0	240.0	—	31.3	—	—	—	—	—	—	36.0	0	—
0	0	0	—	—	5.0	—	0	—	—	—	—	—	—	2.4	—	—
0	7	0	—	—	5.0	—	0	—	—	—	—	—	—	2.0	—	—
0	41	0.07	7.1	112.2	13.9	0.04	54.4	0.03	0.34	0.04	0.07	0.04	3.1	14.6	0	0.3
0	56	0.56	44.6	119.7	36.3	0.53	0	0.01	3.87	0.15	0.50	0.02	8.5	0	0	0.4
0	56	0.56	44.6	119.7	1.1	0.53	0	0.01	3.87	0.15	0.50	0.02	8.5	0	0	0.4
0	86	1.19	97.2	238.9	6.9	1.08	0	0.07	8.61	0.26	1.27	0.04	17.8	0	0	1.2
0	92	1.32	96.9	245.6	1.0	1.14	0	0.03	8.21	0.33	1.23	0.04	18.3	0	0	0.8
0	92	1.32	96.9	245.6	226.3	1.14	0	0.03	8.21	0.33	1.23	0.04	18.3	0	0	0.8
0	114	1.44	107.5	274.4	133.1	1.20	0	0.04	10.19	0.31	1.44	0.05	10.6	0	0	1.1
0	71	1.00	72.4	190.4	0.3	0.83	0	0.06	7.08	0.27	0.91	0.04	13.5	0	0	0.7
0	1	1.40	0	579.7	21.7	0.21	0	0.17	—	0.21	0.50	0.39	64.4	8.8	0	4.0
0	53	0.81	125.0	219.1	1.0	1.35	0	0.21	1.91	0.01	0.10	0.03	7.3	0.2	0	637.4
0	49	0.51	35.3	616.7	16.0	0.59	8.6	0.23	—	0.14	4.22	0.24	33.6	4.3	0	8.0
0	16	1.21	71.1	126.3	0.3	0.94	1.8	0.11	—	0.04	0.31	0.17	19.8	1.0	0	5.2
0	7	0.80	41.3	87.4	65.0	0.83	0	0.05	0.15	0.03	0.26	0.04	10.9	0	0	1.8
0	7	0.80	41.3	87.4	2.4	0.83	0	0.05	—	0.03	0.26	0.04	10.9	0	0	1.8
0	15	2.06	89.1	193.5	5.5	1.92	0	0.07	0.32	0.07	0.48	0.09	23.6	0	0	4.0
0	14	1.95	88.0	203.8	4.2	1.73	0	0.12	0.30	0.07	0.56	0.10	8.1	0.1	0	6.5
0	6	0.75	20.4	123.2	8.4	0.46	0	0.01	0.10	0.02	0.14	0.07	2.0	0.3	0	4.2
0	3	0.45	11.6	78.4	60.9	0.42	0	0.01	0.09	0	0.11	0.06	1.9	0.2	0	3.9
0	3	0.49	6.4	71.2	4.0	0.22	0	0.01	0.05	0	0.11	0.01	5.2	0.7	0	2.0
0	14	1.07	64.3	341.0	2.9	0.66	0	0.11	—	0.06	1.07	0.31	51.5	27.5	0	5.0
0	21	0.78	24.5	324.3	12.2	0.11	0.5	0.07	—	0.05	0.33	0.11	17.2	12.1	0	—
0	10	0.33	11.8	211.6	0.7	0.20	0.4	0.09	0.18	0.06	0.48	0.18	25.0	9.3	0	0.4
0	4	0.19	6.4	42.2	1.8	0.14	0.4	0.04	—	0.02	0.19	0.04	6.0	3.4	0	—
0	13	0.75	22.9	152.7	6.8	0.51	1.4	0.16	—		0.25	0.15	21.1	10.0	0	—
0	94	1.40	102.6	232.7	7.8	1.20	0	0.46	0.09	0.05	0.86	0.13	24.4	0.2	0	7.1
0	8	0.62	20.4	384.7	5.0	0.26	21.2	0.17	—	0.07	4.52	0.25	40.9	11.3	0	—
0	68	1.50	72.6	298.4	0	1.00	0.9	0.22	7.94	0.05	0.70	0.27	35.4	0.9	0	1.9
0	35	1.25	49.4	215.8	0	0.71	0.9	0.10	4.37	0.04	0.59	0.18	25.2	1.1	0	1.2
0	18	0.64	51.9	130.8	0.3	1.29	2.1	0.26	—	0.04	0.27	0.06	12.0	0.6	0	2.4
0	23	0.89	39.5	121.6	1.3	0.43	0	0.24	0.19	0.03	0.76	0.12	3.3	0.2	0	3.9
0	23	0.89	39.5	121.6	118.3	0.43	0	0.24	0.19	0.03	0.76	0.12	3.3	0.2	0	3.9
0	28	1.24	43.5	123.3	1.7	0.44	0	0.40	0.18	0.05	0.83	0.09	3.7	0.4	0	1.2
0	24	1.27	77.1	204.5	4.1	1.30	0.3	0.07	—	0.07	1.61	0.10	17.1	0.1	0	1.0
0	24	1.27	77.1	237.4	118.2	1.30	0	0.07	3.75	0.07	1.61	0.10	17.1	0.1	0	2.6

DA+ Code	Food Description	Quantity	Measure	Wt (g)	H_2O (g)	Ener (kcal)	Prot (g)	Carb (g)	Fiber (g)	Fat (g)	Fat Breakdown (g) Sat	Mono	Poly
	Nuts, Seeds, and Products—*continued*												
32906	Without peanuts, oil roasted, no salt added	¼	cup(s)	36	1.1	221	5.6	8.0	2.0	20.2	3.3	11.9	4.1
	Peanuts												
2807	Dry roasted	¼	cup(s)	37	0.6	214	8.6	7.9	2.9	18.1	2.5	9.0	5.7
2806	Dry roasted, salted	¼	cup(s)	37	0.6	214	8.6	7.9	2.9	18.1	2.5	9.0	5.7
1763	Oil roasted, salted	¼	cup(s)	36	0.5	216	10.1	5.5	3.4	18.9	3.1	9.4	5.5
1884	Peanut butter, chunky	1	tablespoon(s)	16	0.2	94	3.8	3.5	1.3	8.0	1.2	3.7	2.2
30303	Peanut butter, low sodium	1	tablespoon(s)	16	0.3	94	4.0	3.1	1.0	8.1	1.6	3.8	2.2
30421	Peanut butter, natural	1	tablespoon(s)	16	—	100	3.5	3.0	1.0	8.0	1.3	4.0	2.3
30422	Peanut butter, natural, no salt added	1	tablespoon(s)	16	—	105	3.5	3.0	1.0	8.0	1.3	—	—
30305	Peanut butter, reduced fat	1	tablespoon(s)	18	0.2	94	4.7	6.4	0.9	6.1	1.0	2.9	1.7
524	Peanut butter, smooth	1	tablespoon(s)	16	0.3	94	4.0	3.1	1.0	8.1	1.7	3.9	2.3
2804	Raw	¼	cup(s)	37	2.4	207	9.4	5.9	3.1	18.0	2.5	8.9	5.7
	Pecans												
32907	Dry roasted, no salt added	¼	cup(s)	28	0.3	195	2.6	3.7	2.6	20.4	1.7	12.1	5.7
32936	Dry roasted, with salt added	¼	cup(s)	28	0.3	195	2.6	3.7	2.6	20.4	1.7	12.1	5.7
1162	Oil roasted	¼	cup(s)	28	0.3	197	2.5	3.6	2.6	20.7	2.0	11.3	6.5
526	Raw	¼	cup(s)	27	1.0	188	2.5	3.8	2.6	19.6	1.7	11.1	5.9
12973	**Pine nuts or pignolia, dried**	1	tablespoon(s)	9	0.2	58	1.2	1.1	0.3	5.9	0.4	1.6	2.9
	Pistachios												
1164	Dry roasted	¼	cup(s)	31	0.6	174	6.4	9.0	3.0	13.8	1.7	7.3	4.1
32938	Dry roasted, with salt added	¼	cup(s)	32	0.6	180	6.7	9.2	3.2	14.3	1.7	7.6	4.3
1167	**Pumpkin or squash seeds, roasted**	¼	cup(s)	57	1.2	326	16.9	8.3	3.7	27.8	4.8	8.9	11.3
	Sesame												
32912	Sesame butter paste	1	tablespoon(s)	16	0.3	94	2.9	3.8	0.9	8.1	1.1	3.1	3.6
32941	Tahini or sesame butter	1	tablespoon(s)	15	0.4	89	2.6	3.2	0.7	8.0	1.1	3.0	3.5
1169	Whole, roasted, toasted	3	tablespoon(s)	27	0.9	153	4.6	6.9	3.8	13.0	1.8	4.9	5.7
	Soy nuts												
34173	Deep sea salted	¼	cup(s)	28	—	130	11.0	9.0	6.0	6.0	1.0	1.0	3.5
34174	Unsalted	¼	cup(s)	28	—	130	11.0	9.0	6.0	6.0	1.0	1.0	3.5
	Sunflower seeds												
528	Kernels, dried	1	tablespoon(s)	9	0.4	53	1.9	1.8	0.8	4.6	0.4	1.7	2.1
29721	Kernels, dry roasted, salted	1	tablespoon(s)	8	0.1	47	1.5	1.9	0.7	4.0	0.4	0.8	2.6
29723	Kernels, toasted, salted	1	tablespoon(s)	8	0.1	52	1.4	1.7	1.0	4.8	0.5	0.9	3.1
32928	Sunflower seed butter with salt added	1	tablespoon(s)	16	0.1	99	2.8	3.7	0.9	8.8	0.7	6.2	1.6
	Trail mix												
4646	Trail mix	¼	cup(s)	38	3.5	173	5.2	16.8	2.0	11.0	2.1	4.7	3.6
4647	Trail mix with chocolate chips	¼	cup(s)	38	2.5	182	5.3	16.8	—	12.0	2.3	5.1	4.2
4648	Tropical trail mix	¼	cup(s)	35	3.2	155	2.2	23.0	—	6.0	3.0	0.9	1.8
	Walnuts												
529	Dried black, chopped	¼	cup(s)	31	1.4	193	7.5	3.1	2.1	18.4	1.1	4.7	11.0
531	English or Persian	¼	cup(s)	29	1.2	191	4.5	4.0	2.0	19.1	1.8	2.6	13.8
	Vegetarian Foods												
	Prepared												
34222	Brown rice & tofu stir-fry (vegan)	8	ounce(s)	227	183.7	227	12.3	12.6	2.8	16.3	1.3	4.0	9.5
34368	Cheese enchilada casserole (lacto)	8	ounce(s)	227	88.3	400	17.6	37.3	3.8	19.5	10.3	6.6	1.5
34247	Five bean casserole (vegan)	8	ounce(s)	227	164.0	224	4.8	40.3	4.6	5.0	0.9	2.3	1.6
34261	Lentil stew (vegan)	8	ounce(s)	227	150.6	127	7.3	24.2	7.3	0.5	0.1	0.1	0.2
34397	Macaroni and cheese (lacto)	8	ounce(s)	227	163.3	182	8.2	17.3	0.6	8.8	4.5	3.0	0.9
34238	Steamed rice and vegetables (vegan)	8	ounce(s)	227	99.7	263	4.9	39.2	2.5	10.3	1.8	4.2	3.9
34308	Tofu rice burgers (ovo-lacto)	1	piece(s)	218	78.2	446	22.5	67.0	6.0	10.4	2.2	2.5	4.7
34276	Vegan spinach enchiladas (vegan)	1	piece(s)	80	59.1	86	4.8	12.7	2.1	2.3	0.4	0.6	1.0
34243	Vegetable chow mein (vegan)	8	ounce(s)	227	163.5	164	6.3	22.2	2.0	6.2	0.7	2.8	2.4
34454	Vegetable lasagna (lacto)	8	ounce(s)	227	154.8	178	11.6	25.4	2.3	3.6	2.0	0.9	0.3
34339	Vegetable marinara (vegan)	8	ounce(s)	227	180.6	93	2.8	14.9	1.4	2.8	0.4	1.3	0.9
34356	Vegetable rice casserole (lacto)	8	ounce(s)	227	172.6	222	9.0	23.5	3.8	11.3	4.4	3.4	2.0
34311	Vegetable strudel (ovo-lacto)	8	ounce(s)	227	99.9	754	18.8	50.9	3.9	53.5	18.2	26.4	6.1
34371	Vegetable taco (lacto)	1	item(s)	85	54.6	140	4.9	16.7	3.0	6.3	2.9	1.8	1.3
34282	Vegetarian chili (vegan)	8	ounce(s)	227	195.6	115	5.6	21.3	6.8	1.5	0.3	0.3	0.7

KEY: H-4 = Breads/Baked Goods H-8 = Cereal/Rice/Pasta H-14 = Fruit H-18 = Vegetables/Legumes H-28 = Nuts/Seeds H-30 = Vegetarian H-32 = Dairy H-40 = Eggs H-40 = Seafood H-42 = Meats H-46 = Poultry
= Processed Meats H-50 = Beverages H-52 = Fats/Oils H-54 = Sweets H-56 = Spices/Condiments/Sauces H-60 = Mixed Foods/Soups/Sandwiches H-66 = Fast Food H-84 = Convenience H-86 = Baby Foods

Chol (mg)	Calc (mg)	Iron (mg)	Magn (mg)	Pota (mg)	Sodi (mg)	Zinc (mg)	Vit A (µg)	Thia (mg)	Vit E (mg α)	Ribo (mg)	Niac (mg)	Vit B_6 (mg)	Fola (µg)	Vit C (mg)	Vit B_{12} (µg)	Sele (µg)
0	38	0.93	90.4	195.8	4.0	1.68	0.4	0.18	—	0.17	0.71	0.06	20.2	0.2	0	—
0	20	0.82	64.2	240.2	2.2	1.21	0	0.16	2.53	0.04	4.94	0.09	52.9	0	0	2.7
0	20	0.82	64.2	240.2	247.8	1.21	0	0.16	2.85	0.04	4.94	0.09	52.9	0	0	2.7
0	22	0.55	63.4	261.4	115.2	1.18	0	0.03	2.50	0.03	4.98	0.17	43.2	0.3	0	1.2
0	7	0.30	25.6	119.2	77.8	0.45	0	0.02	1.01	0.02	2.19	0.07	14.7	0	0	1.3
0	7	0.30	24.6	103.8	2.7	0.47	0	0.01	1.44	0.02	2.14	0.09	11.8	0	0	0.9
0	0	0.18	—	—	52.5	—	0	—	—	—	—	—	—	0	—	—
0	0	0.18	—	—	0	—	0	—	—	—	—	—	—	0	—	—
0	6	0.34	30.6	120.4	97.2	0.50	0	0.05	1.63	0.01	2.63	0.06	10.8	0	0	1.4
0	7	0.30	24.6	103.8	73.4	0.47	0	0.01	1.44	0.02	2.14	0.09	11.8	0	0	0.9
0	34	1.67	61.3	257.3	6.6	1.19	0	0.23	3.04	0.05	4.40	0.13	87.6	0	0	2.6
0	20	0.77	36.3	116.6	0.3	1.39	1.9	0.12	0.36	0.03	0.32	0.05	4.4	0.2	0	1.1
0	20	0.77	36.3	116.6	105.4	1.39	1.9	0.12	0.36	0.03	0.32	0.05	4.4	0.2	0	1.1
0	18	0.68	33.3	107.8	0.3	1.23	1.4	0.13	0.70	0.03	0.33	0.05	4.1	0.2	0	1.6
0	19	0.69	33.0	111.7	0	1.23	0.8	0.18	0.38	0.04	0.32	0.06	6.0	0.3	0	1.0
0	1	0.48	21.6	51.3	0.2	0.55	0.1	0.03	0.80	0.02	0.38	0.01	2.9	0.1	0	0.1
0	33	1.24	33.5	309.7	1.8	0.72	4.0	0.21	0.74	0.07	0.42	0.35	15.7	0.9	0	3.1
0	34	1.29	34.9	322.2	137.0	0.75	4.2	0.22	0.77	0.07	0.44	0.36	16.3	1.0	0	3.2
0	30	4.58	312.1	447.2	10.2	4.34	0	0.04	0.32	0.09	2.51	0.06	32.3	1.0	0	5.3
0	154	3.07	57.9	93.1	1.9	1.17	0.5	0.04	—	0.03	1.07	0.13	16.0	0	0	5.7
0	21	0.66	14.3	68.8	5.3	0.69	0.4	0.24		0.02	0.85	0.02	14.7	0.6	0	5.2
0	267	3.99	96.1	128.3	3.0	1.93	0	0.22	—	0.07	1.24	0.22	26.5	0	0	9.3
0	40	1.80	—	—	95.0	—	0	—	—	—	—	—	—	1.2	—	—
0	40	1.80	—	—	2.0	—	0	—	—	—	—	—	—	1.2	—	—
0	7	0.47	29.3	58.0	0.8	0.45	0.3	0.13	3.17	0.03	0.75	0.12	20.4	0.1	0	4.8
0	6	0.30	10.3	68.0	29.4	0.42	0	0.01	2.09	0.02	0.56	0.06	19.0	0.1	0	6.3
0	5	0.57	10.8	41.1	51.3	0.44	0	0.03	—	0.02	0.35	0.07	19.9	0.1	0	5.2
0	10	0.66	49.8	92.2	53.0	0.78	0.5	0.01	3.66	0.03	1.08	0.09	37.9	0.4	0	16.7
0	29	1.14	59.3	256.9	85.9	1.21	0.4	0.17	—	0.07	1.77	0.11	26.6	0.5	0	—
2	41	1.27	60.4	243.0	45.4	1.18	0.8	0.15	—	0.08	1.65	0.10	24.4	0.5	0	—
0	20	0.92	33.6	248.1	33.3	0.41	0.7	0.16	—	0.04	0.52	0.11	14.7	2.7	0	—
0	19	0.98	62.8	163.4	0.6	1.05	0.6	0.02	0.56	0.04	0.15	0.18	9.7	0.5	0	5.3
0	29	0.85	46.2	129.0	0.6	0.90	0.3	0.10	0.20	0.04	0.33	0.16	28.7	0.4	0	1.4
0	268	4.67	88.0	379.7	111.4	1.53	0	0.13	0.68	0.11	1.07	0.28	39.0	15.5	0	10.9
43	478	2.52	34.7	215.7	1350.3	1.87	0	0.33	0.48	0.36	2.28	0.12	128.6	22.2	0.4	20.7
0	45	1.25	37.2	376.6	776.2	0.73	0	0.08	1.01	0.08	0.67	0.10	64.5	4.6	0	4.0
0	25	2.09	33.9	388.5	288.8	1.08	0	0.18	1.05	0.09	1.47	0.16	134.2	12.3	0	8.9
22	193	0.68	20.4	126.3	772.5	1.14	0	0.14	0.29	0.24	0.98	0.05	75.4	0.1	0.5	15.6
0	42	1.40	67.5	355.8	1397.4	0.92	175.8	0.16	1.66	0.11	2.75	0.29	31.3	13.1	0	8.3
51	528	5.83	96.8	426.9	1800.8	2.46	0	0.85	0.64	0.45	5.83	0.31	167.7	3.2	0.2	35.1
0	106	1.12	37.2	161.3	104.4	0.68	0	0.06	0.21	0.05	0.54	0.11	19.8	1.4	0	5.3
0	187	3.47	28.5	305.1	367.0	0.75	0	0.13	0.85	0.12	1.37	0.14	76.8	8.1	0	6.4
10	146	1.82	34.5	396.7	647.7	1.12	0	0.19	1.03	0.26	2.02	0.22	107.4	15.2	0.4	19.1
0	17	0.77	17.1	182.0	376.5	0.38	18.2	0.12	0.86	0.08	1.20	0.11	71.6	17.7	0	10.0
16	172	2.01	29.4	393.3	579.0	1.28	0	0.17	1.70	0.28	2.33	0.20	148.5	53.2	0.2	11.6
46	317	3.36	39.0	298.5	815.8	1.98	0	0.45	1.47	0.50	4.51	0.16	175.8	27.1	0.3	31.1
8	79	0.85	26.5	205.7	331.4	0.68	0	0.09	0.26	0.07	0.60	0.08	32.7	4.2	0.1	2.3
0	68	2.42	40.9	531.0	358.9	1.23	0	0.14	1.43	0.13	1.25	0.22	48.6	16.6	0	3.6

DA+ Code	Food Description	Quantity	Measure	Wt (g)	H_2O (g)	Ener (kcal)	Prot (g)	Carb (g)	Fiber (g)	Fat (g)	Fat Breakdown (g) Sat	Mono	Poly
Vegetarian Foods—*continued*													
34367	Vegetarian vegetable soup (vegan)	8	ounce(s)	227	204.6	92	2.5	13.6	2.5	4.0	0.7	1.8	1.2
	Boca												
68284	All American Classic patty w/ organic soy	1	item(s)	71	—	140	15.0	9.0	4.0	5.0	1.5	—	—
32072	Breakfast links	2	item(s)	45	—	70	8.0	5.0	2.0	3.0	1.0	—	—
68285	Bruschetta tomato basil parmesan patty	1	item(s)	71	—	70	10.0	9.0	3.5	1.5	0.5	0.5	—
35780	Cheeseburger meatless burger patty	1	item(s)	71	—	100	13.0	6.0	4.0	4.5	1.5	—	—
68290	Chik'n nuggets	1	item(s)	22	—	45	3.5	4.3	0.8	1.8	0.1	1.3	—
68289	Chik'n patty, original	1	item(s)	71	—	160	11.0	15.0	2.0	6.0	0	—	—
68291	Chik'n patty, spicy	1	item(s)	71	—	160	11.0	15.0	2.0	6.0	0	—	—
35781	Grilled vegetable patty	1	item(s)	71	—	80	12.0	7.0	4.0	1.0	0	—	—
68287	Meatless ground crumbles	½	cup(s)	57	—	60	13.0	6.0	3.0	0.5	0	—	—
68282	Original vegan patty	1	item(s)	71	—	70	13.0	6.0	4.0	0.5	0	—	—
	Gardenburger												
39661	Black bean chipotle burger	1	item(s)	71	45.8	100	5.0	16.0	5.0	3.0	0	1.6	0.8
29913	Original	1	item(s)	71	43.7	100	5.0	18.0	5.0	3.0	1.0	1.2	0.7
29920	Portabella veggie burger	1	item(s)	71	44.9	100	4.0	17.0	5.0	2.5	1.0	0.7	0.5
39662	Sun-dried tomato basil burger	1	item(s)	71	46.3	100	4.0	17.0	4.0	2.5	0.5	0.9	0.6
29915	Veggie medley	1	item(s)	71	46.5	100	3.0	17.0	5.0	2.5	0	1.0	1.0
	Loma Linda												
9311	Big franks, canned	1	item(s)	51	30.1	110	11.0	3.0	2.0	6.0	1.0	1.5	3.5
9323	Fried Chik'n with gravy	2	piece(s)	80	—	150	12.0	5.0	2.0	10.0	1.5	2.5	5.0
9326	Linketts, canned	1	item(s)	35	21.4	70	7.0	1.0	1.0	4.0	0.5	1.0	2.5
9336	Redi-Burger patties, canned	1	slice(s)	85	55.1	120	18.0	7.0	4.0	2.5	0.5	0.5	1.5
9354	Tender Rounds meatball substitute, canned in gravy	6	piece(s)	80	55.3	120	13.0	6.0	1.0	4.5	0.5	1.5	2.5
9356	Vege-Burger, canned	¼	cup(s)	55	39.6	60	12.0	2.0	2.0	0.5	0	0	0.5
	Morningstar Farms												
9371	Breakfast bacon strips	2	item(s)	16	6.7	60	2.0	2.0	1.0	4.5	0.5	1.0	3.0
9368	Breakfast sausage links	2	item(s)	45	28.3	80	9.0	3.0	2.0	3.0	0.5	1.0	1.5
33705	Chik'n nuggets	4	piece(s)	86	43.5	190	12.0	19.0	4.0	9.0	1.5	2.5	4.5
11587	Chik patties	1	item(s)	71	38.3	140	8.0	16.0	2.0	5.0	0.5	1.0	3.5
2531	Garden veggie patties	1	item(s)	67	40.1	110	10.0	9.0	3.0	3.5	0.5	0.5	1.5
9376	Grillers patties, original	1	item(s)	64	35.6	130	15.0	5.0	2.0	6.0	1.0	2.0	3.0
50552	Meal Starters Chik'n strips	12	piece(s)	85	50.6	140	23.0	6.0	1.0	3.5	0.5	1.5	1.5
33715	Meal Starters Grillers recipe crumbles	½	cup(s)	42	26.9	61	7.6	3.8	2.3	1.9	0	0.4	1.1
33702	Spicy black bean veggie burger	1	item(s)	67	37.7	120	11.0	13.0	4.0	4.0	0.5	1.0	2.0
	Worthington												
9418	Chic-ketts, frozen	2	slice(s)	55	31.7	110	14.0	3.0	2.0	5.0	1.0	1.0	3.0
9424	Chili, canned	1	cup(s)	230	167.1	280	24.0	25.0	8.0	10.0	1.5	1.5	7.0
9436	Diced Chik, canned	¼	cup(s)	55	43.0	50	9.0	2.0	1.0	0	0	0	0.0
9440	Dinner roast, frozen	1	slice(s)	85	52.4	180	14.0	6.0	3.0	11.0	1.5	4.5	5.0
9446	Fripats patties, frozen	1	item(s)	64	36.4	130	15.0	5.0	3.0	6.0	1.0	1.5	3.5
9452	Leanies links, frozen	1	item(s)	40	21.6	100	8.0	2.0	1.0	7.0	1.0	1.5	4.5
36702	Meatless chicken style roll, frozen	1	slice(s)	55	—	90	9.0	2.0	1.0	4.5	0.5	1.0	2.5
9428	Meatless corned beef, sliced, frozen	3	slice(s)	57	30.8	145	10.4	5.2	0	8.3	1.0	2.1	5.2
9462	Prosage links	2	item(s)	45	28.9	80	9.0	3.0	2.0	3.0	0.5	0.5	2.0
9484	Stakelets patty beef steak substitute, frozen	1	piece(s)	71	40.8	150	14.0	7.0	2.0	7.0	1.0	2.5	3.5
9486	Stripples bacon substitute	2	item(s)	16	6.7	60	2.0	2.0	0.5	4.5	0.5	1.0	3.0
9496	Vegetable Skallops meat substitute, canned	½	cup(s)	85	61.8	90	17.0	4.0	3.0	1.0	0	0	0.5
Dairy													
	Cheese												
1433	Blue, crumbled	1	ounce(s)	28	12.0	100	6.1	0.7	0	8.1	5.3	2.2	0.2
884	Brick	1	ounce(s)	28	11.7	105	6.6	0.8	0	8.4	5.3	2.4	0.2
885	Brie	1	ounce(s)	28	13.7	95	5.9	0.1	0	7.8	4.9	2.3	0.2
34821	Camembert	1	ounce(s)	28	14.7	85	5.6	0.1	0	6.9	4.3	2.0	0.2
888	Cheddar or colby	1	ounce(s)	28	10.8	112	6.7	0.7	0	9.1	5.7	2.6	0.3
32096	Cheddar or colby, low fat	1	ounce(s)	28	17.9	49	6.9	0.5	0	2.0	1.2	0.6	0.1
32121	Cheddar or colby, low sodium	1	ounce(s)	28	11.1	113	6.9	0.5	0	9.2	5.9	2.6	0.3

E KEY: H-4 = Breads/Baked Goods H-8 = Cereal/Rice/Pasta H-14 = Fruit H-18 = Vegetables/Legumes H-28 = Nuts/Seeds H-30 = Vegetarian H-32 = Dairy H-40 = Eggs H-40 = Seafood H-42 = Meats H-46 = Poultry 8 = Processed Meats H-50 = Beverages H-52 = Fats/Oils H-54 = Sweets H-56 = Spices/Condiments/Sauces H-60 = Mixed Foods/Soups/Sandwiches H-66 = Fast Food H-84 = Convenience H-86 = Baby Foods

Chol (mg)	Calc (mg)	Iron (mg)	Magn (mg)	Pota (mg)	Sodi (mg)	Zinc (mg)	Vit A (μg)	Thia (mg)	Vit E (mg α)	Ribo (mg)	Niac (mg)	Vit B_6 (mg)	Fola (μg)	Vit C (mg)	Vit B_{12} (μg)	Sele (μg)
0	38	1.32	27.9	444.6	504.1	0.45	0	0.11	0.73	0.08	1.55	0.21	39.7	23.8	0	1.0
5	150	1.44	—	—	500.0	—	0	—	—	—	—	—	—	0	—	—
0	20	1.44	—	—	330.0	—	0	—	—	—	—	—	—	0	—	—
5	150	2.70	—	—	290.0	—	0	—	—	—	—	—	—	0	—	—
10	100	1.44	—	—	320.0	—	—	—	—	—	—	—	—	0	—	—
0	10	0.36	—	—	125.0	—	—	—	—	—	—	—	—	0	—	—
0	40	1.80	—	—	430.0	—	—	—	—	—	—	—	—	0	—	—
0	40	1.80	—	—	560.0	—	—	—	—	—	—	—	—	0	—	—
0	60	1.80	—	—	300.0	—	—	—	—	—	—	—	—	0	—	—
0	60	1.80	—	—	270.0	—	0	—	—	—	—	—	—	0	—	—
0	60	1.80	—	—	280.0	—	—	—	—	—	—	—	—	0	—	—
0	20	1.44	18.5	140.0	390.0	0.35	10.0	—	—	—	—	—	—	6.0	—	—
10	40	1.08	2.8	110.2	400.7	0.78	—	—	—	—	—	—	—	3.6	—	—
3	40	0.72	6.4	105.2	490.9	0.07	—	—	—	—	—	—	—	1.2	—	—
3	20	0.72	2.8	55.0	270.0	0.07	—	—	—	—	—	—	—	2.4	—	—
0	20	0.72	12.8	125.2	380.7	0.21	62.6	—	—	—	—	—	—	12.0	0	—
0	0	0.77	—	50.0	220.0	1.17	0	0.22	—	0.10	2.00	0.70	—	0	2.4	—
0	20	1.80	—	70.0	430.0	—	0	1.05	—	0.34	4.00	0.30	—	0	2.4	—
0	0	0.36	—	20.0	160.0	0.52	0	0.12	—	0.20	0.80	0.16	—	0	0.9	—
0	0	1.06	—	140.1	450.3	1.45	0	0.15	—	0.26	4.00	0.40	—	0	1.2	—
0	20	1.08	—	80.0	340.0	0.64	0	0.75	—	0.17	2.00	0.16	—	0	1.2	—
0	0	0.36	—	40.0	130.0	0.71	0	0.12	—	0.10	0.78	0.30	—	0	2.4	—
0	0	0.36	—	15.0	230.0	0.10	0	0.75	—	0.04	1.20	0.07	—	0	0.2	—
0	0	1.80	—	50.0	300.0	—	0	0.38	—	0.17	7.00	0.50	—	0	3.0	—
0	60	1.80	3.4	320.0	600.0	0.69	0	0.38	—	0.10	4.00	0.20	—	0	1.8	—
0	20	1.80	—	280.0	590.0	0.35	0	0.22	—	0.10	3.00	0.16	—	0	1.2	—
0	40	0.72	—	180.0	350.0	0.67	—	7.50	—	0.20	0.94	0.60	—	0	—	—
0	43	1.80	—	130.0	260.0	0.77	0	1.80	—	0.17	4.00	0.40	—	0	2.7	—
0	40	5.40	24.0	109.9	499.8	4.50	0	0.45	—	0.25	7.00	0.40	—	0	1.8	—
0	0	1.36	—	75.8	174.2	0.46	0	0.23	—	0.08	3.03	0.23	0	0	2.3	—
0	60	1.44	34.2	250.0	350.0	0.67	0	9.11	—	0.20	1.21	0.11	32.8	0	0	—
0	0	1.80	—	85.0	390.0	0.88	0	0.22	—	0.14	2.00	0.11	3.8	0	1.2	—
0	40	3.60	—	330.0	1130.0	1.84	0	0.30	—	0.14	2.00	0.70	—	0	1.5	—
0	0	1.08	—	100.0	220.0	0.38	0	0.06	—	0.10	4.00	0.08	—	0	0.2	—
0	20	1.80	—	120.1	580.3	0.77	0	1.80	—	0.26	6.00	0.60	—	0	1.5	—
0	60	1.80	—	120.0	320.0	0.77	0	1.80	—	0.17	3.00	0.60	—	0	1.2	—
0	20	0.72	—	40.0	430.0	0.32	0	0.22	—	0.14	0.80	0.20	—	0	0.9	—
0	100	1.08	—	240.0	240.0	—	0	0.38	—	0.14	4.00	0.30	—	0	1.8	—
0	0	1.87	—	134.7	466.4	0.46	0	1.87	—	0.18	5.18	0.31	—	0	1.9	—
0	0	1.44	—	50.0	320.0	0.45	0	1.80	—	0.17	2.00	0.30	—	0	3.0	—
0	40	1.08	—	130.0	480.0	0.85	0	1.20	—	0.14	3.00	0.30	—	0	1.5	—
0	0	0.36	—	15.0	220.0	0.10	0	0.75	—	0.03	0.40	0.08	—	0	0.2	—
0	0	0.36	—	10.0	390.2	0.85	0	—	—	—	—	—	—	0	0	—
21	150	0.09	6.5	72.6	395.5	0.75	56.1	0.01	0.07	0.11	0.29	0.05	10.2	0	0.3	4.1
27	191	0.12	6.8	38.6	158.8	0.74	82.8	0	0.07	0.10	0.03	0.02	5.7	0	0.4	4.1
28	52	0.14	5.7	43.1	178.3	0.67	49.3	0.02	0.07	0.15	0.11	0.07	18.4	0	0.5	4.1
20	110	0.09	5.7	53.0	238.7	0.67	68.3	0.01	0.06	0.14	0.18	0.06	17.6	0	0.4	4.1
27	194	0.22	7.4	36.0	171.2	0.87	74.8	0	0.08	0.11	0.03	0.02	5.1	0	0.2	4.1
6	118	0.12	4.5	18.7	173.5	0.52	17.0	0	0.02	0.06	0.01	0.01	3.1	0	0.1	4.1
28	199	0.20	7.7	31.8	6.0	0.88	74.8	0.01	0.08	0.11	0.02	0.02	5.1	0	0.2	4.1

TABLE H-1 Table of Food Composition (*continued*) (Computer code is for Cengage Diet Analysis program) (For purposes of calculations, use "0" for t, <1, <0.1, 0.01)

DA+ Code	Food Description	Quantity	Measure	Wt (g)	H_2O (g)	Ener (kcal)	Prot (g)	Carb (g)	Fiber (g)	Fat (g)	Fat Breakdown (g)		
											Sat	Mono	Poly
	Dairy—*continued*												
5	Cheddar, shredded	¼	cup(s)	28	10.4	114	7.0	0.4	0	9.4	6.0	2.7	0.3
889	Edam	1	ounce(s)	28	11.8	101	7.1	0.4	0	7.9	5.0	2.3	0.2
890	Feta	1	ounce(s)	28	15.7	75	4.0	1.2	0	6.0	4.2	1.3	0.2
891	Fontina	1	ounce(s)	28	10.8	110	7.3	0.4	0	8.8	5.4	2.5	0.5
8527	Goat cheese, soft	1	ounce(s)	28	17.2	75	5.3	0	0	6.0	4.1	1.4	0.1
893	Gouda	1	ounce(s)	28	11.8	101	7.1	0.6	0	7.8	5.0	2.2	0.2
894	Gruyere	1	ounce(s)	28	9.4	117	8.5	0.1	0	9.2	5.4	2.8	0.5
895	Limburger	1	ounce(s)	28	13.7	93	5.7	0.1	0	7.7	4.7	2.4	0.1
896	Monterey jack	1	ounce(s)	28	11.6	106	6.9	0.2	0	8.6	5.4	2.5	0.3
42324	Mozarella, low sodium	1	ounce(s)	28	14.1	79	7.8	0.9	0	4.8	3.1	1.4	0.1
13	Mozzarella, part skim milk	1	ounce(s)	28	15.2	72	6.9	0.8	0	4.5	2.9	1.3	0.1
12	Mozzarella, whole milk	1	ounce(s)	28	14.2	85	6.3	0.6	0	6.3	3.7	1.9	0.2
897	Muenster	1	ounce(s)	28	11.8	104	6.6	0.3	0	8.5	5.4	2.5	0.2
898	Neufchatel	1	ounce(s)	28	17.9	72	2.6	1.0	0	6.5	3.6	1.6	0.3
14	Parmesan, grated	1	tablespoon(s)	5	1.0	22	1.9	0.2	0	1.4	0.9	0.4	0.1
17	Provolone	1	ounce(s)	28	11.6	100	7.3	0.6	0	7.5	4.8	2.1	0.2
19	Ricotta, part skim milk	¼	cup(s)	62	45.8	85	7.0	3.2	0	4.9	3.0	1.4	0.2
18	Ricotta, whole milk	¼	cup(s)	62	44.1	107	6.9	1.9	0	8.0	5.1	2.2	0.2
20	Romano	1	tablespoon(s)	5	1.5	19	1.6	0.2	0	1.3	0.9	0.4	0
900	Roquefort	1	ounce(s)	28	11.2	105	6.1	0.6	0	8.7	5.5	2.4	0.4
21	Swiss	1	ounce(s)	28	10.5	108	7.6	1.5	0	7.9	5.0	2.1	0.3
53952	Swiss, low sodium	1	ounce(s)	28	10.7	106	8.1	1.0	0	7.8	5.0	2.1	0.3
	Imitation cheese												
42245	Imitation American cheddar	1	ounce(s)	28	15.1	68	4.7	3.3	0	4.0	2.5	1.2	0.1
53914	Imitation cheddar	1	ounce(s)	28	15.1	68	4.7	3.3	0	4.0	2.5	1.2	0.1
	Cottage cheese												
9	Low fat, 1% fat	½	cup(s)	113	93.2	81	14.0	3.1	0	1.2	0.7	0.3	0
42265	Low fat, 1% fat, no sodium added	½	cup(s)	113	94.4	81	14.0	3.1	0	1.1	0.7	0.3	0
8	Low fat, 2% fat	½	cup(s)	113	91.2	97	13.4	4.1	0	2.8	1.1	0.5	0.1
	Cream cheese												
11	Cream cheese	2	tablespoon(s)	29	15.8	99	1.7	1.2	0	9.9	5.6	2.5	0.4
17366	Cream cheese, fat free	2	tablespoon(s)	30	21.6	32	4.7	2.3	0	0.3	0.2	0.1	0
10438	Tofutti Better than Cream Cheese	2	tablespoon(s)	30	—	85	1.0	9.0	0	5.0	2.0	—	—
	Processed cheese												
24	American cheese food, processed	1	ounce(s)	28	12.5	94	4.8	2.4	0	7.3	4.3	1.9	0.3
25	American cheese spread, processed	1	ounce(s)	28	13.5	82	4.7	2.5	0	6.0	3.8	1.8	0.2
22	American cheese, processed	1	ounce(s)	28	11.2	104	5.1	1.4	0	8.7	5.1	2.3	0.4
42285	Cheddar or American, pasteurized process, low sodium	1	ounce(s)	28	12.1	107	6.3	0.5	0	8.8	5.6	2.5	0.3
9110	Kraft Deluxe Singles pasteurized process American cheese	1	ounce(s)	28	—	108	5.4	0	0	9.5	5.4	—	—
23	Swiss cheese, processed	1	ounce(s)	28	12.0	95	7.0	0.6	0	7.1	4.5	2.0	0.2
	Soy cheese												
65625	Galaxy Foods vegan American cheese slices alternative	1	slice(s)	19	—	40	1.0	5.0	0	2.0	0	0.5	1.5
10437	Galaxy Foods vegan grated parmesan cheese alternative	1	tablespoon(s)	8	—	23	3.0	1.5	0	0	0	0	0
	Cream												
26	Half and half cream	1	tablespoon(s)	15	12.2	20	0.4	0.7	0	1.7	1.1	0.5	0.1
32	Heavy whipping cream, liquid	1	tablespoon(s)	15	8.7	52	0.3	0.4	0	5.6	3.5	1.6	0.2
28	Light coffee or table cream, liquid	1	tablespoon(s)	15	11.1	29	0.4	0.5	0	2.9	1.8	0.8	0.1
30	Light whipping cream, liquid	1	tablespoon(s)	15	9.5	44	0.3	0.4	0	4.6	2.9	1.4	0.1
34	Whipped cream topping, pressurized	1	tablespoon(s)	3	1.8	8	0.1	0.4	0	0.7	0.4	0.2	0
	Sour cream												
36	Sour cream	2	tablespoon(s)	24	17.9	46	0.5	0.7	0	4.7	2.8	1.2	0.2
30556	Sour cream, fat free	2	tablespoon(s)	32	25.8	24	1.0	5.0	0	0	0	0	0
	Imitation cream												
3659	Coffeemate nondairy creamer, liquid	1	tablespoon(s)	15	—	20	0	2.0	0	1.0	0	0	0
40	Cream substitute, powder	1	teaspoon(s)	2	0	11	0.1	1.1	0	0.7	0.7	0	0
904	Imitation sour cream	2	tablespoon(s)	29	20.5	60	0.7	1.9	0	5.6	5.1	0.2	0

KEY: H-4 = Breads/Baked Goods H-8 = Cereal/Rice/Pasta H-14 = Fruit H-18 = Vegetables/Legumes H-28 = Nuts/Seeds H-30 = Vegetarian H-32 = Dairy H-40 = Eggs H-40 = Seafood H-42 = Meats H-46 = Poultry = Processed Meats H-50 = Beverages H-52 = Fats/Oils H-54 = Sweets H-56 = Spices/Condiments/Sauces H-60 = Mixed Foods/Soups/Sandwiches H-66 = Fast Food H-84 = Convenience H-86 = Baby Foods

Chol (mg)	Calc (mg)	Iron (mg)	Magn (mg)	Pota (mg)	Sodi (mg)	Zinc (mg)	Vit A (µg)	Thia (mg)	Vit E (mg α)	Ribo (mg)	Niac (mg)	Vit B_6 (mg)	Fola (µg)	Vit C (mg)	Vit B_{12} (µg)	Sele (µg)
30	204	0.19	7.9	27.7	175.4	0.88	74.9	0.01	0.08	0.11	0.02	0.02	5.1	0	0.2	3.9
25	207	0.12	8.5	53.3	273.6	1.06	68.9	0.01	0.07	0.11	0.02	0.02	4.5	0	0.4	4.1
25	140	0.18	5.4	17.6	316.4	0.82	35.4	0.04	0.05	0.24	0.28	0.12	9.1	0	0.5	4.3
33	156	0.07	4.0	18.1	226.8	0.99	74.0	0.01	0.08	0.06	0.04	0.02	1.7	0	0.5	4.1
13	40	0.54	4.5	7.4	104.3	0.26	81.6	0.02	0.05	0.11	0.12	0.07	3.4	0	0.1	0.8
32	198	0.07	8.2	34.3	232.2	1.11	46.8	0.01	0.07	0.09	0.02	0.02	6.0	0	0.4	4.1
31	287	0.05	10.2	23.0	95.3	1.11	76.8	0.02	0.08	0.08	0.03	0.02	2.8	0	0.5	4.1
26	141	0.04	6.0	36.3	226.8	0.60	96.4	0.02	0.07	0.14	0.04	0.02	16.4	0	0.3	4.1
25	211	0.20	7.7	23.0	152.0	0.85	56.1	0	0.07	0.11	0.03	0.02	5.1	0	0.2	4.1
15	207	0.07	7.4	26.9	4.5	0.89	38.8	0.01	0.04	0.10	0.03	0.02	2.6	0	0.3	4.5
18	222	0.06	6.5	23.8	175.5	0.78	36.0	0.01	0.04	0.09	0.03	0.02	2.6	0	0.2	4.1
22	143	0.12	5.7	21.5	177.8	0.83	50.7	0.01	0.05	0.08	0.03	0.01	2.0	0	0.6	4.8
27	203	0.12	7.7	38.0	178.0	0.80	84.5	0	0.07	0.09	0.03	0.02	3.4	0	0.4	4.1
21	33	0.04	2.8	43.1	94.7	0.23	68.3	0.01	0.11	0.04	0.06	0.01	4.0	0	0.1	0.9
4	55	0.05	1.9	6.3	76.4	0.19	11.4	0	0.01	0.02	0.01	0	0.5	0	0.1	0.9
20	214	0.15	7.9	39.1	248.3	0.92	66.9	0.01	0.07	0.09	0.04	0.02	2.8	0	0.4	4.1
19	167	0.27	9.2	76.9	76.9	0.82	65.8	0.01	0.04	0.11	0.05	0.01	8.0	0	0.2	10.3
31	127	0.23	6.8	64.6	51.7	0.71	73.8	0.01	0.07	0.12	0.06	0.03	7.4	0	0.2	8.9
5	53	0.04	2.0	4.3	60.0	0.13	4.8	0	0.01	0.02	0	0	0.3	0	0.1	0.7
26	188	0.16	8.5	25.8	512.9	0.59	83.3	0.01	—	0.17	0.21	0.04	13.9	0	0.2	4.1
26	224	0.06	10.8	21.8	54.4	1.24	62.4	0.02	0.11	0.08	0.03	0.02	1.7	0	0.9	5.2
26	272	0.05	10.2	31.5	4.0	1.11	61.2	0.01	0.10	0.10	0.03	0.02	1.7	0	0.5	3.5
10	159	0.09	8.2	68.6	381.3	0.73	32.3	0.01	0.08	0.12	0.04	0.03	2.0	0	0.1	4.3
10	159	0.09	8.2	68.6	381.3	0.73	32.3	0.01	0.08	0.12	0.04	0.03	2.0	0	0.1	4.3
5	69	0.16	5.7	97.2	458.8	0.43	12.4	0.02	0.01	0.19	0.14	0.08	13.6	0	0.7	10.2
5	69	0.16	5.7	97.2	14.7	0.43	12.4	0.02	0.01	0.18	0.15	0.08	13.6	0	0.7	9.5
11	103	0.17	7.9	94.9	372.9	0.46	22.6	0.05	0.05	0.22	0.12	0.02	11.3	0	0.5	11.2
32	28	0.11	2.6	40.0	93.1	0.15	106.1	0.01	0.08	0.04	0.04	0.01	3.2	0	0.1	0.7
4	105	0.06	6.6	83.4	210.6	0.45	3.3	0.01	0.01	0.08	0.07	0.01	10.5	0	0.3	1.5
0	0	0	—	—	160.0	—	—	—	—	—	—	—	—	0	—	—
28	193	0.07	7.7	72.3	364.0	0.65	57.0	0.01	0.18	0.10	0.04	0.03	2.0	0	0.4	5.6
16	159	0.09	8.2	68.6	460.7	0.73	49.0	0.01	0.05	0.12	0.04	0.03	2.0	0	0.1	3.2
28	296	0.18	7.4	37.4	473.7	0.71	89.9	0	0.23	0.07	0.02	0.01	2.3	0	0.4	5.7
27	175	0.11	6.2	45.9	2.0	0.85	72.0	0.01	0.08	0.10	0.02	0.02	2.3	0	0.2	3.6
27	338	0	—	33.8	459.0	—	—	—	—	—	—	—	—	0	—	—
24	219	0.17	8.2	61.2	388.4	1.02	56.1	0	0.10	0.08	0.01	0.01	1.7	0	0.3	4.5
0	200	0	—	—	120.0	—	0	—	—	—	—	—	—	0	—	—
0	60	0	—	75.0	97.5	—	15.0	—	—	—	—	—	—	0	—	—
6	16	0.01	1.5	19.7	6.2	0.08	14.7	0.01	0.05	0.02	0.01	0.01	0.5	0.1	0	0.3
21	10	0	1.0	11.3	5.7	0.03	61.7	0	0.16	0.02	0.01	0	0.6	0.1	0	0.1
10	14	0.01	1.4	18.3	6.0	0.04	27.1	0	0.08	0.02	0.01	0	0.3	0.1	0	0.1
17	10	0	1.0	14.6	5.1	0.04	41.8	0	0.13	0.02	0.01	0	0.6	0.1	0	0.1
2	3	0	0.3	4.4	0.2	0.01	5.6	0	0.02	0	0	0	0.1	0	0	0
12	26	0.04	2.4	33.8	19.2	0.09	42.2	0.01	0.11	0.04	0.03	0.01	1.7	0.2	0.1	0.6
3	40	0	3.2	41.3	45.1	0.16	23.4	0.01	0	0.05	0.02	0.01	3.5	0	0.1	1.7
0	0	0	—	—	0	—	0	—	—	—	—	—	—	0	—	—
0	0	0.02	0.1	16.2	3.6	0.01	0	0	0.01	0	0	0	0	0	0	0
0	1	0.11	1.7	46.3	29.3	0.34	0	0	0.21	0	0	0	0	0	0	0.7

TABLE H-1 Table of Food Composition (*continued*) (Computer code is for Cengage Diet Analysis program) (For purposes of calculations, use "0" for t, <1, <0.1, 0.01)

DA+ Code	Food Description	Quantity	Measure	Wt (g)	H_2O (g)	Ener (kcal)	Prot (g)	Carb (g)	Fiber (g)	Fat (g)	Fat Breakdown (g) Sat	Mono	Poly
	Dairy—*continued*												
35972	Nondairy coffee whitener, liquid, frozen	1	tablespoon(s)	15	11.5	20	0.1	1.7	0	1.5	0.3	1.1	0
35976	Nondairy dessert topping, frozen	1	tablespoon(s)	5	2.4	15	0.1	1.1	0	1.2	1.0	0.1	0
35975	Nondairy dessert topping, pressurized	1	tablespoon(s)	4	2.6	12	0	0.7	0	1.0	0.8	0.1	0
	Fluid milk												
60	Buttermilk, low fat	1	cup(s)	245	220.8	98	8.1	11.7	0	2.2	1.3	0.6	0.1
54	Low fat, 1%	1	cup(s)	244	219.4	102	8.2	12.2	0	2.4	1.5	0.7	0.1
55	Low fat, 1%, with nonfat milk solids	1	cup(s)	245	220.0	105	8.5	12.2	0	2.4	1.5	0.7	0.1
57	Nonfat, skim or fat free	1	cup(s)	245	222.6	83	8.3	12.2	0	0.2	0.1	0.1	0
58	Nonfat, skim or fat free with nonfat milk solids	1	cup(s)	245	221.4	91	8.7	12.3	0	0.6	0.4	0.2	0
51	Reduced fat, 2%	1	cup(s)	244	217.7	122	8.1	11.7	0	4.8	3.1	1.4	0.2
52	Reduced fat, 2%, with nonfat milk solids	1	cup(s)	245	217.7	125	8.5	12.2	0	4.7	2.9	1.4	0.2
50	Whole, 3.3%	1	cup(s)	244	215.0	149	7.7	11.7	0	7.9	4.6	2.0	0.5
	Canned milk												
62	Nonfat or skim evaporated	2	tablespoon(s)	32	25.3	25	2.4	3.6	0	0.1	0	0	0
63	Sweetened condensed	2	tablespoon(s)	38	10.4	123	3.0	20.8	0	3.3	2.1	0.9	0.1
61	Whole evaporated	2	tablespoon(s)	32	23.3	42	2.1	3.2	0	2.4	1.4	0.7	0.1
	Dried milk												
64	Buttermilk	¼	cup(s)	30	0.9	117	10.4	14.9	0	1.8	1.1	0.5	0.1
65	Instant nonfat with added vitamin A	¼	cup(s)	17	0.7	61	6.0	8.9	0	0.1	0.1	0	0
5234	Skim milk powder	¼	cup(s)	17	0.7	61	6.0	8.9	0	0.1	0.1	0	0
907	Whole	¼	cup(s)	32	0.8	159	8.4	12.3	0	8.5	5.4	2.5	0.2
909	**Goat milk**	1	cup(s)	244	212.4	168	8.7	10.9	0	10.1	6.5	2.7	0.4
	Chocolate milk												
33155	Chocolate syrup, prepared with milk	1	cup(s)	282	227.0	254	8.7	36.0	0.8	8.3	4.7	2.1	0.5
33184	Cocoa mix with aspartame, added sodium and vitamin A, no added calcium or phosphorus, prepared with water	1	cup(s)	192	177.4	56	2.3	10.8	1.2	0.4	0.3	0.1	0
908	Hot cocoa, prepared with milk	1	cup(s)	250	206.1	193	8.8	26.9	2.5	5.8	3.6	1.7	0.2
69	Low fat	1	cup(s)	250	205.9	178	8.1	31.5	1.3	2.5	1.5	0.8	0.1
68	Reduced fat	1	cup(s)	250	205.4	190	7.5	30.3	1.8	4.8	2.9	1.1	0.2
67	Whole	1	cup(s)	250	205.8	208	7.9	25.9	2.0	8.5	5.3	2.5	0.3
70	**Eggnog**	1	cup(s)	254	209.7	224	11.6	20.4	0	10.6	6.6	3.3	0.5
	Breakfast drinks												
10089	Carnation Breakfast Essentials classic chocolate malt, prepared with skim milk	1	cup(s)	273	—	220	12.5	39.0	0.8	1.0	0.8	—	—
10092	Carnation Breakfast Essentials classic French vanilla, prepared with skim milk, no sugar added	1	cup(s)	257	—	150	12.9	24.0	3.0	0.6	0.2	—	—
57630	Carnation Breakfast Essentials milk chocolate, ready to drink, no sugar added	1	cup(s)	237	—	109	9.5	11.6	1.5	3.6	1.1	—	—
10091	Carnation Breakfast Essentials Strawberry Sensation, prepared with skim milk	1	cup(s)	273	—	220	12.5	39.0	0	0.6	0.4	—	—
1417	Ovaltine rich chocolate flavor, prepared with skim milk	1	cup(s)	258	—	170	8.5	31.0	0	0	0	0	0
8539	**Malted milk, chocolate mix, fortified, prepared with milk**	1	cup(s)	265	215.3	231	8.7	29.7	1.1	8.6	5.0	2.2	0.5
	Milkshakes												
73	Chocolate	1	cup(s)	227	164.0	270	6.9	48.1	0.7	6.1	3.8	1.8	0.2
3163	Strawberry	1	cup(s)	226	167.8	256	7.7	42.8	0.9	6.3	3.9	—	—
74	Vanilla	1	cup(s)	227	169.2	254	8.8	40.3	0	6.9	4.3	2.0	0.3
	Ice cream												
4776	Chocolate	½	cup(s)	66	36.8	143	2.5	18.6	0.8	7.3	4.5	2.1	0.3
12137	Chocolate fudge, no sugar added	½	cup(s)	71	—	100	3.0	16.0	2.0	3.0	1.5	—	—
16514	Chocolate, soft serve	½	cup(s)	87	51.7	192	3.5	19.2	0.6	11.2	6.5	3.0	0.4
16523	Sherbet, all flavors	½	cup(s)	97	63.8	139	1.1	29.3	1.3	1.9	1.1	0.5	0.1
4778	Strawberry	½	cup(s)	66	39.6	127	2.1	18.2	0.6	5.5	3.4	—	—

GE KEY: H-4 = Breads/Baked Goods H-8 = Cereal/Rice/Pasta H-14 = Fruit H-18 = Vegetables/Legumes H-28 = Nuts/Seeds H-30 = Vegetarian H-32 = Dairy H-40 = Eggs H-40 = Seafood H-42 = Meats H-46 = Poultry
18 = Processed Meats H-50 = Beverages H-52 = Fats/Oils H-54 = Sweets H-56 = Spices/Condiments/Sauces H-60 = Mixed Foods/Soups/Sandwiches H-66 = Fast Food H-84 = Convenience H-86 = Baby Foods

Chol (mg)	Calc (mg)	Iron (mg)	Magn (mg)	Pota (mg)	Sodi (mg)	Zinc (mg)	Vit A (μg)	Thia (mg)	Vit E (mg α)	Ribo (mg)	Niac (mg)	Vit B_6 (mg)	Fola (μg)	Vit C (mg)	Vit B_{12} (μg)	Sele (μg)
0	1	0	0	28.5	11.8	0.0	0.1	0	0.12	0	0	0	0	0	0	0.2
0	0	0.01	0.1	0.8	1.2	0.0	0.3	0	0.05	0	0	0	0	0	0	0.1
0	0	0	0	0.8	2.7	0.0	0.2	0	0.04	0	0	0	0	0	0	0.1
10	284	0.12	27.0	370.0	257.3	1.03	34.3	0.08	0.12	0.38	0.14	0.08	12.3	2.5	0.5	4.9
12	305	0.07	26.8	366.0	107.4	1.02	141.5	0.05	0.02	0.45	0.23	0.09	12.2	0	1.1	8.1
10	314	0.12	34.3	396.9	127.4	0.98	144.6	0.10		0.42	0.22	0.11	12.3	2.5	0.9	5.6
5	299	0.07	27.0	382.2	102.9	1.03	149.4	0.11	0.02	0.45	0.23	0.09	12.3	0	1.2	7.6
5	316	0.12	36.8	419.0	129.9	1.00	156.8	0.10	0.02	0.43	0.22	0.11	12.3	2.5	1.0	5.4
20	293	0.05	26.8	341.6	114.7	1.17	134.2	0.10	0.07	0.45	0.22	0.09	12.2	0.5	1.3	6.1
20	314	0.12	34.3	396.9	127.4	0.98	137.2	0.10	—	0.42	0.22	0.11	12.3	2.5	0.9	5.6
24	276	0.07	24.4	322.1	104.9	0.90	112.2	0.11	0.17	0.41	0.22	0.09	12.2	0	1.1	9.0
1	93	0.09	8.6	105.9	36.7	0.29	37.6	0.01	0	0.10	0.06	0.02	2.9	0.4	0.1	0.8
13	109	0.07	9.9	141.9	48.6	0.36	28.3	0.03	0.06	0.16	0.08	0.02	4.2	1.0	0.2	5.7
9	82	0.06	7.6	95.4	33.4	0.24	20.5	0.01	0.04	0.10	0.06	0.02	2.5	0.6	0.1	0.7
21	359	0.09	33.3	482.5	156.7	1.22	14.9	0.12	0.03	0.48	0.27	0.10	14.2	1.7	1.2	6.2
3	209	0.05	19.9	289.9	93.3	0.75	120.5	0.07	0	0.30	0.15	0.06	8.5	1.0	0.7	4.6
3	211	0.05	20.0	291.9	94.0	0.75	114.5	0.07	0	0.30	0.15	0.06	8.6	1.0	0.7	4.7
31	292	0.15	27.2	425.6	118.7	1.07	82.6	0.09	0.19	0.39	0.21	0.10	11.8	2.8	1.0	5.2
27	327	0.12	34.2	497.8	122.0	0.73	139.1	0.12	0.17	0.34	0.68	0.11	2.4	3.2	0.2	3.4
25	251	0.90	50.8	408.9	132.5	1.21	70.5	0.11	0.14	0.47	0.39	0.09	14.1	0	1.1	9.6
0	92	0.75	32.6	405.1	138.2	0.52	0	0.04	0	0.21	0.16	0.05	1.9	0	0.2	2.5
20	285	1.05	57.5	492.5	110.0	1.58	127.5	0.10	0.08	0.46	0.33	0.10	12.5	0.5	1.2	6.8
8	290	0.68	32.5	425.0	152.5	1.02	145.0	0.09	0.05	0.41	0.32	0.10	12.5	2.3	0.8	4.8
20	273	0.60	35.0	422.5	165.0	0.98	160.0	0.11	0.10	0.46	0.41	0.06	5.0	0	0.8	8.5
30	280	0.60	32.5	417.5	150.0	1.02	67.5	0.09	0.17	0.41	0.31	0.10	12.5	2.3	0.8	4.8
150	330	0.51	48.3	419.1	137.2	1.17	149.9	0.09	0.53	0.48	0.27	0.13	2.5	3.8	1.1	10.7
6	500	4.47	100.0	665.0	240.0	3.75	675.7	0.38	3.38	0.51	5.07	0.50	—	30.0	1.5	—
9	500	4.50	100.0	595.0	168.0	3.75	675.7	0.38	3.38	0.51	5.00	0.50	—	30.0	1.5	—
7	364	3.28	87.4	393.1	174.7	2.73	491.9	0.27	2.46	0.31	3.64	0.36	—	21.8	1.1	—
9	500	4.47	100.0	665.0	288.0	3.75	675.7	0.38	3.38	0.51	5.07	0.50	—	30.0	1.5	8.8
5	350	3.60	100.0	—	240.0	3.75	—	0.38	—	0.43	4.00	0.40	—	12.0	1.2	—
27	368	3.76	45.0	575.0	230.6	1.14	946.0	0.76	0.19	1.28	11.03	1.01	13.3	31.8	1.1	9.5
25	300	0.70	36.4	508.9	252.2	1.09	40.9	0.11	0.11	0.50	0.28	0.06	11.4	0	0.7	4.3
25	256	0.25	29.4	412.0	187.9	0.82	58.9	0.10	—	0.44	0.40	0.10	6.8	1.8	0.7	4.8
27	332	0.23	27.3	415.8	215.8	0.89	56.8	0.07	0.11	0.44	0.33	0.10	15.9	0	1.2	5.2
22	72	0.61	19.1	164.3	50.2	0.38	77.9	0.03	0.20	0.13	0.15	0.04	10.6	0.5	0.2	1.6
10	100	0.36	—	—	65.0	—	—	—	—	—	—	—	—	0	—	—
79	113	0.18	10.4	153.1	52.8	0.45	140.1	0.04	0.53	0.16	0.08	0.04	7.8	0.7	0.4	2.6
1	52	0.14	7.7	92.6	44.4	0.46	11.6	0.03	0.01	0.09	0.06	0.02	3.9	2.2	0.1	1.4
19	79	0.14	9.2	124.1	39.6	0.22	63.4	0.03	—	0.17	0.11	0.03	7.9	5.1	0.2	1.3

TABLE H-1 Table of Food Composition (*continued*) (Computer code is for Cengage Diet Analysis program) (For purposes of calculations, use "0" for t, <1, <0.1, 0.01)

DA+ Code	Food Description	Quantity	Measure	Wt (g)	H_2O (g)	Ener (kcal)	Prot (g)	Carb (g)	Fiber (g)	Fat (g)	Fat Breakdown (g) Sat	Mono	Poly
	Dairy—*continued*												
76	Vanilla	½	cup(s)	72	43.9	149	2.5	17.0	0.5	7.9	4.9	2.1	0.3
12146	Vanilla chocolate swirl, fat free, no sugar added	½	cup(s)	71	—	100	3.0	14.0	2.0	3.0	2.0	—	—
82	Vanilla, light	½	cup(s)	76	45.5	137	3.6	22.4	0.2	3.7	2.2	1.0	0.2
78	Vanilla, light, soft serve	½	cup(s)	88	61.2	111	4.3	19.2	0	2.3	1.4	0.7	0.1
	Soy desserts												
15726	Tofutti premium Better Pecan nondairy frozen dessert	½	cup(s)	70	—	210	1.0	21.0	0	13.0	2.0	—	—
15721	Tofutti premium Chocolate Supreme nondairy frozen dessert	½	cup(s)	70	—	180	3.0	18.0	0	11.0	2.0	—	—
15720	Tofutti premium vanilla non-dairy frozen dessert	½	cup(s)	70	—	210	2.0	21.0	0	13.0	2.0	—	—
	Ice milk												
16517	Chocolate	½	cup(s)	74	45.5	138	3.7	19.0	0.6	5.3	3.2	1.5	0.2
16516	Flavored, not chocolate	½	cup(s)	74	44.3	133	3.5	21.8	0.2	3.6	2.2	0.9	0.2
	Pudding												
25032	Chocolate	½	cup(s)	144	109.8	153	5.2	22.7	0.8	5.3	3.1	2.2	0.3
1923	Chocolate, sugar free, prepared with 2% milk	½	cup(s)	133	—	100	5.0	14.0	0.3	3.0	1.5	—	—
1722	Rice	½	cup(s)	113	75.5	151	4.1	30.0	0.4	1.9	1.1	0.5	0.1
4747	Tapioca, ready to eat	1	item(s)	142	102.0	185	2.8	30.8	0	5.5	1.4	3.6	0.1
25031	Vanilla	½	cup(s)	136	109.7	116	4.6	17.6	0	2.9	1.7	1.5	0.3
1924	Vanilla, sugar free, prepared with 2% milk	½	cup(s)	133	—	90	4.0	12.0	0.2	2.0	1.5	—	—
	Frozen yogurt												
4785	Chocolate, soft serve	½	cup(s)	72	45.9	115	2.9	17.9	1.6	4.3	2.6	1.3	0.2
29649	Flavors other than chocolate, nonfat	½	cup(s)	80	52.1	103	3.5	22.2	5.9	0	0	0	0
4786	Vanilla, soft serve	½	cup(s)	72	47.0	114	2.9	17.4	0	4.0	2.5	1.1	0.2
	Milk substitutes												
	Lactose free												
16081	Fat free, calcium fortified milk	1	cup(s)	240	—	90	8.0	13.0	0	0	0	0	0
36486	Low fat milk	1	cup(s)	240	—	110	8.0	13.0	0	2.5	1.5	—	—
36487	Reduced fat milk	1	cup(s)	240	—	130	8.0	13.0	0	5.0	3.0	—	—
36488	Whole milk	1	cup(s)	240	—	160	8.0	13.0	0	8.0	5.0	—	—
	Rice												
10083	Rice Dream carob rice beverage	1	cup(s)	240	—	150	1.0	30.0	0.5	2.5	0	1.5	0.5
17089	Rice Dream original rice beverage, enriched	1	cup(s)	240	—	120	1.0	23.0	0	2.5	0	1.5	0.5
10087	Rice Dream vanilla enriched rice beverage	1	cup(s)	240	—	130	1.0	26.0	0	2.5	0	1.5	0.5
	Soy												
66705	Silk chocolate soymilk	1	cup(s)	243	209.9	140	5.0	23.0	2.0	3.0	0.5	1.0	1.5
66710	Silk DHA omega-3 enriched soymilk	1	cup(s)	243	221.4	110	7.0	8.0	1.0	5.0	0.5	1.0	3.0
66703	Silk soymilk, unsweetened	1	cup(s)	243	226.4	80	7.0	4.0	1.0	4.0	0.5	1.0	2.5
66704	Silk vanilla soymilk	1	cup(s)	243	221.9	100	6.0	10.0	1.0	3.5	0.5	1.0	2.0
34750	Soy Dream chocolate enriched soy beverage	1	cup(s)	240	205.5	150	7.0	21.0	3.0	4.0	0.5	1.0	2.5
34749	Soy Dream vanilla enriched soy beverage	1	cup(s)	240	213.5	120	7.0	14.0	2.0	4.0	0.5	1.0	2.5
	Yogurt												
3615	Custard style, fruit flavors	6	ounce(s)	170	—	180	7.0	31.0	0	2.5	1.5	—	—
3617	Custard style, vanilla	6	ounce(s)	170	—	180	7.0	31.0	0	2.5	1.5	—	—
32101	Fruit, low fat	1	cup(s)	245	184.5	243	9.8	45.7	0	2.8	1.8	0.8	0.1
29638	Fruit, non fat, sweetened with low calorie sweetener	1	cup(s)	241	210.3	108	9.0	19.0	1.0	0.4	0.2	0.1	0
68613	Greek style, vanilla	1	cup(s)	245	—	173	23.0	18.7	0	0	0	0	0
93	Plain, low fat	1	cup(s)	245	208.4	154	12.9	17.2	0	3.8	2.5	1.0	0.1
94	Plain, nonfat	1	cup(s)	245	208.8	137	14.0	18.8	0	0.4	0.3	0.1	0
32100	Vanilla, low fat	1	cup(s)	245	193.6	208	12.1	33.8	0	3.1	2.0	0.8	0.1
5242	Yogurt beverage	1	cup(s)	245	199.8	172	5.9	28.7	0	3.7	2.5	0.6	0.1
	Soy yogurt												
29767	Silk blueberry cultured soy yogurt	5.3	ounce(s)	150	117.5	132	3.5	25.6	0.9	1.8	0	0.4	0.9

E KEY: H-4 = Breads/Baked Goods H-8 = Cereal/Rice/Pasta H-14 = Fruit H-18 = Vegetables/Legumes H-28 = Nuts/Seeds H-30 = Vegetarian H-32 = Dairy H-40 = Eggs H-40 = Seafood H-42 = Meats H-46 = Poultry
8 = Processed Meats H-50 = Beverages H-52 = Fats/Oils H-54 = Sweets H-56 = Spices/Condiments/Sauces H-60 = Mixed Foods/Soups/Sandwiches H-66 = Fast Food H-84 = Convenience H-86 = Baby Foods

Chol (mg)	Calc (mg)	Iron (mg)	Magn (mg)	Pota (mg)	Sodi (mg)	Zinc (mg)	Vit A (μg)	Thia (mg)	Vit E (mg α)	Ribo (mg)	Niac (mg)	Vit B_6 (mg)	Fola (μg)	Vit C (mg)	Vit B_{12} (μg)	Sele (μg)
32	92	0.06	10.1	143.3	57.6	0.50	85.0	0.03	0.22	0.17	0.08	0.03	3.6	0.4	0.3	1.3
10	100	0	—	—	65.0	—	—	—	—	—	—	—	—	0	—	—
21	122	0.14	10.6	158.1	56.2	0.55	97.3	0.04	0.09	0.19	0.10	0.03	4.6	0.9	0.4	1.5
11	138	0.05	12.3	194.5	61.6	0.47	25.5	0.05	0.05	0.17	0.10	0.04	4.4	0.8	0.4	3.2
0	0	0	—	22.0	220.0	—	—	—	—	—	—	—	—	0	—	—
0	0	0	—	—	180.0	—	—	—	—	—	—	—	—	0	—	—
0	0	0	—	—	130.0	—	—	—	—	—	—	—	—	0	—	—
21	118	0.51	14.8	125.8	52.5	0.32	52.5	0.02	0.15	0.09	0.09	0.02	3.0	0.9	0.1	1.6
20	119	0.14	10.4	153.9	54.8	0.54	94.7	0.04	0.09	0.19	0.10	0.03	4.4	0.9	0.3	1.5
35	149	0.95	28.6	211.0	134.8	1.07	0	0.06	0.11	0.25	0.18	0.05	9.9	0.2	0.7	5.4
10	150	0.72	—	330.0	310.0	—	—	0.06	—	0.26	—	—	—	0	—	—
7	115	0.27	15.8	194.6	72.0	0.58	24.8	0.04	0.05	0.18	0.34	0.06	4.5	0.2	0.3	4.3
1	101	0.16	8.5	130.6	205.9	0.31	0	0.03	0.21	0.14	0.09	0.03	4.3	0.4	0.3	0
35	144	0.16	13.8	173.2	133.7	0.63	0	0.05	0.09	0.24	0.11	0.05	8.7	0.2	0.7	5.0
10	150	0	—	190.0	380.0	—	—	0.03	—	0.17	—	—	—	0	—	—
4	106	0.90	19.4	187.9	70.6	0.35	31.7	0.03	—	0.15	0.22	0.05	7.9	0.2	0.2	1.7
0	117	0	7.2	155.8	87.4	0.25	105.7	0.02	0	0.10	0.06	0.02	3.2	0	0.4	1.5
1	103	0.22	10.1	151.9	62.6	0.30	42.5	0.03	0.08	0.16	0.21	0.06	4.3	0.6	0.2	2.4
3	500	0	—	410.0	125.0	—	150.1	—	—	0.43	—	—	—	0	0.9	—
15	300	0	—	410.0	125.0	—	150.1	—	—	0.43	—	—	—	0	0.9	—
20	300	0	—	410.0	125.0	—	150.1	—	—	0.43	—	—	—	0	0.9	—
35	300	0	—	410.0	125.0	—	90.1	—	—	0.43	—	—	—	0	0.9	—
0	0	0	—	0	80.0	—	0	—	0.80	—	—	—	—	0	—	—
0	300	0.72	—	0	100.0	—	25.0	—	—	—	—	—	—	0	1.5	—
0	300	0.36	—	0	105.0	—	25.0	—	—	—	—	—	—	0	1.5	—
0	300	1.44	40.0	350.0	100.0	0.60	25.0	—	—	0.51	—	—	—	0	3.0	4.2
0	350	1.08	40.0	350.0	120.0	1.50	50.0	—	—	0.51	—	0.60	—	21.0	3.0	5.6
0	300	1.08	40.0	300.0	85.0	0.60	25.0	—	—	0.51	—	—	—	0	3.0	5.6
0	300	1.08	40.0	300.0	95.0	0.60	25.0	—	—	0.51	—	—	—	0	3.0	5.6
0	400	1.80	60.0	290.0	125.0	0.75	25.0	0.15	5.03	0.63	1.20	0.20	—	0	3.0	11.2
0	350	8.10	60.0	250.0	135.0	0.62	25.0	0.15	5.03	0.44	1.02	0.20	21.6	0	3.0	5.5
15	300	0	—	290.0	110.0	—	—	—	—	—	—	—	—	0	—	—
15	300	0	—	290.0	110.0	—	—	—	—	—	—	—	—	0	—	—
12	338	0.15	31.9	433.6	129.9	1.64	27.0	0.08	0.05	0.40	0.21	0.09	22.0	1.5	1.1	6.9
5	323	0.58	33.7	470.0	127.7	1.57	4.8	0.09	0.14	0.38	0.42	0.10	26.5	21.9	1.0	6.7
0	288	0	—	—	108.0	—	—	—	—	—	—	—	—	0	—	—
15	448	0.20	41.7	573.3	171.5	2.18	34.3	0.11	0.07	0.52	0.28	0.12	27.0	2.0	1.4	8.1
5	488	0.22	46.5	624.8	188.6	2.38	4.9	0.12	0	0.57	0.30	0.13	29.4	2.2	1.5	8.8
12	419	0.17	39.2	536.5	161.7	2.03	29.4	0.10	0.05	0.49	0.26	0.11	27.0	2.0	1.3	12.0
15	225	0.22	27.0	303.8	95.6	1.10	14.7	0.11	0	0.27	0.30	0.15	29.4	2.1	0.7	—
0	265	0.95	—	—	22.1	—	—	—	—	—	—	—	—	26.5	—	—

DA+ Code	Food Description	Quantity	Measure	Wt (g)	H_2O (g)	Ener (kcal)	Prot (g)	Carb (g)	Fiber (g)	Fat (g)	Fat Breakdown (g)		
											Sat	Mono	Poly
Dairy—*continued*													
34617	Stonyfield Farm O'Soy strawberry-peach pack organic cultured soy yogurt	1	item(s)	113	—	100	5.0	15.0	1.0	2.0	0	—	—
34616	Stonyfield Farm O'Soy vanilla organic cultured soy yogurt	1	item(s)	170	—	150	7.0	24.0	1.0	3.0	0	—	—
Eggs													
	Eggs												
99	Fried	1	item(s)	46	32.0	90	6.3	0.4	0	6.8	2.0	2.8	1.5
100	Hard boiled	1	item(s)	50	37.3	78	6.3	0.6	0	5.3	1.6	2.0	0.7
101	Poached	1	item(s)	50	37.9	72	6.3	0.4	0	4.7	1.6	1.8	1.0
97	Raw, white	1	item(s)	33	28.9	17	3.6	0.2	0	0.1	0	0	0
96	Raw, whole	1	item(s)	50	38.1	72	6.3	0.4	0	4.8	1.6	1.8	1.0
98	Raw, yolk	1	item(s)	17	8.9	55	2.7	0.6	0	4.5	1.6	2.0	0.7
102	Scrambled, prepared with milk and butter	2	item(s)	122	93.2	182	12.2	2.0	0	13.4	4.1	5.4	3.0
	Egg substitutes												
4028	Egg Beaters	¼	cup(s)	61	—	30	6.0	1.0	0	0	0	0	0
920	Frozen	¼	cup(s)	60	43.9	96	6.8	1.9	0	6.7	1.2	1.5	3.7
918	Liquid	¼	cup(s)	63	51.9	53	7.5	0.4	0	2.1	0.4	0.6	1.0
Seafood													
	Cod												
1573	Atlantic cod, cooked, dry heat	3	ounce(s)	85	64.6	89	19.4	0	0	0.7	0.1	0.1	0.2
6040	Atlantic cod or scrod, baked or broiled	3	ounce(s)	85	64.6	89	19.4	0	0	0.7	0.1	0.1	0.2
2905	**Eel, raw**	3	ounce(s)	85	58.0	156	15.7	0	0	9.9	2.0	6.1	0.8
	Fish fillets												
25079	Baked	3	ounce(s)	85	79.9	99	21.7	0	0	0.7	0.1	0.1	0.3
8615	Batter coated or breaded, fried	3	ounce(s)	85	45.6	197	12.5	14.4	0.4	10.5	2.4	2.2	5.3
25082	Broiled fish steaks	3	ounce(s)	85	68.1	128	24.2	0	0	2.6	0.4	0.9	0.8
25083	Poached fish steaks	3	ounce(s)	85	67.1	111	21.1	0	0	2.3	0.3	0.8	0.7
25084	Steamed	3	ounce(s)	85	72.2	79	17.2	0	0	0.6	0.1	0.1	0.2
25089	**Flounder, baked**	3	ounce(s)	85	64.4	113	14.8	0.4	0.1	5.5	1.1	2.2	1.4
1825	**Grouper, cooked, dry heat**	3	ounce(s)	85	62.4	100	21.1	0	0	1.1	0.3	0.2	0.3
	Haddock												
6049	Baked or broiled	3	ounce(s)	85	63.1	95	20.6	0	0	0.8	0.1	0.1	0.3
1578	Cooked, dry heat	3	ounce(s)	85	67.7	77	17.0	0	0	0.5	0.1	0.1	0.2
1886	**Halibut, Atlantic and Pacific, cooked, dry heat**	3	ounce(s)	85	64.7	94	19.2	0	0	1.4	0.3	0.5	0.3
1582	**Herring, Atlantic, pickled**	4	piece(s)	60	33.1	157	8.5	5.8	0	10.8	1.4	7.2	1.0
1587	**Jack mackerel, solids, canned, drained**	2	ounce(s)	57	39.2	88	13.1	0	0	3.6	1.1	1.3	0.9
8580	**Octopus, common, cooked, moist heat**	3	ounce(s)	85	51.4	139	25.4	3.7	0	1.8	0.4	0.3	0.4
1831	**Perch, mixed species, cooked, dry heat**	3	ounce(s)	85	62.3	99	21.1	0	0	1.0	0.2	0.2	0.4
1592	**Pacific rockfish, cooked, dry heat**	3	ounce(s)	85	63.5	93	18.9	0	0	1.4	0.4	0.4	0.4
	Salmon												
1594	Broiled or baked with butter	3	ounce(s)	85	53.9	155	22.9	0	0	6.3	1.2	2.3	2.3
2938	Coho, farmed, raw	3	ounce(s)	85	59.9	136	18.1	0	0	6.5	1.5	2.8	1.6
75533	Pink, canned, boneless, drained	3	ounce(s)	85	60.1	116	20.9	0	0	3.6	0.6	0.8	1.1
50124	Pink, canned, with bones, drained	3	ounce(s)	85	60.1	117	19.6	0.0	0	4.3	0.8	1.0	1.3
75532	Red (sockeye), canned, boneless, drained	3	ounce(s)	85	57.6	134	22.4	0	0	5.0	1.0	1.6	1.3
33210	Red (sockeye), canned, with bones, no salt, drained	3	ounce(s)	85	58.4	130	17.4	0	0	6.2	1.4	2.4	1.9
29727	Smoked chinook (lox)	2	ounce(s)	57	40.8	66	10.4	0	0.0	2.4	0.5	1.1	0.6
154	**Sardines, Atlantic with bones, canned in oil**	3	ounce(s)	85	50.7	177	20.9	0	0	9.7	1.3	3.3	4.4
	Scallops												
155	Mixed species, breaded, fried	3	item(s)	47	27.2	100	8.4	4.7	—	5.1	1.2	2.1	1.3
1599	Steamed	3	ounce(s)	85	69.7	59	10.2	2.7	0	0.4	0.1	0	0.1
1839	**Snapper, mixed species, cooked, dry heat**	3	ounce(s)	85	59.8	109	22.4	0	0	1.5	0.3	0.3	0.5
	Squid												
1868	Mixed species, fried	3	ounce(s)	85	54.9	149	15.3	6.6	0	6.4	1.6	2.3	1.8
16617	Steamed or boiled	3	ounce(s)	85	63.3	89	15.2	3.0	0	1.3	0.3	0.1	0.5

KEY: H-4 = Breads/Baked Goods H-8 = Cereal/Rice/Pasta H-14 = Fruit H-18 = Vegetables/Legumes H-28 = Nuts/Seeds H-30 = Vegetarian H-32 = Dairy H-40 = Eggs H-40 = Seafood H-42 = Meats H-46 = Poultry 3 = Processed Meats H-50 = Beverages H-52 = Fats/Oils H-54 = Sweets H-56 = Spices/Condiments/Sauces H-60 = Mixed Foods/Soups/Sandwiches H-66 = Fast Food H-84 = Convenience H-86 = Baby Foods

Chol (mg)	Calc (mg)	Iron (mg)	Magn (mg)	Pota (mg)	Sodi (mg)	Zinc (mg)	Vit A (µg)	Thia (mg)	Vit E (mg α)	Ribo (mg)	Niac (mg)	Vit B_6 (mg)	Fola (µg)	Vit C (mg)	Vit B_{12} (µg)	Sele (µg)
0	100	1.08	32.0	220.0	25.0	—	—	0.22	—	0.10	—	0.08	—	0	0	—
0	150	1.44	40.0	310.0	40.0	—	—	0.38	—	0.17	—	0.08	—	0	0	—
184	29	0.87	6.0	69.9	95.2	0.64	100.7	0.02	0.60	0.23	0.04	0.08	23.5	0	0.4	15.2
187	25	0.60	5.0	63.0	62.0	0.52	74.5	0.03	0.51	0.26	0.03	0.06	22.0	0	0.6	15.4
185	28	0.88	6.0	69.0	148.5	0.64	80.0	0.02	0.52	0.19	0.03	0.07	17.5	0	0.4	15.3
0	2	0.03	3.6	53.8	54.8	0.01	0.0	0	0	0.14	0.03	0	1.3	0	0	6.6
186	28	0.88	6.0	69.0	71.0	0.64	80.0	0.02	0.52	0.23	0.04	0.09	23.5	0	0.4	15.4
184	22	0.46	0.9	18.5	8.2	0.39	64.8	0.03	0.44	0.09	0.00	0.06	24.8	0	0.3	9.5
338	81	1.60	13.4	161.0	176.9	1.27	196.4	0.05	1.40	0.46	0.09	0.16	43.9	0	0.9	28.7
0	20	1.08	—	95.0	115.0	0.60	225.0	0.15	—	0.85	—	0.08	—	0	1.2	
1	44	1.19	9.0	127.8	119.4	0.59	6.6	0.07	0.95	0.23	0.08	0.08	9.6	0.3	0.2	24.8
1	33	1.32	5.6	207.1	111.1	0.82	11.3	0.07	0.17	0.19	0.07	0	9.4	0	0.2	15.6
47	12	0.42	35.7	207.5	66.3	0.49	11.9	0.07	0.69	0.07	2.14	0.24	6.8	0.9	0.9	32.0
47	12	0.42	35.7	207.5	66.3	0.49	11.9	0.07	0.69	0.07	2.14	0.24	6.8	0.9	0.9	32.0
107	17	0.43	17.0	231.3	43.4	1.38	886.9	0.13	3.40	0.03	2.98	0.06	12.8	1.5	2.6	5.5
44	8	0.32	29.1	489.0	86.1	0.49	0	0.03	0.78	0.05	2.48	0.46	8.5	3.0	1.0	44.3
29	15	1.79	20.4	272.1	452.4	0.37	9.4	0.09	—	0.09	1.79	0.09	17.0	0	0.9	7.7
37	55	0.98	96.7	524.3	62.9	0.49	0	0.06	0.99	0.08	6.81	0.36	14.0	0	1.2	42.5
32	48	0.85	84.0	455.6	54.7	0.43	0	0.06	0.86	0.08	5.92	0.33	12.1	0	1.1	37.0
41	12	0.29	24.7	319.3	41.8	0.35	0	0.07	0.62	0.06	1.89	0.21	6.8	0.8	0.8	32.0
44	19	0.35	47.3	224.7	280.2	0.21	0	0.06	0.42	0.08	2.03	0.19	7.8	2.8	1.6	33.5
40	18	0.97	31.5	403.9	45.1	0.43	42.5	0.07	—	0.01	0.32	0.30	8.5	0	0.6	39.8
63	36	1.15	42.5	339.3	74.0	0.41	16.2	0.03	0.43	0.04	3.94	0.29	6.8	0	1.2	34.4
56	12	0.18	22.1	298.5	222.0	0.34	17.9	0.02	0.47	0.06	3.50	0.28	11.1	0	1.8	27.0
51	8	0.17	23.8	449.0	69.7	0.37	20.4	0.05	0.63	0.03	6.73	0.54	11.9	0	1.1	47.1
8	46	0.73	4.8	41.4	522.0	0.32	154.8	0.02	1.03	0.08	1.98	0.10	1.2	0	2.6	35.1
45	137	1.16	21.0	110.0	214.9	0.58	73.7	0.02	0.58	0.12	3.50	0.12	2.8	0.5	3.9	21.4
82	90	8.11	51.0	535.8	391.2	2.86	76.5	0.05	1.02	0.06	3.21	0.55	20.4	6.8	30.6	76.2
98	87	0.99	32.3	292.5	67.2	1.22	8.5	0.07	—	0.10	1.62	0.12	5.1	1.4	1.9	13.7
52	14	0.31	28.1	397.1	75.7	0.37	4.3	0.02	0.37	0.19	2.46	0.20	8.5	0	1.4	64.8
40	15	1.02	26.9	376.5	98.6	0.56		0.14	1.15	0.05	8.33	0.19	—	1.8	2.3	41.0
43	10	0.29	26.4	382.7	40.0	0.37	47.6	0.08	—	0.09	5.79	0.56	11.1	0.9	2.3	10.7
71	51	0.48	20.4	277.3	321.5	0.55	17.0	0.02	1.09	0.17	6.32	0.09	3.4	0	4.2	33.7
71	241	0.65	27.2	283.2	324.0	0.82	17.0	0.02	1.09	0.17	6.30	0.09	3.4	0	4.2	33.6
56	31	0.41	20.4	265.4	328.3	0.49	47.6	0.03	1.78	0.18	6.54	0.10	3.4	0	4.7	29.4
37	203	0.90	24.7	320.6	63.8	0.87	45.1	0.01	—	0.16	4.66	0.26	8.5	0	0.3	30.1
13	6	0.48	10.2	99.2	1133.8	0.18	14.7	0.01	—	0.06	2.68	0.16	1.1	0	1.8	21.6
121	325	2.48	33.2	337.6	429.5	1.11	27.2	0.07	1.74	0.19	4.46	0.14	8.5	0	7.6	44.8
25	20	0.38	27.4	154.8	215.8	0.49	10.2	0.02	—	0.05	0.70	0.07	23.3	1.1	0.6	12.5
20	5	0.29	18.7	155.6	547.7	0.76	0.8	0.01	0	0.01	0.53	0.06	10.2	0	1.1	10.8
40	34	0.20	31.5	443.9	48.5	0.37	29.8	0.05	—	0	0.29	0.39	5.1	1.4	3.0	41.7
221	33	0.86	32.3	237.3	260.2	1.48	9.4	0.05	—	0.39	2.21	0.05	17.0	3.6	1.0	44.1
227	31	0.63	28.9	192.2	356.3	1.50	8.5	0.01	1.17	0.32	1.70	0.04	3.4	3.2	1.0	43.7

TABLE H-1 Table of Food Composition (*continued*)

(Computer code is for Cengage Diet Analysis program) (For purposes of calculations, use "0" for t, <1, <0.1, 0.01)

DA+ Code	Food Description	Quantity	Measure	Wt (g)	H_2O (g)	Ener (kcal)	Prot (g)	Carb (g)	Fiber (g)	Fat (g)	Fat Breakdown (g)		
											Sat	Mono	Poly
	Seafood—*continued*												
1570	**Striped bass, cooked, dry heat**	3	ounce(s)	85	62.4	105	19.3	0	0	2.5	0.6	0.7	0.9
1601	**Sturgeon, steamed**	3	ounce(s)	85	59.6	111	17.0	0	0	4.3	1.0	2.0	0.7
1840	**Surimi, formed**	3	ounce(s)	85	64.9	84	12.9	5.8	0	0.8	0.2	0.1	0.4
1842	**Swordfish, cooked, dry heat**	3	ounce(s)	85	58.0	146	19.9	0	0	6.7	1.6	3.0	1.2
1846	**Tuna, yellowfin or ahi, raw**	3	ounce(s)	85	63.0	93	20.7	0	0	0.4	0.1	0.1	0.1
	Tuna, canned												
159	Light, canned in oil, drained	2	ounce(s)	57	33.9	112	16.5	0	0	4.7	0.9	1.7	1.6
355	Light, canned in water, drained	2	ounce(s)	57	44.3	49	11.0	0	0	0.5	0.1	0.1	0.2
33211	Light, no salt, canned in oil, drained	2	ounce(s)	57	33.9	112	16.5	0	0	4.7	0.9	1.7	1.6
33212	Light, no salt, canned in water, drained	2	ounce(s)	57	42.6	66	14.5	0	0	0.5	0.1	0.1	0.2
2961	White, canned in oil, drained	2	ounce(s)	57	36.3	105	15.0	0	0	4.6	0.7	1.8	1.7
351	White, canned in water, drained	2	ounce(s)	57	41.5	73	13.4	0	0	1.7	0.4	0.4	0.6
33213	White, no salt, canned in oil, drained	2	ounce(s)	57	36.3	105	15.0	0	0	4.6	0.9	1.4	1.9
33214	White, no salt, canned in water, drained	2	ounce(s)	57	42.0	73	13.4	0	0	1.7	0.4	0.4	0.6
	Yellowtail												
8548	Mixed species, cooked, dry heat	3	ounce(s)	85	57.3	159	25.2	0	0	5.7	1.4	2.2	1.5
2970	Mixed species, raw	2	ounce(s)	57	42.2	83	13.1	0	0	3.0	0.7	1.1	0.8
	Shellfish, meat only												
1857	Abalone, mixed species, fried	3	ounce(s)	85	51.1	161	16.7	9.4	0	5.8	1.4	2.3	1.4
16618	Abalone, steamed or poached	3	ounce(s)	85	40.7	177	28.9	10.1	0	1.3	0.3	0.2	0.2
	Crab												
1851	Blue crab, canned	2	ounce(s)	57	45.2	47	10.1	0	0	0.4	0.1	0.1	0.1
1852	Blue crab, cooked, moist heat	3	ounce(s)	85	67.8	71	15.2	0	0	0.6	0.2	0.1	0.2
8562	Dungeness crab, cooked, moist heat	3	ounce(s)	85	62.3	94	19.0	0.8	0	1.1	0.1	0.2	0.3
1860	**Clams, cooked, moist heat**	3	ounce(s)	85	54.1	126	21.7	4.4	0	1.7	0.2	0.1	0.5
1853	**Crayfish, farmed, cooked, moist heat**	3	ounce(s)	85	68.7	74	14.9	0	0	1.1	0.2	0.2	0.4
	Oysters												
8720	Baked or broiled	3	ounce(s)	85	71.6	77	4.5	2.2	0	5.4	1.1	2.1	1.6
152	Eastern, farmed, raw	3	ounce(s)	85	73.3	50	4.4	4.7	0	1.3	0.4	0.1	0.5
8715	Eastern, wild, cooked, moist heat	3	ounce(s)	85	66.5	87	9.7	4.6	0	2.9	0.8	0.4	0.9
8584	Pacific, cooked, moist heat	3	ounce(s)	85	54.5	139	16.1	8.4	0	3.9	0.9	0.7	1.5
1865	Pacific, raw	3	ounce(s)	85	69.8	69	8.0	4.2	0	2.0	0.4	0.3	0.8
1854	**Lobster, northern, cooked, moist heat**	3	ounce(s)	85	66.4	76	16.2	0	0	0.7	0.2	0.2	0.3
1862	**Mussels, blue, cooked, moist heat**	3	ounce(s)	85	52.0	146	20.2	6.3	0	3.8	0.7	0.9	1.0
	Shrimp												
158	Mixed species, breaded, fried	3	ounce(s)	85	45.0	206	18.2	9.8	0.3	10.4	1.8	3.2	4.3
1855	Mixed species, cooked, moist heat	3	ounce(s)	85	60.9	101	19.4	1.3	0	1.4	0.4	0.3	0.5
	Beef, Lamb, Pork												
	Beef												
4450	Breakfast strips, cooked	2	slice(s)	23	5.9	101	7.1	0.3	0	7.8	3.2	3.8	0.4
174	Corned beef, canned	3	ounce(s)	85	49.1	213	23.0	0	0	12.7	5.3	5.1	0.5
33147	Cured, thin siced	2	ounce(s)	57	32.9	100	15.9	3.2	0	2.2	0.9	1.0	0.1
4581	Jerky	1	ounce(s)	28	6.6	116	9.4	3.1	0.5	7.3	3.1	3.2	0.3
	Ground beef												
5898	Lean, broiled, medium	3	ounce(s)	85	50.4	202	21.6	0	0	12.2	4.8	5.3	0.5
5899	Lean, broiled, well done	3	ounce(s)	85	48.4	214	23.8	0	0	12.5	5.0	5.7	0.3
5914	Regular, broiled, medium	3	ounce(s)	85	46.1	246	20.5	0	0	17.6	6.9	7.7	0.7
5915	Regular, broiled, well done	3	ounce(s)	85	43.8	259	21.6	0	0	18.4	7.5	8.5	0.5
	Beef rib												
4241	Rib, small end, separable lean, 0" fat, broiled	3	ounce(s)	85	53.2	164	25.0	0.0	0	6.4	2.4	2.6	0.2
4183	Rib, whole, lean and fat, 1/4" fat, roasted	3	ounce(s)	85	39.0	320	18.9	0.0	0	26.6	10.7	11.4	0.9
	Beef roast												
16981	Bottom round, choice, separable lean and fat, 1/8" fat, braised	3	ounce(s)	85	46.2	216	27.9	0	0	10.7	4.1	4.6	0.4

Chol (mg)	Calc (mg)	Iron (mg)	Magn (mg)	Pota (mg)	Sodi (mg)	Zinc (mg)	Vit A (µg)	Thia (mg)	Vit E (mg α)	Ribo (mg)	Niac (mg)	Vit B_6 (mg)	Fola (µg)	Vit C (mg)	Vit B_{12} (µg)	Sele (µg)
88	16	0.92	43.4	278.9	74.8	0.43	26.4	0.10	—	0.03	2.18	0.29	8.5	0	3.8	39.8
64	11	0.59	29.8	239.8	316.3	0.36	199.8	0.07	0.53	0.07	8.33	0.19	14.5	0	2.2	13.3
26	8	0.22	36.6	95.2	121.6	0.28	17.0	0.02	0.54	0.02	0.19	0.03	1.7	0	1.4	23.9
66	5	0.38	29.8	424.3	82.5	0.66	36.6	0.08	2.05	0.05	7.87	0.52	1.7	0	1.4	58.3
33	3	0.65	29.8	375.0	38.3	0.31	15.3	0.10	0.20	0.10	15.71	0.79	1.7	0	1.8	77.0
10	7	0.79	17.6	117.3	200.6	0.51	13.0	0.02	0.49	0.07	7.03	0.06	2.8	0	1.2	43.1
20	10	0.92	13.0	101.4	140.0	0.39	9.6	0.02	0.19	0.05	5.74	0.18	2.3	0	1.4	40.0
10	7	0.79	17.6	117.3	28.3	0.51	—	0.02	—	0.07	7.03	0.06	2.8	0	1.2	43.1
17	6	0.87	15.3	134.4	28.3	0.44	—	0.02	—	0.04	7.53	0.20	2.3	0	1.7	45.6
18	2	0.37	19.3	188.8	224.5	0.27	2.8	0.01	1.30	0.04	6.63	0.24	2.8	0	1.2	34.1
24	8	0.55	18.7	134.3	213.6	0.27	3.4	0	0.48	0.02	3.29	0.12	1.1	0	0.7	37.2
18	2	0.37	19.3	188.8	28.3	0.27	—	0.01	—	0.04	6.63	0.24	2.8	0	1.2	34.1
24	8	0.55	18.7	134.4	28.3	0.27	3.4	0	—	0.02	3.29	0.12	1.1	0	0.7	37.2
60	25	0.54	32.3	457.5	42.5	0.57	26.4	0.15		0.04	7.41	0.16	3.4	2.5	1.1	39.8
31	13	0.28	17.0	238.1	22.1	0.29	16.4	0.08	—	0.02	3.85	0.09	2.3	1.6	0.7	20.7
80	31	3.23	47.6	241.5	502.6	0.81	1.7	0.19	—	0.11	1.62	0.13	17.0	1.5	0.6	44.1
144	50	4.85	68.9	295.1	980.6	1.39	3.4	0.29	6.74	0.13	1.90	0.22	6.0	2.6	0.7	75.6
55	52	0.28	20.4	146.8	223.9	2.16	0.6	0.01	1.04	0.05	1.56	0.09	28.9	1.9	1.9	24.3
82	77	0.43	30.6	220.3	335.9	3.24	0.9	0.02	1.56	0.08	2.34	0.13	43.4	2.8	2.8	36.5
65	50	0.37	49.3	347.0	321.5	4.65	26.4	0.05	—	0.17	3.08	0.15	35.7	3.1	8.8	40.5
57	78	23.78	15.3	534.1	1022.2	2.32	145.4	0.13	—	0.36	2.85	0.09	24.7	18.8	84.1	54.4
117	43	0.94	28.1	202.4	82.5	1.26	12.8	0.04	—	0.07	1.42	0.11	9.4	0.4	2.6	29.1
31	48	3.67	14.5	125.0	308.7	31.26	49.3	0.01	1.12	0.06	0.70	0.02	5.1	0	6.6	15.6
21	37	4.92	28.1	105.5	151.4	32.25	6.8	0.09	—	0.06	1.08	0.05	15.3	4.0	13.8	54.2
67	99	7.83	29.8	118.2	141.2	66.84	22.1	0.03	1.45	0.15	1.57	0.05	11.9	0	14.9	33.6
85	14	7.82	37.4	256.8	180.3	28.27	124.2	0.11	0.72	0.38	3.08	0.08	12.8	10.9	24.5	131.0
43	7	4.35	18.7	142.9	90.1	14.13	68.9	0.06	—	0.20	1.71	0.04	8.5	6.8	13.6	65.5
124	82	0.25	36.6	195.6	413.3	3.44	0.8	0.02	0.85	0.01	1.56	0.10	9.4	0	1.2	62.2
48	28	5.71	31.5	227.9	313.8	2.27	77.4	0.26	—	0.36	2.55	0.09	64.6	11.6	20.4	76.2
117	57	1.07	34.0	191.4	292.6	1.17	47.6	0.11	1.11	0.12	2.61	0.08	33.2	1.3	1.6	35.5
179	77	0.27	31.5	144.6	805.3	1.39	76.5	0.03	1.87	0.02	2.28	0.21	20.4	0	1.4	42.1
27	2	0.71	6.1	93.1	509.2	1.44	0	0.02	0.07	0.06	1.46	0.07	1.8	0	0.8	6.1
73	10	1.77	11.9	115.7	762.8	3.04	0	0.02	0.13	0.13	2.07	0.11	7.7	0	1.4	36.5
23	6	1.53	10.8	243.2	815.8	2.26	0	0.05	0	0.11	2.99	0.19	6.2	0	1.5	16.0
14	6	1.54	14.5	169.2	590.0	2.30	0	0.04	0.14	0.04	0.49	0.05	38.0	0	0.3	3.0
58	6	2.00	17.9	266.2	59.5	4.64	0	0.05	—	0.23	4.22	0.23	7.7	0	1.8	16.0
69	12	2.21	18.5	250.0	62.4	5.87	0	0.09	—	0.24	5.10	0.16	9.4	0	1.7	19.1
62	9	2.08	17.0	248.3	70.6	4.41	0	0.03	—	0.16	4.91	0.23	7.7	0	2.5	16.2
71	12	2.30	18.5	242.4	72.4	5.19	0	0.09	—	0.23	4.93	0.18	8.5	0	1.6	18.0
77	16	1.59	21.3	319.8	51.9	4.64	0	0.07	0.34	0.13	7.16	0.54	8.5	0	1.4	29.2
72	9	1.96	16.2	251.7	53.6	4.46	0	0.06	—	0.14	2.86	0.20	6.0	0	2.1	18.7
86	6	2.30	17.9	223.7	35.7	4.59	0	0.06	0.42	0.16	5.05	0.37	8.5	0	1.7	29.3

DA+ Code	Food Description	Quantity	Measure	Wt (g)	H_2O (g)	Ener (kcal)	Prot (g)	Carb (g)	Fiber (g)	Fat (g)	Fat Breakdown (g) Sat	Mono	Poly
	Beef, Lamb, Pork—continued												
16979	Bottom round, separable lean and fat, 1/8" fat, roasted	3	ounce(s)	85	52.4	185	22.5	0	0	9.9	3.8	4.2	0.4
16924	Chuck, arm pot roast, separable lean and fat, 1/8" fat, braised	3	ounce(s)	85	42.9	257	25.6	0	0	16.3	6.5	7.0	0.6
16930	Chuck, blade roast, separable lean and fat, 1/8" fat, braised	3	ounce(s)	85	40.5	290	22.8	0	0	21.4	8.5	9.2	0.8
5853	Chuck, blade roast, separable lean, 0" trim, pot roasted	3	ounce(s)	85	47.4	202	26.4	0	0	10.0	3.9	4.3	0.3
4296	Eye of round, choice, separable lean, 0" fat, roasted	3	ounce(s)	85	56.5	138	24.4	0.0	0	3.7	1.3	1.5	0.1
16989	Eye of round, separable lean and fat, 1/8" fat, roasted	3	ounce(s)	85	52.2	180	24.2	0	0	8.5	3.2	3.6	0.3
	Beef steak												
4348	Short loin, t-bone steak, lean and fat, 1/4" fat, broiled	3	ounce(s)	85	43.2	274	19.4	0.0	0	21.2	8.3	9.6	0.8
4349	Short loin, t-bone steak, lean, 1/4" fat, broiled	3	ounce(s)	85	52.3	174	22.8	0.0	0	8.5	3.1	4.2	0.3
4360	Top loin, prime, lean and fat, 1/4" fat, broiled	3	ounce(s)	85	42.7	275	21.6	0.0	0	20.3	8.2	8.6	0.7
	Beef variety												
188	Liver, pan fried	3	ounce(s)	85	52.7	149	22.6	4.4	0	4.0	1.3	0.6	0.5
4447	Tongue, simmered	3	ounce(s)	85	49.2	242	16.4	0.0	0	19.0	6.9	8.6	0.6
	Lamb chop												
3275	Loin, domestic, lean and fat, 1/4" fat, broiled	3	ounce(s)	85	43.9	269	21.4	0	0	19.6	8.4	8.2	1.4
	Lamb leg												
3264	Domestic, lean and fat, 1/4" fat, cooked	3	ounce(s)	85	45.7	250	20.9	0	0	17.8	7.5	7.5	1.3
	Lamb rib												
182	Domestic, lean and fat, 1/4" fat, broiled	3	ounce(s)	85	40.0	307	18.8	0	0	25.2	10.8	10.3	2.0
183	Domestic, lean, 1/4" fat, broiled	3	ounce(s)	85	50.0	200	23.6	0	0	11.0	4.0	4.4	1.0
	Lamb shoulder												
186	Shoulder, arm and blade, domestic, choice, lean and fat, 1/4" fat, roasted	3	ounce(s)	85	47.8	235	19.1	0	0	17.0	7.2	6.9	1.4
187	Shoulder, arm and blade, domestic, choice, lean, 1/4" fat, roasted	3	ounce(s)	85	53.9	174	21.2	0	0	9.2	3.5	3.7	0.8
3287	Shoulder, arm, domestic, lean and fat, 1/4" fat, braised	3	ounce(s)	85	37.6	294	25.8	0	0	20.4	8.4	8.7	1.5
3290	Shoulder, arm, domestic, lean, 1/4" fat, braised	3	ounce(s)	85	41.9	237	30.2	0	0	12.0	4.3	5.2	0.8
	Lamb variety												
3375	Brain, pan fried	3	ounce(s)	85	51.6	232	14.4	0	0	18.9	4.8	3.4	1.9
3406	Tongue, braised	3	ounce(s)	85	49.2	234	18.3	0	0	17.2	6.7	8.5	1.1
	Pork, cured												
29229	Bacon, Canadian style, cured	2	ounce(s)	57	37.9	89	11.7	1.0	0	4.0	1.3	1.8	0.4
161	Bacon, cured, broiled, pan fried or roasted	2	slice(s)	16	2.0	87	5.9	0.2	0	6.7	2.2	3.0	0.7
42274	Bacon, cured, broiled, pan fried or roasted, reduced sodium	2	slice(s)	16	2.0	87	5.9	0.2	0	6.7	2.2	3.0	0.7
35422	Breakfast strips, cured, cooked	3	slice(s)	34	9.2	156	9.8	0.4	0	12.5	4.3	5.6	1.9
189	Ham, cured, boneless, 11% fat, roasted	3	ounce(s)	85	54.9	151	19.2	0	0	7.7	2.7	3.8	1.2
29215	Ham, cured, extra lean, 4% fat, canned	2	ounce(s)	57	41.7	68	10.5	0	0	2.6	0.9	1.3	0.2
1316	Ham, cured, extra lean, 5% fat, roasted	3	ounce(s)	85	57.5	123	17.8	1.3	0	4.7	1.5	2.2	0.5
16561	Ham, smoked or cured, lean, cooked	1	slice(s)	42	28.8	58	9.1	0.4	0	2.1	0.7	1.0	0.3
42257	Ham, smoked or cured, lean, cooked, low sodium	1	slice(s)	42	28.4	61	8.8	0.6	0	2.3	0.8	1.1	0.2
	Pork chop												
32671	Loin, blade, chops, lean and fat, pan fried	3	ounce(s)	85	49.3	218	21.3	0	0	14.1	3.8	4.3	1.7
32672	Loin, center cut, chops, lean and fat, pan fried	3	ounce(s)	85	49.7	202	23.5	0	0	11.3	4.1	4.7	1.8

Chol (mg)	Calc (mg)	Iron (mg)	Magn (mg)	Pota (mg)	Sodi (mg)	Zinc (mg)	Vit A (μg)	Thia (mg)	Vit E (mg α)	Ribo (mg)	Niac (mg)	Vit B_6 (mg)	Fola (μg)	Vit C (mg)	Vit B_{12} (μg)	Sele (μg)
72	5	1.84	14.5	182.0	29.8	3.77	0	0.05	0.35	0.12	3.93	0.30	6.8	0	1.3	23.0
102	14	2.15	17.0	205.8	42.5	5.94	0	0.05	0.45	0.15	3.63	0.25	7.7	0	1.9	24.1
88	11	2.66	16.2	198.1	55.3	7.15	0	0.06	0.17	0.20	2.07	0.22	4.3	0	1.9	20.9
73	11	3.13	19.6	223.7	60.4	8.73	0	0.07	—	0.24	2.27	0.25	5.1	0	2.1	22.7
63	5	2.17	16.2	200.7	32.3	4.29	0	0.05	0.31	0.15	4.70	0.34	8.5	0	1.4	28.0
73	5	1.98	15.3	193.0	31.5	3.95	0	0.05	0.35	0.14	4.38	0.32	7.7	0	1.5	25.2
58	7	2.56	17.9	233.9	57.8	3.56	0	0.08	0.19	0.18	3.29	0.28	6.0	0	1.8	10.0
50	5	3.11	22.1	278.1	65.5	4.35	0	0.09	0.12	0.21	3.94	0.33	6.8	0	1.9	8.5
67	8	1.89	19.6	294.2	53.6	3.85	0	0.07	—	0.15	3.96	0.31	6.0	0	1.6	19.5
324	5	5.25	18.7	298.5	65.5	4.45	6586.3	0.15	0.39	2.91	14.86	0.87	221.1	0.6	70.7	27.9
112	4	2.22	12.8	156.5	55.3	3.48	0	0.02	0.26	0.25	2.97	0.13	6.0	1.1	2.7	11.2
85	17	1.54	20.4	278.1	65.5	2.96	0	0.09	0.11	0.21	6.04	0.11	15.3	0	2.1	23.3
82	14	1.60	19.6	263.6	61.2	3.79	0	0.09	0.12	0.21	5.66	0.11	15.3	0	2.2	22.5
84	16	1.60	19.6	229.6	64.6	3.40	0	0.08	0.10	0.19	5.95	0.09	11.9	0	2.2	20.3
77	14	1.88	24.7	266.2	72.3	4.48	0	0.09	0.15	0.21	5.57	0.13	17.9	0	2.2	26.4
78	17	1.68	19.6	213.5	56.1	4.45	0	0.08	0.12	0.20	5.23	0.11	17.9	0	2.2	22.3
74	16	1.81	21.3	225.4	57.8	5.14	0	0.08	0.15	0.22	4.90	0.13	21.3	0	2.3	24.2
102	21	2.03	22.1	260.2	61.2	5.17	0	0.06	0.13	0.21	5.66	0.09	15.3	0	2.2	31.6
103	22	2.30	24.7	287.4	64.6	6.21	0	0.06	0.15	0.23	5.38	0.11	18.7	0	2.3	32.1
2129	18	1.73	18.7	304.4	133.5	1.70	0	0.14	—	0.31	3.87	0.20	6.0	19.6	20.5	10.2
161	9	2.24	13.6	134.4	57.0	2.54	0	0.07	—	0.36	3.14	0.14	2.6	6.0	5.4	23.8
28	5	0.39	9.6	195.0	512.5	0.79	0	0.43	0.12	0.10	3.53	0.22	2.3	0	0.4	14.2
18	2	0.23	5.3	90.4	274.7	0.56	1.8	0.06	0.05	0.04	1.78	0.06	0.3	0	0.2	9.9
18	2	0.23	5.3	90.4	164.8	0.56	1.8	0.06	0.05	0.04	1.78	0.06	0.3	0	0.2	9.9
36	5	0.67	8.8	158.4	713.7	1.25	0	0.25	0.09	0.13	2.58	0.12	1.4	0	0.6	8.4
50	7	1.14	18.7	347.9	1275.8	2.10	0	0.62	0.26	0.28	5.23	0.26	2.6	0	0.6	16.8
22	3	0.53	9.6	206.4	711.5	1.09	0	0.47	0.10	0.13	3.01	0.26	3.4	0	0.5	8.2
45	7	1.26	11.9	244.1	1023.0	2.45	0	0.64	0.21	0.17	3.42	0.34	2.6	0	0.6	16.6
22	3	0.37	8.4	131.5	540.1	0.94	2.5	0.23	0.10	0.09	2.18	0.18	1.3	0	0.2	11.9
22	3	0.62	5.9	120.5	407.0	1.21	0	0.31	0.11	0.08	1.69	0.17	1.3	0	0.3	8.2
70	41	0.71	17.0	270.4	72.3	2.45	4.3	0.41	0.17	0.28	7.07	0.40	0	0	0.6	31.2
67	45	0.79	19.6	300.2	79.9	2.72	4.3	0.46	0.17	0.31	7.81	0.45	0	0	0.7	34.7

TABLE H-1 Table of Food Composition (*continued*) (Computer code is for Cengage Diet Analysis program) (For purposes of calculations, use "0" for t, <1, <0.1, 0.01)

DA+ Code	Food Description	Quantity	Measure	Wt (g)	H_2O (g)	Ener (kcal)	Prot (g)	Carb (g)	Fiber (g)	Fat (g)	Fat Breakdown (g) Sat	Mono	Poly
Beef, Lamb, Pork—*continued*													
32682	Loin, center rib, chops, boneless, lean and fat, braised	3	ounce(s)	85	49.5	217	22.4	0	0	13.4	5.2	6.1	1.1
32603	Loin, center rib, chops, lean, broiled	3	ounce(s)	85	55.4	158	21.9	0	0	7.1	2.4	3.0	0.8
32478	Loin, whole, lean and fat, braised	3	ounce(s)	85	49.6	203	23.2	0	0	11.6	4.3	5.2	1.0
32481	Loin, whole, lean, braised	3	ounce(s)	85	52.2	173	24.3	0	0	7.8	2.9	3.5	0.6
	Pork leg or ham												
32471	Rump portion, lean and fat, roasted	3	ounce(s)	85	52.7	178	23.0	0	0	8.8	2.9	3.7	1.9
32468	Whole, lean and fat, roasted	3	ounce(s)	85	46.8	232	22.8	0	0	15.0	5.5	6.7	1.4
	Pork ribs												
32693	Loin, country style, lean and fat, roasted	3	ounce(s)	85	41.1	305	18.5	0	0	25.1	9.1	10.9	2.5
32696	Loin, country style ribs, lean, roasted	3	ounce(s)	85	49.9	193	24.8	0	0	9.7	3.2	3.7	1.2
	Pork shoulder												
32626	Shoulder, arm picnic, lean and fat, roasted	3	ounce(s)	85	44.3	270	20.0	0	0	20.4	7.5	9.1	2.0
32629	Shoulder, arm picnic, lean, roasted	3	ounce(s)	85	51.3	194	22.7	0	0	10.7	3.7	5.1	1.0
	Rabbit												
3366	Domesticated, roasted	3	ounce(s)	85	51.5	168	24.7	0	0	6.8	2.0	1.8	1.3
3367	Domesticated, stewed	3	ounce(s)	85	50.0	175	25.8	0	0	7.2	2.1	1.9	1.4
	Veal												
3391	Liver, braised	3	ounce(s)	85	50.9	163	24.2	3.2	0	5.3	1.7	1.0	0.9
3319	Rib, lean only, roasted	3	ounce(s)	85	55.0	151	21.9	0	0	6.3	1.8	2.3	0.6
1732	Deer or venison, roasted	3	ounce(s)	85	55.5	134	25.7	0	0	2.7	1.1	0.7	0.5
Poultry													
	Chicken												
29562	Flaked, canned	2	ounce(s)	57	39.3	97	10.3	0.1	0	5.8	1.6	2.3	1.3
	Chicken, fried												
73336	Breast, meat and skin, breaded, fried, fast food	3	ounce(s)	85	45.1	214	18.6	6.6	0.4	12.6	3.3	4.7	3.4
36413	Broiler breast, meat and skin, flour coated, fried	3	ounce(s)	85	48.1	189	27.1	1.4	0.1	7.5	2.1	3.0	1.7
35327	Broiler breast, meat only, fried	3	ounce(s)	85	51.2	159	28.4	0.4	0	4.0	1.1	1.5	0.9
36414	Broiler drumstick, meat and skin, flour coated, fried	3	ounce(s)	85	48.2	208	22.9	1.4	0.1	11.7	3.1	4.6	2.7
35389	Broiler drumstick, meat only, fried	3	ounce(s)	85	52.9	166	24.3	0	0	6.9	1.8	2.5	1.7
35406	Broiler leg, meat only, fried	3	ounce(s)	85	51.5	177	24.1	0.6	0	7.9	2.1	2.9	1.9
35484	Broiler wing, meat only, fried	3	ounce(s)	85	50.9	179	25.6	0	0	7.8	2.1	2.6	1.8
29580	Patty, fillet or tenders, breaded, cooked	3	ounce(s)	85	39.1	246	15.9	13.4	0.7	14.2	2.3	5.4	5.8
	Chicken, roasted, meat only												
35409	Broiler leg, meat only, roasted	3	ounce(s)	85	55.0	162	23.0	0	0	7.2	1.9	2.6	1.7
35486	Broiler wing, meat only, roasted	3	ounce(s)	85	53.4	173	25.9	0	0	6.9	1.9	2.2	1.5
35138	Roasting chicken, dark meat, meat only, roasted	3	ounce(s)	85	57.0	151	19.8	0	0	7.4	2.1	2.8	1.7
35136	Roasting chicken, light meat, meat only, roasted	3	ounce(s)	85	57.7	130	23.1	0	0	3.5	0.9	1.3	0.8
35132	Roasting chicken, meat only, roasted	3	ounce(s)	85	57.3	142	21.3	0	0	5.6	1.5	2.1	1.3
	Chicken, stewed												
1268	Gizzard, simmered	3	ounce(s)	85	57.8	131	25.8	0.0	0	2.3	0.6	0.4	0.3
1270	Liver, simmered	3	ounce(s)	85	56.8	142	20.8	0.7	0	5.5	1.8	1.2	1.7
3174	Meat only, stewed	3	ounce(s)	85	56.8	151	23.2	0	0	5.7	1.6	2.0	1.3
	Duck												
1286	Domesticated, meat and skin, roasted	3	ounce(s)	85	44.1	287	16.1	0	0	24.1	8.2	11.0	3.1
1287	Domesticated, meat only, roasted	3	ounce(s)	85	54.6	171	20.0	0	0	9.5	3.4	3.3	1.3
	Goose												
35507	Domesticated, meat and skin, roasted	3	ounce(s)	85	44.2	259	21.4	0	0	18.6	5.8	8.7	2.1
35524	Domesticated, meat only, roasted	3	ounce(s)	85	48.7	202	24.6	0	0	10.8	3.9	3.7	1.3
1297	Liver pate, smoked, canned	4	tablespoon(s)	52	19.3	240	5.9	2.4	0	22.8	7.5	13.3	0.4

KEY: H-4 = Breads/Baked Goods H-8 = Cereal/Rice/Pasta H-14 = Fruit H-18 = Vegetables/Legumes H-28 = Nuts/Seeds H-30 = Vegetarian H-32 = Dairy H-40 = Eggs H-40 = Seafood H-42 = Meats H-46 = Poultry …8 = Processed Meats H-50 = Beverages H-52 = Fats/Oils H-54 = Sweets H-56 = Spices/Condiments/Sauces H-60 = Mixed Foods/Soups/Sandwiches H-66 = Fast Food H-84 = Convenience H-86 = Baby Foods

Chol (mg)	Calc (mg)	Iron (mg)	Magn (mg)	Pota (mg)	Sodi (mg)	Zinc (mg)	Vit A (µg)	Thia (mg)	Vit E (mg α)	Ribo (mg)	Niac (mg)	Vit B_6 (mg)	Fola (µg)	Vit C (mg)	Vit B_{12} (µg)	Sele (µg)
62	4	0.78	14.5	329.1	34.0	1.76	1.7	0.45	—	0.21	3.67	0.26	3.4	0.3	0.4	28.4
56	22	0.58	21.3	291.7	48.5	1.91	0	0.48	0.09	0.19	6.68	0.57	0	0	0.4	38.6
68	18	0.91	16.2	318.0	40.8	2.02	1.7	0.54	0.20	0.22	3.76	0.31	2.6	0.5	0.5	38.5
67	15	0.96	17.0	329.1	42.5	2.11	1.7	0.56	0.18	0.23	3.90	0.33	3.4	0.5	0.5	41.0
72	14	0.77	21.3	353.8	65.5	1.96	2.6	0.42	0.23	0.32	6.33	0.43	0	0	0.6	21.3
80	12	0.86	18.7	299.3	51.0	2.52	2.6	0.54	0.19	0.27	3.89	0.34	8.5	0.3	0.6	38.5
77	21	0.85	18.7	273.8	44.2	1.87	1.7	0.70	0	0.28	3.57	0.36	3.4	0.3	0.6	29.3
84	26	0.83	18.7	331.7	77.4	3.35	0.9	0.49	0.23	0.39	6.65	0.44	0	0	0.8	40.5
80	16	1.00	14.5	276.4	59.5	2.93	1.7	0.44	—	0.26	3.33	0.30	3.4	0.2	0.6	28.6
81	8	1.21	17.0	298.5	68.0	3.46	0	0.49	—	0.30	3.67	0.35	4.3	0.3	0.7	32.7
70	16	1.93	17.9	325.7	40.0	1.93	0	0.08	—	0.18	7.17	0.40	9.4	0	7.1	32.7
73	17	2.02	17.0	255.1	31.5	2.02	0	0.05	0.37	0.14	6.09	0.29	7.7	0	5.5	32.7
435	5	4.35	17.0	279.8	66.3	9.55	17981.7	0.15	0.58	2.43	11.18	0.78	281.5	0.9	71.9	16.4
98	10	0.82	20.4	264.5	82.5	3.82	0	0.05	0.31	0.25	6.38	0.23	11.9	0	1.3	9.4
95	6	3.80	20.4	284.9	45.9	2.34	0	0.15	—	0.51	5.71		—	0	—	11.0
35	8	0.90	6.8	147.4	408.2	0.80	19.3	0.01	—	0.07	3.59	0.20	2.3	0	0.2	—
75	23	0.56	21.3	232.2	468.6	0.66	16.2	0.06	0.22	0.12	7.55	0.31	25.3	0	0.3	21.9
76	14	1.01	25.5	220.3	64.6	0.94	12.8	0.07	0.39	0.11	11.69	0.49	6.3	0	0.3	20.3
77	14	0.97	26.4	234.7	67.2	0.92	6.0	0.07	0.36	0.11	12.57	0.54	3.4	0	0.3	22.3
77	10	1.14	19.6	194.7	75.7	2.46	21.3	0.07	0.66	0.19	5.13	0.30	9.7	0	0.3	15.6
80	10	1.12	20.4	211.7	81.6	2.74	15.3	0.07	—	0.20	5.23	0.33	7.7	0	0.3	16.7
84	11	1.19	21.3	216.0	81.6	2.53	17.0	0.07	0.38	0.21	5.69	0.33	7.7	0	0.3	16.0
71	13	0.97	17.9	176.9	77.4	1.80	15.4	0.04	0.41	0.11	6.16	0.50	3.4	0	0.3	21.6
38	20	0.55	23.8	265.3	728.8	0.51	4.3	0.06	0.76	0.06	7.22	0.42	37.4	0	0.2	15.4
80	10	1.11	20.4	205.8	77.4	2.43	16.2	0.06	0.23	0.20	5.37	0.31	6.8	0	0.3	18.8
72	14	0.99	17.9	178.6	78.2	1.82	15.3	0.04	0.23	0.11	6.22	0.50	3.4	0	0.3	21.0
64	9	1.13	17.0	190.5	80.8	1.81	13.6	0.05	—	0.16	4.88	0.26	6.0	0	0.2	16.7
64	11	0.92	19.6	200.7	43.4	0.66	6.8	0.05	0.23	0.08	8.90	0.46	2.6	0	0.3	21.9
64	10	1.03	17.9	194.7	63.8	1.29	10.2	0.05	—	0.13	6.70	0.35	4.3	0	0.2	20.9
315	14	2.71	2.6	152.2	47.6	3.76	0	0.02	0.17	0.18	2.65	0.06	4.3	0	0.9	35.0
479	9	9.89	21.3	223.7	64.6	3.38	3385.4	0.25	0.70	1.69	9.39	0.64	491.5	23.7	14.3	70.1
71	12	0.99	17.9	153.1	59.5	1.69	12.8	0.04	0.23	0.14	5.20	0.22	5.1	0	0.2	17.8
71	9	2.30	13.6	173.5	50.2	1.58	53.6	0.15	0.60	0.23	4.10	0.15	5.1	0	0.3	17.0
76	10	2.30	17.0	214.3	55.3	2.21	19.6	0.22	0.60	0.40	4.34	0.21	8.5	0	0.3	19.0
77	11	2.41	18.7	279.8	59.5	2.23	17.9	0.07	1.48	0.27	3.54	0.31	1.7	0	0.3	18.5
82	12	2.44	21.3	330.0	64.6	2.70	10.2	0.08	—	0.33	3.47	0.40	10.2	0	0.4	21.7
78	36	2.86	6.8	71.8	362.4	0.48	520.5	0.05	—	0.16	1.31	0.03	31.2	0	4.9	22.9

APPENDIX H

DA+ Code	Food Description	Quantity	Measure	Wt (g)	H_2O (g)	Ener (kcal)	Prot (g)	Carb (g)	Fiber (g)	Fat (g)	Fat Breakdown (g)		
											Sat	Mono	Poly
Poultry—*continued*													
	Turkey												
3256	Ground, cooked	3	ounce(s)	85	52.8	173	23.3	0	0	8.8	2.3	2.9	2.5
3263	Patty, batter coated, breaded, fried	1	item(s)	94	46.7	266	13.2	14.8	0.5	16.9	4.4	7.0	4.4
219	Roasted, dark meat, meat only	3	ounce(s)	85	55.5	147	23.6	0	0	5.1	1.5	1.8	1.4
222	Roasted, fryer roaster breast, meat only	3	ounce(s)	85	58.2	115	25.6	0	0	0.6	0.2	0.1	0.2
220	Roasted, light meat, meat only	3	ounce(s)	85	57.7	125	25.6	0	0	1.8	0.5	0.5	0.4
1303	Turkey roll, light and dark meat	2	slice(s)	57	39.8	84	10.3	1.2	0	4.0	1.2	1.3	1.0
1302	Turkey roll, light meat	2	slice(s)	57	42.9	56	9.2	1.4	0	1.2	0.3	0.3	0.3
Processed Meats													
	Beef												
1331	Corned beef loaf, jellied, sliced	2	slice(s)	57	39.2	87	13.0	0	0	3.5	1.5	1.5	0.2
	Bologna												
13459	Beef	1	slice(s)	28	15.4	90	3.0	1.0	0	8.0	3.5	2.4	0.2
13461	Light, made with pork and chicken	1	slice(s)	28	—	60	3.0	2.0	0	4.0	1.0	2.0	0.4
13458	Made with chicken and pork	1	slice(s)	28	15.0	90	3.0	1.0	0	8.0	3.0	2.6	0.7
3260	Turkey	1	slice(s)	57	36.6	119	6.5	2.7	0.3	9.1	2.5	3.9	2.2
	Chicken												
56941	Deli-sliced, oven roasted	1	slice(s)	9	6.3	13	1.2	0.3	0	0.8	0.3	0.2	0.1
	Ham												
7127	Deli-sliced, honey	1	slice(s)	10	—	10	1.5	0.5	0	0.3	0	—	—
7126	Deli-sliced, smoked	1	slice(s)	9	—	10	1.5	0.2	0	0.2	0.1	—	—
8614	**Mortadella, beef & pork, sliced**	2	slice(s)	46	24.1	143	7.5	1.4	0	11.7	4.4	5.2	1.4
1323	**Pork olive loaf**	2	slice(s)	57	33.1	133	6.7	5.2	0	9.4	3.3	4.5	1.1
1324	**Pork pickle & pimento loaf**	2	slice(s)	57	34.2	128	6.4	4.8	0.9	9.1	3.0	4.0	1.6
	Sausages & frankfurters												
37296	Beerwurst beef, beer salami (bierwurst)	1	slice(s)	29	16.6	74	4.1	1.2	0	5.7	2.5	2.7	0.2
37257	Beerwurst pork beer salami	1	slice(s)	21	12.9	50	3.0	0.4	0	4.0	1.3	1.9	0.5
35338	Berliner, pork & beef	1	ounce(s)	28	17.3	65	4.3	0.7	0	4.9	1.7	2.3	0.4
37298	Bratwurst pork, cooked	1	piece(s)	74	42.3	181	10.4	1.9	0	14.3	5.1	6.7	1.5
37299	Braunschweiger pork liver sausage	1	slice(s)	15	7.7	50	2.2	0.5	0	4.3	1.4	1.9	0.5
1329	Cheesefurter or cheese smokie, beef & pork	1	item(s)	43	22.6	141	6.1	0.6	0	12.5	4.5	5.9	1.3
1330	Chorizo, beef & pork	2	ounce(s)	57	18.1	258	13.7	1.1	0	21.7	8.2	10.4	2.0
8600	Frankfurter, beef	1	item(s)	45	24.3	141	5.0	1.7	0	12.5	4.9	5.4	0.3
202	Frankfurter, beef & pork	1	item(s)	45	25.2	137	5.2	0.8	0	12.4	4.8	6.2	1.2
1293	Frankfurter, chicken	1	item(s)	45	28.1	100	7.0	1.2	0.2	7.3	1.7	2.7	1.7
42303	Frankfurter, low sodium	1	item(s)	57	32.3	178	6.8	1.0	0	16.3	6.9	7.8	0.8
3261	Frankfurter, turkey	1	item(s)	45	28.3	100	5.5	1.7	0	7.8	1.8	2.6	1.8
37275	Italian sausage, pork, cooked	1	item(s)	68	32.0	235	13.0	2.9	0.1	18.6	6.6	8.7	2.4
37307	Kielbasa, kolbassa, pork & beef	1	slice(s)	30	16.6	94	3.7	0.9	0	8.3	2.8	3.6	1.2
1333	Knockwurst or knackwurst, beef & pork	2	ounce(s)	57	31.3	174	6.3	1.8	0	15.7	5.8	7.3	1.7
37285	Pepperoni, beef & pork	1	slice(s)	11	3.4	54	2.5	0	0	4.8	1.6	1.9	0.4
37313	Polish sausage, pork	1	slice(s)	21	11.1	68	2.9	0.3	0	6.0	2.2	2.8	0.6
206	Salami, beef, cooked, sliced	2	slice(s)	52	31.2	136	6.6	1.0	0	11.5	5.1	5.5	0.5
54045	Salami, pork & beef, dry, sliced, 50% less sodium	1	slice(s)	6	2.3	20	1.2	0.4	0	1.5	0.5	0.7	0.1
37272	Salami, pork, dry or hard	1	slice(s)	13	4.6	52	2.9	0.2	0	4.3	1.5	2.0	0.5
40987	Sausage, turkey, cooked	2	ounce(s)	57	36.9	111	13.5	0.0	0	5.9	1.3	1.7	1.5
8620	Smoked sausage, beef & pork	2	ounce(s)	57	30.6	181	6.8	1.4	0	16.3	5.5	6.9	2.2
8619	Smoked sausage, pork	2	ounce(s)	57	32.0	175	6.8	0.5	0	16.0	5.3	6.4	2.1
37273	Smoked sausage, pork link	1	piece(s)	76	42.8	233	9.1	0.1	0	21.4	7.1	8.5	2.7
1336	Summer sausage, thuringer, or cervelat, beef & pork	2	ounce(s)	57	25.6	205	9.9	1.9	0	17.3	6.5	7.4	0.7
37294	Vienna sausage, cocktail, beef & pork, canned	1	piece(s)	16	10.4	37	1.7	0.4	0	3.1	1.1	1.5	0.2
	Spreads												
1318	Ham salad spread	¼	cup(s)	60	37.6	130	5.2	6.4	0	9.3	3.0	4.3	1.6
32419	Pork and beef sandwich spread	4	tablespoon(s)	60	36.2	141	4.6	7.2	0.1	10.4	3.6	4.6	1.5

E KEY: H-4 = Breads/Baked Goods H-8 = Cereal/Rice/Pasta H-14 = Fruit H-18 = Vegetables/Legumes H-28 = Nuts/Seeds H-30 = Vegetarian H-32 = Dairy H-40 = Eggs H-40 = Seafood H-42 = Meats H-46 = Poultry
8 = Processed Meats H-50 = Beverages H-52 = Fats/Oils H-54 = Sweets H-56 = Spices/Condiments/Sauces H-60 = Mixed Foods/Soups/Sandwiches H-66 = Fast Food H-84 = Convenience H-86 = Baby Foods

Chol (mg)	Calc (mg)	Iron (mg)	Magn (mg)	Pota (mg)	Sodi (mg)	Zinc (mg)	Vit A (μg)	Thia (mg)	Vit E (mg α)	Ribo (mg)	Niac (mg)	Vit B_6 (mg)	Fola (μg)	Vit C (mg)	Vit B_{12} (μg)	Sele (μg)
79	24	1.29	25.5	250.0	66.3	2.64	20.4	0.07	0.09	0.18	7.42	0.54	6.0	0	1.1	26.4
71	13	2.07	14.1	258.5	533.0	1.35	9.4	0.09	0.87	0.18	2.16	0.19	57.3	0	0.2	20.8
109	14	1.22	23.0	193.0	88.4	2.98	4.3	0.05	0.06	0.32	5.69	0.37	7.7	0	1.4	26.7
71	10	1.30	24.7	248.3	44.2	1.48	0	0.04	0.08	0.11	6.37	0.48	5.1	0	0.3	27.3
68	8	0.60	27.2	211.7	84.2	1.46	2.6	0.03	0.05	0.17	9.99	0.69	8.5	0	0.3	25.7
31	18	0.77	10.2	153.1	270.5	1.13	0	0.05	0.19	0.16	2.72	0.15	2.8	0	0.1	16.6
28	5	0.20	11.3	281.8	526.2	0.48	0	0.01	0.07	0.03	4.23	0.11	2.3	0	0.3	10.8
27	6	1.16	6.2	57.3	540.4	2.32	0	0	—	0.06	1.00	0.07	4.5	0	0.7	9.8
20	0	0.36	4.0	47.6	310.0	0.58	0	0.01	—	0.03	0.69	0.05	3.7	0	0.4	—
20	40	0.36	—	45.6	300.0	—	0	—	—	—	—	—	—	0	—	—
30	20	0.36	6.0	43.1	300.0	0.40	—	—	—	—	—	—	—	0	—	—
43	70	1.70	9.1	76.5	607.3	0.74	5.1	0.03	0.26	0.05	1.48	0.14	5.1	7.5	0.1	8.7
5	0	0.06	2.2	27.2	108.3	0.10	0.8	—	—	—	—	—	—	0	—	—
5	0	0.06	—	—	125.0	—	0	—	—	—	—	—	—	0	—	—
5	0	0.06	—	—	111.6	—	0	—	—	—	—	—	—	0	—	—
26	8	0.64	5.1	75.0	573.2	0.97	0	0.05	0.10	0.07	1.23	0.06	1.4	0	0.7	10.4
22	62	0.31	10.8	168.7	547.6	0.78	34.1	0.17	0.14	0.15	1.04	0.13	1.1	0	0.7	9.3
33	62	0.76	19.3	210.7	590.7	0.95	44.3	0.22	0.23	0.07	1.41	0.24	21.0	4.4	0.3	4.5
18	3	0.44	3.5	66.5	264.9	0.71	0	0.02	0.06	0.04	0.99	0.05	0.9	0	0.6	4.7
12	2	0.16	2.7	53.3	261.0	0.36	0	0.12	0.04	0.04	0.68	0.07	0.6	0	0.2	4.4
13	3	0.33	4.3	80.2	367.7	0.70	0	0.11	—	0.06	0.88	0.06	1.4	0	0.8	4.0
44	33	0.95	11.1	156.9	412.2	1.70	0	0.37	0.01	0.14	2.37	0.16	1.5	0.7	0.7	15.7
27	1	1.70	1.7	30.2	176.2	0.43	641.0	0.04	0.05	0.23	1.27	0.05	6.7	0	3.1	8.8
29	25	0.46	5.6	88.6	465.3	0.97	2.6	0.11	0.10	0.07	1.25	0.06	1.3	0	0.7	6.8
50	5	0.90	10.2	225.6	700.1	1.93	0	0.36	0.12	0.17	2.91	0.30	1.1	0	1.1	12.0
25	6	0.56	4.9	130.5	466.6	0.93	0	0.01	0.09	0.02	0.94	0.08	4.5	0	0.6	5.0
23	5	0.52	4.5	75.2	368.5	0.83	8.1	0.09	0.11	0.05	1.18	0.06	1.8	0	0.6	6.2
43	33	0.53	9.0	90.9	340.2	0.50	0	0.03	0.10	0.12	2.11	0.15	4.9	0	0.2	10.4
35	11	0.82	1.7	94.6	177.3	1.24	0	0.03	0.10	0.06	1.38	0.07	2.3	0	0.9	6.8
35	67	0.66	6.3	176.4	410.0	0.83	0	0.02	0.28	0.08	1.66	0.06	4.5	0	0.4	6.8
39	14	0.97	12.2	206.7	820.8	1.63	6.8	0.42	0.17	0.16	2.83	0.22	3.4	0.1	0.9	15.0
20	5	0.25	4.0	91.4	275.4	0.48	0	0.06	0.07	0.06	1.00	0.06	0.3	0	0.2	5.9
34	6	0.37	6.2	112.8	527.2	0.94	0	0.19	0.32	0.08	1.55	0.10	1.1	0	0.7	7.7
12	2	0.18	2.3	30.7	181.8	0.28	0	0.04	0	0.03	0.51	0.04	0.6	0.1	0.2	3.8
15	2	0.30	2.9	49.4	182.5	0.40	0	0.10	0.05	0.03	0.72	0.04	0.4	0.2	0.2	3.7
37	3	1.14	6.8	97.8	592.8	0.92	0	0.05	0.10	0.10	1.68	0.09	1.0	0	1.6	7.6
5	0	0.08	1.0	21.2	52.4	0.18	0	0.03	0.02	0.02	0.27	0.03	0.1	0	0.1	1.5
10	2	0.17	2.8	48.4	289.3	0.54	0	0.12	0.03	0.04	0.72	0.07	0.3	0	0.4	3.3
52	12	0.84	11.9	169.0	377.1	2.20	7.4	0.05	0.10	0.14	3.24	0.18	3.4	0.4	0.7	0
33	7	0.43	7.4	101.5	516.4	0.71	7.4	0.11	0.07	0.06	1.67	0.09	1.1	0	0.3	0
35	6	0.33	6.2	273.8	468.8	0.74	0	0.12	0.14	0.10	1.59	0.10	0.6	0	0.4	10.4
46	8	0.45	8.3	366.0	626.6	0.99	0	0.16	0.19	0.14	2.13	0.14	0.8	0	0.5	13.9
42	5	1.16	7.9	147.4	737.0	1.45	0	0.09	0.12	0.19	2.44	0.15	1.1	9.4	3.1	11.5
14	2	0.14	1.1	16.2	155.0	0.26	0	0.01	0.04	0.02	0.26	0.02	0.6	0	0.2	2.7
22	5	0.35	6.0	90.0	645.0	0.66	0	0.26	1.04	0.07	1.26	0.09	0.6	0	0.5	10.7
23	7	0.47	4.8	66.0	607.8	0.61	15.6	0.10	1.04	0.08	1.04	0.07	1.2	0	0.7	5.8

DA+ Code	Food Description	Quantity	Measure	Wt (g)	H_2O (g)	Ener (kcal)	Prot (g)	Carb (g)	Fiber (g)	Fat (g)	Fat Breakdown (g) Sat	Mono	Poly
Processed Meats—*continued*													
	Turkey												
71632	Breast, honey roasted & smoked, presliced	1	slice(s)	28	—	30	5.0	2.0	0	0.5	0	—	—
71612	Breast, oven roasted deli slices, lower sodium	1	slice(s)	28	—	25	5.0	0.5	0	0.5		—	—
71631	Breast, oven roasted, presliced	1	slice(s)	28	—	30	5.0	1.0	0	0.5	0	—	—
7124	Breast, oven-roasted	1	slice(s)	9	—	8	1.5	0.3	0	0.1	0	—	—
71633	Breast, smoked, presliced	1	slice(s)	28	—	30	5.0	1.0	0	0.5	0	—	—
71629	Ham	1	slice(s)	28	—	40	5.0	0.5	0	2.0	0.5	—	—
37270	Pastrami	1	slice(s)	28	20.3	38	4.6	0.5	0	1.8	0.5	0.6	0.5
3262	Salami	2	slice(s)	57	39.1	98	10.9	0.9	0.1	5.2	1.6	1.8	1.4
37318	Salami, cooked	1	slice(s)	28	19.5	49	5.5	0.4	0	2.6	0.8	0.9	0.7
Beverages													
	Beer												
866	Ale, mild	12	fluid ounce(s)	360	331.1	155	1.7	12.8	0	0	0	0.0	0
686	Beer	12	fluid ounce(s)	356	327.7	153	1.6	12.7	0	0	0	0	0
16886	Beer, non alcoholic	12	fluid ounce(s)	360	328.1	133	0.8	29.0	0	0.4	0.1	0.1	0.2
31609	Bud Light beer	12	fluid ounce(s)	355	337.3	110	0.9	6.6	0	0	0	0	0
31608	Budweiser beer	12	fluid ounce(s)	355	329.3	145	1.3	10.6	0	0	0	0	0
869	Light beer	12	fluid ounce(s)	354	335.9	103	0.8	5.8	0	0	0	0.0	0
31613	Michelob Beer	12	fluid ounce(s)	355	326.5	164	1.7	15.0	0	0	0	0	0
31614	Michelob Light beer	12	fluid ounce(s)	355	336.8	123	1.4	8.8	0	0	0	0	0
	Gin, rum, vodka, whiskey												
687	Distilled alcohol, 80 proof	1	fluid ounce(s)	28	18.5	64	0	0	0	0	0	0	0
688	Distilled alcohol, 86 proof	1	fluid ounce(s)	28	17.8	70	0	0	0	0	0	0	0
689	Distilled alcohol, 90 proof	1	fluid ounce(s)	28	17.3	73	0	0	0	0	0	0	0
856	Distilled alcohol, 94 proof	1	fluid ounce(s)	28	16.8	76	0	0	0	0	0	0.0	0
857	Distilled alcohol, 100 proof	1	fluid ounce(s)	28	16.0	82	0	0	0	0	0	0.0	0
	Liqueurs												
33187	Coffee liqueur, 53 proof	1	fluid ounce(s)	35	10.8	113	0	16.3	0	0.1	0	0	0
3142	Coffee liqueur, 63 proof	1	fluid ounce(s)	35	14.4	107	0	11.2	0	0.1	0	0	0
736	Cordials, 54 proof	1	fluid ounce(s)	30	8.9	104	0	13.3	0	0.1	0	0	0
	Wine												
861	California red wine	5	fluid ounce(s)	150	133.4	125	0.3	3.7	0	0	0	0.0	0
858	Domestic champagne	5	fluid ounce(s)	150	—	105	0.3	3.8	0	0	0	0.0	0
690	Sweet dessert wine	5	fluid ounce(s)	147	103.7	235	0.3	20.1	0	0	0	0	0
1481	White wine	5	fluid ounce(s)	148	128.1	121	0.1	3.8	0	0	0.0	0	0
1811	Wine cooler	10	fluid ounce(s)	300	266.8	165	0.2	19.6	0	0.1	0	0	0
	Carbonated												
31898	7 Up	12	fluid ounce(s)	360	320.4	150	0	39.0	0	0	0	0	0
692	Club soda	12	fluid ounce(s)	355	354.8	0	0	0	0	0	0	0	0
12010	Coca-Cola Classic cola soda	12	fluid ounce(s)	360	325.1	210	0	58.5	0	0	0	0	0
693	Cola	12	fluid ounce(s)	368	332.7	136	0.3	35.2	0	0.1	0	0	0
2391	Cola or pepper-type soda, low calorie with saccharin	12	fluid ounce(s)	355	354.5	0	0	0.4	0	0	0	0	0
9522	Cola soda, decaffeinated	12	fluid ounce(s)	372	333.4	153	0.0	39.4	0	0	0	0	0
9524	Cola, decaffeinated, low calorie with aspartame	12	fluid ounce(s)	355	354.3	4	0.4	0.5	0	0	0	0	0
1415	Cola, low calorie with aspartame	12	fluid ounce(s)	355	353.6	7	0.4	1.0	0	0.1	0	0	0
1412	Cream soda	12	fluid ounce(s)	371	321.5	189	0	49.3	0	0	0	0	0
31899	Diet 7 Up	12	fluid ounce(s)	360	—	0	0	0	0	0	0	0	0
12031	Diet Coke cola soda	12	fluid ounce(s)	360	358.3	2	0	0.2	0	0	0	0	0
29392	Diet Mountain Dew soda	12	fluid ounce(s)	354	—	0	0	0	0	0	0	0	0
29389	Diet Pepsi cola soda	12	fluid ounce(s)	354	352.8	0	0	0	0	0	0	0	0
12034	Diet Sprite soda	12	fluid ounce(s)	360	—	4	0	0	0	0	0	0	0
695	Ginger ale	12	fluid ounce(s)	366	333.9	124	0	32.1	0	0	0	0	0
694	Grape soda	12	fluid ounce(s)	372	330.3	160	0	41.7	0	0	0	0	0
1876	Lemon lime soda	12	fluid ounce(s)	368	330.7	147	0.2	37.4	0	0.1	0	0	0
29391	Mountain Dew soda	12	fluid ounce(s)	354	—	170	0	46.0	0	0	0	0	0
3145	Orange soda	12	fluid ounce(s)	372	325.9	179	0	45.8	0	0	0	0	0
1414	Pepper-type soda	12	fluid ounce(s)	368	329.3	151	0	38.3	0	0.4	0.3	0	0
29388	Pepsi regular cola soda	12	fluid ounce(s)	354	313.3	150	0	41.0	0	0	0	0	0
696	Root beer	12	fluid ounce(s)	370	330.1	152	0	39.2	0	0	0	0	0
12044	Sprite soda	12	fluid ounce(s)	360	323.2	144	0	39.0	0	0	0	0	0

KEY: H-4 = Breads/Baked Goods H-8 = Cereal/Rice/Pasta H-14 = Fruit H-18 = Vegetables/Legumes H-28 = Nuts/Seeds H-30 = Vegetarian H-32 = Dairy H-40 = Eggs H-40 = Seafood H-42 = Meats H-46 = Poultry H-48 = Processed Meats H-50 = Beverages H-52 = Fats/Oils H-54 = Sweets H-56 = Spices/Condiments/Sauces H-60 = Mixed Foods/Soups/Sandwiches H-66 = Fast Food H-84 = Convenience H-86 = Baby Foods

Chol (mg)	Calc (mg)	Iron (mg)	Magn (mg)	Pota (mg)	Sodi (mg)	Zinc (mg)	Vit A (μg)	Thia (mg)	Vit E (mg α)	Ribo (mg)	Niac (mg)	Vit B_6 (mg)	Fola (μg)	Vit C (mg)	Vit B_{12} (μg)	Sele (μg)
10	0	0	—	—	240.0	—	0	—	—	—	—	—	—	0	—	—
15	0	0.18	—	—	175.0	—	0	—	—	—	—	—	—	0	—	—
10	0	0	—	—	240.0	—	0	—	—	—	—	—	—	0	—	—
3	0	0.06	—	—	103.3	—	0	—	—	—	—	—	—	0	—	—
10	0	0	—	—	240.0	—	0	—	—	—	—	—	—	0	—	—
18	0	0.72	—	—	315.0	—	0	—	—	—	—	—	—	0	—	—
19	3	1.19	4.0	97.8	278.1	0.61	1.1	0.02	0.06	0.07	1.00	0.08	1.4	2.3	0.1	4.6
43	23	0.71	12.5	122.5	627.7	1.32	1.1	0.24	0.14	0.17	2.26	0.24	5.7	0	0.6	15.0
22	11	0.35	6.2	61.2	284.6	0.66	0.6	0.12	0.07	0.09	1.13	0.12	2.8	0	0.3	7.5
0	14	0.07	21.6	97.2	14.4	0.04	0	0.02	0	0.09	1.85	0.17	21.6	0	0.1	2.2
0	14	0.07	21.4	96.2	14.3	0.04	0	0.02	0	0.09	1.83	0.16	21.4	0	0.1	2.1
0	25	0.22	25.2	28.8	46.8	0.07	0	0.06	0	0.17	4.01	0.10	50.4	1.8	0.1	4.3
0	14	0.11	24.9	92.3	10.6	0	0	0.02	0	0.05	1.39	0.12	21.3	0	0.1	1.4
0	14	0	24.9	117.2	10.6	0	0	0.02	0	0.09	1.82	0.16	21.3	0	0.1	2.1
0	14	0.11	17.7	74.3	14.2	0.04	0	0.02	0	0.05	1.38	0.12	21.2	0	0.1	1.4
0	14	0.07	21.3	95.8	9.0	0.04	0	0.02	0	0.09	1.82	0.16	21.3	0	0.1	2.1
0	14	0.11	17.8	74.6	9.0	0.04	0	0.02	0	0.05	1.39	0.12	21.3	0	0.1	1.4
0	0	0.01	0	0.6	0.3	0.01	0	0	0	0	0	0	0	0	0	0
0	0	0.01	0	0.6	0.3	0.01	0	0	0	0	0	0	0	0	0	0
0	0	0.01	0	0.6	0.3	0.01	0	0	0	0	0	0	0	0	0	0
0	0	0.01	0	0.6	0.3	0.01	0	0	—	0	0	0	0	0	0	0
0	0	0.01	0	0.6	0.3	0.01	0	0	—	0	0	0	0	0	0	0
0	0	0.02	1.0	10.4	2.8	0.01	0	0	0	0	0.05	0	0	0	0	0.1
0	0	0.02	1.0	10.4	2.8	0.01	0	0	—	0	0.05	0	0	0	0	0.1
0	0	0.02	0.6	4.5	1.8	0.01	0	0	0	0	0.02	0	0	0	0	0.1
0	12	1.43	16.2	170.6	15.0	0.15	0	0.02	0	0.04	0.12	0.05	—	0	0	—
0	—	—	—	—	—	—	—	—	—	—	—	—	—	—	0	—
0	12	0.35	13.2	135.4	13.2	0.10	0	0.03	0	0.03	0.31	0	0	0	0	0.7
0	13	0.40	14.8	104.7	7.4	0.18	0	0.01	0	0.02	0.16	0.07	1.5	0	0	0.1
0	18	0.78	18.0	147.0	21.0	0.24	0	0.02	0.03	0.03	0.25	0.08	3.0	5.4	0	0.3
0	7	0.07	3.6	3.6	37.5	0.04	0	0	0	0	0.05	0	0	0	0	0
0	18	0.04	3.6	7.1	74.6	0.36	0	0	0	0	0	0	0	0	0	0
0	7	0.00	0	0	67.5	0.07	0	0	0	0	0	0	0	0	0	0.4
0	7	0.41	0	7.4	14.7	0.07	0	0	0	0	0	0	0	0	0	0.4
0	14	0.07	3.6	14.2	56.8	0.11	0	0	0	0	0	0	0	0	0	0.4
0	7	0.07	0	11.2	14.9	0.04	0	0	0	0	0	0	0	0	0	0.4
0	11	0.07	0	24.9	14.2	0.04	0	0.02	0	0.08	0	0	0	0	0	0.4
0	11	0.39	3.6	28.4	28.4	0.04	0	0.02	0	0.08	0	0	0	0	0	0
0	19	0.19	3.7	3.7	44.5	0.26	0	0	0	0	0	0	0	0	0	0
0	—	—	—	—	45.0	—	—	—	—	—	—	—	—	—	—	—
0	11	0.40	3.6	18.0	42.0	0.04	0	0.02	0	0.08	0	0	0	0	0	0
0	0	0	—	80.0	50.0	—	0	—	—	—	—	—	—	0	—	—
0	0	0	3.6	30.0	35.0	0.04	0	0.02	0	0.08	0	0	0	0	0	0
0	0	0.00	—	109.5	36.0	—	0	—	—	—	—	—	—	0	—	—
0	11	0.66	3.7	3.7	25.6	0.18	0	0	0	0	0	0	0	0	0	0.4
0	11	0.30	3.7	3.7	55.8	0.26	0	0	—	0	0	0	0	0	0	0
0	7	0.41	3.7	3.7	33.2	0.15	0	0	0	0	0.06	0	0	0	0	0
0	0	0	—	5.0	65.0	—	0	—	—	—	—	—	—	0	—	—
0	19	0.22	3.7	7.4	44.6	0.37	0	0	—	0	0	0	0	0	0	0
0	11	0.15	0	3.7	36.8	0.15	0	0	—	0	0	0	0	0	0	0.4
0	0	0	0.0	10.0	30.0	0.07	0	0	0	0	0	0	0	0	0	0.4
0	18	0.18	3.7	3.7	48.0	0.26	0	0	0	0	0	0	0	0	0	0.4
0	7	0.40	3.6	0	70.5	0.14	0	0	0	0	0.05	0	0	0	0	0

TABLE H-1 Table of Food Composition (*continued*)

(Computer code is for Cengage Diet Analysis program) (For purposes of calculations, use "0" for t, <1, <0.1, 0.01)

DA+ Code	Food Description	Quantity	Measure	Wt (g)	H_2O (g)	Ener (kcal)	Prot (g)	Carb (g)	Fiber (g)	Fat (g)	Fat Breakdown (g)		
											Sat	Mono	Poly
Beverages—*continued*													
	Coffee												
731	Brewed	8	fluid ounce(s)	237	235.6	2	0.3	0	0	0	0	0	0
9520	Brewed, decaffeinated	8	fluid ounce(s)	237	234.3	5	0.3	1.0	0	0	0	0	0
16882	Cappuccino	8	fluid ounce(s)	240	224.5	77	4.0	6.2	0.2	4.0	2.3	1.0	0.2
16883	Cappuccino, decaffeinated	8	fluid ounce(s)	240	224.4	74	4.0	6.2	0.2	4.0	2.3	1.0	0.2
16880	Espresso	8	fluid ounce(s)	237	231.8	5	0.3	0	0	0.4	0.2	0	0.2
16881	Espresso, decaffeinated	8	fluid ounce(s)	237	231.8	0	0.2	0	0	0.4	0.2	0	0.2
732	Instant, prepared	8	fluid ounce(s)	239	236.5	5	0.2	0.8	0	0	0	0	0
67526	Starbucks Doubleshot Energy, coffee, canned	15	fluid ounce(s)	443	—	210	12.0	36.0	0	2.0	2.5	—	—
67525	Starbucks Doubleshot, canned	6.5	fluid ounce(s)	192	—	138	4.1	17.9	—	5.7	3.7	—	—
32561	Starbucks Frappuccino, bottled, coffee	9.5	fluid ounce(s)	281	—	200	6.0	37.0	0	3.0	2.0	—	—
32562	Starbucks Frappuccino, bottled, mocha	9.5	fluid ounce(s)	281	—	180	7.0	33.0	0	3.0	2.0	—	—
	Fruit drinks												
29357	Crystal Light sugar-free lemonade drink	8	fluid ounce(s)	237	—	592	0	0	0	0	0	0	0
6012	Fruit punch drink with added vitamin C, canned	8	fluid ounce(s)	248	218.2	119	0	29.7	0	0	0	0	0
31143	Gatorade Thirst Quencher, all flavors	8	fluid ounce(s)	240	—	50	0	14.0	0	0	0	0	0
260	Grape drink, canned	8	fluid ounce(s)	250	210.5	153	0	39.4	0	0	0	0	0
17372	Kool-Aid (lemonade/punch/fruit drink)	8	fluid ounce(s)	248	220.0	108	0.1	27.8	0.2	0	0	0	0
17225	Kool-Aid sugar-free, low-calorie tropical punch drink mix, prepared	8	fluid ounce(s)	240	—	5	0	0	0	0	0	0	0
266	Lemonade, prepared from frozen concentrate	8	fluid ounce(s)	248	221.6	99	0.2	25.8	0	0.1	0	0	0
268	Limeade, prepared from frozen concentrate	8	fluid ounce(s)	247	212.6	128	0	34.1	0	0	0	0	0
57054	Odwalla Pomegranate Limeade	8	fluid ounce(s)	240	—	122	0	29.7	0	0	0	0	0
14266	Odwalla Strawberry C Monster smoothie blend	8	fluid ounce(s)	240	—	240	0	56.0	1.0	0	0	0	0
10099	Snapple fruit punch fruit drink	8	fluid ounce(s)	240	—	110	0	27.0	0	0	0	0	0
10096	Snapple kiwi strawberry fruit drink	8	fluid ounce(s)	240	211.2	110	0	27.0	0	0	0	0	0
14818	SunnyD Tangy Original	6 ¾	fluid ounce(s)	203	—	76	0	18.6	0	0	0	0	0
	Slim Fast ready-to-drink shake												
16054	French Vanilla	10	fluid ounce(s)	325	—	220	10.0	40.0	5.0	2.5	0.5	1.5	0.5
10095	Rich Chocolate Royale	10	fluid ounce(s)	325	—	220	10.0	40.0	5.0	3.0	1.0	1.5	0.5
16055	Strawberries 'n' Cream	10	fluid ounce(s)	325	—	220	10.0	40.0	5.0	2.5	0.5	1.5	0.5
	Tea												
33179	Decaffeinated, prepared	8	fluid ounce(s)	237	236.3	2	0	0.7	0	0	0	0	0
1877	Herbal, prepared	8	fluid ounce(s)	237	236.1	2	0	0.5	0	0	0	0	0
735	Instant tea mix, lemon flavored with sugar, prepared	8	fluid ounce(s)	259	236.2	91	0	22.3	0.3	0.2	0	0	0
734	Instant tea mix, unsweetened, prepared	8	fluid ounce(s)	238	237.1	2	0.1	0.4	0	0	0	0	0
16097	Nestea with lemon, canned	12	fluid ounce(s)	360	328.2	125	0	34.5	0	0	0	0	0
733	Prepared	8	fluid ounce(s)	237	236.3	2	0	0.7	0	0	0	0	0
	Water												
1413	Mineral water, carbonated	8	fluid ounce(s)	237	236.8	0	0	0	0	0	0	0	0
33183	Poland spring water, bottled	8	fluid ounce(s)	237	237.0	0	0	0	0	0	0	0	0
1821	Tap water	8	fluid ounce(s)	237	236.8	0	0	0	0	0	0	0	0
1879	Tonic water	8	fluid ounce(s)	244	222.3	83	0	21.5	0	0	0	0	0
Fats and Oils													
	Butter												
104	Butter	1	tablespoon(s)	14	2.3	102	0.1	0	0	11.5	7.3	3.0	0.4
2522	Butter Buds, dry butter substitute	1	teaspoon(s)	2	0.1	7	0	1.6	0	0.1	0.1	—	—
921	Unsalted	1	tablespoon(s)	14	2.5	102	0.1	0	0	11.5	7.3	3.0	0.4
107	Whipped	1	tablespoon(s)	9	1.5	67	0.1	0	0	7.6	4.7	2.2	0.3
944	Whipped, unsalted	1	tablespoon(s)	9	1.7	67	0.1	0	0	7.6	4.8	2.0	0.3

E KEY: H-4 = Breads/Baked Goods H-8 = Cereal/Rice/Pasta H-14 = Fruit H-18 = Vegetables/Legumes H-28 = Nuts/Seeds H-30 = Vegetarian H-32 = Dairy H-40 = Eggs H-40 = Seafood H-42 = Meats H-46 = Poultry
8 = Processed Meats H-50 = Beverages H-52 = Fats/Oils H-54 = Sweets H-56 = Spices/Condiments/Sauces H-60 = Mixed Foods/Soups/Sandwiches H-66 = Fast Food H-84 = Convenience H-86 = Baby Foods

Chol (mg)	Calc (mg)	Iron (mg)	Magn (mg)	Pota (mg)	Sodi (mg)	Zinc (mg)	Vit A (µg)	Thia (mg)	Vit E (mg α)	Ribo (mg)	Niac (mg)	Vit B_6 (mg)	Fola (µg)	Vit C (mg)	Vit B_{12} (µg)	Sele (µg)
0	5	0.02	7.1	116.1	4.7	0.05	0	0.03	0.02	0.18	0.45	0	4.7	0	0	0
0	9	0.09	9.5	85.2	9.5	0.02	0	0	0	0.03	0.67	0	0	0	0	0.5
12	144	0.10	16.8	220.8	55.2	0.48	55.2	0.07	0.10	0.29	0.34	0.04	7.2	0	0.4	4.6
12	144	0.14	19.2	225.6	55.2	0.48	55.2	0.05	0.10	0.21	0.38	0.04	4.8	0	0.4	4.6
0	5	0.31	189.6	272.5	33.2	0.12	0	0	0.02	0.42	12.34	0	2.4	0.5	0	0
0	5	0.31	189.6	272.5	33.2	0.12	0	0	0	0.42	12.34	0	2.4	0.5	0	0
0	10	0.10	9.5	71.6	9.5	0.02	0	0	0	0	0.56	0	0	0	0	0.2
15	4	0	—	—	170.0	—	0	—	—	1.70	20.00	2.00	—	0.3	3.0	—
20	162	0	—	20.3	69.1	—	0	—	—	—	—	—	—	0	—	—
15	3	0	—	—	100.0	—	0	—	—	—	—	—	—	0	—	—
15	2	0	—	—	95.0	—	0	—	—	—	—	—	—	0	—	—
0	0	0	—	—	4140.5	—	—	—	—	—	—	—	—	0	—	—
0	20	0.22	7.4	62.0	24.8	0.03	1.7	0.05	0.05	0.06	0.05	0.03	9.9	89.3	0	0.5
0	2	0	—	30.0	110.0	—	0	—	—	—	—	—	—	0	—	—
0	130	0.17	2.5	30.0	40.0	0.30	0	0	0	0.01	0.03	0	0	78.5	0	0.3
0	14	0.46	5.0	49.6	31.0	0.20	—	0.04	—	0.05	0.05	0.01		41.6	0	1.0
0	0	0	—	10.1	10.1	—	0	—	—	—	—	—	—	6.0	—	—
0	10	0.40	5.0	37.2	9.9	0.05	0	0.01	0.02	0.05	0.04	0.01	2.5	9.7	0	0.2
0	5	0	4.9	24.7	7.4	0.02	0	0	0	0.01	0.02	0.01	2.5	7.7	0	0.2
0	0	0	—	—	10.1	—	0	—	—	—	—	—	—	0	—	—
0	40	1.08	—	600.0	30.0	—	0	—	—	—	—	—	—	900.0	—	—
0	0	0	—	20.0	5.0	—	0	—	—	—	—	—	—	0	—	—
0	0	0	—	40.0	10.0	—	0	—	—	—	—	—	—	0	—	—
0	0	0	—	—	143.4	—	0	0.19	—	—	—	—	—	50.6	—	—
5	400	2.70	140.0	600.0	220.0	2.25	525.1	0.52	—	0.60	7.00	0.70	—	60.0	2.1	17.5
5	400	2.70	140.0	600.0	220.0	2.25	525.1	0.53	—	0.60	7.00	0.70	—	60.0	2.1	17.5
5	400	2.70	140.0	600.0	220.0	2.25	525.1	0.52	—	0.60	7.00	0.70	—	60.0	2.1	17.5
0	0	0.05	7.1	87.7	7.1	0.05	0	0	0	0.03	0	0	11.9	0	0	0
0	5	0.19	2.4	21.3	2.4	0.09	0	0.02	0	0.01	0	0	2.4	0	0	0
0	5	0.05	2.6	38.8	5.2	0.03	0	0	0	0	0.03	0	0	0	0	0.3
0	7	0.02	4.8	42.8	9.5	0.02	0	0	0	0.01	0.08	0	0	0	0	0
0	11	0	3.6	68.4	46.5	0.22	0	—	—	—	—	—	—	—	—	—
0	0	0.05	7.1	87.7	7.1	0.05	0	0	0	0.03	0	0	11.9	0	0	0
0	33	0	0	0.0	2.4	0	0	0	—	0	0	0	0	0	0	0
0	2	0.02	2.4	0	2.4	0	0	0	—	0	0	0	0	0	0	0
0	7	0	2.4	2.4	7.1	0	0	0	0	0	0	0	0	0	0	0
0	2	0.02	0	0	29.3	0.24	0	0	0	0	0	0	0	0	0	0
31	3	0.00	0.3	3.4	101.4	0.01	97.1	0	0.33	0	0.01	0	0.4	0	0	0.1
0	8	0	0	—	80.2	0	0	0	0	0	0	0	—	0	0	0
31	3	0	0.3	3.4	1.6	0.01	97.1	0	0.33	0	0.01	0	0.4	0	0	0.1
21	2	0.02	0.2	2.4	77.7	0	64.3	0	0.22	0	0	0	0.3	0	0	0.1
20	2	0	0.2	2.3	1.0	0.01	64.3	0	0.22	0	0	0	0.3	0	0	0.1

TABLE H-1 Table of Food Composition (*continued*) (Computer code is for Cengage Diet Analysis program) (For purposes of calculations, use "0" for t, <1, <0.1, 0.01)

DA+ Code	Food Description	Quantity	Measure	Wt (g)	H_2O (g)	Ener (kcal)	Prot (g)	Carb (g)	Fiber (g)	Fat (g)	Fat Breakdown (g) Sat	Mono	Poly
	Fats and Oils—*continued*												
	Fats, cooking												
2671	Beef tallow, semisolid	1	tablespoon(s)	13	0	115	0	0	0	12.8	6.4	5.4	0.5
922	Chicken fat	1	tablespoon(s)	13	0	115	0	0	0	12.8	3.8	5.7	2.7
5454	Household shortening with vegetable oil	1	tablespoon(s)	13	0	115	0	0	0	13.0	3.4	5.5	3.5
111	Lard	1	tablespoon(s)	13	0	115	0	0	0	12.8	5.0	5.8	1.4
	Margarine												
114	Margarine	1	tablespoon(s)	14	2.3	101	0	0.1	0	11.4	2.1	5.5	3.4
5439	Soft	1	tablespoon(s)	14	2.3	103	0.1	0.1	0	11.6	1.7	4.4	2.1
928	Unsalted	1	tablespoon(s)	14	2.6	101	0.1	0.1	0	11.3	2.1	5.2	3.5
119	Whipped	1	tablespoon(s)	9	1.5	67	0	0.1	0	7.5	1.3	3.3	2.4
	Spreads												
54657	I Can't Believe It's Not Butter!, tub, soya oil (non-hydrogenated)	1	tablespoon(s)	14	2.3	102	0.1	0.1	0	11.4	2.8	2.0	5.1
2708	Mayonnaise with soybean and safflower oils	1	tablespoon(s)	14	2.1	99	0.2	0.4	0	11.0	1.2	1.8	7.6
57582	Promise buttery spread	1	tablespoon(s)	14	—	80	0	0	0	8.0	1.5	2.5	4.0
	Oils												
2681	Canola	1	tablespoon(s)	14	0	120	0	0	0	13.6	1.0	8.6	3.8
120	Corn	1	tablespoon(s)	14	0	122	0	0	0	13.6	1.8	3.8	7.4
122	Olive	1	tablespoon(s)	14	0	119	0	0	0	13.5	1.9	9.8	1.4
124	Peanut	1	tablespoon(s)	14	0	119	0	0	0	13.5	2.3	6.2	4.3
2693	Safflower	1	tablespoon(s)	14	0	120	0	0	0	13.6	1.0	10.2	1.7
923	Sesame	1	tablespoon(s)	14	0	120	0	0	0	13.6	1.9	5.4	5.7
128	Soybean, hydrogenated	1	tablespoon(s)	14	0	120	0	0	0	13.6	2.0	5.8	5.1
130	Soybean, with soybean and cottonseed oil	1	tablespoon(s)	14	0	120	0	0	0	13.6	2.4	4.0	6.5
2700	Sunflower	1	tablespoon(s)	14	0	120	0	0	0	13.6	1.8	6.3	5.0
357	**Pam original no stick cooking spray**	1	serving(s)	0	—	0	0	0	0	0	0	0	0
	Salad dressing												
132	Blue cheese	2	tablespoon(s)	30	11.9	143	0.4	1.4	0.1	15.3	2.5	4.0	8.3
133	Blue cheese, low calorie	2	tablespoon(s)	31	25.4	32	1.6	0.9	0	2.3	0.8	0.6	0.8
1764	Caesar	2	tablespoon(s)	30	10.3	163	0.7	1.0	0.2	17.4	2.6	4.1	9.9
29654	Creamy, reduced calorie, fat free, cholesterol free, sour cream and/or buttermilk and oil	2	tablespoon(s)	33	24.7	35	0.5	6.6	0	0.9	0.2	0.2	0.5
29617	Creamy, reduced calorie, sour cream and/or buttermilk and oil	2	tablespoon(s)	30	22.2	48	0.4	2.1	0	4.2	0.6	1.0	2.4
134	French	2	tablespoon(s)	32	11.7	146	0.2	5.0	0	14.3	1.8	2.7	6.7
135	French, low fat	2	tablespoon(s)	32	17.4	71	0.2	10.0	0.5	3.7	0.3	1.4	1.2
136	Italian	2	tablespoon(s)	29	18.6	71	0.1	3.6	0	6.2	0.9	1.7	3.2
137	Italian, diet	2	tablespoon(s)	30	24.0	31	0.1	3.0	0	2.0	0.2	0.5	1.0
139	Mayonnaise-type	2	tablespoon(s)	29	11.7	115	0.3	7.0	0	9.8	1.4	2.6	5.3
942	Oil and vinegar	2	tablespoon(s)	32	15.2	144	0	0.8	0	16.0	2.9	4.7	7.7
1765	Ranch	2	tablespoon(s)	30	11.5	145	0.3	2.0	0.2	15.4	2.4	3.4	8.5
3666	Ranch, reduced calorie	2	tablespoon(s)	30	20.5	63	0.1	2.0	0	6.1	1.6	3.6	0.6
940	Russian	2	tablespoon(s)	30	11.6	107	0.2	9.6	0.2	7.9	0.7	1.8	4.4
939	Russion, low calorie	2	tablespoon(s)	32	20.8	45	0.2	8.8	0.1	1.3	0.2	0.3	0.7
941	Sesame seed	2	tablespoon(s)	30	11.8	133	0.9	2.6	0.3	13.6	1.9	3.6	7.5
142	Thousand Island	2	tablespoon(s)	32	14.9	118	0.3	4.7	0.3	11.2	1.6	2.5	5.8
143	Thousand Island, low calorie	2	tablespoon(s)	30	18.2	59	0.2	7.2	0.4	3.4	0.2	1.9	0.8
	Sandwich spreads												
140	Mayonnaise, low calorie	1	tablespoon(s)	16	8.9	52	0.1	1.3	0	5.3	0.8	1.3	2.9
138	Mayonnaise with soybean oil	1	tablespoon(s)	14	3.0	94	0.1	0.1	0	10.3	1.6	2.3	6.2
141	Tartar sauce	2	tablespoon(s)	29	18.8	59	0.3	3.7	0.1	4.7	0.9	1.0	2.5
	Sweets												
4799	**Butterscotch or caramel topping**	2	tablespoon(s)	41	13.1	103	0.6	27.0	0.4	0	0	0	0
	Candy												
1786	Almond Joy candy bar	1	item(s)	45	3.7	220	2.0	26.0	2.0	13.0	8.0	2.4	0.5
1785	Bit-O-Honey candy	6	item(s)	40	—	150	1.0	32.0	0	3.0	2.0	—	—
33375	Butterscotch candy	2	piece(s)	12	0.6	47	0	10.8	0	0.4	0.2	0.1	0
1701	Chewing gum, stick	1	item(s)	3	0.1	11	0	2.9	0.1	0	0	0	0
33378	Chocolate fudge with nuts, prepared	2	piece(s)	38	2.9	175	1.7	25.8	0.9	7.2	2.5	1.5	2.9

Chol (mg)	Calc (mg)	Iron (mg)	Magn (mg)	Pota (mg)	Sodi (mg)	Zinc (mg)	Vit A (µg)	Thia (mg)	Vit E (mg α)	Ribo (mg)	Niac (mg)	Vit B_6 (mg)	Fola (µg)	Vit C (mg)	Vit B_{12} (µg)	Sele (µg)
14	0	0	0	0	0	0	0	0	0.35	0	0	0	0	0	0	0
11	0	0	0	0	0	0	0	0	0.35	0	0	0	0	0	0	0
0	0	0	0	0	0	0	0	0	0	0	0	0	0	0	0	0
12	0	0	0	0	0	0.01	0	0	0.08	0	0	0	0	0	0	0
0	4	0.01	0.4	5.9	133.0	0	115.5	0	1.27	0.01	0	0	0.1	0	0	0
0	4	0	0.3	5.5	155.4	0	142.7	0	1.01	0	0	0	0.1	0	0	0
0	2	0	0.3	3.5	0.3	0	115.5	0	1.80	0	0	0	0.1	0	0	0
0	0	0	0.1	1.5	59.1	0	73.7	0	1.39	0	0	0	0.1	0	0	0
0	4	0	0.3	5.4	153.1	0	140.6	0	0.71	0	0	0	0.1	0	0	0
8	2	0.07	0.1	4.7	78.4	0.02	11.6	0	3.04	0	0	0.08	1.1	0	0	0.2
0	0	0	—	—	85.0	—	—	—	2.01	—	—	0.70	—	0	1.2	—
0	0	0	0	0	0	0	0	0	2.37	0	0	0	0	0	0	0
0	0	0	0	0	0	0	0	0	1.94	0	0	0	0	0	0	0
0	0	0.08	0	0.1	0.3	0	0	0	1.94	0	0	0	0	0	0	0
0	0	0	0	0	0	0	0	0	2.12	0	0	0	0	0	0	0
0	0	0	0	0	0	0	0	0	4.64	0	0	0	0	0	0	0
0	0	0	0	0	0	0	0	0	0.19	0	0	0	0	0	0	0
0	0	0	0	0	0	0	0	0	1.10	0	0	0	0	0	0	0
0	0	0	0	0	0	0	0	0	1.65	0	0	0	0	0	0	0
0	0	0	0	0	0	0	0	0	5.59	0	0	0	0	0	0	0
0	0	0	—	—	0	—	—	—	—	—	—	—	—	0	—	—
9	11	0.03	2.4	26.4	312.3	0.06	5.7	0	1.28	0.03	0.03	0.01	2.4	0.2	0	0.3
0	28	0.16	2.2	1.6	300.5	0.08	0	0.01	0.08	0.03	0.02	0.01	1.0	0.1	0.1	0.5
12	14	0.32	0.6	8.7	362.7	0.03	2.7	0	1.42	0	0.01	0.01	0.6	0.1	0	0.5
0	12	0.08	1.6	43.9	296.0	0.06	0.3	0	0.22	0.02	0.01	0.01	2.0	0	0	0.5
0	2	0.04	0.6	10.8	336.0	0.01	0	0	0.72	0	0.01	0.01	0	0.1	0	0.5
0	8	0.26	1.6	21.4	267.5	0.09	7.4	0.01	1.60	0.02	0.06	0	0	1.2	0	0
0	4	0.23	2.6	34.2	268.2	0.06	8.6	0.01	0.32	0.02	0.15	0.02	0.6	1.5	0	0.5
0	4	0.08	1.5	24.7	291.9	0.02	0.6	0.01	0.64	0	0.04	0.02	0	0.1	0	0.6
0	5	0.08	1.2	27.0	300.9	0.02	0.3	0	1.28	0	0.03	0.02	0.9	0	0	0.5
8	4	0.06	0.6	2.6	209.0	0.05	6.2	0	0.61	0.01	0	0	1.8	0	0.1	0.5
0	0	0	0	2.6	0.3	0	0	0	1.48	0	0	0	0	0	0	0.5
10	9	0.19	1.5	18.6	328.2	0.12	3.0	0.03	1.27	0.02	0	0.01	1.2	1.0	0.1	0.6
0	5	0.01	0.9	8.1	414.0	0.02	0.6	0	0.73	0.01	0	0	0.3	0.1	0	0.1
0	4	0.18	3.0	51.9	339.9	0.07	8.7	0.01	1.00	0.01	0.18	0.03	1.5	1.8	0	0.5
2	6	0.19	0	50.2	277.8	0.03	0.6	0	0.13	0	0	0	1.0	1.9	0	0.5
0	6	0.18	0	47.1	300.0	0.03	0.6	0	1.50	0	0	0	0	0	0	0.5
8	5	0.38	2.6	34.2	276.2	0.08	4.5	0.46	1.28	0.02	0.13	0	0	0	0	0.5
3	8	0.27	2.1	60.6	286.5	0.06	4.8	0.01	0.30	0.01	0.13	0	0	0.4	0	0
6	1	0.05	0.3	6.4	107.7	0.03	3.4	0	0.49	0	0	0	0.6	0	0	0.4
6	1	0.03	0.1	2.8	87.6	0.02	2.2	0	0.45	0	0	0	0.7	0	0	0.3
2	7	0.07	1.7	19.0	186.8	0.03	3.1	0	0.47	0.01	0.03	0.01	1.4	0.6	0	0.3
0	22	0.08	2.9	34.4	143.1	0.08	11.1	0	—	0.04	0.02	0.01	0.8	0.1	0	0
0	18	0.33	—	114.3	50.0	—	0	—	—	—	—	—	—	0	—	—
0	20	0	—	—	120.0	—	0	—	—	—	—	—	—	0	—	—
1	0	0	0	0.4	46.9	0.01	3.4	0	0.01	0	0	0	0	0	0	0.1
0	0	0	0	0.1	0	0	0	0	0	0	0	0	0	0	0	0
5	22	0.75	20.9	69.5	14.8	0.54	14.4	0.03	0.10	0.04	0.12	0.03	6.1	0.1	0	1.1

APPENDIX H

DA+ Code	Food Description	Quantity	Measure	Wt (g)	H_2O (g)	Ener (kcal)	Prot (g)	Carb (g)	Fiber (g)	Fat (g)	Fat Breakdown (g) Sat	Mono	Poly
	Sweets—*continued*												
1787	Jelly beans	15	item(s)	43	2.7	159	0	39.8	0.1	0	0	0	0
1784	Kit Kat wafer bar	1	item(s)	42	0.7	210	3.0	27.0	1.0	11.0	7.0	2.5	0.4
4674	Krackel candy bar	1	item(s)	41	0.6	210	2.0	28.0	0.5	10.0	6.0	3.9	0.4
4934	Licorice	4	piece(s)	44	7.3	154	1.1	35.1	0	1.0	0	0.1	0
1780	Life Savers candy	1	item(s)	2	—	6	0	1.4	—	0	0	0	0
1790	Lollipop	1	item(s)	28	—	108	0	28.0	0	0	0	0	0
4679	M & Ms peanut chocolate candy, small bag	1	item(s)	49	1.2	250	5.0	30.0	2.0	13.0	5.0	4.0	1.7
1781	M & Ms plain chocolate candy, small bag	1	item(s)	48	0.8	240	2.0	34.0	1.0	10.0	6.0	2.5	0.4
4673	Milk chocolate bar, Symphony	1	item(s)	91	0.9	483	7.7	52.8	1.5	27.8	16.7	7.2	0.6
1783	Milky Way bar	1	item(s)	58	3.7	260	2.0	41.0	1.0	10.0	7.0	1.3	0.2
1788	Peanut brittle	1 ½	ounce(s)	43	0.3	207	3.2	30.3	1.1	8.1	1.8	3.4	1.9
1789	Reese's peanut butter cups	2	piece(s)	42	0.6	210	5.0	24.0	1.0	13.0	4.5	5.5	2.3
4689	Reese's pieces candy, small bag	1	item(s)	43	0.4	200	5.0	25.0	2.0	9.0	8.0	1.9	0.8
33399	Semisweet chocolate candy, made with butter	½	ounce(s)	14	0.1	68	0.6	9.0	0.8	4.2	2.5	1.4	0.1
1782	Snickers bar	1	item(s)	59	3.3	280	4.0	35.0	1.0	14.0	5.0	4.6	1.8
4694	Special Dark chocolate bar	1	item(s)	41	—	190	2.0	25.0	3.0	12.0	8.0	—	—
4695	Starburst fruit chews, original fruits	1	package(s)	40	3.5	160	0	33.0	0	3.5	3.0	0	0
4698	Taffy	3	piece(s)	45	2.2	179	0	41.2	0	1.5	0.9	0.4	0.1
4699	Three Musketeers bar	1	item(s)	60	3.5	260	2.0	46.0	1.0	8.0	5.0	1.4	0.2
11764	Turtles	1	piece(s)	17	—	86	1.0	10.1	0.5	5.0	2.0	—	—
4702	Twix caramel cookie bars	2	item(s)	51	2.4	250	2.0	33.0	1.0	12.0	9.0	1.7	0.4
4705	York Peppermint Pattie	1	item(s)	39	3.5	140	1.0	31.0	1.0	2.5	1.5	0.2	0
	Frosting, icing												
4760	Chocolate frosting, ready to eat	2	tablespoon(s)	31	5.2	122	0.3	19.4	0.3	5.4	1.7	2.8	0.7
4771	Creamy vanilla frosting, ready to eat	2	tablespoon(s)	35	5.3	146	0	23.8	0	5.7	1.0	1.7	2.8
536	White icing	2	tablespoon(s)	40	6.0	167	0	27.2	0	6.5	1.2	1.9	3.2
	Gelatin												
13697	Gelatin snack, all flavors	1	item(s)	96	—	70	1.0	17.0	0	0	0	0	0
2616	Sugar-free, low-calorie mixed fruit gelatin mix, prepared	½	cup(s)	121	—	10	1.0	0	0	0	0	0	0
548	**Honey**	1	tablespoon(s)	21	3.6	64	0.1	17.3	0	0	0	0	0
	Jams, jellies												
550	Jam or preserves	1	tablespoon(s)	20	6.1	56	0.1	13.8	0.2	0	0	0	0
42199	Jams, preserves, dietetic, all flavors, w/sodium saccarin	1	tablespoon(s)	14	6.4	18	0	7.5	0.3	0	0	0	0
552	Jelly	1	tablespoon(s)	21	6.3	56	0	14.7	0.2	0	0	0	0
545	**Marshmallows**	4	item(s)	29	4.7	92	0.5	23.4	0	0.1	0	0	0
4800	**Marshmallow cream topping**	2	tablespoon(s)	40	7.9	129	0.3	31.6	0	0.1	0	0	0
555	**Molasses**	1	tablespoon(s)	20	4.4	58	0	14.9	0	0	0	0	0
4780	**Popsicle or ice pop**	1	item(s)	59	47.5	47	0.0	11.3	0	0.1	0	0	0
	Sugar												
559	Brown sugar, packed	1	teaspoon(s)	5	0.1	17	0	4.5	0	0	0	0	0
563	Powdered sugar, sifted	⅓	cup(s)	33	0.1	130	0	33.2	0	0	0	0	0
561	White granulated sugar	1	teaspoon(s)	4	0	16	0	4.2	0	0	0	0	0
	Sugar substitute												
1760	Equal sweetener, packet size	1	item(s)	1	—	0	0	0.5	0	0	0	0	0
13029	Splenda granular no-calorie sweetener	1	teaspoon(s)	1	—	0	0	0.5	0	0	0	0	0
1759	Sweet N Low sugar substitute, packet	1	item(s)	1	0.1	4	0	0.5	0	0	0	0	0
	Syrup												
3148	Chocolate syrup	2	tablespoon(s)	39	12.1	109	0.8	25.4	1.0	0.4	0.2	0.1	0
29676	Maple syrup	¼	cup(s)	79	25.5	205	0	52.8	0	0	0	0	0
4795	Pancake syrup	¼	cup(s)	80	30.4	187	0	49.2	0	0	0	0	0
	Spices, Condiments, Sauces												
	Spices												
807	Allspice, ground	1	teaspoon(s)	2	0.2	5	0.1	1.4	0.4	0.2	0	0	0
1171	Anise seeds	1	teaspoon(s)	2	0.2	7	0.4	1.1	0.3	0.3	0	0.2	0.1
729	Bakers' yeast, active	1	teaspoon(s)	4	0.2	13	1.6	1.6	1.1	0.3	0	0.2	0
683	Baking powder, double acting with phosphate	1	teaspoon(s)	5	0.2	2	0	1.1	0	0	0	0	0

E KEY: H-4 = Breads/Baked Goods H-8 = Cereal/Rice/Pasta H-14 = Fruit H-18 = Vegetables/Legumes H-28 = Nuts/Seeds H-30 = Vegetarian H-32 = Dairy H-40 = Eggs H-40 = Seafood H-42 = Meats H-46 = Poultry
8 = Processed Meats H-50 = Beverages H-52 = Fats/Oils H-54 = Sweets H-56 = Spices/Condiments/Sauces H-60 = Mixed Foods/Soups/Sandwiches H-66 = Fast Food H-84 = Convenience H-86 = Baby Foods

Chol (mg)	Calc (mg)	Iron (mg)	Magn (mg)	Pota (mg)	Sodi (mg)	Zinc (mg)	Vit A (µg)	Thia (mg)	Vit E (mg α)	Ribo (mg)	Niac (mg)	Vit B_6 (mg)	Fola (µg)	Vit C (mg)	Vit B_{12} (µg)	Sele (µg)
0	1	0.06	0.9	15.7	21.3	0.02	0	0	0	0	0	0	0	0	0	0.5
5	60	0.36	15.5	97.0	30.0	0.04	0	0.05	0.14	0.09	0.21	0.01	7.6	0	0.2	2.1
3	40	0.37	—	168.8	50.0	—	0	—	—	—	—	—	—	0	—	—
0	0	0.22	2.6	28.2	126.3	0.07	0	0.01	0.08	0.02	0.04	0		0	0	
0	0	0	—	—	0	—	0	—	—	—	—	—	—	0	—	—
0	0	0	—	—	10.8	—	0	0	—	0	0	—	—	0	—	1.0
5	40	0.36	34.0	171.1	25.0	0.87	—	0.03	1.40	0.07	1.60	0.04	27.1	0.6	0.2	2.0
5	40	0.36	21.1	125.0	30.0	0.77	13.3	0.04	0.17	0.07	0.13	0.01	3.8	0.6	0.3	1.6
22	228	0.83	61.0	398.6	91.9	1.00	—	0.06	—	0.25	0.15	0.10	—	2.0	0.4	—
5	60	0.18	11.6	72.1	95.0	0.40	14.0	0.03	0.52	0.07	0.09	0.01	2.3	0.6	0.1	1.2
5	11	0.52	17.9	71.4	189.2	0.37	16.6	0.06	1.09	0.02	1.13	0.03	19.6	0	0	1.1
5	20	0.72	26.0	144.1	150.0	0.54	0	0.07	0.06	0.05	1.89	0.04	21.0	0	0.1	0.6
0	0	0.72	37.8	154.4	55.0	0.50	0	0.08	0.43	0.09	2.61	0.05	23.6	0	0	0.3
3	5	0.44	16.3	51.7	1.6	0.23	0.4	0.01	—	0.01	0.06	0.01	0.4	0	0	0.5
5	40	0.36	42.3	189.6	140.0	1.47		0.03	0.88	0.08	2.11	0.05	18.2	0	0.1	4.6
5	0	1.80	—	—	15.0	—	0	—	—	—	—	—	—	0	—	—
0	0	0	0.6	1.2	0	0	0	0	0.19	0	0	0	0.6	23.5	0	0.5
4	4	0	0	1.4	23.4	0.09	12.1	0.01	0.04	0.01	0	0	0	0	0	0.3
5	20	0.36	17.5	80.3	110.0	0.33	14.9	0.02	0.59	0.03	0.14	0.01	2.4	0.6	0.1	1.1
0	20	0.36	—	—	15.1	—	0	—	—	—	—	—	—	0	—	—
5	39	0.35	15.2	104.5	100.0	0.60	—	0.08	0.42	0.11	0.57	0.01	19.9	0.6	0.2	2.4
0	0	0.33	—	43.3	10.0	—	0	—	—	—	—	—	—	0	—	—
0	2	0.43	6.4	60.0	56.1	0.09	0	0	0.48	0.01	0.04	0	0.3	0	0	0.2
0	1	0.06	0.3	11.9	64.4	0.02	0	0	0.54	0.11	0.08	0	2.8	0	0	0
0	1	0.06	0.4	13.6	73.6	0.03	0	0	0.61	0.12	0.09	0	3.2	0	0	0
0	0	0	—	0	40.0	—	0	—	—	—	—	—	—	0	—	—
0	0	0	0	0	45.0	0	0	0	0	0	0	0	—	0	0	—
0	1	0.09	0.4	10.9	0.8	0.05	0	0	0	0.01	0.03	0.01	0.4	0.1	0	0.2
0	4	0.10	0.8	15.4	6.4	0.01	0	0	0.02	0.02	0.01	0	2.2	1.8	0	0.4
0	1	0.06	0.7	9.7	0	0.01	0	0	0.01	0	0	0	1.3	0	0	0.2
0	1	0.04	1.3	11.3	6.3	0.01	0	0	0	0.01	0.01	0	0.4	0.2	0	0.1
0	1	0.07	0.6	1.4	23.0	0.01	0	0	0	0	0.02	0	0.3	0	0	0.5
0	1	0.09	0.8	2.0	32.0	0.02	0	0	0	0	0.03	0	0.4	0	0	0.8
0	41	0.94	48.4	292.8	7.4	0.06	0	0.01	0	0	0.19	0.13	0	0	0	3.6
0	0	0.32	0.6	8.9	4.1	0.09	0	0	0	0	0	0	0	0.4	0	0.1
0	4	0.03	0.4	6.1	1.3	0	0	0	0	0	0.01	0	0	0	0	0.1
0	0	0.02	0.0	0.7	0.7	0	0	0	0	0.01	0	0	0	0	0	0.2
0	0	0	0.0	0.1	0	0	0	0	0	0	0	0	0	0	0	0
0	0	0	—	0	0	—	—	—	—	—	—	—	—	0	—	—
0	0	0	—	—	0	—	0	—	—	—	—	—	—	0	—	—
0	0	0	—	—	0	—	—	—	—	—	—	—	—	0	—	—
0	5	0.82	25.4	87.4	28.1	0.28	0	0	0.01	0.02	0.13	0	0.8	0.1	0	0.5
0	80	0.09	16.5	166.9	9.4	1.16	0	0.05	0	1.00	0.06	0	0	0	0	0.5
0	2	0.02	1.6	12.0	65.6	0.06	0	0.02	0	0.01	0	0	0	0	0	0
0	13	0.13	2.6	19.8	1.5	0.02	0.5	0	—	0	0.05	0	0.7	0.7	0	0.1
0	14	0.78	3.6	30.3	0.3	0.11	0.3	0.01	—	0.01	0.06	0.01	0.2	0.4	0	0.1
0	1	0.09	2.2	38.2	2.0	0.32	0	0.44	0	0.16	1.61	0.06	93.6	0	0	0.3
0	339	0.52	1.8	0.2	363.1	0	0	0	0	0	0	0	0	0	0	0

TABLE H-1 Table of Food Composition (*continued*) (Computer code is for Cengage Diet Analysis program) (For purposes of calculations, use "0" for t, <1, <0.1, 0.01)

DA+ Code	Food Description	Quantity	Measure	Wt (g)	H_2O (g)	Ener (kcal)	Prot (g)	Carb (g)	Fiber (g)	Fat (g)	Fat Breakdown (g)		
											Sat	Mono	Poly
Spices, Condiments, Sauces—*continued*													
1611	Baking soda	1	teaspoon(s)	5	0	0	0	0	0	0	0	0	0
8552	Basil	1	teaspoon(s)	1	0.8	0	0	0	0	0	0	0	0
34959	Basil, fresh	1	piece(s)	1	0.5	0	0	0	0	0	0	0	0
808	Basil, ground	1	teaspoon(s)	1	0.1	3	0.3	0.7	0.5	0.1	0	0	0
809	Bay leaf	1	teaspoon(s)	1	0	2	0	0.4	0.2	0.1	0	0	0
11720	Betel leaves	1	ounce(s)	28	—	17	1.8	2.4	0	0	—	—	—
11710	Capers	1	teaspoon(s)	5	—	0	0	0	0	0	0	0	0
1172	Caraway seeds	1	teaspoon(s)	2	0.2	7	0.4	1.0	0.8	0.3	0	0.1	0.1
1173	Celery seeds	1	teaspoon(s)	2	0.1	8	0.4	0.8	0.2	0.5	0	0.3	0.1
1174	Chervil, dried	1	teaspoon(s)	1	0	1	0.1	0.3	0.1	0	0	0	0
810	Chili powder	1	teaspoon(s)	3	0.3	7	0.3	1.3	0.9	0.4	0.1	0.1	0.2
8553	Chives, chopped	1	teaspoon(s)	1	0.9	0	0	0	0	0	0	0	0
51420	Cilantro (coriander)	1	teaspoon(s)	0	0.3	0	0	0	0	0	0	0	0
811	Cinnamon, ground	1	teaspoon(s)	2	0.2	6	0.1	1.9	1.2	0	0	0	0
812	Cloves, ground	1	teaspoon(s)	2	0.2	6	0.1	1.4	0.7	0.3	0.1	0	0.2
1175	Coriander leaf, dried	1	teaspoon(s)	1	0	2	0.1	0.3	0.1	0	0	0	0
1176	Coriander seeds	1	teaspoon(s)	2	0.2	5	0.2	1.0	0.8	0.3	0	0.2	0
1706	Cornstarch	1	tablespoon(s)	8	0.7	30	0	7.3	0.1	0	0	0	0
1177	Cumin seeds	1	teaspoon(s)	2	0.2	8	0.4	0.9	0.2	0.5	0	0.3	0.1
11729	Cumin, ground	1	teaspoon(s)	5	—	11	0.4	0.8	0.8	0.4	—	—	—
1178	Curry powder	1	teaspoon(s)	2	0.2	7	0.3	1.2	0.7	0.3	0	0.1	0.1
1179	Dill seeds	1	teaspoon(s)	2	0.2	6	0.3	1.2	0.4	0.3	0	0.2	0
1180	Dill weed, dried	1	teaspoon(s)	1	0.1	3	0.2	0.6	0.1	0	0	0	0
34949	Dill weed, fresh	5	piece(s)	1	0.9	0	0	0.1	0	0	0	0	0
1181	Fennel seeds	1	teaspoon(s)	2	0.2	7	0.3	1.0	0.8	0.3	0	0.2	0
1182	Fenugreek seeds	1	teaspoon(s)	4	0.3	12	0.9	2.2	0.9	0.2	0.1	—	—
11733	Garam masala, powder	1	ounce(s)	28	—	107	4.4	12.8	0	4.3	—	—	—
1067	Garlic clove	1	item(s)	3	1.8	4	0.2	1.0	0.1	0	0	0	0
813	Garlic powder	1	teaspoon(s)	3	0.2	9	0.5	2.0	0.3	0	0	0	0
1068	Ginger root	2	teaspoon(s)	4	3.2	3	0.1	0.7	0.1	0	0	0	0
1183	Ginger, ground	1	teaspoon(s)	2	0.2	6	0.2	1.3	0.3	0.1	0	0	0
35497	Leeks, bulb and lower-leaf, freeze-dried	¼	cup(s)	1	0	3	0.1	0.6	0.1	0	0	0	0
1184	Mace, ground	1	teaspoon(s)	2	0.1	8	0.1	0.9	0.3	0.6	0.2	0.2	0.1
1185	Marjoram, dried	1	teaspoon(s)	1	0	2	0.1	0.4	0.2	0.0	0	0	0
1186	Mustard seeds, yellow	1	teaspoon(s)	3	0.2	17	0.9	0.9	0.4	1.2	0.1	0.7	0.3
814	Nutmeg, ground	1	teaspoon(s)	2	0.1	12	0.1	1.1	0.5	0.8	0.6	0.1	0
2747	Onion flakes, dehydrated	1	teaspoon(s)	2	0.1	6	0.1	1.4	0.2	0	0	0	0
1187	Onion powder	1	teaspoon(s)	2	0.1	7	0.2	1.7	0.3	0	0	0	0
815	Oregano, ground	1	teaspoon(s)	2	0.2	5	0.2	1.2	0.8	0.1	0	0	0
816	Paprika	1	teaspoon(s)	2	0.2	6	0.3	1.1	0.7	0.3	0	0	0.2
817	Parsley, dried	1	teaspoon(s)	0	0	1	0.1	0.2	0.1	0	0	0	0
818	Pepper, black	1	teaspoon(s)	2	0.3	5	0.2	1.3	0.5	0.1	0	0	0
819	Pepper, cayenne	1	teaspoon(s)	2	0.1	6	0.2	1.0	0.5	0.3	0.1	0	0.2
1188	Pepper, white	1	teaspoon(s)	2	0.3	7	0.2	1.6	0.6	0.1	0	0	0
1189	Poppy seeds	1	teaspoon(s)	3	0.2	15	0.5	0.8	0.5	1.2	0.1	0.2	0.8
1190	Poultry seasoning	1	teaspoon(s)	2	0.1	5	0.1	1.0	0.2	0.1	0	0	0
1191	Pumpkin pie spice, powder	1	teaspoon(s)	2	0.1	6	0.1	1.2	0.3	0.2	0.1	0	0
1192	Rosemary, dried	1	teaspoon(s)	1	0.1	4	0.1	0.8	0.5	0.2	0.1	0	0
11723	Rosemary, fresh	1	teaspoon(s)	1	0.5	1	0	0.1	0.1	0	0	0	0
2722	Saffron powder	1	teaspoon(s)	1	0.1	2	0.1	0.5	0	0	0	0	0
11724	Sage	1	teaspoon(s)	1	—	1	0	0.1	0	0	—	—	—
1193	Sage, ground	1	teaspoon(s)	1	0.1	2	0.1	0.4	0.3	0.1	0	0	0
30189	Salt substitute	¼	teaspoon(s)	2	—	0	0	0	0	0	0	0	0
30195	Salt, kosher	¼	teaspoon(s)	2	—	0	0	0	0	0	0	0	0
822	Salt, table	¼	teaspoon(s)	2	0	0	0	0	0	0	0	0	0
1194	Savory, ground	1	teaspoon(s)	1	0.1	4	0.1	1.0	0.6	0.1	0	—	—
820	Sesame seed kernels, toasted	1	teaspoon(s)	3	0.1	15	0.5	0.7	0.5	1.3	0.2	0.5	0.6
11725	Sorrel	1	teaspoon(s)	3	—	1	0.1	0.1	0	0	0	—	—
11721	Spearmint	1	teaspoon(s)	2	1.6	1	0.1	0.2	0.1	0	0	0	0
35498	Sweet green peppers, freeze-dried	¼	cup(s)	2	0	5	0.3	1.1	0.3	0	0	0	0
11726	Tamarind leaves	1	ounce(s)	28	—	33	1.6	5.2	0	0.6	—	—	—
11727	Tarragon	1	ounce(s)	28	—	14	1.0	1.8	0	0.3	—	—	—
1195	Tarragon, ground	1	teaspoon(s)	2	0.1	5	0.4	0.8	0.1	0.1	0	0	0.1
11728	Thyme, fresh	1	teaspoon(s)	1	0.5	1	0	0.2	0.1	0	0	0	0

Chol (mg)	Calc (mg)	Iron (mg)	Magn (mg)	Pota (mg)	Sodi (mg)	Zinc (mg)	Vit A (µg)	Thia (mg)	Vit E (mg α)	Ribo (mg)	Niac (mg)	Vit B_6 (mg)	Fola (µg)	Vit C (mg)	Vit B_{12} (µg)	Sele (µg)
0	0	0	0	0	1258.6	0	0	0	0	0	0	0	0	0	0	0
0	2	0.03	0.6	2.6	0	0.01	2.3	0	0.01	0	0.01	0	0.6	0.2	0	0
0	1	0.02	0.3	1.5	0	0	1.3	0	—	0	0	0	0.3	0.1	0	0
0	31	1.26	10.0	36.8	1.1	0.10	0.5	0	0.15	0.02	0.07	0.02	4.3	0	0	0
0	5	0.26	0.7	3.2	0.1	0.02	1.9	0	—	0	0.01	0.01	1.1	0.3	0	0
0	110	2.29	—	155.9	2.0	—	—	0.04	—	0.07	0.20	—	—	0.9	0	—
0	—	—	—	—	105.0	—	—	—	—	—	—	—	—	—	0	—
0	14	0.34	5.4	28.4	0.4	0.12	0.4	0.01	0.05	0.01	0.08	0.01	0.2	0.4	0	0.3
0	35	0.90	8.8	28.0	3.2	0.14	0.1	0.01	0.02	0.01	0.06	0.02	0.2	0.3	0	0.2
0	8	0.19	0.8	28.4	0.5	0.05	1.8	0	—	0	0.03	0.01	1.6	0.3	0	0.2
0	9	0.45	3.9	50.7	42.6	0.11	38.6	0.01	0.99	0.02	0.30	0.05	0.7	0	0	0.5
0	1	0.02	0.4	3.0	0	0.01	2.2	0	0	0	0.01	0	1.0	0.6	0	0
0	0	0.01	0.1	1.7	0.2	0	1.1	0	0.01	0	0	0	0.2	0.1	0	0
0	23	0.19	1.4	9.9	0.2	0.04	0.3	0	0.05	0	0.03	0	0.1	0.1	0	0.1
0	13	0.25	5.4	21.4	5.8	0.05	0.2	0	0.19	0	0.03	0.01	0.5	0	0	0.2
0	7	0.25	4.2	26.8	1.3	0.03	1.8	0.01	0.01	0.01	0.06	0	1.6	3.4	0	0.2
0	13	0.29	5.9	22.8	0.6	0.08	0	0	—	0.01	0.04	—	0	0.4	0	0.5
0	0	0.04	0.2	0.2	0.7	0	0	0	0	0	0	0	0	0	0	0.2
0	20	1.39	7.7	37.5	3.5	0.10	1.3	0.01	0.07	0.01	0.10	0.01	0.2	0.2	0	0.1
0	20	—	—	43.6	4.8	—	—	—	—	—	—	—	—	—	—	—
0	10	0.59	5.1	30.9	1.0	0.08	1.0	0.01	0.44	0.01	0.07	0.02	3.1	0.2	0	0.3
0	32	0.34	5.4	24.9	0.4	0.11	0.1	0.01	—	0.01	0.06	0.01	0.2	0.4	0	0.3
0	18	0.49	4.5	33.1	2.1	0.03	2.9	0	—	0	0.03	0.02	—	0.5	0	—
0	2	0.07	0.6	7.4	0.6	0.01	3.9	0	0.02	0	0.02	0	1.5	0.9	0	—
0	24	0.37	7.7	33.9	1.8	0.07	0.1	0.01	—	0.01	0.12	0.01	—	0.4	0	—
0	7	1.24	7.1	28.5	2.5	0.09	0.1	0.01	—	0.01	0.06	0.02	2.1	0.1	0	0.2
0	215	9.24	93.6	411.1	27.5	1.07	—	0.10	—	0.09	0.71	—	—	0	0	—
0	5	0.05	0.8	12.0	0.5	0.03	0	0.01	0	0	0.02	0.04	0.1	0.9	0	0.4
0	2	0.16	2.2	33.4	1.7	0.08	0	0.01	0.02	0	0.02	0.05	1.3	0	0	0.7
0	1	0.02	1.7	16.6	0.5	0.01	0	0	0.01	0	0.03	0.01	0.4	0.2	0	0
0	2	0.36	3.9	23.8	0.5	0.07	0	0	0	0	0.17	0.01	0.2	0	0	1.0
0	3	0.06	1.3	19.2	0.3	0.01	0.1	0.01	—	0	0.03	0.01	2.9	0.9	0	0
0	4	0.24	2.8	7.9	1.4	0.04	0.7	0.01	—	0.01	0.02	0	1.3	0.4	0	0
0	12	0.50	2.1	9.1	0.5	0.02	2.4	0	0.01	0	0.02	0.01	1.6	0.3	0	0
0	9	0.30	12.2	24.4	0.4	0.20	0.1	0.03	0.17	0.01	0.16	0.01	5.3	0.2	0	6.9
0	4	0.07	4.0	7.7	0.4	0.05	0.1	0.01	0	0	0.03	0	1.7	0.1	0	0
0	4	0.03	1.5	27.1	0.4	0.03	0	0.01	0	0	0.02	0.03	2.8	1.3	0	0.1
0	8	0.08	2.4	20.7	1.5	0.09	0	0.01	0.01	0	0.01	0.02	1.3	0.5	0	0.3
0	29	0.66	4.9	22.7	0.5	0.05	1.5	0	0.33	0.01	0.08	0.02	4.3	0	0	0.1
0	5	0.44	3.7	47.9	1.4	0.09	51.7	0.01	0.61	0.03	0.21	0.04	1.0	0	0	0.1
0	3	0.07	1.2	8.0	1.4	0.02	0.3	0	0.03	0.01	0.03	0	0.5	0.4	0	0
0	9	0.20	3.6	27.9	0.4	0.02	0.6	0	0.02	0	0.02	0.01	0.4	0	0	0.1
0	3	0.14	2.7	36.3	0.5	0.04	37.5	0.01	0.54	0.02	0.16	0.04	1.9	1.4	0	0.2
0	6	0.34	2.2	1.8	0.1	0.03	0	0	—	0	0.01	0	0.2	0.5	0	0.1
0	40	0.27	9.7	20.1	0.7	0.22	0	0.02	0.05	0	0.03	0.01	2.3	0	0	0.4
0	15	0.53	3.4	10.3	0.4	0.05	2.0	0	0.02	0	0.04	0.02	2.1	0.2	0	0.1
0	12	0.34	2.3	11.3	0.9	0.04	0.2	0	0.03	0	0.04	0.01	0.4	0.4	0	0.2
0	15	0.35	2.6	11.5	0.6	0.04	1.9	0.01	—	0.01	0.01	0.02	3.7	0.7	0	0.1
0	2	0.05	0.6	4.7	0.2	0.01	1.0	0	—	0	0.01	0	0.8	0.2	0	—
0	1	0.08	1.8	12.1	1.0	0.01	0.2	0	—	0	0.01	0.01	0.7	0.6	0	0
0	4	—	1.1	2.7	0	0.01	—	0	—	—	—	—	—	—	0	—
0	12	0.20	3.0	7.5	0.1	0.03	2.1	0.01	0.05	0	0.04	0.02	1.9	0.2	0	0
0	8	0	0	754.5	0.1	—	0	—	—	—	—	—	—	0	—	—
0	0	0	—	—	600.0	—	0	—	—	—	—	—	—	0	—	—
0	0	0	0	0.1	581.4	0	0	0	0	0	0	0	0	0	0	0
0	30	0.53	5.3	14.7	0.3	0.06	3.6	0.01	—	—	0.06	0.03	—	0.7	0	0.1
0	3	0.21	9.2	10.8	1.0	0.27	0.1	0.03	0.01	0.01	0.15	0	2.6	0	0	0.9
0	—	—	—	—	0.1	—	—	—	—	—	—	—	—	—	—	—
0	4	0.23	1.2	8.7	0.6	0.02	3.9	0	—	0	0.02	0	2.0	0.3	0	—
0	2	0.17	3.0	50.7	3.1	0.04	4.5	0.02	0.06	0.02	0.12	0.04	3.7	30.4	0	0.1
0	85	1.48	20.2	—	—	—	—	0.07	—	0.03	1.16	—	—	0.9	0	—
0	48	—	14.5	128.1	2.6	0.17	—	0.04	—	—	—	—	—	0.6	0	—
0	18	0.52	5.6	48.3	1.0	0.06	3.4	0	—	0.02	0.14	0.04	4.4	0.8	0	0.1
0	3	0.14	1.3	4.9	0.1	0.01	1.9	0	—	0	0.01	0	0.4	1.3	0	—

DA+ Code	Food Description	Quantity	Measure	Wt (g)	H_2O (g)	Ener (kcal)	Prot (g)	Carb (g)	Fiber (g)	Fat (g)	Fat Breakdown (g) Sat	Mono	Poly
Spices, Condiments, Sauces—*continued*													
821	Thyme, ground	1	teaspoon(s)	1	0.1	4	0.1	0.9	0.5	0.1	0	0	0
1196	Turmeric, ground	1	teaspoon(s)	2	0.2	8	0.2	1.4	0.5	0.2	0.1	0	0
11995	Wasabi	1	tablespoon(s)	14	10.7	10	0.7	2.3	0.2	0	—	—	—
	Condiments												
674	Catsup or ketchup	1	tablespoon(s)	15	10.4	17	0.2	3.9	0	0	0	0	0
5812	Catsup or ketchup, low sodium	1	tablespoon(s)	15	10.4	15	0.3	3.8	0.3	0	0	0	0
703	Dill pickle	1	ounce(s)	28	26.7	3	0.2	0.7	0.3	0	0	0	0
32128	Guacamole	2	tablespoon(s)	32	25.1	42	0.7	2.1	1.1	3.8	0.6	2.4	0.4
1814	Hummus	½	cup(s)	123	79.8	218	6.0	24.7	4.9	10.6	1.4	6.0	2.6
138	Mayonnaise with soybean oil	1	tablespoon(s)	14	3.0	94	0.1	0.1	0	10.3	1.6	2.3	6.2
140	Mayonnaise, low calorie	1	tablespoon(s)	16	8.9	52	0.1	1.3	0	5.3	0.8	1.3	2.9
1682	Mustard, brown	1	teaspoon(s)	5	4.1	5	0.3	0.3	0	0.3	—	—	—
700	Mustard, yellow	1	teaspoon(s)	5	4.1	3	0.2	0.3	0.2	0.2	0	0.1	0
706	Sweet pickle relish	1	tablespoon(s)	15	9.3	20	0.1	5.3	0.2	0.1	0	0	0
141	Tartar sauce	2	tablespoon(s)	29	18.8	59	0.3	3.7	0.1	4.7	0.9	1.0	2.5
	Sauces												
685	Barbecue sauce	2	tablespoon(s)	31	17.1	54	0.3	12.7	0.3	0.2	0	0	0
40849	Barbecue sauce, low sodium	2	tablespoon(s)	31	17.1	54	0.3	12.7	0.3	0.2	0	0	0
834	Cheese sauce	¼	cup(s)	63	44.4	110	4.2	4.3	0.3	8.4	3.8	2.4	1.6
32123	Chili enchilada sauce, green	2	tablespoon(s)	57	53.0	15	0.6	3.1	0.7	0.3	0	0	0.1
32122	Chili enchilada sauce, red	2	tablespoon(s)	32	24.5	27	1.1	5.0	2.1	0.8	0.1	0	0.4
29688	Hoisin sauce	1	tablespoon(s)	16	7.1	35	0.5	7.1	0.4	0.5	0.1	0.2	0.3
1641	Horseradish sauce, prepared	1	teaspoon(s)	5	3.5	9	0.1	0.1	0	0.9	0.5	0.2	0
16670	Mole poblano sauce	½	cup(s)	133	102.8	156	5.4	10.9	2.7	11.6	2.7	5.2	3.0
29689	Oyster sauce	1	tablespoon(s)	16	12.8	8	0.2	1.7	0	0	0	0	0
1655	Pepper sauce or Tabasco	1	teaspoon(s)	5	4.5	1	0.1	0	0	0	0	0	0
347	Salsa	2	tablespoon(s)	32	28.5	9	0.5	2.2	0.6	0.1	0	0	0
2835	Soy sauce, low sodium	1	tablespoon(s)	18	12.8	10	0.9	1.5	0.1	0	0	0	0
52206	Soy sauce, tamari	1	tablespoon(s)	18	11.8	11	1.9	1.0	0.1	0	0	0	0
25292	Sweet and sour sauce	2	tablespoon(s)	35	29.0	22	0.5	5.0	0.1	0.1	0	0	0
1613	Teriyaki sauce	1	tablespoon(s)	18	12.2	16	1.1	2.8	0	0	0	0	0
25294	Tomato sauce	½	cup(s)	150	133.4	61	2.4	11.2	2.7	1.6	0.2	0.4	0.8
42233	Tomato sauce, no salt added	½	cup(s)	122	111.2	35	1.6	8.2	1.8	0.2	0	0	0.1
5187	White sauce, medium-thick	¼	cup(s)	59	44.3	87	2.3	5.4	0.1	6.3	1.7	2.6	1.7
1654	Worcestershire sauce	1	teaspoon(s)	6	4.5	4	0	1.1	0	0	0	0	0
	Vinegar												
30853	Balsamic	1	tablespoon(s)	15	—	10	0	2.0	0	0	0	0	0
727	Cider	1	tablespoon(s)	15	14.0	3	0	0.1	0	0	0	0	0
5176	Distilled	1	tablespoon(s)	15	14.0	3	0	0	0	0	0	0	0
12948	Tarragon	1	tablespoon(s)	15	14.3	3	0	0.1	0	0	0	0	0
Mixed Foods, Sandwiches, and Soups													
	Mixed dishes												
16652	Almond chicken	1	cup(s)	242	187.5	283	20.4	15.9	3.4	15.6	2.1	7.1	5.2
25224	Barbecued chicken	1	serving(s)	177	100.1	325	27.2	15.1	0.1	17.1	4.8	6.8	3.8
25227	Bean burrito	1	item(s)	147	81.7	318	16.2	30.9	5.7	14.9	8.3	4.7	1.0
9516	Beef and vegetable fajita	1	item(s)	223	145.3	377	23.3	34.9	2.7	15.7	5.1	6.9	2.5
16796	Beef or pork egg roll	2	item(s)	128	59.6	355	12.0	35.6	2.6	18.3	4.2	8.6	4.1
73314	Beef stew w/potatoes & vegetables	1	cup(s)	252	214.4	161	18.0	12.9	1.7	4.0	1.6	1.9	0.3
30233	Beef stroganoff with noodles	1	cup(s)	256	192.9	330	19.7	22.1	1.5	18.0	6.6	5.5	3.2
16651	Cashew chicken	1	cup(s)	242	187.5	283	20.4	15.9	3.4	15.6	2.1	7.1	5.2
30274	Cheese pizza with vegetables, thin crust	2	slice(s)	224	101.7	603	25.4	63.0	5.4	27.8	12.2	7.2	6.0
30330	Cheese quesadilla	1	item(s)	142	51.9	484	20.0	37.3	1.8	28.2	13.8	9.7	3.5
25240	Chicken and noodles	1	cup(s)	227	163.7	176	18.3	15.2	0.8	4.2	1.0	1.7	1.0
30239	Chicken and vegetables with broccoli, onion, bamboo shoots in soy based sauce	1	cup(s)	217	164.8	289	22.9	10.6	2.8	17.2	3.0	6.6	6.4
25093	Chicken cacciatore	1	cup(s)	244	176.2	283	29.8	5.4	1.3	15.3	4.3	6.2	3.3
28020	Chicken fried turkey steak	3	ounce(s)	85	62.7	115	12.7	11.3	0.7	1.8	0.5	0.3	0.7
218	Chicken pot pie	1	cup(s)	252	147.9	539	15.3	58.0	3.0	27.3	9.1	9.3	3.5
30240	Chicken teriyaki	1	cup(s)	244	153.2	451	66.5	4.7	0	16.6	4.6	5.9	3.8
25119	Chicken waldorf salad	½	cup(s)	100	67.5	179	14.0	6.5	1.0	10.9	1.8	3.2	5.0
25099	Chili con carne	¾	cup(s)	215	174.7	196	13.7	20.9	6.6	6.9	2.6	3.0	0.5
1062	Coleslaw	¾	cup(s)	90	73.4	70	1.2	11.2	1.3	2.3	0.3	0.6	1.2
1574	Crab cakes, from blue crab	1	item(s)	60	42.6	93	12.1	0.3	0	4.5	0.9	1.7	1.4

E KEY: H-4 = Breads/Baked Goods H-8 = Cereal/Rice/Pasta H-14 = Fruit H-18 = Vegetables/Legumes H-28 = Nuts/Seeds H-30 = Vegetarian H-32 = Dairy H-40 = Eggs H-40 = Seafood H-42 = Meats H-46 = Poultry
8 = Processed Meats H-50 = Beverages H-52 = Fats/Oils H-54 = Sweets H-56 = Spices/Condiments/Sauces H-60 = Mixed Foods/Soups/Sandwiches H-66 = Fast Food H-84 = Convenience H-86 = Baby Foods

Chol (mg)	Calc (mg)	Iron (mg)	Magn (mg)	Pota (mg)	Sodi (mg)	Zinc (mg)	Vit A (µg)	Thia (mg)	Vit E (mg α)	Ribo (mg)	Niac (mg)	Vit B_6 (mg)	Fola (µg)	Vit C (mg)	Vit B_{12} (µg)	Sele (µg)
0	26	1.73	3.1	11.4	0.8	0.09	2.7	0.01	0.10	0.01	0.07	0.01	3.8	0.7	0	0.1
0	4	0.91	4.2	55.6	0.8	0.10	0	0	0.07	0.01	0.11	0.04	0.9	0.6	0	0.1
0	13	0.11	—	—	—	—	—	0.02	—	0.01	0.07	—	—	11.2	0	—
0	2	0.06	2.3	47.3	136.1	0.04	3.9	0	0.22	0.03	0.22	0.02	1.4	0.6	0	0
0	3	0.08	2.8	57.3	3.0	0.04	7.0	0	0.22	0.02	0.21	0.02	1.5	2.3	0	0
0	12	0.10	2.0	26.1	248.1	0.03	2.6	0.01	0.03	0.01	0.03	0.01	0.3	0.2	0	0
1	12	0.27	10.2	152.1	79.1	0.13	—	0.03	0.28	0.04	0.43	0.07	—	2.5	0	0
0	60	1.92	35.7	212.8	297.7	1.34	0	0.11	0.92	0.06	0.49	0.49	72.6	9.7	0	3.0
6	1	0.03	0.1	2.8	87.6	0.02	2.2	0	0.45	0	0	0	0.7	0	0	0.3
6	1	0.05	0.3	6.4	107.7	0.03	3.4	0	0.49	0	0	0	0.6	0	0	0.4
0	6	0.09	0.9	6.8	68.1	0.02	0	0	0.09	0	0.01	0	—	0.1	0	—
0	3	0.08	2.5	6.9	56.8	0.03	0.2	0.02	0.02	0	0.03	0	0.3	0.1	0	1.6
0	0	0.13	0.8	3.8	121.7	0.02	9.1	0	0.09	0	0.03	0	0.2	0.2	0	0
2	7	0.07	1.7	19.0	186.8	0.03	3.1	0	0.47	0.01	0.03	0.01	1.4	0.6	0	0.3
0	10	0.20	4.1	72.5	320.9	0.05	3.4	0.01	0.25	0.02	0.19	0.02	0.6	0.2	0	0.4
0	10	0.20	4.1	72.5	41.6	0.05	3.4	0.01	0.25	0.02	0.19	0.02	2.5	0.2	0	0.4
18	116	0.13	5.7	18.9	521.6	0.62	50.4	0	—	0.07	0.02	0.01	2.5	0.3	0.1	2.0
0	5	0.36	9.5	125.7	61.9	0.11	—	0.03	0	0.02	0.63	0.06	—	43.9	0	0
0	7	1.05	11.1	231.3	113.8	0.14	—	0.02	0	0.22	0.61	0.34	—	0.3	0	0.3
0	5	0.16	3.8	19.0	258.4	0.05	0	0	0.04	0.03	0.19	0.01	3.7	0.1	0	0.3
2	5	0.01	0.5	6.6	15.8	0.02	8.0	0	0.02	0.01	0	0	0.3	0.1	0	0.1
1	36	1.56	58.3	278.3	294.1	1.06	13.3	0.07	1.76	0.09	1.95	0.09	14.6	3.6	0.1	2.1
0	5	0.03	0.6	8.6	437.3	0.01	0	0	0	0.02	0.24	0	2.4	0	0.1	0.7
0	1	0.05	0.6	6.0	29.8	0.01	3.9	0	0	0	0.01	0.01	0.1	0.2	0	0
0	10	0.13	4.8	91.2	225.6	0.06	7.7	0.01	0.39	0.01	0.36	0.06	1.3	0.6	0	0.3
0	3	0.36	6.1	32.4	599.9	0.07	0	0.01	0	0.02	0.60	0.03	2.9	0	0	0.1
0	4	0.43	7.2	37.9	999.3	0.08	0	0.01	0	0.03	0.71	0.04	3.2	0	0	0.1
0	5	0.20	3.1	51.2	183.6	0.05	0	0.01	0.09	0.01	0.33	0.02	2.3	1.4	0	1.4
0	5	0.31	11.0	40.5	689.9	0.02	0	0.01	0	0.01	0.23	0.02	1.4	0	0	0.2
0	28	1.36	26.2	573.3	265.2	0.40	0	0.06	2.11	0.07	1.58	0.16	20.4	19.6	0	1.9
0	16	1.24	19.5	403.8	13.4	0.24	26.8	0.03	1.73	0.08	1.19	0.12	13.4	8.5	0	0.2
4	70	0.20	8.3	92.3	209.4	0.24	61.5	0.04	0.17	0.11	0.24	0.02	6.0	0.5	0.2	2.4
0	6	0.30	0.7	45.4	55.6	0.01	0.3	0	0	0.01	0.04	0	0.5	0.7	0	0
—	0	0	—	—	0	—	—	—	—	—	—	—	—	0	—	—
0	1	0.03	0.7	10.9	0.7	0.01	0	0	0	0	0	0	0	0	0	0
0	1	0	0.1	0.3	0.3	0	0	0	0	0	0	0	0	0.0	0	0.1
0	0	0.08	—	2.4	0.8	—	—	0.08	—	0.08	0.08	—	—	0.3	0	—
44	63	1.55	55.7	617.1	532.4	1.33	33.9	0.07	3.97	0.24	9.03	0.53	29.0	5.8	0.2	23.2
120	26	1.56	30.0	372.8	476.7	2.68	0	0.07	1.12	0.26	6.89	0.39	25.8	5.0	0.3	19.3
38	331	2.91	47.3	451.1	548.1	1.85	0	0.27	1.42	0.27	1.80	0.20	132.3	4.4	0.3	15.3
58	98	3.46	35.7	468.3	876.4	3.66	17.8	0.35	1.07	0.17	7.01	0.44	133.8	23.0	0.8	33.9
17	41	1.87	24.3	256.0	633.6	1.09	471.0	0.29	0.41	0.13	2.72	0.21	124.2	35.3	0.2	27.5
38	30	2.20	32.8	484.2	589.5	4.31	178.4	0.13	0.24	0.23	5.02	0.24	25.1	8.7	1.5	15.6
74	77	2.82	35.8	378.9	829.4	3.58	66.6	0.24	1.36	0.25	6.39	0.28	87.0	1.0	0.7	33.5
44	63	1.55	55.7	617.1	532.4	1.33	33.9	0.07	3.97	0.24	9.03	0.53	29.0	5.8	0.2	23.2
54	569	3.65	49.3	436.8	1480.6	3.18	143.4	0.41	2.64	0.33	5.32	0.17	266.6	12.5	1.1	39.6
60	487	2.77	31.2	215.8	1036.6	2.17	154.8	0.28	0.89	0.30	2.42	0.08	102.2	6.2	0.3	24.9
49	45	1.34	25.3	275.7	399.5	0.96	58.2	0.18	0.41	0.18	8.21	0.31	71.4	0.7	0.4	25.4
61	54	1.59	34.7	429.7	557.7	1.87	342.9	0.10	2.52	0.21	5.54	0.41	54.3	26.9	0.2	16.9
109	49	2.35	39.4	471.4	488.9	2.14	0	0.11	1.39	0.22	9.75	0.59	25.3	8.6	0.3	22.2
25	64	1.21	17.7	205.8	129.7	1.03	4.0	0.14	0.06	0.17	3.28	0.20	29.1	0.4	0.3	14.8
60	73	2.77	35.3	312.5	957.6	1.41	138.6	0.58	0.40	0.28	5.62	0.30	126.0	0.8	0.8	17.9
200	41	3.22	75.6	612.4	1361.5	4.73	36.6	0.16	0.61	0.42	20.90	1.03	14.6	0	0.7	49.5
42	20	0.78	23.7	196.1	245.7	1.13	0	0.04	0.58	0.10	4.05	0.25	13.1	1.7	0.2	10.6
27	44	3.17	50.0	645.1	788.7	3.44	0	0.13	1.38	0.24	3.02	0.24	31.0	10.2	0.6	6.6
7	41	0.53	9.0	162.9	20.7	0.18	47.7	0.06	—	0.06	0.24	0.11	24.3	29.4	0	0.6
90	63	0.65	19.8	194.4	198.0	2.45	34.2	0.05	—	0.05	1.74	0.10	36.6	1.7	3.6	24.4

TABLE H-1 Table of Food Composition (*continued*) (Computer code is for Cengage Diet Analysis program) (For purposes of calculations, use "0" for t, <1, <0.1, 0.01)

DA+ Code	Food Description	Quantity	Measure	Wt (g)	H_2O (g)	Ener (kcal)	Prot (g)	Carb (g)	Fiber (g)	Fat (g)	Fat Breakdown (g) Sat	Mono	Poly
	Mixed Foods, Sandwiches, and Soups—*continued*												
32144	Enchiladas with green chili sauce (enchiladas verdes)	1	item(s)	144	103.8	207	9.3	17.6	2.6	11.7	6.4	3.6	1.0
2793	Falafel patty	3	item(s)	51	17.7	170	6.8	16.2	—	9.1	1.2	5.2	2.1
28546	Fettuccine Alfredo	1	cup(s)	240	87.2	267	12.3	45.8	1.8	3.5	1.8	0.8	0.4
32146	Flautas	3	item(s)	162	78.0	438	24.9	36.3	4.1	21.6	8.2	8.8	2.3
29629	Fried rice with meat or poultry	1	cup(s)	198	122.0	323	17.1	52.2	1.8	4.9	1.1	1.4	1.8
16649	General Tso chicken	1	cup(s)	146	65.9	431	18.8	35.0	1.3	23.9	4.0	5.7	11.0
1826	Green salad	¾	cup(s)	104	98.9	17	1.3	3.3	2.2	0.1	0	0	0
16650	Kung Pao chicken	1	cup(s)	162	87.1	436	28.9	11.4	2.3	30.7	4.5	13.0	11.8
16622	Lamb curry	1	cup(s)	236	157.6	474	25.6	11.1	2.6	37.1	6.7	14.9	13.3
25253	Lasagna with ground beef	1	cup(s)	238	157.2	288	17.6	22.2	2.5	14.6	7.6	4.8	0.8
442	Macaroni and cheese, prepared	1	cup(s)	243	144.7	484	18.5	54.2	2.7	21.0	8.4	7.2	3.7
29637	Meat filled ravioli with tomato or meat sauce, canned	1	cup(s)	251	196.5	248	8.6	34.5	4.0	8.6	3.6	4.0	0.6
25105	Meat loaf	1	slice(s)	115	84.6	244	17.0	6.6	0.4	15.9	6.1	6.9	0.8
16646	Moo shi pork	1	cup(s)	151	77.6	504	18.9	5.2	0.6	45.4	6.8	18.2	18.6
16788	Nachos with beef, beans, cheese, tomatoes and onions	1	serving(s)	195	102.8	505	23.0	35.4	4.9	30.8	12.2	10.2	5.6
6116	Pepperoni pizza	2	slice(s)	142	66.1	362	20.2	39.7	2.9	13.9	4.5	6.3	2.3
29601	Pizza with meat and vegetables, thin crust	2	slice(s)	232	97.7	698	30.0	60.5	4.9	37.2	15.5	11.3	6.7
655	Potato salad	½	cup(s)	125	95.0	179	3.3	14.0	1.6	10.3	1.8	3.1	4.7
25109	Salisbury steaks with mushroom sauce	1	serving(s)	135	101.8	250	17.0	9.5	0.5	15.4	6.0	6.7	0.8
16637	Shrimp creole with rice	1	cup(s)	243	178.2	296	24.7	27.6	1.7	8.9	1.6	3.6	3.0
41866	Spaghetti and meatballs, canned	1	cup(s)	248	196.7	241	11.1	27.0	—	9.9	3.6	4.0	1.2
28585	Spicy thai noodles (pad thai)	8	ounce(s)	227	72.7	218	8.8	35.1	3.0	6.4	0.8	3.4	1.7
33073	Stir fried pork and vegetables with rice	1	cup(s)	236	173.9	351	15.4	33.7	1.8	16.3	5.6	7.0	2.6
28588	Stuffed shells	2 ½	item(s)	249	157.6	242	15.1	27.7	2.7	8.2	3.1	3.0	1.3
16821	Sushi with egg in seaweed	6	piece(s)	156	116.7	192	8.9	20.0	0.3	7.8	2.1	3.2	1.9
16819	Sushi with vegetables and fish	6	piece(s)	156	97.6	236	6.9	48.1	0.6	0.8	0.2	0.2	0.2
16820	Sushi with vegetables in seaweed	6	piece(s)	156	109.4	187	3.5	41.0	0.8	0.4	0.1	0.1	0.1
25266	Sweet and sour pork	¾	cup(s)	249	206.0	265	29.3	16.9	1.0	8.1	2.7	3.6	1.4
16824	Tabouli, tabbouleh or tabuli	1	cup(s)	160	124.1	198	2.6	15.5	3.7	15.0	2.1	10.7	1.7
25276	Three bean salad	½	cup(s)	99	82.3	96	1.9	9.6	2.6	6.0	0.8	1.6	3.2
160	Tuna salad	½	cup(s)	103	64.7	192	16.4	9.6	0	9.5	1.6	3.0	4.2
25241	Turkey and noodles	1	cup(s)	227	162.4	193	17.1	15.2	0.8	6.6	1.7	2.5	1.6
16794	Vegetable egg roll	2	item(s)	128	63.3	323	8.0	38.6	3.3	15.3	3.2	7.3	3.8
16818	Vegetable sushi, no fish	6	piece(s)	156	92.1	256	4.2	56.7	0.9	0.4	0.1	0.1	0.1
	Sandwiches												
1744	Bacon, lettuce and tomato with mayonnaise	1	item(s)	164	95.8	346	11.7	35.7	2.5	17.4	3.7	5.4	6.6
30287	Bologna and cheese with margarine	1	item(s)	111	45.7	339	13.6	29.9	1.4	18.0	7.0	5.7	3.3
30286	Bologna with margarine	1	item(s)	83	33.4	251	8.8	27.2	1.4	11.6	3.3	3.9	2.9
16546	Cheese	1	item(s)	83	31.2	254	9.4	27.9	1.4	11.5	4.5	2.9	3.1
8789	Cheeseburger, large, plain	1	item(s)	166	70.8	506	28.7	34.5	2.3	28.3	11.2	9.2	0.9
8624	Cheeseburger, large, with bacon, vegetables and condiments	1	item(s)	195	91.4	550	30.8	36.8	2.5	30.9	11.9	10.6	1.3
1745	Club with bacon, chicken, tomato, lettuce and mayonnaise	1	item(s)	246	137.8	546	40.4	40.1	2.7	24.0	5.6	7.6	8.5
1908	Cold cut submarine with cheese and vegetables	1	item(s)	228	131.8	456	21.8	51.0	2.0	18.6	6.8	8.2	2.3
30247	Corned beef	1	item(s)	130	74.1	268	18.8	25.6	1.7	9.4	3.6	3.4	1.2
25283	Egg salad	1	item(s)	126	72.0	278	10.4	28.5	1.5	13.4	3.0	4.0	4.8
16686	Fried egg	1	item(s)	96	49.2	225	10.7	26.2	1.4	8.1	2.2	3.0	2.3
16547	Grilled cheese	1	item(s)	83	27.8	282	9.4	28.0	1.4	14.6	5.2	5.2	3.2
16659	Gyro with onion and tomato	1	item(s)	390	255.6	593	44.2	73.7	3.9	12.2	4.4	4.3	1.6
1906	Ham and cheese	1	item(s)	146	74.2	352	20.7	33.3	2.0	15.5	6.4	6.7	1.4
31890	Ham with mayonnaise	1	item(s)	112	55.8	272	13.7	28.0	2.1	11.4	2.7	3.9	4.0
756	Hamburger, double patty, large, with condiments and vegetables	1	item(s)	226	121.5	540	34.3	40.3	—	26.6	10.5	10.3	2.8
8793	Hamburger, large, plain	1	item(s)	137	57.7	426	22.6	31.7	1.5	22.9	8.4	9.9	2.1

E KEY: H-4 = Breads/Baked Goods H-8 = Cereal/Rice/Pasta H-14 = Fruit H-18 = Vegetables/Legumes H-28 = Nuts/Seeds H-30 = Vegetarian H-32 = Dairy H-40 = Eggs H-40 = Seafood H-42 = Meats H-46 = Poultry
8 = Processed Meats H-50 = Beverages H-52 = Fats/Oils H-54 = Sweets H-56 = Spices/Condiments/Sauces H-60 = Mixed Foods/Soups/Sandwiches H-66 = Fast Food H-84 = Convenience H-86 = Baby Foods

Chol (mg)	Calc (mg)	Iron (mg)	Magn (mg)	Pota (mg)	Sodi (mg)	Zinc (mg)	Vit A (µg)	Thia (mg)	Vit E (mg α)	Ribo (mg)	Niac (mg)	Vit B_6 (mg)	Fola (µg)	Vit C (mg)	Vit B_{12} (µg)	Sele (µg)
27	266	1.08	38.5	251.4	276.3	1.27	—	0.07	0.03	0.16	1.28	0.18	—	59.3	0.2	6.0
0	28	1.74	41.8	298.4	149.9	0.76	0.5	0.07	—	0.08	0.53	0.06	53.0	0.8	0	0.5
10	181	1.55	36.3	167.2	412.1	1.36	0	0.34	0.09	0.34	2.69	0.10	221.3	0.8	0.5	38.4
73	146	2.66	61.3	222.9	885.7	3.44	0	0.10	0.10	0.17	3.00	0.27	—	0	1.2	36.7
63	28	1.52	25.7	223.7	689.0	1.58	17.8	0.05	0.34	0.08	5.14	0.23	11.9	0	0.1	22.2
77	18	1.69	26.3	293.5	635.1	1.90	16.1	0.04	1.77	0.17	4.16	0.29	21.9	2.3	0.3	21.0
0	13	0.65	11.4	178.0	26.9	0.22	59.0	0.03	—	0.05	0.57	0.08	38.3	24.0	0	0.4
65	50	1.94	63.2	432.5	895.9	1.52	38.9	0.15	3.73	0.15	13.05	0.58	42.1	7.5	0.3	23.0
78	45	3.68	54.3	835.4	1064.4	6.04	30.7	0.10	5.90	0.31	7.52	0.28	30.7	14.6	2.5	28.1
66	226	2.22	39.6	438.3	495.6	2.87	0	0.20	1.14	0.29	3.07	0.20	91.1	9.6	1.1	26.1
39	671	2.55	48.6	301.3	928.3	1.99	226.0	0.40	1.36	0.52	2.73	0.12	126.4	0	0.6	44.2
13	33	2.63	32.6	424.2	888.5	1.13	37.7	0.14	1.38	0.15	3.23	0.16	70.3	0	0.4	24.1
85	63	1.95	21.8	295.6	422.2	3.42	0	0.08	0.09	0.29	3.77	0.14	29.0	0.4	1.6	17.2
157	32	1.40	27.2	350.3	1051.0	1.78	54.4	0.51	5.54	0.41	4.04	0.44	18.1	7.9	0.5	31.0
74	310	2.89	93.6	481.6	520.7	4.60	115.1	0.09	2.42	0.26	2.92	0.37	50.7	5.7	1.6	17.5
28	129	1.87	17.0	305.3	533.9	1.04	105.1	0.27	—	0.47	6.09	0.11	92.7	3.3	0.4	26.1
79	554	3.83	51.0	471.0	1719.1	3.85	136.9	0.47	2.55	0.38	6.20	0.20	257.5	9.0	1.4	45.0
85	24	0.81	18.8	317.5	661.3	0.39	40.0	0.10	—	0.08	1.11	0.18	8.8	12.5	0	5.1
60	77	2.00	23.7	308.4	369.1	3.47	0	0.11	0.03	0.30	4.00	0.14	33.3	0.3	1.7	16.9
262	192	4.59	51.0	291.6	984.2	2.48	75.3	0.24	2.45	0.09	3.19	0.24	136.1	14.8	0.8	58.3
17	89	3.03	34.7	498.5	781.2	1.36	47.1	0.24	1.17	0.21	5.54	0.18	—	5.5	0.6	23.6
37	32	1.55	49.2	183.9	587.1	1.06	0	0.17	1.29	0.13	1.85	0.17	55.7	16.0	0.1	3.2
46	40	2.66	32.8	400.0	569.4	2.08	0	0.51	0.60	0.20	5.00	0.30	163.1	18.3	0.4	22.5
30	194	2.50	54.3	382.8	466.6	1.48	0	0.24	1.87	0.30	3.77	0.28	161.0	9.8	0.2	29.9
187	45	1.79	18.7	137.3	455.5	1.06	115.4	0.12	0.89	0.28	1.31	0.15	82.7	1.9	0.5	20.0
12	23	2.12	18.7	115.4	424.3	0.65	7.8	0.23	0.23	0.04	2.37	0.11	135.7	0.9	0.3	14.8
0	17	1.54	17.2	85.8	154.4	0.69	10.9	0.20	0.08	0.04	1.89	0.13	120.1	2.2	0	10.1
74	41	1.72	34.0	612.1	623.9	2.52	0	0.80	0.73	0.37	6.69	0.65	14.6	9.8	0.7	49.7
0	32	1.20	35.2	246.4	798.4	0.48	54.4	0.07	2.43	0.04	1.12	0.11	32.0	25.3	0	0.5
0	27	0.96	15.5	145.0	207.4	0.53	0	0.04	0.94	0.06	0.26	0.06	25.0	9.2	0	2.5
13	17	1.02	19.5	182.4	412.0	0.57	24.6	0.03	—	0.07	6.87	0.08	8.2	2.3	1.2	42.2
53	50	1.74	23.3	283.1	396.6	1.85	84.2	0.17	0.30	0.22	4.60	0.22	78.0	0.8	0.8	27.1
0	55	2.36	32.0	302.1	677.1	0.67	199.7	0.30	0.73	0.18	2.40	0.17	130.6	16.5	0.1	15.6
0	20	2.43	17.2	90.5	425.9	0.70	0	0.27	0.06	0.04	2.47	0.10	156.0	0.2	0	9.7
21	82	2.43	29.5	344.4	944.6	1.08	42.6	0.34	1.16	0.26	4.42	0.21	108.2	10.2	0.2	27.9
39	518	2.47	26.6	213.1	894.7	1.64	73.3	0.35	0.57	0.29	3.25	0.18	96.6	0.2	0.9	22.8
17	159	2.21	17.4	143.6	534.5	1.05	10.0	0.34	0.34	0.18	3.17	0.15	91.3	0.2	0.5	18.1
22	486	2.11	21.6	126.2	627.5	1.00	66.4	0.29	0.58	0.23	2.53	0.10	93.8	0	0.4	15.9
93	277	4.02	39.8	360.2	884.8	5.16	—	0.32	—	0.69	7.42	0.44	129.5	0.0	2.5	34.9
98	267	4.04	44.8	464.1	1314.3	5.21	—	0.34	—	0.68	8.25	0.47	122.8	1.4	2.4	6.6
96	221	4.08	54.1	511.7	949.6	2.24	36.9	0.57	1.35	0.35	17.36	0.74	147.6	4.7	0.6	51.7
36	189	2.51	68.4	394.4	1650.7	2.58	70.7	1.00	—	0.80	5.49	0.14	109.4	12.3	1.1	30.8
44	139	3.02	20.8	135.2	1099.8	2.28	2.6	0.28	0.21	0.20	3.69	0.11	92.3	0.3	0.8	33.4
217	106	2.58	18.6	145.0	494.1	0.94	0	0.27	1.10	0.44	2.27	0.16	112.1	0.7	0.6	24.5
174	164	2.71	19.2	126.7	348.5	1.05	95.0	0.30	0.68	0.34	2.56	0.13	112.3	0	0.4	25.9
21	491	2.13	21.6	128.6	669.0	1.00	131.1	0.22	1.09	0.22	2.30	0.06	62.3	0	0.2	15.9
98	179	5.66	78.0	799.5	873.6	7.99	35.1	0.85	1.09	0.69	14.11	0.62	234.0	12.5	2.5	70.2
58	130	3.24	16.1	290.5	770.9	1.37	96.4	0.31	0.29	0.48	2.69	0.20	78.8	2.8	0.5	23.1
32	150	2.44	24.6	213.9	986.7	1.16	5.6	0.61	0.49	0.22	4.05	0.26	94.1	2.1	0.2	22.6
122	102	5.85	49.7	569.5	791.0	5.67	—	0.36	—	0.38	7.57	0.54	110.7	1.1	4.1	25.5
71	74	3.58	27.4	267.1	474.0	4.11	0	0.29	—	0.29	6.25	0.23	80.8	0	2.1	27.1

TABLE H-1 Table of Food Composition (*continued*) (Computer code is for Cengage Diet Analysis program) (For purposes of calculations, use "0" for t, <1, <0.1, 0.01)

DA+ Code	Food Description	Quantity	Measure	Wt (g)	H_2O (g)	Ener (kcal)	Prot (g)	Carb (g)	Fiber (g)	Fat (g)	Fat Breakdown (g)		
											Sat	Mono	Poly
Mixed Foods, Sandwiches, and Soups—*continued*													
8795	Hamburger, large, with vegetables and condiments	1	item(s)	218	121.4	512	25.8	40.0	3.1	27.4	10.4	11.4	2.2
25134	Hot chicken salad	1	item(s)	98	48.8	239	15.6	23.4	1.1	8.8	2.8	2.6	2.8
25133	Hot turkey salad	1	item(s)	98	50.4	221	16.0	23.4	1.1	6.6	2.2	1.8	2.3
1411	Hotdog with bun, plain	1	item(s)	98	52.9	242	10.4	18.0	1.6	14.5	5.1	6.9	1.7
30249	Pastrami	1	item(s)	134	82.6	221	16.5	26.6	1.7	4.8	1.8	1.4	0.9
16701	Peanut butter	1	item(s)	93	24.2	337	13.0	37.4	3.4	16.1	3.4	7.1	5.0
30306	Peanut butter and jelly	1	item(s)	93	24.7	323	11.0	41.6	3.1	13.7	2.9	6.1	4.2
1909	Roast beef submarine with mayonnaise and vegetables	1	item(s)	216	127.4	410	28.6	44.3	—	13.0	7.1	1.8	2.6
1910	Roast beef, plain	1	item(s)	139	67.6	346	21.5	33.4	1.2	13.8	3.6	6.8	1.7
1907	Steak with mayonnaise and vegetables	1	item(s)	204	104.2	459	30.3	52.0	2.3	14.1	3.8	5.3	3.3
25288	Tuna salad	1	item(s)	179	102.2	415	24.1	28.9	1.6	22.2	3.6	5.5	11.4
30283	Turkey submarine with cheese, lettuce, tomato and mayonnaise	1	item(s)	277	167.2	529	29.3	50.9	3.0	22.9	6.5	5.8	8.3
31891	Turkey with mayonnaise	1	item(s)	143	73.9	330	29.1	26.7	1.4	11.1	2.4	2.5	4.9
	Soups												
25296	Bean	1	cup(s)	243	204.8	153	10.8	23.2	8.2	1.9	0.5	0.7	0.6
711	Bean with pork, condensed, prepared with water	1	cup(s)	266	227.0	168	7.7	22.1	7.7	5.7	1.5	2.1	1.8
713	Beef noodle, condensed, prepared with water	1	cup(s)	244	224.9	83	4.7	8.7	0.7	3.0	1.1	1.2	0.5
825	Cheese, condensed, prepared with milk	1	cup(s)	251	206.9	231	9.5	16.2	1.0	14.6	9.1	4.1	0.5
826	Chicken broth, condensed, prepared with water	1	cup(s)	244	234.1	39	4.9	0.9	0	1.4	0.4	0.6	0.3
25297	Chicken noodle soup	1	cup(s)	241	218.2	99	9.1	9.2	0.8	2.5	0.7	0.9	0.6
827	Chicken noodle, condensed, prepared with water	1	cup(s)	248	232.7	62	3.1	7.3	0.5	2.4	0.6	1.0	0.7
724	Chicken noodle, dehydrated, prepared with water	1	cup(s)	245	230.7	56	2.1	9.0	0.2	1.3	0.3	0.5	0.4
1769	Chicken noodle, low sodium, condensed, prepared with water	1	cup(s)	248	232.7	62	3.1	7.3	0.5	2.4	0.6	1.0	0.7
823	Cream of asparagus, condensed, prepared with milk	1	cup(s)	248	213.3	161	6.3	16.4	0.7	8.2	3.3	2.1	2.2
824	Cream of celery, condensed, prepared with milk	1	cup(s)	248	214.4	164	5.7	14.5	0.7	9.7	3.9	2.5	2.7
708	Cream of chicken, condensed, prepared with milk	1	cup(s)	248	210.4	191	7.5	15.0	0.2	11.5	4.6	4.5	1.6
715	Cream of chicken, condensed, prepared with water	1	cup(s)	244	221.1	117	3.4	9.3	0.2	7.4	2.1	3.3	1.5
709	Cream of mushroom, condensed, prepared with milk	1	cup(s)	252	219.3	161	5.9	14.5	0.8	9.0	2.8	2.2	3.6
716	Cream of mushroom, condensed, prepared with water	1	cup(s)	248	229.3	97	1.6	8.3	0.7	6.4	1.2	1.5	3.5
9558	Cream of mushroom, low sodium, canned, ready to serve	1	cup(s)	244	218.1	139	2.5	15.6	0	7.4	2.0	1.6	3.3
25298	Cream of vegetable	1	cup(s)	260	229.2	151	6.4	13.8	1.7	7.9	1.4	4.2	1.8
16689	Egg drop	1	cup(s)	244	226.6	66	2.8	10.5	1.0	1.5	0.4	0.5	0.3
25138	Golden squash	1	cup(s)	258	224.0	144	7.5	20.6	1.5	3.9	0.7	2.1	0.9
16663	Hot and sour	1	cup(s)	244	221.2	95	6.3	10.6	1.2	3.0	0.6	0.7	0.8
28054	Lentil chowder	1	cup(s)	248	204.1	168	10.8	30.9	13.2	0.6	0.1	0.1	0.3
28560	Macaroni and bean	1	cup(s)	246	138.8	147	6.6	23.3	5.0	3.5	0.5	2.2	0.5
714	Manhattan clam chowder, condensed, prepared with water	1	cup(s)	249	229.7	75	2.1	11.9	1.5	2.1	0.4	0.4	1.3
28561	Minestrone	1	cup(s)	240	184.6	105	5.2	17.3	4.8	2.2	0.3	1.4	0.3
717	Minestrone, condensed, prepared with water	1	cup(s)	241	220.1	82	4.3	11.2	1.0	2.5	0.6	0.7	1.1
53690	Minestrone, reduced sodium, canned, ready to serve	1	cup(s)	241	210.4	120	4.8	21.7	5.8	1.9	0.3	0.7	0.6
28038	Mushroom & wild rice	1	cup(s)	241	196.6	88	4.7	13.3	1.6	0.3	0.1	0	0.1
828	New England clam chowder, condensed, prepared with milk	1	cup(s)	252	215.4	154	8.2	18.8	0.8	5.1	2.8	0.7	1.3
75714	New England clam chowder, reduced sodium, canned, ready to serve	1	cup(s)	256	221.5	179	6.0	14.5	2.0	10.8	1.8	2.3	5.1
28036	New England style clam chowder	1	cup(s)	254	235.0	67	3.0	11.5	1.2	0.1	0	0	0
28566	Old country pasta	1	cup(s)	245	175.9	151	6.5	21.0	3.4	3.4	1.6	2.1	0.7

Chol (mg)	Calc (mg)	Iron (mg)	Magn (mg)	Pota (mg)	Sodi (mg)	Zinc (mg)	Vit A (µg)	Thia (mg)	Vit E (mg α)	Ribo (mg)	Niac (mg)	Vit B_6 (mg)	Fola (µg)	Vit C (mg)	Vit B_{12} (µg)	Sele (µg)
87	96	4.93	43.6	479.6	824.0	4.88	—	0.41	—	0.37	7.28	0.33	115.5	2.6	2.4	33.6
39	114	1.93	20.4	150.3	469.7	1.22	0	0.20	0.31	0.23	4.94	0.20	79.5	0.2	0.3	16.9
37	113	2.04	21.8	166.9	459.2	1.09	0	0.19	0.25	0.21	4.36	0.23	79.6	0.2	0.3	20.3
44	24	2.31	12.7	143.1	670.3	1.98	0	0.24	—	0.27	3.65	0.05	60.8	0.1	0.5	26.0
36	142	3.19	22.8	178.2	1069.3	3.10	4.0	0.31	0.20	0.22	4.78	0.17	93.8	0.4	1.0	21.0
0	181	2.86	59.5	255.8	447.3	1.36	0	0.37	2.65	0.19	6.85	0.21	132.1	0	0	15.9
0	154	2.45	51.2	225.1	384.1	1.16	0	0.31	2.25	0.16	5.82	0.18	112.5	0.1	0	13.6
73	41	2.81	67.0	330.5	844.6	4.38	30.2	0.41	—	0.41	5.96	0.32	88.6	5.6	1.8	25.7
51	54	4.23	30.6	315.5	792.3	3.39	11.1	0.38	—	0.31	5.87	0.26	68.1	2.1	1.2	29.2
73	92	5.16	49.0	524.3	797.6	4.53	—	0.41	—	0.37	7.30	0.37	128.5	5.5	1.6	42.0
53	97	3.23	35.6	296.5	794.9	1.09	0	0.27	1.76	0.27	12.29	0.48	99.6	1.1	2.4	71.5
66	521	4.68	52.6	567.8	1795.0	2.63	105.3	0.70	1.36	0.60	4.38	0.33	166.2	11.6	0.7	44.9
64	162	3.42	34.3	307.5	471.9	3.00	5.7	0.34	0.74	0.28	7.05	0.46	98.7	0	0.3	42.2
4	63	2.35	45.2	491.2	539.4	1.12	28.0	0.24	0.23	0.13	3.00	0.16	116.2	2.1	0.2	4.3
3	82	2.00	45.2	391.0	928.3	1.01	45.2	0.09	1.14	0.03	0.55	0.04	31.9	1.6	0	8.2
5	20	1.07	7.3	97.6	793.0	1.51	12.2	0.07	1.22	0.06	1.04	0.04	29.3	0.5	0.2	7.3
48	289	0.80	20.1	341.4	1019.1	0.68	358.9	0.06	—	0.33	0.50	0.08	10.0	1.3	0.4	7.0
0	10	0.51	2.4	209.8	746.6	0.24	0	0.01	0.05	0.07	3.35	0.02	4.9	0	0.2	0
19	22	1.03	13.6	283.4	631.4	0.68	54.2	0.13	0.18	0.13	4.74	0.12	46.8	1.1	0.3	10.3
12	15	1.64	9.9	54.6	865.5	0.40	27.3	0.14	0.07	0.11	1.34	0.05	29.8	0	0	11.9
10	5	0.49	7.3	31.9	561.0	0.20	2.5	0.20	0.12	0.07	1.06	0.02	27.0	0	0	9.3
12	15	1.64	9.9	54.6	429.0	0.40	27.3	0.14	0.07	0.11	1.34	0.05	29.8	0	0	11.9
22	174	0.87	19.8	359.6	1041.6	0.92	62.0	0.10	—	0.28	0.88	0.06	29.8	4.0	0.5	8.0
32	186	0.69	22.3	310.0	674.6	0.20	114.1	0.07	—	0.25	0.44	0.06	7.4	1.5	0.5	4.7
27	181	0.67	17.4	272.8	897.8	0.67	178.6	0.07	—	0.26	0.92	0.07	7.4	1.2	0.5	8.0
10	34	0.61	2.4	87.8	846.7	0.63	163.5	0.03	—	0.06	0.82	0.02	2.4	0.2	0.1	7.0
10	171	0.25	17.6	259.6	899.6	0.78	75.6	0.07	0.65	0.26	0.54	0.07	7.6	0.3	0.7	6.8
0	17	0.22	5.0	76.9	843.2	0.15	2.5	0.01	0.60	0.02	0.42	0.02	2.5	0	0	3.5
8	33	0	—	155.6	61.4	—	0	—	—	—	—	—	—	0	—	—
1	71	1.10	16.3	311.2	694.3	0.55	202.3	0.10	1.35	0.19	2.99	0.10	49.2	9.2	0.3	4.5
56	17	0.63	4.9	53.7	902.8	0.22	48.8	0.05	0.32	0.05	0.38	0.05	17.1	15.9	0.1	1.0
4	261	0.76	42.4	522.3	496.7	0.92	0	0.18	1.39	0.38	1.15	0.16	42.9	10.5	0.9	7.9
51	46	1.56	22.0	134.2	917.4	0.54	22.0	0.06	0.95	0.08	1.24	0.16	19.5	0	0.2	1.0
0	54	3.86	64.9	660.5	28.3	2.00	0	0.38	0.98	0.11	1.82	0.33	195.9	13.1	0	3.7
0	70	1.92	35.6	270.1	519.7	0.89	0	0.14	1.33	0.14	1.42	0.13	92.3	4.9	0	9.3
2	27	1.59	10.0	184.3	562.7	0.90	49.8	0.03	1.25	0.04	0.79	0.10	10.0	4.0	3.9	9.2
0	71	1.80	31.8	264.9	434.9	0.74	0	0.10	1.12	0.10	0.69	0.10	61.8	10.9	0	4.0
2	34	0.92	7.2	313.3	612.1	0.75	118.1	0.05	—	0.04	0.94	0.10	50.6	1.2	0	8.0
0	48	1.73	31.3	448.2	518.1	0.77	79.5	0.14	1.69	0.10	1.54	0.14	37.8	13.7	0	5.1
0	29	1.11	27.3	347.4	281.1	0.93	0	0.06	0.16	0.22	3.03	0.15	26.9	3.8	0.1	4.9
18	176	3.05	30.2	451.1	688.0	1.08	93.2	0.20	0.55	0.44	2.00	0.18	22.7	5.3	12.2	11.1
8	36	1.43	33.3	862.7	496.6	0.69	20.5	0.04	1.02	0.04	1.08	0.33	15.4	8.4	2.4	11.0
4	74	1.06	29.6	465.3	349.9	0.45	0	0.07	0.41	0.11	0.93	0.17	16.1	10.0	6.1	6.2
7	55	2.44	50.7	472.7	346.8	0.76	0	0.20	0.94	0.16	2.55	0.26	102.3	18.8	0.1	9.2

TABLE H-1 Table of Food Composition (*continued*) (Computer code is for Cengage Diet Analysis program) (For purposes of calculations, use "0" for t, <1, <0.1, 0.01)

DA+ Code	Food Description	Quantity	Measure	Wt (g)	H_2O (g)	Ener (kcal)	Prot (g)	Carb (g)	Fiber (g)	Fat (g)	Fat Breakdown (g)		
											Sat	Mono	Poly
Mixed Foods, Sandwiches, and Soups—*continued*													
725	Onion, dehydrated, prepared with water	1	cup(s)	230	220.3	28	0.7	6.4	0.7	0	0	0	0
16667	Shrimp gumbo	1	cup(s)	244	207.2	163	8.9	18.3	2.9	6.8	3.9	1.6	0.6
28037	Southwestern corn chowder	1	cup(s)	240	211.2	109	4.8	19.7	2.2	0.5	0.1	0.1	0.2
30282	Soybean (miso)	1	cup(s)	240	218.8	84	6.0	7.8	1.9	3.4	0.6	1.2	1.3
25140	Split pea	1	cup(s)	165	116.6	83	4.5	18.5	1.5	0.4	0.1	0	0.2
718	Split pea with ham, condensed, prepared with water	1	cup(s)	253	206.9	190	10.3	28.0	2.3	4.4	1.8	1.8	0.6
32411	Split pea with ham, reduced sodium & fat, ready to serve	1	cup(s)	243	196.8	185	12.6	27.5	—	2.7	0.7	1.0	0.5
726	Tomato vegetable, dehydrated, prepared with water	1	cup(s)	245	230.9	54	1.9	9.9	0.7	0.8	0.4	0.3	0.1
710	Tomato, condensed, prepared with milk	1	cup(s)	252	216.7	139	6.3	22.6	1.5	3.3	1.8	0.8	0.3
719	Tomato, condensed, prepared with water	1	cup(s)	248	226.6	74	2.0	16.3	1.5	0.7	0.2	0.2	0.2
40840	Tomato, low sodium, prepared wtih water	1	cup(s)	244	223.0	73	1.9	16.0	1.5	0.7	0.2	0.2	0.2
28595	Turkey noodle	1	cup(s)	244	217.0	113	8.1	14.9	1.9	2.4	0.3	1.2	0.7
28051	Turkey vegetable	1	cup(s)	241	215.4	106	12.1	9.0	1.9	1.1	0.3	0.2	0.3
25141	Vegetable	1	cup(s)	252	225.3	92	4.5	19.6	4.3	0.4	0.1	0	0.2
720	Vegetable beef, condensed, prepared with water	1	cup(s)	244	224.0	76	5.4	9.9	2.0	1.9	0.8	0.8	0.1
28598	Vegetable gumbo	1	cup(s)	244	179.4	162	4.2	27.5	3.4	4.6	0.7	3.1	0.6
40841	Vegetable, low sodium, prepared with water	1	cup(s)	253	231.1	83	2.8	15.3	2.8	1.1	0.2	0.3	0.5
721	Vegetarian vegetable, condensed, prepared with water	1	cup(s)	241	222.7	67	2.1	11.8	0.7	1.9	0.3	0.8	0.7
Fast Food													
	Arby's												
751	Beef 'n cheddar sandwich	1	item(s)	195	—	440	23.0	47.0	2.0	18.0	5.0	—	
36131	Chocolate shake, regular	1	serving(s)	468	—	570	14.0	99.0	1.0	15.0	10.0	—	—
80611	Cravin' chicken sandwich, crispy	1	item(s)	221	—	510	26.0	51.0	4.0	22.0	4.0	—	—
36045	Curly fries, large size	1	serving(s)	210	—	658	7.3	77.3	8.4	36.6	5.2	—	—
36044	Curly fries, medium size	1	serving(s)	170	—	540	6.0	62.0	7.0	29.0	4.0	—	—
57171	French dip & Swiss sandwich w/ au jus sauce	1	item(s)	286	—	430	26.0	52.0	2.0	14.0	6.0	—	—
34778	Jalapeno bites, 5-piece	1	serving(s)	110	—	280	5.0	31.0	2.0	16.0	6.0	—	—
9296	Jamocha shake, regular	1	serving(s)	468	—	560	14.0	98.0	1.0	15.0	10.0	—	—
9249	Junior roast beef sandwich	1	item(s)	87	—	210	12.0	25.0	1.0	6.0	2.0	—	—
9251	Large roast beef sandwich	1	item(s)	281	—	580	45.0	49.0	3.0	22.0	9.0	—	—
56537	Market Fresh crispy chicken farmhouse chopped salad	1	serving(s)	337	—	430	29.0	26.0	4.0	24.0	9.0	—	—
34769	Market Fresh roast turkey & Swiss sandwich	1	serving(s)	326	—	700	39.0	77.0	5.0	27.0	7.0	—	—
80607	Market Fresh roast turkey & Swiss wrap	1	item(s)	272	—	490	34.0	39.0	7.0	25.0	6.0	—	—
80608	Market Fresh roast turkey farmhouse chopped salad	1	serving(s)	300	—	240	22.0	10.0	3.0	13.0	7.0	—	—
9267	Market Fresh roast turkey ranch & bacon sandwich	1	serving(s)	344	—	800	45.0	78.0	5.0	36.0	9.0	—	—
34780	Mozzarella sticks, 4-piece	1	serving(s)	137	—	420	21.0	35.0	2.0	21.0	9.0	—	—
9275	Potato cakes	1	serving(s)	100	—	230	2.0	25.0	3.0	14.0	2.0	—	—
750	Roast beef sandwich, regular	1	item(s)	154	—	350	23.0	39.0	2.0	12.0	4.0	—	
2009	Super roast beef sandwich	1	item(s)	229	—	430	23.0	45.0	3.0	17.0	5.0	—	—
36130	Vanilla shake, regular	1	serving(s)	425	—	470	14.0	75.0	0	15.0	10.0	—	—
	Auntie Anne's												
35351	Almond soft pretzel	1	item(s)	127	—	350	8.0	74.0	2.0	2.0	1.0	—	—
35371	Cheese dipping sauce	1	serving(s)	31	—	78	2.3	1.6	0	6.2	2.3	—	—
35353	Cinnamon sugar soft pretzel	1	item(s)	136	—	380	8.0	84.0	2.0	1.0	0	—	—
35354	Cinnamon sugar soft pretzel with butter	1	item(s)	147	—	470	8.0	84.0	2.0	12.0	7.0	—	—
56651	Garlic soft pretzel	1	item(s)	119	—	310	8.0	65.0	2.0	1.0	0	—	—
35372	Marinara dipping sauce	1	serving(s)	37	—	45	2.0	6.0	1.0	2.0	0	—	—
35357	Original soft pretzel	1	serving(s)	119	—	310	8.0	65.0	2.0	1.0	0	—	—
35358	Original soft pretzel with butter	1	item(s)	123	—	340	8.0	65.0	2.0	5.0	3.0	—	—
56653	Original soft preztel without salt	1	item(s)	117	—	310	8.0	65.0	2.0	1.0	0	—	—

E KEY: H-4 = Breads/Baked Goods H-8 = Cereal/Rice/Pasta H-14 = Fruit H-18 = Vegetables/Legumes H-28 = Nuts/Seeds H-30 = Vegetarian H-32 = Dairy H-40 = Eggs H-40 = Seafood H-42 = Meats H-46 = Poultry
8 = Processed Meats H-50 = Beverages H-52 = Fats/Oils H-54 = Sweets H-56 = Spices/Condiments/Sauces H-60 = Mixed Foods/Soups/Sandwiches H-66 = Fast Food H-84 = Convenience H-86 = Baby Foods

Chol (mg)	Calc (mg)	Iron (mg)	Magn (mg)	Pota (mg)	Sodi (mg)	Zinc (mg)	Vit A (µg)	Thia (mg)	Vit E (mg α)	Ribo (mg)	Niac (mg)	Vit B_6 (mg)	Fola (µg)	Vit C (mg)	Vit B_{12} (µg)	Sele (µg)
0	21	0.12	9.2	71.3	795.8	0.12	0	0.03	0.02	0.03	0.14	0.06	0	0.2	0	0.5
90	132	2.90	46.4	429.4	646.6	1.12	65.9	0.17	1.63	0.13	2.21	0.24	104.9	18.5	0.2	17.6
1	83	0.94	26.1	417.2	208.9	0.58	0	0.09	0.28	0.15	1.75	0.24	32.9	35.9	0.3	2.1
0	62	1.82	38.4	367.2	976.8	0.77	230.4	0.06	0.96	0.16	2.62	0.16	55.2	4.6	0.2	1.4
0	30	1.25	32.7	352.3	607.9	0.57	0	0.12	0.14	0.09	1.67	0.21	72.0	8.8	0	0.4
8	23	2.28	48.1	399.7	1006.9	1.32	22.8	0.15	—	0.08	1.47	0.07	2.5	1.5	0.3	8.0
15	—	2.24	—	—	833.5	—	318.3	—	—	—	—	—	—	10.2	—	—
0	20	0.59	9.8	164.1	323.4	0.20	9.8	0.06	0.42	0.09	1.22	0.06	12.3	2.9	0	2.0
10	174	1.39	30.2	461.2	529.2	0.93	95.8	0.10	0.45	0.32	1.37	0.15	5.0	15.9	0.7	9.3
0	20	1.34	17.4	277.8	471.2	0.30	24.8	0.05	0.42	0.08	1.25	0.10	0	15.6	0	6.2
0	20	1.32	17.1	273.3	80.5	0.29	24.4	0.05	0.41	0.08	1.23	0.10	0	15.4	0	6.1
25	31	1.44	23.7	217.1	398.4	0.76	0	0.22	0.63	0.11	2.91	0.16	65.1	5.9	0.1	16.1
21	38	1.37	23.5	405.4	347.8	0.96	0	0.09	0.21	0.09	3.55	0.30	26.1	10.5	0.2	10.0
0	41	2.44	39.4	684.8	720.6	0.67	0	0.12	1.82	0.13	2.37	0.27	38.0	23.5	0.1	1.8
5	20	1.10	7.3	168.4	851.6	1.51	190.3	0.04	0.59	0.05	1.01	0.07	9.8	2.4	0.3	2.7
0	56	2.05	37.3	334.5	501.9	0.60	0	0.18	1.13	0.08	1.72	0.16	104.1	18.8	0	3.9
0	30	0.83	32.9	549.0	490.8	0.51	108.8	0.14	1.82	0.12	1.95	0.21	15.2	1.0	0	5.1
0	24	1.06	7.2	207.3	814.6	0.46	171.1	0.05	1.40	0.05	0.90	0.06	9.6	1.4	0	4.3
45	150	4.50	—	—	1290.0	—	—	—	—	—	—	—	—	1.2	—	—
50	500	1.08	—	—	450.0	—	—	—	—	—	—	—	—	4.8	—	—
50	100	2.70	—	—	1110.0	—	—	—	—	—	—	—	—	9.0	—	—
0	42	2.82	—	—	1483.6	—	0	—	—	—	—	—	—	0	—	—
0	20	1.80	—	—	1200.0	—	0	—	—	—	—	—	—	0	—	—
55	150	4.50	—	—	2120.0	—	—	—	—	—	—	—	—	4.8	—	—
25	40	0.72	—	—	600.0	—	—	—	—	—	—	—	—	0	—	—
50	500	0.72	—	—	440.0	—	—	—	—	—	—	—	—	4.8	—	—
25	40	2.70	—	—	520.0	—	0	—	—	—	—	—	—	0	—	—
110	80	8.10	—	—	1870.0	—	0	—	—	—	—	—	—	0	—	—
65	250	1.44	—	—	1000.0	—	—	—	—	—	—	—	—	12.0	—	—
80	450	5.40	—	—	1770.0	—	—	—	—	—	—	—	—	6.0	—	—
80	350	3.60	—	—	1550.0	—	—	—	—	—	—	—	—	6.0	—	—
60	250	1.44	—	—	760.0	—	—	—	—	—	—	—	—	12.0	—	—
105	450	5.40	—	—	2200.0	—	—	—	—	—	—	—	—	6.0	—	—
50	600	0.72	—	—	1690.0	—	—	—	—	—	—	—	—	0	—	—
0	20	0.36	—	—	460.0	—	0	—	—	—	—	—	—	0	—	—
45	60	4.50	—	—	950.0	—	0	—	—	—	—	—	—	0	—	—
45	80	4.50	—	—	1060.0	—	—	—	—	—	—	—	—	6.0	—	—
50	500	0.36	—	—	390.0	—	—	—	—	—	—	—	—	4.8	—	—
0	20	0.72	—	—	400.0	—	0	—	—	—	—	—	—	0	—	—
12	78	0	—	—	364.3	—	23.3	—	—	—	—	—	—	0	—	—
0	20	0.72	—	—	400.0	—	0	—	—	—	—	—	—	0	—	—
25	20	0.72	—	—	400.0	—	—	—	—	—	—	—	—	0	—	—
0	20	0.72	—	—	990.0	—	0	—	—	—	—	—	—	0	—	—
0	0	1.08	—	—	140.0	—	20.0	—	—	—	—	—	—	36.0	—	—
0	20	0.72	—	—	990.0	—	0	—	—	—	—	—	—	0	—	—
10	20	0.72	—	—	990.0	—	—	—	—	—	—	—	—	0	—	—
0	20	0.72	—	—	400.0	—	0	—	—	—	—	—	—	0	—	—

APPENDIX H

DA+ Code	Food Description	Quantity	Measure	Wt (g)	H_2O (g)	Ener (kcal)	Prot (g)	Carb (g)	Fiber (g)	Fat (g)	Fat Breakdown (g)		
											Sat	Mono	Poly
	Fast Food—*continued*												
35361	Sesame soft pretzel	1	item(s)	128	—	360	10.0	67.0	3.0	6.0	1.0	—	—
35362	Sesame soft pretzel with butter	1	item(s)	132	—	400	10.0	67.0	3.0	10.0	3.5	—	—
35364	Sour cream & onion soft pretzel	1	item(s)	123	—	330	9.0	68.0	2.0	1.5	0	—	—
35366	Sour cream & onion soft pretzel with butter	1	item(s)	127	—	360	9.0	68.0	2.0	5.0	3.0	—	—
35373	Sweet mustard dipping sauce	1	serving(s)	35	—	60	2.0	10.0	0	2.0	1.0	—	—
	Boston Market												
51194	Apple pie	1	slice(s)	163	—	580	43.0	74.0	3.0	30.0	13.0	—	—
35058	Brownie, chocolate	1	item(s)	85	—	320	5.0	49.0	3.0	13.0	3.0	—	—
35013	Chicken Carver sandwich with cheese and sauce	1	item(s)	321	—	750	57.0	64.0	3.0	29.0	8.0	—	—
34979	Chicken gravy	4	ounce(s)	113	—	50	0	7.0	0	2.0	0.5	—	—
35053	Chicken noodle soup	¾	cup(s)	171	—	103	9.1	9.5	0.8	3.3	1.0	—	—
34973	Chicken pot pie	1	item(s)	425	—	800	32.0	59.0	4.0	48.0	18.0	—	—
35054	Chicken tortilla soup with toppings	¾	cup(s)	171	—	193	8.0	14.1	0.9	12.2	3.3	—	—
35064	Chocolate cake	1	slice(s)	145	—	580	5.0	67.0	3.0	34.0	11.0	—	—
35057	Cornbread	1	item(s)	57	—	180	2.0	31.0	0	5.0	1.5	—	—
35008	Cranberry walnut relish	¾	cup(s)	210	—	350	3.0	75.0	3.0	4.5	0	—	—
34980	Creamed spinach	¾	cup(s)	191	—	280	9.0	12.0	4.0	23.0	15.0	—	—
34998	Fresh vegetable stuffing	1	cup(s)	136	—	190	3.0	25.0	2.0	8.0	1.0	—	—
34991	Garlic dill new potatoes	¾	cup(s)	156	—	140	3.0	24.0	3.0	3.0	1.0	—	—
34982	Green beans	¾	cup(s)	91	—	60	2.0	7.0	3.0	3.5	1.5	—	—
34984	Homestyle mashed potatoes	¾	cup(s)	221	—	270	5.0	36.0	4.0	11.0	5.0	—	—
34985	Homestyle mashed potatoes and gravy	1	cup(s)	227	—	153	3.4	22.4	2.0	6.4	4.1	—	—
34988	Hot cinnamon apples	¾	cup(s)	145	—	210	0	47.0	3.0	3.0	0	—	—
34989	Macaroni and cheese	¾	cup(s)	221	—	300	11.0	35.0	2.0	11.0	7.0	—	—
34970	Meatloaf	1	serving(s)	218	—	520	29.0	21.0	0	36.0	16.0	—	—
39383	Nestle Toll House chocolate chip cookie	1	item(s)	78	—	370	4.0	49.0	2.0	19.0	9.0	—	—
34963	Quarter chicken, white meat, no skin or wing	1	item(s)	173	—	250	41.0	4.0	0	8.0	2.5	—	—
34964	Quarter chicken, white meat, with skin and wing	1	item(s)	110	—	330	50.0	3.0	0	12.0	4.0	—	—
34968	Roasted turkey breast	5	ounce(s)	141	—	188	38.8	0	0	3.1	1.3	—	—
35011	Seasonal fresh fruit salad	1	serving(s)	142	—	60	1.0	15.0	1.0	0	0	0	0
51192	Spinach with garlic butter sauce	1	serving(s)	170	—	130	5.0	9.0	5.0	9.0	6.0	—	—
34999	Squash casserole	¾	cup(s)	187	—	330	7.0	20.0	3.0	24.0	13.0	—	—
35003	Steamed vegetables	1	cup(s)	136	—	60	2.0	8.0	3.0	2.0	0	—	—
35005	Sweet corn	¾	cup(s)	176	—	170	6.0	37.0	2.0	4.0	1.0	—	—
35004	Sweet potato casserole	¾	cup(s)	198	—	460	4.0	77.0	3.0	16.0	4.5	—	—
	Burger King												
29731	Biscuit with sausage, egg & cheese	1	item(s)	191	—	550	20.0	34.0	1.0	37.0	19.0	—	—
14249	Cheeseburger	1	item(s)	121	—	310	16.0	28.0	1.0	15.0	7.0	—	—
14251	Chicken sandwich	1	item(s)	218	—	630	24.0	46.0	3.0	39.0	7.0	—	—
14259	Chocolate shake, 12 ounces	1	item(s)	340	—	340	7.0	60.0	1.0	9.0	7.0	—	—
29732	Croissanwich with sausage & cheese	1	item(s)	106	37.2	380	14.0	26.0	0	24.0	10.0	12.7	3.3
14261	Croissanwich with sausage, egg & cheese	1	item(s)	159	71.4	460	19.0	27.0	0	31.0	11.0	15.8	6.1
3809	Double cheeseburger	1	item(s)	171	—	460	27.0	28.0	1.0	27.0	13.0	—	—
14244	Double Whopper sandwich	1	item(s)	373	—	920	48.0	51.0	3.0	58.0	19.0	—	—
14245	Double Whopper with cheese sandwich	1	item(s)	398	—	1010	53.0	53.0	3.0	65.0	24.0	—	—
14250	Fish sandwich	1	item(s)	248	—	640	23.0	67.0	3.0	31.0	5.0	—	—
14255	French fries, medium, salted	1	serving(s)	148	—	440	5.0	56.0	5.0	22.0	4.5	—	—
14262	French toast sticks (5)	1	serving(s)	109	37.6	380	5.0	49.0	2.0	18.0	3.0	10.6	2.9
14248	Hamburger	1	item(s)	110	—	260	14.0	27.0	1.0	11.0	4.0	—	—
14263	Hash brown rounds, small	1	serving(s)	78	27.1	240	2.0	23.0	3.0	15.0	3.5	—	—
14256	Onion rings, medium	1	serving(s)	117	—	400	6.0	47.0	4.0	21.0	3.5	—	—
39000	Tendercrisp chicken sandwich	1	item(s)	284	—	800	32.0	68.0	3.0	46.0	8.0	—	—
37514	TenderGrill chicken sandwich	1	item(s)	259	—	410	38.0	49.0	2.0	7.0	1.5	—	—
14258	Vanilla shake, 12 ounces	1	item(s)	340	—	290	7.0	46.0	0	9.0	7.0	—	—
1736	Whopper sandwich	1	item(s)	290	—	670	29.0	51.0	3.0	40.0	11.0	—	—
14243	Whopper with cheese sandwich	1	item(s)	315	—	770	33.0	52.0	3.0	48.0	16.0	—	—

Chol (mg)	Calc (mg)	Iron (mg)	Magn (mg)	Pota (mg)	Sodi (mg)	Zinc (mg)	Vit A (µg)	Thia (mg)	Vit E (mg α)	Ribo (mg)	Niac (mg)	Vit B_6 (mg)	Fola (µg)	Vit C (mg)	Vit B_{12} (µg)	Sele (µg)
0	100	1.80	—	—	990.0	—	0	—	—	—	—	—	—	0	—	—
10	100	1.80	—	—	990.0	—	—	—	—	—	—	—	—	0	—	—
0	60	0.72	—	—	1180.0	—	0	—	—	—	—	—	—	0	—	—
10	60	0.72	—	—	1180.0	—	—	—	—	—	—	—	—	0	—	—
35	0	0	—	—	0	—	0	—	—	—	—	—	—	0	—	—
0	—	—	—	—	690.0	—	—	—	—	—	—	—	—	—	—	—
50	—	—	—	—	220.1	—	—	—	—	—	—	—	—	—	—	—
160	211	2.85	—	—	1960.0	—	—	—	—	—	—	—	—	15.8	—	—
0	0	0	—	—	690.0	—	—	—	—	—	—	—	—	0	—	—
39	—	—	—	—	584.8	—	—	—	—	—	—	—	—	—	—	—
140	40	4.50	—	—	1090.0	—	—	—	—	—	—	—	—	1.2	—	—
33	—	—	—	—	986.4	—	—	—	—	—	—	—	—	—	—	—
45	36	1.64	—	—	360.0	—	—	—	—	—	—	—	—	0	—	—
10	0	0.71	—	—	320.0	—	—	—	—	—	—	—	—	0	—	—
0	0	5.40	—	—	0	—	0	—	—	—	—	—	—	0	—	—
70	264	2.85	—	—	580.0	—	—	—	—	—	—	—	—	9.5	—	—
0	—	—	—	—	580.0	—	—	—	—	—	—	—	—	—	—	—
0	0	0.86	—	—	120.0	—	—	—	—	—	—	—	—	14.3	—	—
0	43	0.38	—	—	180.0	—	—	—	—	—	—	—	—	5.1	—	—
25	51	0.46	—	—	820.0	—	—	—	—	—	—	—	—	19.2	—	—
17	68	0.41	—	—	834.1	—	—	—	—	—	—	—	—	16.9	—	—
0	16	0.29	—	—	15.0	—	—	—	—	—	—	—	—	0	—	—
30	345	1.66	—	—	1100.0	—	—	—	—	—	—	—	—	0	—	—
145	140	3.78	—	—	1030.0	—	—	—	—	—	—	—	—	1.8	—	—
20	0	1.32	—	—	340.0	—	—	—	—	—	—	—	—	0	—	—
125	0	0.89	—	—	480.0	—	0	—	—	—	—	—	—	0	—	—
165	0	0.78	—	—	960.0	—	0	—	—	—	—	—	—	0	—	—
69	25	2.25	—	—	625.0	—	—	—	—	—	—	—	—	0	—	—
0	16	0.29	—	—	20.0	—	—	—	—	—	—	—	—	29.5	—	—
20	—	—	—	—	200.0	—	—	—	—	—	—	—	—	—	—	—
70	200	0.72	—	—	1110.0	—	—	—	—	—	—	—	—	4.8	—	—
0	53	0.47	—	—	40.0	—	—	—	—	—	—	—	—	24.0	—	—
0	0	0.43	—	—	95.0	—	—	—	—	—	—	—	—	5.8	—	—
5	44	1.18	—	—	270.0	—	—	—	—	—	—	—	—	9.8	—	—
210	250	2.70	—	—	1520.0	—	—	—	—	—	—	—	—	0	—	—
40	150	2.70	—	—	740.0	—	—	0.25	—	0.32	4.18	—	—	1.2	—	—
65	64	2.90	—	—	1390.0	—	—	0.50	—	0.32	10.29	—	—	0	—	—
30	333	0.80	—	—	270.0	—	—	0.12	—	0.62	0.26	—	—	2.7	0	—
50	99	1.78	20.1	—	780.0	1.52	—	0.35	1.04	0.34	4.34	—	—	0	0.6	22.2
215	146	2.63	28.6	—	1000.0	2.08	—	0.39	1.67	0.52	4.72	0.29	—	0	1.1	38.0
80	250	4.50	—	—	990.0	—	—	0.26	—	0.45	6.37		—	1.2	—	—
140	150	8.08	—	—	1090.0	—	—	0.40	—	0.60	11.05	—	—	9.0	—	—
160	299	8.08	—	—	1530.0	—	—	0.40	—	0.67	11.04	—	—	9.0	—	—
45	101	3.63	—	—	1560.0	—	—	—	—			—	—	3.6	—	—
0	20	0.71	—	—	670.0	—	0	0.16	—	0.48	2.30	—	—	8.9	—	—
0	60	1.80	21.3	—	430.0	0.57	0	0.32	0.99	0.20	2.88	0.06	—	0	0	13.7
30	80	2.70	—	—	520.0	—	—	0.25	—	0.28	4.26	—	—	1.2	—	—
0	0	0.36	—	—	380.0	—	0	0.12	0.83	0.06	1.36	0.17	—	1.2	—	—
0	100	0	—	—	630.0	—	0	0.14	—	0.09	2.33	—	—	0	—	—
70	79	4.44	—	—	1640.0	—	—	—	—	—	—	—	—	8.9	—	—
75	57	6.83	—	—	1310.0	—	—	—	—	—	—	—	—	5.7	—	—
30	348	0	—	—	230.0	—	—	0.11	—	0.63	0.21	—	—	2.4	0	—
75	100	5.38	—	—	1020.0	—	—	0.39	—	0.44	7.30	—	—	9.0	—	—
100	249	5.38	—	—	1450.0	—	—	0.39	—	0.51	7.29	—	—	9.0	—	—

APPENDIX H

DA+ Code	Food Description	Quantity	Measure	Wt (g)	H_2O (g)	Ener (kcal)	Prot (g)	Carb (g)	Fiber (g)	Fat (g)	Fat Breakdown (g)		
											Sat	Mono	Poly
Fast Food—*continued*													
	Carl's Jr.												
33962	Carl's bacon Swiss crispy chicken sandwich	1	item(s)	330	—	800	39.0	67.0	5.0	41.0	10.0	—	—
10801	Carl's Catch Fish sandwich	1	item(s)	298	—	730	20.0	77.0	5.0	37.0	6.0	—	—
10862	Carl's Famous Star hamburger	1	item(s)	269	—	620	25.0	56.0	3.0	34.0	10.0	—	—
10785	Charbroiled chicken club sandwich	1	item(s)	269	—	570	42.0	45.0	3.0	26.0	7.0	—	—
10866	Charbroiled chicken salad	1	item(s)	417	—	260	32.0	15.0	5.0	8.0	3.0	—	—
10855	Charbroiled Santa Fe Chicken sandwich	1	item(s)	273	—	640	39.0	45.0	3.0	33.0	8.0	—	—
10790	Chicken stars (6 pieces)	6	item(s)	84	—	320	12.0	14.0	2.0	24.0	6.0	—	—
34864	Chocolate shake, small	1	serving(s)	397	260.7	710	14.0	86.0	1.0	33.0	23.0	4.3	0.6
10797	Crisscut fries	1	serving(s)	139	—	450	5.0	42.0	4.0	29.0	5.0	—	—
10799	Double Western Bacon cheeseburger	1	item(s)	326	—	980	52.0	73.0	3.0	53.0	23.0	—	—
14238	French fries, small	1	serving(s)	119	—	320	4.0	42.0	4.0	15.0	3.0	—	—
10798	French toast dips without syrup, 5 pieces	1	serving(s)	110	—	430	8.0	51.0	2.0	22.0	4.0	—	—
10802	Onion rings	1	serving(s)	128	—	530	8.0	61.0	3.0	28.0	4.5	—	—
34858	Spicy chicken sandwich	1	item(s)	206	—	550	17.0	61.0	4.0	28.0	5.0	—	—
34867	Strawberry shake, small	1	serving(s)	397	—	700	14.0	85.0	0	33.0	23.0	—	—
10865	Super Star hamburger	1	item(s)	358	—	820	41.0	58.0	3.0	49.0	17.0	—	—
38925	The Six Dollar burger	1	item(s)	406	—	910	46.0	63.0	3.0	54.0	20.0	—	—
10818	Vanilla shake, small	1	item(s)	397	260.9	710	14.0	86.0	0	33.0	23.0	7.1	1.3
10770	Western Bacon cheeseburger	1	item(s)	225	—	667	30.6	67.6	2.8	30.6	12.0	—	—
10770	Western Bacon cheeseburger	1	item(s)	243	—	720	33.0	73.0	3.0	33.0	13.0	—	—
	Chick-Fil-A												
38746	Biscuit with bacon, egg & cheese	1	item(s)	159	—	500	21.0	43.0	2.0	27.0	12.0	—	—
38747	Biscuit with egg	1	item(s)	127	—	420	14.0	42.0	2.0	21.0	8.5	—	—
38748	Biscuit with egg & cheese	1	item(s)	154	—	470	17.0	43.0	2.0	25.0	11.0	—	—
38752	Biscuit with sausage, egg & cheese	1	item(s)	204	—	760	28.0	43.0	2.0	52.0	20.0	—	—
72643	Chargrilled chicken and fruit salad	1	item(s)	347	—	230	22.0	23.0	4.0	6.0	3.5	—	—
38760	Chargrilled chicken club sandwich	1	item(s)	258	—	410	37.0	39.0	3.0	12.0	5.0	—	—
38761	Chargrilled chicken Cool Wrap	1	item(s)	291	—	410	33.0	50.0	9.0	12.0	4.0	—	—
38758	Chargrilled chicken sandwich	1	item(s)	228	—	300	29.0	38.0	3.0	3.5	1.0	—	—
38763	Chick-n-Strips	4	item(s)	218	—	500	47.0	24.0	1.0	24.0	4.5	—	—
38742	Chicken biscuit	1	item(s)	143	—	440	17.0	47.0	3.0	20.0	8.0	—	—
38743	Chicken biscuit with cheese	1	item(s)	157	—	490	20.0	48.0	3.0	24.0	10.5	—	—
38764	Chicken salad sandwich on wheat bun	1	item(s)	233	—	500	29.0	52.0	4.0	20.0	3.5	—	—
38756	Chicken sandwich	1	item(s)	179	—	430	31.0	39.0	3.0	17.0	3.5	—	—
38757	Chicken sandwich, deluxe	1	item(s)	257	—	490	35.0	43.0	3.0	21.0	6.0	—	—
38770	Cole slaw	1	item(s)	298	—	580	3.0	31.0	5.0	50.0	8.0	—	—
38776	Diet lemonade, small	1	cup(s)	226	—	11	0	4.2	0	0.0	0	0	0
50867	Fruit cup, large	1	item(s)	194	—	100	1.0	27.0	3.0	0.0	0	0	0
38755	Hashbrowns	1	serving(s)	77	—	280	3.0	25.0	2.0	19.0	4.0	—	—
38765	Hearty breast of chicken soup	1	cup(s)	226	—	114	5.7	15.4	1.6	3.3	0.8	—	—
38741	Hot buttered biscuit	1	item(s)	86	—	310	5.0	41.0	2.0	13.0	6.0	—	—
38778	IceDream, small cone	1	item(s)	135	—	170	5.0	31.0	0	4.0	2.0	—	—
38774	IceDream, small cup	1	serving(s)	227	—	290	8.0	50.0	0	7.0	4.5	—	—
38775	Lemonade, small	1	cup(s)	226	—	120	0	32.5	0	0.0	0	0	0
38777	Nuggets	8	item(s)	113	—	270	28.0	12.0	1.0	12.0	2.5	—	—
38769	Side salad	1	item(s)	113	—	70	5.0	5.0	2.0	4.5	3.0	—	—
72642	Spicy chicken sandwich	1	item(s)	196	—	490	31.0	46.0	4.0	20.0	4.0	—	—
72626	Spicy chicken sandwich, deluxe	1	item(s)	281	—	580	36.0	48.0	4.0	27.0	8.0	—	—
38772	Waffle potato fries, small, salted	1	serving(s)	85	—	290	3.0	34.0	3.0	16.0	3.0	—	—
72633	Yogurt parfait w/ granola	1	item(s)	227	—	290	7.0	54.0	2.0	5.0	2.0	—	—
	Cinnabon												
39571	Cinnabon Bites	1	serving(s)	149	—	510	8.0	77.0	2.0	19.0	5.0	—	—
39570	Cinnabon Stix	5	item(s)	85	—	379	6.0	41.0	1.0	21.0	6.0	—	—
39567	Classic roll	1	item(s)	221	—	813	15.0	117.0	4.0	32.0	8.0	—	—
39568	Minibon	1	item(s)	92	—	339	6.0	49.0	2.0	13.0	3.0	—	—

Chol (mg)	Calc (mg)	Iron (mg)	Magn (mg)	Pota (mg)	Sodi (mg)	Zinc (mg)	Vit A (µg)	Thia (mg)	Vit E (mg α)	Ribo (mg)	Niac (mg)	Vit B_6 (mg)	Fola (µg)	Vit C (mg)	Vit B_{12} (µg)	Sele (µg)
75	200	4.50	—	—	2130.0	—	—	—	—	—	—	—	—	4.8	—	—
40	100	3.60	—	—	1320.0	—	—	—	—	—	—	—	—	4.8	—	—
65	100	4.50	—	—	1060.0	—	—	—	—	—	—	—	—	6.0	—	—
90	150	3.60	—	—	1310.0	—	—	—	—	—	—	—	—	6.0	—	—
70	200	2.70	—	—	620.0	—	—	—	—	—	—	—	—	27.0	—	—
95	200	3.60	—	—	1440.0	—	—	—	—	—	—	—	—	6.0	—	—
35	19	0.72	—	—	460.0	—	0	—	—	—	—	—	—	0	—	—
100	500	0.72	67.5	794.0	300.0	1.63	419.4	0.23	0.44	0.97	0.64	0.20	19.9	0	1.4	6.7
0	20	1.08	—	—	900.0	—	—	—	—	—	—	—	—	0	—	—
140	250	5.40	—	—	1790.0	—	—	—	—	—	—	—	—	0	—	—
0	20	1.08	—	—	830.0	—	0	—	—	—	—	—	—	1.2	—	—
0	80	1.44	—	—	480.0	—	0	—	—	—	—	—	—	0	—	—
0	20	1.08	—	—	590.0	—	—	—	—	—	—	—	—	1.2	—	—
25	100	3.60	—	—	1220.0	—	—	—	—	—	—	—	—	1.2	—	—
100	500	0	—	—	250.0	—	—	—	—	—	—	—	—	0	—	—
115	100	5.40	—	—	1120.0	—	—	—	—	—	—	—	—	9.0	—	—
130	250	5.40	—	—	2080.0	—	—	—	—	—	—	—	—	9.0	—	—
100	500	0.00	51.6	659.2	240.1	2.26	449.1	0.10	0.99	2.62	0.85	0.24	0	0	0.9	12.7
69	185	4.17	—	—	1342.6	—	—	—	—	—	—	—	—	0	—	—
75	200	4.50	—	—	1450.0	—	—	—	—	—	—	—	—	0	—	—
230	150	3.60	—	—	1370.0	—	—	—	—	—	—	—	—	0	—	—
260	—	—	—	—	830.0	—	—	—	—	—	—	—	—	—	—	—
275	—	—	—	—	1070.0	—	—	—	—	—	—	—	—	—	—	—
325	—	—	—	—	1620.0	—	—	—	—	—	—	—	—	—	—	—
55	150	1.80	—	—	650.0	—	—	—	—	—	—	—	—	96.0	—	—
80	250	3.60	—	—	1460.0	—	—	—	—	—	—	—	—	12.0	—	—
55	200	4.50	—	—	1300.0	—	—	—	—	—	—	—	—	24.0	—	—
55	100	3.60	—	—	1120.0	—	—	—	—	—	—	—	—	12.0	—	—
95	60	3.60	—	—	1630.0	—	—	—	—	—	—	—	—	0	—	—
25	80	1.80	—	—	1240.0	—	—	—	—	—	—	—	—	0	—	—
40	—	—	—	—	1480.0	—	—	—	—	—	—	—	—	—	—	—
80	200	4.50	—	—	1240.0	—	—	—	—	—	—	—	—	4.8	—	—
65	150	2.70	—	—	1370.0	—	0	—	—	—	—	—	—	0	—	—
75	250	2.70	—	—	1620.0	—	—	—	—	—	—	—	—	9.0	—	—
35	80	1.08	—	—	450.0	—	—	—	—	—	—	—	—	72.0	—	—
0	—	—	—	—	7.1	—	—	—	—	—	—	—	—	—	—	—
0	20	0.36	—	—	0	—	0	—	—	—	—	—	—	186.0	—	—
0	20	0.72	—	—	410.0	—	0	—	—	—	—	—	—	6.0	—	—
20	—	—	—	—	902.4	—	—	—	—	—	—	—	—	—	—	—
0	60	1.08	—	—	700.0	—	—	—	—	—	—	—	—	0	—	—
15	150	0.36	—	—	115.0	—	—	—	—	—	—	—	—	1.2	—	—
25	—	—	—	—	200.0	—	—	—	—	—	—	—	—	—	—	—
0	—	—	—	—	3.5	—	—	—	—	—	—	—	—	—	—	—
70	—	—	—	—	990.0	—	—	—	—	—	—	—	—	—	—	—
15	150	0.72	—	—	110.0	—	—	—	—	—	—	—	—	24.0	—	—
60	150	4.50	—	—	1730.0	—	—	—	—	—	—	—	—	0	—	—
80	300	4.50	—	—	1880.0	—	—	—	—	—	—	—	—	9.0	—	—
0	—	—	—	—	140.1	—	—	—	—	—	—	—	—	—	—	—
10	200	0.72	—	—	70.0	—	—	—	—	—	—	—	—	30.0	—	—
35	—	—	—	—	530.0	—	—	—	—	—	—	—	—	—	—	—
16	—	—	—	—	413.2	—	—	—	—	—	—	—	—	—	—	—
67	—	—	—	—	801.0	—	—	—	—	—	—	—	—	—	—	—
27	—	—	—	—	337.0	—	—	—	—	—	—	—	—	—	—	—

DA+ Code	Food Description	Quantity	Measure	Wt (g)	H_2O (g)	Ener (kcal)	Prot (g)	Carb (g)	Fiber (g)	Fat (g)	Fat Breakdown (g)		
											Sat	Mono	Poly
Fast Food—*continued*													
39573	Mochalatta Chill with whipped cream	16	fluid ounce(s)	473	—	425	10.0	63.0	2.0	17.0	11.0	—	—
39569	Pecanbon	1	item(s)	272	—	1100	16.0	141.0	8.0	56.0	10.0	—	—
	Dairy Queen												
1466	Banana split	1	item(s)	374	—	520	9.0	94.0	3.0	13.0	10.0	—	—
38561	Chocolate chip cookie dough Blizzard, small	1	item(s)	319	—	710	13.0	103.0	1.0	27.0	14.0	—	—
1464	Chocolate malt, small	1	item(s)	427	—	650	15.0	110.0	0	16.0	10.0	—	—
38541	Chocolate shake, small	1	item(s)	406	—	570	13.0	92.0	0	15.0	10.0	—	—
1463	Chocolate sundae, small	1	item(s)	163	—	280	5.0	48.0	0	7.0	4.5	—	—
1462	Dipped cone, small	1	item(s)	156	—	330	6.0	36.0	0	15.0	6.0	—	—
58376	Mint Oreo Blizzard, small	1	item(s)	297	—	580	12.0	89.0	1.0	20.0	10.0	—	—
38552	Oreo Brownie Earthquake	1	serving(s)	304	—	760	11.0	117.0	2.0	27.0	16.0	—	—
38555	Oreo cookies Blizzard, small	1	item(s)	283	—	550	12.0	81.0	1.0	20.0	10.0	—	—
38547	Royal Treats Peanut Buster Parfait	1	item(s)	304	—	700	16.0	94.0	2.0	30.0	16.0	—	—
17256	Vanilla soft serve	½	cup(s)	94	—	145	4.0	21.5	0	4.5	3.0	—	—
	Domino's												
31604	Breadsticks	1	item(s)	30	—	110	2.0	11.0	0	6.0	1.5	—	—
31605	Cheesy bread	1	item(s)	36	—	120	4.0	11.0	0	6.0	2.0	—	—
37548	CinnaStix	1	item(s)	33	—	120	2.0	14.0	1.0	6.0	1.0	—	—
31606	Wings w/ barbecue sauce	1	item(s)	30	—	63	4.3	3.5	0.3	3.3	0.9	—	—
31607	Wings w/ hot sauce	1	item(s)	30	—	50	4.3	1.3	0.3	3.3	0.9	—	—
	Domino's Artisan pizza												
81942	Chicken & Bacon Carbonara	1	slice(s)	76	—	150	8.0	18.0	1.0	6.0	2.5	—	—
81939	Italian Sausage & Pepper Trio	1	slice(s)	74	—	160	7.0	18.0	1.0	7.0	2.5	—	—
81940	Spinach & Feta	1	slice(s)	62	—	150	6.0	17.0	1.0	7.0	3.0	—	—
81941	Tuscan Salami & Roasted Veggie	1	slice(s)	64	—	150	5.0	17.0	1.0	6.0	2.0	—	—
	Domino's hand-tossed pizza												
31573	America's favorite feast, 12"	1	slice(s)	109	—	250	10.0	27.0	2.0	12.0	5.0	—	—
31574	America's favorite feast, 14"	1	slice(s)	151	—	350	14.0	36.0	2.0	17.0	7.0	—	—
37543	Bacon Cheeseburger Feast, 12"	1	slice(s)	106	—	270	12.0	26.0	2.0	13.0	5.5	—	—
37545	Bacon Cheeseburger Feast, 14"	1	slice(s)	146	—	380	17.0	36.0	2.0	19.0	9.0	—	—
81919	Cali Chicken Bacon Ranch, 12"	1	slice(s)	114	—	320	14.0	25.0	1.0	18.0	6.5	—	—
81920	Cali Chicken Bacon Ranch, 14"	1	slice(s)	154	—	430	19.0	33.0	1.0	25.0	9.0	—	—
31569	Cheese, 12"	1	slice(s)	93	—	210	8.0	25.0	1.0	8.0	3.5	—	—
31570	Cheese, 14"	1	slice(s)	128	57.4	290	12.0	35.0	2.0	11.0	5.5	2.8	2.3
31685	Deluxe Feast, 12"	1	slice(s)	106	—	226	9.0	26.0	2.0	9.5	3.5	—	—
31694	Deluxe Feast, 14"	1	slice(s)	145	—	320	13.0	36.0	2.0	14.0	6.0	—	—
31686	ExtravaganZZa Feast, 12"	1	slice(s)	132	—	290	13.0	28.0	2.0	14.0	6.5	—	—
31695	ExtravaganZZa Feast, 14"	1	slice(s)	176	89.4	390	17.0	37.0	2.0	19.0	8.0	6.4	2.5
81931	Fiery Hawaiian, 12"	1	slice(s)	118	—	250	12.0	27.0	2.0	11.0	5.0	—	—
81932	Fiery Hawaiian, 14"	1	slice(s)	160	—	350	15.0	36.0	2.0	16.0	6.5	—	—
39033	Ham and pineapple, 12"	1	slice(s)	100	—	200	8.0	26.0	1.0	6.5	2.5	—	—
39034	Ham and pineapple, 14"	1	slice(s)	128	—	290	12.0	35.0	2.0	11.0	5.5	—	—
31687	MeatZZa Feast, 12"	1	slice(s)	117	—	280	12.0	27.0	2.0	14.0	5.5	—	—
31696	MeatZZa Feast, 14"	1	slice(s)	160	—	380	18.0	36.0	2.0	19.0	8.0	—	—
81923	Memphis BBQ Chicken, 12"	1	slice(s)	103	—	260	13.0	28.0	1.0	12.0	5.5	—	—
81924	Memphis BBQ Chicken, 14"	1	slice(s)	140	—	360	16.0	37.0	1.0	15.0	7.5	—	—
31571	Pepperoni Feast, 12"	1	slice(s)	99	—	260	11.0	25.0	1.0	13.0	5.5	—	—
31572	Pepperoni Feast, 14"	1	slice(s)	136	—	360	15.0	34.0	2.0	18.0	8.0	—	—
81927	Philly Cheese Steak, 12"	1	slice(s)	101	—	260	11.0	24.0	1.0	12.0	6.0	—	—
81928	Philly Cheese Steak, 14"	1	slice(s)	135	—	330	15.0	32.0	1.0	16.0	8.0	—	—
81935	Wisconsin 6 Cheese, 12"	1	slice(s)	101	—	250	12.0	25.0	1.0	12.0	6.0	—	—
81936	Wisconsin 6 Cheese, 14"	1	slice(s)	137	—	340	15.0	34.0	2.0	16.0	7.5	—	—
	Domino's thin crust pizza												
31583	America's Favorite Feast, 12"	1	slice(s)	81	—	210	8.0	15.0	1.0	13.0	5.0	—	—
31584	America's Favorite Feast, 14"	1	slice(s)	112	—	280	11.0	21.0	2.0	17.5	6.5	—	—
31579	Cheese, 12"	1	slice(s)	64	—	165	7.0	15.0	1.5	9.0	3.5	—	—
31580	Cheese, 14"	1	slice(s)	88	36.6	230	9.0	20.0	1.0	11.5	5.0	3.3	3.3
31688	Deluxe Feast, 12"	1	slice(s)	79	—	190	7.0	15.5	1.0	11.0	4.0	—	—
31697	Deluxe Feast, 14"	1	slice(s)	106	—	250	10.0	21.0	2.0	14.5	5.5	—	—
31689	ExtravaganZZa Feast, 12"	1	slice(s)	103	—	240	10.5	16.0	1.5	15.0	6.0	—	—
31698	ExtravaganZZa Feast, 14"	1	slice(s)	137	—	320	14.0	22.0	2.0	19.5	7.5	—	—
39037	Ham and pineapple, 12"	1	slice(s)	71	—	155	6.5	16.0	1.0	7.5	2.8	—	—
39038	Ham and pineapple, 14"	1	slice(s)	97	—	220	8.0	21.0	1.0	10.0	3.5	—	—

Chol (mg)	Calc (mg)	Iron (mg)	Magn (mg)	Pota (mg)	Sodi (mg)	Zinc (mg)	Vit A (µg)	Thia (mg)	Vit E (mg α)	Ribo (mg)	Niac (mg)	Vit B_6 (mg)	Fola (µg)	Vit C (mg)	Vit B_{12} (µg)	Sele (µg)
63	—	—	—	—	287.0	—	—	—	—	—	—	—	—	—	—	—
63	—	—	—	—	600.0	—	—	—	—	—	—	—	—	—	—	—
30	250	2.70	—	—	160.0	—	—	—	—	—	—	—	—	18.0	—	—
55	350	2.70	—	—	350.0	—	—	—	—	—	—	—	—	0	—	—
55	500	3.60	—	—	310.0	—	—	—	—	—	—	—	—	0	—	—
50	500	1.80	—	—	250.0	—	—	—	—	—	—	—	—	0	—	—
25	200	1.80	—	—	115.0	—	—	—	—	—	—	—	—	0	—	—
25	200	1.44	—	—	105.0	—	—	—	—	—	—	—	—	0	—	—
40	350	3.60	—	—	410.0	—	—	—	—	—	—	—	—	0	—	—
60	250	3.60	—	—	400.0	—	—	—	—	—	—	—	—	0	—	—
40	350	2.70	—	—	410.0	—	—	—	—	—	—	—	—	0	—	—
35	400	3.60	—	—	360.0	—	—	—	—	—	—	—	—	0	—	—
15	125	0.90	—	—	65.0	—	112.6	—	—	—	—	—	—	0	—	—
0	0	0.72	—	—	100.0	—	0	—	—	—	—	—	—	1.2	—	—
5	40	0.72	—	—	140.0	—	—	—	—	—	—	—	—	1.2	—	—
0	0	0.72	—	—	85.0	—	0	—	—	—	—	—	—	1.2	—	—
21	5	0.36	—	—	162.5	—	—	—	—	—	—	—	—	0.6	—	—
21	5	0.27	—	—	340.0	—	—	—	—	—	—	—	—	0.9	—	—
20	60	1.44	—	—	360.0	—	—	—	—	—	—	—	—	3.6	—	—
15	60	1.44	—	—	330.0	—	—	—	—	—	—	—	—	9.0	—	—
10	80	1.08	—	—	250.0	—	—	—	—	—	—	—	—	2.4	—	—
10	60	1.08	—	—	280.0	—	—	—	—	—	—	—	—	6.0	—	—
25	100	2.16	—	—	630.0	—	—	—	—	—	—	—	—	3.6	—	—
35	150	2.52	—	—	870.0	—	—	—	—	—	—	—	—	6.0	—	—
35	150	1.80	—	—	590.0	—	—	—	—	—	—	—	—	6.0	—	—
45	203	2.56	—	—	830.0	—	—	—	—	—	—	—	—	8.5	—	—
40	190	1.80	—	—	660.0	—	—	—	—	—	—	—	—	4.8	—	—
55	260	2.52	—	—	900.0	—	—	—	—	—	—	—	—	7.2	—	—
20	150	1.44	—	—	460.0	—	—	—	—	—	—	—	—	3.6	—	—
25	220	1.80	30.7	206.1	640.0	1.59	78.1	0.41	1.27	0.22	4.29	0.10	—	6.0	0.6	29.4
15	80	1.80	—	—	505.0	—	—	—	—	—	—	—	—	6.0	—	—
30	150	2.52	—	—	730.0	—	—	—	—	—	—	—	—	11.4	—	—
35	150	2.52	—	—	770.0	—	—	—	—	—	—	—	—	7.2	—	—
45	200	2.88	38.7	306.2	1020.0	2.23	89.8	0.24	1.41	0.39	5.72	—	—	11.4	1.0	42.2
25	170	1.80	—	—	760.0	—	—	—	—	—	—	—	—	10.2	—	—
35	240	2.52	—	—	1030.0	—	—	—	—	—	—	—	—	14.4	—	—
20	100	1.47	—	—	490.0	—	—	—	—	—	—	—	—	4.9	—	—
25	220	1.80	—	—	640.0	—	—	—	—	—	—	—	—	6.0	—	—
35	150	2.16	—	—	760.0	—	—	—	—	—	—	—	—	3.6	—	—
50	200	2.52	—	—	1030.0	—	—	—	—	—	—	—	—	6.0	—	—
30	210	1.80	—	—	500.0	—	—	—	—	—	—	—	—	2.4	—	—
40	260	2.16	—	—	680.0	—	—	—	—	—	—	—	—	4.8	—	—
30	150	1.80	—	—	650.0	—	—	—	—	—	—	—	—	3.6	—	—
40	200	2.52	—	—	880.0	—	—	—	—	—	—	—	—	6.0	—	—
30	190	1.80	—	—	540.0	—	—	—	—	—	—	—	—	4.8	—	—
40	260	2.16	—	—	690.0	—	—	—	—	—	—	—	—	6.0	—	—
25	220	1.80	—	—	500.0	—	—	—	—	—	—	—	—	3.6	—	—
35	290	2.16	—	—	690.0	—	—	—	—	—	—	—	—	6.0	—	—
25	120	0.72	—	—	500.0	—	—	—	—	—	—	—	—	3.0	—	—
35	170	1.08	—	—	690.0	—	—	—	—	—	—	—	—	3.6	—	—
20	170	0.54	—	—	330.0	—	—	—	—	—	—	—	—	2.4	—	—
25	240	0.72	21.1	177.8	460.0	1.36	—	0.05	1.31	0.07	0.89	0.06	—	3.6	0.6	17.4
20	120	0.72	—	—	410.0	—	—	—	—	—	—	—	—	6.0	—	—
30	170	1.08	—	—	550.0	—	—	—	—	—	—	—	—	9.0	—	—
35	170	1.08	—	—	640.0	—	—	—	—	—	—	—	—	6.0	—	—
45	220	1.44	—	—	840.0	—	—	—	—	—	—	—	—	9.0	—	—
15	120	0.36	—	—	350.0	—	—	—	—	—	—	—	—	3.0	—	—
25	190	0.72	—	—	485.0	—	—	—	—	—	—	—	—	4.8	—	—

TABLE H-1 Table of Food Composition (*continued*) (Computer code is for Cengage Diet Analysis program) (For purposes of calculations, use "0" for t, <1, <0.1, 0.01)

DA+ Code	Food Description	Quantity	Measure	Wt (g)	H_2O (g)	Ener (kcal)	Prot (g)	Carb (g)	Fiber (g)	Fat (g)	Fat Breakdown (g)		
											Sat	Mono	Poly
Fast Food—*continued*													
31690	MeatZZa Feast, 12"	1	slice(s)	89	—	235	10.5	15.5	1.0	14.5	6.0	—	—
31699	MeatZZa Feast, 14"	1	slice(s)	121	—	310	15.0	21.0	2.0	19.5	7.5	—	—
31581	Pepperoni Feast, 12"	1	slice(s)	71	—	215	9.0	14.0	1.0	13.5	5.5	—	—
31582	Pepperoni Feast, 14"	1	slice(s)	97	—	290	12.0	19.0	2.0	18.5	7.5	—	—
	In-n-Out Burger												
34391	Cheesburger with mustard & ketchup	1	serving(s)	268	—	400	22.0	41.0	3.0	18.0	9.0	—	—
34374	Cheeseburger	1	serving(s)	268	—	480	22.0	39.0	3.0	27.0	10.0	—	—
34390	Cheeseburger, lettuce leaves instead of buns	1	serving(s)	300	—	330	18.0	11.0	3.0	25.0	9.0	—	—
34377	Chocolate shake	1	serving(s)	425	—	690	9.0	83.0	0	36.0	24.0	—	—
34375	Double-Double cheeseburger	1	serving(s)	330	—	670	37.0	39.0	3.0	41.0	18.0	—	—
34393	Double-Double cheeseburger with mustard & ketchup	1	serving(s)	330	—	590	37.0	41.0	3.0	32.0	17.0	—	—
34392	Double-Double cheeseburger, lettuce leaves instead of buns	1	serving(s)	362	—	520	33.0	11.0	3.0	39.0	17.0	—	—
34376	French fries	1	serving(s)	125	—	400	7.0	54.0	2.0	18.0	5.0	—	—
34373	Hamburger	1	item(s)	243	—	390	16.0	39.0	3.0	19.0	5.0	—	—
34389	Hamburger with mustard & ketchup	1	serving(s)	243	—	310	16.0	41.0	3.0	10.0	4.0	—	—
34388	Hamburger, lettuce leaves instead of buns	1	serving(s)	275	—	240	13.0	11.0	3.0	17.0	4.0	—	—
34379	Strawberry shake	1	serving(s)	425	—	690	9.0	91.0	0	33.0	22.0	—	—
34378	Vanilla shake	1	serving(s)	425	—	680	9.0	78.0	0	37.0	25.0	—	—
	Jack in the Box												
30392	Bacon ultimate cheeseburger	1	item(s)	315	—	980	43.0	52.0	2.0	67.0	27.0	—	—
1740	Breakfast Jack	1	item(s)	113	—	300	16.0	29.0	1.0	14.0	5.0	—	—
14074	Cheeseburger	1	item(s)	118	—	320	16.0	30.0	1.0	15.0	7.0	—	—
14106	Chicken breast strips, 4 piece	4	piece(s)	201	—	500	35.0	36.0	3.0	25.0	6.0	—	—
37241	Chicken club salad, plain, without salad dressing	1	serving(s)	415	—	480	33.0	28.0	6.0	27.0	10.0	—	—
14064	Chicken sandwich	1	item(s)	145	—	400	15.0	38.0	2.0	21.0	4.5	—	—
14111	Chocolate ice cream shake, small	1	serving(s)	351	—	750	12.0	95.0	1.0	36.0	24.0	—	—
14073	Hamburger	1	item(s)	106	—	280	14.0	29.0	1.0	12.0	4.5	—	—
14090	Hash browns	1	serving(s)	73	—	230	2.0	20.0	2.0	16.0	4.0	—	—
14072	Jack's Spicy Chicken sandwich	1	item(s)	251	—	550	24.0	59.0	4.0	24.0	5.0	—	—
1468	Jumbo Jack hamburger	1	item(s)	249	—	580	20.0	51.0	2.0	33.0	11.0	—	—
1469	Jumbo Jack hamburger with cheese	1	item(s)	274	—	670	24.0	53.0	2.0	40.0	15.0	—	—
14099	Natural cut french fries, large	1	serving(s)	229	—	620	9.0	75.0	8.0	32.0	7.0	—	—
14098	Natural cut french fries, medium	1	serving(s)	169	—	460	6.0	55.0	6.0	24.0	6.0	—	—
1470	Onion rings	1	serving(s)	119	—	500	6.0	51.0	3.0	30.0	6.0	—	—
33141	Sausage, egg & cheese biscuit	1	item(s)	184	—	590	20.0	38.0	2.0	40.0	16.0	—	—
14095	Seasoned curly fries, medium	1	serving(s)	130	—	420	6.0	46.0	5.0	24.0	5.0	—	—
14077	Sourdough Jack	1	item(s)	228	—	680	26.0	41.0	2.0	46.0	17.0	—	—
37249	Southwest grilled chicken salad, plain, w/o salad dressing	1	serving(s)	442	—	310	31.0	28.0	7.0	12.0	5.0	—	—
14112	Strawberry ice cream shake, small	1	serving(s)	349	—	730	11.0	90.0	0	35.0	24.0	—	—
14078	Ultimate cheeseburger	1	item(s)	304	—	920	38.0	52.0	2.0	63.0	26.0	—	—
14110	Vanilla ice cream shake, small	1	serving(s)	314	—	650	11.0	70.0	0	35.0	24.0	—	—
	Jamba Juice												
55682	Acai Super-Antioxidant smoothie	24	fluid ounce(s)	680	—	415	5.5	85.1	5.5	6.5	2.2	—	—
31645	Aloha Pineapple smoothie	24	fluid ounce(s)	680	—	447	6.5	105.8	4.4	1.6	0.5	—	—
31646	Banana Berry smoothie	24	fluid ounce(s)	680	—	436	4.4	102.5	4.4	1.6	0.5	—	—
31647	Carribean Passion smoothie	24	fluid ounce(s)	680	—	393	3.3	89.5	3.3	1.6	0.5	—	—
38422	Carrot juice	16	fluid ounce(s)	473	—	130	4.0	30.0	0	0.5	0	—	—
31648	Chocolate Moo'd smoothie	24	fluid ounce(s)	680	—	622	16.4	126.5	3.3	5.5	2.7	—	—
31657	Mango-a-go-go smoothie	24	fluid ounce(s)	680	—	436	3.3	102.5	3.3	1.6	0.5	—	—
55684	Matcha Green Tea Blast smoothie	24	fluid ounce(s)	680	—	458	10.9	99.3	2.2	0	0	0	0
55673	Mega Mango smoothie	24	fluid ounce(s)	680	—	371	4.4	92.7	5.5	0.5	0	—	—
36945	Orange Dream Machine smoothie	24	fluid ounce(s)	680	—	513	10.9	112.4	1.1	1.6	1.1	—	—
38424	Orange juice, freshly squeezed	16	fluid ounce(s)	473	—	200	3.0	52.0	1.0	1.0	0	—	—
31660	Orange-a-peel smoothie	24	fluid ounce(s)	680	—	404	7.6	92.7	3.3	0	0	—	—

SE KEY: H-4 = Breads/Baked Goods H-8 = Cereal/Rice/Pasta H-14 = Fruit H-18 = Vegetables/Legumes H-28 = Nuts/Seeds H-30 = Vegetarian H-32 = Dairy H-40 = Eggs H-40 = Seafood H-42 = Meats H-46 = Poultry
8 = Processed Meats H-50 = Beverages H-52 = Fats/Oils H-54 = Sweets H-56 = Spices/Condiments/Sauces H-60 = Mixed Foods/Soups/Sandwiches H-66 = Fast Food H-84 = Convenience H-86 = Baby Foods

Chol (mg)	Calc (mg)	Iron (mg)	Magn (mg)	Pota (mg)	Sodi (mg)	Zinc (mg)	Vit A (μg)	Thia (mg)	Vit E (mg α)	Ribo (mg)	Niac (mg)	Vit B_6 (mg)	Fola (μg)	Vit C (mg)	Vit B_{12} (μg)	Sele (μg)
35	170	0.90	—	—	630.0	—	—	—	—	—	—	—	—	3.0	—	—
50	220	1.08	—	—	850.0	—	—	—	—	—	—	—	—	3.6	—	—
30	145	0.72	—	—	510.0	—	—	—	—	—	—	—	—	3.0	—	—
40	220	1.08	—	—	700.0	—	—	—	—	—	—	—	—	3.6	—	—
60	200	3.60	—	—	1080.0	—	—	—	—	—	—	—	—	12.0	—	—
60	200	3.60	—	—	1000.0	—	—	—	—	—	—	—	—	9.0	—	—
60	200	2.70	—	—	720.0	—	—	—	—	—	—	—	—	12.0	—	—
95	300	0.72	—	—	350.0	—	—	—	—	—	—	—	—	0	—	—
120	350	5.40	—	—	1440.0	—	—	—	—	—	—	—	—	9.0	—	—
115	350	5.40	—	—	1520.0	—	—	—	—	—	—	—	—	12.0	—	—
120	350	4.50	—	—	1160.0	—	—	—	—	—	—	—	—	12.0	—	—
0	20	1.80	—	—	245.0	—	0	—	—	—	—	—	—	0	—	—
40	40	3.60	—	—	650.0	—	—	—	—	—	—	—	—	9.0	—	—
35	40	3.60	—	—	730.0	—	—	—	—	—	—	—	—	12.0	—	—
40	40	2.70	—	—	370.0	—	—	—	—	—	—	—	—	12.0	—	—
85	300	0	—	—	280.0	—	—	—	—	—	—	—	—	0	—	—
90	300	0	—	—	390.0	—	—	—	—	—	—	—	—	0	—	—
135	308	7.39	—	490.0	1880.0	—	—	—	—	—	—	—	—	0.6	—	—
215	145	3.49	—	180.0	730.0	—	—	—	—	—	—	—	—	3.5	—	—
45	151	3.61	—	230.0	730.0	—	—	—	—	—	—	—	—	0	—	—
80	18	1.60	—	530.0	1260.0	—	—	—	—	—	—	—	—	1.1	—	—
75	280	3.36	—	790.0	1050.0	—	—	—	—	—	—	—	—	50.4	—	—
35	100	2.70	—	240.0	740.0	—	—	—	—	—	—	—	—	4.8	—	—
115	460	0.47	—	740.0	280.0	—	—	—	—	—	—	—	—	0	—	—
30	100	3.60	—	210.0	540.0	—	0	—	—	—	—	—	—	0	—	—
0	10	0.18	—	160.0	330.0	—	0	—	—	—	—	—	—	0	—	—
50	150	1.80	—	420.0	1050.0	—	—	—	—	—	—	—	—	9.0	—	—
50	164	4.92	—	350.0	920.0	—	—	—	—	—	—	—	—	9.8	—	—
75	234	4.21	—	380.0	1290.0	—	—	—	—	—	—	—	—	8.4	—	—
0	20	1.42	—	1580.0	1150.0	—	0	—	—	—	—	—	—	8.9	—	—
0	19	1.01	—	1160.0	850.0	—	0	—	—	—	—	—	—	5.6	—	—
0	40	2.70	—	140.0	420.0	—	9.8	—	—	—	—	—	—	18.0	—	—
245	88	2.37	—	260.0	1140.0	—	—	—	—	—	—	—	—	0	—	—
0	40	1.80	—	610.0	920.0	—	—	—	—	—	—	—	—	0	—	—
75	200	4.50	—	390.0	1200.0	—	—	—	—	—	—	—	—	9.0	—	—
90	274	4.11	—	930.0	820.0	—	—	—	—	—	—	—	—	43.8	—	—
115	466	0	—	630.0	240.0	—	—	—	—	—	—	—	—	0	—	—
120	308	7.39	—	440.0	1530.0	—	—	—	—	—	—	—	—	0.6	—	—
115	532	0	—	630.0	230.0	—	—	—	—	—	—	—	—	0	—	—
5	109	1.96	—	—	60.0	—	—	—	—	—	—	—	—		—	—
5	164	1.96	—	—	60.0	—	—	—	—	—	—	—	—	98.2	—	—
5	164	1.18	—	—	98.2	—	—	—	—	—	—	—	—	16.2	—	—
5	106	1.57	—	—	54.5	—	—	—	—	—	—	—	—	72.0	—	—
0	100	2.72	—	—	230.0	—	2325.0	—	—	—	—	—	—	18.1	—	—
16	545	—	—	—	414.5	—	—	—	—	—	—	—	—	1.3	—	—
5	112	0.79	—	—	49.1	—	—	—	—	—	—	—	—	72.0	—	—
0	164	1.57	—	—	229.1	—	—	—	—	—	—	—	—	9.8	—	—
0	44	1.96	—	—	10.9	—	354.5	—	—	—	—	—	—	183.3	—	—
11	218	0.79	—	—	218.2	—	—	—	—	—	—	—	—	52.4	—	—
0	57	1.03	—	—	0	—	49.8	—	—	—	—	—	—	246.0	—	—
0	218	1.57	—	—	136.4	—	—	—	—	—	—	—	—	150.5	—	—

APPENDIX H

TABLE H-1 Table of Food Composition (*continued*)

(Computer code is for Cengage Diet Analysis program) (For purposes of calculations, use "0" for t, <1, <0.1, 0.01)

DA+ Code	Food Description	Quantity	Measure	Wt (g)	H_2O (g)	Ener (kcal)	Prot (g)	Carb (g)	Fiber (g)	Fat (g)	Fat Breakdown (g)		
											Sat	Mono	Poly
	Fast Food—*continued*												
55675	Peach Perfection smoothie	24	fluid ounce(s)	680	—	327	2.2	81.8	5.5	0.5	0	—	—
31662	Peach Pleasure smoothie	24	fluid ounce(s)	680	—	404	3.3	96.0	4.4	1.6	1.1	—	—
55676	Pomegranate Paradise smoothie	24	fluid ounce(s)	680	—	371	2.2	92.7	5.5	0.5	0	—	—
55665	Protein Berry Workout smoothie w/ soy protein	24	fluid ounce(s)	680	—	412	18.2	84.3	4.8	1.4	0	—	—
31668	Razzmatazz smoothie	24	fluid ounce(s)	680	—	425	3.3	99.3	4.4	1.6	1.1	—	—
31669	Strawberries Wild smoothie	24	fluid ounce(s)	680	—	404	5.5	94.9	3.3	0	0	—	—
38421	Strawberry Surf Rider smoothie	24	fluid ounce(s)	680	—	469	3.3	112.4	4.4	1.6	0.5	—	—
55674	Strawberry Whirl smoothie	24	fluid ounce(s)	680	—	327	2.2	81.8	6.5	0.5	0	—	—
38428	Wheatgrass juice, freshly squeezed	1	ounce(s)	28	—	5	1.0	1.0	0	0	0	0	0
	Kentucky Fried Chicken (KFC)												
31850	BBQ baked beans	1	serving(s)	130	—	200	8.0	39.0	9.0	1.5	0	—	—
31853	Biscuit	1	item(s)	57	—	220	4.0	24.0	1.0	11.0	2.5	—	—
31851	Cole slaw	1	serving(s)	130	—	180	1.0	22.0	3.0	10.0	1.5	—	—
31849	Corn on the cob	1	item(s)	146	—	140	5.0	33.0	4.0	1.0	0	—	—
31842	Crispy strips	3	item(s)	151	—	370	28.0	17.0	1.0	20.0	4.0	—	—
74456	Doublicious chicken sandwich, Original Recipe	1	item(s)	188	—	520	32.0	40.0	2.0	25.0	7.0	—	—
3761	Extra Crispy chicken, breast	1	item(s)	176	—	510	39.0	16.0	0	33.0	7.0	—	—
3762	Extra Crispy chicken, drumstick	1	item(s)	60	—	150	12.0	4.0	0	10.0	2.5	—	—
3763	Extra Crispy chicken, thigh	1	item(s)	114	—	290	17.0	16.0	1.0	18.0	4.0	—	—
3764	Extra Crispy chicken, whole wing	1	item(s)	52	—	150	11.0	11.0	1.0	7.0	1.5	—	—
51218	Famous Bowls mashed potatoes with gravy	1	serving(s)	525	—	680	26.0	74.0	6.0	31.0	8.0	—	—
39387	Green beans	1	serving(s)	86	—	20	1.0	3.0	1.0	0	0	—	—
31841	Honey BBQ chicken sandwich	1	item(s)	162	—	310	23.0	42.0	1.0	4.0	1.0	—	—
10859	Hot wings	6	piece(s)	132	—	420	24.0	24.0	0	24.0	3.0	—	—
51223	Hot wings, fiery buffalo	6	item(s)	204	—	480	30.0	36.0	6.0	21.0	3.0	—	—
39386	Hot wings, honey BBQ	6	item(s)	198	—	480	30.0	42.0	6.0	21.0	3.0	—	—
31848	Macaroni & cheese	1	serving(s)	135	—	160	5.0	19.0	1.0	7.0	2.5	—	—
31847	Mashed potatoes with gravy	1	serving(s)	145	—	120	2.0	19.0	1.0	4.0	1.0	—	—
74460	Original Recipe chicken filet	1	item(s)	100	—	200	22.0	8.0	1.0	9.0	1.5	—	—
10825	Original Recipe chicken, breast	1	item(s)	161	—	340	38.0	9.0	2.0	17.0	4.0	—	—
10826	Original Recipe chicken, drumstick	1	item(s)	59	—	140	13.0	3.0	0	8.0	2.0	—	—
10827	Original Recipe chicken, thigh	1	item(s)	126	—	350	19.0	7.0	1.0	27.0	7.0	—	—
10828	Original Recipe chicken, whole wing	1	item(s)	47	—	140	10.0	4.0	0	9.0	2.0	—	—
31844	Popcorn chicken, small or individual	1	item(s)	114	—	370	19.0	21.0	2.0	24.0	4.5	—	—
31852	Potato salad	1	serving(s)	128	—	200	2.0	24.0	3.0	10.0	2.0	—	—
10845	Potato wedges, small	1	serving(s)	102	—	250	4.0	32.0	3.0	12.0	2.0	—	—
	Long John Silver's												
3777	Batter dipped fish sandwich	1	item(s)	176	—	470	18.0	49.0	3.0	23.0	5.0	—	—
37568	Battered fish	1	item(s)	92	—	260	12.0	17.0	0	16.0	4.0	—	—
37569	Breaded clams	1	serving(s)	85	—	320	9.0	29.0	2.0	19.0	4.5	—	—
39398	Cocktail sauce	1	ounce(s)	28	—	25	0	6.0	0	0	0	0	0
3770	Coleslaw	1	serving(s)	113	—	200	1.0	15.0	3.0	15.0	2.5	—	—
39401	Crab cake, lobster stuffed	1	item(s)	62	—	170	6.0	16.0	1.0	9.0	2.0	—	—
78975	Fish taco	1	item(s)	117	—	360	9.0	30.0	3.0	23.0	4.5	—	—
39400	French fries, large	1	item(s)	113	—	310	3.0	45.0	4.0	14.0	3.5	—	—
3774	Fries, regular	1	serving(s)	85	—	230	3.0	34.0	3.0	10.0	2.5	—	—
3779	Hushpuppy	1	piece(s)	23	—	60	1.0	9.0	1.0	2.5	0.5	—	—
56963	Shrimp scampi	1	serving(s)	130	—	200	17.0	3.0	0	13.0	2.5	—	—
3781	Shrimp, batter-dipped, 1 piece	1	piece(s)	14	—	43	1.7	2.7	0	3.0	0.8	—	—
39399	Tartar sauce	1	ounce(s)	28	—	100	0	4.0	0	9.0	1.5	—	—
39395	Ultimate Fish sandwich	1	item(s)	206	—	530	21.0	50.0	3.0	27.0	8.0	—	—
	McDonald's												
2262	Baked apple pie	1	item(s)	77	28.5	250	2.0	32.0	4.0	13.0	7.0	7.1	0.8
2247	Barbecue sauce	1	item(s)	28	16.1	50	0	12.0	0	0	0	0	0
737	Big Mac hamburger	1	item(s)	215	112.3	550	25.0	46.0	3.0	29.0	10.0	7.5	0.7
738	Cheeseburger	1	item(s)	114	45.0	300	15.0	33.0	2.0	12.0	6.0	4.1	0.4
1873	Chicken McNuggets 6 piece	6	item(s)	97	44.8	280	13.0	18.0	1.0	18.0	3.0	7.7	5.3
3792	Chicken McNuggets, 4 piece	4	item(s)	65	30.2	190	9.0	12.0	1.0	12.0	2.0	5.2	3.6
2264	Chocolate shake, large	1	item(s)	356	223.2	580	13.0	102.0	1.0	14.0	8.0	4.0	0.8

APPENDIX H

E KEY: H-4 = Breads/Baked Goods H-8 = Cereal/Rice/Pasta H-14 = Fruit H-18 = Vegetables/Legumes H-28 = Nuts/Seeds H-30 = Vegetarian H-32 = Dairy H-40 = Eggs H-40 = Seafood H-42 = Meats H-46 = Poultry
8 = Processed Meats H-50 = Beverages H-52 = Fats/Oils H-54 = Sweets H-56 = Spices/Condiments/Sauces H-60 = Mixed Foods/Soups/Sandwiches H-66 = Fast Food H-84 = Convenience H-86 = Baby Foods

Chol (mg)	Calc (mg)	Iron (mg)	Magn (mg)	Pota (mg)	Sodi (mg)	Zinc (mg)	Vit A (μg)	Thia (mg)	Vit E (mg α)	Ribo (mg)	Niac (mg)	Vit B_6 (mg)	Fola (μg)	Vit C (mg)	Vit B_{12} (μg)	Sele (μg)
0	65	1.18	—	—	32.7	—	245.5	—	—	—	—	—	—	65.5	—	—
5	87	0.77	—	—	54.5	—	—	—	—	—	—	—	—	16.4	—	—
0	109	1.96	—	—	38.2	—	245.5	—	—	—	—	—	—	85.1	—	—
0	1054	3.45	76.7	690.0	220.4	0.86	—	0.11	0.39	0.16	1.15	0.67	76.7	51.7	0	5.4
5	109	1.57	—	—	60.0	—	—	—	—	—	—	—	—	58.9	—	—
5	218	1.92	—	—	152.7	—	—	—	—	—	—	—	—	52.4	—	—
5	87	1.13	—	—	10.9	—	—	—	—	—	—	—	—	85.1	—	—
0	87	1.96	—	—	27.3	—	5.5	—	—	—	—	—	—	78.5	—	—
0	—	1.73	—	—	0	—	—	—	—	—	—	—	—	3.7	—	—
0	—	—	—	—	680.0	—	—	—	—	—	—	—	—	—	—	—
0	40	1.80	—	—	640.0	—	—	—	—	—	—	—	—	0	—	—
5	40	0.72	—	—	270.0	—	—	—	—	—	—	—	—	12.0	—	—
0	—	—	—	—	5.0	—	—	—	—	—	—	—	—	—	—	—
65	40	1.44	—	—	1220.0	—	0	—	—	—	—	—	—	1.2	—	—
85	—	—	—	—	1300.0	—	—	—	—	—	—	—	—	—	—	—
110		—	—	—	1010.0	—	—	—	—	—	—	—	—	—	—	—
55	0	1.44	—	—	300.0	—	0	—	—	—	—	—	—	0	—	—
95	20	2.70	—	—	700.0	—	—	—	—	—	—	—	—	—	—	—
45	20	1.08	—	—	340.0	—	—	—	—	—	—	—	—	0	—	—
45	—	—	—	—	2130.0	—	—	—	—	—	—	—	—	—	—	—
0	—	—	—	—	290.0	—	—	—	—	—	—	—	—	—	—	—
70	—	—	—	—	810.0	—	—	—	—	—	—	—	—	—	—	—
120	—	—	—	—	840.0	—	—	—	—	—	—	—	—	—	—	—
60	—	—	—	—	2340.0	—	—	—	—	—	—	—	—	—	—	—
60	—	—	—	—	2040.0	—	—	—	—	—	—	—	—	—	—	—
5	—	—	—	—	720.0	—	—	—	—	—	—	—	—	—	—	—
0	—	—	—	—	530.0	—	—	—	—	—	—	—	—	—	—	—
55	—	—	—	—	670.0	—	—	—	—	—	—	—	—	—	—	—
135	20	2.70	—	—	960.0	—	—	—	—	—	—	—	—	6.0	—	—
70	20	1.08	—	—	340.0	—	—	—	—	—	—	—	—	0	—	—
110	20	2.70	—	—	870.0	—	—	—	—	—	—	—	—	1.2	—	—
50	20	1.44	—	—	350.0	—	0	—	—	—	—	—	—	1.2	—	—
25	40	1.80	—	—	1110.0	—	0	—	—	—	—	—	—	0	—	—
5	—	—	—	—	540.0	—	—	—	—	—	—	—	—	—	—	—
0	20	1.08	—	—	700.0	—	0	—	—	—	—	—	—	0	—	—
40	60	1.80	—	—	1180.0	—	—	—	—	—	—	—	—	1.2	—	—
35	0	0	—	—	790.0	—	0	—	—	—	—	—	—	0	—	—
35	20	1.44	—	—	1190.7	—	0	—	—	—	—	—	—	0	—	—
0	0	0	—	—	250.0	—	—	—	—	—	—	—	—	0	—	—
20	40	0.36	—	—	340.0	—	—	—	—	—	—	—	—	18.0	—	—
30	60	0.72	—	—	390.0	—	0	—	—	—	—	—	—	0	—	—
25	60	1.44	—	—	810.0	—	0	—	—	—	—	—	—	0	—	—
0	0	0	—	—	460.0	—	0	—	—	—	—	—	—	18.0	—	—
0	0	0	—	370.2	350.2	—	0	—	—	—	—	—	—	15.0	—	—
0	20	0.36	—	—	200.0	—	0	—	—	—	—	—	—	0	—	—
135	60	0.72	—	—	650.0	—	—	—	—	—	—	—	—	0	—	—
15	0	0	—	—	160.0	—	0	—	—	—	—	—	—	0	—	—
15	0	0	—	—	250.0	—	0	—	—	—	—	—	—	0	—	—
55	100	1.80	—	—	1500.0	—	—	—	—	—	—	—	—	1.2	—	—
0	20	1.08	5.4	48.5	170.0	0.18	—	0.23	1.49	0.16	2.03	0.04	—	15.0	—	—
0	0	0	3.6	55.2	260.0	0.05	3.4	0.01	0.30	0.01	0.19	0.02	—	0	—	—
75	250	4.50	43.0	396.0	970.0	4.11	—	0.38	—	0.45	7.28	—	—	1.2	1.9	—
40	202	2.72	22.8	200.0	680.0	2.18	—	0.25	—	0.30	4.59	—	—	1.2	1.0	—
40	20	0.72	23.0	239.0	540.0	0.56	0	0.15	—	0.10	7.03	0.38	—	1.2	0.3	—
25	0	0.36	15.0	161.0	360.0	0.38	0	0.10	—	0.07	4.74	0.25	—	1.2	0.2	—
50	450	1.80	57.0	804.6	250.0	1.78	324.0	0.14	0	0.76	0.47	0.18	—	0	1.9	—

TABLE H-1 Table of Food Composition (*continued*) (Computer code is for Cengage Diet Analysis program) (For purposes of calculations, use "0" for t, <1, <0.1, 0.01)

DA+ Code	Food Description	Quantity	Measure	Wt (g)	H_2O (g)	Ener (kcal)	Prot (g)	Carb (g)	Fiber (g)	Fat (g)	Fat Breakdown (g)		
											Sat	Mono	Poly
Fast Food—*continued*													
29774	Crispy chicken sandwich	1	item(s)	213	110.7	510	24.0	55.0	3.0	22.0	3.5	6.8	7.9
743	Egg McMuffin	1	item(s)	138	72.6	300	18.0	30.0	2.0	12.0	5.0	3.8	2.4
742	Filet-O-Fish sandwich	1	item(s)	142	65.0	390	15.0	39.0	2.0	19.0	4.0	5.7	8.5
2257	French fries, large	1	serving(s)	154	58.0	500	6.0	63.0	6.0	25.0	3.5	12.0	7.2
1872	French fries, small	1	serving(s)	71	27.1	230	3.0	29.0	3.0	11.0	1.5	5.5	3.3
33822	Fruit 'n Yogurt Parfait	1	item(s)	149	110.9	150	4.0	30.0	1.0	2.0	1.0	0.2	0.1
739	Hamburger	1	item(s)	100	44.5	250	12.0	31.0	2.0	9.0	3.5	3.8	1.4
2003	Hash browns	1	item(s)	56	29.5	150	1.0	15.0	2.0	9.0	1.5	4.8	2.8
2260	Hot fudge sundae	1	item(s)	179	105.3	330	8.0	53.0	1.0	9.0	7.0	1.9	0.4
1874	Plain Hotcakes with syrup and margarine	3	item(s)	221	89.7	570	8.0	105.0	3.0	13.0	3.5	1.9	4.6
38388	Premium Bacon Ranch salad with grilled chicken, no dressing	1	serving(s)	306	249.1	230	30.0	10.0	4.0	9.0	4.0	3.1	1.3
38391	Premium Caesar salad with grilled chicken, no dressing	1	serving(s)	296	245.5	190	27.0	10.0	4.0	5.0	3.0	1.5	0.6
38393	Premium Caesar salad, no dressing	1	serving(s)	213	191.1	90	7.0	9.0	3.0	4.0	2.5	1.0	0.3
29775	Premium Grilled Chicken Classic sandwich	1	item(s)	200	114.6	350	28.0	42.0	3.0	9.0	2.0	2.3	4.1
57683	Premium Southwest salad w/grilled chicken	1	item(s)	335	—	290	27.0	28.0	7.0	8.0	2.5	—	—
740	Quarter Pounder hamburger	1	item(s)	173	87.1	420	25.0	38.0	2.0	19.0	7.0	7.3	0.5
741	Quarter Pounder hamburger with cheese	1	item(s)	202	98.8	520	30.0	41.0	3.0	26.0	12.0	9.3	0.9
2005	Sausage McMuffin with egg	1	item(s)	164	81.9	450	21.0	30.0	2.0	27.0	10.0	10.8	4.5
50831	Side salad	1	item(s)	87	81.7	20	1.0	4.0	1.0	0.0	0	0	0
	Pizza Hut												
39009	Hot chicken wings	2	item(s)	44	—	100	10.0	1.0	0	6.0	2.0	—	—
14025	Meat Lovers hand-tossed pizza	1	slice(s)	105	—	300	14.0	26.0	1.0	16.0	7.0	—	—
14026	Meat Lovers pan pizza	1	slice(s)	113	—	330	14.0	27.0	1.0	18.0	7.0	—	—
31009	Meat Lovers stuffed crust pizza	1	slice(s)	165	—	480	22.0	39.0	2.0	26.0	11.0	—	—
14024	Meat Lovers thin 'n crispy pizza	1	slice(s)	85	—	280	13.0	22.0	1.0	16.0	6.0	—	—
14031	Pepperoni Lovers hand-tossed pizza	1	slice(s)	95	—	270	13.0	26.0	1.0	13.0	6.0	—	—
14032	Pepperoni Lovers pan pizza	1	slice(s)	101	—	290	13.0	27.0	1.0	14.0	6.0	—	—
31011	Pepperoni Lovers stuffed crust pizza	1	slice(s)	149	—	430	20.0	40.0	2.0	21.0	10.0	—	—
14030	Pepperoni Lovers thin 'n crispy pizza	1	slice(s)	75	—	250	12.0	22.0	1.0	13.0	6.0	—	—
10834	Personal Pan pepperoni pizza	1	slice(s)	50	—	153	6.5	16.8	0.8	6.5	2.5	—	—
10842	Personal Pan supreme pizza	1	slice(s)	64	—	180	7.5	17.3	1.0	9.0	3.5	—	—
39013	Personal Pan Veggie Lovers pizza	1	slice(s)	58	—	138	5.5	17.5	1.0	5.0	2.0	—	—
14028	Veggie Lovers hand-tossed pizza	1	slice(s)	102	—	200	9.0	27.0	2.0	6.0	3.0	—	—
14029	Veggie Lovers pan pizza	1	slice(s)	107	—	230	9.0	28.0	2.0	9.0	3.5	—	—
31010	Veggie Lovers stuffed crust pizza	1	slice(s)	155	—	330	15.0	41.0	2.0	12.0	6.0	—	—
14027	Veggie Lovers thin 'n crispy pizza	1	slice(s)	86	—	180	8.0	23.0	1.0	6.0	3.0	—	—
39012	Wing blue cheese dipping sauce	1	item(s)	43	—	230	1.0	2.0	0	24.0	4.5	—	—
39011	Wing ranch dipping sauce	1	item(s)	43	—	220	0	2.0	0	23.0	3.5	—	—
	Starbucks												
33107	Caffè mocha, tall nonfat, w/o whipped cream	12	fluid ounce(s)	354	—	170	10.0	32.0	0.5	2.0	1.0	—	—
33108	Caffè mocha, tall whole milk, w/whipped cream	12	fluid ounce(s)	354	—	290	10.0	34.0	0.5	16.0	9.0	—	—
38052	Cappuccino, tall	12	fluid ounce(s)	354	—	110	6.0	9.0	0	6.0	3.0	—	—
38053	Cappuccino, tall nonfat	12	fluid ounce(s)	354	—	60	6.0	9.0	0	0	0	0	0
38054	Cappuccino, tall soymilk	12	fluid ounce(s)	354	—	100	5.0	12.0	0.5	3.0	0	—	—
68043	Caramel Apple Spice, tall, w/o whipped cream	12	fluid ounce(s)	354	—	210	0	53.0	0	0	0	0	0
68256	Espresso, single shot	1	fluid ounce(s)	30	—	5	0	0.5	0	0	0	0	0
38088	Flavored syrup, 1 pump	1	serving(s)	10	—	20	0	5.0	0	0	0	0	0
38067	Frappuccino, tall caramel w/o whipped cream	12	fluid ounce(s)	354	—	200	3.0	42.0	0	2.5	1.5	—	—
39891	Frappuccino, tall caramel, light	12	fluid ounce(s)	354	—	130	4.0	25.0	2.0	1.0	0	—	—
67330	Frappuccino, tall Cinnamon Dolce, light	12	fluid ounce(s)	354	—	105	3.7	21.7	2.2	0.4	0.0	—	—

Chol (mg)	Calc (mg)	Iron (mg)	Magn (mg)	Pota (mg)	Sodi (mg)	Zinc (mg)	Vit A (μg)	Thia (mg)	Vit E (mg α)	Ribo (mg)	Niac (mg)	Vit B_6 (mg)	Fola (μg)	Vit C (mg)	Vit B_{12} (μg)	Sele (μg)
45	150	3.60	57.5	483.5	990.0	1.41	38.3	0.42	—	0.36	11.80	—	—	3.6	—	—
260	300	2.70	27.6	238.7	780.0	1.78	—	0.36	0.81	0.51	4.28	0.20	—	0	—	—
40	150	1.80	38.3	312.4	590.0	0.82	—	0.30	1.66	0.19	3.15	—	—	0	1.5	36.2
0	20	1.44	49.3	862.4	350.0	0.68	0	0.50	—	0.05	4.25	0.80	—	12.0	—	—
0	20	0.72	22.7	397.6	160.0	0.31	0	0.23	—	0.03	1.96	0.37	—	4.8	—	—
5	100	0.67	20.9	248.8	70.0	0.54	—	0.07	—	0.17	0.35	—	—	9.0	0.3	—
25	100	2.70	21.0	192.0	480.0	1.95	—	0.25	—	0.24	4.54	—	—	1.2	0.8	26.2
0	0	0.36	11.8	219.0	310.0	0.19	0	0.06	—	0.01	1.26	0.14	—	1.2	—	—
25	249	1.44	34.0	440.3	170.0	1.00	145.0	0.08	0.34	0.41	0.27	0.09	—	0	1.0	—
20	150	2.70	28.7	276.3	660.0	0.64	—	0.45	—	0.40	3.23	0.12	—	0	0	—
85	150	1.80	—	—	700.0	—	—	0.17	—	0.25	11.33	—	—	21.0	—	—
70	200	1.78	—	754.8	580.0	—	—	0.17	—	0.20	11.31	—	—	21.0	—	—
10	200	1.44	19.2	460.1	180.0	—	—	0.09	—	0.08	0.45	—	—	18.0	0	0.4
65	150	3.60	56.0	456.0	820.0	1.38	—	0.39	1.06	0.38	13.04	0.61	—	4.8	0.3	—
70	150	2.70	—	—	650.0	—	—	—	—	—	—	—	—	21.0	—	—
65	150	4.50	38.1	392.7	700.0	4.65	—	0.32	—	0.60	7.70	—	—	1.2	2.2	—
95	300	4.50	44.4	442.4	1100.0	5.31	—	0.33	—	0.71	7.78	—	—	1.2	2.5	—
285	300	3.60	29.5	280.4	890.0	2.00	—	0.43	0.82	0.56	4.80	0.24	—	1.2	1.1	—
0	20	0.72	—	191.4	10.0	—	—	0.04	—	0.03	0.18	—	—	15.0	0	—
55	—	—	—	—	430.0	—	—	—	—	—	—	—	—	—	—	—
40	—	—	—	—	860.0	—	—	—	—	—	—	—	—	—	—	—
40	—	—	—	—	830.0	—	—	—	—	—	—	—	—	—	—	—
70	—	—	—	—	1380.0	—	—	—	—	—	—	—	—	—	—	—
40	—	—	—	—	860.5	—	—	—	—	—	—	—	—	—	—	—
35	—	—	—	—	770.0	—	—	—	—	—	—	—	—	—	—	—
35	—	—	—	—	730.0	—	—	—	—	—	—	—	—	—	—	—
60	—	—	—	—	1230.0	—	—	—	—	—	—	—	—	—	—	—
35	—	—	—	—	760.0	—	—	—	—	—	—	—	—	—	—	—
14	—	—	—	—	352.5	—	—	—	—	—	—	—	—	—	—	—
20	—	—	—	—	420.0	—	—	—	—	—	—	—	—	—	—	—
9	—	—	—	—	297.5	—	—	—	—	—	—	—	—	—	—	—
15	—	—	—	—	530.0	—	—	—	—	—	—	—	—	—	—	—
15	—	—	—	—	500.0	—	—	—	—	—	—	—	—	—	—	—
35	—	—	—	—	880.0	—	—	—	—	—	—	—	—	—	—	—
15	—	—	—	—	530.0	—	—	—	—	—	—	—	—	—	—	—
20	—	—	—	—	420.0	—	—	—	—	—	—	—	—	—	—	—
10	—	—	—	—	420.0	—	—	—	—	—	—	—	—	—	—	—
2	300	2.70	—	—	0	—	—	—	—	—	—	—	—	0	—	—
45	300	2.70	—	—	0	—	—	—	—	—	—	—	—	0	—	—
15	200	0	—	—	0	—	—	—	—	—	—	—	—	0	—	—
2	200	0	—	—	0	—	—	—	—	—	—	—	—	0	—	—
0	200	1.08	—	—	0	—	—	—	—	—	—	—	—	0	—	—
0	0	0	—	—	0	—	0	—	—	—	—	—	—	0	—	—
0	0	0	—	—	0	—	0	—	—	—	—	—	—	0	—	—
0	0	0	—	—	0	—	0	—	—	—	—	—	—	0	0	—
10	100	0	—	—	0	—	—	—	—	—	—	—	—	0	—	—
2	100	0	—	—	180.0	—	0	—	—	—	—	—	—	0	—	—
0	112	0	—	—	0	—	0	—	—	—	—	—	—	0	—	—

DA+ Code	Food Description	Quantity	Measure	Wt (g)	H_2O (g)	Ener (kcal)	Prot (g)	Carb (g)	Fiber (g)	Fat (g)	Fat Breakdown (g) Sat	Mono	Poly
Fast Food—*continued*													
67329	Frappuccino, tall Cinnamon Dolce, w/whipped cream	12	fluid ounce(s)	354	—	270	3.0	42.0	0	11.0	6.0	—	—
38070	Frappuccino, tall coffee	12	fluid ounce(s)	354	—	180	3.0	36.0	0	2.5	1.5	—	—
39894	Frappuccino, tall coffee, light	12	fluid ounce(s)	354	—	90	3.0	18.0	0	0	0	—	—
67339	Frappuccino, tall Double Chocolaty Chip, w/whipped cream	12	fluid ounce(s)	354	—	300	5.0	42.0	0.5	14.0	9.0	—	—
38071	Frappuccino, tall espresso	12	fluid ounce(s)	354	—	150	2.0	34.0	0	1.0	0	—	—
39883	Frappuccino, tall Java Chip, w/o whipped cream	12	fluid ounce(s)	354	—	240	4.0	47.0	0.5	5.0	3.5	—	—
38073	Frappuccino, tall mocha w/o whipped cream	12	fluid ounce(s)	354	—	200	3.0	42.0	0.5	3.0	2.0	—	—
39897	Frappuccino, tall mocha, light	12	fluid ounce(s)	354	—	110	3.0	23.0	0.5	0.5	0	—	—
39887	Frappuccino, tall Strawberries & Creme, w/o whipped cream	12	fluid ounce(s)	354	—	190	3.0	38.0	0	3.0	1.5	—	—
38063	Frappuccino, tall Tazo chai creme w/o whipped cream	12	fluid ounce(s)	354	—	160	3.0	32.0	0	2.0	1.0	—	—
38080	Frappuccino, tall vanilla w/o whipped cream	12	fluid ounce(s)	354	—	200	3.0	39.0	0	3.5	2.0	—	—
39898	Frappuccino, tall white chocolate mocha, light blend	12	fluid ounce(s)	354	—	210	4.0	37.0	0	5.0	3.0	—	—
38074	Frappuccino, tall white chocolate w/o whipped cream	12	fluid ounce(s)	354	—	240	4.0	48.0	0	4.0	2.5	—	—
68822	Hot chocolate, tall soy, w/o whipped cream	12	fluid ounce(s)	354	—	230	9.0	40.0	2.0	6.0	1.5	—	—
67421	Iced mocha, tall white chocolate, nonfat, w/whipped cream	12	fluid ounce(s)	354	—	230	8.0	42.0	0	4.5	3.5	—	—
33111	Latte, tall w/nonfat milk	12	fluid ounce(s)	354	—	100	10.0	15.0	0	0	0	0	0
33112	Latte, tall w/whole milk	12	fluid ounce(s)	354	—	180	10.0	14.0	0	9.0	5.0	—	—
33109	Macchiato, tall caramel w/nonfat milk	12	fluid ounce(s)	354	—	140	7.0	25.0	0	1.0	1.0	—	—
33110	Macchiato, tall caramel w/whole milk	12	fluid ounce(s)	354	—	200	8.0	25.0	0	8.0	5.0	—	—
38089	Mocha syrup	1	serving(s)	17	—	25	1.0	6.0	0	0.5	0	—	—
67546	Tazo black shaken iced tea lemonade, tall	12	fluid ounce(s)	354	—	100	0	25.0	0	0	0	0	0
38076	Tazo black shaken iced tea, tall	12	fluid ounce(s)	354	—	60	0	15.0	0	0	0	0	0
67551	Tazo iced chai tea latte, tall w/nonfat milk	12	fluid ounce(s)	354	—	150	6.0	33.0	0	0	0	0	0
67417	Tazo iced green tea latte, tall w/nonfat milk	12	fluid ounce(s)	354	—	180	7.0	37.0	0.5	0	0	0	0
38090	Whipped cream	1	serving(s)	30	—	90	1.0	3.0	0	9.0	5.0	—	—
38062	White chocolate mocha, tall nonfat w/o whipped cream	12	fluid ounce(s)	354	—	270	12.0	47.0	0	4.5	3.5	—	—
38061	White chocolate mocha, tall w/ whipped cream	12	fluid ounce(s)	354	—	390	11.0	48.0	0	18.0	11.0	—	—
38048	White hot chocolate, tall nonfat w/o whipped cream	12	fluid ounce(s)	354	—	270	12.0	47.0	0	4.5	3.5	—	—
38050	White hot chocolate, tall soymilk w/whipped cream	12	fluid ounce(s)	354	—	380	11.0	52.0	0.5	14.0	8.0	—	—
38047	White hot chocolate, tall w/whipped cream	12	fluid ounce(s)	354	—	410	12.0	48.0	0	19.0	12.0	—	—
	Subway												
80576	Breakfast BMT Melt	1	item(s)	142	—	240	16.0	25.0	6.0	10.0	4.0	—	—
80594	Buffalo chicken sandwich, 6", wheat bread	1	item(s)	268	—	420	25.0	46.0	5.0	15.0	3.0	—	—
15842	Cheese steak sandwich, 6", wheat bread	1	item(s)	297	—	500	38.0	51.0	6.0	17.0	9.0	—	—
40478	Chicken & bacon ranch sandwich, 6", white or wheat bread	1	serving(s)	292	—	570	35.0	47.0	5.0	28.0	10.0	—	—
32045	Chocolate chip cookie	1	item(s)	45	—	220	2.0	30.0	1.0	10.0	5.0	—	—
32048	Chocolate chip M&M cookie	1	item(s)	45	—	210	2.0	32.0	0.5	10.0	5.0	—	—
32049	Chocolate chunk cookie	1	item(s)	45	—	220	2.0	30.0	0.5	10.0	5.0	—	—
4024	Classic Italian B.M.T. sandwich, 6", white bread	1	item(s)	221	—	400	19.0	44.0	2.0	16.0	6.0	—	—
15838	Classic tuna sandwich, 6", wheat bread	1	item(s)	233	—	470	20.0	44.0	5.0	24.0	4.0	—	—
15837	Classic tuna sandwich, 6", white bread	1	item(s)	228	—	460	19.0	42.0	2.0	24.0	4.0	—	—

GE KEY: H-4 = Breads/Baked Goods H-8 = Cereal/Rice/Pasta H-14 = Fruit H-18 = Vegetables/Legumes H-28 = Nuts/Seeds H-30 = Vegetarian H-32 = Dairy H-40 = Eggs H-40 = Seafood H-42 = Meats H-46 = Poultry 48 = Processed Meats H-50 = Beverages H-52 = Fats/Oils H-54 = Sweets H-56 = Spices/Condiments/Sauces H-60 = Mixed Foods/Soups/Sandwiches H-66 = Fast Food H-84 = Convenience H-86 = Baby Foods

Chol (mg)	Calc (mg)	Iron (mg)	Magn (mg)	Pota (mg)	Sodi (mg)	Zinc (mg)	Vit A (µg)	Thia (mg)	Vit E (mg α)	Ribo (mg)	Niac (mg)	Vit B_6 (mg)	Fola (µg)	Vit C (mg)	Vit B_{12} (µg)	Sele (µg)
35	100	0	—	—	0	—	—	—	—	—	—	—	—	0	—	—
10	100	0	—	—	0	—	—	—	—	—	—	—	—	0	—	—
0	100	0	—	—	0	—	—	—	—	—	—	—	—	0	—	—
40	150	2.70	—	—	0	—	—	—	—	—	—	—	—	0	—	—
2	60	0	—	—	0	—	—	—	—	—	—	—	—	0	—	—
10	100	2.70	—	—	0	—	—	—	—	—	—	—	—	0	—	—
10	100	0.72	—	—	0	—	—	—	—	—	—	—	—	0	—	—
0	100	0.72	—	—	0	—	—	—	—	—	—	—	—	0	—	—
10	100	0.36	—	—	0	—	—	—	—	—	—	—	—	3.6	—	—
10	100	0	—	—	0	—	—	—	—	—	—	—	—	0	—	—
10	100	0	—	—	0	—	—	—	—	—	—	—	—	0	—	—
10	150	0	—	—	0	—	—	—	—	—	—	—	—	0	—	—
10	2	0	—	—	0	—	—	—	—	—	—	—	—	0	—	—
0	300	3.60	—	—	0	—	—	—	—	—	—	—	—	0	—	—
2	300	0	—	—	0	—	—	—	—	—	—	—	—	1.2	—	—
2	350	0	—	—	0	—	—	—	—	—	—	—	—	0	—	—
30	300	0	—	—	0	—	—	—	—	—	—	—	—	0	—	—
2	250	0	—	—	0	—	—	—	—	—	—	—	—	0	—	—
25	250	0	—	—	0	—	—	—	—	—	—	—	—	0	—	—
0	0	0.72	—	—	0	—	0	—	—	—	—	—	—	0	—	—
0	0	0	—	—	10.0	—	0	—	—	—	—	—	—	6.0	—	—
0	0	0	—	—	0	—	0	—	—	—	—	—	—	0	—	—
2	200	0.36	—	—	0	—	—	—	—	—	—	—	—	0	—	—
2	250	0.36	—	—	0	—	—	—	—	—	—	—	—	6.0	—	—
30	20	0.36	—	—	10.0	—	90.1	—	—	—	—	—	—	0	—	—
2	400	0	—	—	0	—	—	—	—	—	—	—	—	1.2	0	—
50	400	0	—	—	0	—	—	—	—	—	—	—	—	1.2	—	—
2	450	0	—	—	0	—	—	—	—	—	—	—	—	1.2	—	—
25	400	1.44	—	—	0	—	—	—	—	—	—	—	—	1.2	—	—
50	400	0	—	—	0	—	—	—	—	—	—	—	—	1.2	—	—
130	200	1.44	—	—	830.0	—	—	—	—	—	—	—	—	1.2	—	—
55	300	3.60	—	—	1190.0	—	—	—	—	—	—	—	—	15.0	—	—
85	500	4.50	—	—	1310.0	—	—	—	—	—	—	—	—	12.0	—	—
95	500	3.60	—	—	1080.0	—	—	—	—	—	—	—	—	15.0	—	—
15	0	1.08	—	—	130.0	—	—	—	—	—	—	—	—	0	—	—
15	20	1.00	—	—	100.0	—	0	—	—	—	—	—	—	0	—	—
10	0	1.00	—	—	100.0	—	0	—	—	—	—	—	—	0	—	—
45	300	3.60	—	—	1280.0	—	—	—	—	—	—	—	—	12.0	—	—
35	300	3.60	—	—	620.0	—	—	—	—	—	—	—	—	12.0	—	—
35	300	3.60	—	—	600.0	—	—	—	—	—	—	—	—	12.0	—	—

DA+ Code	Food Description	Quantity	Measure	Wt (g)	H_2O (g)	Ener (kcal)	Prot (g)	Carb (g)	Fiber (g)	Fat (g)	Fat Breakdown (g)		
											Sat	Mono	Poly
	Fast Food—*continued*												
32043	Club sandwich, 6", wheat bread	1	item(s)	347	—	420	39.0	50.0	4.0	8.0	3.5	—	—
4030	Cold cut combo sandwich, 6", white bread	1	item(s)	228	—	360	17.0	44.0	2.0	13.0	4.0	—	—
385	Ham sandwich, 6", wheat bread	1	item(s)	219	—	290	18.0	46.0	5.0	4.5	1.0	—	—
3888	Meatball marinara sandwich, 6", wheat bread	1	item(s)	301	—	480	21.0	59.0	8.0	18.0	7.0	—	—
4651	Meatball sandwich, 6", white bread	1	item(s)	296	—	470	20.0	57.0	5.0	18.0	7.0	—	—
80596	Melt sandwich, 6", wheat bread	1	item(s)	240	—	370	23.0	47.0	5.0	11.0	5.0	—	—
32046	Oatmeal raisin cookie	1	item(s)	45	—	200	3.0	30.0	1.0	8.0	4.0	—	—
16379	Oven-roasted chicken breast sandwich, 6", wheat bread	1	item(s)	233	—	320	23.0	47.0	5.0	5.0	1.5	—	—
32047	Peanut butter cookie	1	item(s)	45	—	220	4.0	26.0	1.0	12.0	5.0	—	—
4655	Roast beef sandwich, 6", wheat bread	1	item(s)	233	—	320	24.0	45.0	5.0	5.0	1.5	—	—
3957	Roast beef sandwich, 6", white bread	1	item(s)	228	—	310	23.0	43.0	2.0	5.0	1.5	—	—
16378	Roasted chicken breast sandwich, 6", white bread	1	item(s)	228	—	310	22.0	45.0	2.0	5.0	1.5	—	—
4032	Spicy Italian sandwich, 6", white bread	1	item(s)	216	—	470	19.0	44.0	2.0	24.0	9.0	—	—
4031	Steak & cheese sandwich, 6", white bread	1	item(s)	239	—	370	25.0	46.0	2.0	10.0	4.5	—	—
32050	Sugar cookie	1	item(s)	45	—	220	2.0	28.0	0.5	12.0	6.0	—	—
80579	Sunrise Melt with egg	1	item(s)	149	—	230	18.0	26.0	6.0	8.0	3.0	—	—
40477	Sweet onion chicken teriyaki sandwich, 6", white or wheat bread	1	serving(s)	276	—	380	26.0	59.0	5.0	4.5	1.0	—	—
15834	Turkey breast & ham sandwich, 6", white bread	1	item(s)	214	—	270	17.0	44.0	2.0	4.0	1.0	—	—
16376	Turkey breast sandwich, 6", white bread	1	item(s)	214	—	270	17.0	44.0	2.0	3.5	1.0	—	—
15843	Veggie Delite salad	1	item(s)	271	—	50	3.0	9.0	4.0	1.0	0	—	—
15841	Veggie Delite sandwich, 6", wheat bread	1	item(s)	162	—	230	8.0	44.0	5.0	2.5	0.5	—	—
16375	Veggie Delite sandwich, 6", white bread	1	item(s)	157	—	220	7.0	42.0	2.0	2.5	0	—	—
32051	White chip macadamia nut cookie	1	item(s)	45	—	220	2.0	29.0	0.5	11.0	5.0	—	—
	Taco Bell												
29906	7-Layer burrito	1	item(s)	283	—	510	18.0	68.0	12.0	18.0	6.0	—	—
744	Bean burrito	1	item(s)	198	105.3	370	13.0	56.0	10.0	10.0	3.5	2.1	3.7
749	Beef burrito supreme	1	item(s)	248	—	420	17.0	52.0	9.0	15.0	7.0	—	—
33417	Beef Chalupa Supreme	1	item(s)	153	—	370	14.0	31.0	3.0	21.0	6.0	—	—
29910	Beef Gordita Supreme	1	item(s)	153	—	300	13.0	31.0	4.0	13.0	5.0	—	—
2014	Beef soft taco	1	item(s)	99	—	210	10.0	21.0	3.0	9.0	4.0	—	—
10860	Beef soft taco supreme	1	item(s)	135	—	240	11.0	24.0	3.0	11.0	5.0	—	—
66167	Cheesy Fiesta potatoes	1	serving(s)	135	—	270	4.0	28.0	3.0	16.0	2.5	—	—
34472	Chicken burrito supreme	1	item(s)	248	—	390	21.0	51.0	7.0	12.0	5.0	—	—
33418	Chicken Chalupa Supreme	1	item(s)	153	—	350	17.0	30.0	2.0	18.0	4.0	—	—
29909	Chicken quesadilla	1	item(s)	184	—	520	28.0	41.0	4.0	28.0	12.0	—	—
50171	Chicken soft taco	1	item(s)	99	57.8	187	13.2	19.5	1.2	6.3	2.5	1.6	1.6
29907	Chili cheese burrito	1	item(s)	156	—	370	16.0	40.0	4.0	16.0	8.0	—	—
10794	Cinnamon twists	1	serving(s)	35	—	170	1.0	26.0	1.0	7.0	0.0	—	—
66033	Fresco bean burrito	1	item(s)	213	—	340	12.0	56.0	11.0	8.0	2.5	—	—
66025	Fresco chicken burrito supreme	1	item(s)	241	—	340	18.0	50.0	8.0	8.0	2.5	—	—
66020	Fresco crunchy taco	1	item(s)	92	—	150	7.0	13.0	3.0	7.0	2.5	—	—
66026	Fresco steak burrito supreme	1	item(s)	241	—	330	16.0	49.0	8.0	8.0	3.0	—	—
29911	Grilled chicken Gordita Supreme	1	item(s)	153	—	270	17.0	29.0	2.0	10.0	3.5	—	—
29912	Grilled Steak Gordita Supreme	1	item(s)	153	—	270	14.0	29.0	2.0	11.0	4.0	—	—
29904	Grilled steak soft taco	1	item(s)	128	—	250	11.0	20.0	2.0	14.0	4.0	—	—
2021	Mexican pizza	1	serving(s)	213	—	540	21.0	47.0	8.0	30.0	8.0	—	—
10772	Meximelt	1	serving(s)	128	—	280	15.0	23.0	4.0	14.0	7.0	—	—
2011	Nachos	1	serving(s)	99	33.9	330	4.0	31.0	2.0	20.0	2.0	12.6	2.6
2012	Nachos BellGrande	1	serving(s)	305	—	770	20.0	78.0	15.0	42.0	7.0	—	—
2023	Pintos 'n cheese	1	serving(s)	128	—	180	10.0	19.0	9.0	7.0	3.0	—	—

GE KEY: H-4 = Breads/Baked Goods H-8 = Cereal/Rice/Pasta H-14 = Fruit H-18 = Vegetables/Legumes H-28 = Nuts/Seeds H-30 = Vegetarian H-32 = Dairy H-40 = Eggs H-40 = Seafood H-42 = Meats H-46 = Poultry
18 = Processed Meats H-50 = Beverages H-52 = Fats/Oils H-54 = Sweets H-56 = Spices/Condiments/Sauces H-60 = Mixed Foods/Soups/Sandwiches H-66 = Fast Food H-84 = Convenience H-86 = Baby Foods

Chol (mg)	Calc (mg)	Iron (mg)	Magn (mg)	Pota (mg)	Sodi (mg)	Zinc (mg)	Vit A (μg)	Thia (mg)	Vit E (mg α)	Ribo (mg)	Niac (mg)	Vit B_6 (mg)	Fola (μg)	Vit C (mg)	Vit B_{12} (μg)	Sele (μg)
70	80	7.20	—	—	2100.0	—	—	—	—	—	—	—	—	18.0	—	—
50	350	4.50	—	—	1120.0	—	—	—	—	—	—	—	—	12.0	—	—
25	300	2.70	—	—	830.0	—	—	—	—	—	—	—	—	12.0	—	—
30	350	4.50	—	—	950.0	—	—	—	—	—	—	—	—	21.0	—	—
30	350	4.50	—	—	930.0	—	—	—	—	—	—	—	—	21.0	—	—
45	400	2.70	—	—	1210.0	—	—	—	—	—	—	—	—	12.0	—	—
15	20	1.08	—	—	130.0	—	0	—	—	—	—	—	—	0	—	—
45	300	2.70	—	—	640.0	—	—	—	—	—	—	—	—	18.0	—	—
10	20	1.08	—	—	130.0	—	—	—	—	—	—	—	—	0	—	—
45	300	4.50	—	—	700.0	—	—	—	—	—	—	—	—	12.0	—	—
45	300	4.50	—	—	680.0	—	—	—	—	—	—	—	—	12.0	—	—
45	300	2.70	—	—	620.0	—	—	—	—	—	—	—	—	18.0	—	—
50	300	3.60	—	—	1500.0	—	—	—	—	—	—	—	—	12.0	—	—
50	400	4.50	—	—	1040.0	—	—	—	—	—	—	—	—	12.0	—	—
15	0	0.72	—	—	130.0	—	0	—	—	—	—	—	—	0	—	—
130	200	1.44	—	—	810.0	—	—	—	—	—	—	—	—	1.2	—	—
50	350	3.60	—	—	900.0	—	—	—	—	—	—	—	—	18.0	—	—
20	300	3.60	—	—	800.0	—	—	—	—	—	—	—	—	12.0	—	—
20	300	3.60	—	—	790.0	—	—	—	—	—	—	—	—	12.0	—	—
0	40	1.08	—	—	65.0	—	—	—	—	—	—	—	—	27.0	—	—
0	300	2.70	—	—	310.0	—	—	—	—	—	—	—	—	12.0	—	—
0	300	2.70	—	—	290.0	—	—	—	—	—	—	—	—	12.0	—	—
15	20	0.72	—	—	130.0	—	—	—	—	—	—	—	—	0	—	—
20	—	—	—	—	1410.0	—	—	—	—	—	—	—	—	—	—	—
5	246	4.69	67.3	516.8	980.0	1.70	5.9	0.38	0.99	0.20	4.00	0.20	134.6	0.8	0.3	20.6
35	—	—	—	—	1380.0	—	—	—	—	—	—	—	—	—	—	—
35	—	—	—	—	610.0	—	—	—	—	—	—	—	—	—	—	—
35	—	—	—	—	590.0	—	—	—	—	—	—	—	—	—	—	—
30	—	—	—	—	620.0	—	—	—	—	—	—	—	—	—	—	—
35	—	—	—	—	650.0	—	—	—	—	—	—	—	—	—	—	—
5	—	—	—	—	840.0	—	—	—	—	—	—	—	—	—	—	—
40	—	—	—	—	1420.0	—	—	—	—	—	—	—	—	—	—	—
40	—	—	—	—	650.0	—	—	—	—	—	—	—	—	—	—	—
75	—	—	—	—	1420.0	—	—	—	—	—	—	—	—	—	—	—
29	121	1.57	23.8	214.8	606.9	0.75	1.0	0.16	0.35	0.11	5.12	0.11	68.3	0.2	0.1	12.6
40	—	—	—	—	1080.0	—	—	—	—	—	—	—	—	—	—	—
0	—	—	—	—	200.0	—	—	—	—	—	—	—	—	—	—	—
0	—	—	—	—	1290.0	—	—	—	—	—	—	—	—	—	—	—
25	—	—	—	—	1410.0	—	—	—	—	—	—	—	—	—	—	—
20	—	—	—	—	350.0	—	—	—	—	—	—	—	—	—	—	—
15	—	—	—	—	1340.0	—	—	—	—	—	—	—	—	—	—	—
35	—	—	—	—	620.0	—	—	—	—	—	—	—	—	—	—	—
30	—	—	—	—	550.0	—	—	—	—	—	—	—	—	—	—	—
30	—	—	—	—	710.0	—	—	—	—	—	—	—	—	—	—	—
45	—	—	—	—	1020.0	—	—	—	—	—	—	—	—	—	—	—
45	—	—	—	—	870.0	—	—	—	—	—	—	—	—	—	—	—
5	88	1.11	51.5	180.2	370.0	1.14	1.0	0.12	1.04	0.13	0.90	0.18	12.9	—	—	3.4
30	—	—	—	—	1300.0	—	—	—	—	—	—	—	—	—	—	—
15	—	—	—	—	720.0	—	—	—	—	—	—	—	—	—	—	—

APPENDIX H

TABLE H-1 Table of Food Composition (*continued*) (Computer code is for Cengage Diet Analysis program) (For purposes of calculations, use "0" for t, <1, <0.1, 0.01)

DA+ Code	Food Description	Quantity	Measure	Wt (g)	H_2O (g)	Ener (kcal)	Prot (g)	Carb (g)	Fiber (g)	Fat (g)	Fat Breakdown (g) Sat	Mono	Poly
Fast Food—*continued*													
34473	Steak burrito supreme	1	item(s)	248	—	380	18.0	51.0	7.0	12.0	5.0	—	—
33419	Steak Chalupa Supreme	1	item(s)	153	—	340	15.0	29.0	2.0	18.0	4.0	—	—
747	Taco	1	item(s)	78	—	170	8.0	12.0	3.0	10.0	3.5	—	—
2015	Taco salad with salsa, with shell	1	serving(s)	463	—	770	27.0	75.0	12.0	41.0	10.0	—	—
748	Tostada	1	item(s)	170	—	250	11.0	29.0	10.0	10.0	3.5	—	—
Convenience Meals													
	Banquet												
14788	Boneless white fried chicken meal	1	item(s)	286	—	350	12.0	35.0	5.0	17.0	4.0	—	—
14773	Chicken pasta marinara meal	1	item(s)	184	—	290	12.0	29.0	3.0	14.0	3.0	—	—
29960	Fish sticks meal	1	item(s)	207	—	310	11.0	44.0	4.0	10.0	2.5	—	—
29957	Lasagna with meat sauce meal	1	item(s)	227	—	250	12.0	34.0	4.0	7.0	2.5	—	—
14777	Macaroni and cheese meal	1	item(s)	227	—	260	10.0	39.0	3.0	6.0	3.0	—	—
1741	Meatloaf meal	1	item(s)	269	—	280	12.0	28.0	4.0	13.0	5.0	—	—
39418	Pepperoni pizza meal	1	item(s)	163	—	340	11.0	47.0	4.0	12.0	3.5	—	—
1743	Salisbury steak meal	1	item(s)	269	—	290	11.0	25.0	4.0	16.0	7.0	—	—
14772	Turkey meal	1	item(s)	262	—	250	13.0	32.0	5.0	7.0	2.0	—	—
	Healthy Choice												
9337	Beef pot roast complete meal	1	item(s)	312	—	290	17.0	45.0	6.0	4.5	1.5	2.0	1.0
57075	Café Steamers Cajun style chicken & shrimp	1	item(s)	295	—	250	17.0	33.0	5.0	5.0	1.0	—	—
57078	Café Steamers chicken linguini with red pepper Alfredo	1	item(s)	292	—	280	22.0	35.0	5.0	6.0	2.5	—	—
57074	Café Steamers sweet sesame chicken	1	item(s)	292	—	330	17.0	50.0	6.0	6.0	1.0	2.5	2.0
9316	Lemon pepper fish meal	1	item(s)	303	—	310	14.0	50.0	5.0	5.0	1.0	—	—
9322	Traditional salisbury steak meal	1	item(s)	354	—	310	18.0	46.0	9.0	6.0	2.5	2.0	1.0
9359	Traditional turkey breast meal	1	item(s)	298	—	290	18.0	44.0	8.0	4.5	1.0	2.0	1.5
	Lean Cuisine												
11043	Culinary Collection baked chicken	1	item(s)	245	—	240	15.0	34.0	3.0	4.5	1.0	1.0	2.0
360	Simple Favorites chicken chow mein	1	item(s)	255	—	260	14.0	41.0	3.0	4.0	1.0	1.5	1.5
11054	Simple Favorites chicken enchilada suiza	1	serving(s)	255	190.9	270	12.0	47.0	3.0	4.0	1.5	1.0	1.0
9467	Simple Favorites fettuccini Alfredo	1	item(s)	262	—	280	14.0	42.0	1.0	6.0	3.0	1.5	1.0
9479	Simple Favorites French bread deluxe pizza	1	item(s)	174	—	340	16.0	46.0	4.0	10.0	3.5	2.5	1.5
11055	Simple Favorites lasagna with meat sauce	1	item(s)	298	—	320	20.0	43.0	4.0	7.0	3.5	2.0	1.0
58267	Spa Collection ginger garlic stir fry with chicken	1	item(s)	280	—	290	17.0	46.0	4.0	4.0	1.0	1.0	1.5
	Michelina's												
55332	Cheese manicotti with marinara sauce entrée	1	item(s)	227	—	270	11.0	34.0	3.0	11.0	5.0	—	—
1915	Fettuccini Alfredo with chicken & broccoli entrée	1	item(s)	241	—	310	15.0	38.0	2.0	10.0	6.0	—	—
55320	Lean Gourmet five cheese lasagna entrée	1	item(s)	227	—	290	13.0	50.0	8.0	5.0	2.0	—	—
55329	Lean Gourmet Meatloaf entrée	1	item(s)	227	—	180	11.0	21.0	2.0	6.0	3.0	—	—
55325	Lean Gourmet Santa Fe style rice & beans entrée	1	item(s)	255	—	320	10.0	52.0	3.0	8.0	3.5	—	—
	Stouffer's												
36564	Beef pot roast entrée	1	item(s)	255	—	210	14.0	30.0	2.0	4.0	1.5	—	—
2313	Cheese French bread pizza	1	serving(s)	294	—	370	14.0	44.0	4.0	15.0	6.0	—	—
2366	Chicken pot pie entrée	1	item(s)	454	—	590	19.0	54.0	1.0	34.0	13.0	—	—
11116	Homestyle baked chicken breast with mashed potatoes and gravy entrée	1	item(s)	252	—	250	20.0	20.0	1.0	10.0	3.0	—	—
11152	Homestyle roast turkey breast with stuffing and mashed potatoes entrée	1	item(s)	273	—	290	16.0	30.0	2.0	12.0	3.5	—	—
41781	Lasagna with meat & sauce entrée	1	item(s)	595	441.9	690	47.8	74.8	6.5	22.4	11.3	7.6	1.4
	Weight Watchers												
11164	Smart Ones chicken enchiladas suiza entrée	1	item(s)	255	—	290	11.0	49.0	3.0	5.0	2.0	1.5	1.0
39763	Smart Ones chicken oriental entrée	1	item(s)	255	—	230	14.0	41.0	2.0	1.5	0	0	0

GE KEY: H-4 = Breads/Baked Goods H-8 = Cereal/Rice/Pasta H-14 = Fruit H-18 = Vegetables/Legumes H-28 = Nuts/Seeds H-30 = Vegetarian H-32 = Dairy H-40 = Eggs H-40 = Seafood H-42 = Meats H-46 = Poultry
48 = Processed Meats H-50 = Beverages H-52 = Fats/Oils H-54 = Sweets H-56 = Spices/Condiments/Sauces H-60 = Mixed Foods/Soups/Sandwiches H-66 = Fast Food H-84 = Convenience H-86 = Baby Foods

Chol (mg)	Calc (mg)	Iron (mg)	Magn (mg)	Pota (mg)	Sodi (mg)	Zinc (mg)	Vit A (µg)	Thia (mg)	Vit E (mg α)	Ribo (mg)	Niac (mg)	Vit B_6 (mg)	Fola (µg)	Vit C (mg)	Vit B_{12} (µg)	Sele (µg)
30	—	—	—	—	1340.0	—	—	—	—	—	—	—	—	—	—	—
30	—	—	—	—	580.0	—	—	—	—	—	—	—	—	—	—	—
30	—	—	—	—	330.0	—	—	—	—	—	—	—	—	—	—	—
60	—	—	—	—	1650.0	—	—	—	—	—	—	—	—	—	—	—
15	—	—	—	—	730.0	—	—	—	—	—	—	—	—	—	—	—
35	100	1.08	40.0	450.0	930.0	1.50	0	0.09	—	0.14	1.20	0.12	—	4.8	0.5	—
15	60	1.80	40.0	380.0	550.0	0.90	—	—	—	0.10	1.60	0.08	—	2.4	1.8	—
25	100	1.80	40.0	290.0	540.0	0.60	—	0.12	—	0.17	0.80	—	—	0	3.0	—
10	60	2.70	40.0	420.0	510.0	1.20	—	0.30	—	0.25	3.00	—	—	1.2	2.7	—
15	100	1.44	32.0	220.0	760.0	0.90	—	0.30	—	0.51	0.80	—	—	0	0.4	—
40	20	1.08	32.0	420.0	1000.0	1.50	0	—	—	—	—	0.16	—	0	0.6	—
10	150	1.80	40.0	310.0	730.0	1.50	—	0.12	—	0.34	0.80	0.12	—	0	—	—
30	20	1.44	32.0	380.0	1100.0	1.50	0	0.06	—	0.14	1.60		—	0	0.9	—
25	40	1.80	32.0	360.0	1060.0	1.20	—	0.15	—	0.17	3.00	0.12	—	6.0	0.9	—
40	40	1.80	40.0	720.0	500.0	3.00	—	0.03	—	0.17	3.00	0.20	—	30.0	1.5	21.0
45	40	1.08	40.0	480.0	590.0	1.20	—	0.22	—	0.25	6.00	0.20	—	6.0	0.5	0
35	100	1.80	40.0	440.0	570.0	1.50	—	0.22	—	0.34	5.00	0.20	—	30.0	0.6	63.0
30	40	0.72	40.0	440.0	400.0	0.90	—	0.09	—	0.14	4.00	0.30	—	1.2	0.6	0
25	60	1.08	40.0	480.0	450.0	0.60	—	0.22	—	0.07	2.00	0.40	—	24.0	1.2	14.0
35	100	2.70	60.0	880.0	590.0	3.00	—	0.15	—	0.17	3.00	0.16	—	24.0	1.2	21.0
25	60	1.80	40.0	680.0	450.0	1.20	—	0.22	—	0.25	5.00	0.20	—	4.8	0.5	31.5
25	40	1.17	—	500.0	650.0	—	—	—	—	—	—	—	—	3.6	—	—
25	60	1.08	—	380.0	550.0	—	—	—	—	—	—	—	—	3.6	—	—
20	150	1.08	—	380.0	550.0	—	—	0.20	—	0.15	1.68	—	—	1.2	—	—
15	200	0.72	—	270.0	690.0	—	0	—	—	—	—	—	—	0	—	—
20	150	2.70	—	330.0	760.0	—	—	—	—	—	—	—	—	12.0	—	—
30	200	2.70	—	710.0	590.0	—	—	—	—	—	—	—	—	3.6	—	—
30	60	1.44	—	550.0	640.0	—	—	—	—	—	—	—	—	15.0	—	—
30	200	1.08	—	—	980.0	—	—	—	—	—	—	—	—	12.0	—	—
45	150	1.80	—	—	700.0	—	—	—	—	—	—	—	—	9.0	—	—
10	150	3.60	—	—	560.0	—	—	—	—	—	—	—	—	12.0	—	—
35	40	1.44	—	—	860.0	—	—	—	—	—	—	—	—	6.0	—	—
20	150	1.44	—	—	670.0	—	—	—	—	—	—	—	—	6.0	—	—
25	20	1.80	—	—	710.0	—	—	—	—	—	—	—	—	4.8	—	—
20	250	1.80	—	—	600.0	—	—	—	—	—	—	—	—	2.4	—	—
50	100	3.60	—	—	930.0	—	—	—	—	—	—	—	—	1.2	—	—
60	40	0.36	—	—	730.0	—	0	—	—	—	—	—	—	0	—	—
45	40	1.08	—	490.0	970.0	—	—	—	—	—	—	—	—	3.6	—	—
77	411	3.63	—	940.1	1856.4	—	—	0.36	—	0.30	3.81	—	—	3.6	—	—
25	100	0.72	—	—	640.0	—	—	—	—	—	—	—	—	6.0	—	—
25	20	0.36	—	—	700.0	—	—	—	—	—	—	—	—	2.4	—	—

DA+ Code	Food Description	Quantity	Measure	Wt (g)	H_2O (g)	Ener (kcal)	Prot (g)	Carb (g)	Fiber (g)	Fat (g)	Fat Breakdown (g) Sat	Mono	Poly
Convenience Meals—*continued*													
11187	Smart Ones pepperoni pizza	1	item(s)	173	—	410	19.0	63.0	4.0	9.0	3.0	2.5	1.5
58556	Smart Ones spaghetti with meat sauce entrée	1	item(s)	326	—	290	14.0	44.0	5.0	6.0	1.5	2.0	1.0
31512	Smart Ones spicy szechuan style vegetables & chicken	1	item(s)	255	—	240	11.0	38.0	4.0	5.0	1.0	2.0	2.5
Baby Foods													
787	Apple juice	4	fluid ounce(s)	127	111.6	60	0	14.8	0.1	0.1	0	0	0
778	Applesauce, strained	4	tablespoon(s)	64	56.7	26	0.1	6.9	1.1	0.1	0	0	0
779	Bananas with tapioca, strained	4	tablespoon(s)	60	50.4	34	0.2	9.2	1.0	0.1	0	0	0
604	Carrots, strained	4	tablespoon(s)	56	51.7	15	0.4	3.4	1.0	0.1	0	0	0
770	Chicken noodle dinner, strained	4	tablespoon(s)	64	54.8	42	1.7	5.8	1.3	1.3	0.4	0.5	0.3
801	Green beans, strained	4	tablespoon(s)	60	55.1	16	0.7	3.8	1.3	0.1	0	0	0.1
910	Human milk, mature	2	fluid ounce(s)	62	53.9	43	0.6	4.2	0	2.7	1.2	1.0	0.3
760	Mixed cereal, prepared with whole milk	4	ounce(s)	113	89.8	109	4.7	13.9	0.9	3.8	2.0	1.0	0.4
772	Mixed vegetable dinner, strained	2	ounce(s)	57	50.3	23	0.7	5.4	0.9	0.1	—	—	0.1
762	Rice cereal, prepared with whole milk	4	ounce(s)	113	92.9	96	3.9	11.7	0	3.8	2.0	1.0	0.4
758	Teething biscuits	1	item(s)	11	0.7	43	1.2	8.4	0.2	0.5	0.1	0.2	0.1

Chol (mg)	Calc (mg)	Iron (mg)	Magn (mg)	Pota (mg)	Sodi (mg)	Zinc (mg)	Vit A (µg)	Thia (mg)	Vit E (mg α)	Ribo (mg)	Niac (mg)	Vit B_6 (mg)	Fola (µg)	Vit C (mg)	Vit B_{12} (µg)	Sele (µg)
30	100	1.44	—	—	730.0	—	—	—	—	—	—	—	—	0	—	—
10	100	2.70	—	—	520.0	—	—	—	—	—	—	—	—	12.0	—	—
10	60	2.70	—	—	710.0	—	—	—	—	—	—	—	—	0	—	—
0	5	0.72	3.8	115.4	10.1	0.04	1.3	0.01	0.76	0.02	0.11	0.04	0	73.4	0	0.1
0	3	0.14	1.9	45.4	0	0.01	0.6	0.01	0.38	0.02	0.04	0.02	1.3	24.5	0	0.2
0	3	0.12	6.0	52.8	0	0.04	1.2	0.01	0.36	0.02	0.11	0.07	3.6	10.0	0	0.4
0	12	0.21	5.0	109.8	38.6	0.08	320.9	0.01	0.29	0.02	0.26	0.04	8.4	3.2	0	0.1
10	17	0.41	9.0	89.0	24.3	0.35	70.4	0.03	0.13	0.04	0.46	0.04	8.3	0.1	0	2.4
0	23	0.40	12.0	87.6	4.2	0.13	10.8	0.02	0.04	0.05	0.22	0.02	14.4	0.2	0	0.1
9	20	0.02	1.8	31.4	10.5	0.10	37.6	0.01	0.05	0.02	0.11	0.01	3.1	3.1	0	1.1
10	249	11.83	22.7	188.2	47.6	0.67	46.5	0.35	0.53	0.51	4.40	0.06	10.2	0.3	0.5	6.9
—	12	0.19	6.2	68.6	21.5	0.09	77.1	0.01	—	0.02	0.28	0.04	4.5	1.6	0	0.4
11	191	4.12	28.4	171.2	47.6	0.56	47.6	0.28	0.50	0.37	2.78	0.08	6.8	0.2	0.5	4.9
1	29	0.39	3.8	35.5	25.0	0.10	3.1	0.03	0.12	0.06	0.48	0.01	7.6	1.0	0	2.6

Appendix I WHO Nutrition Recommendations

The World Health Organization (WHO) has assessed the relationships between diet and the development of chronic diseases. This appendix presents its nutrition recommendations for adults:

- Energy: sufficient to support growth, physical activity, and a healthy body weight (BMI between 18.5 and 24.9) and to avoid weight gain greater than 11 pounds (5 kilograms) during adult life
- Total fat: 15 to 30 percent of total energy
- Saturated fatty acids: <10 percent of total energy
- Polyunsaturated fatty acids: 6 to 10 percent of total energy
- Omega-6 polyunsaturated fatty acids: 5 to 8 percent of total energy
- Omega-3 polyunsaturated fatty acids: 1 to 2 percent of total energy
- *Trans*-fatty acids: <1 percent of total energy
- Total carbohydrate: 55 to 75 percent of total energy
- Sugars: <10 percent of total energy, preferably <5 percent of total energy
- Protein: 10 to 15 percent of total energy
- Cholesterol: <300 mg per day
- Salt (sodium): <5 g salt per day (<2 g sodium per day), appropriately iodized
- Potassium: ≥3510 mg per day
- Fruits and vegetables: ≥400 g per day (about 1 pound)
- Total dietary fiber: >25 g per day from foods
- Physical activity: one hour of moderate-intensity activity, such as walking, on most days of the week

Appendix J Healthy People 2020

Table 1-4 (p. 25) lists the objectives from the Nutrition and Weight Status section of the Healthy People 2020 initiative. Table J-1 presents additional nutrition-related objectives from other topic areas.

TABLE J-1 Nutrition-Related Objectives from Other Topic Areas

Access to Health Services

- Increase the proportion of persons who receive appropriate evidence-based clinical preventive services.

Adolescent Health

- Increase the proportion of schools with a school breakfast program.

Arthritis, Osteoporosis, and Chronic Back Conditions

- Reduce hip fractures among older adults.
- Reduce the proportion of adults with osteoporosis.

Cancer

- Reduce the cancer death rate.
- Increase the mental and physical health-related quality of life of cancer survivors.

Diabetes

- Reduce the annual number of new cases of diagnosed diabetes in the population.
- Reduce the death rate among the population with diabetes.
- Reduce the diabetes death rate.
- Improve glycemic control among the population with diagnosed diabetes.
- Improve lipid control among persons with diagnosed diabetes.
- Increase the proportion of the population with diagnosed diabetes whose blood pressure is under control.
- Increase the proportion of persons with diagnosed diabetes who receive formal diabetes education.
- Increase prevention behaviors in persons at high risk for diabetes with prediabetes.

Early and Middle Childhood

- Increase the proportion of elementary, middle, and senior high schools that require school health education.

Educational and Community-Based Programs

- Increase the proportion of preschool Early Head Start and Head Start programs that provide health education to prevent health problems in the following areas: unintentional injury; violence; tobacco use and addiction; alcohol and drug use, unhealthy dietary patterns; and inadequate physical activity, dental health, and safety.
- Increase the proportion of elementary, middle, and senior high schools that provide comprehensive school health education to prevent health problems in the following areas: unintentional injury; violence; suicide; tobacco use and addiction; alcohol or other drug use; unintended pregnancy, human immunodeficiency virus/acquired immune deficiency syndrome (HIV/AIDS), and STD (sexually transmitted diseases) infection; unhealthy dietary patterns; and inadequate physical activity.
- Increase the proportion of college and university students who receive information from their institution on each of the priority health risk behavior areas (all priority areas; unintentional injury; violence; suicide; tobacco use and addiction; alcohol and other drug use; unintended pregnancy, human immunodeficiency virus/acquired immune deficiency syndrome (HIV/AIDS), and STD (sexually transmitted diseases) infection,; unhealthy dietary patterns; and inadequate physical activity).
- Increase the proportion of worksites that offer an employee health promotion program to their employees.
- Increase the number of community-based organizations (including local health departments, tribal health services, nongovernmental organizations, and state agencies) providing population-based primary prevention services.

Environmental Health

- Reduce blood lead levels in children.
- Reduce the number of US homes that are found to have lead-based paint or related hazards.

(continued)

TABLE J-1 Nutrition-Related Objectives from Other Topic Areas (*continued*)

Food Safety
• Reduce infections caused by key pathogens transmitted commonly through food. • Reduce the number of outbreak-associated infections due to Shiga toxin-producing *Escherichia coli* O157:H7, or *Campylobacter, Listeria*, or *Salmonella* species associated with food commodity groups. • Reduce severe allergic reactions to food among adults with a food allergy diagnosis. • Increase the proportion of consumers who follow key food safety practices. • Improve food safety practices associated with foodborne illness in foodservice and retail establishments.
Heart Disease and Stroke
• Increase overall cardiovascular health in the US population. • Reduce coronary heart disease deaths. • Reduce stroke deaths. • Reduce the proportion of persons in the population with hypertension. • Reduce the proportion of adults with high total blood cholesterol levels. • Reduce the mean total blood cholesterol levels among adults. • Increase the proportion of adults with prehypertension who meet the recommended guidelines. • Increase the proportion of adults with hypertension who meet the recommended guidelines. • Increase the proportion of adults with elevated LDL cholesterol who have been advised by a health-care provider regarding cholesterol-lowering management including lifestyle changes and, if indicated, medication. • Increase the proportion of adults with elevated LDL-cholesterol who adhere to the prescribed LDL cholesterol–lowering management lifestyle changes and, if indicated, medication.
Maternal, Infant, and Child Health
• Reduce low birth weight (LBW) and very low birth weight (VLBW). • Reduce preterm births. • Increase the proportion of pregnant women who receive early and adequate prenatal care. • Increase the proportion of mothers who achieve a recommended weight gain during their pregnancies. • Increase the proportion of women of childbearing potential with intake of at least 400 micrograms of folic acid from fortified foods or dietary supplements. • Reduce the proportion of women of childbearing potential who have low red blood cell folate concentrations. • Increase the proportion of women delivering a live birth who received preconception care services and practiced key recommended preconception health behaviors. • Increase the proportion of infants who are breastfed. • Increase the proportion of employers that have worksite lactation support programs. • Reduce the proportion of breastfed newborns who receive formula supplementation within the first 2 days of life. • Reduce the occurrence of fetal alcohol syndrome (FAS). • Reduce occurrence of neural tube defects.
Mental Health and Mental Disorders
• Reduce the proportion of adolescents who engage in disordered eating behaviors in an attempt to control their weight.
Older Adults
• Increase the proportion of the health-care workforce (including dietitians) with geriatric certification.
Oral Health
• Increase the proportion of the US population served by community water systems with optimally fluoridated water.
Physical Activity
• Reduce the proportion of adults who engage in no leisure-time physical activity. • Increase the proportion of adolescents and adults who meet current federal physical activity guidelines for aerobic physical activity and for muscle-strengthening activity. • Increase the proportion of the nation's public and private schools that require daily physical education for all students. • Increase the proportion of adolescents who participate in daily school physical education. • Increase regularly scheduled elementary school recess in the United States. • Increase the proportion of children and adolescents who do not exceed recommended limits for screen time.

SOURCE: Adapted from Healthy people 2020: www.healthypeople.gov.

Appendix K Aids to Calculation

Many mathematical problems have been worked out in the "How To" features of the text. This appendix offers additional help and examples.

Conversions

A conversion factor is a fraction that converts a measurement expressed in one unit to another unit—for example, from pounds to kilograms or from feet to meters. To create a conversion factor, an equality (such as 1 kilogram = 2.2 pounds) is expressed as a fraction:

$$\frac{1\text{ kg}}{2.2\text{ lb}} \text{ and } \frac{2.2\text{ lb}}{1\text{ kg}}$$

To convert the units of a measurement, use the fraction with the desired unit in the numerator.

Example 1 Convert a weight of 130 pounds to kilograms. Multiply 130 pounds by the conversion factor that includes both pounds and kilograms, with the desired unit (kilograms) in the numerator:

$$130\text{ lb} \times \frac{1\text{ kg}}{2.2\text{ lb}} = \frac{130\text{ kg}}{2.2} = 59\text{ kg}$$

Alternatively, to convert a measurement from one unit of measure to another, multiply the given measurement by the appropriate equivalent found on the next page of weights and measures.

Example 2 Convert 64 fluid ounces to liters. Locate the equivalent measure from the volume section on the next page (1 ounce = 0.03 liter) and multiply the number of ounces by 0.03:

$$64\text{ oz} \times 0.03\text{ oz/L} = 1.9\text{ L}$$

Percentages

A percentage is a fraction whose denominator is 100. For example:

$$50\% = \frac{50}{100}$$

Like other fractions, percentages are used to express a portion of a quantity. Fractions whose denominators are numbers other than 100 can be converted to percentages by first dividing the numerator by the denominator and then multiplying the result by 100.

Example 3 Express 5/8 as a percent.

$$\frac{5}{8} = 5 \div 8 = 0.625$$

$$0.625 \times 100 = 62.5\%$$

The following examples show how to calculate specific percentages.

Example 4 Suppose your energy intake for the day is 2000 kcalories (kcal) and your recommended energy intake is 2400 kcalories. What percent of the recommended energy intake did you consume?

Divide your intake by the recommended intake.
2000 kcal (intake) ÷ 2400 kcal (recommended) = 0.83
Multiply by 100 to express the decimal as a percent.
0.83 × 100 = 83%

Example 5 Suppose a man's intake of vitamin C is 120 milligrams and his RDA is 90 milligrams. What percent of the RDA for vitamin C did he consume?

Divide the intake by the recommended intake.
120 mg (intake) ÷ 90 mg (RDA) = 1.33
Multiply by 100 to express the decimal as a percent.
1.33 × 100 = 133%

Example 6 Dietary recommendations suggest that carbohydrates provide 45 to 65 percent of the day's energy intake. If your energy intake is 2000 kcalories, how much carbohydrate should you eat?

Because this question has a range of acceptable answers, work the problem twice. First, use 45% to find the least amount you should eat.

Divide 45 by 100 to convert to a decimal.
45 ÷ 100 = 0.45
Multiply kcalories by 0.45.
2000 kcal × 0.45 = 900 kcal
Divide kcalories by 4 to convert carbohydrate kcal to grams.
900 kcal ÷ 4 kcal/g = 225 g

Now repeat the process using 65% to find the maximum number of grams of carbohydrates you should eat.

Divide 65 by 100 to convert it to a decimal.

65 ÷ 100 = 0.65

Multiply kcalories by 0.65.

2000 kcal × 0.65 = 1300 kcal

Divide kcalories by 4 to convert carbohydrate kcal to grams.

1300 kcal ÷ 4 kcal/g = 325 g

If you plan for between 45% and 65% of your 2000-kcalorie intake to be from carbohydrates, you should eat between 225 grams and 325 grams of carbohydrates.

Weights and Measures

Length

1 centimeter (cm) = 0.39 inches (in)
1 foot (ft) = 30 centimeters (cm)
1 inch (in) = 2.54 centimeters (cm)
1 meter (m) = 39.37 inches (in)

Weight

1 gram (g) = 0.001 kilograms (kg)
= 1000 milligrams (mg)
= 0.035 ounces (oz)
1 kilogram (kg) = 1000 grams (g)
= 2.2 pounds (lb)
1 microgram (μg) = 0.001 milligrams (mg)
1 milligram (mg) = 0.001 grams (g)
= 1000 micrograms (μg)
1 ounce (oz) = 28 grams (g)
= 0.03 kilograms (kg)
= 1/16 or 0.0625 pound (lb)
1 pound (lb) = 454 grams (g)
= 0.45 kilograms (kg)
= 16 ounces (oz)

Volume

1 cup = 16 tablespoons (tbs or T)
= 0.25 liters (L)
= 236 milliliters (mL, commonly rounded to 250 mL)
= 8 ounces (oz)
1 liter (L) = 33.8 fluid ounces (fl oz)
= 0.26 gallons (gal)
= 2.1 pints (pt)
= 1.06 quarts (qt)
= 1000 milliliters (mL)
1 milliliter (mL) = 0.001 liters (L)
= 0.03 fluid ounces (fl oz)
= 1/5 teaspoon (tsp)
1 ounce (oz) = 0.03 liters (L)
= 30 milliliters (mL)
= 2 tablespoons (tbs)
1 pint (pt) = 2 cups (c)
= 0.47 liters (L)
= 16 ounces (oz)
= 0.5 quarts (qt)
1 quart (qt) = 4 cups (c)
= 0.95 liters (L)
= 32 ounces (oz)
= 1/4 or 0.25 gallon (gal)
= 2 pints (pt)
1 tablespoon (tbs or T) = 3 teaspoons (tsp)
= 15 milliliters (mL)
1 teaspoon (tsp) = 5 milliliters (mL)
1 gallon (gal) = 16 cups (c)
= 3.8 liters (L)
= 128 ounces (oz)
= 8 pints (pt)
= 4 quarts (qt)
1 cup (c) = 8 ounces (oz)
= 16 tablespoons (tbs)
= 250 milliliters (mL)

Energy

1 megajoule (MJ) = 240 kcalories (kcal)
1 kilojoule (kJ) = 0.24 kcalories (kcal)
1 kcalorie (kcal) = 4.2 kilojoule (kJ)
1 g alcohol = 7 kcal = 29 kJ
1 g carbohydrate = 4 kcal = 17 kJ
1 g fat = 9 kcal = 37 kJ
1 g protein = 4 kcal = 17 kJ

Temperature

To change from Fahrenheit (°F) to Celsius (°C), subtract 32 from the Fahrenheit measure and then multiply that result by 0.56.

To change from Celsius (°C) to Fahrenheit (°F), multiply the Celsius measure by 1.8 and add 32 to that result.

A comparison of some useful temperatures is given below.

	Celsius	Fahrenheit
Boiling point	100°C	212°F
Body temperature	37°C	98.6°F
Freezing point	0°C	32°F

Glossary

Many medical terms have their origins in Latin or Greek. By learning a few common derivations, you can glean the meaning of words you have never heard of before. For example, once you know that "hyper" means above normal, "glyc" means glucose, and "emia" means blood, you can easily determine that "hyperglycemia" means high blood glucose. The derivations below will help you to learn many terms presented in this glossary.

General

a- or **an-** = not, without
ana- = (build) up
ant- or **anti-** = against
ante- or **pre-** = before
bi- or **di-** = two, twice
bio- or **-biotic** = life
bovine = of cattle
calor = heat
cata- or **kata-** = (break) down
chele = claw
chroma = color
co- = with, together
dys- or **mal-** = bad, difficult, painful
endo- = inner, within, inside
epi- = upon (over)
erythro- = red
exo- = outside of, without
extra- = outside of, beyond, in addition
gen or **genesis** = producing, arising, making
homeo- = like, similar, the same, constant unchanging state
hyper- = over, above, excessive
hypo- = below, under, beneath, too little
in- = not
inter- = between, in the midst
intra- = within
lac- or **lacto-** = milk
-lysis = breaking, breakdown
macro- = large, great
malacia = softening
metallo- = metal
micro- = small
mono- = one, single
neo- = new, recent
oligo- = few, small
-osis or **-asis** = condition
para- = near
peri- = around, about
phag- or **phago-** = eat
-philia, -phil, -philic = love
-phobia = fear
phyto- = plant
poly- = many, much
pro- = for, in front of
re- = back, again
semi- = half
-stat or **-stasis-** = stationary, staying
sub- = beneath
tri- = three
xero- = dry

Body

angi- or **vaso-** = vessel
arterio- = artery
cardi-, cardiac, cardio-, or **cardial** = heart
cerebro = brain
cyst = closed sac
-cyte or **–cytic** = cell
encephalic = brain
entero- or **enteric** = intestine
fibro- = fibrous tissue
gastro- = stomach
globin = globular protein
hema-, hemo-, or **-emia** = blood
hepatic = liver
myo- = muscle
nephr- or **renal** = kidney
neuro- = nerve
osteo- = bone
pulmo- = lung
sarco- = flesh
soma = body
ure- or **-uria** = urine
vascular = blood vessels
vena = vein

Chemistry

-al = aldehyde
amino- or **amine** = containing nitrogen
-ase = enzyme
-ate = salt
carbo- = carbon (C)
glyc-, glyco-, gluc-, or **gluco-** = sweet (glucose)
glyceride = of glycerol
hydro- or **hydrate** = water
lipo- = lipid
-ol = alcohol
-ose = carbohydrate
peptide = referring to amino acids
saccha- or **sucro-** = sugar

Disease

athero- = porridge, fatty plaque
carcin- = cancer
-itis = infection, inflammation
-osis or **-asis** = condition
thrombo = clot

24-hour dietary recall: a record of foods eaten by a person for one 24-hour period.

A

A1C: a test that measures the percentage of hemoglobin that has glucose attached, which helps to diagnose diabetes and evaluate long-term glycemic control.

absorption: the uptake of nutrients by the cells of the small intestine for transport into either the blood or the lymph.

Academy of Nutrition and Dietetics: the professional organization of dietitians in the United States; formerly the American Dietetic Association.

Acceptable Daily Intake (ADI): the estimated amount of a sweetener that individuals can safely consume each day over the course of a lifetime without adverse effect.

Acceptable Macronutrient Distribution Ranges (AMDR): ranges of intakes for the energy nutrients that provide adequate energy and nutrients and reduce the risk of chronic diseases.

accredited: approved; in the case of medical centers or universities, certified by an agency recognized by the US Department of Education.

acetaldehyde (ass-et-AL-duh-hide)**:** an intermediate in alcohol metabolism.

acetyl CoA (ASS-eh-teel or ah-SEET-il, coh-AY)**:** a 2-carbon compound (acetate, or acetic acid) to which a molecule of CoA is attached.

acid controllers: medications used to prevent or relieve indigestion by suppressing production of acid in the stomach; also called *H2 blockers.*

acid-base balance: the equilibrium in the body between acid and base concentrations.

acidosis (assi-DOE-sis)**:** higher-than-normal acidity in the blood and body fluids.

acids: compounds that release hydrogen ions in a solution.

acne: a chronic inflammation of the skin's follicles and oil-producing glands, which leads to an accumulation of oils inside the ducts that surround hairs; usually associated with the maturation of young adults.

acupuncture (AK-you-PUNK-cher)**:** a technique that involves piercing the skin with long thin needles at specific anatomical points to relieve pain or illness. Acupuncture sometimes uses heat, pressure, friction, suction, or electromagnetic energy to stimulate the points.

acute malnutrition: malnutrition caused by recent severe food restriction; characterized in children by underweight for height (*wasting*).

adaptive thermogenesis: adjustments in energy expenditure related to changes in environment such as extreme cold and to physiological events such as overfeeding, trauma, and changes in hormone status.

added sugars: sugars and other kcaloric sweeteners that are added to foods during processing, preparation, or at the table. Added sugars do not include the naturally occurring sugars found in fruits and milk products.

additives: substances not normally consumed as foods but added to food either intentionally or by accident.

adequacy (dietary): providing all the essential nutrients, fiber, and energy in amounts sufficient to maintain health.

Adequate Intake (AI): the average daily amount of a nutrient that appears sufficient to maintain a specified criterion; a value used as a guide for nutrient intake when an RDA cannot be determined.

adipokines (ADD-ih-poe-kines)**:** proteins synthesized and secreted by adipose cells.

adiponectin: a protein produced by adipose cells that inhibits inflammation and protects against insulin resistance, type 2 diabetes, and cardiovascular disease.

adipose (ADD-ih-poce) **tissue:** the body's fat tissue; consists of masses of triglyceride-storing cells.

adolescence: the period from the beginning of puberty until maturity.

adrenal glands: glands adjacent to, and just above, each kidney.

adverse reactions: unusual responses to food (including intolerances and allergies).

aerobic (air-ROE-bic)**:** requiring oxygen.

aerobic physical activity: activity in which the body's large muscles move in a rhythmic manner for a sustained period of time. Aerobic activity, also called *endurance activity,* improves cardiorespiratory fitness. Brisk walking, running, swimming, and bicycling are examples.

AIDS (acquired immune deficiency syndrome): the late stage of HIV infection, in which severe complications of opportunistic infections and cancers develop.

alcohol: a class of organic compounds containing hydroxyl (OH) groups.

alcohol abuse: a pattern of drinking that includes failure to fulfill work, school, or home responsibilities; drinking in situations that are physically dangerous (as in driving while intoxicated); recurring alcohol-related legal problems (as in aggravated assault charges); or continued drinking despite ongoing social problems that are caused by or worsened by alcohol.

alcohol dehydrogenase (dee-high-DROJ-eh-nayz)**:** an enzyme active in the stomach and the liver that converts ethanol to acetaldehyde.

alcoholism: a pattern of drinking that includes a strong craving for alcohol, a loss of control and an inability to stop drinking once begun, withdrawal symptoms (nausea, sweating, shakiness, and anxiety) after heavy drinking, and the need for increasing amounts of alcohol to feel "high."

alcohol-related birth defects (ARBD): malformations in the skeletal and organ systems (heart, kidneys, eyes, ears) associated with prenatal alcohol exposure.

alcohol-related neurodevelopmental disorder (ARND): abnormalities in the central nervous system and cognitive development associated with prenatal alcohol exposure.

aldosterone (al-DOS-ter-own)**:** a hormone secreted by the adrenal glands that regulates blood pressure by increasing the reabsorption of sodium by the kidneys. Aldosterone also regulates chloride and potassium concentrations.

alkalosis (alka-LOE-sis)**:** higher-than-normal alkalinity (base) in the blood and body fluids.

alpha cells: cells of the pancreas that secrete glucagon in response to low blood glucose concentration.

alpha-lactalbumin (lact-AL-byoo-min)**:** a major protein in human breast milk, as opposed to *casein* (CAY-seen), a major protein in cow's milk.

alpha-tocopherol: the active vitamin E compound.

Alzheimer's (AHLZ-high-merz) **disease:** a degenerative disease of the brain involving memory loss and major structural changes in neuron networks; also known as *senile dementia of the Alzheimer's type (SDAT), primary degenerative dementia of senile onset,* or *chronic brain syndrome.*

amenorrhea (ay-MEN-oh-REE-ah)**:** the absence of or cessation of menstruation. *Primary amenorrhea* is menarche delayed beyond 16 years of age. *Secondary amenorrhea* is the absence of three to six consecutive menstrual cycles.

amino (a-MEEN-oh) **acids:** building blocks of proteins. Each contains an amino group, an acid group, a hydrogen atom, and a distinctive side group, all attached to a central carbon atom.

amino acid pool: the supply of amino acids derived from either food proteins or body proteins that collect in the cells and circulating blood and stand ready to be incorporated in proteins and other compounds or used for energy.

amino acid score: a measure of protein quality assessed by comparing a protein's amino acid pattern with that of a reference protein; also called the *chemical score.*

ammonia: a compound with the chemical formula NH_3, produced during the deamination of amino acids.

amniotic (am-nee-OTT-ic) **sac:** the "bag of waters" in the uterus, in which the fetus floats.

amylase (AM-ih-lace): an enzyme that hydrolyzes amylose (a form of starch). Amylase is a *carbohydrase,* an enzyme that breaks down carbohydrates.

anabolic steroids: drugs related to the male sex hormone, testosterone, that stimulate the development of lean body mass.

anabolism (an-AB-o-lism): reactions in which small molecules are put together to build larger ones. Anabolic reactions require energy.

anaerobic (AN-air-ROE-bic): not requiring oxygen.

anaphylactic (ana-fill-LAC-tic) **shock:** a life-threatening, whole-body allergic reaction to an offending substance.

androstenedione: hormones made in the adrenal glands that serve as precursors to the male sex hormone, testosterone; falsely promoted as burning fat, building muscle, and slowing aging.

anecdote: a personal account of an experience or event; not reliable scientific information.

anemia (ah-NEE-me-ah): literally, "too little blood." Anemia is any condition in which too few red blood cells are present, or the red blood cells are immature (and therefore large) or too small or contain too little hemoglobin to carry the normal amount of oxygen to the tissues. Anemia is not a disease itself but can be a symptom of many different disease conditions, including many nutrient deficiencies, bleeding, excessive red blood cell destruction, and defective red blood cell formation.

anencephaly (AN-en-SEF-a-lee): an uncommon and always fatal type of neural tube defect, characterized by the absence of a brain.

aneurysm (AN-you-rizm): an abnormal enlargement or bulging of a blood vessel (usually an artery) caused by damage to or weakness in the blood vessel wall.

angina (an-JYE-nah or AN-ji-nah): a painful feeling of tightness or pressure in and around the heart, often radiating to the back, neck, and arms; caused by a lack of oxygen to an area of heart muscle.

angiotensin I (AN-gee-oh-TEN-sin): an inactive precursor that is converted by an enzyme to yield active angiotensin II.

angiotensin II: a hormone involved in blood pressure regulation.

angiotensinogen: a precursor protein that is hydrolyzed to angiotensin I by renin.

anions (AN-eye-uns): negatively charged ions.

anorexia (an-oh-RECK-see-ah) **nervosa:** an eating disorder characterized by a refusal to maintain a minimally normal body weight and a distortion in perception of body shape and weight.

antacids: medications used to relieve indigestion by neutralizing acid in the stomach.

antagonist: a competing factor that counteracts the action of another factor. When a drug displaces a vitamin from its site of action, the drug renders the vitamin ineffective and thus acts as a vitamin antagonist.

anthropometric (AN-throw-poe-MET-rick): relating to measurement of the physical characteristics of the body, such as height and weight.

antibodies: large proteins of the blood and body fluids, produced by the immune system in response to the invasion of the body by foreign molecules (usually proteins called *antigens*). Antibodies combine with and inactivate the foreign invaders, thus protecting the body.

antidiuretic hormone (ADH): a hormone produced by the pituitary gland in response to dehydration (or a high sodium concentration in the blood) that stimulates the kidneys to reabsorb more water and therefore to excrete less. In addition to its antidiuretic effect, ADH elevates blood pressure and so is also called *vasopressin* (VAS-oh-PRES-in).

antigens: substances that elicit the formation of antibodies or an inflammation reaction from the immune system. A bacterium, a virus, a toxin, and a protein in food that causes allergy are all examples of antigens.

antioxidants: in the body, substances that significantly decrease the adverse effects of free radicals on normal physiological functions.

antioxidants: as a food additive, preservatives that delay or prevent rancidity of fats in foods and other damage to food caused by oxygen.

antipromoters: factors that oppose the development of cancer.

antiscorbutic (AN-tee-skor-BUE-tik) **factor:** the original name for vitamin C.

anus (AY-nus): the terminal outlet of the GI tract.

aorta (ay-OR-tuh): the large, primary artery that conducts blood from the heart to the body's smaller arteries.

apoptosis: cell death.

appendix: a narrow blind sac extending from the beginning of the colon that contains bacteria and lymph cells.

appetite: the integrated response to the sight, smell, thought, or taste of food that initiates or delays eating.

aquaculture: the practice of fish farming.

arachidonic (a-RACK-ih-DON-ic) **acid:** an omega-6 polyunsaturated fatty acid with 20 carbons and four double bonds; present in small amounts in meat and other animal products and synthesized in the body from linoleic acid.

ariboflavinosis (ay-RYE-boh-FLAY-vin-oh-sis): riboflavin deficiency.

aroma therapy: a technique that uses oil extracts from plants and flowers (usually applied by massage or baths) to enhance physical, psychological, and spiritual health.

arteries: vessels that carry blood from the heart to the tissues.

artesian water: water drawn from a well that taps a confined aquifer in which the water is under pressure.

arthritis: inflammation of a joint, usually accompanied by pain, swelling, and structural changes.

artificial fats: zero-energy fat replacers that are chemically synthesized to mimic the sensory and cooking qualities of naturally occurring fats but are totally or partially resistant to digestion.

artificial sweeteners: sugar substitutes that provide negligible, if any, energy; sometimes called *nonnutritive sweeteners.*

ascorbic acid: one of the two active forms of vitamin C. Many people refer to vitamin C by this name.

-ase (ACE): a suffix denoting an enzyme. The root of the word often identifies the compounds the enzyme works on. Examples include: *carbohydrase* (KAR-boe-HIGH-drase), an enzyme that hydrolyzes carbohydrates; *lipase* (LYE-pase), an enzyme that hydrolyzes lipids (fats); and *protease* (PRO-tee-ase), an enzyme that hydrolyzes proteins.

atherogenic: able to initiate or promote atherosclerosis.

atherosclerosis (ATH-er-oh-scler-OH-sis): a type of artery disease characterized by plaques (accumulations of lipid-containing material) on the inner walls of the arteries.

atoms: the smallest components of an element that have all of the properties of the element.

ATP, or **adenosine** (ah-DEN-oh-seen) **triphosphate** (try-FOS-fate): a common high-energy compound composed of a purine (adenine), a sugar (ribose), and three phosphate groups. ATP = A–P~P~P, with each ~ denoting a "high-energy" bond.

atrophic (a-TRO-fik) **gastritis** (gas-TRY-tis): chronic inflammation of the stomach accompanied by a diminished size and functioning of the mucous membranes and glands. This condition is also characterized by inadequate hydrochloric acid and intrinsic factor—two substances needed for vitamin B_{12} absorption.

atrophy (AT-ro-fee): becoming smaller; with regard to muscles, a decrease in size (and strength) because of disuse, undernutrition, or wasting diseases.

autoimmune disorder: a condition in which the body develops antibodies to its own proteins and then proceeds to destroy cells containing these proteins. In type 1 diabetes, the body develops antibodies to its insulin and destroys the pancreatic cells that produce the insulin, creating an insulin deficiency.

autonomic nervous system: the division of the nervous system that controls the body's automatic responses. Its two branches are the *sympathetic* branch, which helps the body respond to stressors from the outside environment, and the *parasympathetic* branch, which regulates normal body activities between stressful times.

avidin (AV-eh-din): the protein in egg whites that binds biotin.

ayurveda (AH-your-VAY-dah): a traditional Hindu system of improving health by using herbs, diet, meditation, massage, and yoga to stimulate the body, mind, and spirit to prevent and treat disease.

B

bacteriophages (bak-TIR-ee-oh-fayjz): viruses that infect bacteria.

balance (dietary): providing foods in proportion to one another and in proportion to the body's needs.

bariatric: pertaining to the field of medicine that specializes in treating obesity.

basal metabolic rate (BMR): the rate of energy use for metabolism under specified conditions: after a 12-hour fast and restful sleep, without any physical activity or emotional excitement, and in a comfortable setting. It is usually expressed as kcalories per kilogram body weight per hour.

basal metabolism: the energy needed to maintain life when a body is at complete digestive, physical, and emotional rest.

bases: compounds that accept hydrogen ions in a solution.

B-cells: lymphocytes that produce antibodies. *B* stands for *bone marrow,* where the B-cells develop and mature.

beer: an alcoholic beverage traditionally brewed by fermenting malted barley and adding hops for flavor.

behavior modification: the changing of behavior by the manipulation of antecedents (cues or environmental factors that trigger behavior), the behavior itself, and consequences (the penalties or rewards attached to the behavior).

belching: the release of air or gas from the stomach through the mouth.

benign: an abnormal mass of cells that is noncancerous.

beriberi: the thiamin-deficiency disease characterized by muscle weakness, edema, or both.

beta-carotene (BAY-tah KARE-oh-teen): one of the carotenoids; an orange pigment and vitamin A precursor found in plants.

beta cells: cells in the pancreas that secrete insulin in response to elevated blood glucose concentration.

beta-alanine: a nonessential amino acid that is the rate-limiting precursor for the synthesis of the dipeptide carnosine. Carnosine acts primarily as a buffer in skeletal muscle. Beta-alanine supplements raise carnosine concentrations, which enhance the muscles' buffering capacity.

beta-hydroxymethylbutryate (HMB): a metabolite of the amino acid leucine promoted to increase muscle mass and strength.

BHA and **BHT:** preservatives commonly used to slow the development of off-flavors, odors, and color changes caused by oxidation; BHA is butylated hydroxyanisole and BHT is butylated hydroxytoluene.

bicarbonate: an alkaline compound with the formula HCO_3 that is secreted from the pancreas as part of the pancreatic juice. Bicarbonate is also produced in all cell fluids from the dissociation of carbonic acid to help maintain the body's acid-base balance.

bile: an emulsifier that prepares fats and oils for digestion; an exocrine secretion made by the liver, stored in the gallbladder, and released into the small intestine when needed.

binders: chemical compounds in foods that combine with nutrients (especially minerals) to form complexes the body cannot absorb. Examples include *phytates* (FYE-tates) and *oxalates* (OCK-sa-lates).

binge drinking: pattern of drinking that raises blood alcohol concentration to 0.08 percent or higher; usually corresponds to four or more drinks for women and five or more drinks for men on a single occasion, generally within a couple of hours.

binge-eating disorder: an eating disorder characterized by recurring episodes of eating a significant amount of food in a short period of time with marked feelings of lack of control.

bioaccumulation: the accumulation of contaminants in the flesh of animals high on the food chain.

bioavailability: the rate at and the extent to which a nutrient is absorbed and used.

bioelectromagnetic medical applications: the use of electrical energy, magnetic energy, or both to stimulate bone repair, wound healing, and tissue regeneration.

biofeedback: the use of special devices to convey information about heart rate, blood pressure, skin temperature, muscle relaxation, and the like to enable a person to learn how to consciously control these medically important functions.

biofield therapeutics: a manual healing method that directs a healing force from an outside source (commonly God or another supernatural being) through the practitioner and into the client's body; commonly known as "laying on of hands."

biological value (BV): a measure of protein quality assessed by measuring the amount of protein nitrogen that is retained from a given amount of protein nitrogen absorbed.

biotechnology: the use of biological systems or organisms to create or modify products. Examples include the use of bacteria to make yogurt, yeast to make beer, and cross-breeding to enhance crop production.

biotin (BY-oh-tin): a B vitamin that functions as a coenzyme in metabolism.

blastocyst (BLASS-toe-sist): the developmental stage of the zygote when it is about 5 days old and ready for implantation.

blind experiment: an experiment in which the subjects do not know whether they are members of the experimental group or the control group.

bloating: uncomfortable abdominal fullness or distention.

blood lipid profile: results of blood tests that reveal a person's total cholesterol, triglycerides, and various lipoproteins.

body composition: the proportions of muscle, bone, fat, and other tissue that make up a person's total body weight.

body mass index (BMI): a measure of a person's weight relative to height; determined by dividing the weight (in kilograms) by the square of the height (in meters).

bolus (BOH-lus): a portion; with respect to food, the amount swallowed at one time.

bomb calorimeter (KAL-oh-RIM-eh-ter): an instrument that measures the heat energy released when foods are burned, thus providing an estimate of the potential energy (kcalories) of the foods.

bone density: a measure of bone strength. When minerals fill the bone matrix (making it dense), they give it strength.

bone meal: crushed or ground bone preparations intended to supply calcium to the diet. Calcium from bone is not well absorbed and is often contaminated with toxic minerals such as arsenic, mercury, lead, and cadmium.

bottled water: drinking water sold in bottles.

botulism (BOT-chew-lism): an often fatal foodborne illness caused by the ingestion of foods containing a toxin produced by bacteria that grow without oxygen.

bovine growth hormone (BGH): a hormone produced naturally in the pituitary gland of a cow that promotes growth and milk production; now produced for agricultural use by bacteria.

bovine spongiform encephalopathy (BOH-vine SPON-jih-form in-SEF-eh-LOP-eh-thee) or **BSE:** an often fatal illness of cattle and wild game that affects the nervous system and is transmitted to people by eating infected meats; commonly called *mad cow disease.*

bran: the protective coating around the kernel of grain, rich in nutrients and fiber.

branched-chain amino acids: the essential amino acids leucine, isoleucine, and valine, which are present in large amounts in skeletal muscle tissue; falsely promoted as fuel for exercising muscles.

breast milk bank: a service that collects, screens, processes, and distributes donated human milk.

brite adipocytes: white fat cells with brown fat cell characteristics; also called *beige adipocytes.*

brown adipose tissue: masses of specialized fat cells packed with pigmented mitochondria that produce heat instead of ATP.

brown sugar: refined white sugar crystals to which manufacturers have added molasses syrup with natural flavor and color; 91 to 96 percent pure sucrose.

buffers: compounds that keep a solution's pH constant when acids or bases are added.

bulimia (byoo-LEEM-ee-ah) **nervosa:** an eating disorder characterized by repeated episodes of binge eating usually followed by self-induced vomiting, misuse of laxatives or diuretics, fasting, or excessive exercise.

C

caffeine: a natural stimulant found in many common foods and beverages, including coffee, tea, and chocolate; may enhance endurance by stimulating fatty acid release. High doses cause headaches, trembling, rapid heart rate, and other undesirable side effects.

calbindin: a calcium-binding transport protein that requires vitamin D for its synthesis.

calcidiol: vitamin D found in the blood that is made from the hydroxylation of calciol in the liver; also called *25-hydroxyvitamin D.*

calciferol (kal-SIF-er-ol): vitamin D.

calciol: vitamin D derived from animals in the diet or made in the skin from 7-dehydrocholesterol, a precursor of cholesterol, with the help of sunlight; also called *cholecalciferol* or *vitamin* D_3.

calcitonin (KAL-seh-TOE-nin): a hormone secreted by the thyroid gland that regulates blood calcium by lowering it when levels rise too high.

calcitriol: vitamin D that is made from the hydroxylation of calcidiol in the kidneys; the biologically active hormone; also called *1,25-dihydroxyvitamin D* or *active vitamin D.*

calcium: the most abundant mineral in the body; found primarily in the body's bones and teeth.

calcium-binding protein: a protein in the intestinal cells, made with the help of vitamin D, that facilitates calcium absorption.

calcium rigor: hardness or stiffness of the muscles caused by high blood calcium concentrations.

calcium tetany (TET-ah-nee): intermittent spasm of the extremities due to nervous and muscular excitability caused by low blood calcium concentrations.

calmodulin (cal-MOD-you-lin): a calcium-binding protein that regulates such cell activities as muscle contractions.

calories: a measure of *heat* energy. Energy provided by foods and beverages is measured in *kilocalories* (1000 calories equal 1 kilocalorie), abbreviated *kcalories* or *kcal.* One kcalorie is the amount of heat necessary to raise the temperature of 1 kilogram (kg) of water 1°C. The scientific use of the term *kcalorie* is the same as the popular use of the term *calorie.*

cancers: malignant growths or tumors that result from abnormal and uncontrolled cell division.

capillaries (CAP-ill-aries): small vessels that branch from an artery. Capillaries connect arteries to veins. Exchange of oxygen, nutrients, and waste materials takes place across capillary walls.

carbohydrase (KAR-boe-HIGH-drase): an enzyme that hydrolyzes carbohydrates.

carbohydrate loading: a regimen of moderate exercise followed by the consumption of a high-carbohydrate diet that enables muscles to store glycogen beyond their normal capacities; also called *glycogen loading* or *glycogen super compensation.*

carbohydrates: compounds composed of carbon, oxygen, and hydrogen arranged as monosaccharides or multiples of monosaccharides. Most, but not all, carbohydrates have a ratio of one carbon molecule to one water molecule: $(CH_2O)_n$.

carbonated water: water that contains carbon dioxide gas, either naturally occurring or added, that causes bubbles to form in it; also called *bubbling* or *sparkling water.* The FDA defines seltzer, soda, and tonic waters as soft drinks; they are not regulated as water.

carbonic acid: a compound with the formula H_2CO_3 that results from the combination of carbon dioxide (CO_2) and water (H_2O); of particular importance in maintaining the body's acid-base balance.

carcinogenesis (CAR-sin-oh-JEN-eh-sis): the process of cancer development.

carcinogen (CAR-sin-oh-jen or car-SIN-oh-jen): a substance that can cause cancer; the adjective is *carcinogenic.*

cardiac output: the volume of blood discharged by the heart each minute; determined by multiplying the stroke volume by the heart rate. The stroke volume is the amount of oxygenated blood the heart ejects toward the tissues at each beat. Cardiac output (volume/minute) = stroke volume (volume/beat) × heart rate (beats/minute).

cardiorespiratory conditioning: improvements in heart and lung function and increased blood volume, brought about by aerobic training.

cardiorespiratory endurance: the ability to perform large-muscle, dynamic exercise of moderate to high intensity for prolonged periods.

cardiovascular disease (CVD): diseases of the heart and blood vessels throughout the body. Atherosclerosis is the main cause of CVD. When the arteries that carry blood to the heart muscle become blocked, the heart suffers damage known as *coronary heart disease (CHD).*

carnitine (CAR-neh-teen): a nonessential, nonprotein amino acid made in the body from lysine that helps transport fatty acids across the mitochondrial membrane. As a supplement, carnitine supposedly "burns" fat and spares glycogen during endurance events, but in reality it does neither.

carotenoids (kah-ROT-eh-noyds): pigments commonly found in plants and animals, some of which have vitamin A activity. The carotenoid with the greatest vitamin A activity is beta-carotene.

cartilage therapy: the use of cleaned and powdered connective tissue, such as collagen, to improve health.

catabolism (ca-TAB-o-lism): reactions in which large molecules are broken down to smaller ones. Catabolic reactions release energy.

catalyst (CAT-uh-list): a compound that facilitates chemical reactions without itself being changed in the process.

cataracts (KAT-ah-rakts): clouding of the eye lenses that impairs vision and can lead to blindness.

cathartic (ka-THAR-tik): a strong laxative.

cations (CAT-eye-uns): positively charged ions.

CDC (Centers for Disease Control and Prevention): a branch of the Department of Health and Human Services that is responsible for, among other things, monitoring foodborne diseases.

celiac disease: an intestinal disorder in which the inability to absorb the protein portion of gluten results in an immune response that damages intestinal cells; also called *celiac sprue* or *gluten-sensitive enteropathy.*

cell: the basic structural unit of all living things.

cell differentiation (DIF-er-EN-she-AY-shun): the process by which immature cells develop specific functions different from those of the original that are characteristic of their mature cell type.

cell membrane: the thin layer of tissue that surrounds the cell and encloses its contents, made primarily of lipid and protein.

central nervous system: the central part of the nervous system; the brain and spinal cord.

central obesity: excess fat around the trunk of the body; also called *abdominal fat* or *upper-body fat.*

cerebral thrombosis: a clot that blocks blood flow through an artery that feeds the brain.

certified lactation consultants: health-care providers who specialize in helping new mothers establish a healthy breastfeeding relationship with their newborn. These consultants are often registered nurses with specialized training in breast and infant anatomy and physiology.

certified nutritionist or **certified nutritional consultant** or **certified nutrition therapist**: a person who has been granted a document declaring his or her authority as a nutrition professional.

cesarean (si-ZAIR-ee-un) **delivery**: a surgically assisted birth involving removal of the fetus by an incision into the uterus, usually by way of the abdominal wall.

chaff: the outer inedible part of a grain; also called the *husk.*

CHD risk equivalents: disorders that raise the risk of heart attacks, strokes, and other complications associated with cardiovascular disease to the same degree as existing CHD. These disorders include symptomatic carotid artery disease, peripheral arterial disease, abdominal aortic aneurysm, and diabetes mellitus.

cheilosis (kye-LOH-sis or kee-LOH-sis): a condition of reddened lips with cracks at the corners of the mouth.

chelate (KEY-late): a substance that can grasp the positive ions of a mineral.

chelation (kee-LAY-shun) **therapy**: the use of ethylene diamine tetraacetic acid (EDTA) to bind with metallic ions, thus healing the body by removing toxic metals.

chiropractic (KYE-roh-PRAK-tik): a manual healing method of manipulating the spine to restore health.

chloride (KLO-ride): the major anion in the extracellular fluids of the body. Chloride is the ionic form of chlorine, Cl^-.

chlorophyll (KLO-row-fil): the green pigment of plants, which absorbs light and transfers the energy to other molecules, thereby initiating photosynthesis.

cholecalciferol (KO-lee-kal-SIF-er-ol): vitamin D derived from animals in the diet and made in the skin from 7-dehydrocholesterol, a precursor of cholesterol, with the help of sunlight; also called *vitamin* D_3.

cholecystokinin (COAL-ee-SIS-toe-KINE-in), or **CCK**: a hormone produced by cells of the intestinal wall. Target organ: the gallbladder. Response: release of bile and slowing of GI motility.

cholesterol (koh-LESS-ter-ol): one of the sterols containing a four-ring carbon structure with a carbon side chain.

cholesterol-free: less than 2 milligrams of cholesterol per serving and 2 grams or less of saturated fat and *trans* fat combined per serving.

choline (KOH-leen): a nitrogen-containing compound found in foods and made in the body from the amino acid methionine. Choline is part of the phospholipid lecithin and the neurotransmitter acetylcholine.

chromium: an essential trace mineral that enhances the activity of insulin.

chromium picolinate (CROW-mee-um pick-oh-LYN-ate): a trace mineral supplement; falsely promoted as building muscle, enhancing energy, and burning fat. *Picolinate* is a derivative of the amino acid tryptophan, which seems to enhance chromium absorption.

chromosomes: structures within the nucleus of a cell made of DNA and associated proteins. Human beings have 46 chromosomes in 23 pairs. Each chromosome has many genes.

chronic diseases: diseases characterized by slow progression and long duration. Examples include heart disease, diabetes, and some cancers.

chronic malnutrition: malnutrition caused by long-term food deprivation; characterized in children by short height for age (*stunting*).

chronological age: a person's age in years from his or her date of birth.

chylomicrons (kye-lo-MY-cronz): the class of lipoproteins that transport lipids from the intestinal cells to the rest of the body.

chyme (KIME): the semiliquid mass of partly digested food expelled by the stomach into the duodenum.

cirrhosis (seer-OH-sis): advanced liver disease in which liver cells turn orange, die, and harden, permanently losing their function; often associated with alcoholism.

cis: on the near side of; refers to a chemical configuration in which the hydrogen atoms are located on the same side of a double bond.

citric acid cycle: a series of metabolic reactions that break down molecules of acetyl CoA to carbon dioxide and hydrogen atoms; also called the *TCA cycle, tricarboxylic acid cycle,* or the *Krebs cycle.*

clinically severe obesity: a BMI of 40 or greater or a BMI of 35 or greater with additional medical problems. A less preferred term used to describe the same condition is *morbid obesity.*

clone: a genetic copy of an organism created without sexual reproduction; similar to identical twins, but born at different times.

CoA (coh-AY): coenzyme A; the coenzyme derived from the B vitamin pantothenic acid and central to energy metabolism.

coenzymes: complex organic molecules that work with enzymes to facilitate the enzymes' activity. Many coenzymes have B vitamins as part of their structures.

cofactor: a small, inorganic or organic substance that facilitates the action of an enzyme.

colitis (ko-LYE-tis): inflammation of the colon.

collagen (KOL-ah-jen): the structural protein from which connective tissues such as scars, tendons, ligaments, and the foundations of bones and teeth are made.

colonic irrigation: the popular, but potentially harmful practice of "washing" the large intestine with a powerful enema machine; also called *colonic hydrotherapy.*

colostrum (ko-LAHS-trum): a milklike secretion from the breast, present during the first few days after delivery before milk appears; rich in protective factors.

complementary and alternative medicine (CAM): diverse medical and health-care systems, practices, and products that are not currently considered part of conventional medicine; also called *adjunctive, unconventional,* or *unorthodox therapies.*

complementary proteins: two or more dietary proteins whose amino acid assortments complement each other in such a way that the essential amino acids limited in one are supplied by the other.

complex carbohydrates: polysaccharides (starches and fibers).

compound: a substance composed of two or more different atoms—for example, water (H_2O).

conception: the union of the male sperm and the female ovum; fertilization.

condensation: a chemical reaction in which water is released as two molecules combine to form one larger product.

conditionally essential amino acid: an amino acid that is normally nonessential, but must be supplied by the diet in special circumstances when the need for it exceeds the body's ability to make it.

conditionally essential nutrient: a nutrient that is normally nonessential, but must be supplied by the diet in special circumstances when the need for it exceeds the body's ability to make it.

confectioners' sugar: finely powdered sucrose, 99.9 percent pure.

congregate meals: nutrition programs that provide food for the elderly in conveniently located settings such as community centers.

conjugated linoleic acids: several fatty acids that have the same chemical formula as linoleic acid (18 carbons, two double bonds) but with different configurations (the double bonds occur on adjacent carbons).

constipation: the condition of having infrequent or difficult bowel movements.

contaminants: substances that make a food impure and unsuitable for ingestion.

contamination iron: iron found in foods as the result of contamination by inorganic iron salts from iron cookware, iron-containing soils, and the like.

control group: a group of individuals similar in all possible respects to the experimental group except for the treatment. Ideally, the control group receives a placebo while the experimental group receives a real treatment.

convenient dietary supplements: liquid mean replacers, energy drinks, energy bars, and energy gels that athletes and active people use to replenish energy and nutrients when time is limited.

conventional medicine: diagnosis and treatment of diseases as practiced by medical doctors (M.D.), doctors of osteopathy (D.O.), and allied health professionals such as physical therapists and registered nurses; also called *allopathy; Western, mainstream, orthodox,* or *regular medicine;* and *biomedicine.*

cool-down: 5 to 10 minutes of light activity, such as walking or stretching, following a vigorous workout to gradually return the body's core to near-normal temperature.

copper: an essential trace mineral that is part of many enzymes.

Cori cycle: the pathway in which glucose is metabolized to lactate (by anaerobic glycolysis) in the muscle, lactate is converted back to glucose in the liver, then glucose is returned to the muscle; named after the scientist who elucidated this pathway.

corn sweeteners: corn syrup and sugars derived from corn.

corn syrup: a syrup made from cornstarch that has been treated with acid, high temperatures, and enzymes to produce glucose, maltose, and dextrins. It may be dried and used as *corn syrup solids.* See also *high-fructose corn syrup (HFCS).*

cornea (KOR-nee-uh): the transparent membrane covering the outside of the eye.

coronary arteries: blood vessels that supply blood to the heart.

coronary heart disease (CHD): the damage that occurs when the blood vessels carrying blood to the heart (the *coronary arteries*) become narrow and occluded.

coronary thrombosis: a clot that blocks blood flow through an artery that feeds the heart muscle.

correlation (CORE-ee-LAY-shun): the simultaneous increase, decrease, or change in two variables. If A increases as B increases, or if A decreases as B decreases, the correlation is *positive.* (This does not mean that A causes B or vice versa.) If A increases as B decreases, or if A decreases as B increases, the correlation is *negative.* (This does not mean that A prevents B or vice versa.) Some third factor may account for both A and B.

cortical bone: the very dense bone tissue that forms the outer shell surrounding trabecular bone and comprises the shaft of a long bone.

coupled reactions: pairs of chemical reactions in which some of the energy released from the breakdown of one compound is used to create a bond in the formation of another compound.

covalent bonds: strong chemical bonds formed between atoms by sharing electrons.

covert (KOH-vert): hidden, as if under covers.

C-reactive protein (CRP): a protein released during the acute phase of infection or inflammation that enhances immunity by promoting phagocytosis and activating platelets. Its presence may be used to assess a person's risk of an impending heart attack or stroke.

creatine (KREE-ah-tin): a nitrogen-containing compound that combines with phosphate to form the high-energy compound creatine phosphate (or phosphocreatine) in muscles.

creatine phosphate (CP): a high-energy compound in muscle cells that acts as a reservoir of energy that can maintain a steady supply of ATP. CP provides the energy for short bursts of activity; also called *phosphocreatine.*

cretinism (CREE-tin-ism): a congenital disease characterized by mental and physical retardation and commonly caused by maternal iodine deficiency during pregnancy.

critical periods: finite periods during development in which certain events occur that will have irreversible effects on later developmental stages; usually a period of rapid cell division.

cross-contamination: the contamination of food by bacteria that occurs when the food comes into contact with surfaces previously touched by raw meat, poultry, or seafood.

cruciferous vegetables: vegetables of the cabbage family, including cauliflower, broccoli, and brussels sprouts.

crypts (KRIPTS): tubular glands that lie between the intestinal villi and secrete intestinal juices into the small intestine.

cultural competence: having an awareness and acceptance of cultures and the ability to interact effectively with people of diverse cultures.

cytokines (SIGH-toe-kines): special proteins that direct immune and inflammatory responses.

cytoplasm (SIGH-toh-plazm): the cell contents, except for the nucleus.

cytosol: the fluid of cytoplasm that contains water, ions, nutrients, and enzymes.

D

Daily Values (DV): reference values developed by the FDA specifically for use on food labels.

dead zones: oxygen-depleted areas of bodies of water in which marine life cannot survive; often caused by algae overgrowth that occurs when agricultural fertilizers and wastes enter the waterways.

deamination (dee-AM-ih-NAY-shun): removal of the amino (NH_2) group from a compound such as an amino acid.

defecate (DEF-uh-cate): to move the bowels and eliminate waste.

deficient: inadequate; a nutrient amount that fails to meet the body's needs and eventually results in deficiency symptoms.

dehydration: the condition in which body water output exceeds water input. Symptoms include thirst, dry skin and mucous membranes, rapid heartbeat, low blood pressure, and weakness.

Delaney Clause: a 1958 amendment to the Food, Drugs, and Cosmetic Act of 1938, named after Congressman James Delaney of New York that states that no substance that is known to cause cancer in animals or human beings at any dose level shall be added to foods.

***de minimis* rule:** a guideline that defines risk as a cancer rate of less than one cancer per million people exposed to a contaminant over a 70-year lifetime.

denaturation (dee-NAY-chur-AY-shun): the change in a protein's shape and consequent loss of its function brought about by heat, agitation, acid, base, alcohol, heavy metals, or other agents.

dental caries: decay of teeth.

dental plaque: a gummy mass of bacteria that grows on teeth and can lead to dental caries and gum disease.

dextrose: the name food manufacturers use for the sugar that is chemically the same as glucose; *anhydrous dextrose* is similar, differing primarily in the temperature of crystallization.

DHEA (dehydroepiandrosterone) and **androstenedione:** hormones made in the adrenal glands that serve as precursors to the male sex hormone, testosterone; falsely promoted as burning fat, building muscle, and slowing aging.

DHF (dihydrofolate): a coenzyme form of folate.

DIAAS (digestible indispensable amino acid score): a measure of protein quality similar to PDCAAS, except it determines protein digestibility at the end of the small intestine, which more accurately reflects the extent of amino acid absorption.

diabetes (DYE-uh-BEE-teez): metabolic disorders characterized by elevated blood glucose resulting from insufficient insulin, ineffective insulin, or both; the complete medical term is *diabetes mellitus* (meh-LIE-tus).

diarrhea: the frequent passage of watery bowel movements.

diet: the foods and beverages a person eats and drinks.

diet history: a record of eating behaviors and the foods a person eats.

dietary fibers: in plant foods, the *nonstarch polysaccharides* that are not digested by human digestive enzymes, although some are digested by GI tract bacteria.

dietary folate equivalents (DFE): the amount of folate available to the body from naturally occurring sources, fortified foods, and supplements, accounting for differences in the bioavailability from each source. DFE = μg food folate + (1.7 × μg synthetic folate).

Dietary Reference Intakes (DRI): a set of nutrient intake values for healthy people in the United States and Canada. These values are used for planning and assessing diets and include: Estimated Average Requirements (EAR), Recommended Dietary Allowances (RDA), Adequate Intakes (AI), and Tolerable Upper Intake Levels (UL).

dietary supplement: any pill, capsule, tablet, liquid, or powder that contains vitamins, minerals, herbs, or amino acids intended to increase dietary intake of these substances.

dietetic technician: a person who has completed a minimum of an associate's degree from an accredited university or college and an approved dietetic technician program that includes a supervised practice experience. See also *dietetic technician, registered (DTR).*

dietetic technician, registered (DTR): a dietetic technician who has passed a national examination and maintains registration through continuing professional education.

dietitian: a person trained in nutrition, food science, and diet planning. See also *registered dietitian nutritionist.*

digestion: the process by which food is broken down into absorbable units.

digestive enzymes: proteins found in digestive juices that act on food substances, causing them to break down into simpler compounds.

digestive system: all the organs and glands associated with the ingestion and digestion of food.

dioxins (dye-OCK-sins): a class of chemical pollutants created as by-products of chemical manufacturing, incineration, chlorine bleaching of paper pulp, and other industrial processes. Dioxins persist in the environment and accumulate in the food chain.

dipeptide (dye-PEP-tide): two amino acids bonded together.

diploma mills: entities without valid accreditation that provide worthless degrees.

direct calorimetry: a means of estimating energy expenditure by measuring the amount of heat released.

disaccharides (dye-SACK-uh-rides): pairs of monosaccharides linked together.

discretionary kcalories: the kcalories remaining in a person's energy allowance after consuming enough nutrient-dense foods to meet all nutrient needs for a day.

disordered eating: eating behaviors that are neither normal nor healthy, including restrained eating, fasting, binge eating, and purging.

dispensable amino acids: nonessential amino acids.

dissociates (dis-SO-see-aites): physically separates.

distilled water: water that has been vaporized and recondensed, leaving it free of dissolved minerals.

diverticula (dye-ver-TIC-you-la): sacs or pouches that develop in the weakened areas of the intestinal wall (like bulges in an inner tube where the tire wall is weak).

diverticulitis (DYE-ver-tic-you-LYE-tis): infected or inflamed diverticula.

diverticulosis (DYE-ver-tic-you-LOH-sis): the condition of having diverticula.

DNA (deoxyribonucleic acid): the double helix molecules of which genes are made.

docosahexaenoic (DOE-cossa-HEXA-ee-NO-ick) **acid (DHA):** an omega-3 polyunsaturated fatty acid with 22 carbons and six double bonds; present in fatty fish and synthesized in limited amounts in the body from linolenic acid.

dolomite: a compound of minerals (calcium magnesium carbonate) found in limestone and marble. Dolomite is powdered and is sold as a calcium-magnesium supplement. However, it may be contaminated with toxic minerals, is not well absorbed, and interferes with absorption of other essential minerals.

double-blind experiment: an experiment in which neither the subjects nor the researchers know which subjects are members of the experimental group and which are serving as control subjects, until after the experiment is over.

Down syndrome: a genetic abnormality that causes mental retardation, short stature, and flattened facial features.

drink: a dose of any alcoholic beverage that delivers ½ ounce of pure ethanol: 5 ounces of wine, 10 ounces of wine cooler, 12 ounces of beer, or 1½ ounces of liquor (80 proof whiskey, scotch, rum, or vodka).

drug: a substance that can modify one or more of the body's functions.

drug history: a record of all the drugs, over-the-counter and prescribed, that a person takes routinely.

DTR: see *dietetic technician, registered.*

duodenum (doo-oh-DEEN-um or doo-ODD-num): the top portion of the small intestine (about "12 fingers' breadth" long in ancient terminology).

dysphagia (dis-FAY-jah): difficulty swallowing.

E

eating disorders: disturbances in eating behavior that jeopardize a person's physical or psychological health.

eating pattern: customary intake of foods and beverages over time.

eclampsia (eh-KLAMP-see-ah): a condition characterized by extremely high blood pressure, elevated protein in the urine, seizures, and possibly coma.

edema (eh-DEEM-uh): the swelling of body tissue caused by excessive amounts of fluid in the interstitial spaces; seen in protein deficiency (among other conditions).

edentulous (ee-DENT-you-lus): lack of teeth.

eicosanoids (eye-COSS-uh-noyds): derivatives of 20-carbon fatty acids; biologically active compounds that help to regulate blood pressure, blood clotting, and other body functions. They include *prostaglandins* (PROS-tah-GLAND-ins), *thromboxanes* (throm-BOX-ains), and *leukotrienes* (LOO-ko-TRY-eens).

eicosapentaenoic (EYE-cossa-PENTA-ee-NO-ick) **acid** (EPA): an omega-3 polyunsaturated fatty acid with 20 carbons and five double bonds; present in fatty fish and synthesized in limited amounts in the body from linolenic acid.

electrolyte solutions: solutions that can conduct electricity.

electrolytes: salts that dissolve in water and dissociate into charged particles called ions.

electron transport chain: the final pathway in energy metabolism that transports electrons from hydrogen to oxygen and captures the energy released in the bonds of ATP; also called the *respiratory chain.*

element: a substance composed of atoms that are alike—for example, iron (Fe).

embolism (EM-boh-lizm): the obstruction of a blood vessel by an *embolus* (EM-boh-luss), or traveling clot, causing sudden tissue death.

embryo (EM-bree-oh): the developing infant from 2 to 8 weeks after conception.

emetic (em-ETT-ic): an agent that causes vomiting.

empty-kcalorie foods: a popular term used to denote foods that contribute energy but lack protein, vitamins, and minerals.

emulsifier (ee-MUL-sih-fire): a substance with both water-soluble and fat-soluble portions that promotes the mixing of oils and fats in a watery solution.

endogenous (en-DODGE-eh-nus): from within the body.

endoplasmic reticulum (en-doh-PLAZ-mic reh-TIC-you-lum): a complex network of intracellular membranes. The *rough endoplasmic reticulum* is dotted with ribosomes, where protein synthesis takes place. The *smooth endoplasmic reticulum* bears no ribosomes.

endosperm: the inner edible part of a kernel of grain, rich in starch and proteins.

enema: solution inserted into the rectum and colon to stimulate a bowel movement and empty the lower large intestine.

energy: the capacity to do work. The energy in food is chemical energy. The body can convert this chemical energy to mechanical, electrical, or heat energy.

energy balance: the energy (kcalories) consumed from foods and beverages compared with the energy expended through metabolic processes and physical activities.

energy density: a measure of the energy a food provides relative to the weight of the food (kcalories per gram).

energy-yielding nutrients: the nutrients that break down to yield energy the body can use (carbohydrate, fat, and protein).

enhanced water: water that is fortified with ingredients such as vitamins, minerals, protein, oxygen, or herbs. Enhanced water is marketed as *vitamin water, sports water, oxygenated water,* and *protein water.*

enriched: the addition to a food of specific nutrients to replace losses that occur during processing so that the food will meet a specified standard.

enteropancreatic (EN-ter-oh-PAN-kree-AT-ik) **circulation:** the circulatory route from the pancreas to the intestine and back to the pancreas.

enzymes: proteins that facilitate chemical reactions without being changed in the process; protein catalysts.

EPA (Environmental Protection Agency): a federal agency that is responsible for, among other things, regulating pesticides and establishing water quality standards.

epidemic (ep-ih-DEM-ick): the appearance of a disease (usually infectious) or condition that attacks many people at the same time in the same region.

epigenetics: the study of heritable changes in gene function that occur without a change in the DNA sequence.

epiglottis (epp-ih-GLOTT-iss): cartilage in the throat that guards the entrance to the trachea and prevents fluid or food from entering it when a person swallows.

epinephrine (EP-ih-NEFF-rin): a hormone of the adrenal gland that modulates the stress response; formerly called *adrenaline.* When administered by injection, epinephrine counteracts anaphylactic shock by opening the airways and maintaining heartbeat and blood pressure.

epithelial (ep-i-THEE-lee-ul) **cells:** cells on the surface of the skin and mucous membranes.

epithelial tissue: the layer of the body that serves as a selective barrier between the body's interior and the environment. Examples are the cornea of the eyes, the skin, the respiratory lining of the lungs, and the lining of the digestive tract.

ergocalciferol (ER-go-kal-SIF-er-ol): vitamin D derived from plants in the diet; also called *vitamin* D_2.

ergogenic (ER-go-JEN-ick) **aids:** substances or techniques used in an attempt to enhance physical performance.

erythrocyte (eh-RITH-ro-cite) **hemolysis** (he-MOLL-uh-sis): the breaking open of red blood cells (erythrocytes); a symptom of vitamin E–deficiency disease in human beings.

erythrocyte protoporphyrin (PRO-toe-PORE-fe-rin): a precursor to hemoglobin.

erythropoietin (eh-RITH-ro-POY-eh-tin): a hormone that stimulates red blood cell production.

esophageal (ee-SOFF-ah-GEE-al) **sphincter:** a sphincter muscle at the upper or lower end of the esophagus. The *lower esophageal sphincter* is also called the *cardiac sphincter* because of its proximity to the heart.

esophagus (ee-SOFF-ah-gus): the food pipe; the conduit from the mouth to the stomach.

essential amino acids: amino acids that the body requires but cannot make, and so must be obtained from the diet; also called *indispensable amino acids.*

essential fatty acids: fatty acids that the body requires but cannot make, and so must be obtained from the diet; both linoleic acid and linolenic acid are essential fatty acids.

essential nutrients: nutrients a person must obtain from food because the body cannot make them for itself in sufficient quantity to meet physiological needs; also called *indispensable nutrients.* About 40 nutrients are currently known to be essential for human beings.

Estimated Average Requirement (EAR): the average daily amount of a nutrient that will maintain a specific biochemical or physiological function in half the healthy people of a given age and gender group.

Estimated Energy Requirement (EER): the average dietary energy intake that maintains energy balance and good health in a person of a given age, gender, weight, height, and level of physical activity.

estrogens: hormones responsible for the menstrual cycle and other female characteristics.

ethanol: a particular type of alcohol found in beer, wine, and liquor; also called *ethyl alcohol.*

ethnic foods: foods associated with particular cultural groups.

excessive drinking: heavy drinking, binge drinking, or both.

exchange lists: diet-planning tools that organize foods by their proportions of carbohydrate, fat, and protein. Foods on any single list can be used interchangeably.

exercise: planned, structured, and repetitive body movements that promote or maintain physical fitness.

exogenous (eks-ODGE-eh-nus): from outside the body.

experimental group: a group of individuals similar in all possible respects to the control group except for the treatment. The experimental group receives the real treatment.

extra lean: less than 5 grams of fat, 2 grams of saturated fat and *trans* fat combined, and 95 milligrams of cholesterol per serving and per 100 grams of meat, poultry, and seafood.

extracellular fluid: fluid outside the cells. Extracellular fluid includes two main components—the interstitial fluid between cells and the intravascular fluid inside blood vessels. Extracellular fluid accounts for approximately one-third of the body's water.

F

FAD (flavin adenine dinucleotide): a coenzyme form of riboflavin.

fad diets: popular eating plans that promise quick weight loss. Most fad diets severely limit certain foods or overemphasize others (for example, never eat potatoes or pasta, or eat cabbage soup daily).

faith healing: healing by invoking divine intervention without the use of medical, surgical, or other traditional therapy.

false negative: a test result indicating that a condition is not present (negative) when in fact it is present (therefore false).

false positive: a test result indicating that a condition is present (positive) when in fact it is not (therefore false).

famine: widespread and extreme scarcity of food in an area that causes starvation and death in a large portion of the population.

FAO (Food and Agriculture Organization): an international agency (part of the United Nations) that has adopted standards to regulate pesticide use among other responsibilities.

fasting plasma glucose: a test that measures plasma glucose after a person has fasted (no food or kcaloric beverages) for at least 8 hours.

fat replacers: ingredients that replace some or all of the functions of fat and may or may not provide energy.

fat-free: less than 0.5 gram of fat per serving (and no added fat or oil); synonyms include *zero-fat, no fat,* and *nonfat.*

fats: lipids that are solid at room temperature (77°F, or 25°C).

fatty acid oxidation: the metabolic breakdown of fatty acids to acetyl CoA; also called *beta oxidation.*

fatty acids: organic compounds composed of a carbon chain with hydrogens attached and an acid group (COOH) at one end and a methyl group (CH_3) at the other end.

fatty liver: an early stage of liver deterioration seen in several diseases, including obesity and alcoholic liver disease. Fatty liver is characterized by an accumulation of fat in the liver cells.

fatty streaks: accumulations of cholesterol and other lipids along the walls of the arteries.

FDA (Food and Drug Administration): the federal agency responsible for ensuring the safety and wholesomeness of all dietary supplements and foods processed and sold in interstate commerce except meat, poultry, and eggs (which are under the jurisdiction of the USDA); inspecting food plants and imported foods; and setting standards for food composition and product labeling.

female athlete triad: a potentially fatal combination of three medical problems—disordered eating, amenorrhea, and osteoporosis.

fermentable: the extent to which bacteria in the GI tract can break down fibers to fragments that the body can use.

ferritin (FAIR-ih-tin): the iron storage protein.

fertility: the capacity of a woman to produce a normal ovum periodically and of a man to produce normal sperm; the ability to reproduce.

fetal alcohol spectrum disorder: a range of physical, behavioral, and cognitive abnormalities caused by prenatal alcohol exposure.

fetal alcohol syndrome (FAS): a cluster of physical, behavioral, and cognitive abnormalities associated with prenatal alcohol exposure, including facial malformations, growth retardation, and central nervous disorders.

fetal programming: the influence of substances during fetal growth on the development of diseases in later life.

fetus (FEET-us): the developing infant from 8 weeks after conception until term.

fibrocystic (FYE-bro-SIS-tik) **breast disease:** a harmless condition in which the breasts develop lumps, sometimes associated with caffeine consumption. In some, it responds to abstinence from caffeine; in others, it can be treated with vitamin E.

fibrosis (fye-BROH-sis): an intermediate stage of liver deterioration seen in several diseases, including viral hepatitis and alcoholic liver disease. In fibrosis, the liver cells lose their function and assume the characteristics of connective tissue cells (fibers).

filtered water: water treated by filtration, usually through *activated carbon filters* that reduce the lead in tap water, or by *reverse osmosis* units that force pressurized water across a membrane removing lead, arsenic, and some microorganisms from tap water.

fitness: the characteristics that enable the body to perform physical activity; more broadly, the ability to meet routine physical demands with enough reserve energy to rise to a physical challenge; or the body's ability to withstand stress of all kinds.

flatulence: passage of excessive amounts of intestinal gas.

flavonoids (FLAY-von-oyds): yellow pigments in foods; phytochemicals that may exert physiological effects on the body.

flaxseeds: the small brown seeds of the flax plant; valued in nutrition as a source of fiber, lignans, and omega-3 fatty acids.

flexibility: the capacity of the joints to move through a full range of motion; the ability to bend and recover without injury.

fluid balance: maintenance of the proper types and amounts of fluid in each compartment of the body fluids.

fluorapatite (floor-APP-uh-tite): the stabilized form of tooth crystal, in which fluoride has replaced the hydroxyl groups of hydroxyapatite.

fluoride: an essential trace mineral that makes teeth stronger and more resistant to decay.

fluorosis (floor-OH-sis): discoloration and pitting of tooth enamel caused by excess fluoride during tooth development.

FMN (flavin mononucleotide): a coenzyme form of riboflavin.

folate (FOLE-ate): a B vitamin; also known as folic acid, folacin, or pteroylglutamic (tare-o-EEL-glue-TAM-ick) acid (PGA). The coenzyme forms are *DHF* (*dihydrofolate*) and *THF* (*tetrahydrofolate*).

follicle-stimulating hormone (FSH): a hormone that stimulates maturation of the ovarian follicles in females and the production of sperm in males. (The ovarian follicles are part of the female reproductive system where the eggs are produced.) The release of FSH is mediated by *follicle-stimulating hormone releasing hormone (FSH–RH).*

food allergy: an adverse reaction to food that involves an immune response; also called *food-hypersensitivity reaction.*

food and nutrition history: a record of eating behaviors and the foods a person eats.

food aversions: strong desires to avoid particular foods.

food banks: facilities that collect and distribute food donations to authorized organizations feeding the hungry.

food chain: the sequence in which living things depend on other living things for food.

food cravings: strong desires to eat particular foods.

food crisis: a sharp rise in the rates of hunger and malnutrition, usually set off by a shock to either the supply of, or demand for, food and a sudden spike in food prices.

food deserts: neighborhoods and communities characterized by limited access to nutritious and affordable foods.

food frequency questionnaire: a checklist of foods on which a person can record the frequency with which he or she eats each food.

food group plans: diet-planning tools that sort foods into groups based on nutrient content and then specify that people should eat certain amounts of foods from each group.

food insecurity: limited or uncertain access to foods of sufficient quality or quantity to sustain a healthy and active life.

food insufficiency: an inadequate amount of food due to a lack of resources.

food intolerances: adverse reactions to foods that do not involve the immune system.

food poverty: hunger resulting from inadequate access to available food for various reasons, including inadequate resources, political obstacles, social disruptions, poor weather conditions, and lack of transportation.

food record: an extensive, accurate log of all foods eaten over a period of several days or weeks. A food record that includes associated information such as when, where, and with whom each food is eaten is sometimes called a *food diary.*

food recovery: collecting wholesome food for distribution to low-income people who are hungry.

food security: access to enough food to sustain a healthy and active life.

food substitutes: foods that are designed to replace other foods.

foodborne illness: an illness transmitted to human beings through food and water, caused by either an infectious agent (foodborne infection) or a poisonous substance (food intoxication); commonly known as *food poisoning.*

foods: products derived from plants or animals that can be taken into the body to yield energy and nutrients for the maintenance of life and the growth and repair of tissues.

fortified: the addition to a food of nutrients that were either not originally present or present in insignificant amounts. Fortification can be used to correct or prevent a widespread nutrient deficiency or to balance the total nutrient profile of a food.

fossil fuels: coal, oil, and natural gas.

fraudulent: the promotion, for financial gain, of devices, treatments, services, plans, or products (including diets and supplements) that alter or claim to alter a human condition without proof of safety or effectiveness.

free: "nutritionally trivial" and unlikely to have a physiological consequence; synonyms include *without, no,* and *zero.* A food that does not contain a nutrient naturally may make such a claim, but only as it applies to all similar foods (for example, "applesauce, a fat-free food").

free radical: an unstable molecule with one or more unpaired electrons.

fructose (FRUK-tose or FROOK-tose): a monosaccharide; sometimes known as *fruit sugar* or *levulose.* Fructose is found abundantly in fruits, honey, and saps.

fuel: compounds that cells can use for energy. The major fuels include glucose, fatty acids, and amino acids; other fuels include ketone bodies, lactate, glycerol, and alcohol.

full term: births occurring at 39 through 40 weeks of gestation.

functional foods: foods that have a potentially beneficial effect on health when consumed as part of a varied diet on a regular basis at effective levels.

G

g: grams; a unit of weight equivalent to about 0.03 ounces.

galactose (ga-LAK-tose): a monosaccharide; part of the disaccharide lactose.

gallbladder: the organ that stores and concentrates bile. When it receives the signal that fat is present in the duodenum, the gallbladder contracts and squirts bile through the bile duct into the duodenum.

gastric glands: exocrine glands in the stomach wall that secrete gastric juice into the stomach.

gastric juice: the digestive secretion of the gastric glands of the stomach.

gastrin: a hormone secreted by cells in the stomach wall. Target organ: the glands of the stomach. Response: secretion of gastric acid.

gastroesophageal reflux: the backflow of stomach acid into the esophagus, causing damage to the cells of the esophagus and the sensation of heartburn; commonly known as *heartburn* or *acid indigestion.*

gastroesophageal reflux disease (GERD): a condition characterized by symptoms of reflux occurring two or more times a week.

gastrointestinal (GI) tract: the digestive tract. The principal organs are the stomach and intestines.

gatekeepers: with respect to nutrition, key people who control other people's access to foods and thereby exert profound impacts on their nutrition. Examples are the spouse who buys and cooks the food, the parent who feeds the children, and the caregiver in a day-care center.

gene expression: the process by which a cell converts the genetic code into RNA and protein.

gene pool: all the genetic information of a population at a given time.

generally recognized as safe (GRAS): food additives that have long been in use and are believed to be safe. First established by the FDA in 1958, the GRAS list is subject to revision as new facts become known.

genes: sections of chromosomes that contain the instructions needed to make one or more proteins.

genetic engineering: the use of biotechnology to modify the genetic material of living cells so that they will produce new substances or perform new functions. Foods produced via this technology are called *genetically modified (GM)* or *genetically engineered (GE) foods.*

genetics: the study of genes and inheritance.

genome (GEE-nome): the complete set of genetic material (DNA) in an organism or a cell. The study of genomes is called *genomics.*

genomics: the study of all the genes in an organism and their interactions with environmental factors.

genotoxicant: a substance that mutates or damages genetic material.

geophagia: the specific craving for nonfood items such as clay, baby powder, chalk, ash, ceramics, paper, paint chips, charcoal, or dirt.

germ: the seed that grows into a mature plant, especially rich in vitamins and minerals.

gestation (jes-TAY-shun): the period from conception to birth. For human beings, the average length of a healthy gestation is 40 weeks. Pregnancy is often divided into 3-month periods, called *trimesters.*

gestational diabetes: glucose intolerance with onset or first recognition during pregnancy.

gestational hypertension: high blood pressure that develops in the second half of pregnancy and resolves after childbirth, usually without affecting the outcome of the pregnancy.

ghrelin (GRELL-in): a protein produced by the stomach cells that enhances appetite and decreases energy expenditure.

glands: cells or groups of cells that secrete materials for special uses in the body. Glands may be *exocrine* (EKS-oh-crin) *glands,* secreting their materials "out" (into the digestive tract or onto the surface of the skin), or *endocrine* (EN-doe-crin) *glands,* secreting their materials "in" (into the blood).

glossitis (gloss-EYE-tis): an inflammation of the tongue.

glucagon (GLOO-ka-gon): a hormone secreted by special cells in the pancreas in response to low blood glucose concentration. Glucagon elicits release of glucose from liver glycogen stores.

glucocorticoids: hormones from the adrenal cortex that affect the body's management of glucose.

glucogenic amino acids: amino acids that can make glucose via either pyruvate or TCA cycle intermediates.

gluconeogenesis (gloo-ko-nee-oh-JEN-ih-sis): the making of glucose from a noncarbohydrate source such as amino acids or glycerol.

glucose (GLOO-kose): a monosaccharide; sometimes known as *blood sugar* in the body or *dextrose* in foods.

glucose polymers: compounds that supply glucose, not as single molecules, but linked in chains somewhat like starch. The objective is to attract less water from the body into the digestive tract (osmotic attraction depends on the number, not the size, of particles).

glucose tolerance factors (GTF): small organic compounds that enhance insulin's actions.

gluten-free: a food that contains less that 20 parts per million of gluten from any source; synonyms include *no gluten, free of gluten*, or *without gluten.*

glycemic (gly-SEEM-ic) **index:** a method of classifying foods according to their potential for raising blood glucose.

glycemic response: the extent to which a food raises the blood glucose concentration and elicits an insulin response.

glycerol (GLISS-er-ol): an alcohol composed of a three-carbon chain, which can serve as the backbone for a triglyceride.

glycobiology: the study of sugars and their derivatives.

glycogen (GLY-ko-jen): an animal polysaccharide composed of glucose; a storage form of glucose manufactured and stored in the liver and muscles. Glycogen is not a significant food source of carbohydrate and is not counted as a dietary carbohydrate in foods.

glycolipids: sugars attached to lipids in a cell's membrane.

glycolysis (gly-COLL-ih-sis): the metabolic breakdown of glucose to pyruvate. Glycolysis does not require oxygen (anaerobic).

glycoproteins: sugars attached to a protein.

goblet cells: cells of the GI tract (and lungs) that secrete mucus.

goiter (GOY-ter): an enlargement of the thyroid gland due to an iodine deficiency, malfunction of the gland, or overconsumption of a goitrogen. Goiter caused by iodine deficiency is sometimes called *simple goiter.*

goitrogen (GOY-troh-jen): a substance that enlarges the thyroid gland and causes *toxic goiter.* Goitrogens occur naturally in such foods as cabbage, kale, brussels sprouts, cauliflower, broccoli, and kohlrabi.

Golgi (GOAL-gee) **apparatus:** a set of membranes within the cell where secretory materials are packaged for export.

good source of: the product provides between 10 and 19 percent of the Daily Value for a given nutrient per serving.

gout (GOWT): a common form of arthritis characterized by deposits of uric acid crystals in the joints.

growth hormone (GH): a hormone secreted by the pituitary that regulates the cell division and protein synthesis needed for normal growth; also called *somatotropin.* The release of GH is mediated by *GH-releasing hormone (GHRH)* and *GH-inhibiting hormone.*

H

hard water: water with a high calcium and magnesium content.

hazard: a source of danger; used to refer to circumstances in which harm is possible under normal conditions of use.

Hazard Analysis Critical Control Points (HACCP): a systematic plan to identify and correct potential microbial hazards in the manufacturing, distribution, and commercial use of food products; commonly referred to as "HASS-ip."

HDL (high-density lipoprotein): the type of lipoprotein that transports cholesterol back to the liver from the cells; composed primarily of protein.

health claims: statements that characterize the relationship between a nutrient or other substance in a food and a disease or health-related condition.

health history: an account of a client's current and past health status and disease risks.

healthy: on food labels, a food that is low in fat, saturated fat, cholesterol, and sodium and that contains at least 10 percent of the Daily Values for vitamin D, potassium, iron, calcium, protein, or fiber.

Healthy Eating Index: a measure that assesses how well a diet meets the recommendations of the *Dietary Guidelines for Americans.*

Healthy People: a national public health initiative under the jurisdiction of the US Department of Health and Human Services (DHHS) that identifies the most significant preventable threats to health and focuses efforts toward eliminating them.

heart attack: sudden tissue death caused by blockages of vessels that feed the heart muscle; also called *myocardial* (my-oh-KAR-dee-al) *infarction* (in-FARK-shun) or *cardiac arrest.*

heartburn: a burning sensation in the chest area caused by backflow of stomach acid into the esophagus; medically known as *gastroesophageal reflux.*

heat stroke: a dangerous accumulation of body heat with accompanying loss of body fluid.

heavy drinking: more than three drinks on any day for women and more than four drinks on any day for men.

heavy metals: mineral ions such as mercury and lead, so called because of their relatively high atomic weight; many heavy metals are poisonous.

Heimlich (HIME-lick) **maneuver (abdominal thrusts):** a technique for dislodging an object from the trachea of a choking person; named for the physician who developed it.

hematocrit (hee-MAT-oh-krit): the percentage of total blood volume that consists of red blood cells.

heme (HEEM) **iron:** the iron in foods that is bound to the hemoglobin and myoglobin proteins; found only in meat, fish, and poultry.

hemochromatosis (HE-moh-KRO-ma-toe-sis): a genetically determined failure to prevent absorption of unneeded dietary iron that is characterized by iron overload and tissue damage.

hemoglobin (HE-moh-GLO-bin): the globular protein of the red blood cells that transports oxygen from the lungs to tissues throughout the body; hemoglobin accounts for 80 percent of the body's iron.

hemolytic (HE-moh-LIT-ick) **anemia:** the condition of having too few red blood cells as a result of erythrocyte hemolysis.

hemophilia (HE-moh-FEEL-ee-ah): a hereditary disease in which the blood is unable to clot because it lacks the ability to synthesize certain clotting factors.

hemorrhagic (hem-oh-RAJ-ik) **disease:** a disease characterized by excessive bleeding.

hemorrhoids (HEM-oh-royds): painful swelling of the veins surrounding the rectum.

hemosiderin (heem-oh-SID-er-in): an iron-storage protein primarily made in times of iron overload.

hepatic portal vein: the vein that collects blood from the GI tract and conducts it to the liver.

hepatic vein: the vein that collects blood from the liver and returns it to the heart.

hepcidin: a hormone produced by the liver that regulates iron balance.

herbal (ERB-al) **medicine:** the use of plants to treat disease or improve health; also known as *botanical medicine* or *phytotherapy*.

hGH (human growth hormone): a hormone produced by the brain's pituitary gland that regulates normal growth and development; also called *somatotropin*.

high: on food labels, 20 percent or more of the Daily Value for a given nutrient per serving; synonyms include *rich in* or *excellent source*.

high fiber: 5 grams or more of fiber per serving. A high-fiber claim made on a food that contains more than 3 grams of fat per serving and per 100 grams of food must also declare total fat.

high food security: no indications of food-access problems or limitations.

high potency: 100% or more of the Daily Value for the nutrient in a single supplement and for at least two-thirds of the nutrients in a multinutrient supplement.

high-fructose corn syrup (HFCS): a syrup made from cornstarch that has been treated with an enzyme that converts some of the glucose to the sweeter fructose; made especially for use in processed foods and beverages, where it is the predominant sweetener. With a chemical structure similar to sucrose, HFCS has a fructose content of 42 or 55 percent, with glucose making up the remainder.

high-quality proteins: dietary proteins containing all the essential amino acids in relatively the same amounts that human beings require. They may also contain nonessential amino acids.

high-risk pregnancy: a pregnancy characterized by indicators that make it likely the birth will be surrounded by problems such as premature delivery, difficult birth, restricted growth, birth defects, and early infant death.

histamine (HISS-tah-mean or HISS-tah-men): a substance produced by cells of the immune system as part of a local immune reaction to an antigen.

HIV (human immunodeficiency virus): the virus that destroys lymphocytes and impairs immunity, eventually causing AIDS.

HMB (beta-hydroxybetamethylbutyrate): a metabolite of the branched-chain amino acid leucine promoted to increase muscle mass and strength.

homeopathy (hoh-me-OP-ah-thee): a practice based on the theory that "like cures like," that is, that substances that cause symptoms in healthy people can cure those symptoms when given in very dilute amounts.

homeostasis (HOME-ee-oh-STAY-sis): the maintenance of constant internal conditions (such as blood chemistry, temperature, and blood pressure) by the body's control systems. A homeostatic system is constantly reacting to external forces to maintain limits set by the body's needs.

honey: sugar (mostly sucrose) formed from nectar gathered by bees. Composition and flavor vary, but honey always contains a mixture of sucrose, fructose, and glucose.

hormones: chemical messengers. Hormones are secreted by a variety of glands in response to altered conditions in the body. Each hormone travels to one or more specific target tissues or organs, where it elicits a specific response to maintain homeostasis. The study of hormones and their actions is called *endocrinology*.

hormone-sensitive lipase: an enzyme inside adipose cells that responds to the body's need for fuel by hydrolyzing triglycerides so that their parts (glycerol and fatty acids) enter the general circulation and thus become available to other cells for fuel. The signals to which this enzyme responds include epinephrine and glucagon, which oppose insulin.

hourly sweat rate: the amount of weight lost plus fluid consumed during exercise per hour. One pound equals roughly 2 cups (500 milliliters) of fluid.

human carrying capacity: the maximum number of people the earth can support over time.

human genome (GEE-nome): the complete set of genetic material (DNA) in a human being.

human microbiome: the collection of microbes found in or on the human body.

hunger: the painful sensation caused by a lack of food that initiates food-seeking behavior; a consequence of food insecurity that, because of prolonged, involuntary lack of food, results in discomfort, illness, weakness, or pain that goes beyond the usual uneasy sensation.

husk: the outer inedible part of a grain; also called the *chaff*.

hydrochloric acid: an acid composed of hydrogen and chloride atoms (HCl) that is normally produced by the gastric glands.

hydrogenation (HIGH-dro-jen-AY-shun or high-DROJ-eh-NAY-shun): a chemical process by which hydrogens are added to monounsaturated or polyunsaturated fatty acids to reduce the number of double bonds, making the fats more saturated (solid) and more resistant to oxidation (protecting against rancidity). Hydrogenation produces *trans*-fatty acids.

hydrolysis (high-DROL-ih-sis): a chemical reaction in which one molecule is split into two molecules, with hydrogen (H) added to one and a hydroxyl group (OH) added to the other (from water, H_2O). The noun is *hydrolysis;* the verb is *hydrolyze*.

hydrophilic (high-dro-FIL-ick): a term referring to water-loving, or water-soluble, substances.

hydrophobic (high-dro-FOE-bick): a term referring to water-fearing, or non-water-soluble, substances; also known as *lipophilic* (fat loving).

hydrotherapy: the use of water (in whirlpools, as douches, or packed as ice, for example) to promote relaxation and healing.

hydroxyapatite (high-drox-ee-APP-ah-tite): crystals made of calcium and phosphorus.

hyperactivity: inattentive and impulsive behavior that is more frequent and severe than is typical of others a similar age; professionally called *attention-deficit/hyperactivity disorder (ADHD)*.

hypercalcemia: high blood calcium that may develop from a variety of disorders, including vitamin D toxicity. It does *not* develop from a high calcium intake.

hyperglycemia: elevated blood glucose concentrations.

hyperplastic obesity: obesity due to an increase in the *number* of fat cells.

hypertension: consistently higher-than-normal blood pressure. Hypertension that develops without an identifiable cause is known as *essential* or *primary hypertension;* hypertension that is caused by a specific disorder such as kidney disease is known as *secondary hypertension*.

hyperthermia: an above-normal body temperature.

hypertrophic obesity: obesity due to an increase in the *size* of fat cells.

hypertrophy (high-PER-tro-fee): growing larger; with regard to muscles, an increase in size (and strength) in response to use.

hypnotherapy: a technique that uses hypnosis and the power of suggestion to improve health behaviors, relieve pain, and heal.

hypoglycemia (HIGH-po-gly-SEE-me-ah): an abnormally low blood glucose concentration.

hyponatremia (HIGH-poe-na-TREE-mee-ah): a decreased concentration of sodium in the blood.

hypothalamus (high-po-THAL-ah-mus): a brain center that controls activities such as maintenance of water balance, regulation of body temperature, and control of appetite.

hypothermia: a below-normal body temperature.

hypothesis (hi-POTH-eh-sis): an unproven statement that tentatively explains the relationships between two or more variables.

hypothyroidism: underactivity of the thyroid gland that may be caused by iodine deficiency or any number of other causes.

I

ileocecal (ill-ee-oh-SEEK-ul) **valve:** the sphincter separating the small and large intestines.

ileum (ILL-ee-um): the last segment of the small intestine.

imagery: a technique that guides clients to achieve a desired physical, emotional, or spiritual state by visualizing themselves in that state.

imitation foods: foods that substitute for and resemble another food, but are nutritionally inferior to it with respect to vitamin, mineral, or protein content. If the substitute is not inferior to the food it resembles and if its name provides an accurate description of the product, it need not be labeled "imitation."

immune response: the body's reaction to foreign antigens, which neutralizes or eliminates them, thus preventing damage.

immune system: the body's natural defense against foreign materials that have penetrated the skin or mucous membranes.

immunity: the body's ability to defend itself against diseases.

immunoglobulins (IM-you-noh-GLOB-you-linz): proteins capable of acting as antibodies.

implantation (IM-plan-TAY-shun): the embedding of the blastocyst in the inner lining of the uterus.

indigestion: incomplete or uncomfortable digestion, usually accompanied by pain, nausea, vomiting, heartburn, intestinal gas, or belching.

indirect calorimetry: a means of estimating energy expenditure by measuring the amount of oxygen consumed.

indirect or **incidental additives:** substances that can get into food as a result of contact during growing, processing, packaging, storing, cooking, or some other stage before the foods are consumed; sometimes called *accidental additives.*

indispensable amino acids: essential amino acids.

indispensable nutrients: nutrients a person must obtain from food because the body cannot synthesize them in amounts sufficient to meet physiological needs; also called *essential nutrients.*

infectious diseases: diseases caused by bacteria, viruses, parasites, or other microorganisms that can be transmitted from one person to another through air, water, or food; by contact; or through vector organisms such as mosquitoes.

inflammation: an immunological response to cellular injury characterized by an increase in white blood cells.

initiators: factors that cause mutations that give rise to cancer, such as radiation and carcinogens.

inorganic: not containing carbon or pertaining to living organisms. The two classes of nutrients that are inorganic are minerals and water.

inositol (in-OSS-ih-tall): a nonessential nutrient that can be made in the body from glucose. Inositol is a part of cell membrane structures.

insoluble fibers: nonstarch polysaccharides that do not dissolve in water. Examples include the tough, fibrous structures found in the strings of celery and the skins of corn kernels.

insulin (IN-suh-lin): a hormone secreted by special cells in the pancreas in response to (among other things) elevated blood glucose concentration. Insulin controls the transport of glucose from the bloodstream into the muscle and fat cells.

insulin resistance: the condition in which a normal amount of insulin produces a subnormal effect in muscle, adipose, and liver cells, resulting in an elevated fasting glucose; a metabolic consequence of obesity that precedes type 2 diabetes.

integrative medicine: care that combines conventional and complementary therapies for which there is some high-quality scientific evidence of safety and effectiveness. Integrative medicine emphasizes the importance of the relationship between the practitioner and the patient and focuses on wellness, healing, and the whole person.

intentional food additives: additives intentionally added to foods, such as nutrients, colors, and preservatives.

intermittent claudication (klaw-dih-KAY-shun): severe calf pain caused by inadequate blood supply. It occurs when walking and subsides during rest.

Internet (the Net): a worldwide network of millions of computers linked together to share information.

interstitial (IN-ter-STISH-al) **fluid:** fluid between the cells (intercellular), usually high in sodium and chloride. Interstitial fluid is a large component of extracellular fluid.

intestinal ischemia (is-KEY-me-ah): a diminished blood flow to the intestines that is characterized by abdominal pain, forceful bowel movements, and blood in the stool.

intra-abdominal fat: fat stored within the abdominal cavity in association with the internal abdominal organs, as opposed to the fat stored directly under the skin (subcutaneous fat); also called *visceral fat.*

intracellular fluid: fluid within the cells, usually high in potassium and phosphate. Intracellular fluid accounts for approximately two-thirds of the body's water.

intravascular fluid: fluid within blood vessels.

intrinsic factor: a glycoprotein (a protein with short polysaccharide chains attached) secreted by the stomach cells that binds with vitamin B_{12} in the small intestine to aid in the absorption of vitamin B_{12}.

invert sugar: a mixture of glucose and fructose formed by the hydrolysis of sucrose in a chemical process; sold only in liquid form and sweeter than sucrose. Invert sugar is used as a food additive to help preserve freshness and prevent shrinkage.

iodide: the ion form of iodine.

iodine: an essential trace mineral that is needed for the synthesis of thyroid hormones.

ions (EYE-uns): atoms or molecules that have gained or lost electrons and therefore have electrical charges. Examples include the positively charged sodium ion (Na^+) and the negatively charged chloride ion (Cl^-).

iridology: the study of changes in the iris of the eye and their relationships to disease.

iron: an essential trace mineral that is needed for the transport of oxygen and the metabolism of energy nutrients.

iron deficiency: the state of having depleted iron stores.

iron-deficiency anemia: severe depletion of iron stores that results in low hemoglobin and small, pale red blood cells. Iron-deficiency anemia is a *microcytic* (my-cro-SIT-ic) *hypochromic* (high-po-KROME-ic) *anemia.*

iron overload: toxicity from excess iron.

irradiation: sterilizing a food by exposure to energy waves, similar to ultraviolet light and microwaves; sometimes called *ionizing radiation.*

irritable bowel syndrome: an intestinal disorder of unknown cause. Symptoms include abdominal discomfort and cramping, diarrhea, constipation, or alternating diarrhea and constipation.

IU: international units; an old measure of vitamin activity determined by biological methods (as opposed to new measures that are determined by direct chemical analyses). Many fortified foods and supplements use IU on their labels.

J

jejunum (je-JOON-um): the first two-fifths of the small intestine beyond the duodenum.

joule: a measure of *work* energy; the amount of energy expended when 1 kilogram is moved 1 meter by a force of 1 newton.

K

kcal: abbreviation of kcalories; a unit by which energy is measured.

kcalorie: a unit by which energy is measured. One kcalorie is the amount of heat necessary to raise the temperature of 1 kilogram (kg) of water 1°C. The scientific use of the term *kcalorie* is the same as the popular use of the term *calorie.*

kcalorie (energy) control: management of food energy intake.

kcalorie-free: fewer than 5 kcalories per serving.

kefir (keh-FUR): a fermented milk created by adding *Lactobacillus acidophilus* and other bacteria that break down lactose to glucose and galactose, producing a sweet, lactose-free product.

keratin (KARE-uh-tin): a water-insoluble protein; the normal protein of hair and nails.

keratinization: accumulation of keratin in a tissue; a sign of vitamin A deficiency.

keratomalacia (KARE-ah-toe-ma-LAY-shuh): softening of the cornea that leads to irreversible blindness; a sign of severe vitamin A deficiency.

Keshan (KESH-an or ka-SHAWN) **disease:** the heart disease associated with selenium deficiency; named for one of the provinces of China where it was first studied. Keshan disease is characterized by heart enlargement and insufficiency; fibrous tissue replaces the muscle tissue that normally composes the middle layer of the walls of the heart.

keto (KEY-toe) **acid:** an organic acid that contains a carbonyl group (C=O).

ketogenic amino acids: amino acids that are degraded to acetyl CoA.

ketone (KEE-tone) **bodies:** acidic compounds produced by the liver during the incomplete breakdown of fat when carbohydrate is not available.

ketosis (kee-TOE-sis): an undesirably high concentration of ketone bodies in the blood and urine.

Krebs cycle: named after the scientist who elucidated this biochemistry, a series of metabolic reactions that break down molecules of acetyl CoA to carbon dioxide and hydrogen atoms; also called the *citric acid cycle* or the *TCA cycle.*

kwashiorkor (kwash-ee-OR-core or kwash-ee-or-CORE): severe malnutrition characterized by failure to grow and develop, edema, changes in the pigmentation of hair and skin, fatty liver, anemia, and apathy.

L

lactase: an enzyme that hydrolyzes lactose.

lactase deficiency: a lack of the enzyme required to digest the disaccharide lactose into its component monosaccharides (glucose and galactose).

lactate: a 3-carbon compound produced from pyruvate during anaerobic metabolism.

lactation: production and secretion of breast milk for the purpose of nourishing an infant.

lacteals (LACK-tee-als): the lymphatic vessels of the intestine that take up nutrients and pass them to the lymph circulation.

lacto-ovo-vegetarian diet: an eating pattern that includes milk, milk products, and eggs, but excludes meat, poultry, and seafood from the diet.

lactose (LAK-tose): a disaccharide composed of glucose and galactose; commonly known as *milk sugar.*

lactose intolerance: a condition that results from the inability to digest the milk sugar lactose; characterized by bloating, gas, abdominal discomfort, and diarrhea. Lactose intolerance differs from milk allergy, which is caused by an immune reaction to the protein in milk.

lactovegetarian diet: an eating pattern that includes milk and milk products, but excludes meat, poultry, seafood, and eggs from the diet.

large intestine or colon (COAL-un): the lower portion of intestine that completes the digestive process. Its segments are the *ascending colon*, the *transverse colon*, the *descending colon*, and the *sigmoid colon.*

larynx (LAIR-inks): the entryway to the trachea that contains the vocal cords; also called the *voice box.*

laxatives: substances that loosen the bowels and thereby prevent or treat constipation.

LDL (low-density lipoprotein): the type of lipoprotein derived from very-low-density lipoproteins (VLDL) as triglycerides are removed and broken down; composed primarily of cholesterol.

lean: less than 10 grams of fat, 4.5 grams of saturated fat and *trans* fat combined, and 95 milligrams of cholesterol per serving and per 100 grams of meat, poultry, and seafood. For mixed dishes such as burritos and sandwiches, less than 8 grams of fat, 3.5 grams of saturated fat, and 80 milligrams of cholesterol per reference amount customarily consumed.

lean body mass: the body minus its fat.

lecithin (LESS-uh-thin): one of the phospholipids. Both nature and the food industry use lecithin as an emulsifier to combine water-soluble and fat-soluble ingredients that do not ordinarily mix, such as water and oil.

legumes (lay-GYOOMS or LEG-yooms): plants of the bean and pea family, with seeds that are rich in protein compared with other plant-derived foods.

leptin: a protein produced by fat cells under direction of the *ob* gene that decreases appetite and increases energy expenditure.

less: on food labels, at least 25 percent less of a given nutrient or kcalories than the comparison food; synonyms include *fewer* and *reduced.*

less cholesterol: 25 percent or less cholesterol than the comparison food (reflecting a reduction of at least 20 milligrams per serving), and 2 grams or less of saturated fat and *trans* fat combined per serving.

less fat: 25 percent or less fat than the comparison food.

less saturated fat: 25 percent or less saturated fat and *trans* fat combined than the comparison food.

let-down reflex: the reflex that forces milk to the front of the breast when the infant begins to nurse.

levulose: an older name for fructose.

license to practice: permission under state or federal law, granted on meeting specified criteria, to use a certain title (such as dietitian) and offer certain services. *Licensed dietitians* may use the initials *LD* after their names.

life expectancy: the average number of years lived by people in a given society.

life span: the maximum number of years of life attainable by a member of a species.

light or **lite:** one-third fewer kcalories than the comparison food; 50 percent or less of the fat or sodium than the comparison food; any use of the term other than as defined must specify what it is referring to (for example, "light in color" or "light in texture").

lignans: phytochemicals present in flaxseed that are converted to phytosterols by intestinal bacteria and are under study as possible anticancer agents.

limiting amino acid: the essential amino acid found in the shortest supply relative to the amounts needed for protein synthesis in the body. Four amino acids are most likely to be limiting: lysine, methionine, threonine, and tryptophan.

lingual: pertaining to the tongue.

linoleic (lin-oh-LAY-ick) **acid:** an essential fatty acid with 18 carbons and two double bonds.

linolenic (lin-oh-LEN-ick) **acid:** an essential fatty acid with 18 carbons and three double bonds.

lipases (LYE-pasez): enzymes that hydrolyze lipids (fats). *Lingual lipase* is a fat-digesting enzyme secreted from the salivary gland at the base of the tongue; *gastric lipase* is a fat-digesting enzyme secreted from the cells of the stomach.

lipids: a family of compounds that includes triglycerides, phospholipids, and sterols. Lipids are characterized by their insolubility in water. (Lipids also include the fat-soluble vitamins.)

lipoprotein-associated phospholipase A(2) or **Lp-PLA(2):** a lipoprotein-bound enzyme that generates potent proinflammatory and proatherogenic products such as oxidized free fatty acids and lysophosphatidylcholine. Lp-PLA(2) is a specific marker of plaque inflammation.

lipoprotein lipase (LPL): an enzyme that hydrolyzes triglycerides passing by in the bloodstream and directs their parts into the cells, where they can be metabolized for energy or reassembled for storage.

lipoproteins (LIP-oh-PRO-teenz): clusters of lipids associated with proteins that serve as transport vehicles for lipids in the lymph and blood.

lipotoxicity: the adverse effects of fat in nonadipose tissues.

liquor or **distilled spirits:** an alcoholic beverage traditionally made by fermenting and distilling a carbohydrate source such as molasses, potatoes, rye, beets, barley, or corn.

Listeriosis (lis-TEAR-ee-OH-sis): an infection caused by eating food contaminated with the bacterium *Listeria monocytogenes*, which can be killed by pasteurization and cooking but can survive at refrigerated temperatures; certain ready-to-eat foods, such as hot dogs and deli meats, may become contaminated after cooking or processing, but before packaging.

liver: the organ that manufactures bile, among many other functions.

longevity: long duration of life.

low: on food labels, an amount that would allow frequent consumption of a food without exceeding the Daily Value for the nutrient. A food that is naturally low in a nutrient may make such a claim, but only as it applies to all similar foods (for example, "fresh cauliflower, a low-sodium food"); synonyms include *little, few,* and *low source of.*

low birthweight (LBW): a birthweight of 5½ pounds (2500 grams) or less; indicates probable poor health in the newborn and poor nutrition status in the mother during pregnancy, before pregnancy, or both. Optimal birthweight for a full-term baby is 6½ to 8 pounds.

low cholesterol: 20 milligrams or less of cholesterol per serving and 2 grams or less of saturated fat and *trans* fat combined per serving.

low fat: 3 grams or less of fat per serving.

low food security: reduced quality of life with little or no indication of reduced food intake; formerly known as *food insecurity without hunger.*

low kcalorie: 40 kcalories or less per serving.

low saturated fat: 1 gram or less of saturated fat and less than 0.5 gram of *trans* fat per serving.

low sodium: 140 milligrams or less per serving.

low-risk pregnancy: a pregnancy characterized by factors that make it likely the birth will be normal and the infant healthy.

lumen (LOO-men): the space within a vessel such as the intestine.

lutein (LOO-teen): a plant pigment of yellow hue; a phytochemical believed to play roles in eye functioning and health.

luteinizing (LOO-tee-in-EYE-zing) **hormone (LH):** a hormone that stimulates ovulation and the development of the corpus luteum (the small tissue that develops from a ruptured ovarian follicle and secretes hormones); so called because the follicle turns yellow as it matures. In men, LH stimulates testosterone secretion. The release of LH is mediated by *luteinizing hormone–releasing hormone (LH–RH).*

lycopene (LYE-koh-peen): a pigment responsible for the red color of tomatoes and other red-hued vegetables; a phytochemical that may act as an antioxidant in the body.

lymph (LIMF): a clear yellowish fluid that is similar to blood except that it contains no red blood cells or platelets. Lymph from the GI tract transports fat and fat-soluble vitamins to the bloodstream via lymphatic vessels.

lymphatic (lim-FAT-ic) **system:** a loosely organized system of vessels and ducts that convey fluids toward the heart. The GI part of the lymphatic system carries the products of fat digestion into the bloodstream.

lymphocytes (LIM-foh-sites): white blood cells that participate in acquired immunity; B cells and T cells.

lysosomes (LYE-so-zomes): cellular organelles; membrane-enclosed sacs of degradative enzymes.

M

macrobiotic diet: a philosophical eating pattern based on mostly plant foods such as whole grains, legumes, and vegetables, with small amounts of fish, fruits, nuts, and seeds.

macrocytic: abnormally large blood cells.

macronutrients: carbohydrate, fat, and protein; the nutrients the body requires in relatively large amounts (many grams daily).

macrophages (MAK-roe-fay-jez): large phagocytic cells that serve as scavengers of the blood, clearing it of old or abnormal cells, cellular debris, and antigens.

macrosomia (mak-roh-SO-me-ah): abnormally large body size. In the case of infants, a birthweight at the 90th percentile or higher for gestational age (roughly 9 lb—or 4000 g—or more); macrosomia results from prepregnancy obesity, excessive weight gain during pregnancy, or uncontrolled gestational diabetes.

macular (MACK-you-lar) **degeneration:** deterioration of the macular area of the eye that can lead to loss of central vision and eventual blindness. The *macula* is a small, oval, yellowish region in the center of the retina that provides the sharp, straight-ahead vision so critical to reading and driving.

magnesium: a cation within the body's cells, active in many enzyme systems.

major minerals: essential mineral nutrients the human body requires in relatively large amounts (greater than 100 milligrams per day); sometimes called *macrominerals.*

malignant (ma-LIG-nant): describes a cancerous cell or tumor, which can injure healthy tissue and spread cancer to other regions of the body.

malnutrition: any condition caused by excess or deficient food energy or nutrient intake or by an imbalance of nutrients.

malt syrup: a sweetener made from sprouted barley and containing mostly maltose.

maltase: an enzyme that hydrolyzes maltose.

maltose (MAWL-tose): a disaccharide composed of two glucose units; sometimes known as *malt sugar.*

mammary glands: glands of the female breast that secrete milk.

manganese: an essential trace mineral that acts as a cofactor for many enzymes.

maple sugar: a sugar (mostly sucrose) purified from the concentrated sap of the sugar maple tree.

marasmus (ma-RAZ-mus): severe malnutrition characterized by poor growth, dramatic weight loss, loss of body fat and muscle, and apathy.

margin of safety: when speaking of food additives, a zone between the concentration normally used and that at which a hazard exists. For common table salt, for example, the margin of safety is 1/5 (five times the amount normally used would be hazardous).

marginal food security: one or two indications of food-access problems but with little or no change in food intake.

massage therapy: a healing method in which the therapist manually kneads muscles to reduce tension, increase blood circulation, improve joint mobility, and promote healing of injuries.

mastication: the process of chewing.

matrix (MAY-tricks): the basic substance that gives form to a developing structure; in the body, the formative cells from which teeth and bones grow.

matter: anything that takes up space and has mass.

Meals on Wheels: a nutrition program that delivers food for the elderly to their homes.

meat replacements: products formulated to look and taste like meat, fish, or poultry; usually made of textured vegetable protein.

medical history: an account of a patient's current and past health status and disease risks.

medication and supplement history: a record of all the drugs, over-the-counter and prescribed, as well as dietary and herbal supplements that a person takes routinely.

meditation: a self-directed technique of relaxing the body and calming the mind.

megaloblastic: abnormally large blood cells.

menadione (men-uh-DYE-own): the synthetic form of vitamin K.

menaquinone (men-ah-KWYN-own): the bacteria-produced form of vitamin K; also called *vitamin* K_2.

Menkes disease: a genetic disorder of copper transport that creates a copper deficiency and results in mental retardation, poor muscle tone, seizures, brittle kinky hair, and failure to thrive.

MEOS or **microsomal** (my-krow-SO-mal) **ethanol oxidizing system:** a system of enzymes in the liver that oxidize not only alcohol but also several classes of drugs.

metabolic syndrome: a combination of risk factors—elevated fasting blood glucose, hypertension, abnormal blood lipids, and abdominal obesity—that greatly increase a person's risk of developing coronary heart disease; also called *Syndrome X, insulin resistance syndrome,* or *dysmetabolic syndrome.*

metabolic water: water generated during metabolism.

metabolism: the sum total of all the chemical reactions that go on in living cells. *Energy metabolism* includes all the reactions by which the body obtains and expends the energy from food.

metalloenzymes (meh-TAL-oh-EN-zimes): enzymes that contain one or more minerals as part of their structures.

metallothionein (meh-TAL-oh-THIGH-oh-neen): a sulfur-rich protein that avidly binds with and transports metals such as zinc.

metastasize (me-TAS-tah-size): the spread of cancer from one part of the body to another.

methylation: the addition of a methyl group (CH_3).

MFP factor: a peptide released during the digestion of meat, fish, and poultry that enhances nonheme iron absorption.

mg: milligrams; one-thousandth of a gram.

mg NE: milligrams of niacin equivalents; a measure of niacin activity.

micelles (MY-cells): tiny spherical complexes of emulsified fat that arise during digestion; most contain bile salts and the products of lipid digestion, including fatty acids, monoglycerides, and cholesterol.

microangiopathies: disorders of the small blood vessels.

microarray technology: research tools that analyze the expression of thousands of genes simultaneously and search for particular gene changes associated with a disease. DNA microarrays are also called *DNA chips.*

microbes (MY-krobes): microscopically small organisms including bacteria, viruses, fungi, and protozoa; also called *microorganisms.*

microcytic (my-cro-SIT-ic) **hypochromic** (high-po-KROME-ic) **anemia:** small, pale red blood cells that develop in iron-deficiency anemia.

microgram (μg): one millionth of a gram.

microgram DFE (μg DFE): micrograms dietary folate equivalents; a measure of folate activity.

microgram RAE (μg RAE): micrograms retinol activity equivalents; a measure of vitamin A activity.

micronutrients: vitamins and minerals; the nutrients the body requires in relatively small amounts (milligrams or micrograms daily).

microvilli (MY-cro-VILL-ee or MY-cro-VILL-eye): tiny, hairlike projections on each cell of every villus that can trap nutrient particles and transport them into the cells; singular *microvillus.*

milk anemia: iron-deficiency anemia that develops when an excessive milk intake displaces iron-rich foods from the diet.

milliequivalents per liter (mEq/L): the concentration of electrolytes in a volume of solution. Milliequivalents reveal characteristics about the solution that are not evident when the concentration is expressed in terms of weight.

mineral oil: a purified liquid derived from petroleum and used to treat constipation.

mineral water: water from a spring or well that naturally contains at least 250 parts per million (ppm) of minerals. Minerals give water a distinctive flavor. Many mineral waters are high in sodium.

mineralization: the process in which calcium, phosphorus, and other minerals crystallize on the collagen matrix of a growing bone, hardening the bone.

minerals: inorganic elements. Some minerals are essential nutrients required in small amounts by the body for health.

misinformation: false or misleading information.

mitochondria (my-toh-KON-dree-uh): the cellular organelles responsible for producing ATP aerobically; made of membranes with enzymes mounted on them. (The singular is *mitochondrion.*)

mmol: millimoles; one thousandth of a mole, the molecular weight of a substance. To convert mmol to mg, multiply by the atomic weight of the substance.

moderate-intensity physical activity: physical activity that requires some increase in breathing and/or heart rate and expends 3.5 to 7 kcalories per minute. Walking at a speed of 3 to 4.5 miles per hour (about 15 to 20 minutes to walk 1 mile) is an example.

moderation (alcohol): up to one drink per day for women and up to two drinks per day for men.

moderation (dietary): providing enough but not too much of a substance.

molasses: the thick brown syrup produced during sugar refining. Molasses retains residual sugar and other by-products and a few minerals; blackstrap molasses contains significant amounts of calcium and iron.

molecule: two or more atoms of the same or different elements joined by chemical bonds. Examples are molecules of the element oxygen, composed of two oxygen atoms (O_2), and molecules of the compound water, composed of two hydrogen atoms and one oxygen atom (H_2O).

molybdenum (mo-LIB-duh-num): an essential trace mineral that acts as a cofactor for many enzymes.

monoglycerides: molecules of glycerol with one fatty acid attached. A molecule of glycerol with two fatty acids attached is a *diglyceride.*

monosaccharides (mon-oh-SACK-uh-rides): carbohydrates of the general formula $C_nH_{2n}O_n$ that typically form a single ring. The monosaccharides important in nutrition are *hexoses,* sugars with six atoms of carbon and the formula $C_6H_{12}O_6$.

monosodium glutamate (MSG): a sodium salt of the amino acid glutamic acid commonly used as a flavor enhancer. The FDA classifies MSG as a "generally recognized as safe" ingredient.

monounsaturated fatty acid: a fatty acid that lacks two hydrogen atoms and has one double bond between carbons; abbreviated *MUFA.* Examples include palmitoleic acid and oleic acid. A *monounsaturated fat* is composed of triglycerides in which most of the fatty acids are monounsaturated.

more: on food labels, at least 10 percent more of the Daily Value for a given nutrient than the comparison food; synonyms include *added* and *extra.*

motility (moh-TIL-ih-tee): the spontaneous movement of the GI tract muscles.

mouth: the oral cavity containing the tongue and teeth.

MSG symptom complex: an acute, temporary intolerance reaction that may occur after the ingestion of the additive MSG (monosodium glutamate). Symptoms include burning sensations, chest and facial flushing and pain, and throbbing headaches.

mucous (MYOO-kus) **membranes:** the membranes, composed of mucus-secreting cells, that line the surfaces of body tissues.

mucus (MYOO-kus): a slippery substance secreted by cells of the GI lining (and other body linings) that protects the cells from exposure to digestive juices (and other destructive agents). The lining of the GI tract with its coat of mucus is a *mucous membrane.* (The noun is *mucus;* the adjective is *mucous.*)

muscle dysmorphia (dis-MORE-fee-ah): a psychiatric disorder characterized by a preoccupation with building body mass.

muscle endurance: the ability of a muscle to contract repeatedly without becoming exhausted.

muscle power: the product of force generation (strength) and movement velocity (speed); the speed at which a given amount of exertion is completed.

muscle strength: the ability of muscles to work against resistance.

mutations: permanent changes in the DNA that can be inherited.

myoglobin: the oxygen-holding protein of the muscle cells.

N

NAD (nicotinamide adenine dinucleotide): the main coenzyme form of the vitamin niacin. Its reduced form is NADH.

NADP (the phosphate form of NAD): a coenzyme form of niacin.

nanoceuticals: substances with extremely small particles that have been manufactured by nanotechnology.

nanotechnology: a manufacturing technology that manipulates atoms to change the structure of matter.

narcotic (nar-KOT-ic): a drug that dulls the senses, induces sleep, and becomes addictive with prolonged use.

natural water: water obtained from a spring or well that is certified to be safe and sanitary. The mineral content may not be changed, but the water may be treated in other ways such as with ozone or by filtration.

naturopathic (nay-chur-oh-PATH-ick) **medicine:** a system that taps the natural healing forces within the body by integrating several practices, including traditional medicine, herbal medicine, clinical nutrition, homeopathy, acupuncture, East Asian medicine, hydrotherapy, and manipulative therapy.

nectar: a sugary fluid secreted by plants to encourage pollination by insects.

neotame (NEE-oh-tame): an artificial sweetener composed of two amino acids (phenylalanine and aspartic acid); approved for use in the United States.

net protein utilization (NPU): a measure of protein quality assessed by measuring the amount of protein nitrogen that is retained from a given amount of protein nitrogen eaten.

neural tube: the embryonic tissue that forms the brain and spinal cord.

neural tube defects: malformations of the brain, spinal cord, or both during embryonic development that often result in lifelong disability or death. The two main types of neural tube defects are *spina bifida* (literally "split spine") and *anencephaly* ("no brain").

neurofibrillary tangles: snarls of the threadlike strands that extend from the nerve cells, commonly found in the brains of people with Alzheimer's dementia.

neurons: nerve cells; the structural and functional units of the nervous system. Neurons initiate and conduct nerve impulse transmissions.

neuropeptide Y: a chemical produced in the brain that stimulates appetite, diminishes energy expenditure, and increases fat storage.

neurotransmitters: chemicals that are released at the end of a nerve cell when a nerve impulse arrives there. They diffuse across the gap to the next cell and alter the membrane of that second cell to either inhibit or excite it.

neutrophils (NEW-tro-fills): the most common of white blood cell. Neutrophils destroy antigens by phagocytosis.

niacin (NIGH-a-sin): a B vitamin. The coenzyme forms are *NAD (nicotinamide adenine dinucleotide)* and *NADP (the phosphate form of NAD).* Niacin can be eaten preformed or made in the body from its precursor, tryptophan, an essential amino acid.

niacin equivalents (NE): the amount of niacin present in food, including the niacin that can theoretically be made from its precursor, tryptophan, present in the food. 1 NE = 1 mg niacin or 60 mg tryptophan.

niacin flush: a temporary burning, tingling, and itching sensation that occurs when a person takes a large dose of nicotinic acid; often accompanied by a headache and reddened face, arms, and chest.

night blindness: slow recovery of vision after flashes of bright light at night or an inability to see in dim light; an early symptom of vitamin A deficiency.

nitrites (NYE-trites): salts added to food to prevent botulism. One example is sodium nitrite, which is used to preserve meats.

nitrogen balance: the amount of nitrogen consumed (N in) as compared with the amount of nitrogen excreted (N out) in a given period of time.

nitrosamines (nye-TROHS-uh-meens): derivatives of nitrites that may be formed in the stomach when nitrites combine with amines. Nitrosamines are carcinogenic in animals.

nonessential amino acids: amino acids that the body can make; also called *dispensable amino acids.*

nonexercise activity thermogenesis (NEAT): energy expended in everyday spontaneous activities.

nonheme iron: the iron in foods that is not bound to proteins; found in both plant-derived and animal-derived foods.

nonnutritive sweeteners: sweeteners that yield no energy (or insignificant energy in the case of aspartame).

nucleotide bases: the nitrogen-containing building blocks of DNA and RNA—cytosine (C), thymine (T), uracil (U), guanine (G), and adenine (A). In DNA, the base pairs are A–T and C–G and in RNA, the base pairs are A–U and C–G.

nucleotides: the subunits of DNA and RNA molecules, composed of a phosphate group, a 5-carbon sugar (deoxyribose for DNA and ribose for RNA), and a nitrogen-containing base.

nucleus: a major membrane-enclosed body within cells, which contains the cell's genetic material (DNA), embedded in chromosomes.

nursing bottle tooth decay: extensive tooth decay due to prolonged tooth contact with formula, milk, fruit juice, or other carbohydrate-rich liquid offered to an infant in a bottle.

nutrient claims: statements that characterize the quantity of a nutrient in a food.

nutrient density: a measure of the nutrients a food provides relative to the energy it provides. The more nutrients and the fewer kcalories, the higher the nutrient density.

nutrient profiling: ranking foods based on their nutrient composition.

nutrients: chemical substances obtained from food and used in the body to provide energy, structural materials, and regulating agents to support growth, maintenance, and repair of the body's tissues. Nutrients may also reduce the risks of some diseases.

nutrigenetics: the science of how genes affect the activities of nutrients.

nutrigenomics: the science of how nutrients affect the activities of genes.

nutrition: the science of the nutrients in foods and of their actions within the body. A broader definition includes the study of human behaviors related to food and eating.

nutrition assessment: a comprehensive analysis of a person's nutrition status that uses health, socioeconomic, drug, and diet histories; anthropometric measurements; physical examinations; and laboratory tests.

nutrition screening: the use of preliminary nutrition assessment techniques to identify people who are malnourished or are at risk for malnutrition.

nutritional genomics: the science of how nutrients affect the activities of genes (*nutrigenomics*) and how genes affect the activities of nutrients (*nutrigenetics*).

nutritionist: a person who specializes in the study of nutrition. Note that this definition does not specify qualifications and may apply not only to registered dietitian nutritionists but also to self-described experts whose training is questionable. Most states have licensing laws that define the scope of practice for those calling themselves nutritionists.

nutritive sweeteners: sweeteners that yield energy, including both sugars and sugar alcohols.

O

obese: too much body fat with adverse health effects; BMI 30 or more.

obesogenic (oh-BES-oh-JEN-ick) **environment:** all the factors surrounding a person that promote weight gain, such as increased food intake, especially of unhealthy choices, and decreased physical activity.

obligatory (ah-BLIG-ah-TORE-ee) **water excretion:** the minimum amount of water the body has to excrete each day to dispose of its wastes—about 500 milliliters (about 2 cups, or 1 pint).

oils: lipids that are liquid at room temperature (77°F, or 25°C).

olestra: a synthetic fat made from sucrose and fatty acids that provides 0 kcalories per gram; also known as *sucrose polyester.*

oligopeptide (OL-ee-go-PEP-tide): string of four to nine amino acids.

omega: the last letter of the Greek alphabet (ω), used by chemists to refer to the position of the closest double bond to the methyl (CH_3) end of a fatty acid.

omega-3 fatty acid: a polyunsaturated fatty acid in which the closest double bond to the methyl (CH_3) end of the carbon chain is three carbons away.

omega-6 fatty acid: a polyunsaturated fatty acid in which the closest double bond to the methyl (CH_3) end of the carbon chain is six carbons away.

omnivorous: an eating pattern that includes foods derived from both animals and plants.

opsin (OP-sin): the protein portion of visual pigment molecules.

oral rehydration therapy (ORT): the administration of a simple solution of sugar, salt, and water, taken by mouth, to treat dehydration caused by diarrhea.

organelles: subcellular structures such as ribosomes, mitochondria, and lysosomes.

organic: in agriculture, crops grown and processed according to USDA regulations defining the use of fertilizers, herbicides, insecticides, fungicides, preservatives, and other chemical ingredients.

organic: in chemistry, substances or molecules containing carbon-carbon bonds or carbon-hydrogen bonds that are characteristic of living organisms. The four classes of nutrients that are organic are carbohydrates, lipids (fats), proteins, and vitamins.

organic: on food labels, that at least 95 percent of the product's ingredients have been grown and processed according to USDA regulations defining the use of fertilizers, herbicides, insecticides, fungicides, preservatives, and other chemical ingredients.

organic halogens: an organic compound containing one or more atoms of a halogen—fluorine, chlorine, iodine, or bromine.

orthomolecular medicine: the use of large doses of vitamins to treat chronic disease.

osmosis: the movement of water across a membrane *toward* the side where the solutes are more concentrated.

osmotic pressure: the amount of pressure needed to prevent the movement of water across a membrane.

osteoarthritis: a painful, degenerative disease of the joints that occurs when the cartilage in a joint deteriorates; joint structure is damaged, with loss of function; also called *degenerative arthritis.*

osteoblasts: cells that build bone during growth.

osteocalcin (os-teo-KAL-sen): a calcium-binding protein in bones, essential for normal mineralization.

osteoclasts: cells that destroy bone during growth.

osteomalacia (OS-tee-oh-ma-LAY-shuh): a bone disease characterized by softening of the bones. Symptoms include bending of the spine and bowing of the legs. The disease occurs most often in adult women.

osteoporosis (OS-tee-oh-pore-OH-sis): a disease in which the bones become porous and fragile due to a loss of minerals; also called *adult bone loss.*

outbreaks: two or more cases of a similar illness resulting from the ingestion of a common food.

overload: an extra physical demand placed on the body; an increase in the frequency, duration, or intensity of an activity. A principle of training that states for a body system to improve, it must be worked at frequencies, durations, or intensities that increase by increments.

overnutrition: excess energy or nutrients.

overt (oh-VERT): out in the open and easy to observe.

overweight: body weight greater than the weight range that is considered healthy; BMI 25 to 29.9.

ovum (OH-vum): the female reproductive cell, capable of developing into a new organism upon fertilization; commonly referred to as an egg.

oxaloacetate (OKS-ah-low-AS-eh-tate): a carbohydrate intermediate of the TCA cycle.

oxidants (OKS-ih-dants): compounds (such as oxygen itself) that oxidize other compounds. Compounds that prevent oxidation are called *antioxidants,* whereas those that promote it are called *prooxidants.*

oxidation (OKS-ee-DAY-shun): the process of a substance combining with oxygen; oxidation reactions involve the loss of electrons.

oxidative stress: a condition in which the production of oxidants and free radicals exceeds the body's ability to handle them and prevent damage.

oxytocin (OCK-see-TOH-sin): a hormone that stimulates the mammary glands to eject milk during lactation and the uterus to contract during childbirth.

oyster shell: a product made from the powdered shells of oysters that is sold as a calcium supplement, but it is not well absorbed by the digestive system.

ozone therapy: the use of ozone gas to enhance the body's immune system.

P

pancreas: a gland that secretes digestive enzymes and juices into the duodenum. (The pancreas also secretes hormones into the blood that help to maintain glucose homeostasis.)

pancreatic (pank-ree-AT-ic) **juice:** the exocrine secretion of the pancreas that contains enzymes for the digestion of carbohydrate, fat, and protein as well as bicarbonate, a neutralizing agent. The juice flows from the pancreas into the small intestine through the pancreatic duct. (The pancreas also has an endocrine function, the secretion of insulin and other hormones.)

pantothenic (PAN-toe-THEN-ick) **acid:** a B vitamin. The principal active form is part of coenzyme A, called "CoA" throughout Chapter 7.

parasympathetic nervous system: the part of the autonomic nervous system that dominates during nonstressful conditions and includes such effects as normal heart rate, pupil dilation, and peristalsis.

parathyroid hormone: a hormone from the parathyroid glands that regulates blood calcium by raising it when levels fall too low; also known as *parathormone* (PAIR-ah-THOR-moan).

pasteurization: heat processing of food that inactivates some, but not all, microorganisms in the food; not a sterilization process. Bacteria that cause spoilage are still present.

pathogens (PATH-oh-jenz): microorganisms capable of producing disease.

PBB (polybrominated biphenyl) and **PCB (polychlorinated biphenyl):** toxic organic halogens used in pesticides, paints, and flame retardants.

PDCAAS (protein digestibility–corrected amino acid score): a measure of protein quality assessed by comparing the amino acid score of a food protein with the amino acid requirements of preschool-age children and then correcting for the true digestibility of the protein.

peak bone mass: the highest attainable bone density for an individual, developed during the first three decades of life.

peer review: a process in which a panel of scientists rigorously evaluates a research study to ensure that the scientific method was followed.

pellagra (pell-AY-gra): the niacin-deficiency disease, characterized by diarrhea, dermatitis, dementia, and eventually death.

pepsin: a gastric enzyme that hydrolyzes protein. Pepsin is secreted in an inactive form, *pepsinogen,* which is activated by hydrochloric acid in the stomach.

pepsinogen: an inactive compound that is activated by hydrochloric acid in the stomach to form pepsin.

peptic ulcer: a lesion in the mucous membrane of either the stomach (a *gastric ulcer*) or the duodenum (a *duodenal ulcer*).

peptidase: a digestive enzyme that hydrolyzes peptide bonds. *Tripeptidases* cleave tripeptides; *dipeptidases* cleave dipeptides.

peptide bond: a bond that connects the acid end of one amino acid with the amino end of another, forming a link in a protein chain.

percent Daily Value (%DV): the percentage of a Daily Value recommendation found in a specified serving of food for key nutrients based on a 2000-kcalorie diet.

percent fat-free: may be used only if the product meets the definition of *low fat* or *fat-free* and must reflect the amount of fat in 100 grams (for example, a food that contains 2.5 grams of fat per 50 grams can claim to be "95 percent fat-free").

perinatal: referring to the time between the twenty-eighth week of gestation and 1 month after birth.

peripheral (puh-RIFF-er-ul) **nervous system:** the peripheral (outermost) part of the nervous system; the vast complex of wiring that extends from the central nervous system to the body's outermost areas. It contains both *somatic* and *autonomic* components.

peripheral resistance: the resistance to pumped blood in the small arterial branches (arterioles) that carry blood to the tissues.

peristalsis (per-ih-STALL-sis): wavelike muscular contractions of the GI tract that push its contents along.

pernicious (per-NISH-us) **anemia:** a blood disorder that reflects a vitamin B_{12} deficiency caused by lack of intrinsic factor and characterized by abnormally large and immature red blood cells. Other symptoms include muscle weakness and irreversible neurological damage.

persistence: stubborn or enduring continuance; with respect to food contaminants, the quality of persisting, rather than breaking down, in the bodies of animals and human beings.

personal and social history: a record of a person's economic and social background, including such factors as education, income, and ethnic identity.

pesticides: chemicals used to control insects, weeds, fungi, and other pests on plants, vegetables, fruits, and animals. Used broadly, the term includes herbicides (to kill weeds), insecticides (to kill insects), and fungicides (to kill fungi).

pH: the unit of measure expressing a substance's acidity or alkalinity. The lower the pH, the higher the H^+ ion concentration and the stronger the acid. A pH above 7 is alkaline, or base (a solution in which OH^- ions predominate).

phagocytes (FAG-oh-sites): white blood cells (neutrophils and macrophages) that have the ability to ingest and destroy foreign substances.

phagocytosis (FAG-oh-sigh-TOH-sis): the process by which phagocytes engulf and destroy foreign materials.

pharmacological effect: the body's response to a large dose of a nutrient (levels commonly available only from supplements) that overwhelms some body system and acts like a drug.

pharynx (FAIR-inks): the passageway leading from the nose and mouth to the larynx and esophagus, respectively.

phenylketonuria (FEN-il-KEY-toe-NEW-ree-ah) or **PKU:** an inherited disorder characterized by failure to metabolize the amino acid phenylalanine to tyrosine.

phlebotomy: the withdrawal of blood from the body.

phosphocreatine (PC): a high-energy compound in muscle cells that acts as a reservoir of energy that can maintain a steady supply of ATP and provides the energy for short bursts of activity; also called *creatine phosphate (CP).*

phospholipid (FOS-foe-LIP-id): a compound similar to a triglyceride but having a phosphate group (a phosphorus-containing salt) and choline (or another nitrogen-containing compound) in place of one of the fatty acids.

phosphorus: a major mineral found mostly in the body's bones and teeth.

photosynthesis: the process by which green plants use the sun's energy to make carbohydrates from carbon dioxide and water.

phylloquinone (FILL-oh-KWYN-own): the plant form of vitamin K; also called *vitamin* K_1.

physical activity: bodily movement produced by muscle contractions that substantially increase energy expenditure.

physiological age: a person's age as estimated from her or his body's health and probable life expectancy.

physiological effect: the body's response to a normal dose of a nutrient (levels commonly found in foods) that provides a normal blood concentration.

physiological fuel value: the number of kcalories that the body derives from a food, in contrast to the number of kcalories determined by calorimetry.

phytic (FYE-tick) **acid:** a nonnutrient component of plant seeds; also called *phytate* (FYE-tate). Phytic acid occurs in the husks of grains, legumes, and seeds and is capable of binding minerals such as zinc, iron, calcium, magnesium, and copper in insoluble complexes in the intestine, which the body excretes unused.

phytochemicals (FIE-toe-KEM-ih-cals): nonnutrient compounds found in plants. Some phytochemicals have biological activity in the body.

phytoestrogens: phytochemicals structurally similar to human estrogen that weakly mimic or modulate estrogen's action in the body. Phytoestrogens include the isoflavones *genistein, daidzein,* and *glycitein.*

pica (PIE-ka): a craving for and consumption of nonfood substances. Pica is known as *geophagia* (gee-oh-FAY-gee-uh) when referring to eating clay, baby powder, chalk, ash, ceramics, paper, paint chips, or charcoal; *pagophagia* (pag-oh-FAY-gee-uh) when referring to eating large quantities of ice; and *amylophagia* (AM-ee-low-FAY-gee-ah) when referring to eating uncooked starch (flour, laundry starch, or raw rice).

pigment: a molecule capable of absorbing certain wavelengths of light so that it reflects only those that we perceive as a certain color.

placebo (pla-SEE-bo): an inert, harmless medication given to provide comfort and hope; a sham treatment used in controlled research studies.

placebo effect: a change that occurs in response to expectations about the effectiveness of a treatment that actually has no pharmaceutical effects.

placenta (plah-SEN-tuh): the organ that develops inside the uterus early in pregnancy, through which the fetus receives nutrients and oxygen and returns carbon dioxide and other waste products to be excreted.

plant-based diets: an eating pattern that derives most of its protein from plant products (although some animal products may be included).

plant-pesticides: pesticides made by the plants themselves.

plant sterols: phytochemicals that have structural similarities to cholesterol and lower blood cholesterol by interfering with cholesterol absorption. Plant sterols include *sterol esters* and *stanol esters.*

plaque (PLACK): an accumulation of fatty deposits, smooth muscle cells, and fibrous connective tissue that develops in the artery walls in atherosclerosis. Plaque associated with atherosclerosis is known as *atheromatous* (ATH-er-OH-ma-tus) *plaque.*

platelets: tiny, disc-shaped bodies in the blood, important in blood clot formation.

PLP (pyridoxal phosphate): the primary active coenzyme form of vitamin B_6.

point of unsaturation: the double bond of a fatty acid, where hydrogen atoms can easily be added to the structure.

polar: characteristic of a neutral molecule, such as water, that has opposite charges spatially separated within the molecule.

polypeptide: many (10 or more) amino acids bonded together.

polysaccharides: compounds composed of many monosaccharides linked together. An intermediate string of 3 to 10 monosaccharides is an *oligosaccharide.*

polyunsaturated fatty acid: a fatty acid that lacks four or more hydrogen atoms and has two or more double bonds between carbons; abbreviated *PUFA*. Examples include linoleic acid (two double bonds) and linolenic acid (three double bonds). A *polyunsaturated fat* is composed of triglycerides in which most of the fatty acids are polyunsaturated.

portion sizes: the quantity of a food served or eaten at one meal or snack; *not* a standard amount.

postpartum amenorrhea (ay-MEN-oh-REE-ah): the normal temporary absence of menstrual periods immediately following childbirth.

potable (POT-ah-bul): suitable for drinking.

potassium: the principal cation within the body's cells; critical to the maintenance of fluid balance, nerve impulse transmissions, and muscle contractions.

powdered bone: crushed or ground bone preparations intended to supply calcium to the diet. Calcium from bone is not well absorbed and is often contaminated with toxic minerals such as arsenic, mercury, lead, and cadmium.

prebiotics: food components (such as fibers) that are not digested by the human body but are used as food by the GI bacteria to promote their growth and activity.

precursors: substances that precede others; with regard to vitamins, compounds that can be converted into active vitamins; also known as *provitamins.*

prediabetes: condition in which blood glucose levels are higher than normal, but below the diagnosis of diabetes; formerly called *impaired glucose tolerance.* Prediabetes is considered a major risk factor for future diabetes and cardiovascular diseases.

preeclampsia (PRE-ee-KLAMP-see-ah): a condition characterized by high blood pressure and some protein in the urine.

preformed vitamin A: dietary vitamin A in its active form.

prehypertension: slightly higher-than-normal blood pressure, but not as high as hypertension.

prenatal alcohol exposure: subjecting a fetus to a pattern of excessive alcohol intake characterized by substantial regular use or heavy episodic drinking.

preservatives: antimicrobial agents, antioxidants, and other additives that retard spoilage or maintain desired qualities, such as softness in baked goods.

pressure ulcers: damage to the skin and underlying tissues as a result of compression and poor circulation; commonly seen in people who are bedridden or chair-bound.

preterm (premature): births occurring before 37 weeks of gestation; births occurring at 37 to 38 weeks of gestation are designated *early term.*

primary deficiency: a nutrient deficiency caused by inadequate dietary intake of a nutrient.

probiotics: living microorganisms found in foods and dietary supplements that, when consumed in sufficient quantities, are beneficial to health.

processed foods: foods that have been treated to change their physical, chemical, microbiological, or sensory properties.

proenzyme: the inactive form of an enzyme; also called a *zymogen.*

progesterone: the hormone of gestation (pregnancy).

prolactin (pro-LAK-tin): a hormone secreted from the anterior pituitary gland that acts on the mammary glands to promote the production of milk. The release of prolactin is mediated by *prolactin-inhibiting hormone (PIH).*

promoters: factors that favor the development of cancers once they have begun.

proof: a way of stating the percentage of alcohol in distilled liquor. Liquor that is 100 proof is 50 percent alcohol; 90 proof is 45 percent, and so forth.

prooxidants: substances that significantly induce oxidative stress.

proteases (PRO-tee-aces): enzymes that hydrolyze proteins.

protein digestibility: a measure of the amount of amino acids absorbed from a given protein intake.

protein efficiency ratio (PER): a measure of protein quality assessed by determining how well a given protein supports weight gain in growing rats; used to establish the protein quality for infant formulas and baby foods.

protein turnover: the degradation and synthesis of protein.

protein-sparing action: the action of carbohydrate (and fat) in providing energy that allows protein to be used for other purposes.

proteins: compounds composed of carbon, hydrogen, oxygen, and nitrogen atoms, arranged into amino acids linked in a chain. Some amino acids also contain sulfur atoms.

proteome: all proteins in a cell. The study of all proteins produced by a species is called *proteomics.*

puberty: the period in life in which a person becomes physically capable of reproduction.

public health dietitians: dietitians who specialize in providing nutrition services through organized community efforts.

public water: water from a municipal or county water system that has been treated and disinfected.

purified water: water that has been treated by distillation or other physical or chemical processes that remove dissolved solids. Because purified water contains no minerals or contaminants, it is useful for medical and research purposes.

purines: compounds of nitrogen-containing bases such as adenine, guanine, and caffeine. Purines that originate from the body are *endogenous* and those that derive from foods are *exogenous.*

pyloric (pie-LORE-ic) **sphincter:** the circular muscle that separates the stomach from the small intestine and regulates the flow of partially digested food into the small intestine; also called *pylorus* or *pyloric valve.*

pyruvate (PIE-roo-vate): a 3-carbon compound that plays a key role in energy metabolism.

Q

qi gong (chée GUNG): a Chinese system that combines movement, meditation, and breathing techniques to enhance the flow of *qi* (vital energy) in the body.

quality of life: a person's perceived physical and mental well-being.

R

rachitic (ra-KIT-ik) **rosary:** the poorly formed rib attachments that may develop in a vitamin D deficiency; literally, "the rosary of rickets."

radura: an international symbol used to identify retail foods that have been irradiated.

randomization (RAN-dom-ih-ZAY-shun): a process of choosing the members of the experimental and control groups without bias.

raw sugar: the first crop of crystals harvested during sugar processing. Raw sugar cannot be sold in the United States because it contains too much filth (dirt, insect fragments, and the like). Sugar sold as "raw sugar" domestically has actually gone through more than half of the refining steps.

RDN: see *registered dietitian nutritionist.*

Recommended Dietary Allowance (RDA): the average daily amount of a nutrient considered adequate to meet the known nutrient needs of practically all healthy people; a goal for dietary intake by individuals.

rectum: the muscular terminal part of the intestine, extending from the sigmoid colon to the anus.

reduced kcalorie: at least 25 percent fewer kcalories per serving than the comparison food.

reference protein: a standard against which to measure the quality of other proteins.

refined: the process by which the coarse parts of a food are removed. When wheat is refined into flour, the bran, germ, and husk are removed, leaving only the endosperm.

refined flour: finely ground endosperm that is usually enriched with nutrients and bleached for whiteness; sometimes called *white flour.*

reflux: a backward flow.

registered dietitian (RD): an alternative term for an RDN.

registered dietitian nutritionist (RDN): a person who has completed a minimum of a bachelor's degree from an accredited university or college, has completed approved course work and a supervised practice program, has passed a national examination, and maintains registration through continuing professional education; also called *registered dietitian (RD).*

registration: listing; with respect to health professionals, listing with a professional organization that requires specific course work, experience, and passing of an examination.

relaxin: the hormone of late pregnancy.

remodeling: the dismantling and re-formation of a structure.

renin (REN-in): an enzyme from the kidneys that hydrolyzes the protein angiotensinogen to angiotensin I, which results in the kidneys reabsorbing sodium.

rennin: an enzyme that coagulates milk; found in the gastric juice of cows, but not human beings.

replication (REP-lih-KAY-shun): repeating an experiment and getting the same results.

requirement: the lowest continuing intake of a nutrient that will maintain a specified criterion of adequacy.

residues: whatever remains. In the case of pesticides, those amounts that remain on or in foods when people buy and use them.

resistance training: the use of free weights or weight machines to provide resistance for developing muscle strength, power, and endurance; also called *weight training.* A person's own body weight may also be used to provide resistance such as when a person does push-ups, pull-ups, or abdominal crunches.

resistant starches: starches that escape digestion and absorption in the small intestine of healthy people.

resistin (ree-ZIS-tin): a protein produced by adipose cells that promotes inflammation and causes insulin resistance.

respiratory chain: the final pathway in energy metabolism that transports electrons from hydrogen to oxygen and captures the energy released in the bonds of ATP; also called the *electron transport chain.*

resting metabolic rate (RMR): similar to the basal metabolic rate (BMR), a measure of the energy use of a person at rest in a comfortable setting, but with less stringent criteria for recent food intake and physical activity. Consequently, the RMR is slightly higher than the BMR.

retina (RET-in-uh): the innermost membrane of the eye, composed of several layers, including one that contains the rods and cones.

retinal (RET-ih-nal): the aldehyde form of vitamin A.

retinoic (RET-ih-NO-ick) **acid:** the acid form of vitamin A.

retinoids (RET-ih-noyds): chemically related compounds with biological activity similar to that of retinol; metabolites of retinol.

retinol (RET-ih-nol): the alcohol form of vitamin A.

retinol activity equivalents (RAE): a measure of vitamin A activity; the amount of retinol that the body will derive from a food containing preformed retinol or its precursor, beta-carotene.

retinol-binding protein (RBP): the specific protein responsible for transporting retinol.

rheumatoid (ROO-ma-toyd) **arthritis:** a disease of the immune system involving painful inflammation of the joints and related structures.

rhodopsin (ro-DOP-sin): a light-sensitive pigment of the retina that contains the retinal form of vitamin A and the protein opsin.

riboflavin (RYE-boh-flay-vin): a B vitamin. The coenzyme forms are *FMN (flavin mononucleotide)* and *FAD (flavin adenine dinucleotide).*

ribose: a naturally occurring 5-carbon sugar needed for the synthesis of ATP.

ribosomes (RYE-boh-zomes): protein-making organelles in cells that are composed of RNA and protein.

rickets: the vitamin D–deficiency disease in children characterized by inadequate mineralization of bone (manifested in bowed legs or knock-knees, outward-bowed chest, and "beads" on ribs). A rare type of rickets, not caused by vitamin D deficiency, is known as *vitamin D–refractory rickets.*

risk: a measure of the probability and severity of harm.

risk factor: a condition or behavior associated with an elevated frequency of a disease but not proved to be causal. Leading risk factors for chronic diseases include obesity, cigarette smoking, high blood pressure, high blood cholesterol, physical inactivity, and a diet high in saturated fats and low in vegetables, fruits, and whole grains.

RNA (ribonucleic acid): a compound similar to DNA, but RNA is a single strand with a ribose sugar instead of a deoxyribose sugar and uracil instead of thymine as one of its bases.

S

safety: the condition of being free from harm or danger.

saliva: the secretion of the salivary glands. Its principal enzyme begins carbohydrate digestion.

salivary glands: exocrine glands that secrete saliva into the mouth.

salt: a compound composed of a positive ion other than H^+ and a negative ion other than OH^-. An example is sodium chloride (Na^+Cl^-).

sarcopenia (SAR-koh-PEE-nee-ah): loss of skeletal muscle mass, strength, and quality.

satiating: having the power to suppress hunger and inhibit eating.

satiation (say-she-AY-shun): the feeling of satisfaction and fullness that occurs during a meal and halts eating. Satiation determines how much food is consumed during a meal.

satiety (sah-TIE-eh-tee): the feeling of fullness and satisfaction that occurs after a meal and inhibits eating until the next meal. Satiety determines how much time passes between meals.

saturated fat-free: less than 0.5 gram of saturated fat and 0.5 gram of *trans* fat per serving.

saturated fatty acid: a fatty acid carrying the maximum possible number of hydrogen atoms—for example, stearic acid. A *saturated fat* is composed of triglycerides in which most of the fatty acids are saturated.

scurvy: the vitamin C–deficiency disease.

secondary deficiency: a nutrient deficiency caused by something other than an inadequate intake such as a disease condition or drug interaction that reduces absorption, accelerates use, hastens excretion, or destroys the nutrient.

secretin (see-CREET-in): a hormone produced by cells in the duodenum wall. Target organ: the pancreas. Response: secretion of bicarbonate-rich pancreatic juice.

sedentary: physically inactive (literally, "sitting down a lot").

segmentation (SEG-men-TAY-shun): a periodic squeezing or partitioning of the intestine at intervals along its length by its circular muscles.

selenium (se-LEEN-ee-um): an essential trace mineral that is part of an antioxidant enzyme.

senile dementia: the loss of brain function beyond the normal loss of physical adeptness and memory that occurs with aging.

senile plaques: clumps of the protein fragment beta-amyloid on the nerve cells, commonly found in the brains of people with Alzheimer's dementia.

serotonin (SER-oh-TONE-in): a neurotransmitter important in sleep regulation, appetite control, and sensory perception, among other roles. Serotonin is synthesized in the body from the amino acid tryptophan with the help of vitamin B_6.

serving sizes: the standardized quantity of a food; such information allows comparisons when reading food labels and consistency when following the *Dietary Guidelines.*

set point: the point at which controls are set (for example, on a thermostat). The set-point theory that relates to body weight proposes that the body tends to maintain a certain weight by means of its own internal controls.

sickle-cell anemia: a hereditary form of anemia characterized by abnormal sickle- or crescent-shaped red blood cells. Sickled cells interfere with oxygen transport and blood flow. Symptoms are precipitated by dehydration and insufficient oxygen (as may occur at high altitudes) and include hemolytic anemia (red blood cells burst), fever, and severe pain in the joints and abdomen.

simple carbohydrates: monosaccharides and disaccharides (the sugars).

small for gestational age (SGA): term describing an infant whose birthweight is low compared with the number of weeks in utero, often reflecting growth failure.

small intestine: a 10-foot length of small-diameter intestine that is the major site of digestion of food and absorption of nutrients. Its segments are the *duodenum, jejunum,* and *ileum.*

sodium: the principal cation in the extracellular fluids of the body; critical to the maintenance of fluid balance, nerve impulse transmissions, and muscle contractions.

sodium bicarbonate (baking soda): a white crystalline powder that is used to buffer acid that accumulates in the muscles and blood during high-intensity exercise.

sodium-free and **salt-free:** less than 5 milligrams of sodium per serving.

soft water: water with a high sodium or potassium content.

solanine (SOH-lah-neen): a poisonous narcotic-like substance present in potato skins and sprouts.

solid fats: fats that are not usually liquid at room temperature; commonly found in most foods derived from animals and vegetable oils that have been hydrogenated. Solid fats typically contain more saturated and *trans* fats than most oils.

soluble fibers: nonstarch polysaccharides that dissolve in water to form a gel. An example is pectin from fruit, which is used to thicken jellies.

solutes (SOLL-yutes): the substances that are dissolved in a solution. The number of molecules in a given volume of fluid is the *solute concentration.*

somatic (so-MAT-ick) **nervous system:** the division of the nervous system that controls the voluntary muscles, as distinguished from the autonomic nervous system, which controls involuntary functions.

somatostatin (GHIH): a hormone that inhibits the release of growth hormone; the opposite of *somatotropin (GH).*

sperm: the male reproductive cell, capable of fertilizing an ovum.

sphincter (SFINK-ter): a circular muscle surrounding, and able to close, a body opening. Sphincters are found at specific points along the GI tract and regulate the flow of food particles.

spina (SPY-nah) **bifida** (BIFF-ih-dah): one of the most common types of neural tube defects, characterized by the incomplete closure of the spinal cord and its bony encasement.

sports anemia: a transient condition of low hemoglobin in the blood, associated with the early stages of sports training or other strenuous activity.

spring water: water originating from an underground spring or well. It may be bubbly (carbonated), or "flat" or "still," meaning not carbonated. Brand names such as "Spring Pure" do not necessarily mean that the water comes from a spring.

starches: plant polysaccharides composed of many glucose molecules.

sterile: free of microorganisms, such as bacteria.

sterols (STARE-ols or STEER-ols): compounds containing a four-ring carbon structure with any of a variety of side chains attached.

stomach: a muscular, elastic, saclike portion of the digestive tract that grinds and churns swallowed food, mixing it with acid and enzymes to form chyme.

stools: waste matter discharged from the colon; also called *feces* (FEE-seez).

stress: any threat to a person's well-being; a demand placed on the body to adapt.

stress fractures: bone damage or breaks caused by stress on bone surfaces during exercise.

stress response: the body's response to stress, mediated by both nerves and hormones.

stressors: environmental elements, physical or psychological, that cause stress.

stroke: an event in which the blood flow to a part of the brain is cut off; also called *cerebrovascular accident (CVA).*

structure-function claims: statements that characterize the relationship between a nutrient or other substance in a food and its role in the body.

subclavian (sub-KLAY-vee-an) **vein:** the vein that provides passageway from the lymphatic system to the vascular system.

subclinical deficiency: a deficiency in the early stages, before the outward signs have appeared.

subcutaneous fat: fat stored directly under the skin.

subjects: the people or animals participating in a research project.

successful weight-loss maintenance: achieving a weight loss of at least 5 to 10 percent of initial body weight and maintaining the loss for at least 1 year.

sucrase: an enzyme that hydrolyzes sucrose.

sucrose (SUE-krose): a disaccharide composed of glucose and fructose; commonly known as *table sugar, beet sugar,* or *cane sugar.* Sucrose also occurs in many fruits and some vegetables and grains.

sudden infant death syndrome (SIDS): the unexpected and unexplained death of an apparently well infant; the most common cause of death of infants between the second week and the end of the first year of life; also called *crib death.*

sugar alcohols: sugarlike compounds that can be derived from fruits or commercially produced from dextrose; also called *polyols.* Examples include *erythritol, isomalt, lactitol, maltitol, mannitol, sorbitol,* and *xylitol.*

sugar-free: less than 0.5 gram of sugar per serving.

sugars: simple carbohydrates composed of monosaccharides, disaccharides, or both.

sulfate: a salt produced from the oxidation of sulfur.

sulfites: salts containing sulfur that are added to foods to prevent spoilage.

sulfur: a mineral present in the body as part of some proteins.

sushi: vinegar-flavored rice and seafood, typically wrapped in seaweed and stuffed with colorful vegetables. Some sushi is stuffed with raw fish; other varieties contain cooked seafood.

sustainable: able to continue indefinitely; using resources at such a rate that the earth can keep on replacing them and producing pollutants at a rate with which the environment and human cleanup efforts can keep pace, so that no net accumulation of pollution occurs.

sustainable agriculture: ability to produce food indefinitely, with little or no harm to the environment.

sympathetic nervous system: the part of the autonomic nervous system that dominates during stressful conditions and includes such effects as increased heart rate, dilated pupils, slowed peristalsis, and secretion of epinephrine and norepinephrine.

symptomatic allergy: an immune response that produces antibodies and symptoms.

synergistic (SIN-er-JIS-tick): multiple factors operating together in such a way that their combined effects are greater than the sum of their individual effects.

T

tagatose (TAG-ah-tose): poorly absorbed monosaccharide similar in structure to fructose; naturally occurring or derived from lactose.

TCA cycle or **tricarboxylic** (try-car-box-ILL-ick) **acid cycle:** a series of metabolic reactions that break down molecules of acetyl CoA to carbon dioxide and hydrogen atoms; also called the *citric acid cycle* or the *Krebs cycle* after the biochemist who elucidated its reactions.

T-cells: lymphocytes that attack antigens. *T* stands for the *thymus gland,* where the T-cells mature.

tempeh (TEM-pay): a fermented soybean food, rich in protein and fiber.

teratogen (ter-AT-oh-jen): a substance that causes abnormal fetal development and birth defects.

teratogenic (ter-AT-oh-jen-ik): causing abnormal fetal development and birth defects.

testosterone: a steroid hormone from the testicles, or testes. The steroids are chemically related to, and some are derived from, the lipid cholesterol.

textured vegetable protein: processed soybean protein used in vegetarian products such as soy burgers.

theory: a tentative explanation that integrates many and diverse findings to further the understanding of a defined topic.

thermic effect of food (TEF): an estimation of the energy required to process food (digest, absorb, transport, metabolize, and store ingested nutrients); also called the *specific dynamic effect (SDE)* of food or the *specific dynamic activity (SDA)* of food. The sum of the TEF and any increase in the metabolic rate due to overeating is known as *diet-induced thermogenesis (DIT).*

thermogenesis: the generation of heat; used in physiology and nutrition studies as an index of how much energy the body is expending.

THF (tetrahydrofolate): a coenzyme form of folate.

thiamin (THIGH-ah-min): a B vitamin. The coenzyme form is *TPP (thiamin pyrophosphate).*

thirst: a conscious desire to drink.

thoracic (thor-ASS-ic) **duct:** the main lymphatic vessel that collects lymph and drains into the left subclavian vein.

thrombosis (throm-BOH-sis): the formation of a *thrombus* (THROM-bus), or a blood clot, that may obstruct a blood vessel, causing gradual tissue death.

thyroid-stimulating hormone (TSH): a hormone secreted by the pituitary that stimulates the thyroid gland to secrete its hormones—thyroxine and triiodothyronine. The release of TSH is mediated by *TSH-releasing hormone (TRH).*

thyrotropin: another name for thyroid-stimulating hormone (TSH).

tocopherols (tuh-KOFF-uh-rawls): members of the vitamin E family having the chemical structure of a complex ring structure with a long saturated side chain.

tocotrienols (TOE-koh-try-EE-nawls): members of the vitamin E family having the chemical structure of a complex ring structure with a long unsaturated side chain.

tofu (TOE-foo): a curd made from soybeans, rich in protein and often fortified with calcium; used in many Asian and vegetarian dishes in place of meat.

Tolerable Upper Intake Level (UL): the maximum daily amount of a nutrient that appears safe for most healthy people and beyond which there is an increased risk of adverse health effects.

tolerance level: the maximum amount of residue permitted in a food when a pesticide is used according to the label directions.

toxicity: the ability of a substance to harm living organisms. All substances are toxic if high enough concentrations are used.

TPP (thiamin pyrophosphate): the coenzyme form of thiamin.

trabecular (tra-BECK-you-lar) **bone:** the lacy inner structure of calcium crystals that supports the bone's structure and provides a calcium storage bank.

trace minerals: essential mineral nutrients the human body requires in relatively small amounts (less than 100 milligrams per day); sometimes called *microminerals.*

trachea (TRAKE-ee-uh): the air passageway from the larynx to the lungs; also called the *windpipe.*

***trans*:** on the other side of; refers to a chemical configuration in which the hydrogen atoms are located on opposite sides of a double bond.

***trans* fat-free:** less than 0.5 gram of *trans* fat and less than 0.5 gram of saturated fat per serving.

transamination (TRANS-am-ih-NAY-shun): the transfer of an amino group from one amino acid to a keto acid, producing a new nonessential amino acid and a new keto acid.

transcription: the process of messenger RNA being made from a template of DNA.

transcription factors: proteins that bind to specific sites in DNA and alter gene expression.

***trans*-fatty acids:** fatty acids with hydrogens on opposite sides of the double bond.

transferrin (trans-FAIR-in): the iron transport protein.

transient ischemic (is-KEY-mik) **attack (TIA):** a temporary reduction in blood flow to the brain, which causes temporary symptoms that vary depending on the part of the brain affected. Common symptoms include light-headedness, visual disturbances, paralysis, staggering, numbness, and inability to swallow.

translation: the process of messenger RNA directing the sequence of amino acids and synthesis of proteins.

travelers' diarrhea: nausea, vomiting, and diarrhea caused by consuming food or water contaminated by any of several organisms, most commonly, *E. coli, Shigella, Campylobacter jejuni,* and *Salmonella.*

triglycerides (try-GLISS-er-rides): the chief form of fat in the diet and the major storage form of fat in the body; composed of a molecule of glycerol with three fatty acids attached; also called *triacylglycerols* (try-ay-seel-GLISS-er-ols).

tripeptide: three amino acids bonded together.

tumor: an abnormal tissue mass with no physiological function; also called a *neoplasm* (NEE-oh-plazm).

turbinado (ter-bih-NOD-oh) **sugar:** sugar produced using the same refining process as white sugar, but without the bleaching and anticaking treatment. Traces of molasses give turbinado its sandy color.

type 1 diabetes: the less common type of diabetes in which the pancreas produces little to no insulin. Type 1 diabetes usually results from autoimmune destruction of pancreatic beta cells.

type 2 diabetes: the more common type of diabetes in which the cells fail to respond to insulin. Type 2 diabetes usually accompanies obesity and results from insulin resistance coupled with insufficient insulin secretion.

U

ulcer: a lesion of the skin or mucous membranes characterized by inflammation and damaged tissues. See also *peptic ulcer.*

ultrahigh temperature (UHT) treatment: sterilizing a food by brief exposure to temperatures above those normally used.

umbilical (um-BILL-ih-cul) **cord:** the ropelike structure through which the fetus's veins and arteries reach the placenta; the route of nourishment and oxygen to the fetus and the route of waste disposal from the fetus. The scar in the middle of the abdomen that marks the former attachment of the umbilical cord is the *umbilicus* (um-BILL-ih-cus), commonly known as the "belly button."

uncoupled reactions: chemical reactions in which energy is released as heat.

undernutrition: deficient energy or nutrients.

underweight: body weight lower than the weight range that is considered healthy; BMI less than 18.5.

unsaturated fatty acid: a fatty acid that lacks hydrogen atoms and has at least one double bond between carbons (includes monounsaturated and polyunsaturated fatty acids). An *unsaturated fat* is composed of triglycerides in which most of the fatty acids are unsaturated.

urea (you-REE-uh): the principal nitrogen-excretion product of protein metabolism. Two ammonia fragments are combined with carbon dioxide to form urea.

USDA (US Department of Agriculture): the federal agency responsible for enforcing standards for the wholesomeness and quality of meat, poultry, and eggs produced in the United States; conducting nutrition research; and educating the public about nutrition.

uterus (YOU-ter-us): the muscular organ within which the infant develops before birth.

V

validity (va-LID-ih-tee): having the quality of being founded on fact or evidence.

variables: factors that change. A variable may depend on another variable (for example, a child's height depends on his age), or it may be independent (for example, a child's height does not depend on the color of her eyes). Sometimes both variables correlate with a third variable (a child's height and eye color both depend on genetics).

variety (dietary): eating a wide selection of foods within and among the major food groups.

vasoconstrictor (VAS-oh-kon-STRIK-tor): a substance that constricts or narrows the blood vessels.

vasopressin (VAS-oh-PRES-in): another name for antidiuretic hormone, so called because it elevates blood pressure.

vegan (VEE-gan) **diet:** an eating pattern that excludes all animal-derived foods (including meat, poultry, fish, eggs, and dairy products) from the diet; also called *pure vegetarian, strict vegetarian,* or *total vegetarian.*

vegetarian diet: a general term used to describe an eating pattern that excludes meat, poultry, fish, or other animal-derived foods from the diet.

veins (VANES): vessels that carry blood to the heart.

very low food security: multiple indications of disrupted eating patterns and reduced food intake; formerly known as *food insecurity with hunger.*

very low sodium: 35 milligrams or less per serving.

vigorous-intensity physical activity: physical activity that requires a large increase in breathing and/or heart rate and expends more than 7 kcalories per minute. Walking at a very brisk pace (>4.5 miles per hour) or running at a pace of at least 5 miles per hour are examples.

villi (VILL-ee or VILL-eye): fingerlike projections from the folds of the small intestine; singular *villus.*

visceral fat: fat stored within the abdominal cavity in association with the internal abdominal organs; also called *intra-abdominal fat.*

viscous: a gel-like consistency.

vitamin A: all naturally occurring compounds with the biological activity of *retinol,* the alcohol form of vitamin A.

vitamin A activity: a term referring to both the active forms of vitamin A and the precursor forms in foods without distinguishing between them.

vitamin B_6: a family of compounds—pyridoxal, pyridoxine, and pyridoxamine. The primary active coenzyme form is *PLP* (*pyridoxal phosphate*).

vitamin B_{12}: a B vitamin characterized by the presence of cobalt. The active forms of coenzyme B_{12} are *methylcobalamin* and *deoxyadenosylcobalamin.*

vitamin D_2: vitamin D derived from plants in the diet; also called *ergocalciferol* (ER-go-kal-SIF-er-ol).

vitamin D_3: vitamin D derived from animals in the diet or made in the skin from 7-dehydrocholesterol, a precursor of cholesterol, with the help of sunlight; also called *cholecalciferol* (KO-lee-kal-SIF-er-ol) or *calciol.* After hydroxylation in the liver, calciol becomes *calcidiol* and after hydroxylation in the kidneys, calcidiol becomes *calcitriol.*

vitamins: organic, essential nutrients required in small amounts by the body for health. Vitamins regulate body processes that support growth and maintain life.

VLDL (very-low-density lipoprotein): the type of lipoprotein made primarily by liver cells to transport lipids to various tissues in the body; composed primarily of triglycerides.

VO_{2max}: the maximum rate of oxygen consumption by an individual at sea level.

vomiting: expulsion of the contents of the stomach up through the esophagus to the mouth.

vulnerable plaque: plaque that is susceptible to rupture because it has only a thin fibrous barrier between its lipid-rich core and the artery lining.

W

waist circumference: an anthropometric measurement used to assess a person's abdominal fat.

warm-up: 5 to 10 minutes of light activity, such as easy jogging or cycling, prior to a workout to prepare the body for more vigorous activity.

water balance: the balance between water intake and output (losses).

water intoxication: the rare condition in which body water contents are too high in all body fluid compartments.

water stress: intense demands on water resources by human activities such as municipal water supplies, industries, power plants, and agriculture.

wean: to gradually replace breast milk with infant formula or other foods appropriate to an infant's diet.

websites: Internet resources composed of text and graphic files, each with a unique URL (Uniform Resource Locator) that names the site (for example, www.usda.gov).

weight management: maintaining body weight in a healthy range by preventing gradual weight gains over time and losing weight if overweight, and by preventing weight losses and gaining weight if underweight.

well water: water drawn from ground water by tapping into an aquifer.

Wernicke-Korsakoff (VER-nee-key KORE-sah-kof) **syndrome:** a neurological disorder typically associated with chronic alcoholism and caused by a deficiency of the B vitamin thiamin; also called *alcohol-related dementia.*

wheat flour: any flour made from the endosperm of the wheat kernel.

whey protein: a by-product of cheese production; falsely promoted as increasing muscle mass. Whey is the watery part of milk that separates from the curds.

white sugar: granulated sucrose or "table sugar," produced by dissolving, concentrating, and recrystallizing raw sugar.

WHO (World Health Organization): an international agency concerned with promoting health and eradicating disease.

whole grain: a grain that maintains the same relative proportions of starchy endosperm, germ, and bran as the original (all but the husk); not refined.

whole-wheat flour: any flour made from the entire wheat kernel.

Wilson's disease: a genetic disorder of copper metabolism that creates a copper toxicity and results in neurologic symptoms such as tremors, impaired speech, inappropriate behaviors, and personality changes.

wine: an alcoholic beverage traditionally made by fermenting a sugar source such as grape juice.

without appreciable risk: practical certainty that injury will not result even after a lifetime of exposure.

X

xanthophylls (ZAN-tho-fills): pigments found in plants responsible for the color changes seen in autumn leaves.

xerophthalmia (zer-off-THAL-mee-uh): progressive blindness caused by inadequate mucus production due to severe vitamin A deficiency.

xerosis (zee-ROW-sis): abnormal drying of the skin and mucous membranes; a sign of vitamin A deficiency.

Y

yields: production per acre.

yogurt: milk product that results from the fermentation of lactic acid in milk by *Lactobacillus bulgaricus* and *Streptococcus thermophilus.*

Z

zinc: an essential trace mineral that is part of many enzymes and a constituent of insulin.

zygote (ZY-goat): the initial product of the union of ovum and sperm; a fertilized ovum.

zymogen (ZYE-mo-jen): the inactive precursor of an enzyme; sometimes called a *proenzyme.*

Index

- Page numbers in bold indicate definition of term.
- Page numbers followed by the letter "f" indicate figures or photographs.
- Page numbers followed by the letter "n" indicate footnotes.
- Page numbers followed by the letter "t" indicate tables.

A

B

C

D

G

M

T

U

V

W

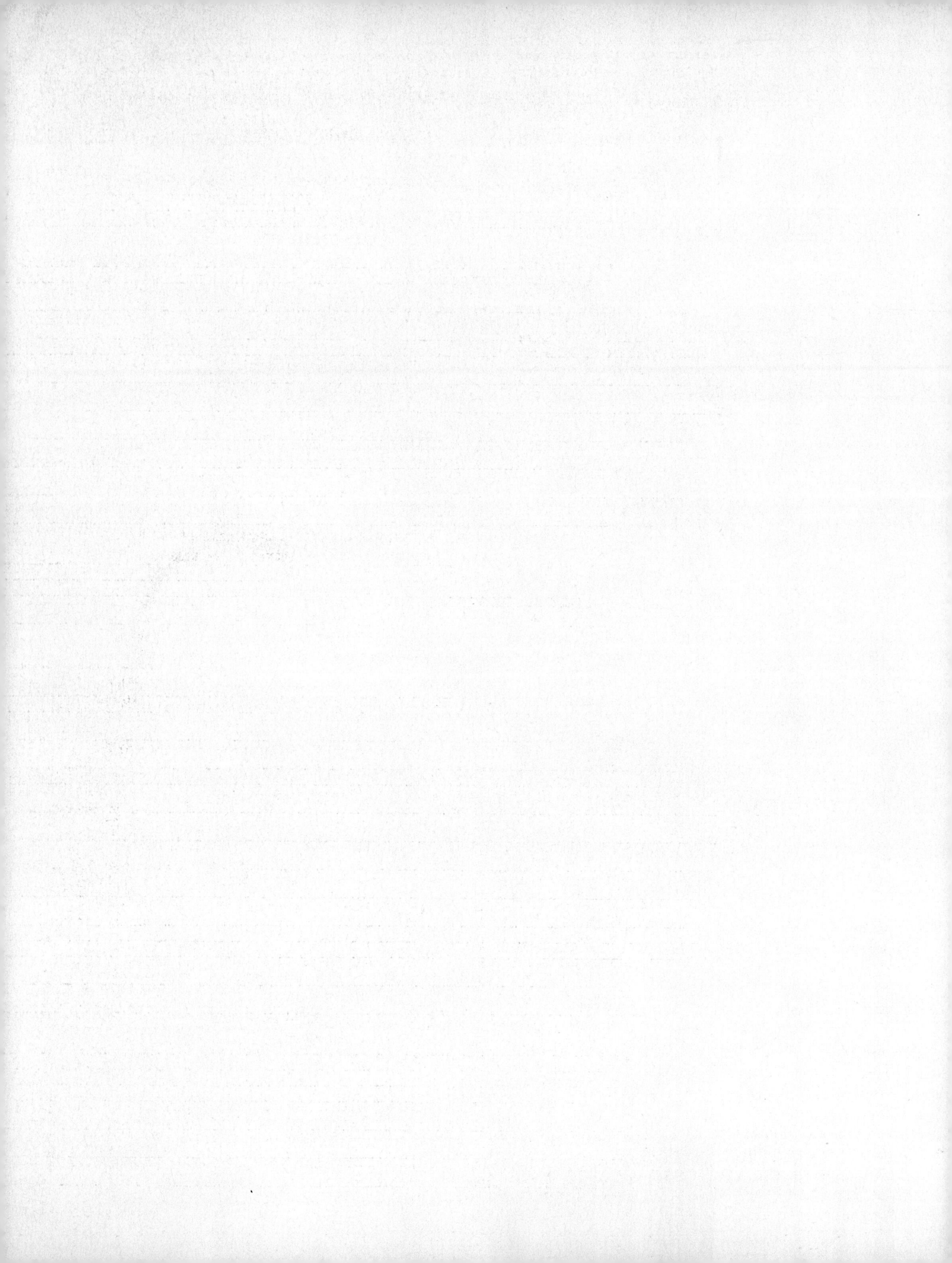

STUDY IT

1 An Overview of Nutrition

Review the key points of this chapter below, learn the definitions of bold terms, and then take the practice quiz on the back of this card.

1.1 Food Choices

- People select **foods** based on such factors as taste and convenience, but **diets** based on **nutrition** knowledge may better support good health.
- Individual foods are neither "good" nor "bad"; daily food choices made over a lifetime may improve health or contribute to **chronic diseases.**

1.2 The Nutrients

- Foods provide **nutrients**—substances that provide **energy,** structural materials, and regulating agents to support the growth, maintenance, and repair of the body's tissues. **Essential nutrients** *must* be obtained from foods.
- The six classes of nutrients include carbohydrates, lipids (fats), proteins, **vitamins, minerals,** and water. Carbohydrates, lipids, proteins, and vitamins are **organic,** meaning they contain carbon; minerals and water are **inorganic,** meaning they do not contain carbon.
- Energy is measured in **kcalories**—a measure of heat energy. One kcalorie is the amount of heat necessary to raise the temperature of 1 kg water 1°C.
- The **energy-yielding nutrients** are carbohydrate (4 kcal/g), fat (9 kcal/g), and protein (4 kcal/g). Alcohol provides 7 kcal/g, but it is not considered a nutrient.
- Vitamins, minerals, and water do not provide energy; instead, they facilitate a variety of activities in the body.

1.3 The Science of Nutrition

- The science of nutrition is the study of nutrients and other substances in foods and the body's handling of them.
- Researchers follow the scientific method (review Figure 1-3, p. 13). They randomly assign **control** and **experimental groups,** use large sample sizes, provide **placebos,** and are **blind** to treatments. Their findings are reviewed and **replicated** by other scientists before being accepted as **valid.**
- **Correlations** indicate an association between **variables,** not a cause.

1.4 Dietary Reference Intakes

- **Dietary Reference Intakes (DRI)** are a set of nutrient intake values used to plan and evaluate diets for healthy people.
- **Estimated Average Requirement (EAR)** defines the amount of a nutrient that supports a specific function in the body for half of the population. **Recommended Dietary Allowance (RDA)** is based on the EAR and establishes a goal for dietary intake that will meet the needs of almost all healthy people. **Adequate Intake (AI)** serves a similar purpose when an RDA cannot be determined.
- **Estimated Energy Requirement (EER)** defines the average amount of energy intake needed to maintain energy balance, and **Acceptable Macronutrient Distribution Ranges (AMDR)** define the proportions contributed by carbohydrate, fat, and protein to a healthy diet. Carbohydrates should consist of 45 to 65 percent of kcalories, fat 20 to 35 percent, and protein 10 to 35 percent.
- **Tolerable Upper Intake Level (UL)** establishes the highest amount that appears safe for regular consumption.

1.5 Nutrition Assessment

- **Malnutrition** develops when people get too little **(undernutrition),** too much **(overnutrition),** or an imbalance of energy or nutrients.
- Four **nutrition assessment** methods include historical information on diet and health, **anthropometric** measurements, physical examinations, and laboratory tests. Together, these methods reveal the stages of a nutrient deficiency (review Figure 1-7, p. 24).
- A **primary deficiency** is caused by an inadequate intake of a nutrient; a **secondary deficiency** is caused by a condition that reduces absorption, accelerates use, increases excretion, or destroys the nutrient.

1.6 Diet and Health

- **Risk factors** such as obesity and cigarette smoking increase the likelihood of disease development (review Table 1-6).
- Some risk factors, such as genetics, are important but cannot be changed. Recommendations focus on changeable, personal life choices such as diet and activity habits.
- Diet has no influence on some diseases but is linked closely to others (review Table 1-5).

TABLE 1-5 Leading Causes of Death in the United States

	Percentage of Total Deaths
1. **Heart disease**	23.7
2. **Cancers**	22.9
3. Chronic lung diseases	5.7
4. **Strokes**	5.1
5. Accidents	4.9
6. Alzheimer's disease	3.4
7. **Diabetes mellitus**	2.9
8. Pneumonia and influenza	2.1
9. Kidney disease	1.8
10. Suicide	1.5

NOTE: The diseases highlighted in bold have relationships with diet.

SOURCE: Deaths: Preliminary data for 2011, *National Vital Statistics Reports*, October 10, 2012, Centers for Disease Control and Prevention, www.cdc.gov/nchs.

TABLE 1-6 Factors Contributing to Deaths in the United States

Factors	Percentage of Deaths
Tobacco	18
Poor diet/inactivity	15
Alcohol	4
Microbial agents	3
Toxic agents	2
Motor vehicles	2
Firearms	1
Sexual behavior	<1
Illicit drugs	<1

SOURCE: A. H. Mokdad and coauthors, Actual causes of death in the United States, 2000, *Journal of the American Medical Association* 291 (2004): 1238–1245, with corrections from *Journal of the American Medical Association* 293 (2005): 298.

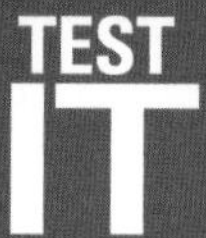

Take the quiz below to test your mastery of the key chapter concepts.

1.1 Food Choices (pp. 4–6)

LEARN IT Describe how various factors influence personal food choices.

1. When people eat the foods typical of their families or geographic region, their choices are influenced by:
   a. habit.
   b. nutrition.
   c. personal preference.
   d. heritage or tradition.

1.2 The Nutrients (pp. 6–12)

LEARN IT Name the six major classes of nutrients and identify which are organic and which yield energy.

2. What is the difference between organic and inorganic?
3. How much energy do carbohydrates, fats, and proteins yield per gram? How is energy measured?
4. Describe how alcohol resembles nutrients. Why is alcohol not considered a nutrient?
5. The nutrient found most abundantly in both the human body and most foods is:
   a. fat.
   b. water.
   c. minerals.
   d. proteins.
6. The inorganic nutrients are:
   a. proteins and fats.
   b. vitamins and minerals.
   c. minerals and water.
   d. vitamins and proteins.
7. The energy-yielding nutrients are:
   a. fats, minerals, and water.
   b. minerals, proteins, and vitamins.
   c. carbohydrates, fats, and vitamins.
   d. carbohydrates, fats, and proteins.

1.3 The Science of Nutrition (pp. 12–18)

LEARN IT Explain the scientific method and how scientists use various types of research studies and methods to acquire nutrition information.

8. What is the science of nutrition?
9. Explain how variables might be correlational but not causal.
10. Studies of populations that reveal correlations between dietary habits and disease incidence are:
    a. clinical trials.
    b. laboratory studies.
    c. case-control studies.
    d. epidemiological studies.
11. An experiment in which neither the researchers nor the subjects know who is receiving the treatment is known as:
    a. double blind.
    b. double control.
    c. blind variable.
    d. placebo control.

1.4 Dietary Reference Intakes (pp. 18–22)

LEARN IT Define the four categories of the DRI and explain their purposes.

12. What judgment factors are involved in setting the energy and nutrient recommendations?
13. An RDA represents the:
    a. highest amount of a nutrient that appears safe for most healthy people.
    b. lowest amount of a nutrient that will maintain a specified criterion of adequacy.
    c. average amount of a nutrient considered adequate to meet the known nutrient needs of practically all healthy people.
    d. average amount of a nutrient that will maintain a specific biochemical or physiological function in half the people.

1.5 Nutrition Assessment (pp. 22–26)

LEARN IT Explain how the four assessment methods are used to detect energy and nutrient deficiencies and excesses.

14. What methods are used in nutrition surveys? What kinds of information can these surveys provide?
15. Historical information, physical examinations, laboratory tests, and anthropometric measurements are:
    a. techniques used in diet planning.
    b. steps used in the scientific method.
    c. approaches used in disease prevention.
    d. methods used in a nutrition assessment.
16. A deficiency caused by an inadequate dietary intake is called a(n):
    a. overt deficiency.
    b. covert deficiency.
    c. primary deficiency.
    d. secondary deficiency.

1.6 Diet and Health (pp. 26–28)

LEARN IT Identify several risk factors and explain their relationships to chronic diseases.

17. Behaviors such as smoking, dietary habits, physical activity, and alcohol consumption that influence the development of disease are known as:
    a. risk factors.
    b. chronic causes.
    c. preventive agents.
    d. disease descriptors.

HIGHLIGHT 1 Nutrition Information and Misinformation (pp. 30–35)

LEARN IT Recognize misinformation and describe how to identify reliable nutrition information.

18. Nutrition misinformation is often based on:
    a. clinical trials.
    b. anecdotal evidence.
    c. double blind studies.
    d. epidemiological research.

Multiple Choice Answers

1.d 5.b 6.c 7.d 10.d 11.a 13.c 15.d 16.c 17.a 18.b

2 Planning a Healthy Diet

Review the key points of this chapter below, learn the definitions of bold terms, and then take the practice quiz on the back of this card.

2.1 Principles and Guidelines

- A well-planned **eating pattern** delivers *adequate* nutrients, a *balanced* array of nutrients, and an appropriate amount of *energy* (*kcalories*). It is based on ***nutrient-dense*** foods, ***moderate*** in substances that can be detrimental to health, and *varied* in its selections.
- The *Dietary Guidelines for Americans* offer practical advice on how to eat for good health (review Table 2-1, p. 41).

2.2 Diet-Planning Guides

- The USDA Food Patterns help consumers select the types and amounts of foods to provide **adequacy, balance,** and **variety** in the diet. It makes it easier to plan a diet that includes a balance of grains, vegetables, fruits, protein foods, and milk products. In making any food choice, remember to view the food in the context of the total diet.
- The combination of many different foods provides the array of nutrients that are essential to a healthy diet (review Figure 2-2, pp. 44–45).
- MyPlate reminds consumers to make healthy choices from the five **food groups** (review Figure 2-4, p. 48).

2.3 Food Labels

- Food labels list ingredients in descending order of predominance by weight, nutrition facts based on standard **serving sizes,** and **Daily Values** based on a 2000-kcalorie diet (review Figure 2-9).
- **Nutrient claims** reflect the quantity of a nutrient (high or low), **health claims** reflect relationships between a nutrient and a disease (potassium reduces risk of hypertension), and **structure-function claims** reflect relationships between a nutrient and its function in the body (calcium builds bones).

> FIGURE 2-9 **Example of a Food Label**

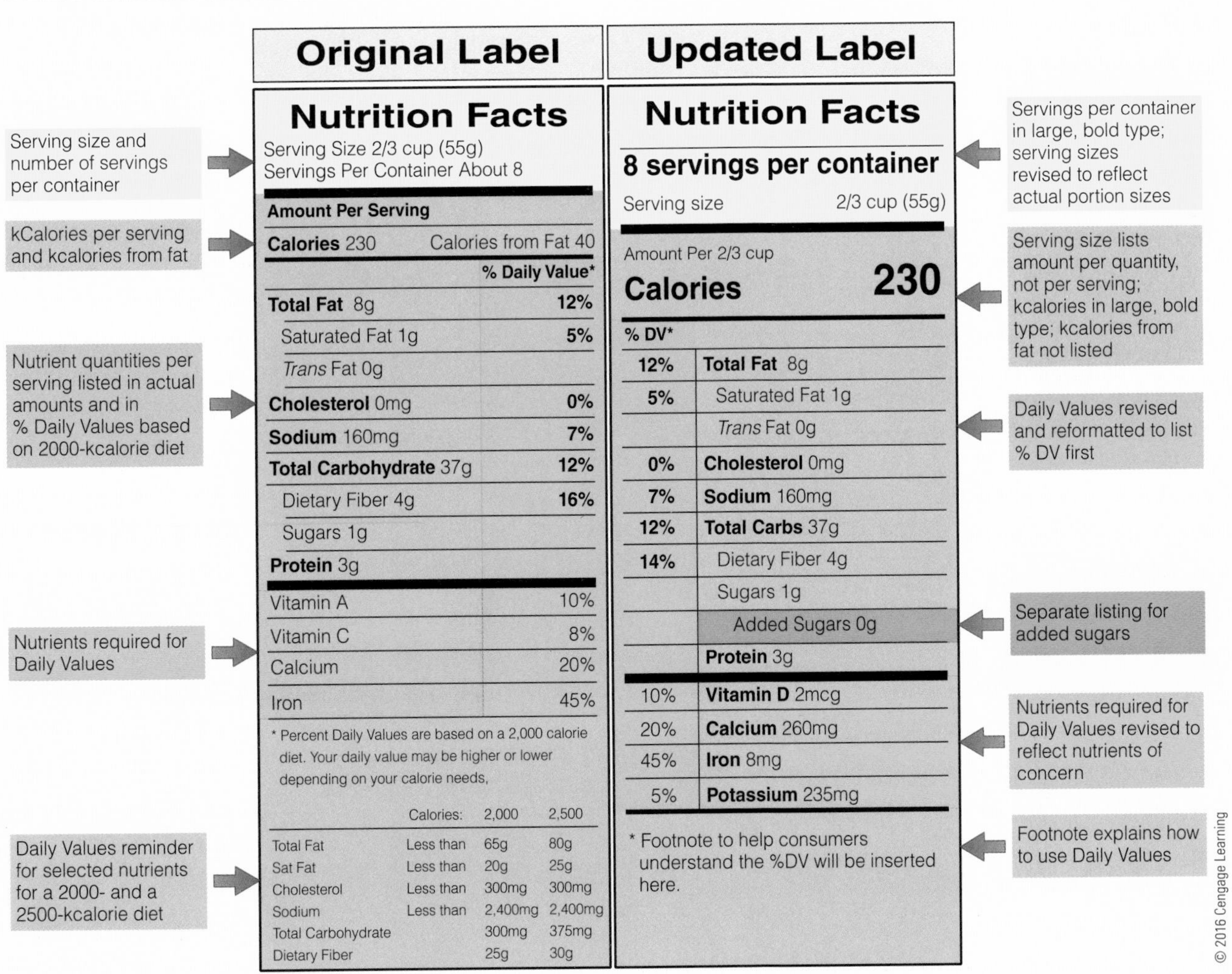

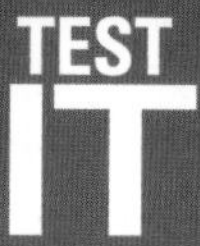

Take the quiz below to test your mastery of the key chapter concepts.

2.1 Principles and Guidelines (pp. 38–42)

LEARN IT Explain how each of the diet-planning principles can be used to plan a healthy diet.

1. What recommendations appear in the *Dietary Guidelines for Americans*?
2. The diet-planning principle that provides all the essential nutrients in sufficient amounts to support health is:
   a. balance.
   b. variety.
   c. adequacy.
   d. moderation.
3. A person who chooses a chicken leg that provides 0.5 milligram of iron and 95 kcalories instead of 2 tablespoons of peanut butter that also provides 0.5 milligram of iron but 188 kcalories is using the principle of nutrient:
   a. control.
   b. density.
   c. adequacy.
   d. moderation.
4. Which of the following is consistent with the *Dietary Guidelines for Americans*?
   a. Choose a diet restricted in fat and cholesterol.
   b. Balance the food you eat with physical activity.
   c. Choose a diet with plenty of milk products and meats.
   d. Eat an abundance of foods to ensure nutrient adequacy.

2.2 Diet-Planning Guides (pp. 42–56)

LEARN IT Use the USDA Food Patterns to develop a meal plan within a specified energy allowance.

5. Review the *Dietary Guidelines*. What types of grocery selections would you make to achieve those recommendations?
6. According to the USDA Food Patterns, cheese is grouped as a:
   a. meat.
   b. protein food.
   c. milk product.
   d. miscellaneous fat.
7. Foods within a given food group of the USDA Food Patterns are similar in their contents of:
   a. energy.
   b. proteins and fibers.
   c. vitamins and minerals.
   d. carbohydrates and fats.
8. In the exchange system, each portion of food on any given list provides about the same amount of:
   a. energy.
   b. satiety.
   c. vitamins.
   d. minerals.
9. Enriched grain products are fortified with:
   a. fiber, folate, iron, niacin, and zinc.
   b. thiamin, iron, calcium, zinc, and sodium.
   c. iron, thiamin, riboflavin, niacin, and folate.
   d. folate, magnesium, vitamin B_6, zinc, and fiber.

2.3 Food Labels (pp. 56–63)

LEARN IT Compare the information on food labels to make selections that meet specific dietary and health goals.

10. What information can you expect to find on a food label? How can this information help you choose between two similar products?
11. What are the Daily Values? How can they help you meet health recommendations?
12. Describe the differences between nutrient claims, health claims, and structure-function claims.
13. Food labels list ingredients in:
    a. alphabetical order.
    b. ascending order of predominance by weight.
    c. descending order of predominance by weight.
    d. manufacturer's order of preference.
14. "Milk builds strong bones" is an example of a:
    a. health claim.
    b. nutrition fact.
    c. nutrient content claim.
    d. structure-function claim.
15. Daily Values on food labels are based on a:
    a. 1500-kcalorie diet.
    b. 2000-kcalorie diet.
    c. 2500-kcalorie diet.
    d. 3000-kcalorie diet.

HIGHLIGHT 2 Vegetarian Diets (pp. 64–69)

LEARN IT Develop a well-balanced vegetarian meal plan.

16. Which of the following nutrients is most likely to be lacking in a vegan diet?
    a. fiber
    b. folate
    c. vitamin C
    d. vitamin B_{12}

Multiple Choice Answers
2. c 3. b 4. b 6. c 7. c 8. a 9. c 13. c 14. d 15. b 16. d

STUDY IT

3 Digestion, Absorption, and Transport

Review the key points of this chapter below, learn the definitions of the bold terms, and then take the practice quiz on the back of this card.

3.1 Digestion

- **Digestion** breaks down foods into nutrients. **Absorption** brings the nutrients into the cells of the **small intestine** for transport to the body's cells.
- Food enters the **mouth** and travels along the **gastrointestinal tract**—down the **esophagus** and through the upper and lower esophageal **sphincters** to the **stomach,** then through the **pyloric sphincter** to the small intestine, on through the **ileocecal valve** to the **large intestine,** past the **appendix** to the **rectum,** ending at the **anus** (review Figure 3-1).
- The wavelike contractions of **peristalsis** and the periodic squeezing of **segmentation** keep things moving at a reasonable pace. Along the way, secretions from the **salivary glands,** stomach, **pancreas, liver** (via the **gallbladder**), and small intestine deliver fluids and **digestive enzymes** (review Table 3-1).

3.2 Absorption

- The many folds and **villi** of the small intestine increase its surface area, making nutrient absorption efficient.
- Nutrients pass through the cells of the intestinal villi and enter either the blood (if they are water soluble or small fat fragments) or the **lymph** (if they are fat soluble).

3.3 The Circulatory Systems

- Nutrients leaving the **digestive system** via the blood are routed directly to the liver before being transported to the body's cells.
- Nutrients leaving via the lymphatic system bypass the liver at first, but eventually enter the vascular system via the **thoracic duct,** which opens into the **subclavian vein.**

3.4 The Health and Regulation of the GI Tract

- A diverse and abundant population of **microbes** supports GI health.
- The regulation of GI processes depends on the coordinated efforts of the hormonal system and the nervous system.
- Together, digestion and absorption break down foods into nutrients for the body's use.
- To function optimally, a healthy GI tract needs a balanced diet, adequate rest, and regular physical activity.

> FIGURE 3-1 **The Gastrointestinal Tract**

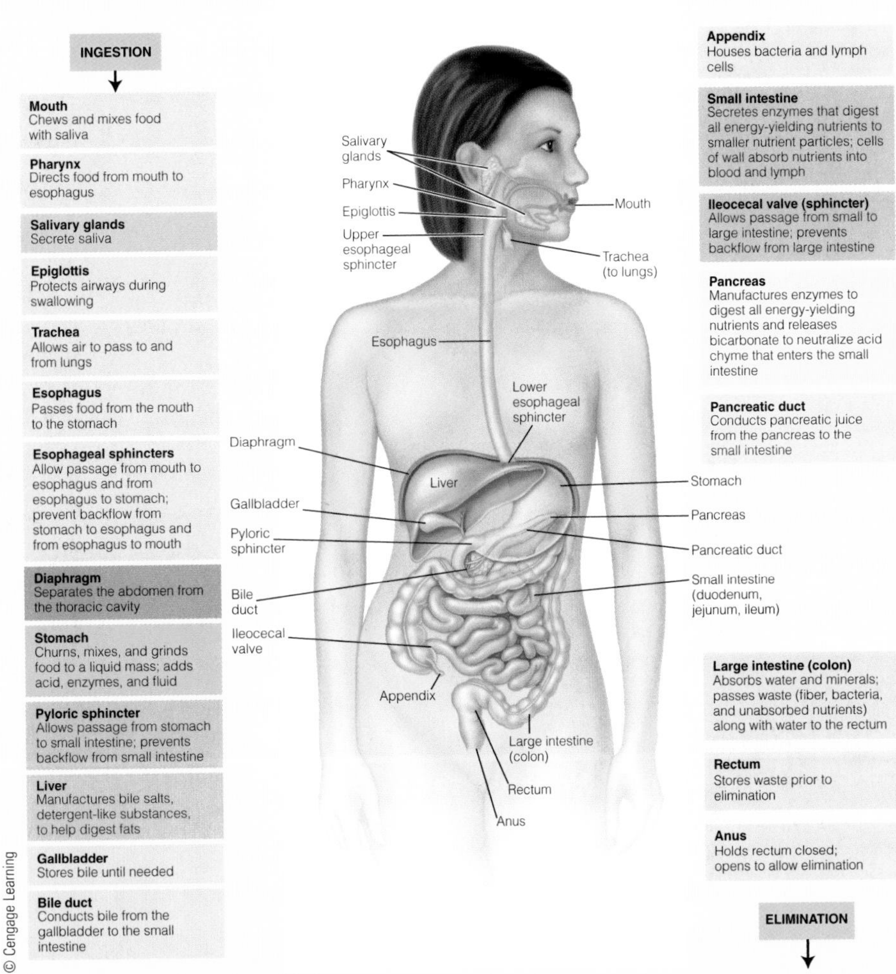

INGESTION
Mouth Chews and mixes food with saliva
Pharynx Directs food from mouth to esophagus
Salivary glands Secrete saliva
Epiglottis Protects airways during swallowing
Trachea Allows air to pass to and from lungs
Esophagus Passes food from the mouth to the stomach
Esophageal sphincters Allow passage from mouth to esophagus and from esophagus to stomach; prevent backflow from stomach to esophagus and from esophagus to mouth
Diaphragm Separates the abdomen from the thoracic cavity
Stomach Churns, mixes, and grinds food to a liquid mass; adds acid, enzymes, and fluid
Pyloric sphincter Allows passage from stomach to small intestine; prevents backflow from small intestine
Liver Manufactures bile salts, detergent-like substances, to help digest fats
Gallbladder Stores bile until needed
Bile duct Conducts bile from the gallbladder to the small intestine
Salivary glands
Pharynx
Epiglottis
Upper esophageal sphincter
Mouth
Trachea (to lungs)
Esophagus
Lower esophageal sphincter
Diaphragm
Liver
Gallbladder
Pyloric sphincter
Bile duct
Ileocecal valve
Appendix
Large intestine (colon)
Rectum
Anus
Stomach
Pancreas
Pancreatic duct
Small intestine (duodenum, jejunum, ileum)
Appendix Houses bacteria and lymph cells
Small intestine Secretes enzymes that digest all energy-yielding nutrients to smaller nutrient particles; cells of wall absorb nutrients into blood and lymph
Ileocecal valve (sphincter) Allows passage from small to large intestine; prevents backflow from large intestine
Pancreas Manufactures enzymes to digest all energy-yielding nutrients and releases bicarbonate to neutralize acid chyme that enters the small intestine
Pancreatic duct Conducts pancreatic juice from the pancreas to the small intestine
Large intestine (colon) Absorbs water and minerals; passes waste (fiber, bacteria, and unabsorbed nutrients) along with water to the rectum
Rectum Stores waste prior to elimination
Anus Holds rectum closed; opens to allow elimination
ELIMINATION

TABLE 3-1 **Summary of Digestive Secretions and Their Major Actions**

Organ or Gland	Target Organ	Secretion	Action
Salivary glands	Mouth	Saliva	Fluid eases swallowing; salivary enzyme breaks down some **carbohydrate.***
Gastric glands	Stomach	Gastric juice	Fluid mixes with bolus; hydrochloric acid uncoils **proteins;** enzymes break down proteins; mucus protects stomach cells.*
Pancreas	Small intestine	Pancreatic juice	Bicarbonate neutralizes acidic gastric juices; pancreatic enzymes break down **carbohydrates, fats,** and **proteins.**
Liver	Gallbladder	Bile	Bile is stored until needed.
Gallbladder	Small intestine	Bile	Bile emulsifies **fat** so that enzymes can have access to break it down.
Intestinal glands	Small intestine	Intestinal juice	Intestinal enzymes break down **carbohydrate, fat,** and **protein** fragments; mucus protects the intestinal wall.

*Saliva and gastric juice also contain lipases, but most fat breakdown occurs in the small intestine.

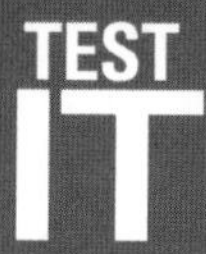

Take the quiz below to test your mastery of the key chapter concepts.

3.1 Digestion (pp. 72–78)

LEARN IT Explain how foods move through the digestive system, describing the actions of the organs, muscles, and digestive secretions along the way.

1. Describe the challenges associated with digesting food and the solutions offered by the human body.
2. Name five organs that secrete digestive juices. How do the juices and enzymes facilitate digestion?
3. The semiliquid, partially digested food that travels through the intestinal tract is called:
   a. bile.
   b. lymph.
   c. chyme.
   d. secretin.
4. The muscular contractions that move food through the GI tract are called:
   a. hydrolysis.
   b. sphincters.
   c. peristalsis.
   d. bowel movements.
5. The main function of bile is to:
   a. emulsify fats.
   b. catalyze hydrolysis.
   c. slow protein digestion.
   d. neutralize stomach acidity.
6. The pancreas neutralizes stomach acid in the small intestine by secreting:
   a. bile.
   b. mucus.
   c. enzymes.
   d. bicarbonate.
7. Which nutrient passes through the GI tract mostly undigested and unabsorbed?
   a. fat
   b. fiber
   c. protein
   d. carbohydrate

3.2 Absorption (pp. 78–82)

LEARN IT Describe the anatomical details of the intestinal cells that facilitate nutrient absorption.

8. The fingerlike projections on the small intestine that dramatically increase its surface area are called:
   a. villi.
   b. crypts.
   c. goblet cells.
   d. chylomicrons.
9. Absorption occurs primarily in the:
   a. mouth.
   b. stomach.
   c. small intestine.
   d. large intestine.

3.3 The Circulatory Systems (pp. 82–84)

LEARN IT Explain how nutrients are routed in the circulatory systems from the GI tract into the body and identify which nutrients enter the blood directly and which must first enter the lymph.

10. All blood leaving the GI tract travels first to the:
    a. heart.
    b. liver.
    c. kidneys.
    d. pancreas.
11. Which nutrients leave the GI tract by way of the lymphatic system?
    a. water and minerals
    b. proteins and minerals
    c. all vitamins and minerals
    d. fats and fat-soluble vitamins

3.4 The Health and Regulation of the GI Tract (pp. 85–89)

LEARN IT Describe how bacteria, hormones, and nerves influence the health and activities of the GI tract.

12. How does the composition of the diet influence the functioning of the GI tract?
13. What steps can you take to help your GI tract function at its best?
14. Digestion and absorption are coordinated by the:
    a. pancreas and kidneys.
    b. liver and gallbladder.
    c. hormonal system and the nervous system.
    d. vascular system and the lymphatic system.
15. Gastrin, secretin, and cholecystokinin are examples of:
    a. crypts.
    b. enzymes.
    c. hormones.
    d. goblet cells.

HIGHLIGHT 3 Common Digestive Problems (pp. 90–96)

LEARN IT Outline strategies to prevent or alleviate common GI problems.

16. Which of the following is most likely to aggravate heartburn?
    a. eat small meals
    b. drink liquids between meals
    c. eat slowly and chew thoroughly
    d. lie down to rest immediately after eating

Multiple Choice Answers

3. c 4. c 5. a 6. d 7. b 8. a 9. c 10. b 11. d 14. c 15. c 16. d

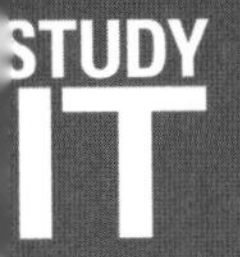

4 The Carbohydrates: Sugars, Starches, and Fibers

Review the key points of this chapter below, learn the definitions of bold terms, and then take the practice quiz on the back of this card.

4.1 The Chemist's View of Carbohydrates

- **Carbohydrates** include **monosaccharides, disaccharides,** and **polysaccharides** (review Table 4-1).
- Carbohydrates are made of carbon (C), oxygen (O), and hydrogen (H); each atom forms a specified number of chemical bonds: carbon forms four, oxygen forms two, and hydrogen forms one (review Figure 4-1, p. 100).
- Monosaccharides (**glucose, fructose,** and **galactose**) all have the same chemical formula ($C_6H_{12}O_6$), but their structures differ. Disaccharides (**maltose, sucrose,** and **lactose**) each contain a glucose paired with one of the three monosaccharides.
- A **condensation** reaction can bond two monosaccharides together to form a disaccharide and water (review Figure 4-4, p. 102). A **hydrolysis** reaction can use water to split a disaccharide into its two monosaccharides (review Figure 4-5, p. 102).
- Chains of monosaccharides are called **polysaccharides** and include **glycogen, starches,** and **dietary fibers.** Both glycogen and starch are storage forms of glucose—glycogen in the body, and starch in plants—and both yield energy.
- Dietary fibers contain glucose (and other monosaccharides), but their bonds cannot be broken by human digestive enzymes; they yield little, if any, energy.
- **Soluble fibers** dissolve in water to form gels and are easily digested by bacteria in the colon. **Insoluble fibers** do not dissolve in water or form gels and are less readily fermented.

TABLE 4-1 The Carbohydrate Family

Monosaccharides	
Glucose	
Fructose	
Galactose	
Disaccharides	
Maltose (glucose + glucose)	
Sucrose (glucose + fructose)	
Lactose (glucose + galactose)	
Polysaccharides	
Glycogen[a]	
Starches (amylose and amylopectin)	
Fibers (soluble and insoluble)	

[a]Glycogen is a polysaccharide, but not a common dietary source of carbohydrate.

4.2 Digestion and Absorption of Carbohydrates

- The body digests starches into the disaccharide maltose. Maltose and the other disaccharides (lactose and sucrose) from foods are broken down into monosaccharides, which are absorbed (review Figure 4-9, p. 107).
- Fibers help to regulate the passage of food through the GI tract and slow the absorption of glucose.
- **Lactose intolerance** occurs when there is insufficient lactase to digest the disaccharide lactose found in milk and milk products. Symptoms include GI distress.

4.3 Glucose in the Body

- Dietary carbohydrates provide glucose that can be used by the cells for energy, stored by the liver and muscles as glycogen, or converted into fat if intakes exceed needs.
- All of the body's cells depend on glucose; those of the central nervous system are especially dependent on it.
- Without glucose, the body is forced to break down its protein tissues to make glucose **(gluconeogenesis)** and to alter energy metabolism to make **ketone bodies** from fats.
- Blood glucose regulation depends on two pancreatic hormones: **insulin** to move glucose from the blood into the cells when levels are high and **glucagon** to free glucose from glycogen stores and release it into the blood when levels are low (review Figure 4-10, p. 111).

4.4 Health Effects and Recommended Intakes of Sugars

- Excessive intakes of **sugars** may increase the risk of dental caries, displace needed nutrients and fiber, and contribute to obesity when energy intake exceeds needs.
- Concentrated sweets are relatively low in nutrients, high in kcalories, and may need to be limited; sugars that occur naturally in fruits, vegetables, and milk are acceptable.
- To control weight gain, blood glucose, and dental caries, consumers may use alternative sweeteners (**artificial sweeteners,** herbal products, and **sugar alcohols**) to limit kcalories and minimize sugar intake (review Table 4-8, p. 119).

4.5 Health Effects and Recommended Intakes of Starch and Fibers

- Adequate intake of fiber fosters weight management, lowers blood cholesterol, and may help prevent colon cancer, diabetes, hemorrhoids, appendicitis, and diverticulosis.
- Excessive intake of fiber displaces energy- and nutrient-dense foods, causes intestinal discomfort and distention, and may interfere with mineral absorption.
- Because starches and fibers help control body weight and prevent heart disease, cancer, diabetes, and GI disorders, the *Dietary Guidelines* suggest plenty of whole grains, vegetables, legumes, and fruits—enough to provide 45 to 65 percent of the daily energy intake from carbohydrate.

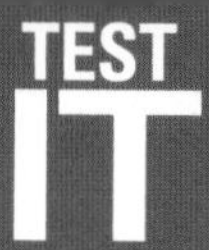

Take the quiz below to test your mastery of the key chapter concepts.

4.1 The Chemist's View of Carbohydrates

(pp. 100–105)

LEARN IT Identify the monosaccharides, disaccharides, and polysaccharides common in nutrition by their chemical structures and major food sources.

1. What happens in a condensation reaction? In a hydrolysis reaction?
2. How are starch and glycogen similar, and how do they differ? How do the fibers differ from the other polysaccharides?
3. Disaccharides include:
   a. starch, glycogen, and fiber.
   b. amylose, pectin, and dextrose.
   c. sucrose, maltose, and lactose.
   d. glucose, galactose, and fructose.
4. The making of a disaccharide from two monosaccharides is an example of:
   a. digestion.
   b. hydrolysis.
   c. condensation.
   d. gluconeogenesis.
5. The significant difference between starch and cellulose is that:
   a. starch is a polysaccharide, but cellulose is not.
   b. animals can store glucose as starch, but not as cellulose.
   c. hormones can make glucose from cellulose, but not from starch.
   d. digestive enzymes can break the bonds in starch, but not in cellulose.

4.2 Digestion and Absorption of Carbohydrates (pp. 105–108)

LEARN IT Summarize carbohydrate digestion and absorption.

6. What role does fiber play in digestion and absorption?
7. Describe lactose intolerance and its symptoms.
8. The ultimate goal of carbohydrate digestion and absorption is to yield:
   a. fibers.
   b. glucose.
   c. enzymes.
   d. amylase.
9. The enzyme that breaks a disaccharide into glucose and galactose is:
   a. amylase.
   b. maltase.
   c. sucrase.
   d. lactase.

4.3 Glucose in the Body (pp. 108–113)

LEARN IT Explain how the body maintains its blood glucose concentration and what happens when blood glucose rises too high or falls too low.

10. What are the possible fates of glucose in the body? What is the protein-sparing action of carbohydrate?
11. The storage form of glucose in the body is:
    a. insulin.
    b. maltose.
    c. glucagon.
    d. glycogen.
12. With insufficient glucose in metabolism, fat fragments combine to form:
    a. dextrins.
    b. mucilages.
    c. phytic acids.
    d. ketone bodies.
13. What does the pancreas secrete when blood glucose rises? When blood glucose falls?
    a. insulin; glucagon
    b. glucagon; insulin
    c. insulin; glycogen
    d. glycogen; epinephrine

4.4 Health Effects and Recommended Intakes of Sugars (pp. 113–120)

LEARN IT Describe how added sugars can contribute to health problems.

14. What are the dietary recommendations regarding concentrated sugar intakes?
15. Describe the risks and benefits of using alternative sweeteners.

4.5 Health Effects and Recommended Intakes of Starch and Fibers (pp. 120–127)

LEARN IT Identify the health benefits of, and recommendations for, starches and fibers.

16. What foods provide starches and fibers?
17. Carbohydrates are found in virtually all foods except:
    a. milks.
    b. meats.
    c. breads.
    d. fruits.
18. What percentage of the daily energy intake should come from carbohydrates?
    a. 15 to 20
    b. 25 to 30
    c. 45 to 50
    d. 45 to 65

HIGHLIGHT 4 Carbs, kCalories, and Controversies (pp. 128–131)

LEARN IT Summarize the key scientific evidence behind some of the current controversies surrounding carbohydrates and their kcalories.

19. Which of the following is true?
    a. High-fructose corn syrup is chemically similar to sucrose.
    b. Diets with a high glycemic index are most effective in fostering weight loss.
    c. Energy intake from carbohydrates has remained stable over the past 40 years.
    d. Some people have a physiological addiction to sugar that makes it impossible for them to moderate use.

Multiple Choice Answers

3. c 4. c 5. d 8. b 9. d 11. d 12. d 13. a 17. b 18. d 19. a

STUDY IT

5 The Lipids: Triglycerides, Phospholipids, and Sterols

Review the key points of this chapter below, learn the definitions of the bold terms, and then take the practice quiz on the back of this card.

5.1 The Chemist's View of Fatty Acids and Triglycerides

- The predominant **lipids** both in foods and in the body are **triglycerides: glycerol** with three **fatty acids** attached by way of condensation reactions (review Figure 5-3, p. 137). Other lipids include phospholipids and sterols (review Table 5-2).
- Fatty acids vary in the length of their carbon chains, their degrees of unsaturation, and the location of their double bond(s). **Saturated fatty acids** are fully loaded with hydrogens; **unsaturated (monounsaturated** or **polyunsaturated)** fatty acids are missing hydrogens and have double bonds.
- **Hydrogenation** protects against oxidation (thereby promoting shelf-life) and alters the texture of foods by making liquid vegetable **oils** more solid. This process makes polyunsaturated **fats** more saturated and creates ***trans*-fatty acids.**

5.2 The Chemist's View of Phospholipids and Sterols

- The chemical structure of **phospholipids,** including **lecithin,** allows them to be soluble in both water and fat. In the body, phospholipids are part of cell membranes; in foods, phospholipids act as emulsifiers to mix fats with water.
- **Sterols** have a multiple-ring structure that differs from the structure of other lipids. In the body, sterols include **cholesterol,** bile, vitamin D, and some hormones. Animal-derived foods contain cholesterol.

5.3 Digestion, Absorption, and Transport of Lipids

- **Bile emulsifies** fats, making them accessible to the **lipases** that dismantle triglycerides to **monoglycerides** and fatty acids for absorption (review Figure 5-12, p. 143).
- Four types of **lipoproteins** carry triglycerides, phospholipids, and cholesterol throughout the body: **chylomicrons** are the largest and contain mostly dietary triglycerides, **VLDL** are smaller and are about half triglycerides, **LDL** are smaller still and contain mostly cholesterol, and **HDL** are the densest and are rich in protein (review Figure 5-16, p. 146).

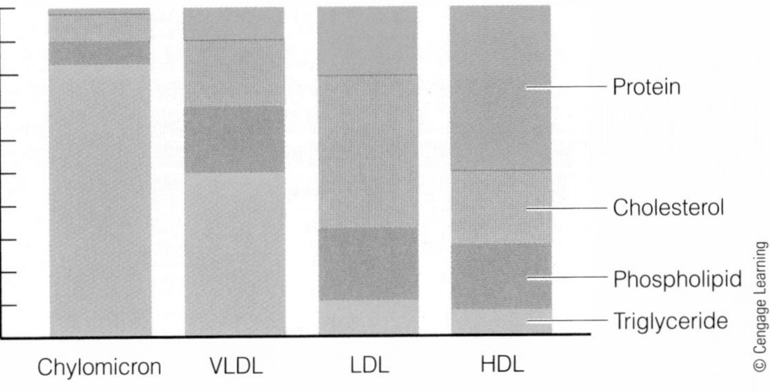

TABLE 5-2 The Lipid Family

Triglycerides

- 1 Glycerol (per triglyceride) and
- 3 Fatty acids (per triglyceride); depending on the number of double bonds, fatty acids may be:
  - *Saturated* (no double bonds)
  - *Monounsaturated* (one double bond)
  - *Polyunsaturated* (more than one double bond); depending on the location of the double bonds, polyunsaturated fatty acids may be:
    - *Omega-3* (double bond closest to methyl end is 3 carbons away)
    - *Omega-6* (double bond closest to methyl end is 6 carbons away)

Phospholipids (such as lecithin)

Sterols (such as cholesterol)

5.4 Lipids in the Body

- In the body, triglycerides provide energy, insulate against temperature extremes, protect against shock, and help the body use carbohydrate and protein efficiently.
- **Linoleic acid** (18 carbons, omega-6) and **linolenic acid** (18 carbons, omega-3) are **essential fatty acids,** serving as structural parts of cell membranes and as precursors to the longer fatty acids that can make **eicosanoids.**
- The body stores fat if given excesses, and uses body fat for energy when needed. (The liver can also convert excess carbohydrate and protein into fat.) Fat breakdown requires carbohydrate for maximum efficiency; without carbohydrate, fatty acids break down to **ketone bodies.**

5.5 Health Effects and Recommended Intakes of Saturated Fats, *Trans* Fats, and Cholesterol

- Some fat in the diet is necessary, but too much fat provides energy (kcalories) without nutrients, which leads to obesity and nutrient inadequacies.
- Too much saturated fat, *trans* fat, and cholesterol increases the risk of heart disease and possibly cancer.
- Recommendations advise that a diet be moderate in total fat and low in saturated fat, *trans* fat, and cholesterol.

5.6 Health Effects and Recommended Intakes of Monounsaturated and Polyunsaturated Fats

- Some fat in the diet has health benefits, especially the monounsaturated and polyunsaturated fats that protect against heart disease and possibly cancer.
- The *Dietary Guidelines* recommend replacing saturated fats with monounsaturated and polyunsaturated fats, particularly **omega-3** fatty acids from foods such as fatty fish, not from supplements.
- Many selection and preparation strategies can help bring these goals within reach, and food labels help to identify foods consistent with these guidelines.

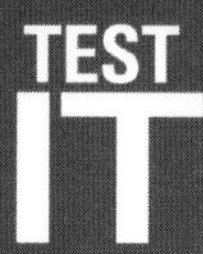

Take the quiz below to test your mastery of the key chapter concepts.

5.1 The Chemist's View of Fatty Acids and Triglycerides (pp. 134–140)

LEARN IT Recognize the chemistry of fatty acids and triglycerides and differences between saturated and unsaturated fats.

1. Name three classes of lipids found in the body and in foods. What are some of their functions in the body? What features do fats bring to foods?
2. What features distinguish fatty acids from each other?
3. What does the term *omega* mean with respect to fatty acids? Describe the roles of the omega fatty acids in disease prevention.
4. Describe the structure of a triglyceride.
5. What does hydrogenation do to fats? What are *trans*-fatty acids, and how do they influence heart disease?
6. Saturated fatty acids:
   a. are always 18 carbons long.
   b. have at least one double bond.
   c. are fully loaded with hydrogens.
   d. are always liquid at room temperature.
7. A triglyceride consists of:
   a. three glycerols attached to a lipid.
   b. three fatty acids attached to a glucose.
   c. three fatty acids attached to a glycerol.
   d. three phospholipids attached to a cholesterol.
8. The difference between *cis*- and *trans*-fatty acids is:
   a. the number of double bonds.
   b. the length of their carbon chains.
   c. the location of the first double bond.
   d. the configuration around the double bond.

5.2 The Chemist's View of Phospholipids and Sterols (pp. 140–141)

LEARN IT Describe the chemistry, food sources, and roles of phospholipids and sterols.

9. Which of the following is *not* true? Lecithin is:
   a. an emulsifier.
   b. a phospholipid.
   c. an essential nutrient.
   d. a constituent of cell membranes.

5.3 Digestion, Absorption, and Transport of Lipids (pp. 142–147)

LEARN IT Summarize fat digestion, absorption, and transport.

10. What do lipoproteins do? What are the differences among the chylomicrons, VLDL, LDL, and HDL?
11. Chylomicrons are produced in the:
    a. liver.
    b. pancreas.
    c. gallbladder.
    d. small intestine.
12. Transport vehicles for lipids are called:
    a. micelles.
    b. lipoproteins.
    c. blood vessels.
    d. monoglycerides.

5.4 Lipids in the Body (pp. 148–150)

LEARN IT Outline the major roles of fats in the body, including a discussion of essential fatty acids and the omega fatty acids.

13. Which of the following is *not* true? Fats:
    a. contain glucose.
    b. provide energy.
    c. protect against organ shock.
    d. carry vitamins A, D, E, and K.
14. The essential fatty acids include:
    a. stearic acid and oleic acid.
    b. oleic acid and linoleic acid.
    c. palmitic acid and linolenic acid.
    d. linoleic acid and linolenic acid.

5.5 Health Effects and Recommended Intakes of Saturated Fats, *Trans* Fats, and Cholesterol (pp. 150–152)

LEARN IT Explain the relationships among saturated fats, *trans* fat, and cholesterol and chronic diseases, noting recommendations.

15. How does excessive fat intake influence health? What factors influence LDL, HDL, and total blood cholesterol?
16. What are the dietary recommendations regarding saturated fat and cholesterol intake? List ways to reduce intake.
17. The lipoprotein most associated with a high risk of heart disease is:
    a. CHD.
    b. HDL.
    c. LDL.
    d. LPL.

5.6 Health Effects and Recommended Intakes of Monounsaturated and Polyunsaturated Fats (pp. 153–162)

LEARN IT Explain the relationships between monounsaturated and polyunsaturated fats and health, noting recommendations.

18. What is the Daily Value for fat (for a 2000-kcalorie diet)?
19. A person consuming 2200 kcalories a day who wants to meet health recommendations should limit daily fat intake to:
    a. 20 to 35 grams.
    b. 50 to 85 grams.
    c. 75 to 100 grams.
    d. 90 to 130 grams.

HIGHLIGHT 5 High-Fat Foods–Friend or Foe? (pp. 164–169)

LEARN IT Identify which fats support health and which impair it.

20. List foods that are high in saturated fats and foods that are high in unsaturated fats that could easily be used to replace them.

Multiple Choice Answers
6. c 7. c 8. d 9. c 11. d 12. b 13. a 14. d 17. c 19. b

Review the key points of this chapter below, learn the definitions of the bold terms, and then take the practice quiz on the back of this card.

6.1 The Chemist's View of Proteins

- **Proteins** are more chemically complex than carbohydrates or lipids; they are made of 20 different **amino acids,** 9 of which the body cannot make. These 9 are the **essential amino acids**—histidine, isoleucine, leucine, lysine, methionine, phenylalanine, threonine, tryptophan, and valine.
- Each amino acid contains an amino group, an acid group, a hydrogen atom, and a distinctive side group, all attached to a central carbon atom.
- Cells link amino acids together by a **peptide bond** in a series of condensation reactions to create proteins (review Figure 6-3, p. 173). The distinctive sequence of amino acids in each protein determines its unique shape and function.

6.2 Digestion and Absorption of Proteins

- The stomach's hydrochloric acid first denatures dietary proteins, then **enzymes** cleave them into smaller polypeptides and some amino acids.
- Pancreatic and intestinal enzymes split **polypeptides** further, to **oligo-, tri-,** and **dipeptides,** and then split most of these to single amino acids that can be absorbed into the intestinal cells (review Figure 6-6, p. 176).

6.3 Proteins in the Body

- Cells synthesize proteins according to the **genetic** information provided by the **DNA** in the nucleus of each cell (review Figure 6-7, p. 178). This information dictates the sequence in which amino acids are linked together to form a given protein. Sequencing errors occasionally occur, sometimes with significant consequences.
- A sampling of protein functions are summarized in Table 6-3.
- Proteins are constantly being synthesized and broken down as needed, a process known as **protein turnover.**
- The body's assimilation of amino acids into proteins and its release of amino acids via protein degradation and excretion can be tracked by measuring **nitrogen balance,** which should be positive during growth and steady in adulthood. An energy deficit or an inadequate protein intake may force the body to break down lean body tissue and use amino acids as fuel, creating a negative nitrogen balance.
- Protein eaten in excess of need is degraded and stored as body fat.

6.4 Protein in Foods

- **High-quality proteins** deliver all of the essential amino acids in adequate amounts, which ensures protein synthesis. Mixtures of foods containing **complementary proteins** can each supply the amino acids missing in the other.
- In addition to its amino acid content, the quality of a protein is measured by its **digestibility** and its ability to support growth.

6.5 Health Effects and Recommended Intakes of Protein

- Protein deficiency impairs the body's ability to grow and function optimally.
- Excess protein offers no advantage and may incur health problems as well.
- The optimal diet is adequate in energy from carbohydrate and fat and delivers 0.8 grams of protein per kilogram of healthy body weight each day.
- Healthy people do not need protein or amino acid supplements.

TABLE 6-3 **Protein Functions in the Body**

Structural materials	Proteins form integral parts of most body tissues and provide strength and shape to skin, tendons, membranes, muscles, organs, and bones.
Enzymes	Proteins facilitate chemical reactions.
Hormones	Proteins regulate body processes. (Some, but not all, hormones are proteins.)
Fluid balance	Proteins help to maintain the volume and composition of body fluids.
Acid-base balance	Proteins help to maintain the acid-base balance of body fluids by acting as **buffers.**
Transportation	Proteins transport substances, such as lipids, vitamins, minerals, and oxygen, around the body.
Antibodies	Proteins inactivate foreign invaders, thus protecting the body against diseases.
Energy and glucose	Proteins provide some fuel, and glucose if needed, for the body's energy needs.
Other	The protein fibrin creates blood clots; the protein **collagen** forms scars; the protein opsin participates in vision.

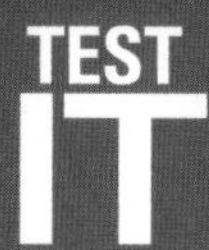

Take the quiz below to test your mastery of the key chapter concepts.

6.1 The Chemist's View of Proteins

(pp. 172–175)

LEARN IT Recognize the chemical structures of amino acids and proteins.

1. Explain how the sequence of amino acids affects protein shape and function.
2. What are essential amino acids?
3. Which part of its chemical structure differentiates one amino acid from another?
   a. its side group
   b. its acid group
   c. its amino group
   d. its double bonds
4. Isoleucine, leucine, and lysine are:
   a. proteases.
   b. polypeptides.
   c. essential amino acids.
   d. complementary proteins.

6.2 Digestion and Absorption of Proteins (pp. 175–176)

LEARN IT Summarize protein digestion and absorption.

5. In the stomach, hydrochloric acid:
   a. denatures proteins and activates pepsin.
   b. hydrolyzes proteins and denatures pepsin.
   c. emulsifies proteins and releases peptidase.
   d. condenses proteins and facilitates digestion.

6.3 Proteins in the Body (pp. 177–184)

LEARN IT Describe how the body makes proteins and uses them to perform various roles.

6. What are enzymes? What roles do they play in chemical reactions? Describe the differences between enzymes and hormones.
7. How does the body use amino acids? What is deamination? Define *nitrogen balance*. What conditions are associated with zero, positive, and negative balance?
8. Proteins that maintain the acid-base balance of the blood and body fluids by accepting and releasing hydrogen ions are:
   a. buffers.
   b. enzymes.
   c. hormones.
   d. antigens.
9. If an essential amino acid that is needed to make a protein is unavailable, the cells must:
   a. deaminate another amino acid.
   b. substitute a similar amino acid.
   c. break down proteins to obtain it.
   d. synthesize the amino acid from glucose and nitrogen.
10. Protein turnover describes the amount of protein:
    a. found in foods and the body.
    b. absorbed from the diet.
    c. synthesized and degraded.
    d. used to make glucose.

6.4 Protein in Foods (pp. 185–186)

LEARN IT Explain the differences between high-quality and low-quality proteins, including notable food sources of each.

11. How can vegetarians meet their protein needs without eating meat?
12. Which of the following foods provides the highest quality protein?
    a. egg
    b. corn
    c. gelatin
    d. whole grains

6.5 Health Effects and Recommended Intakes of Protein (pp. 186–191)

LEARN IT Identify the health benefits of, and recommendations for, protein.

13. How might protein excess, or the type of protein eaten, influence health?
14. What factors are considered in establishing recommended protein intakes?
15. What are the benefits and risks of taking protein and amino acid supplements?
16. The protein RDA for a healthy adult who weighs 180 pounds is:
    a. 50 milligrams/day.
    b. 65 grams/day.
    c. 180 grams/day.
    d. 2000 milligrams/day.
17. Which of these foods has the least protein per ½ cup?
    a. rice
    b. broccoli
    c. pinto beans
    d. orange juice

HIGHLIGHT 6 Nutritional Genomics (pp. 194–199)

LEARN IT Explain how nutrients influence gene activity (nutrigenomics) and how genes influence the activities of nutrients (nutrigenetics).

18. The area of study that examines how environmental factors influence gene expression without changing the DNA is known as:
    a. epigenetics.
    b. chromosomal biology.
    c. methylation translation.
    d. microarray technologies.

Multiple Choice Answers

3. a 4. c 5. a 8. a 9. c 10. c 12. a 16. b 17. d 18. a

Review the key points of this chapter below, learn the definitions of the bold terms, and then take the practice quiz on the back of this card.

7.1 Chemical Reactions in the Body

- During digestion, the energy-yielding nutrients—carbohydrates, lipids, and proteins—are broken down to glucose (and other monosaccharides), glycerol, fatty acids, and amino acids. These compounds may enter metabolic pathways to yield energy (review Figure 7-5).
- **Enzymes** with their **coenzymes** help cells use nutrients to build compounds **(anabolism)** or break them down to release energy **(catabolism)**—review Figure 7-2, p. 203.
- **ATP**—a high-energy compound—captures the energy released during catabolism (review Figure 7-4, p. 204).

7.2 Breaking Down Nutrients for Energy

- Glucose breakdown begins with **glycolysis,** a pathway that produces **pyruvate** (review Figure 7-6, p. 208).
- Pyruvate may be converted to **lactate anaerobically** (without oxygen) or to **acetyl CoA aerobically** (with oxygen).
- Pyruvate can make glucose; acetyl CoA cannot make glucose (review Figure 7-9, p. 210).
- The glycerol part of a triglyceride can make either pyruvate (and then glucose) or acetyl CoA. The fatty acids of a triglyceride *cannot* make glucose; they can provide abundant acetyl CoA (review Figure 7-11, p. 211).
- Some amino acids can be used to make glucose; others can be used either to provide energy or to make fat. Before an amino acid enters these metabolic pathways, its nitrogen-containing amino group must be removed through deamination.
- The digestion of carbohydrate yields glucose (and other monosaccharides); some glucose is stored as glycogen, and some is broken down to pyruvate and acetyl CoA.
- The digestion of fat yields glycerol and fatty acids; some are reassembled and stored as body fat, and others are broken down to acetyl CoA.
- The digestion of protein yields amino acids; most amino acids are used to build body protein or other nitrogen-containing compounds, some are broken down to acetyl CoA, and others enter the **TCA cycle** directly.
- Acetyl CoA may enter the TCA cycle to release energy (review Figure 7-15, p. 214) or combine with other molecules of acetyl CoA to make body fat.

7.3 Feasting and Fasting

- If energy intake exceeds energy needs, the result will be weight gain—regardless of whether the excess is from protein, carbohydrate, or fat (review Table 7-2). The body is most efficient at storing excess energy from dietary fat.
- When fasting, the body adapts to conserve energy and minimize losses by increasing fat breakdown to **fuel** most cells, using glycerol and amino acids to make glucose for the brain and red blood cells, producing **ketone bodies** for the brain, suppressing appetite, and slowing **metabolism.**

> FIGURE 7-5 **Simplified Overview of Energy-Yielding Pathways**

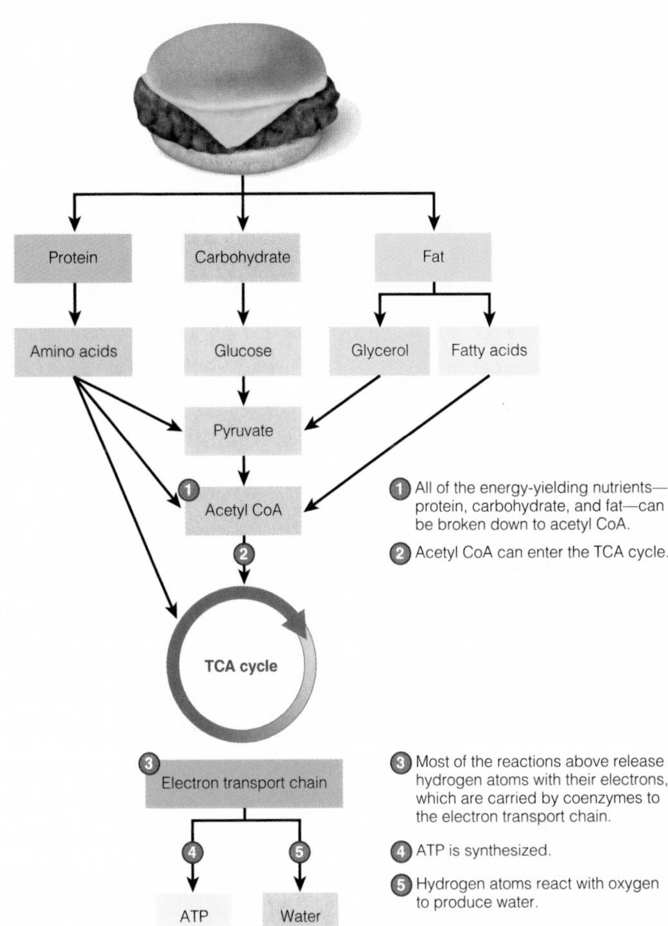
Protein
Carbohydrate
Fat
Amino acids
Glucose
Glycerol
Fatty acids
Pyruvate
1
Acetyl CoA
2
TCA cycle
3
Electron transport chain
4
5
ATP
Water
1 All of the energy-yielding nutrients—protein, carbohydrate, and fat—can be broken down to acetyl CoA.
2 Acetyl CoA can enter the TCA cycle.
3 Most of the reactions above release hydrogen atoms with their electrons, which are carried by coenzymes to the electron transport chain.
4 ATP is synthesized.
5 Hydrogen atoms react with oxygen to produce water.

TABLE 7-2 **Review of Energy-Yielding Nutrient End Points**

Nutrient	Yields energy?	Yields glucose?	Yields amino acids and body proteins?	Yields fat stores?
Carbohydrates (glucose)	Yes	Yes	Yes—when nitrogen is available, can yield *nonessential* amino acids	Yes
Lipids (fatty acids)	Yes	No	No	Yes
Lipids (glycerol)	Yes	Yes—when carbohydrate is unavailable	Yes—when nitrogen is available, can yield *nonessential* amino acids	Yes
Proteins (amino acids)	Yes	Yes—when carbohydrate is unavailable	Yes	Yes

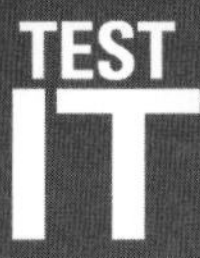

TEST IT

Take the quiz below to test your mastery of the key chapter concepts.

7.1 Chemical Reactions in the Body

(pp. 202–205)

LEARN IT Identify the nutrients involved in energy metabolism and the high-energy compound that captures the energy released during their breakdown.

1. Define *metabolism, anabolism,* and *catabolism*; give an example of each.
2. What are coenzymes, and what service do they provide in metabolism?
3. Hydrolysis is an example of a(n):
   a. coupled reaction.
   b. anabolic reaction.
   c. catabolic reaction.
   d. synthesis reaction.
4. During metabolism, released energy is captured and transferred by:
   a. enzymes.
   b. pyruvate.
   c. acetyl CoA.
   d. adenosine triphosphate.

7.2 Breaking Down Nutrients for Energy

(pp. 205–215)

LEARN IT Summarize the main steps in the energy metabolism of glucose, glycerol, fatty acids, and amino acids.

5. Name the four basic units, derived from foods, that are used by the body in energy metabolism. How many carbons are in the "backbones" of each?
6. Define *aerobic* and *anaerobic*. How does insufficient oxygen influence metabolism?
7. How does the body dispose of excess nitrogen?
8. The body derives most of its energy from:
   a. proteins and fats.
   b. vitamins and minerals.
   c. glucose and fatty acids.
   d. glycerol and amino acids.
9. Glycolysis:
   a. requires oxygen.
   b. generates abundant energy.
   c. converts glucose to pyruvate.
   d. produces ammonia as a by-product.
10. The pathway from pyruvate to acetyl CoA:
    a. produces lactate.
    b. is known as gluconeogenesis.
    c. is metabolically irreversible.
    d. requires more energy than it produces.
11. For complete oxidation, acetyl CoA enters:
    a. glycolysis.
    b. the TCA cycle.
    c. the Cori cycle.
    d. the electron transport chain.
12. Deamination of an amino acid produces:
    a. vitamin B_6 and energy.
    b. pyruvate and acetyl CoA.
    c. ammonia and a keto acid.
    d. carbon dioxide and water.
13. Before entering the TCA cycle, each of the energy-yielding nutrients is broken down to:
    a. ammonia.
    b. pyruvate.
    c. electrons.
    d. acetyl CoA.

7.3 Feasting and Fasting (pp. 216–221)

LEARN IT Explain how an excess of any of the three energy-yielding nutrients contributes to body fat and how an inadequate intake of any of them shifts metabolism.

14. What adaptations does the body make during a fast? What are ketone bodies? Define *ketosis*.
15. Distinguish between a loss of *fat* and a loss of *weight*, and describe how each might happen.
16. The body stores energy for future use in:
    a. proteins.
    b. acetyl CoA.
    c. triglycerides.
    d. ketone bodies.
17. During a fast, when glycogen stores have been depleted, the body begins to synthesize glucose from:
    a. acetyl CoA.
    b. amino acids.
    c. fatty acids.
    d. ketone bodies.
18. During a fast, the body produces ketone bodies by:
    a. hydrolyzing glycogen.
    b. condensing acetyl CoA.
    c. transaminating keto acids.
    d. converting ammonia to urea.

HIGHLIGHT 7 Alcohol in the Body (pp. 222–233)

LEARN IT Describe how alcohol disrupts metabolism and impairs health.

19. Alcohol metabolism occurs primarily in the:
    a. liver.
    b. brain.
    c. kidneys.
    d. muscles.

Multiple Choice Answers

3. c 4. d 8. c 9. c 10. c 11. b 12. c 13. d 16. c 17. b 18. b 19. a

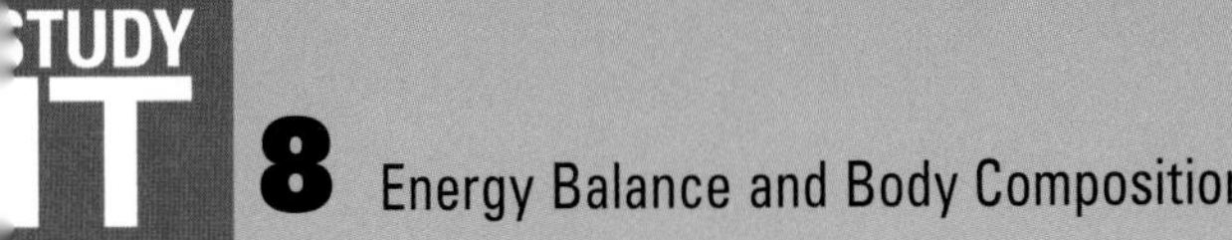

8 Energy Balance and Body Composition

Review the key points of this chapter below, learn the definitions of the bold terms, and then take the practice quiz on the back of this card.

8.1 Energy Balance

- When energy consumed equals energy expended, a person is in **energy balance** and body weight is stable.
- If more energy is taken in than is expended, a person gains weight. If more energy is expended than is taken in, a person loses weight.

8.2 Energy In: The kCalories Foods Provide

- Scientists use a **bomb calorimeter** to estimate the potential energy of foods by measuring the heat energy released when foods are burned.
- **Hunger** and **appetite** initiate eating, whereas **satiation** and **satiety** stop and delay eating, respectively (review Figure 8-2, p. 238). Each responds to messages from the nervous and hormonal systems. Superimposed on these signals are complex factors involving emotions, habits, and other aspects of human behavior.

8.3 Energy Out: The kCalories the Body Expends

- A person in energy balance takes in energy from food and expends much of it on **basal metabolism,** some of it on physical activities, and a little on the **thermic effect of food** (review Figure 8-4).
- Energy requirements vary from person to person based on such factors as gender, age, weight, and height as well as the intensity and duration of physical activity.

8.4 Body Weight and Body Composition

- Body weight standards are based on a person's weight in relation to height, called the **body mass index (BMI),** and reflect disease risks, not **body composition.** BMI does not identify body fat or its distribution, and it may misclassify muscular people as overweight.
- $\text{BMI} = \dfrac{\text{weight (kg)}}{\text{height (m)}^2}$ or $\dfrac{\text{weight (lb)}}{\text{height (in)}^2} \times 703.$

> FIGURE 8-4 **Components of Energy Expenditure**

The amount of energy expended in voluntary physical activities has the greatest variability, depending on a person's activity patterns. For a sedentary person, physical activities may account for less than half as much energy as basal metabolism, whereas an extremely active person may expend as much on activity as for basal metabolism.

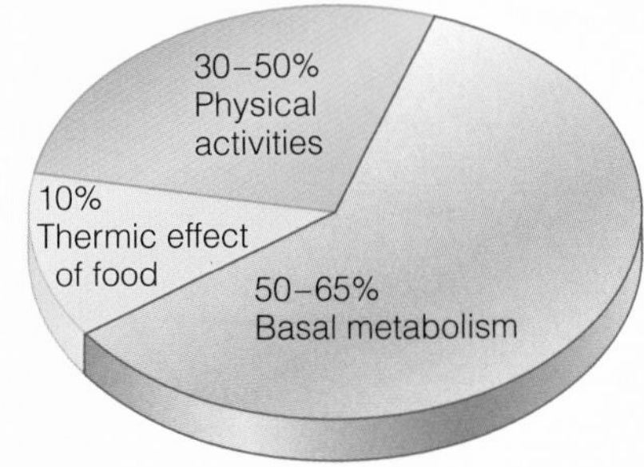

The amount of energy expended in a day differs for each individual, but in general, basal metabolism is the largest component of energy expenditure and thermic effect of food is the smallest.

> FIGURE 8-7 **Distribution of Body Weights in US Adults**

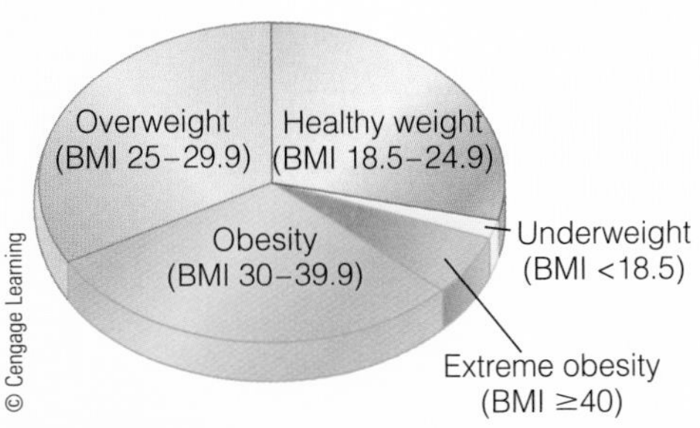

Underweight: BMI <18.5
Healthy: BMI 18.5 to 24.9
Overweight: BMI 25 to 29.9
Obese: BMI ≥30

- Two-thirds of US adults have a BMI greater than 25 (review Figure 8-7).
- The ideal amount of body fat varies from person to person, but excess body fat poses health risks.
- **Central obesity**—excess abdominal fat distributed around the trunk of the body— is more common in men and presents greater health risks than excess fat distributed on the lower body, which is more common in women (review Figure 8-8 and Figure 8-9, p. 250).
- Women with a **waist circumference** greater than 35 inches and men with a waist circumference greater than 40 inches have a high risk of central obesity–related health problems.

8.5 Health Risks Associated with Body Weight and Body Fat

- The healthiest weight for an individual depends on personal factors such as body fat distribution, family health history, and current health status. At the extremes, both overweight and underweight impose health risks (review Figure 8-11).

> FIGURE 8-11 **BMI and Mortality**

This J-shaped curve describes the relationship between body mass index (BMI) and mortality and shows that both underweight and overweight present risks of a premature death.

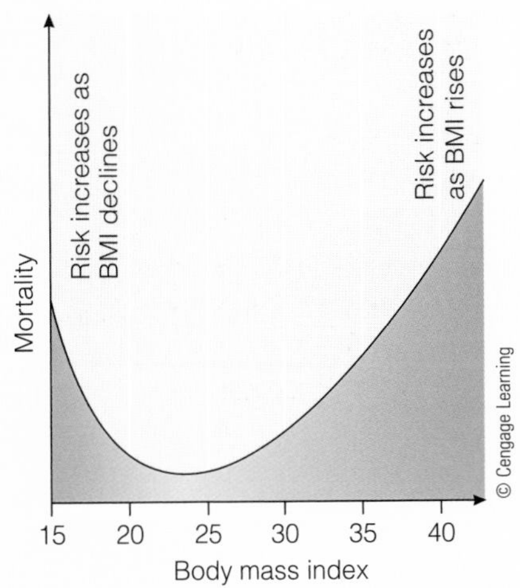

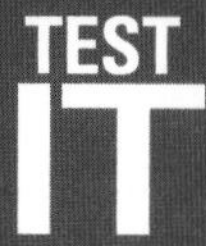

Take the quiz below to test your mastery of the key chapter concepts.

8.1 Energy Balance (p. 236)

LEARN IT Describe energy balance and the consequences of not being in balance.

1. A person who consistently consumes 1700 kcalories a day and expends 2200 kcalories a day for a month would be expected to:
   a. lose ½ to 1 pound.
   b. gain ½ to 1 pound.
   c. lose 4 to 5 pounds.
   d. gain 4 to 5 pounds.

8.2 Energy In: The kCalories Foods Provide (pp. 236–240)

LEARN IT Discuss some of the physical, emotional, and environmental influences on food intake.

2. A bomb calorimeter measures:
   a. physiological fuel.
   b. energy available from foods.
   c. kcalories a person derives from foods.
   d. heat a person releases in basal metabolism.

3. The psychological desire to eat that accompanies the sight, smell, or thought of food is known as:
   a. hunger.
   b. satiety.
   c. appetite.
   d. palatability.

4. A person watching television after dinner reaches for a snack during a commercial in response to:
   a. external cues.
   b. hunger signals.
   c. stress arousal.
   d. satiety factors.

8.3 Energy Out: The kCalories the Body Expends (pp. 240–244)

LEARN IT List the components of energy expenditure and factors that might influence each.

5. The largest component of energy expenditure is:
   a. basal metabolism.
   b. physical activity.
   c. indirect calorimetry.
   d. thermic effect of food.

6. A major factor influencing BMR is:
   a. hunger.
   b. food intake.
   c. body composition.
   d. physical activity.

7. The thermic effect of an 800-kcalorie meal is about:
   a. 8 kcalories.
   b. 80 kcalories.
   c. 160 kcalories.
   d. 200 kcalories.

8.4 Body Weight and Body Composition (pp. 245–251)

LEARN IT Distinguish between body weight and body composition including methods to assess each.

8. What problems are involved in defining "ideal" body weight?

9. What is central obesity, and what is its relationship to disease?

10. For health's sake, a person with a BMI of 21 might want to:
   a. lose weight.
   b. maintain weight.
   c. gain weight.

11. Which of the following reflects height and weight?
   a. body mass index
   b. central obesity
   c. waist circumference
   d. body composition

8.5 Health Risks Associated with Body Weight and Body Fat (pp. 251–254)

LEARN IT Identify relationships between body weight and chronic diseases.

12. Which of the following increases disease risks?
   a. BMI 19–21
   b. BMI 22–25
   c. lower-body fat
   d. central obesity

HIGHLIGHT 8 Eating Disorders (pp. 256–263)

LEARN IT Compare the diagnoses, characteristics, and treatments of the different eating disorders.

13. Which of the following is *not* commonly seen in RED-S
   a. amenorrhea
   b. osteoporosis
   c. disordered eating
   d. muscle dysmorphia

Multiple Choice Answers

1. c 2. b 3. c 4. a 5. a 6. c 7. b 10. b 11. a 12. d 13. d

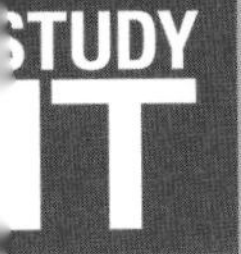

9 Weight Management: Overweight, Obesity, and Underweight

Review the key points of this chapter below, learn the definitions of the bold terms, and then take the practice quiz on the back of this card.

9.1 Overweight and Obesity

- Fat cells develop by increasing in number and size (review Figure 9-2, p. 267).
- Preventing weight gain depends on limiting the number of fat cells; weight loss depends on decreasing the size of fat cells.
- **Lipoprotein lipase (LPL)** removes triglycerides from the blood for storage in both adipose tissue and muscle cells. LPL activity is influenced by weight and gender.
- With weight gains or losses, the body adjusts in an attempt to return to its previous weight (**set point** theory).

9.2 Causes of Overweight and Obesity

- Obesity has multiple causes and different combinations of causes in different people.
- Some environmental causes, such as overeating and physical inactivity, may be within a person's control, and some, such as genetics, may be beyond it.
- Proteins such as **ghrelin** and **leptin** regulate food intake and energy homeostasis. Ghrelin enhances appetite and decreases energy expenditure, whereas leptin suppresses appetite and increases energy expenditure.

9.3 Problems of Overweight and Obesity

- Whether a person should lose weight depends on factors such as the extent of overweight, age, health risks, and genetics.
- Not all obesity will cause disease or shorten life expectancy. Just as there are unhealthy, normal-weight people, there are healthy, overweight people.
- Some people risk more in the process of losing weight than in remaining overweight.
- **Fad diets** and weight-loss supplements can be as physically and psychologically damaging as excess body weight.

9.4 Aggressive Treatments for Obesity

- Obese people with high risks of medical problems may need aggressive treatment, including drugs or surgery.
- Others may benefit most from improving eating and physical activity habits.

9.5 Weight-Loss Strategies

- A person who adopts a lifelong "eating plan for good health" rather than a "diet for weight loss" will be more likely to keep the lost weight off.
- Table 9-3 (p. 281) provides several tips for successful **weight management.**

> FIGURE 9-7 **Influence of Physical Activity on Discretionary kCalories**

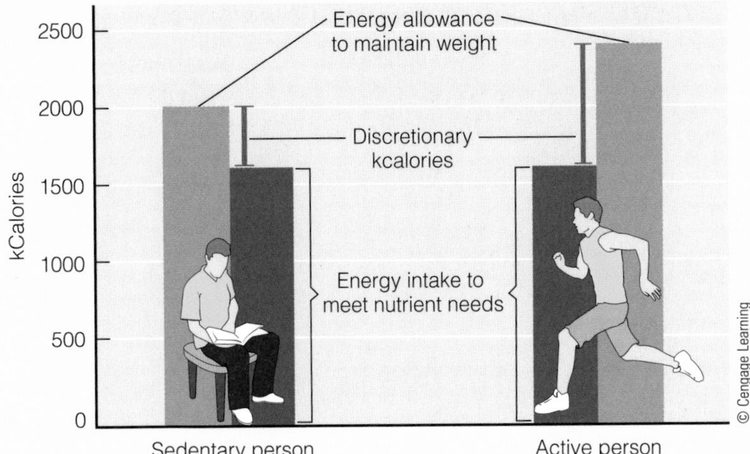

- Physical activity can increase energy expenditure (review Figure 9-7), improve body composition, help control appetite, reduce stress and stress eating, and enhance physical and psychological well-being.
- A surefire remedy for obesity has yet to be found; a combination of approaches is most effective.
- Weight loss depends on adjusting diet and physical activity so that more energy is expended than is taken in.
- For weight loss, energy intake should be reduced by 500 to 750 kcalories per day, depending on starting body weight and usual food intake.
- Safe rate for weight loss is ½ to 2 pounds per week or 5 to 10 percent body weight within 6 months.
- **Behavior modification** and cognitive restructuring retrain habits to support a healthy eating and activity plan.
- Treatment requires time, individualization, and sometimes the assistance of a registered dietitian nutritionist or support group.
- Preventing weight gains and **successful weight-loss maintenance** require vigilant attention to diet and physical activity; taking care of oneself is a lifelong responsibility.

9.6 Underweight

- Both the incidence of **underweight** and the health problems associated with it are less prevalent than overweight and its associated problems.
- To gain weight, a person must train physically and increase energy intake by selecting energy-dense foods, eating regular meals, taking larger portions, and consuming extra snacks and beverages.
- Table 9-5 (p. 291) includes a summary of weight-gain strategies.

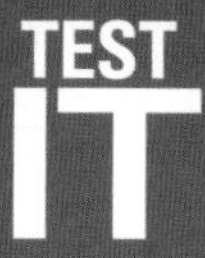

Take the quiz below to test your mastery of the key chapter concepts.

9.1 Overweight and Obesity (pp. 266–268)

LEARN IT Describe how body fat develops and why it can be difficult to maintain weight gains and losses.

1. With weight loss, fat cells:
   a. decrease in size only.
   b. decrease in number only.
   c. decrease in both number and size.
   d. decrease in number, but increase in size.
2. Describe the role of lipoprotein lipase (LPL).

9.2 Causes of Overweight and Obesity (pp. 268–272)

LEARN IT Review some of the causes of obesity.

3. Obesity is caused by:
   a. overeating.
   b. inactivity.
   c. defective genes.
   d. multiple factors.
4. The protein produced by the fat cells under the direction of the *ob* gene is called:
   a. leptin.
   b. serotonin.
   c. sibutramine.
   d. phentermine.

9.3 Problems of Overweight and Obesity (pp. 272–274)

LEARN IT Discuss the physical, social, and psychological consequences of overweight and obesity.

5. Which of the following is *not* used to evaluate the risks to health from obesity?
   a. body mass index
   b. blood leptin levels
   c. waist circumference
   d. disease risk profiles

9.4 Aggressive Treatments for Obesity (pp. 274–276)

LEARN IT Explain the risks and benefits, if any, of aggressive ways to treat obesity.

6. Gastric bypass surgery:
   a. is the best noninvasive treatment for obesity.
   b. limits food intake by reducing the capacity of the stomach.
   c. allows a person to eat unlimited amounts of food without weight gain.
   d. suppresses hunger by increasing production of gastrointestinal hormones.

9.5 Weight-Loss Strategies (pp. 276–289)

LEARN IT Outline reasonable strategies for achieving and maintaining a healthy body weight.

7. What are the benefits of increased physical activity in a weight-loss program?
8. Describe the behavioral strategies for changing an individual's dietary habits. What role does personal attitude play?
9. A realistic goal for weight loss is to reduce body weight:
   a. down to the weight a person was at age 25.
   b. down to the ideal weight in the weight-for-height tables.
   c. by 10 percent over 6 months.
   d. by 15 percent over 3 months.
10. A nutritionally sound weight-loss diet might restrict daily energy intake to create a:
    a. 1000-kcalorie-per-month deficit.
    b. 500-kcalorie-per-month deficit.
    c. 500-kcalorie-per-day deficit.
    d. 3500-kcalorie-per-day deficit.
11. Successful weight loss depends on:
    a. avoiding fats and limiting water.
    b. taking supplements and drinking water.
    c. increasing proteins and restricting carbohydrates.
    d. reducing energy intake and increasing physical activity.
12. Physical activity does *not* help a person to:
    a. lose weight.
    b. retain muscle.
    c. maintain weight loss.
    d. lose fat in trouble spots.
13. Which strategy would *not* help an overweight person to lose weight?
    a. Exercise.
    b. Eat slowly.
    c. Limit high-fat foods.
    d. Eat energy-dense foods regularly.

9.6 Underweight (pp. 289–291)

LEARN IT Summarize strategies for gaining weight.

14. Which strategy would *not* help an underweight person to gain weight?
    a. Exercise.
    b. Drink plenty of water.
    c. Eat snacks between meals.
    d. Eat large portions of foods.

HIGHLIGHT 9 The Latest and Greatest Weight-Loss Diet–Again (pp. 296–299)

LEARN IT Contrast the differences between popular fad diets and weight-loss diets based on sound nutrition.

15. A real benefit typical of many fad diets is:
    a. ketosis.
    b. a diet plan.
    c. changes in metabolism.
    d. quick and permanent weight loss.

Multiple Choice Answers

1. a 3. d 4. a 5. b 6. b 9. c 10. c 11. d 12. d 13. d 14. b 15. b

10 The Water-Soluble Vitamins: B Vitamins and Vitamin C

Review the key points of this chapter below, learn the definitions of the bold terms, and then take the practice quiz on the back of this card.

10.1 The Vitamins—An Overview

- The **vitamins** are organic, essential nutrients needed in tiny amounts in the diet both to prevent deficiency diseases and to support optimal health. The body handles the vitamins differently depending on whether they are water- or fat-soluble (review Table 10-2).
- The water-soluble vitamins are the B vitamins and vitamin C; the fat-soluble vitamins are vitamins A, D, E, and K. The B vitamins include thiamin, niacin, riboflavin, vitamin B_6, folate, vitamin B_{12}, pantothenic acid, and biotin.

10.2 The B Vitamins

- The B vitamins serve as **coenzymes**—small organic molecules closely associated with enzymes that facilitate the work of cells (review Figure 10-2).
- **Thiamin** is part of the coenzyme TPP, which assists in energy metabolism. Deficiency can result in **beriberi.** Thiamin occurs in small quantities in many nutritious foods; pork is an exceptionally good source.
- **Riboflavin** is part of the coenzymes FMN and FAD that accept and donate hydrogens during energy metabolism. Milk and milk products are good sources.
- **Niacin** is part of the coenzymes NAD and NADP that participate in many metabolic reactions. The deficiency disease, **pellagra,** causes diarrhea, dermatitis, dementia, and eventually death ("the 4 Ds"). Toxicity produces **"niacin flush"**—a tingling, painful sensation. The amino acid tryptophan can be converted to niacin in the body: 60 mg tryptophan = 1 **NE (niacin equivalent)**. Good sources of niacin are protein-rich foods.
- **Biotin** plays a critical role in energy metabolism, replenishing oxaloacetate in the TCA cycle. Biotin is widespread in foods; deficiencies and toxicities are rare.
- **Pantothenic acid** is part of coenzyme A that forms acetyl CoA in many metabolic pathways. Pantothenic acid is widespread in foods; deficiencies and toxicities are rare.
- **Vitamin B_6** occurs as pyridoxal, pyridoxine, and pyridoxamine; all can become part of the coenzyme PLP, which is active in amino acid metabolism. Deficiency causes convulsions; toxicity causes nerve damage.
- **Folate** is part of the coenzyme THF that activates vitamin B_{12}, synthesizes DNA, and regenerates the amino acid methionine from homocysteine. Folate helps prevent **neural tube defects.** Excessive folate can mask the **anemia** of a vitamin B_{12} deficiency, but it will not prevent the associated nerve damage. Folate is abundant in legumes, fruits, and vegetables.

TABLE 10-2 Water-Soluble and Fat-Soluble Vitamins Compared

	Water-Soluble Vitamins: B Vitamins and Vitamin C	Fat-Soluble Vitamins: Vitamins A, D, E, and K
Absorption	Directly into the blood	First into the lymph, then the blood
Transport	Travel freely	Many require transport proteins
Storage	Circulate freely in water-filled parts of the body	Stored in the cells associated with fat
Excretion	Kidneys detect and remove excess in urine	Less readily excreted; tend to remain in fat-storage sites
Toxicity	Possible to reach toxic levels when consumed from supplements	Likely to reach toxic levels when consumed from supplements
Requirements	Needed in frequent doses (perhaps 1 to 3 days)	Needed in periodic doses (perhaps weeks or even months)

NOTE: Exceptions occur, but these differences between the water-soluble and fat-solule vitamins are valid generalizations.

- **Vitamin B_{12}** activates folate, synthesizes DNA, regenerates methionine from homocysteine, and maintains the sheath that protects nerve fibers. Deficiencies typically occur when either hydrochloric acid or **intrinsic factor** is lacking. Vitamin B_{12} is found primarily in foods derived from animals.
- Many substances (including **inositol and carnitine**) that people claim as B vitamins are not. Fortunately, a variety of foods from each food group provides an adequate supply of all B vitamins.

10.3 Vitamin C

- Vitamin C acts as an **antioxidant**—a substance that decreases the adverse effects of **free radicals** in the body.
- Vitamin C works as a **cofactor** in the synthesis of **collagen,** neurotransmitters (serotonin and norepinephrine), hormones (thyroxine), and other compounds.
- Vitamin C deficiency causes **scurvy.**

> FIGURE 10-2 Coenzyme Action

Some vitamins form part of the coenzymes that enable enzymes either to synthesize compounds (as illustrated by the lower enzymes in this figure) or to dismantle compounds (as illustrated by the upper enzymes).

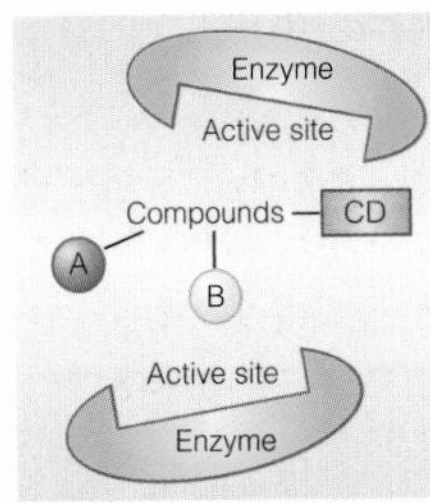

Without coenzymes, compounds A, B, and CD don't respond to their enzymes.

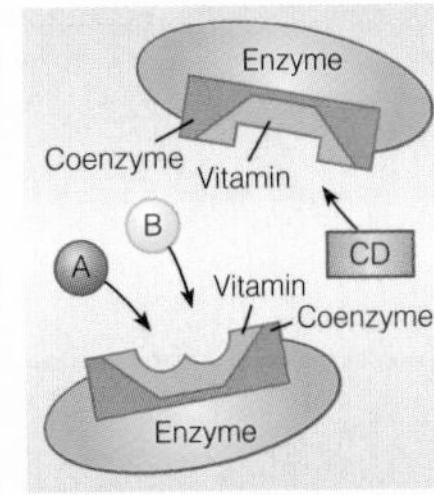

With the coenzymes in place, compounds are attracted to their sites on the enzymes . . .

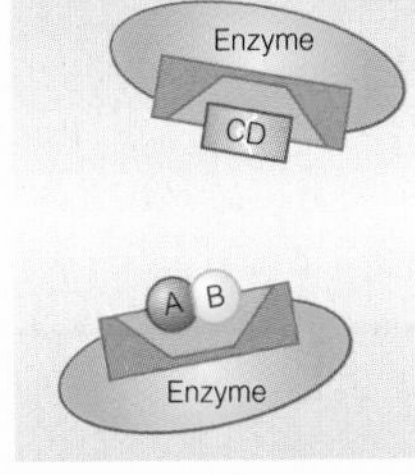

. . . and the reactions proceed instantaneously. The coenzymes often donate or accept electrons, atoms, or groups of atoms.

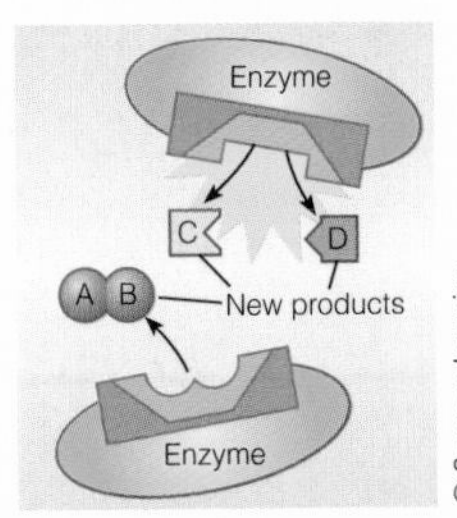

The reactions are completed with either the formation of a new product, AB, or the breaking apart of a compound into two new products, C and D, and the release of energy.

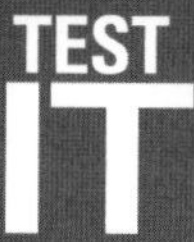

Take the quiz below to test your mastery of the key chapter concepts.

10.1 The Vitamins—An Overview

(pp. 302–304)

LEARN IT Describe how vitamins differ from the energy nutrients and how fat-soluble vitamins differ from water-soluble vitamins.

1. Vitamins:
   a. are inorganic compounds.
   b. yield energy when broken down.
   c. are soluble in either water or fat.
   d. perform best when linked in long chains.
2. The rate at and the extent to which a vitamin is absorbed and used in the body is known as its:
   a. bioavailability.
   b. intrinsic factor.
   c. physiological effect.
   d. pharmacological effect.

10.2 The B Vitamins (pp. 304–327)

LEARN IT Identify the main roles, deficiency symptoms, and food sources for each of the B vitamins (thiamin, riboflavin, niacin, biotin, pantothenic acid, vitamin B_6, folate, and vitamin B_{12}).

3. Which B vitamins are involved in energy metabolism? Protein metabolism? Cell division?
4. What is the relationship of tryptophan to niacin?
5. Describe the relationship between folate and vitamin B_{12}.
6. What risks are associated with high doses of niacin? Vitamin B_6? Vitamin C?
7. Many of the B vitamins serve as:
   a. coenzymes.
   b. antagonists.
   c. antioxidants.
   d. serotonin precursors.
8. With respect to thiamin, which of the following is the most nutrient dense?
   a. 1 slice whole-wheat bread (69 kcalories and 0.1 milligram thiamin)
   b. 1 cup yogurt (144 kcalories and 0.1 milligram thiamin)
   c. 1 cup snow peas (69 kcalories and 0.22 milligram thiamin)
   d. 1 chicken breast (141 kcalories and 0.06 milligram thiamin)
9. The body can make niacin from:
   a. tyrosine.
   b. serotonin.
   c. carnitine.
   d. tryptophan.
10. The vitamin that protects against neural tube defects is:
    a. niacin.
    b. folate.
    c. riboflavin.
    d. vitamin B_{12}.
11. A lack of intrinsic factor may lead to:
    a. beriberi.
    b. pellagra.
    c. pernicious anemia.
    d. atrophic gastritis.
12. Which of the following is a B vitamin?
    a. inositol
    b. carnitine
    c. vitamin B_{15}
    d. pantothenic acid

10.3 Vitamin C (pp. 327–333)

LEARN IT Identify the main roles, deficiency symptoms, and food sources for vitamin C.

13. Vitamin C serves as a(n):
    a. coenzyme.
    b. antagonist.
    c. antioxidant.
    d. intrinsic factor.
14. The requirement for vitamin C is highest for:
    a. smokers.
    b. athletes.
    c. alcoholics.
    d. the elderly.

See p. 332–333 for a summary of the water-soluble vitamins.

HIGHLIGHT Vitamin and Mineral Supplements (pp. 335–341)

LEARN IT Present arguments for and against the use of dietary supplements.

15. The best vitamin and mineral supplements:
    a. are high-potency.
    b. are nanoceuticals.
    c. are made from organic vegetables.
    d. provide 50 to 150 percent of the Daily Value.

Multiple Choice Answers

1.c 2.a 7.a 8.c 9.d 10.b 11.c 12.d 13.c 14.a 15.d

TUDY IT **11** The Fat-Soluble Vitamins: A, D, E, and K

eview the key points of this chapter below, learn the definitions of the bold terms, and then take the practice quiz on the back of this card.

11.1 Vitamin A and Beta-Carotene

- **Vitamin A** is found in the body in three forms: **retinol, retinal,** and **retinoic acid.** Together, they are essential to vision, healthy epithelial tissues, and growth.
- Vitamin A deficiency is a major health problem worldwide, leading to infections, blindness, and **keratinization.**
- Toxicity can also cause problems and is most often associated with supplement abuse.
- Animal-derived foods such as liver and whole or fortified milk provide **retinoids,** whereas brightly colored plant-derived foods such as spinach, carrots, and pumpkins provide **beta-carotene** and other **carotenoids.**
- In addition to serving as a precursor for vitamin A, beta-carotene may act as an antioxidant in the body.

11.2 Vitamin D

- **Vitamin D** can be synthesized in the body with the help of sunlight (see Figure 11-8) or obtained from fortified milk.
- Vitamin D sends signals to three primary target sites: the GI tract to absorb more calcium and phosphorus, the bones to release more, and the kidneys to retain more. These actions maintain blood calcium concentrations and support bone formation.
- A vitamin D deficiency causes **rickets** in childhood and **osteomalacia** in later life.

11.3 Vitamin E

- Vitamin E **(alpha-tocopherol)** acts as an antioxidant, defending lipids and other components of the cells against oxidative damage.
- Deficiencies are rare, but they do occur in premature infants, the primary symptom being **erythrocyte hemolysis** (red blood cell breakage).
- Vitamin E is found predominantly in vegetable oils and appears to be one of the least toxic of the fat-soluble vitamins.

11.4 Vitamin K

- Vitamin K helps with blood clotting (review Figure 11-11, p. 359), and its deficiency causes **hemorrhagic disease** (uncontrolled bleeding).
- Bacteria in the GI tract can make vitamin K; people typically receive about half of their requirements from bacterial synthesis and half from foods such as green vegetables and vegetable oils.
- Because people depend on bacterial synthesis for vitamin K, deficiency is most likely in newborn infants and in people taking antibiotics.

> FIGURE 11-8 **Vitamin D Synthesis and Activation**

The final activation step in the kidneys is tightly regulated by hormones.

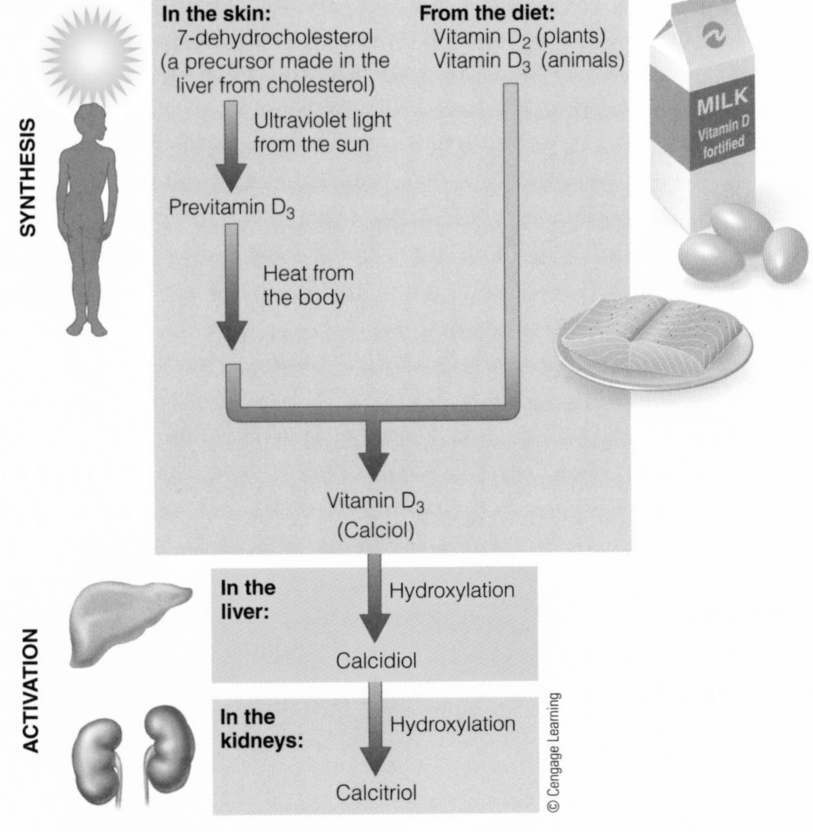

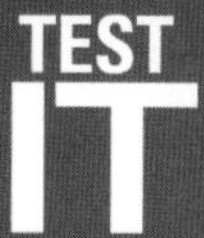

Take the quiz below to test your mastery of the key chapter concepts.

11.1 Vitamin A and Beta-Carotene (pp. 344–351)

LEARN IT Identify the main roles, deficiency symptoms, and food sources for vitamin A.

1. What are vitamin precursors? Name the precursors of vitamin A, and tell in what classes of foods they are found. Give examples of foods with high vitamin A activity.

2. The form of vitamin A active in vision is:
   a. retinal.
   b. retinol.
   c. rhodopsin.
   d. retinoic acid.

3. Vitamin A–deficiency symptoms include:
   a. rickets and osteomalacia.
   b. hemorrhaging and jaundice.
   c. night blindness and keratomalacia.
   d. fibrocystic breast disease and erythrocyte hemolysis.

4. Good sources of vitamin A include:
   a. oatmeal, pinto beans, and ham.
   b. apricots, turnip greens, and liver.
   c. whole-wheat bread, green peas, and tuna.
   d. corn, grapefruit juice, and sunflower seeds.

11.2 Vitamin D (pp. 351–356)

LEARN IT Identify the main roles, deficiency symptoms, and sources for vitamin D.

5. How is vitamin D unique among the vitamins?

6. To keep minerals available in the blood, vitamin D targets:
   a. the skin, the muscles, and the bones.
   b. the kidneys, the liver, and the bones.
   c. the intestines, the kidneys, and the bones.
   d. the intestines, the pancreas, and the liver.

7. Vitamin D can be synthesized from a precursor that the body makes from:
   a. bilirubin.
   b. tocopherol.
   c. cholesterol.
   d. beta-carotene.

11.3 Vitamin E (pp. 357–358)

LEARN IT Identify the main roles, deficiency symptoms, and food sources for vitamin E.

8. Vitamin E's most notable role is to:
   a. protect lipids against oxidation.
   b. activate blood-clotting proteins.
   c. support protein and DNA synthesis.
   d. enhance calcium deposits in the bones.

9. The classic sign of vitamin E deficiency is:
   a. rickets.
   b. xeropthalmia.
   c. muscular dystrophy.
   d. erythrocyte hemolysis.

11.4 Vitamin K (pp. 358–361)

LEARN IT Identify the main roles, deficiency symptoms, and sources for vitamin K.

10. What conditions may lead to vitamin K deficiency?

11. Without vitamin K:
    a. muscles atrophy.
    b. bones become soft.
    c. skin rashes develop.
    d. blood fails to clot.

12. A significant amount of vitamin K comes from:
    a. vegetable oils.
    b. sunlight exposure.
    c. bacterial synthesis.
    d. fortified grain products.

See p. 361 for a summary of the fat-soluble vitamins.

HIGHLIGHT 11 Antioxidant Nutrients in Disease Prevention (pp. 364–368)

LEARN IT Describe how antioxidants defend against free radicals that contribute to diseases.

13. Free radicals:
    a. are highly reactive.
    b. defend against cancer.
    c. act as antioxidants in the body.
    d. are found abundantly in fruits and vegetables.

Multiple Choice Answers

2. a 3. c 4. b 6. c 7. c 8. a 9. d 11. d 12. c 13. a

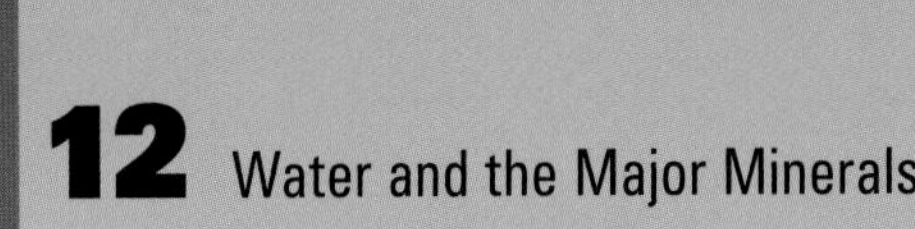

12 Water and the Major Minerals

Review the key points of this chapter below, learn the definitions of the bold terms, and then take the practice quiz on the back of this card.

12.1 Water and the Body Fluids

- Water makes up about 60 percent of an adult's body weight.
- Water assists with the transport of nutrients and waste products throughout the body, participates in chemical reactions, acts as a solvent, serves as a shock absorber, and regulates body temperature.
- To maintain **water balance,** intake from liquids, foods, and metabolism must equal losses from the kidneys, skin, lungs, and GI tract (review Table 12-3, p. 373).
- Whenever the body experiences low blood volume, low blood pressure, or highly concentrated body fluids, the actions of **ADH, renin, angiotensin,** and **aldosterone** restore homeostasis (review Figure 12-3).
- **Electrolytes** (charged minerals) in the fluids help distribute the fluids inside and outside the cells, thus ensuring the appropriate water balance and acid-base balance to support all life processes.
- Excessive losses of fluids and electrolytes upset these balances, and the kidneys play a key role in restoring homeostasis.

FIGURE 12-3 **How the Body Regulates Blood Volume and Blood Pressure**

The renin-angiotensin-aldosterone system helps regulate blood volume and therefore blood pressure.

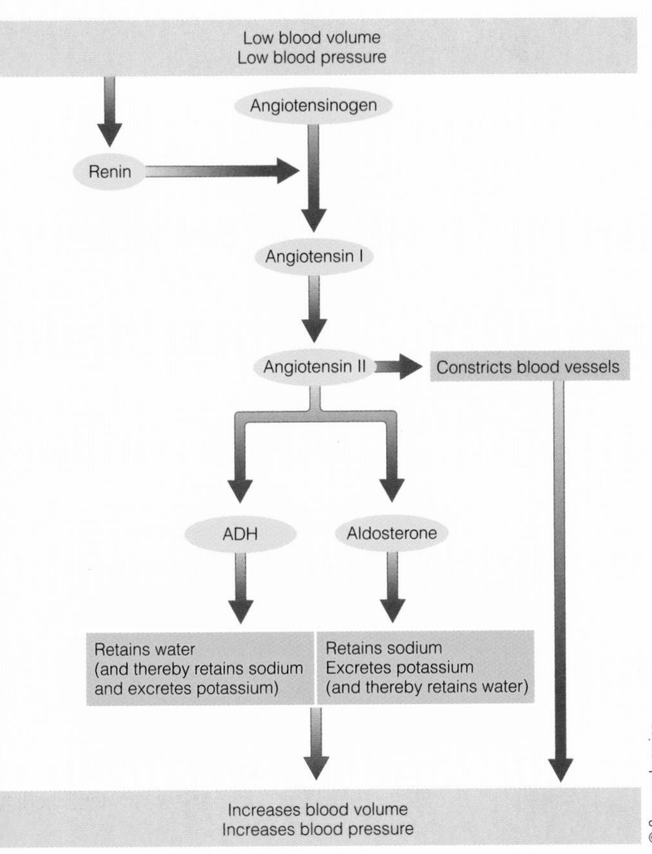

12.2 The Minerals—An Overview

- The **major minerals** are needed in the diet and found in the body in larger quantities than the **trace minerals** (review Figure 12-9, p. 381).
- Minerals are inorganic elements that retain their chemical identities; receive special handling and regulation in the body; and may bind with other substances or interact with other minerals, thus limiting their absorption.
- The major minerals, especially sodium, chloride, and potassium, influence the body's fluid balance; whenever an **anion** moves, a **cation** moves—always maintaining homeostasis.
- Sodium, chloride, potassium, calcium, and magnesium are key members of the team of nutrients that direct nerve impulse transmission and muscle contraction. They are also the primary nutrients involved in regulating blood pressure.
- Phosphorus and magnesium participate in many reactions involving glucose, fatty acids, amino acids, and the vitamins. Calcium, phosphorus, and magnesium combine to form the structure of the bones and teeth. Each major mineral also plays other specific roles in the body.

12.3 The Major Minerals

- **Sodium** is the main cation outside cells and one of the primary electrolytes responsible for maintaining fluid balance. Dietary deficiency is rare; excesses seem to aggravate hypertension, and so health professionals advise a diet moderate in **salt** and sodium.
- **Chloride** is the major anion outside cells, and it associates closely with sodium. In addition to its role in fluid balance, chloride is part of the stomach's hydrochloric acid.
- **Potassium** is the primary cation inside cells and plays an important role in maintaining fluid balance. Fresh foods, notably fruits and vegetables, are its best sources.
- **Calcium** is found primarily in the bones, where it provides a rigid structure and a reservoir of calcium for the blood. Blood calcium participates in muscle contraction, blood clotting, and nerve impulses, and it is closely regulated by a system of hormones and vitamin D (review Figure 12-12, p. 389). Milk and milk products are good sources of calcium, but certain vegetables and tofu also provide calcium. Even when calcium intake is inadequate, blood calcium remains normal, but at the expense of bone loss, which can lead to **osteoporosis.**
- **Phosphorus** accompanies calcium both in the crystals of bone and in many foods such as milk. Phosphorus is also important in energy metabolism, as part of phospholipids, and as part of the genetic materials DNA and RNA.
- **Magnesium** supports bone **mineralization** and participates in numerous enzyme systems and in heart function. It is found abundantly in legumes and dark green, leafy vegetables and, in some areas, in water.
- **Sulfate** is found in all protein-containing foods. Its primary role in amino acids is to stabilize proteins by forming disulfide bridges.

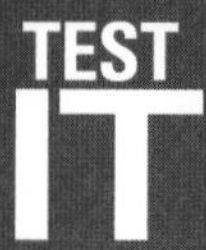

Take the quiz below to test your mastery of the key chapter concepts.

12.1 Water and the Body Fluids (pp. 372–381)

LEARN IT Explain how the body regulates fluid balance.

1. List the roles of water in the body.
2. List the sources of water intake and routes of water excretion.
3. What is ADH? Where does it exert its action? What is aldosterone? How does it work?
4. How does the body use electrolytes to regulate fluid balance?
5. The body generates water during the:
   a. buffering of acids.
   b. dismantling of bone.
   c. metabolism of minerals.
   d. oxidation of energy nutrients through the electron transport chain.
6. Regulation of fluid and electrolyte balance and acid-base balance depends primarily on the:
   a. kidneys.
   b. intestines.
   c. sweat glands.
   d. specialized tear ducts.

12.2 The Minerals—An Overview (pp. 381–382)

LEARN IT List some of the ways minerals differ from vitamins and other nutrients.

7. What do the terms major and trace mean when describing the minerals in the body?
8. Describe some characteristics of minerals that distinguish them from vitamins.
9. The distinction between the major and trace minerals reflects the:
   a. ability of their ions to form salts.
   b. amounts of their contents in the body.
   c. importance of their functions in the body.
   d. capacity to retain their identity after absorption.

12.3 The Major Minerals (pp. 382–398)

LEARN IT Identify the main roles, deficiency symptoms, and food sources for each of the major minerals (sodium, chloride, potassium, calcium, phosphorus, magnesium, and sulfate).

10. What is the major function of sodium in the body? Describe how the kidneys regulate blood sodium. Is a dietary deficiency of sodium likely? Why or why not?
11. List calcium's roles in the body. How does the body keep blood calcium constant regardless of intake?
12. Name significant food sources of calcium. What are the consequences of inadequate intakes?
13. List the roles of phosphorus in the body. Discuss the relation ships between calcium and phosphorus. Is a dietary deficienc of phosphorus likely? Why or why not?
14. State the major functions of chloride, potassium, magnesium and sulfur in the body. Are deficiencies of these nutrient likely to occur in your own diet? Why or why not?
15. The principal cation in extracellular fluids is:
    a. sodium.
    b. chloride.
    c. potassium.
    d. phosphorus.
16. The role of chloride in the stomach is to help:
    a. support nerve impulses.
    b. convey hormonal messages.
    c. maintain a strong acidity.
    d. assist in muscular contractions.
17. Which would provide the most potassium?
    a. bologna
    b. potatoes
    c. pickles
    d. whole-wheat bread
18. Calcium homeostasis depends on:
    a. vitamin K, aldosterone, and renin.
    b. vitamin K, parathyroid hormone, and renin.
    c. vitamin D, aldosterone, and calcitonin.
    d. vitamin D, calcitonin, and parathyroid hormone.
19. Calcium absorption is hindered by:
    a. lactose.
    b. oxalates.
    c. vitamin D.
    d. stomach acid.
20. Phosphorus assists in many activities in the body, but not:
    a. energy metabolism.
    b. the clotting of blood.
    c. the transport of lipids.
    d. bone and teeth formation.
21. Most of the body's magnesium can be found in the:
    a. bones.
    b. nerves.
    c. muscles.
    d. extracellular fluids.

See p. 397 for a summary of the major minerals.

HIGHLIGHT 12 Osteoporosis and Calcium (pp. 400–405)

LEARN IT Describe factors that contribute to the development of osteoporosis and strategies to prevent it.

22. Which of the following is not a risk factor for osteoporosis?
    a. overweight
    b. cigarette smoking
    c. sedentary lifestyle
    d. inadequate dietary calcium and vitamin D

Multiple Choice Answers

5. d 6. a 9. b 15. a 16. c 17. b 18. d 19. b 20. b 21. a 22. a

Review the key points of this chapter below, learn the definitions of the bold terms, and then take the practice quiz on the back of this card.

13.1 The Trace Minerals—An Overview

- The body needs tiny amounts of the **trace minerals.**
- The trace minerals can be toxic at levels not far above estimated requirements—a consideration for supplement users (review Figure 13-1, p. 408).
- Like the other nutrients, the trace minerals are best obtained by eating a variety of foods.

13.2 The Trace Minerals

- **Iron** is found in **hemoglobin** and **myoglobin** where it carries oxygen for energy metabolism; iron also acts as a **cofactor** for some enzymes. **Iron deficiency** is most common among infants and young children, teenagers, women of childbearing age, and pregnant women. Symptoms include fatigue and anemia. **Iron overload** is most common in men. **Heme iron,** which is found only in meat, fish, and poultry, is better absorbed than **nonheme iron,** which occurs in most foods (review Figure 13-4). Nonheme iron absorption is improved by eating iron-containing foods with foods containing the **MFP factor** and vitamin C; absorption is limited by phytates and oxalates.
- Zinc-requiring enzymes participate in reactions affecting growth, vitamin A activity, and pancreatic digestive enzyme synthesis. Both dietary **zinc** and zinc-rich pancreatic secretions (via **enteropancreatic circulation**) are available for absorption. Absorption is monitored by a special binding protein (**metallothionein**) in the small intestine. Protein-rich foods derived from animals are the best sources of bioavailable zinc. Fiber and phytates in cereals bind zinc, limiting absorption. Symptoms of deficiency include growth retardation and sexual immaturity.
- Iodide, the **iodine** ion, is an essential component of the thyroid hormone. A deficiency can lead to **goiter** (enlargement of the thyroid gland) and can impair fetal development, causing **cretinism.** Iodization of salt has largely eliminated iodine deficiency in the United States.
- **Selenium** is an antioxidant nutrient that works closely with the glutathione peroxidase enzyme and vitamin E. Selenium is found with protein in foods. Deficiencies are associated with a predisposition to a type of heart abnormality known as **Keshan disease.**
- **Copper** is a component of several enzymes, all of which are involved with oxygen or oxidation. Some act as antioxidants; others are essential to iron metabolism. Legumes, whole grains, and shellfish are good sources of copper.
- Manganese-dependent enzymes are involved in bone formation and various metabolic processes. Because **manganese** is widespread in plant foods, deficiencies are rare, although regular use of calcium and iron supplements may limit manganese absorption.
- **Fluoride** makes teeth more resistant to decay. Fluoridation of public water reduces the incidence of dental caries; excess fluoride during tooth development can discolor and pit tooth enamel **(fluorosis).**
- **Chromium** enhances insulin's action. Deficiency can result in a diabetes-like condition. Chromium is widely available in unrefined foods including brewer's yeast, whole grains, and liver.
- **Molybdenum** is a part of many **metalloenzymes.** Deficiencies are unknown and toxicity is rare. It is found in a variety of foods.

13.3 Contaminant Minerals

- Contaminant minerals include the **heavy metals** lead, mercury, and cadmium that enter the food supply by way of soil, water, and air pollution.
- Lead typifies the ways all heavy metals behave in the body: they interfere with nutrients that are trying to do their jobs. The "good guy" nutrients are shoved aside by the "bad guy" contaminants. Then, when the contaminants cannot perform the role of the nutrients, health diminishes.
- To safeguard our health, we must defend ourselves against contamination by eating nutrient-rich foods and preserving a clean environment.

> FIGURE 13-4 **Heme and Nonheme Iron in Foods**

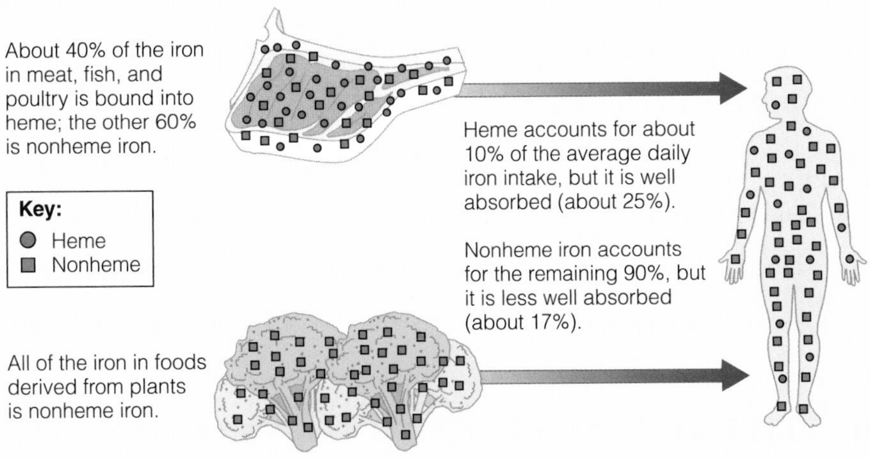

About 40% of the iron in meat, fish, and poultry is bound into heme; the other 60% is nonheme iron.
Key:
Heme
Nonheme
All of the iron in foods derived from plants is nonheme iron.
Heme accounts for about 10% of the average daily iron intake, but it is well absorbed (about 25%).
Nonheme iron accounts for the remaining 90%, but it is less well absorbed (about 17%).

TEST IT

Take the quiz below to test your mastery of the key chapter concepts.

13.1 The Trace Minerals—An Overview (pp. 408–409)

LEARN IT Summarize key factors unique to the trace minerals.

1. Discuss the importance of balanced and varied diets in obtaining the essential minerals and avoiding toxicities.
2. Describe some of the ways trace minerals interact with one another and with other nutrients.

13.2 The Trace Minerals (pp. 410–428)

LEARN IT Identify the main roles, deficiency symptoms, and food sources for each of the essential trace minerals (iron, zinc, iodine, selenium, copper, manganese, fluoride, chromium, and molybdenum).

3. Distinguish between heme and nonheme iron. Discuss the factors that enhance iron absorption.
4. Iron absorption is impaired by:
   a. heme.
   b. phytates.
   c. vitamin C.
   d. MFP factor.
5. Which of these people is *least* likely to develop an iron deficiency?
   a. 3-year-old boy
   b. 52-year-old man
   c. 17-year-old girl
   d. 24-year-old woman
6. Which of the following would *not* describe the blood cells of a severe iron deficiency?
   a. anemic
   b. microcytic
   c. pernicious
   d. hypochromic
7. Which provides the most absorbable iron?
   a. 1 apple
   b. 1 cup milk
   c. 3 ounces steak
   d. ½ cup spinach
8. What causes iron overload? What are its symptoms?
9. Describe the similarities and differences in the absorption and regulation of iron and zinc.
10. Discuss possible reasons for a low intake of zinc. What factors affect the bioavailability of zinc?
11. The intestinal protein that helps to regulate zinc absorption is:
    a. albumin.
    b. ferritin.
    c. hemosiderin.
    d. metallothionein.
12. A classic sign of zinc deficiency is:
    a. anemia.
    b. goiter.
    c. mottled teeth.
    d. growth retardation.
13. What public health measure has been used in preventing simple goiter?
14. Cretinism is caused by a deficiency of:
    a. iron.
    b. zinc.
    c. iodine.
    d. selenium.
15. The mineral best known for its role as an antioxidant is:
    a. copper.
    b. selenium.
    c. manganese.
    d. molybdenum.
16. What measure has been recommended for protection against tooth decay?
17. Fluorosis occurs when fluoride:
    a. is excessive.
    b. is inadequate.
    c. binds with phosphorus.
    d. interacts with calcium.
18. Which mineral enhances insulin activity?
    a. zinc
    b. iodine
    c. chromium
    d. manganese

See p. 430 for a summary of the trace minerals.

13.3 Contaminant Minerals (p. 429)

LEARN IT Describe how contaminant minerals disrupt body processes and impair nutrition status.

19. Which of the following does lead *not* compete with?
    a. iron
    b. zinc
    c. fluoride
    d. calcium

HIGHLIGHT 13 Phytochemicals and Functional Foods (pp. 433–439)

LEARN IT Define *phytochemicals* and explain how they might defend against chronic diseases.

20. Examples of phytochemicals include:
    a. LDL and DNA.
    b. lycopene and lutein.
    c. soybeans and flaxseeds.
    d. carcinogens and goitrogens.

Multiple Choice Answers

4.b 5.b 6.c 7.c 11.d 12.d 14.c 15.b 17.a 18.c 19.c 20.b

STUDY IT

14 Fitness: Physical Activity, Nutrients, and Body Adaptations

Review the key points of this chapter below, learn the definitions of the bold terms, and then take the practice quiz on the back of this card.

14.1 Fitness

- **Physical activity** promotes good health and reduces the risk of developing a number of diseases.
- The components of **fitness** are **flexibility, muscle strength, muscle endurance,** and **cardiorespiratory endurance.**
- Participating in cardiorespiratory, strength, and flexibility activities improves fitness and benefits health (review Table 14-2, p. 444).

14.2 Energy Systems and Fuels to Support Activity

- The high-energy compound ATP provides the energy that powers all the activities of living cells.
- Physical activity uses ATP.
- Three major energy systems enable muscle cells to replenish ATP during activity: the phosphagen system, the lactic acid system, and the aerobic system.
- The phosphagen system relies on the breakdown of another high-energy compound **CP,** to replenish ATP. CP can split anaerobically to release phosphate and restore ATP.

  During rest: ATP + creatine → CP

  During activity: CP → ATP + creatine
- The lactic acid system involves the incomplete oxidation of glucose anaerobically to lactate.
- The aerobic system generates ATP from the oxidation of carbohydrate, fat, and some amino acids.
- Fuel mixture during physical activity depends on diet, the intensity and duration of activity, and training (review Table 14-4).
- During intense activity, the fuel mix is mostly glucose; during less intense activity, fat makes a greater contribution.
- With endurance training, muscle cells adapt to store more glycogen and to rely less on glucose and more on fat for energy.
- Active athletes may need more protein than **sedentary** people do; they typically eat more food and therefore obtain enough protein without supplements (review Table 14-5, p. 455).

14.3 Vitamins and Minerals to Support Activity

- With the possible exception of iron for women, well-nourished active people and athletes do not need dietary supplements.

14.4 Fluids and Electrolytes to Support Activity

- **Heat stroke** and **hypothermia** can be fatal (review Table 14-6, p. 458).
- Active people need to drink plenty of water (review Table 14-7, p. 458).
- Endurance athletes need to drink both water and carbohydrate-containing beverages, especially during training and competition.
- During events lasting longer than 3 hours, athletes may need to replace sodium losses to prevent **hyponatremia.**

14.5 Diets for Physically Active People

- To enhance athletic performance and overall health, a diet should provide ample fluid and a variety of nutrient-dense foods in quantities to meet energy needs.
- Carbohydrate-rich foods that are light and easy to digest are best for pregame and recovery meals.

TABLE 14-4 Primary Fuels Used for Activities of Different Intensities and Durations

Activity Intensity	Activity Duration	Energy System	Preferred Fuel Source	Oxygen Needed?	Activity Example
Extreme	5 to 10 sec	Phosphagen system	ATP-CP (immediate availability)	No	100-meter sprint, shot put, golf or baseball bat swing, tennis or volleyball serve
Very high	20 sec to 2 min	Lactic acid system	ATP from carbohydrate (anaerobic glycolysis)	No	400-meter run, 100-meter swim, gymnastic routines
High	2 min to 20 min	Aerobic system	ATP from carbohydrate (glycolysis and TCA cycle)	Yes	Cycling, swimming, running
Moderate	> 20 min	Aerobic system	ATP from fat (fatty acid-oxidation and TCA cycle)	Yes	Hiking

NOTE: All energy systems function at all times, but depending on the intensity of the activity and the conditioning of the athlete, one system will predominate at any given time.

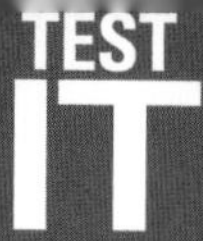

Take the quiz below to test your mastery of the key chapter concepts.

14.1 Fitness (pp. 442–448)

LEARN IT Describe the health benefits of being physically fit and explain how to develop the components of fitness.

1. Explain physical activity overload.
2. Define *cardiorespiratory conditioning* and list some of its benefits.
3. Physical inactivity is linked to all of the following diseases except:
   a. cancer.
   b. diabetes.
   c. emphysema.
   d. hypertension.
4. Physical activity overload can be applied by performing:
   a. an activity less often.
   b. an activity with more intensity.
   c. an activity in a different setting.
   d. a different activity each day of the week.

14.2 Energy Systems and Fuels to Support Activity (pp. 448–455)

LEARN IT Identify the factors that influence fuel use during physical activity and the types of activities that depend more on glucose or fat, respectively.

5. What types of activity are anaerobic? Which are aerobic? Describe the relationships among energy expenditure, type of activity, and oxygen use.
6. The process that regenerates glucose from lactate is known as the:
   a. Cori cycle.
   b. ATP-CP cycle.
   c. adaptation cycle.
   d. cardiac output cycle.
7. "Hitting the wall" is a term runners sometimes use to describe:
   a. dehydration.
   b. competition.
   c. indigestion.
   d. glucose depletion.
8. The technique endurance athletes use to maximize glycogen stores is called:
   a. aerobic training.
   b. muscle conditioning.
   c. carbohydrate loading.
   d. progressive overloading.
9. Conditioned muscles rely less on ________ and more on ________ for energy.
   a. protein; fat
   b. fat; protein
   c. glycogen; fat
   d. fat; glycogen

14.3 Vitamins and Minerals to Support Activity (pp. 455–457)

LEARN IT List which vitamins and mineral supplements, if any, athletes may need and why.

10. Why are some athletes likely to develop iron-deficiency anemia? Compare iron-deficiency anemia and sports anemia, explaining the differences.
11. Vitamin or mineral supplements taken just before an event are useless for improving performance because the:
    a. athlete sweats the nutrients out during the event.
    b. stomach can't digest supplements during physical activity.
    c. nutrients are diluted by all the fluids the athlete drinks.
    d. body needs hours or days for the nutrients to do their work.
12. Physically active young women, especially those who are endurance athletes, are prone to:
    a. energy excess.
    b. iron deficiency.
    c. protein overload.
    d. vitamin A toxicity.

14.4 Fluids and Electrolytes to Support Activity (pp. 457–462)

LEARN IT Identify the factors that influence an athlete's fluid needs and describe the differences between water and sports drinks.

13. Discuss the importance of hydration during training, and list recommendations to maintain fluid balance.
14. The body's need for ________ far surpasses its need for any other nutrient.
    a. water
    b. protein
    c. vitamins
    d. carbohydrate

14.5 Diets for Physically Active People (pp. 462–464)

LEARN IT Discuss an appropriate daily eating pattern for athletes and list one example of a recommended pregame and recovery meal.

15. A recommended pregame meal includes plenty of fluids and provides between:
    a. 300 and 800 kcalories, mostly from fat-rich foods.
    b. 50 and 100 kcalories, mostly from fiber-rich foods.
    c. 1000 and 2000 kcalories, mostly from protein-rich foods.
    d. 300 and 800 kcalories, mostly from carbohydrate-rich foods.

HIGHLIGHT 14 Supplements as Ergogenic Aids (pp. 467–471)

LEARN IT Present arguments for and against the use of ergogenic aids.

16. Discuss two ergogenic aids that seem to perform as claimed and two that are dangerous, banned, or illegal.

Multiple Choice Answers

3.c 4.b 6.a 7.d 8.c 9.c 11.d 12.b 14.a 15.d

STUDY IT

15 Life Cycle Nutrition: Pregnancy and Lactation

Review the key points of this chapter below, learn the definitions of the bold terms, and then take the practice quiz on the back of this card.

15.1 Nutrition prior to Pregnancy

- Prior to pregnancy, the health and behaviors of both men and women can influence **fertility** and fetal development. In preparation, they can achieve and maintain a healthy body weight, choose an adequate and balanced diet, be physically active, receive regular medical care, manage chronic conditions, and avoid harmful influences.

15.2 Growth and Development during Pregnancy

- The infant develops through three stages—the **zygote, embryo,** and **fetus** (review Figure 15-2, p. 476). Each organ and tissue grows on its own schedule (review Figure 15-4, p. 477).
- Times of intense development are **critical periods** that depend on nutrients (review Figure 15-3, p. 477).
- Without folate, the neural tube fails to develop completely during the first month of pregnancy; all women of childbearing age should take folate daily. Common **neural tube defects** include **anencephaly** and **spina bifida.**

15.3 Maternal Weight

- A healthy pregnancy depends on a sufficient weight gain.
- Women who begin their pregnancies at a healthy weight need to gain about 30 pounds to cover the growth and development of the **placenta, uterus,** blood, breasts, and infant (review Figure 15-7, p. 482).
- Physical activity throughout pregnancy can help a woman develop the strength she needs to carry the extra weight and maintain habits that will help her lose it after the birth.

15.4 Nutrition during Pregnancy

- Energy and nutrient needs are high during pregnancy; the diet should include an extra serving from each of the five food groups.
- Supplements of iron and folate are recommended.
- Nausea, constipation, and heartburn commonly accompany pregnancy and can usually be alleviated with a few simple strategies (review Table 15-2, p. 487). **Food cravings** do not typically reflect physiological needs.

15.5 High-Risk Pregnancies

- High-risk pregnancies (review Table 15-3) threaten the life and health of both mother and infant and are likely to produce an infant with a low birth weight.
- Proper nutrition and abstinence from smoking, alcohol, and other drugs improve the outcome as can prenatal care to monitor for **gestational diabetes** and **preeclampsia.**

15.6 Nutrition during Lactation

- During **lactation,** women need extra fluid and enough energy and nutrients to produce about 25 ounces of milk a day.
- Breastfeeding is contraindicated for those with HIV/AIDS.
- Alcohol, other drugs, smoking, and contaminants may reduce milk production or enter breast milk and impair infant development.

TABLE 15-3 High-Risk Pregnancy Factors

Factor	Condition that Raises Risk
Maternal weight	
• Prior to pregnancy	Prepregnancy BMI either <18.5 or ≥25
• During pregnancy	Insufficient or excessive pregnancy weight gain (see Table 15-1, p. 481)
Maternal nutrition	Nutrient deficiencies or toxicities; eating disorders
Socioeconomic status	Poverty, lack of family support, low level of education, limited food available
Lifestyle habits	Smoking, alcohol or other drug use
Age	Teens, especially 15 years or younger; women 35 years or older
Previous pregnancies	
• Number	Many previous pregnancies (3 or more to mothers younger than age 20; 4 or more to mothers age 20 or older)
• Interval	Short or long intervals between pregnancies (<18 months or >59 months)
• Outcomes	Previous history of problems
• Multiple births	Twins or triplets
• Birthweight	Low- or high-birthweight infants
Maternal health	
• High blood pressure	Development of gestational hypertension
• Diabetes	Development of gestational diabetes
• Chronic diseases	Diabetes; heart, respiratory, and kidney disease; certain genetic disorders; special diets and medications

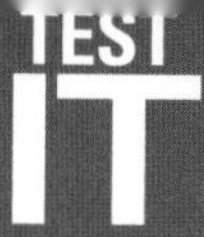

Take the quiz below to test your mastery of the key chapter concepts.

15.1 Nutrition prior to Pregnancy (p. 474)

LEARN IT List the ways men and women can prepare for a healthy pregnancy.

1. The health and behaviors of men and women prior to pregnancy can influence all of the following except:
   a. fertility.
   b. infant's gender.
   c. placenta development.
   d. infant's mental development.

15.2 Growth and Development during Pregnancy (pp. 475–479)

LEARN IT Describe fetal development from conception to birth and explain how maternal malnutrition can affect critical periods.

2. Describe the placenta and its function.
3. Explain why women of childbearing age need folate in their diets. How much is recommended, and how can women ensure that these needs are met?
4. The spongy structure that delivers nutrients to the fetus and returns waste products to the mother is called the:
   a. embryo.
   b. uterus.
   c. placenta.
   d. amniotic sac.

15.3 Maternal Weight (pp. 480–483)

LEARN IT Explain how both underweight and overweight can interfere with a healthy pregnancy and how weight gain and physical activity can support maternal health and infant growth.

5. Which of these strategies is *not* a healthy option for an overweight woman?
   a. Limit weight gain during pregnancy.
   b. Postpone weight loss until after pregnancy.
   c. Follow a weight-loss diet during pregnancy.
   d. Try to achieve a healthy weight before becoming pregnant.
6. A reasonable weight gain during pregnancy for a normal-weight woman is about:
   a. 10 pounds.
   b. 20 pounds.
   c. 30 pounds.
   d. 40 pounds.

15.4 Nutrition during Pregnancy (pp. 483–488)

LEARN IT Summarize the nutrient needs of women during pregnancy.

7. Which nutrients are needed in the greatest amounts during pregnancy? Why are they so important? Describe wise food choices for the pregnant woman.

15.5 High-Risk Pregnancies (pp. 488–496)

LEARN IT Identify factors predicting low-risk and high-risk pregnancies and describe ways to manage them.

8. What is the significance of infant birthweight in terms of the child's future health?
9. Describe some of the special problems of the pregnant adolescent. Which nutrients are needed in increased amounts?
10. What practices should be avoided during pregnancy? Why?
11. To help prevent neural tube defects, grain products are now fortified with:
    a. iron.
    b. folate.
    c. protein.
    d. vitamin C.
12. Pregnant women should *not* take supplements of:
    a. iron.
    b. folate.
    c. vitamin A.
    d. vitamin C.
13. The combination of high blood pressure, protein in the urine, and edema signals:
    a. jaundice.
    b. preeclampsia.
    c. gestational diabetes.
    d. gestational hypertension.

15.6 Nutrition during Lactation (pp. 496–501)

LEARN IT Summarize the nutrient needs of women during lactation.

14. To facilitate lactation, a mother needs:
    a. about 5000 kcalories a day.
    b. adequate nutrition and rest.
    c. vitamin and mineral supplements.
    d. a glass of wine or beer before each feeding.
15. A breastfeeding woman should drink plenty of water to:
    a. produce more milk.
    b. suppress lactation.
    c. prevent dehydration.
    d. dilute nutrient concentration.
16. A woman may need iron supplements during lactation:
    a. to enhance the iron in her breast milk.
    b. to provide iron for the infant's growth.
    c. to replace the iron in her body's stores.
    d. to support the increase in her blood volume.

HIGHLIGHT 15 Fetal Alcohol Syndrome (pp. 505–507)

LEARN IT Explain how drinking alcohol endangers the fetus and how women can prevent fetal alcohol syndrome.

17. Public health recommendations for alcohol consumption during pregnancy advise:
    a. abstinence from alcohol.
    b. beer or wine, but not liquor.
    c. alcohol in moderation (one drink a day).
    d. abstinence in the first trimester, moderation in the second trimester, and no restrictions in the third trimester.

Multiple Choice Answers

1. b 4. c 5. c 6. c 11. b 12. c 13. b 14. b 15. c 16. c 17. a

16 Life Cycle Nutrition: Infancy, Childhood, and Adolescence

Review the key points of this chapter below, learn the definitions of the bold terms, and then take the practice quiz on the back of this card.

16.1 Nutrition during Infancy

- The primary food for infants during the first 12 months is either breast milk or iron-fortified formula. Cow's milk is not appropriate until after age 1.
- Breast milk offers both nutrients and immunological protection.
- Breast milk provides many factors that protect infants from illnesses and support better nutrition (review Table 16-3, p. 514).
- At 4 to 6 months of age, infants should gradually begin eating solid foods, including iron-fortified cereals and vitamin-C rich fruits and vegetables.
- By 1 year, infants are drinking from a cup and eating a variety of foods.
- Infants may benefit from supplements containing vitamin D, iron, and fluoride (review Table 16-2, p. 513).

16.2 Nutrition during Childhood

- Children's appetites and nutrient needs reflect their stage of growth.
- Children who are chronically hungry and malnourished suffer growth retardation; temporary hunger and mild nutrient deficiencies produce more subtle problems—such as poor academic performance.
- Iron deficiency is widespread and has many physical and behavioral consequences.
- **Hyperactivity** is not caused by poor nutrition; misbehavior may be due to lack of sleep, too little physical activity, or too much television, among other factors.
- Some children have **food allergies**—**adverse reactions** that involve an immune response—most often caused by peanuts, tree nuts, milk, eggs, wheat, soybeans, fish, or shellfish.
- Childhood obesity is a major health problem (review Figure 16-9, p. 529).
- Children need to eat nutrient-dense foods and learn how to make healthful diet and activity choices.

16.3 Nutrition during Adolescence

- The need for iron increases during **adolescence** for both males and females; blood losses incurred through menstruation increase iron needs for females further (review Table 16-15, p. 540).
- Sufficient calcium intake during adolescence supports optimal bone growth and density.
- The adolescent growth spurt increases the need for energy and nutrients.
- Adolescents who drink soft drinks regularly have a higher energy intake and a lower calcium intake; they are also more likely to be overweight.

TABLE 16-9 Recommended Eating and Physical Activity Behaviors to Prevent Obesity

The Expert Committee of the American Medical Association recommends the following healthy habits for children 2 to 18 years of age to help prevent childhood obesity:

- Limit consumption of sugar-sweetened beverages, such as soft drinks and fruit-flavored punches.
- Eat the recommended amounts of fruits and vegetables every day (2 to 4.5 cups per day based on age).
- Learn to eat age-appropriate portions of foods.
- Eat foods low in energy density such as those high in fiber and/or water and modest in fat.
- Eat a nutritious breakfast every day.
- Eat a diet rich in calcium.
- Eat a diet balanced in recommended proportions for carbohydrate, fat, and protein.
- Eat a diet high in fiber.
- Eat together as a family as often as possible.
- Limit the frequency of restaurant meals.
- Limit television watching or other screen time to no more than 2 hours per day and do not have televisions or computers in bedrooms.
- Engage in at least 60 minutes of moderate to vigorous physical activity every day.

SOURCE: S. E. Barlow, Expert Committee recommendations regarding the prevention, assessment, and treatment of child and adolescent overweight and obesity: Summary report, *Pediatrics* 120 (2007): S164–S192.

TEST IT

Take the quiz below to test your mastery of the key chapter concepts.

16.1 Nutrition during Infancy (pp. 510–520)

LEARN IT List some of the components of breast milk and describe the appropriate foods for infants during the first year of life.

1. What are the appropriate uses of formula feeding? What criteria would you use in selecting an infant formula?
2. Why are solid foods not recommended for an infant during the first few months of life? When is an infant ready to start eating solid food?
3. Identify foods that are inappropriate for infants and explain why they are inappropriate.
4. A reasonable weight for a healthy 5-month-old infant who weighed 8 pounds at birth might be:
   a. 12 pounds.
   b. 16 pounds.
   c. 20 pounds.
   d. 24 pounds.
5. Dehydration can develop quickly in infants because:
   a. much of their body water is extracellular.
   b. they lose a lot of water through urination and tears.
   c. only a small percentage of their body weight is water.
   d. they drink lots of breast milk or formula, but little water.
6. An infant should begin eating solid foods between:
   a. 2 and 4 weeks.
   b. 1 and 3 months.
   c. 4 and 6 months.
   d. 8 and 10 months.

16.2 Nutrition during Childhood (pp. 520–539)

LEARN IT Explain how children's appetites and nutrient needs reflect their stage of growth and why iron deficiency and obesity are often concerns during childhood.

7. What nutrition problems are most common in children? What strategies can help prevent these problems?
8. Describe the relationships between nutrition and behavior. How does television influence nutrition?
9. Describe a true food allergy. Which foods most often cause allergic reactions? How do food allergies influence nutrition status?
10. Describe the problems associated with childhood obesity and the strategies for prevention and treatment.
11. List strategies for introducing nutritious foods to children.
12. What impact do school meal programs have on the nutrition status of children?
13. Among US children, the most prevalent nutrient deficiency is of:
    a. iron.
    b. folate.
    c. protein.
    d. vitamin D.
14. A true food allergy always:
    a. elicits an immune response.
    b. causes an immediate reaction.
    c. creates an aversion to the offending food.
    d. involves symptoms such as headaches or hives.
15. Which of the following strategies is *not* effective?
    a. Play first, eat later.
    b. Provide small portions.
    c. Encourage children to help prepare meals.
    d. Use dessert as a reward for eating vegetables.

16.3 Nutrition during Adolescence (pp. 539–543)

LEARN IT Discuss some of the challenges in meeting the nutrient needs of adolescents.

16. Describe the changes in nutrient needs from childhood to adolescence. Why is an adolescent girl more likely to develop an iron deficiency than an adolescent boy?
17. How do adolescents' eating habits influence their nutrient intakes?
18. To help teenagers consume a balanced diet, parents can:
    a. monitor the teens' food intake.
    b. give up—parents can't influence teenagers.
    c. keep the pantry and refrigerator well stocked.
    d. forbid snacking and insist on regular, well-balanced meals.
19. During adolescence, energy and nutrient needs:
    a. reach a peak.
    b. fall dramatically.
    c. rise, but do not peak until adulthood.
    d. fluctuate so much that generalizations can't be made.
20. The nutrients most likely to fall short in the adolescent diet are:
    a. sodium and fat.
    b. folate and zinc.
    c. iron and calcium.
    d. protein and vitamin A.
21. To balance the day's intake, an adolescent who eats a hamburger, fries, and cola at lunch might benefit most from a dinner of:
    a. fried chicken, rice, and banana.
    b. ribeye steak, baked potato, and iced tea.
    c. pork chop, mashed potatoes, and apple juice.
    d. spaghetti with meat sauce, broccoli, and milk.

HIGHLIGHT 16 Childhood Obesity and the Early Development of Chronic Diseases (pp. 548–553)

LEARN IT Describe the lifestyle factors that can help prevent childhood obesity and the development of type 2 diabetes and heart disease.

22. Describe the dietary strategies to help prevent the early development of chronic diseases.

Multiple Choice Answers

4. b 5. a 6. c 13. a 14. a 15. d 18. c 19. a 20. c 21. d

17 Life Cycle Nutrition: Adulthood and the Later Years

Review the key points of this chapter below, learn the definitions of the bold terms, and then take the practice quiz on the back of this card.

17.1 Nutrition and Longevity

- **Life expectancy** in the United States increased dramatically in the 20th century.
- Factors that enhance **longevity** include limited or no alcohol use, regular balanced meals, weight control, abstinence from smoking, regular physical activity, and adequate sleep.
- Energy restriction in animals seems to lengthen their lives; whether such dietary intervention in human beings is beneficial remains unknown.
- Nutrition—especially when combined with regular physical activity—can influence aging and longevity by supporting good health and preventing disease.

17.2 The Aging Process

- Changes that accompany aging can impair nutrition status. Among physiological changes, hormone activity alters body composition, immune system changes raise the risk of infections, **atrophic gastritis** interferes with digestion and absorption, and tooth loss limits food choices.
- Psychological changes such as depression, economic changes such as loss of income, and social changes such as loneliness contribute to poor food intake.

17.3 Energy and Nutrient Needs of Older Adults

- Some nutrients need special attention in the diet, but supplements are not routinely recommended.
- Table 17-5 helps determine the risk of malnutrition in older adults.

17.4 Nutrition-Related Concerns of Older Adults

- **Senile dementia** and cognitive losses afflict many older adults; some face loss of vision due to **cataracts** or **macular degeneration** or cope with the pain of **arthritis.**

TABLE 17-5 Risk Factors for Malnutrition in Older Adults

	These questions help *determine* the risk of malnutrition in older adults:
Disease	• Do you have an illness or condition that changes the types or amounts of foods you eat?
Eating poorly	• Do you eat fewer than two meals a day? Do you eat fruits, vegetables, and milk products daily?
Tooth loss or mouth pain	• Is it difficult or painful to eat?
Economic hardship	• Do you have enough money to buy the food you need?
Reduced social contact	• Do you eat alone most of the time?
Multiple medications	• Do you take three or more different prescribed or over-the-counter medications daily?
Involuntary weight loss or gain	• Have you lost or gained 10 pounds or more in the last 6 months?
Needs assistance	• Are you physically able to shop, cook, and feed yourself?
Elderly person	• Are you older than 80?

- Table 17-2 provides a summary of the nutrient concerns of aging.
- Some problems may be inevitable, but others are preventable and good nutrition may play a key role.

17.5 Food Choices and Eating Habits of Older Adults

- **Congregate meals** provide older adults with both nutrients and social interactions; those who are homebound receive delivered meals **(Meals on Wheels).**
- Adults living alone can prepare nutritious, inexpensive meals with a little creativity and careful shopping.

TABLE 17-2 Nutrient Concerns of Aging

Nutrient	Effect of Aging	Comments
Water	Lack of thirst and decreased total body water make dehydration likely.	Mild dehydration is a common cause of confusion. Difficulty obtaining water or getting to the bathroom may compound the problem.
Energy	Need decreases as muscle mass decreases **(sarcopenia).**	Physical activity moderates the decline.
Fiber	Likelihood of constipation increases with low intakes and changes in the GI tract.	Inadequate water intakes and lack of physical activity, along with some medications, compound the problem.
Protein	Needs may stay the same or increase slightly.	Low-fat, high-fiber legumes and grains meet both protein and other nutrient needs.
Vitamin B_{12}	Atrophic gastritis is common.	Deficiency causes neurological damages; supplements may be needed.
Vitamin D	Increased likelihood of inadequate intake; skin synthesis declines.	Daily sunlight exposure in moderation or supplements may be beneficial.
Calcium	Intakes may be low; osteoporosis is common.	Stomach discomfort commonly limits milk intake; calcium substitutes or supplements may be needed.
Iron	In women, status improves after menopause; deficiencies are linked to chronic blood losses and low stomach acid output.	Adequate stomach acid is required for absorption; antacid or other medicine use may aggravate iron deficiency; vitamin C and meat increase absorption.
Zinc	Intakes are often inadequate and absorption may be poor, but needs may also increase.	Medications interfere with absorption; deficiency may depress appetite and sense of taste.

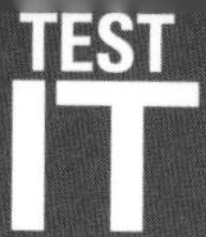

Take the quiz below to test your mastery of the key chapter concepts.

17.1 Nutrition and Longevity (pp. 556–560)

LEARN IT Describe the role nutrition plays in longevity.

1. Life expectancy in the United States is about:
   a. 48 to 60 years.
   b. 58 to 70 years.
   c. 68 to 80 years.
   d. 78 to 90 years.
2. The human life span is about:
   a. 85 years.
   b. 100 years.
   c. 115 years.
   d. 130 years.
3. A 72-year-old person whose physical health is similar to that of people 10 years younger has a(n):
   a. chronological age of 62.
   b. physiological age of 72.
   c. physiological age of 62.
   d. absolute age of minus 10.
4. Rats live longest when given diets that:
   a. eliminate all fat.
   b. provide lots of protein.
   c. allow them to eat freely.
   d. restrict their energy intakes.

17.2 The Aging Process (pp. 560–564)

LEARN IT Summarize how nutrition interacts with the physical, psychological, economic, and social changes involved in aging.

5. Which characteristic is *not* commonly associated with atrophic gastritis?
   a. inflamed stomach
   b. vitamin B_{12} toxicity
   c. bacterial overgrowth
   d. lack of intrinsic factor

17.3 Energy and Nutrient Needs of Older Adults (pp. 564–567)

LEARN IT Explain why the needs for some nutrients increase or decrease during aging.

6. Why does the risk of dehydration increase as people age?
7. Why do energy needs usually decline with advancing age?
8. Identify some factors that complicate the task of setting nutrient standards for older adults.
9. On average, adult energy needs:
   a. decline 5 percent per year.
   b. decline 5 percent per decade.
   c. remain stable throughout life.
   d. rise gradually throughout life.

17.4 Nutrition-Related Concerns of Older Adults (pp. 567–572)

LEARN IT Identify how nutrition might contribute to, or prevent, the development of age-related problems associated with vision, arthritis, the brain, and alcohol use.

10. Which nutrients seem to protect against cataract development?
    a. minerals
    b. lecithins
    c. antioxidants
    d. amino acids
11. The best dietary advice for a person with osteoarthritis might be to:
    a. avoid milk products.
    b. take fish oil supplements.
    c. take vitamin E supplements.
    d. lose weight, if overweight.

17.5 Food Choices and Eating Habits of Older Adults (pp. 572–576)

LEARN IT Instruct an adult on how to shop for groceries and prepare healthy meals for one person on a tight budget.

12. What characteristics contribute to malnutrition in older people?
13. Congregate meal programs are preferable to Meals on Wheels because they provide:
    a. nutritious meals.
    b. referral services.
    c. social interactions.
    d. financial assistance.
14. The OAA Nutrition Program is available to:
    a. all people 65 years and older.
    b. all people 60 years and older.
    c. homebound people only, 60 years and older.
    d. low-income people only, 60 years and older.

HIGHLIGHT 17 Nutrient-Drug Interactions (pp. 579–583)

LEARN IT Explain why certain nutrients and medications interact.

15. Why are elderly people with chronic diseases most vulnerable to interactions that can create nutrient imbalances or interfere with drug effectiveness?

Multiple Choice Answers

1. c 2. d 3. c 4. d 5. b 9. b 10. c 11. d 13. c 14. b

STUDY IT 18 Diet and Health

Review the key points of this chapter below, learn the definitions of the bold terms, and then take the practice quiz on the back of this card.

18.1 Nutrition and Infectious Diseases

- Public health measures such as purification of water and safe handling of food help prevent the spread of infection in populations; immunizations and antibiotics protect individuals.
- Nutrition cannot prevent or cure **infectious diseases,** but adequate intakes of all the nutrients can help support the immune system as the body defends against disease-causing agents.
- If the immune system is impaired because of malnutrition or diseases such as **AIDS,** a person becomes vulnerable to infectious disease.
- Inflammation underlies many chronic diseases.

18.2 Nutrition and Chronic Diseases

- Heart disease, cancers, and strokes are the three leading causes of death in the United States, and diabetes also ranks among the top 10.
- These four chronic diseases have significant links with nutrition and with one another (review Figure 18-2); other lifestyle risk factors and genetics also play a role.

18.3 Cardiovascular Disease

- **Atherosclerosis** is characterized by a build-up of plaque in an artery wall.
- Rupture of **plaque** or abnormal blood clotting can cause heart attacks and strokes.
- Dietary recommendations to lower the risks of **cardiovascular disease** are summarized in Table 18-5 (p. 596); quitting smoking and engaging in regular physical activity also improve heart health.

18.4 Hypertension

- The most effective dietary strategy for preventing **hypertension** is weight control.
- The **DASH eating pattern** is rich in fruits, vegetables, nuts, and low-fat milk products and low in fat, saturated fat, and sodium (review Table 18-7, p. 600).

> FIGURE 18-2 **Interrelationships among Chronic Diseases**

Notice that many chronic diseases are themselves risk factors for other chronic diseases and that all of them are linked to obesity. The risk factors highlighted in blue define the **metabolic syndrome.**

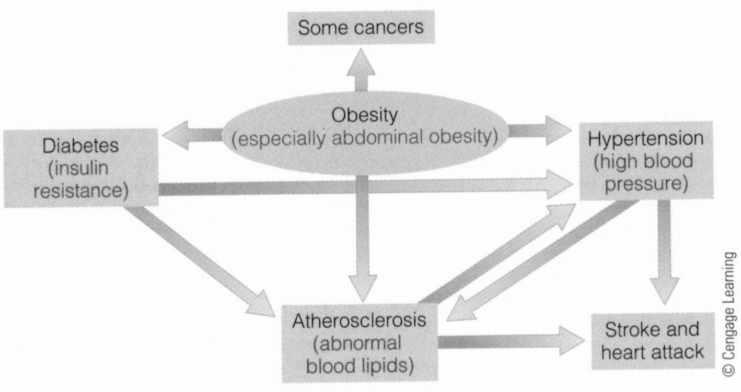

TABLE 18-12 **Dietary Guidelines and Recommendations for Chronic Diseases Compared**

Dietary Guidelines	Heart Disease	Hypertension	Diabetes	Cancer
Prevent and/or reduce overweight and obesity.	✓	✓	✓	✓
Increase physical activity and reduce time spent in sedentary behaviors.	✓	✓	✓	✓
Keep total fat 20 to 35 percent of kcalories.	✓			
Consume less than 10 percent of kcalories from saturated fatty acids and keep *trans*-fatty acid consumption as low as possible.	✓		✓	✓
Increase vegetable and fruit intake. Consume at least half of all grains as whole grains.	✓	✓	✓	✓
Reduce the intake of kcalories from added sugars.	✓		✓	
Reduce daily sodium intake to less than 2300 milligrams.[a]	✓	✓	✓	✓
If alcohol is consumed, it should be consumed in moderation.	✓	✓	✓	✓

[a]Further reduce daily sodium intake to 1500 milligrams among persons who are 51 and older and those of any age who are African American or have hypertension, diabetes, or chronic kidney disease.

18.5 Diabetes Mellitus

- **Diabetes** is characterized by high blood glucose and either insufficient insulin, ineffective insulin, or a combination of the two.
- People with **type 1 diabetes** coordinate diet, insulin, and physical activity to help control their blood glucose.
- People with **type 2 diabetes** benefit most from a diet and physical activity program that controls glucose fluctuations and promotes weight loss.

18.6 Cancer

- Some dietary factors, such as alcohol and heavily smoked foods, may **initiate cancer** development; others, such as animal fats, may **promote** cancer once it develops; and still others, such as fiber, antioxidant nutrients, and phytochemicals, may serve as **antipromoters** that protect against cancer development.
- To obtain the best possible nutrition at the lowest possible cancer risk, eat many fruits, vegetables, legumes, and whole grains and little saturated fat; minimize weight gain through regular physical activity and a healthy diet (review Table 18-11, p. 609).

18.7 Recommendations for Chronic Diseases

- Optimal nutrition keeps people healthy and reduces the risk of chronic diseases.
- Dietary recommendations are aimed at populations and focus on controlling weight; limiting saturated and *trans* fat; increasing fiber-rich fruits, vegetables, and whole grains; and balancing food intake with physical activity (review Table 18-12).

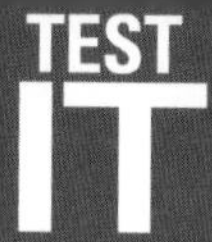

Take the quiz below to test your mastery of the key chapter concepts.

18.1 Nutrition and Infectious Diseases (pp. 586–588)

LEARN IT Identify factors that protect people from the spread of infectious diseases and describe the role of nutrition in immunity.

1. The immune cells of the body do *not* include:
   a. B-cells.
   b. T-cells.
   c. antigens.
   d. phagocytes.

2. Which of the following produce antibodies?
   a. phagocytes
   b. T-cells
   c. antigens
   d. B-cells

18.2 Nutrition and Chronic Diseases (pp. 589–590)

LEARN IT List the leading nutrition-related causes of death in the United States.

3. The leading cause of death in the United States is:
   a. AIDS.
   b. cancer.
   c. diabetes.
   d. heart disease.

18.3 Cardiovascular Disease (pp. 590–597)

LEARN IT Describe how atherosclerosis develops and strategies to lower blood cholesterol levels.

4. Plaques in the arteries contribute to the development of:
   a. cancer.
   b. diabetes.
   c. atherosclerosis.
   d. infectious diseases.

5. Which blood lipid correlates directly with heart disease?
   a. HDL
   b. LDL
   c. VLDL
   d. triglycerides

6. Weight loss and physical activity may protect against heart disease by:
   a. raising LDL and insulin levels.
   b. raising HDL and lowering blood pressure.
   c. lowering LDL and increasing clot formation.
   d. improving insulin sensitivity and raising blood pressure.

18.4 Hypertension (pp. 598–600)

LEARN IT Present strategies to lower blood pressure.

7. What is the most effective strategy for most people to lower their blood pressure?
   a. lose weight
   b. restrict salt
   c. monitor glucose
   d. supplement protein

18.5 Diabetes Mellitus (pp. 600–605)

LEARN IT Compare the dietary strategies to manage type 1 diabetes with those to prevent and treat type 2 diabetes.

8. Describe the differences between type 1 diabetes and type 2 diabetes.

9. All of the following factors increase the risk of type 2 diabetes *except:*
   a. aging.
   b. inactivity.
   c. obesity.
   d. smoking.

10. The most important dietary strategy in diabetes is to:
    a. provide for a consistent carbohydrate intake.
    b. restrict fat to 30 percent of daily kcalories.
    c. limit carbohydrate intake to 300 milligrams a day.
    d. take multiple vitamin and mineral supplements daily.

18.6 Cancer (pp. 605–609)

LEARN IT Differentiate among cancer initiators, promoters, and antipromoters and describe how nutrients or foods might play a role in each category.

11. Describe the characteristics of a diet that might offer the best protection against the onset of cancer.

12. Which of the following help(s) to protect against cancer?
    a. alcohol
    b. pickled foods
    c. phytochemicals
    d. omega-6 fatty acids

18.7 Recommendations for Chronic Diseases (pp. 610–612)

LEARN IT Summarize dietary recommendations to prevent chronic diseases.

13. Describe the dietary choices that best protect against the development of most chronic diseases.

HIGHLIGHT 18 Complementary and Alternative Medicine (pp. 617–625)

LEARN IT Present arguments for and against the use of complementary and alternative medicine.

14. Which of the following is generally considered safe?
    a. chaparral to cleanse blood
    b. aloe to promote wound healing
    c. ephedra to promote weight loss
    d. yohimbe to enhance male sexual performance

Multiple Choice Answers

1. c 2. d 3. d 4. c 5. b 6. b 7. a 9. d 10. a 12. c 14. b

STUDY IT

19 Consumer Concerns about Foods and Water

Review the key points of this chapter below, learn the definitions of the bold terms, and then take the practice quiz on the back of this card.

19.1 Food Safety and Foodborne Illnesses

- Maintaining a safe food supply requires everyone's efforts (review Figure 19-1, p. 631).
- Millions of people suffer mild to life-threatening symptoms caused by **foodborne illnesses** (review Table 19-1, p. 629).
- The "How To" (pp. 632–633) describes how these illnesses can be prevented by storing and cooking foods at their proper temperatures and by preparing them in sanitary conditions.
- **Irradiation** of certain foods protects consumers from foodborne illness, but also raises some concerns.

19.2 Nutritional Adequacy of Foods and Diets

- In the marketplace, food labels, the *Dietary Guidelines for Americans,* and MyPlate all help consumers learn about nutrition and how to plan healthy diets.
- At home, consumers can minimize nutrient losses from fruits and vegetables by refrigerating them, washing them before cutting them, storing them in airtight containers, and cooking them for short times in minimal water.

19.3 Environmental Contaminants

- Environmental contamination of foods is a concern, but so far, the **hazards** appear relatively small.
- Remain alert to the possibility of contamination, and keep an ear open for public health announcements and advice.
- Eat a variety of foods to protect against the accumulation of toxins in the body. Each food eaten dilutes **contaminants** that may be present in other components of the diet.

19.4 Natural Toxicants in Foods

- Natural toxicants include the goitrogens in cabbage, cyanogens in lima beans, and **solanine** in potatoes.
- Any substance can be **toxic** when consumed in excess.
- Poisons are poisons, whether made by people or by nature. The source of a chemical does not make it hazardous; its chemical structure and the quantity consumed do.

19.5 Pesticides

- **Pesticides** can safely improve crop yields when used according to regulations, but they can also be hazardous when used inappropriately.
- The FDA tests both domestic and imported foods for pesticide **residues** in the fields and in market basket surveys of foods prepared table ready.
- Consumers can minimize their ingestion of pesticide residues on foods by following the suggestions in Table 19-3 (p. 644).
- Alternative farming methods may allow farmers to grow crops with few or no pesticides.

19.6 Food Additives

- The benefits of food **additives** seem to justify the **risks** associated with their use.
- The FDA regulates the use of these **intentional additives:** antimicrobial agents (such as **nitrites**) to prevent microbial spoilage; antioxidants (such as vitamins C and E, **sulfites,** and **BHA** and **BHT**) to prevent oxidative changes; colors (such as tartrazine) and flavor enhancers (such as **MSG**) to appeal to senses; and nutrients (such as iodine in salt) to enrich or fortify foods (see Table 19-5).
- **Incidental additives** sometimes get into foods during processing, but rarely present a hazard; some processes such as treating livestock with hormones and antibiotics raise consumer concerns.

19.7 Consumer Concerns about Water

- Like foods, water may contain infectious microorganisms, environmental contaminants, pesticide residues, and additives.
- The EPA monitors the **safety** of the public water system, but many consumers choose home water treatment systems or bottled water instead of tap.

TABLE 19-5 **Intentional Food Additives**

Food Additive	Purpose	Common Examples
Antimicrobials	Prevent food spoilage from microorganisms	Salt, sugar, nitrites and nitrates (such as sodium nitrate), bacteriophages
Antioxidants	Prevent oxidative changes in color, flavor, or texture and delay rancidity and other damage to foods caused by oxygen	Vitamin C (erythorbic acid, sodium ascorbate), vitamin E (tocopherol), sulfites (sulfur dioxide, sodium sulfite, sodium bisulfite, potassium bisulfite, sodium metabisulfite, potassium metabisulfite), BHA and BHT
Colors	Enhance appearance	Artificial: indigotine, erythrosine, tartrazine Natural: annatto (yellow), caramel (yellowish brown), carotenoids (yellowish orange), dehydrated beets (reddish brown), grape skins (red, green)
Flavors	Enhance taste	Salt, sugar, spices, artificial sweeteners, MSG
Emulsifiers and gums	Thicken, stabilize, or otherwise improve consistency and texture	Emulsifiers: lecithin, alginates, mono- and diglycerides Gums: agar, alginates, carrageenan, guar, locust bean, psyllium, pectin, xanthan gum, gum arabic, cellulose derivatives
Nutrients (vitamins and minerals)	Improve the nutritive value by replacing vitamins and minerals lost in processing (enrichment) or adding vitamins or minerals that may be lacking in the diet (fortification)	Thiamin, niacin, riboflavin, folate, iron (in grain products); iodine (in salt); vitamins A and D (in milk); vitamin C and calcium (in fruit drinks); vitamin B_{12} (in vegetarian foods)

TEST IT

Take the quiz below to test your mastery of the key chapter concepts.

19.1 Food Safety and Foodborne Illnesses (pp. 628–637)

LEARN IT Describe how foodborne illnesses can be prevented.

1. Distinguish between the two types of foodborne illnesses and provide an example of each.
2. What special precautions apply to meats? To seafood?
3. Eating a contaminated food such as undercooked poultry or unpasteurized milk might cause a:
   a. food allergy.
   b. food infection.
   c. food intoxication.
   d. botulinum reaction.
4. The temperature danger zone for foods ranges from:
   a. −20°F to 120°F.
   b. 0°F to 100°F.
   c. 20°F to 120°F.
   d. 40°F to 140°F.
5. Examples of foods that frequently cause foodborne illness are:
   a. canned foods.
   b. steaming-hot foods.
   c. fresh fruits and vegetables.
   d. raw milk, seafood, meat, and eggs.
6. Irradiation can help improve our food supply by:
   a. cooking foods quickly.
   b. killing microorganisms.
   c. minimizing the use of preservatives.
   d. improving the nutrient content of foods.

19.2 Nutritional Adequacy of Foods and Diets (pp. 637–638)

LEARN IT Explain how to minimize nutrient losses in the kitchen.

7. Describe which nutrients are most vulnerable to destruction.

19.3 Environmental Contaminants (pp. 638–641)

LEARN IT Explain how environmental contaminants get into foods and how people can protect themselves against contamination.

8. How does bioaccumulation of toxins occur and how does that influence the safety of foods?

19.4 Natural Toxicants in Foods (pp. 641–642)

LEARN IT Identify natural toxicants and determine whether they are hazardous.

9. Solanine is an example of a(n):
   a. heavy metal.
   b. artificial color.
   c. natural toxicant.
   d. animal hormone.

19.5 Pesticides (pp. 642–645)

LEARN IT Debate the risks and benefits of using pesticides.

10. How do pesticides become a hazard to the food supply, and how are they monitored? In what ways can people reduce the concentrations of pesticides in and on foods that they prepare?

19.6 Food Additives (pp. 646–652)

LEARN IT List common food additives, their purposes, and examples.

11. What is the difference between a GRAS substance and a regulated food additive? Give examples of each.
12. The standard that deems additives safe if lifetime use presents no more than a one-in-a-million risk of cancer is known as the:
    a. Delaney Clause.
    b. zero-risk policy.
    c. GRAS list of standards.
    d. *de minimis* rule.
13. Common antimicrobial additives include:
    a. salt and nitrites.
    b. carrageenan and MSG.
    c. dioxins and sulfites.
    d. vitamin C and vitamin E.
14. Common antioxidants include:
    a. BHA and BHT.
    b. tartrazine and MSG.
    c. sugar and vitamin E.
    d. nitrosamines and salt.
15. Incidental additives that may enter foods during processing include:
    a. dioxins and BGH.
    b. dioxins and folate.
    c. beta-carotene and agar.
    d. nitrites and irradiation.

19.7 Consumer Concerns about Water (pp. 652–654)

LEARN IT Discuss consumer concerns about water.

16. Chlorine is added to water to:
    a. protect against dental caries.
    b. destroy harmful minerals such as lead and mercury.
    c. kill pathogenic microorganisms.
    d. remove the sulfur that produces a "rotten egg" odor.

HIGHLIGHT 19 Food Biotechnology (pp. 656–661)

LEARN IT Debate the pros and cons surrounding genetically engineered foods.

17. Describe genetic engineering and how it is similar to, and how it differs from, the way farmers have been breeding their crops for centuries.

Multiple Choice Answers

3. b 4. d 5. d 6. b 9. c 12. d 13. a 14. a 15. a 16. c

20 Hunger and the Global Environment

Review the key points of this chapter below, learn the definitions of the bold terms, and then take the practice quiz on the back of this card.

20.1 Hunger in the United States

- **Food insecurity** and **hunger** are widespread in the United States among those living in poverty (review Figure 20-1).
- Ironically, hunger and malnutrition can occur among obese people (review Figure 20-2).
- Government assistance programs help to relieve poverty and hunger; **food recovery** programs and other community efforts are equally important.

20.2 World Hunger

- Natural causes such as drought, flood, and pests and political causes such as armed conflicts and government policies all contribute to the extreme hunger and poverty seen in developing countries.
- More people means more mouths to feed, which worsens the problems of poverty and hunger.
- Poverty and hunger encourage parents to have more children; breaking this cycle requires improving the economic status of the people and providing them with health care, education, and family planning.
- Hunger leads to **acute malnutrition** and **chronic malnutrition,** which appear most evident in nutrient deficiencies and growth failure.

20.3 Malnutrition

- Inadequate food intake in children leads to poor growth and nutrient deficiencies.
- Children suffering from acute malnutrition (recent severe food deprivation) may be underweight for their height, whereas those experiencing chronic malnutrition (long-term food deprivation) are short for their age.
- Problems resulting from nutrient deficiencies include preterm births and low birth weights (iron), stillbirths and cretinism (iodine), blindness (vitamin A), and growth failure (zinc).
- Treatment for malnutrition should be individualized to ensure rapid weight gain and to correct nutrient deficiencies.

20.4 The Global Environment

- The global environment is deteriorating, largely because of our irresponsible use of resources and energy.
- Environmental degradation reduces our ability to produce enough food to feed the world's people.
- The rapid increase in the world's population exacerbates the situation.
- Governments, businesses, and all individuals can make environmentally conscious choices to help solve the hunger problem, improve the quality of life, and generate jobs.
- Personal choices, made by many people, can have a great impact.

> FIGURE 20-1 **Prevalence of Food Security in US Households**

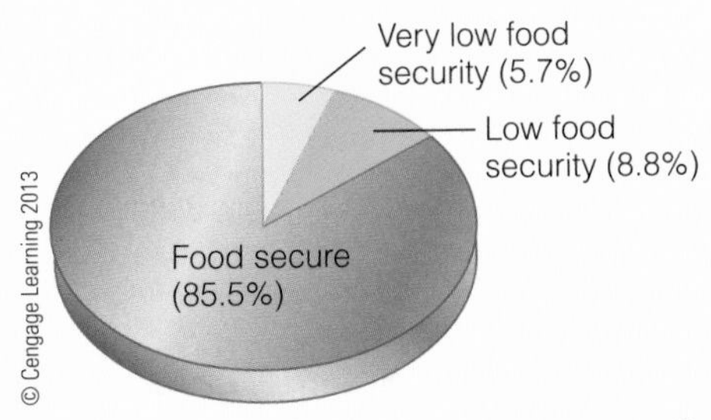

SOURCE: A. Coleman-Jensen, M. Nord, and A. Singh, *Household Food Security in the United States in 2012*, Economic Research Service, U.S. Department of Agriculture, www.ers.usda.gov, September 2013.

> FIGURE 20-2 **The Poverty-Obesity Paradox**

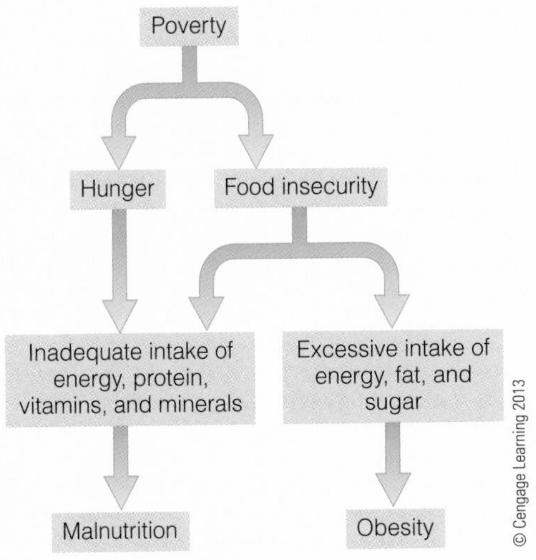

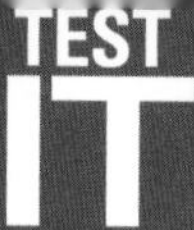

Take the quiz below to test your mastery of the key chapter concepts.

20.1 Hunger in the United States (pp. 664–667)

LEARN IT Identify some reasons why hunger is present in a country as wealthy as the United States.

1. Food insecurity refers to the:
   a. uncertainty of foods' safety.
   b. fear of eating too much food.
   c. limited availability of foods.
   d. reliability of food production.

2. The most common cause of hunger in the United States is:
   a. poverty.
   b. alcohol abuse.
   c. mental illness.
   d. lack of education.

3. SNAP debit cards cannot be used to purchase:
   a. tomato plants.
   b. birthday cakes.
   c. cola beverages.
   d. laundry detergent.

4. Which action is not typical of a food recovery program?
   a. gathering potatoes from a harvested field
   b. collecting overripe tomatoes from a wholesaler
   c. offering SNAP debit cards to low-income people
   d. delivering restaurant leftovers to a community shelter

20.2 World Hunger (pp. 668–670)

LEARN IT Identify some reasons why hunger is present in the developing countries of the world.

5. The primary cause of the worst famine in the 20th century was:
   a. armed conflicts.
   b. natural disasters.
   c. food contaminations.
   d. government policies.

6. Which of the following is most critical in providing food to all the world's people?
   a. decreasing air pollution
   b. increasing water supplies
   c. decreasing population growth
   d. increasing agricultural land

20.3 Malnutrition (pp. 671–673)

LEARN IT Describe the consequences of nutrient and energy inadequacies.

7. The most likely cause of death in malnourished children is:
   a. growth failure.
   b. diarrheal disease.
   c. simple starvation.
   d. vitamin A deficiency.

20.4 The Global Environment (pp. 674–680)

LEARN IT Explain why relieving environmental problems will also help to alleviate hunger and poverty.

8. Discuss the different paths by which rich and poor countries can attack the problems of world hunger and the environment.

HIGHLIGHT 20 Environmentally Friendly Food Choices (pp. 682–687)

LEARN IT Discuss ways consumers can conserve resources when making food-related choices.

9. The most ecologically sound diet is:
   a. animal based and locally produced.
   b. animal based and globally produced.
   c. vegetable based and locally produced.
   d. vegetable based and globally produced.

Multiple Choice Answers

1. c 2. a 3. d 4. c 5. d 6. c 7. b 9. c

Daily Values (DV) for Food Labels

The Daily Values (DV) are standards developed by the Food and Drug Administration (FDA) for use on food labels. The values are based on 2000 kcalories a day for adults and children aged 4 years and older. Chapter 2 provides more details.

Nutrient	Amount
Vitamins	
Biotin	30 μg
Choline	550 mg
Folate	400 μg DFE
Niacin	16 mg NE
Pantothenic acid	5 mg
Riboflavin	1.3 mg
Thiamin	1.2 mg
Vitamin A	900 μg RAE
Vitamin B_6	1.7 mg
Vitamin B_{12}	2.4 μg
Vitamin C	90 mg
Vitamin D	20 μg
Vitamin E (α-tocopherol)	15 mg
Vitamin K	120 μg
Minerals	
Calcium	1300 mg
Chloride	2300 mg
Chromium	35 μg
Copper	0.9 mg
Iodine	150 μg
Iron	18 mg
Magnesium	420 mg
Manganese	2.3 mg
Molybdenum	45 μg
Phosphorus	1250 mg
Potassium	4700 mg
Selenium	55 μg
Sodium	2300 mg
Zinc	11 mg

Food Component	Amount	Calculation Factors
Fat	65 g	30% of kcalories
Saturated fat	20 g	10% of kcalories
Cholesterol	300 mg	Same regardless of kcalories
Carbohydrate (total)	300 g	60% of kcalories
Fiber	28 g	14 g per 1000 kcalories
Protein	50 g	10% of kcalories

GLOSSARY OF NUTRIENT MEASURES

kcal: kcalories; a unit by which energy is measured (Chapter 1 provides more details).

g: grams; a unit of weight equivalent to about 0.03 ounces.

mg: milligrams; one-thousandth of a gram.

μg: micrograms; one-millionth of a gram.

IU: international units; an old measure of vitamin activity determined by biological methods (as opposed to new measures that are determined by direct chemical analyses).For those still using IU, the following factors can be used for conversions.

- For vitamin A, 1 IU = 0.3 μg retinol
- For vitamin D, 1 IU = 0.02 μg cholecalciferol
- For vitamin E, 1 IU = 0.67 mg α-tocopherol

mg NE: milligrams niacin equivalents; a measure of niacin activity (Chapter 10 provides more details).

- 1 NE = 1 mg niacin
  = 60 mg tryptophan (an amino acid)

μg DFE: micrograms dietary folate equivalents; a measure of folate activity (Chapter 10 provides more details).

- 1 μg DFE = 1 μg food folate
  = 0.6 μg folic acid from fortified food or as a supplement taken with food

μg RAE: micrograms retinol activity equivalents; a measure of vitamin A activity (Chapter 11 provides more details).

- 1 μg RAE = 1 μg retinol
  = 12 μg β-carotene
  = 24 μg other vitamin A carotenoids

mmol: millimoles; one-thousanth of a mole, the molecular weight of a substance. To convert mmol to mg, multiply by the atomic weight of the substance.

- For sodium, mmol × 23 = mg Na
- For chloride, mmol × 35.5 = mg Cl
- For sodium chloride, mmol × 58.5 = mg NaCl